HIGH-ACUITY NURSING,

Third Edition

Pamela Stinson Kidd, RN, PhD, ARNP, CEN
Associate Dean for Research & Graduate Studies
College of Nursing
Arizona State University
Tempe, AZ
Formerly: College of Nursing
University of Kentucky
Lexington, KY

Kathleen Dorman Wagner, RN, CS, MSN
College of Nursing
University of Kentucky
Lexington, KY

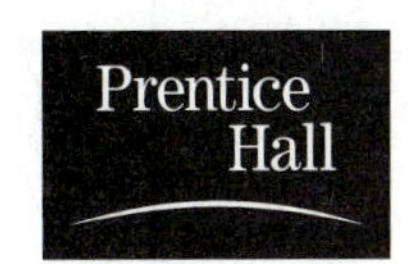

Upper Saddle River, New Jersey 07458

Notice: Care has been taken to confirm the accuracy of information presented in this book. The authors, editors, and the publisher, however, cannot accept any responsibility for errors or omissions or for consequences from application of the information in this book and make no warranty, express or implied, with respect to its contents.

The authors and publisher have exerted every effort to ensure that drug selections and dosages set forth in this text are in accord with current recommendations and practice at time of publication. However, in view of ongoing research, changes in government regulations, and the constant flow of information relating to drug therapy and drug reactions, the reader is urged to check the package inserts of all drugs for any change in indications of dosage and for added warnings and precautions. This is particularly important when the recommended agent is a new and/or infrequently employed drug.

Library of Congress Cataloging-in-Publication Data

Kidd, Pamela Stinson.
High acuity nursing / Pamela Stinson Kidd, Kathleen Dorman Wagner.—3rd ed.
p. ; cm.
Includes bibliographical references and index.
ISBN 0-8385-3745-6
1. Intensive care nursing. I. Wagner, Kathleen Dorman. II. Title.
[DNLM: 1. Critical Care—methods. 2. Critical Illness—nursing. 3. Nursing Process.
WY 154 K46h 2001]
RT120.I5 K53 2001
610.73'61—dc21 00-034017

Publisher: Julie Alexander
Executive Editor: Maura Connor
Acquisitions Editor: Nancy Anselment
Director of Manufacturing and Production: Bruce Johnson
Managing Editor: Patrick Walsh
Production Editor: Linda Begley, Rainbow Graphics
Production Liaison: Cathy O'Connell
Manufacturing Manager: Ilene Sanford
Director of Marketing: Leslie Cavaliere
Editorial Assistant: Beth Ann Romph
Creative Design: Marianne Frasco
Cover Designer: Joe Sengotta
Composition and Interior Design: Rainbow Graphics
Printing and Binding: Banta Harrisonburg

PRENTICE-HALL INTERNATIONAL (UK) LIMITED, *London*
PRENTICE-HALL OF AUSTRALIA PTY. LIMITED, *Sydney*
PRENTICE-HALL CANADA, INC., *Toronto*
PRENTICE-HALL HISPANOAMERICANA, S.A., *Mexico*
PRENTICE-HALL OF INDIA PRIVATE LIMITED, *New Delhi*
PRENTICE-HALL OF JAPAN, INC., *Tokyo*
PRENTICE-HALL SINGAPORE PTE. LTD
EDITORA PRENTICE-HALL DO BRASIL, LTDA., *Rio de Janeiro*

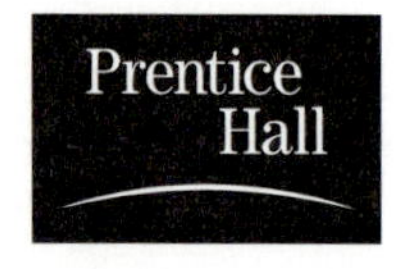

10 9 8 7
ISBN 0-8385-3745-6

CONTENTS

PREFACE

When the first edition of *High-Acuity Nursing* was published in 1992, the term *high acuity* was largely confined to leveling patient acuity for determining hospital staffing needs rather than being applied to nursing education. Our choice of titles was unusual and perhaps a little risky since nursing programs were using medical–surgical nursing texts or sometimes critical care nursing texts for teaching complex care concepts. Today, there is a growing trend to offer a high-acuity nursing course as part of the required undergraduate nursing curriculum. This, we believe, reflects the changing nature of the acute care patient population and the need to adequately prepare new nurses (and retool experienced nurses) to meet these rapidly changing needs.

The term *high acuity* refers to a level of patient problems beyond uncomplicated acute illness on a health–illness continuum. Today, high-acuity patients are increasingly found outside of critical care units or even acute care institutions. The patient population is older and sicker upon entering the health care system, and hospitalized patients are being discharged earlier, often in a poorer state of health. In the home health setting, nurses are providing care to clients with mechanical ventilators, central intravenous lines, IV antibiotic therapy, and complicated injuries. Whereas critical care units are considered specialty areas within the hospital walls, much of the knowledge required to work within that specialty is generalist in nature. It is this generalist knowledge base that is needed by all nurses who work with patients experiencing complex care problems to assure competent and safe nursing practice.

Purpose of the Text

The *High-Acuity Nursing* text delivers information using learner-focused, active learning principles, and concise language and format. The format breaks down complex information into small, understandable chunks for easier understanding. Self-testing is provided throughout the text, using Pretests, short section quizzes, and Posttests. All answers are provided to give learners immediate feedback on their command of section content before proceeding to the next module section.

The self-study modules in this book focus on the relationship between pathophysiology and the nursing process with the following goals in mind:

1. Revisit and translate critical pathophysiologic concepts pertaining to the high-acuity patient in a clinically applicable manner
2. Examine the interrelationships among physiologic concepts
3. Enhance clinical decision-making skills
4. Free class time to focus on clinical application
5. Hold learners accountable for their own learning
6. Provide immediate feedback to the learner regarding assimilation of concepts and principles
7. Provide self-paced learning

Ultimately, the goal for the learner is to be able to approach patient care conceptually, so that care is given with a strong underlying understanding of its rationale.

This book is appropriate for use in multiple educational settings, for example, nursing students, novice nurses, novice critical care nurses, and community health/home health nurse. It is also a review book for the experienced nurse wanting to update knowledge in high-acuity nursing for continuing education purposes. Hospital staff development departments will find it useful as supplemental or required reading for nursing staff high-acuity or critical care classes. It has also been used for teaching basic pathophysiology, and as a review book for the NCLEX exam.

Organization of the Text

The book consists of nine parts: Special Topics, Respiration and Ventilation, Cellular Oxygenation, Perfusion, Neurologic, Metabolic, Gastrointestinal, Injury, and Life Span: Special Needs.

For continuity, the modules in Parts I through VIII

are written in a consistent manner, using a single concept or nursing application format. The single concept modules contain an Introduction, Glossary, Abbreviation List, Objectives, Pretest, Review Questions, and a Posttest. Each module is divided into sections covering one facet of the module's topic (e.g., physiology, pathophysiology, or nursing management).

Parts II through VIII conclude with a nursing care module, which uses a case study problem-solving approach to test the learner's skill in applying the information presented in each part.

Part I, Special Topics, is composed of four modules. The topics included in this part apply to high-acuity patients in general or focus on a special procedure, as is the case with the organ transplantation module. Module 1 addresses the psychosocial needs of high-acuity patients, their families, and the nurses who care for them. Module 2 focuses on acute pain and the unique needs of high-acuity patients in pain assessment and management. Module 3 presents fluid and electrolyte concepts and problems. Finally, Module 4 provides an overview of organ transplantation from two perspectives: the donor and the recipient.

Parts II through *VIII* present topics that represent the complex problems, assessments, and treatments commonly associated with the nursing care of high-acuity patients. Ten modules focus on single organ system dysfunction (e.g., brain, spinal cord, lungs, heart, blood, kidneys, liver, pancreas, gastrointestinal, and skin). Three modules address concepts related to multiple organ dysfunction. Five modules focus on assessment (e.g., arterial blood gas analysis, hemodynamic monitoring, cardiac monitoring, responsiveness, and trauma assessment). Four modules address interventions (mechanical ventilation, management of stroke/brain attack, wound management, and trauma resuscitation). Finally, two modules focus on altered metabolic and immune responses.

Part IX, Life Span: Special Needs, addresses high-acuity pediatric, obstetric, and elderly patient concepts. In reality, the nurse may encounter these special needs patients in multiple settings, including acute care facilities, clinics, or home settings. In the hospital setting, nurses often encounter high-acuity pediatric patients who have been integrated into adult areas because of lack of pediatric bed availability. Obstetric patients who become acutely ill may also be admitted to a nonobstetric hospital area. Obstetric patients have special needs related to the physiologic changes encountered in pregnancy that must be addressed in planning and implementing nursing. The elderly comprise a large percentage of the high-acuity patient population in most settings that provide nursing care. The three modules in this part integrate multiple physiologic concepts with the nursing process.

New to This Edition

The third edition has added three new modules to reflect the needs of our text users, including *Fluid and Electrolyte Balance in the High-Acuity Patient, Acute Hematologic Dysfunction,* and *Acute Gastrointestinal Dysfunction.* In addition, all modules have been updated, and multiple modules have been substantially reorganized or streamlined. Test items have been revised to reflect the changes in content.

Summary

This text is a series of reality-based modules that focus on concepts frequently encountered in high-acuity patients. It is not designed as a comprehensive review of pathophysiology or medical–surgical nursing. The book's format reduces learner feelings of being overwhelmed by complex information. Learners are more apt to feel in command of the concepts, giving them the confidence to proceed to the more complex concepts. The third edition of *High-Acuity Nursing* has maintained the look and feel of the previous editions. Although the third edition has been expanded slightly (there are now 38 modules), we have not compromised on our approach. The ultimate goal of this book continues to be to enhance the preparation of nurses for practice in today's health care settings.

Pamela Stinson Kidd
Kathleen Dorman Wagner

About the Authors

Pamela Kidd is Associate Dean for Research and Graduate Studies in the College of Nursing at Arizona State University. She is the former Director of the KY Injury Prevention and Research Center at the University of Kentucky. Pam is also a Family Nurse Practitioner who works in a mobile health service. A working mother of a 6 year old and a 21 year old, she knows firsthand about stress-related illness and injury prevention across the lifespan!

Kathleen Wagner is a Lecturer in the Undergraduate Program in the College of Nursing at the University of Kentucky. Her background is as a Clinical Nurse Specialist in adult critical care, with over 15 years of experience in diverse critical care and high-acuity settings and 20 years as a nurse educator. As a nurse educator, she teaches pathophysiology and high-acuity nursing. She is also a doctoral student in the College of Education, studying Instructional Systems Design.

CONTRIBUTORS

Sharon Jackson Barton, RN, PhD (Module 36)
Assistant Professor
College of Nursing
Nurse Researcher, UK Children's Hospital
University of Kentucky
Lexington, KY

Diane Orr Chlebowy, RN, MA, MS, Doctoral Candidate (Module 25)
Assistant Professor
College of Nursing
University of Kentucky
Lexington, KY

Dee Ann Day, RN, MSN, ARNP, CCRN (Modules 17, 20)
Assistant Professor
Spalding University
School of Nursing
Louisville, KY

Deborah L. Dobbelhoff, RN
Level III Nurse
Pediatric Intensive Care Unit
University of Kentucky
Children's Hospital
Lexington, KY

Judy Elder, RN, BSN, MDiv (Retired) (Module 1)
Formerly Nurse Liaison
University of Kentucky
Lexington, KY

Julia Fultz, RN, BSN, CFN, CEN (Modules 33, 34, 35)
Flight Nurse
UK Air Medical Service
University of Kentucky
Lexington, KY

Laurie Giovanetti, RN, BSN (Module 37)
Labor and Delivery
Perinatal Nurse Consultant
University Hospital
University of Kentucky
Lexington, KY

Melanie Hardin-Pierce, RN, MSN, ACNP-CS (Modules 28, 29, 30, 31)
Assistant Professor
College of Nursing
University of Kentucky
Lexington, KY

Helen Frisch Hodges, RN, PhD (Module 24)
Associate Professor, RN-BSN Coordinator
Georgia Baptist College of Nursing
Atlanta, GA

Karen Johnson, RN, PhD, CCRN (Modules 9, 10, 11, 12, 32)
Lecturer
University of Arizona
College of Nursing
Tucson, AZ

Debbie Kitchen, RN, MSN, CS (Module 38)
Clinical Nurse Specialist in Gerontology Nursing
St. Joseph Hospital
Lexington, KY

Theresa Loan, RN, PhD (Module 22)
Formerly Nutrition Support Service
University of Kentucky Medical Center
Lexington, KY

Megan C. Switzer, ARNP, MSN, CCRN (Modules 13, 14, 15, 16)
Cardiovascular Clinical Specialist
Genetech, Inc.
Family Nurse Practitioner
St. Joseph Hospital Mobile Health Service
St. Joseph Hospital
Lexington, KY

Diana Thacker, BSN, RN, CPTC (Module 4)
Senior Hospital Services Coordinator
Kentucky Organ Donor Affiliates
Lexington, KY

Barbara L. Vanderveer, RN, MSN (Module 2)
Department of Anesthesiology
University of Kentucky
Lexington, KY

Reviewers

Pamela K. Branson, RN, MSN
Patient and Family Services
University of Kentucky
Lexington, KY

Zara R. Brenner, MS, RN, CS
School of Nursing
SUNY Brockport
Brockport, NY

Mary Lynn Burnett, RN, C, MSN
Instructor/Clinical Educator
School of Nursing
Wichita State University
Wichita, KS

Ruth N. Grendell, DNSc, RN
School of Nursing
Point Loma Nazarene University
San Diego, CA

Carol S. Ladden, MSN, CRNP
School of Nursing
University of Pennsylvania
Philadelphia, PA

Cyndi Logsdon, DNS, ARNC
School of Nursing
Spalding University
Louisville, KY

Gracie Wishnia, PhD, RNC
School of Nursing
Spalding University
Louisville, KY

Kathy Zellner, RN, MSN
Bellin School of Nursing
Green Bay, WI

David Gater, Jr., MD, PhD
Assistant Professor
Physical Medicine & Rehabilitation
University of Kentucky
Lexington, KY

Acknowledgments

I want to thank my dear colleague and friend, Kathy Wagner, for hanging in there with me on this revision. WE ARE A TEAM. The complexity of high-acuity nursing is amazing. It is impossible for one person to keep up to date in everything. If I feel this overwhelmed, I can only imagine what our students go through. My thanks to all of the reviewers! We have tried to reduce the information into critical chunks that can be meaningfully linked. We want to encourage people to enter this wonderful career called nursing. By making the food on the plate digestible, we hope to do what we can to prevent burnout, self-defeat, and broken dreams. Here's to passing the NCLEX on the first try!

PSK

The development of each new edition presents new challenges. In this revision, my personal challenge was juggling the roles as wife and mother, nurse educator, and doctoral student. Pam's solid support and confident "can do" attitude brought me back from the brink many times. Thanks so much, Pam—we do indeed make a good team. My thanks also go out to my two daughters, Becky and Debby, and my husband, Don. Their loving support made all of the juggling doable.

KDW

Part I

Special Topics

Module 1

Caring for the Critically Ill Patient: Patient, Family, and Nursing Considerations

Pamela Stinson Kidd, Judy Elder

This module is written at a core knowledge level for individuals who provide nursing care for critically ill patients, regardless of the practice setting. The focus of the module is the nursing role in caring for critically ill patients and the effect of the critical illness or injury on the patient, family, and nurse. The module is divided into two parts: Patient and Family Considerations and Nursing Considerations. Part One consists of five sections. Section One introduces the critically ill patient. Sections Two and Three address the stages of illness and nursing strategies to assist the patient in coping with being critically ill. Section Four discusses the influence of the environment on the patient's psychological and physical integrity. Section Five examines the educational needs of critically ill patients and their family. The second part, consisting of six sections, discusses the nursing role in caring for critically ill patients. Section Six examines visitation policies and the critically ill patient. Section Seven discusses work design and staffing strategies for the critically ill patient. The interface between technology and caring is discussed in Section Eight. Stressors and satisfying factors associated with nursing the critically ill patient are addressed in Section Nine. Section Ten examines resource allocation issues, and Section Eleven encourages the learner to complete a self-assessment in order to identify potential sources of personal conflict in working with the critically ill. Each section includes a set of review questions to help the learner evaluate his or her understanding of the section's content before moving on to the next section. All Section Reviews and the module Pretest and Posttest include answers. It is suggested that the learner review those concepts answered incorrectly in the review questions before proceeding to the next section.

Objectives

Following completion of this module, the learner will be able to

1. Discuss the evolution of the health care system in regard to caring for critically ill patients.
2. Discuss stages of illness a critically ill patient may experience.
3. Identify ways the nurse can help the critically ill patient to cope with the illness and/or injury.
4. Identify the influence of environment on the critically ill patient's psychological and physical responses.
5. Discuss the educational needs of critically ill patients and their families.
6. Explain the impact of visitation on patients and family members.
7. Identify work design and staffing strategies for the high-acuity patient.
8. Discuss the interface between technology and caring.
9. Describe stressful and satisfying aspects in providing nursing care for the critically ill patient.
10. Describe resource allocation issues as they relate to the critically ill patient.
11. Identify personal values that may contribute to satisfaction or stress in caring for the critically ill patient.

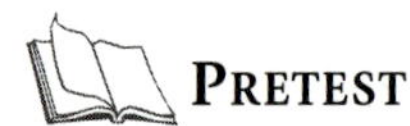

PRETEST

1. Critically ill patients frequently complain about which of the following when hospitalized?
   A. lack of privacy
   B. hospital food
   C. inadequate nursing staff
   D. lack of blankets
2. Denial during critical illness
   A. can have positive effects on health outcomes
   B. increases oxygen consumption
   C. is a maladaptive coping strategy
   D. promotes false hope
3. Hypohugganemia is
   A. a reduction in red blood cells related to social isolation
   B. desaturation of oxyhemoglobin
   C. an adversity to touch
   D. a state of touch deficiency
4. Who of the following is at greatest risk for developing sensory problems?
   A. adolescent patient
   B. unresponsive patient
   C. female patient
   D. transplant patient
5. A major reason that computers are being tested for use in decision making with critically ill patients is
   A. computers are compact
   B. computers are time efficient
   C. any staff member can input available data
   D. there is a large amount of data that must be processed in order to make a decision
6. Nurses who work with critically ill patients cite which of the following as a major stressor?
   A. overtime work
   B. nurse–patient ratio
   C. constant need to reverify skills and procedures
   D. interpersonal conflict with other health team members
7. Of the following patient populations, which population is the least vulnerable in regard to resource allocation?
   A. neonates
   B. elderly
   C. oncology patients
   D. transplant patients
8. Which of the following factors may inhibit learning in critically ill patients?
   A. medications
   B. previous knowledge of illness
   C. educational level
   D. gender
9. Families of critically ill patients desire which of the following needs to be met first by the nurse?
   A. physical
   B. spiritual
   C. cognitive
   D. emotional
10. Mr. Rogers states, "I'm going to have to put up with this scar and make the best of it." This response indicates he is in which of the following states of illness?
    A. awareness
    B. resolution
    C. restitution
    D. denial
11. The purpose of imagery is to
    A. ignore the real situation
    B. replace unpleasant experiences with relaxation
    C. promote use of the senses
    D. increase neurologic stimulation
12. Critically ill patients have which of the following characteristics?
    A. have been hospitalized previously
    B. need extensive rehabilitation
    C. are physically unstable
    D. have chronic illness
13. The use of equipment in the nursing role may
    A. increase the nurse's stress level
    B. decrease nursing surveillance responsibility
    C. decrease the need for patient advocacy
    D. increase patient satisfaction
14. Which of the following is a hazard of technology?
    A. increased fragmentation of care
    B. decreased demand for nursing staff
    C. decreased competition with patient for nursing time
    D. increased patient feeling of independence
15. Which of the following may be a source of burnout?
    A. hourly nursing assessment
    B. nursing care plans
    C. continuing education requirements
    D. primary nursing
16. Which of the following may be a symptom of burnout?
    A. nurse requests to work a holiday
    B. nurse assists coworkers in care
    C. nurse complains of inadequate physician standing orders
    D. nurse states that "females always give in to their pain"
17. Mr. Martin states that he has dreamed of being tortured while in the intensive care unit. The nurse recognizes that this is a symptom of
    A. sensory deprivation
    B. burnout
    C. fatigue
    D. uncontrolled pain
18. Children of critically ill patients
    A. do not want to visit their ill parent
    B. should be given a choice to visit their parent

C. experience emotional distress after visitation
D. want to visit their critically ill fathers but not their critically ill mothers

19. Which of the following have nurses identified as increasing their satisfaction with their role?
A. getting on-call pay
B. orienting new staff
C. working multiple shifts
D. small nurse–patient ratio

20. All of the following have been cited to relieve stress associated with the nursing role EXCEPT
A. discussion with co-workers
B. self-assessment of achievements
C. serving as unit resource person
D. watching television

Pretest answers: 1. A, 2. A, 3. D, 4. B, 5. D, 6. D, 7. D, 8. A, 9. C, 10. B, 11. B, 12. C, 13. A, 14. A, 15. D, 16. D, 17. A, 18. B, 19. D, 20. C

Glossary

Burnout. A crisis state evolving from stress; to become exhausted by making excessive demands on energy, strength, or resources

Delusion. Fixed, irrational belief not consistent with cultural mores; may include persecutory or grandiose ideas

Hallucination. False sensory perception occurring without any external stimulus; a person can see, feel, hear, smell, or taste things that another person cannot

Hypohugganemia. A state of touch deficiency when the need for physical contact increases or when the need remains the same but the opportunities for physical contact are diminished

Illusion. False interpretation of an external sensory stimulus that is usually visual or auditory in nature

Sensory perceptual alterations. The amount, character, or intensity of stimuli exceeds the person's minimum or maximum threshold of tolerance for sensory input; accompanied by a diminished, exaggerated, distorted, or impaired response

Abbreviations

dB. decibel

SPA. sensory perceptual alteration

PATIENT AND FAMILY CONSIDERATIONS

SECTION ONE: Evolution of Patient Care Areas for Critically Ill Patients

At the completion of this section, the learner will be able to discuss briefly the evolution of the health care system in regard to caring for critically ill patients.

The nurse caring for the critically ill patient must be able to analyze clinical situations, make decisions based on this analysis, and act on the decisions made rapidly and precisely. Comfort with uncertainty and patient instability are requirements in this area. The nurse is instrumental in treating patients' health problems as well as their reactions to the health care environment. The nurse is usually the constant in caring for the critically ill patient. The nurse coordinates the care of the other health team members.

Nurses working in critical care units have received respect both within and outside the nursing profession. This respect is related to social events. World wars produced the need for trauma care and intensive nursing both before and after surgery. Polio epidemics provided the motivation for respiratory care. Traditionally, patients were admitted to the intensive care unit for nursing care in combination with technologic capabilities. The perception evolved that good nursing care could be found only in the intensive care unit (Baggs, 1989).

Intensive care units (ICUs) were first developed in the early 1960s. The reasons for their development were (1) the implementation of cardiopulmonary resuscitation so that people might survive sudden death events; (2) better understanding of the treatment of hypovolemic shock related to recent war experiences; (3) implementation of emergency medical services, resulting in improved transport systems; (4) development of technologic inventions that required close observation for effective use (i.e., electrocardiographic monitoring); and (5) initiation of renal transplant surgery.

The first ICUs were recovery rooms. Patients admitted were still anesthetized. Problems resulted, however, when the amount of surgery increased, and recovery rooms were needed for patients to recover from anesthesia. The more acutely ill patient who required extra equipment and observation was placed in the newly created ICU.

Although critically ill patients are viewed historically as being in a critical care unit, this is no longer true because of the shortage of critical care beds and increased patient acuity. The critically ill patient is physically unstable and at risk of developing life-threatening problems. These patients require continuous, intensive assessment and interventions for restoration of physiologic stability (American Association of Critical Care Nurses [AACN], 1994). They also require care that incorporates their hopes, dreams, values, cultural practices, and concerns (Harvey et al., 1993). Patients with chronic illnesses who experience an acute exacerbation, as well as patients with a nonsignificant medical history who are involved in a traumatic event or exhibit an acute problem, fall within this definition. The nursing shortage (particularly the shortage of critical care nurses), an increase in life expectancy, an increase in number of persons with chronic illness, and the number of uninsured/underinsured patients create an increased demand for services. Therefore, critically ill patients may be found in a variety of settings: intensive care units, emergency departments, postanesthesia care units, medical–surgical units, obstetric units, hospice units, and the home. The trend is to use more assistive devices and less surgical procedures. Thus, the demand for advanced practice nurses who can teach home caregivers how to coexist with these assistive devices and deal with the ramifications of living with an acutely ill patient will increase (Wlody, 1998).

Regardless of the setting, patients have complained about the helplessness and embarrassment they have felt when they were critically ill. Some patients fear dying, pain, and the uncertainty of their situation. They are fearful of moving in bed because of tubing, attachments, and incisions. They frequently feel frustrated about their inability to communicate when they are endotracheally intubated. The inability to communicate is the most distressing aspect of mechanical ventilation (Halm & Alpen, 1993). Critically ill patients often are left nude or partially exposed. They are powerless and are stripped of their identity. For many patients, it is the first time they have faced their own mortality (Clark, 1993). They may have an altered appearance (Urban, 1998).

Nurses caring for the critically ill patient can anticipate patient feelings and support patient independence. Education about the nature of machinery can decrease fears of harming oneself and the machinery. Nurses can role-model communication skills. Privacy should not be sacrificed, and the lack of it should not be justified by the intensity of the patient situation.

In summary, the nurse must remember the complexity surrounding critical illness. The physiologic needs of the patient take precedence; however, physiologic and psychological factors both must be considered when analyzing patient responses. For example, sensory alterations may occur because of electrolyte imbalances, drug reactions, or stimuli overload. The aim of this module is to support patient adaptation in a holistic manner using a humanistic approach.

SECTION ONE REVIEW

1. Which of the following factors contributed to the development of ICUs?
   - A. increased number of patients requiring hospitalization
   - B. development of Medicare/Medicaid system
   - C. implementation of cardiopulmonary resuscitation
   - D. movement of nursing education to the collegiate setting
2. Which of the following characteristics best describes critically ill patients?
   - A. physiologically unstable with uncertain health outcomes
   - B. volume depleted and edematous
   - C. frustrated and demanding
   - D. having impaired physical mobility and altered nutritional state

Answers: 1. C, 2. A

SECTION TWO: Stages of Illness

At the completion of this section, the learner will be able to discuss the stages of illness a critically ill patient may experience.

Critical illness produces a loss of the familiar self-image and has an impact on self-esteem. The patient may need to adapt to loss of health, loss of limb, disfigurement, or a necessary change in lifestyle. Change may precipitate grieving. Critically ill patients may respond to these losses by experiencing certain predictable phases. The first stage is shock and disbelief, because the diagnosis does not have an emotional meaning. The patient may be uncooperative because he or she is projecting difficulties onto hospital procedures, equipment, and personnel. In this stage, a patient may worry more about the equipment being used than about the diagnosis, since the diagnosis may be a threat to life. Denial can have positive effects. It may pro-

TABLE 1–1. PHASES OF STRESS FOR FAMILIES

PHASE	DEFINITION	MANIFESTATIONS	INTERVENTIONS
High anxiety	Worry about the ill family member and the family	Fainting, nausea, restlessness	Provide accurate information
Denial	Regression to a comfortable way of thinking	Refusing to discuss reality	Reiterate the facts of the situation
Anger	An attempt to place blame for what has happened	Verbal abuse directed toward heath care staff	Active listening—help to focus on the real cause of anger
Remorse	Families regret they could not or did not prevent the situation	Elements of guilt and sorrow	Interject reality
Grief	Admission that life has changed; reality of the loss processed	Sadness, crying	Allow expression of emotions and provide empathy
Reconciliation	Putting things in place	Planning for the future; speaking about the changes	Provide resources to support family functioning

Adapted from Hopkins, A. (1994). The trauma nurse's role with families in crisis. Crit Care Nurse *14:35–43.*

tect the patient against the emotional impact of the illness and conserve energy by removing worry. The nurse should function as a noncritical listener. Patient statements can be clarified, but reality is not stressed (Suchman, 1965).

The awareness stage is characterized by an attempt to regain control. Patients may express guilt about the illness or injury as a gesture of assuming responsibility for events over which they may or may not have actual control. The patient may be demanding or exhibit signs of withdrawal. Both signs are indicative of anger toward either others or the self. The nurse should not argue with the patient. Consistent, dependable nursing care should be provided.

During the next stage, restitution, the patient may verbalize fears about the future. New behaviors are initiated that reflect new limitations. Sadness is experienced, and crying episodes may be frequent. The patient may reorganize relationships with family and friends. The nurse can assist by building communication to assist with problem solving.

Resolution, the final stage, involves identity change. The patient may begin to think of the illness as a growing experience. Limitations are accepted as consequences and not as defects.

These stages are not fixed but reflect a dynamic process of adjusting to an acute situation. The patient may regress to an earlier stage during periods of heightened anxiety. One aim in caring for the critically ill patient is to foster a feeling of security. A patient may feel vulnerable because of physiologic changes, such as paralysis or traction. Emotional vulnerability may be experienced when restraints are applied as a protective mechanism. Several factors may produce anxiety in the patient even if they mean that the patient is more physiologically stable. The removal of electrodes, weaning from the ventilator, reduction in pain medication, and increasing mobility are among these factors.

Families also progress through phases when experiencing stress related to a critically ill family member (Aultschuler, 1997). Each family varies regarding the sequence of the phases and the rate of progression. The six phases are described in Table 1–1. After progressing through the phases, some families grow stronger while others never return to their previous functioning level. Nursing interventions appropriate for each phase are listed in the table.

In summary, the critically ill patient and his or her family may progress through a series of emotional stages because of losses experienced during the illness event. The stages the patient progresses through are referred to as denial, awareness, restitution, and resolution. The family experiences high anxiety, denial, anger, remorse, grief, and reconciliation. The patient's and family's progression through these stages may not be linear. When an additional stressor occurs, the patient and/or family may regress to a previous stage in which they feel more secure.

Section Two Review

1. A major behavior of a patient in the denial stage of illness is
   A. false humor
   B. crying
   C. anger
   D. projection of difficulties onto objects and staff

2. The awareness stage of illness is characterized by all of the following EXCEPT
   A. increased dependence on others
   B. expression of guilt
   C. withdrawal behavior
   D. being demanding of caregivers

3. Mr. Abe was involved in a motor vehicle crash and sustained multiple lower extremity fractures. He will need additional surgery and prolonged physical therapy. The nurse finds Mr. Abe drawing plans for remodeling his porch to accommodate a wheelchair. This behavior reflects which stage of illness?
   A. denial
   B. awareness
   C. restitution
   D. resolution
4. When interacting with a patient in denial, the nurse should
   A. reinforce reality
   B. function as a noncritical listener
   C. explain the current treatment plan
   D. help the patient to recall the injury event
5. A family of a patient who sustained a spinal cord injury is talking about the college football scholarship the patient will need to return because of the patient's quadriplegia. This family exhibits behavior reflecting which stage of family stress?
   A. remorse
   B. reconciliation
   C. grief
   D. anger
6. An appropriate nursing intervention for a family experiencing high anxiety is
   A. active listening
   B. provide accurate information
   C. exhibit empathy
   D. acknowledge family loss

Answers: 1. D, 2. A, 3. D, 4. B, 5. C, 6. B

SECTION THREE: Coping with Critical Illness

At the completion of this section, the learner will be able to identify ways the nurse can help the critically ill patient to cope with the illness or injury event.

Critically ill patients use strategies to maintain or increase their sense of hope during a life-threatening event (Patel, 1996). They may use pleasant, distracting images of favored activities, or may express a conviction that a positive outcome is possible. The belief that growth results from crisis fosters hope. Spiritual practices and beliefs that allow the patient to transcend suffering facilitate coping. Caregivers who convey positive expectations that the patient will be able to cope with the stresses as well as who assist the patient by gentle pushing support the patient's hope (Miller, 1989).

We are increasingly becoming aware of the importance of the search for meaning in life-changing events. Spirituality, a sense of faith and transcendence, and a sorting out of old life views are frequently part of the experience of the patient and family after critical illness or injury. Questions such as "Why me?", "Why this?", and "Why now?" become part of the patient's/family's quest for meaning. The critical care nurse can provide a sounding board for such questions and a nonjudgmental listener as patients and families sort out their answers.

Because of the increased emphasis on manipulating equipment (discussed further in Section Eight of this module), human contact has received decreased emphasis during critical illness. Touching is a form of communication and a behavior of caring. Fear, pain, and acute stress can increase a person's need for touch (Dominion, 1971), and generally, complex technology increases the need for human touch (Kirchhoff et al., 1985). Although the patient's sex, ethnicity, and age may influence the perception of touch as a caring behavior, most individuals appreciate being touched during a crisis (Clement, 1988). Although limited research has been conducted with adults, neonates who received non–task-oriented touch had greater weight gain and a shorter hospital stay. Back rubs and massage should be nursing interventions. Experts in massage and therapeutic touch should be part of the health care team (Bartz, 1993). A state of touch deficiency may occur, **hypohugganemia,** in which a person's need for physical contact increases or the need remains constant while the opportunities for touch decrease (Clement, 1986). Touch may decrease perceived pain and anxiety, and may accelerate wound healing by decreasing the number of suppressor T cells (Quinn, 1993). However, patients should be warned prior to touching to respect the patient's personal space.

Alternative therapies are now more widely accepted as ways of helping the patient cope with illness. One goal of alternative therapy is to help the patient manage symptoms. It is important to remember that all patients are in need of healing even if they cannot be cured. There are several classifications of alternative therapies. This section will be limited to discussing those therapies that focus on the mind's ability to affect the body (e.g., meditation, imagery, relaxation). Many of these therapies are based on psychoneuroimmunology. Briefly, the limbic system in the brain mediates emotions through regulation of neuropeptides. Neuropeptides affect immune cells and ultimately cell response.

Self-regulation strategies, such as progressive muscle relaxation, biofeedback, and self-hypnosis, may be used to enhance the patient's feeling of control and to foster pain and anxiety relief. These strategies have an impact on the autonomic, endocrine, immune, and neuropeptide systems (Hoekstra, 1994). Relaxation has been associated with decreased premature ventricular contractions. Promoting relaxation decreases sympathetic nervous system activity. This enhances the effect of pain medications; decreases fatigue, anxiety, and muscle tension; increases effective breathing patterns; and helps the patient to dissociate from pain. The use of humor also may help the patient cope with critical illness. Initially, laughter accelerates respiratory and heart rate, but this phase is followed by decreased blood pressure and deep, effective breathing. The relaxation response is stimulated by endorphin release (Hoekstra, 1994).

Imagery and progressive muscle relaxation are self-regulation responses that involve all the senses. Imagery can influence both the voluntary and involuntary nervous systems. Imagery has been associated with decreased pain, decreased cortisol levels, and less wound erythema (Hoekstra, 1994). Healthier images can become blueprints to reframe positive changes at the biochemical cellular level (Guzetta et al., 1998). The patient learns conscious control of his or her sympathetic nervous system. The nurse must individualize the imagery process. Individualization requires an understanding of physiology of the illness; knowledge of medication, procedures, and diagnostic tests; and an understanding of the patient's beliefs (Dossey, 1990). The goal is to create an image of healing or the peacefulness of moving into death (if this is appropriate). Imagery desensitizes potentially anxiety-producing events by replacing fear or pain with relaxation. The following case study demonstrates the use of imagery. The case study is referred to again in Sections Four and Five.

Mr. T is a 79-year-old man who had an exploratory laparotomy for a perforated duodenal ulcer. He has a history of chronic airflow limitation and is steroid dependent. Mr. T's wound is healing by secondary intention. He has been having a great deal of pain during dressing changes.

The nurse prepares the patient care area by dimming lights and decreasing noise. The nurse can place a sign outside the patient's room indicating that an imagery session is taking place. The nurse promotes relaxation by encouraging Mr. T to start at the top of his head and imagine that each muscle is going limp. She describes it as a heavy good feeling. The nurse will go through each body section separately (neck, shoulders, and so on). Mr. T will close his eyes and concentrate on his body.

Nurse: "As the old dressing is being removed, your new tissue is getting fresh nutrients because dead skin and bacteria are being pulled away with the gauze. Imagine a tiny skin cell with hands that reach out to join another skin cell to make a firm chain. Although you are a little uncomfortable, you want the dressing to be removed because the new skin cells cannot grow underneath the debris from the old cells. As the new cells get nutrients, there is less drainage and less discomfort. Now, imagine that the skin is completely together just like it was before surgery. There is no need for more dressing changes.

"Each time your dressing is changed, concentrate on this image of the skin cells joining hands to make a firm chain that is completely together and healed. Imagine the cells getting fresh air and food that make them strong."

The goal of this imagery session was to describe positive aspects of the dressing change, in order to replace Mr. T's fear with a positive image of healing.

Coping skills of families and patients vary and the critical care nurse is challenged to adapt interventions to fit individual families. Using Jalowiec's Coping Scale as a guide, Table 1–2 describes coping responses and the corresponding nursing interventions.

In summary, the nurse can use several strategies to assist the critically ill patient in coping with the illness or injury event. These strategies include instilling hope, supporting spirituality, using physical touch, promoting relaxation, and using guided imagery with progressive muscle relaxation. Regardless of what type of coping response is exhibited, the nurse can intervene to support positive coping.

TABLE 1–2. SAMPLE COPING RESPONSES AND INTERVENTIONS

JCS[a] COPING STYLE	SAMPLE COPING RESPONSE	NURSING INTERVENTIONS
Supportant	Talk with others	• Ask family member to share perceptions of present and future impact of the critical illness. • Use techniques of active listening, reflecting, and clarifying. • Use open-ended questions. • Assit family member to identify support persons (relatives, friends, and professionals). • Role-model listening skills to support persons and positively reinforce. • Encourage family member to set aside regular times with a support person expressly for the purpose of talking about their situation. • Recommend that family member make and receive phone calls from support persons.
	Prayer	• Pray with family member or be present during prayer. • Refer to clergy as appropriate. • Reaffirm verbalized perceptions of a Greater Strength. • Encourage to keep a prayer journal.

(continues)

TABLE 1–2. SAMPLE COPING RESPONSES AND INTERVENTIONS *(continued)*

JCS[a] COPING STYLE	SAMPLE COPING RESPONSE	NURSING INTERVENTIONS
Optimistic	Positive thinking	• Assist family to designate a realistic "Daily Positive Thought" and post in patient's room. • Acknowledge family strengths to increase awareness of personal resources. • Reaffirm family member's ability to manage situation. • Note indicators of personal growth through adversity.
	Hope	• Report signs of patient's improvement to family. • Assist family to visualize and verbalize realistically how the situation could have a positive outcome. • Identify short-term goals for patient or family that can be met each day.
Confrontive	Gain information	• Initiate contact with the family to provide information. • Offer appropriate and specific explanations initially and throughout hospitalization. • Use visual aids and repetition. • Be honest and accurate to increase professional credibility. • Encourage family to ask questions. • Verify understanding and clarify misconceptions. • Arrange a time each day with family for patient updates. • Consider usefulness of regular telephone contacts with family.
	Control/change situation	• Acknowledge family's expressions of powerlessness and identify factors that contribute. • Request suggestions from family about case management. • Enlist family participation in patient care. • Allow flexibility in visiting pattern. • Share with family members that they can control their self-talk processes.
Self-Reliant	Self-talk	• Increase awareness of self-talk content. • Emphasize the relationship between negative self-talk, negative emotions, and decreased physical, mental, and social functioning. • Teach positive self-talk and reframing strategies, using written materials as appropiate to stretch nurses' time.
	Withdraw socially	• Provide quiet space. • Arrange time alone if desired. • Identify potential advantages of contact with others during stress. • Initiate conversation, even if brief.
Fatalistic	Expect the worst outcome	• If the worst outcome is likely, offer emotional support and acknowledge the possibility of a poor outcome. • If the worst outcome is likely, provide accurate information, encourage thought replacement, and reaffirm the benefits of hope.
Palliative	Eat, drink, smoke	• Identify and replace negative thoughts that drive behavior. • Encourage moderation, such as mild foods, nonalcoholic beverages. • Delay modification plan for long-standing behaviors until after crisis stage of critical illness.
	Exercise	• Relate benefits of physical activity. • Encourage to walk indoors or outdoors daily. • Identify community sites for short-term exercise.
	Distraction	• Arrange for recreational diversions in waiting area, such as a television, videocassette player and movies, table for playing cards, and writing supplies.
Evasive	Blaming others	• Label negative emotions, for example "frustration," "anger." • Identify and replace thoughts associated with negative emotion. • Identify thougths to modify or replace negative thought. • Note that disenchantment with others may be a phase in the coping process. • Reaffirm the capacity of people for positive change. • Recall that placing blame externally may be effective coping during the crisis stage of illness.
Emotive	Ventilate negative emotions	• Encouage family to ventilate outside of the unit so as not to convey negative emotions to patient. • Encourage family member to tell the "story" of the illness to diffuse emotions. • Verbalize acceptance of feelings. • Maintain eye contact.
	Worry	• Coach in worrying constructively, as in formulating a worst outcome plan. • Assist family to identify pointless fretting. • Supply thought management guidance to replace unuseful ways of thinking. • Engage family members in holding each other accountable for diminishing nonconstructive worry.

[a]Jalowiec Coping Scale.
Used with permission of Anne Jalowiec, RN, Ph.D., FAAN.

SECTION THREE REVIEW

1. The rationale for using self-regulation techniques with critically ill patients is to
   A. promote feelings of control
   B. decrease parasympathetic nervous system impulses
   C. improve nurse–patient relationships
   D. help the patient associate with personal pain

2. Which of the following factors influences the perception of touch as a caring behavior?
   A. environmental temperature
   B. cultural background
   C. length of the hospitalization
   D. size of caregiver's hands

Answers: 1. A, 2. B

SECTION FOUR: Environmental Stressors

At the completion of this section, the learner will be able to discuss environmental stresses of the critically ill patient.

Sensory input involves all five senses: visual, auditory, olfactory, gustatory, and tactile. Individual perceptions of stimuli to the senses vary. Usually, people select stimuli that are most acceptable to them. However, during critical illness, the patient does not have control over the choice of the environment and its stimuli. The very young, the very old, and the postoperative or unresponsive patients are at greatest risk of experiencing **sensory perceptual alterations (SPAs).**

Sensory deprivation may occur because of either impaired use of the senses or inadequate quality and quantity of sensory input. The patient is not able to relate meaningfully to the environment. Symptoms of sensory deprivation include **illusions, delusions, hallucinations,** restlessness, and loss of sense of time. These symptoms may appear as early as 8 hours after a period of sensory deprivation (Farrimond, 1984). The nurse must assess whether the symptoms have a psychological basis or physical basis, such as hypoxia or increased intracranial pressure. Restricted movement, a windowless patient care area, monotonous light, and lack of stimuli all can provide sensory deprivation. The use of physical or pharmacologic restraints and family visit restrictions may also increase sensory deprivation (Urban, 1998).

A combination of sensory overload and deprivation can exist. The patient is deprived of normal sensory stimuli while being exposed to continuous strange stimuli not normally encountered. The nurse should assess what sounds are in the patient's normal environment and expose the patient to these sounds if possible (through tape recordings). Visitors can be effective by discussing familiar topics with the patient (Smith, 1994). Unresponsive patients are particularly challenging, since information about the patient's normal environment must be collected through a third person. It is difficult to assess whether unresponsive patients are experiencing sensory alterations, because they cannot communicate symptoms.

Sensory overload may occur when the patient is exposed to noise for continuous periods of time without rest. Patients perceive the most annoying sources of noise to be (1) staff conversation, (2) disturbing sounds from other patients, (3) overhead pages, and (4) loud sounds at night causing awakening (Baker, 1993). Certain individuals may be more sensitive to noise and experience greater noise-induced stress (Topf, 1992). Noise produces peripheral vasoconstriction, which can cause increased afterload (see Module 13 for explanation of afterload), especially in patients with hypertension. This response does not diminish on repeated exposure (Williams, 1989). Noise has a potentiating effect on ototoxic drugs (i.e., furosemide, aminoglycoside antibiotics, and salicylates) (Williams, 1989). Noise also stimulates the sympathetic nervous system, resulting in increased heart rate and oxygen consumption. Staff may become habituated to the noise. Noise levels at 40 decibels (dB) supports rest and sleep while the average noise level in critical care units ranges from 55 to 65 dB (Urban, 1998). Thus, staff may underestimate the noise level in the patient care setting. Table 1–3 summarizes physiologic and behavioral responses to noise.

Odors may also distress the patient. Odors may contribute to embarrassment and loss of dignity.

TABLE 1–3. PHYSIOLOGIC AND BEHAVIORAL RESPONSES TO NOISE

PHYSIOLOGIC	BEHAVIORAL
Elevated heart rate	Decreased problem solving
Increased blood pressure	Restlessness
Sodium/water retention	Nervousness
Elevated cortisol	Heightened aggression
Elevated cholesterol	Disturbed sleep, rest, and relaxation

Data from Baker C: Sensory overload and noise in the ICU: Sources of environmental stress. Crit Care Q *6:66–80, 1984; and Hansell H: The behavioral effects of noise on man: The patient with "intensive care unit psychosis."* Heart Lung *13:59–65, 1984.*

Critically ill patients are at risk for SPAs, which occur when either the amount, character, or intensity of stimuli exceeds the person's minimum or maximum threshold of tolerance for sensory input accompanied by a diminished, exaggerated, distorted, or impaired response. Responses may include altered consciousness, cognitive impairment, disturbances in affect, altered perception of reality, altered levels of activity, and sleep disturbances (Wilson, 1993).

SPAs have been noted to occur in 12 percent to 38 percent of conscious ICU patients between the third and seventh day after admission to the intensive care unit (Easton & MacKenzie, 1988). Interestingly, this is the same period of time when sleep deprivation usually occurs (Halm & Alpen, 1993). The highest incidence of this disorder has occurred in general surgical and cardiac surgical patients (Wilson, 1993). Varying degrees of delirium may exist, but usually illusions, delusions, and hallucinations are present. Patients may be experiencing symptoms but are reluctant to share them with the nurse for fear of being labeled crazy. It is important for the nurse to assess whether the delirium is related to physiologic reasons or the misinterpretation of unfamiliar environmental cues. Liver failure, electrolyte abnormalities, septic shock, hypoxia, and drug toxicities all can produce these symptoms. Retrospective research studies have revealed that patients frequently feel that they are being held prisoner and that they were repeatedly trying to escape (Schnaper & Cowley, 1976). SPAs occur more frequently in patients who deny preoperative anxiety and in patients in windowless patient care areas (Easton & MacKenzie, 1988). The increased acuity of patients in medical–surgical floor settings and the need for sophisticated equipment to monitor these critically ill patients may increase the prevalence of SPAs outside the intensive care unit.

Planned rest periods that allow for 2 hours of uninterrupted sleep are essential. Rapid eye movement (REM) sleep requires a 90- to 100-minute total sleep period for its occurrence. Therefore, 2-hour periods promote REM sleep. REM sleep helps to maintain optimism, attention span, and self-confidence. It may also increase levels of growth hormone, promoting anabolism and healing (Wood, 1993; Urban, 1999). There is an increased need for REM sleep after periods of worry. Deprivation of REM sleep can impair memory and learning ability and produce hallucinations (Wood, 1993). Lack of REM sleep increases adrenal hormone production, which suppresses the immune system. Noise has been associated with suppression of REM sleep (Topf & Davis, 1993). Sleep deprivation has been associated with death (Krachman, 1995).

The nurse can implement several interventions to prevent SPAs in critically ill patients. The audible volume of bedside monitors should be decreased to allow greater patient rest and to deemphasize how ill a patient may be. Nurses should provide frequent interpretations of environmental noise. Bedside equipment should be positioned away from the head of the bed. Exit valves on ventilators should face away from the patient's head. Suctioning equipment should be turned off when not in use. Intravenous infusion pumps should be refilled before the alarm sounds (Halm & Alpen, 1993). Phones can be set on low volume. Patient doors can be closed. Posted reminders to speak softly can be placed in high-traffic areas and by telephones. Nurses should ask patients if they have experienced any strange sensory experiences. Wall clocks and calendars may help the patient to remain oriented to time. However, clocks are not helpful if the patient's room does not have a window, since day and night cannot be discriminated (Hansell, 1984).

Darkened eyeshades and earplugs can be used to decrease noise and light. Lights can be dimmed to facilitate discrimination of day from night and promote circadian rhythms. Circadian rhythms influence basal metabolic rate, respiratory and heart rates, and body temperature. Circadian rhythms respond to environmental cues, such as light to dark alteration. Interventions can be spaced to allow rest periods, which should be provided with the same emphasis as that placed on hemodynamic measurements and assessment of vital signs. Nurses should document the amount of uninterrupted sleep the patient experiences (Wood, 1993).

Remember Mr. T from Section Three? Although his primary problem was a perforated ulcer, he also had a history of chronic airflow limitation and was steroid dependent. He had an acute exacerbation of respiratory failure. Arterial blood gases (ABGs) are pH 7.29, P_{CO_2} 55, PO_2 50. He is transferred to the surgical intensive care unit. Mr. T is intubated and placed on a ventilator. Tidal volume is 700, F_{IO_2} is 40 percent, assist/control mode, positive end-expiratory pressure is 5, with a rate of 10.

Mr. T is susceptible to SPAs.

General surgical patients have the highest incidence of ICU psychosis. It is important for the nurse to know his day of admission into the ICU, since SPAs usually occur between the third and seventh days. He is unable to communicate verbally. Being placed on the ventilator may prevent adequate rest periods due to frequent suctioning and noise. In summary, the critically ill patient is at risk for experiencing sensory deprivation, sensory overload, a combination of sensory overload and deprivation, sleep deprivation, and SPAs. The nurse can diminish patient susceptibility to these conditions by decreasing the amplitude of voices and telephones, closing patient doors, promoting orientation to time and place, and helping to discriminate night from day by changing unit lighting. Communication can be improved by using chalkboards or establishing a system of symbols.

SECTION FOUR REVIEW

1. SPAs occur
   A. only in intensive care units
   B. in patients over 65 years of age
   C. most often in coronary care units
   D. between the third and seventh day of admission
2. A frequently cited annoying noise among critically ill patients is
   A. ambulance sirens
   B. hospital paging system
   C. television
   D. equipment noise
3. Lack of REM sleep produces
   A. hypertension
   B. immunosuppression
   C. seizures
   D. aggressive behavior
4. Which of the following nursing interventions would support the patient's circadian rhythm cycle?
   A. dimming lights during normal sleep time
   B. putting a wall clock up in the patient's room
   C. encouraging normal bowel habits
   D. decreasing environmental noise

Answers: 1. D, 2. B, 3. B, 4. A

SECTION FIVE: Educational Needs of Patients and Families

At the completion of this section, the learner will be able to identify educational needs of critically ill patients and their families and strategies to meet these needs.

Critically ill patients have a right to know and understand what procedures are being done to and for them. Health care knowledge may decrease the length of the patient's hospitalization or the number of readmissions for the same condition. Initially, when teaching critically ill patients, the nurse must aim at decreasing stress and promoting comfort rather than increasing knowledge. The patient and family may not recall what the nurse said 10 minutes later, but the patient's blood pressure may be decreased or the pain lessened. As adult learners, critically ill patients focus on learning in order to solve problems. Thus, the nurse must assess what the patient considers to be problematic in order to make learning meaningful. Basic questions about what the patient and family want to know will assist the nurse in focusing content. It is also helpful to identify what the patient already knows. The reduced nurse–patient ratio used in most settings where critically ill patients are placed facilitates teaching. An interpersonal relationship allows for the patient to trust the abilities and knowledge of the nurse. For the critically ill patient to learn, he or she must feel secure.

Several factors inhibit learning in critically ill patients. Patients may be fatigued due to hypoxia, anemia, and being in a hypermetabolic state. They may have barriers to communication, such as endotracheal tubes. They may have a large number of hourly procedures and diagnostic tests that prevent quality teaching time. Pain will diminish a person's ability to concentrate. Drugs may depress the central nervous system and affect memory. The nurse should assess the patient for the presence of these factors. Physiologic needs take precedence over the need to know and the need to understand (Maslow, 1970). Once the patient's condition has stabilized, however, the patient is able to concentrate on learning.

Research has demonstrated that families also have a need for knowledge, and this need remains consistent regardless of the length of time the family member remains in the ICU (Davis-Martin, 1994). Families have consistently rated cognitive needs as being more important than emotional or physical needs. In 100 percent of nine research studies designed to identify the needs of families of critically ill patients, "to have questions answered honestly" and "to know specific facts regarding what is wrong with the patient and the patient's progress" were listed as the most important needs (Hickey, 1990; Miracle & Hovekamp, 1994). The need to know the prognosis and chance for recovery was listed as important in 90 percent of the studies. The need to believe there is hope is also highly rated by families (Davis-Martin, 1994). "To receive information in understandable terms" was identified 80 percent of the time. In addition to the need for knowledge, families indicated needing a mechanism through which they could receive information, such as a consistent nurse whom they could contact or who would contact the family. Being contacted about positive or negative changes in the patient's condition is important. Regardless of whether the family members were blood relatives or significant others, they indicated the same needs (Bouman, 1984). These findings were consistent up to 96 hours after admission. The use of nontechnical terms and written materials may be appropriate, since the family's ability to comprehend and process information may be limited as a result of the crisis of the critical illness.

Compared with general floor settings, families with a

member in an ICU desired (1) for staff to give them direction on what to do at the bedside, (2) to have a place to be alone as a family unit, (3) to be informed in advance of any transfer plan, and (4) to have flexibility in visitation (Foss & Tenholder, 1993). Needs of families change over time. An initial need is to feel that their loved one is receiving quality care. Later, the family has a greater need to spend time with the patient and participate in the patient's care (Urban, 1998).

In situations in which the patient is designated as Do Not Resuscitate (DNR), the nurse must reassure the family that physical and emotional care will be given. Families progress through three stages with health care providers: (1) naive trust, (2) disenchantment, and (3) guarded alliance where trust is on an informed level. Nurses can convey hope as an ever-changing process that adapts to the reality of the situation, even in impending death (Bouley, von Hofe, & Blatt, 1994; Rose, 1995).

Families who have consented to organ and/or tissue donation indicate their need to understand the diagnosis of brain death and the need for follow-up information about the recipients of their loved one's organs and tissue (Pelletier, 1993).

Mr. T, discussed in Sections Three and Four, is improving. His blood gases have improved, and he is being weaned from the ventilator. The ventilator is in synchronized intermittent mandatory ventilation (SIMV) mode at a rate of 8.

The nurse has been teaching Mr. T about his wound care, including the chance for infection related to his wound and the use of steroids. Up to this point, Mr. T has been eager to learn and has asked questions using a writing board. This morning, he appears anxious.

Before teaching Mr. T, the nurse should assess the cause of Mr. T's anxiety. Is it related to hypoxia secondary to weaning? The nurse draws blood for an ABG measurement, and the findings are within normal limits, O_2 saturation is also normal. Mr. T's anxiety may be related to the fear of not being able to breathe without the machine. Patient teaching should center on decreasing Mr. T's anxiety. On questioning, Mr. T admits he is frightened about getting weaned and moving out of the ICU. The nurse concentrates on explaining how the staff is sure Mr. T will be able to breathe. Next, she explains when he will be transferred to the general floor and how he will continue to be monitored.

In summary, both critically ill patients and their family members want to learn about their illness and the hospital environment. Adults use problem-centered learning. Therefore, they are interested in information that is immediately useful and applicable. A person is unable to learn if her or his stress level is high. Therefore, the next step in teaching critically ill patients is to address the issue that is causing the most anxiety. Information should be given in clear, succinct terms. The nurse should assess what the patient and family member already know in order to build on this foundation. Physiologic factors that can interfere with learning also must be assessed.

SECTION FIVE REVIEW

Questions 1 and 2 pertain to Ms. Bee.

Ms. Bee was admitted with a diagnosis of acute myocardial infarction. Her vital signs are respiratory rate 32, heart rate 100, temperature 102°F orally, blood pressure 90/70 mm Hg. She is on a continuous nitroglycerin IV infusion for chest pain.

1. Which of the following factors would NOT interfere with Ms. Bee's ability to learn?
   A. pain
   B. temperature
   C. respiratory rate
   D. heart rate
2. The nurse should focus on teaching Ms. Bee
   A. cardiac rehabilitation plans
   B. how the heart functions
   C. why it is important to state when she is having pain
   D. rationale for the nitroglycerin
3. Families of critically ill patients list which of the following needs as being the most important?
   A. emotional
   B. psychomotor
   C. cognitive
   D. spiritual
4. Families who have consented to organ/tissue donation need to understand
   A. how long the organs are viable
   B. the diagnosis of brain death
   C. how funeral arrangements are made
   D. how tissue is crossmatched

Answers: 1. D, 2. C, 3. C, 4. B

NURSING CONSIDERATIONS

SECTION SIX: Visiting the Critically Ill Patient

At the completion of this section, the learner will be able to identify the rationale for visitation policies and the effects of visitation on critically ill patients.

Nurses do not agree on the benefits of visitation. Unfortunately, little research has been done regarding the physiologic effects of visitation. Some nurses tend to view visitation as psychologically supportive to the patient but physiologically destructive. These nurses believe that visitation disrupts nursing care and has negative family consequences. Exhaustion is one of these negative consequences (Kirchhoff et al., 1993). Other nurses view visitation as a necessary treatment and not as a privilege granted by the hospital (Cleveland, 1994).

Patients also differ in their views toward visitation. The age and setting of the patient may be associated with visitation preferences. In one study, middle-aged patients (35 to 65 years) desired frequent short visits at any time of the day, while elderly patients (older than 65 years) preferred 45-minute afternoon visits (Simpson, 1993). Patients in coronary care wanted two visits daily, while patients in surgical intensive care wanted more daily visits (Simpson, 1993).

As patients differ in their likes and dislikes regarding visitation, they also differ in their physiologic response to visitation. In a study by Kleman et al. (1993), patients with ejection fractions less than 40 percent, who were smokers, and who desired visits displayed some physiologic reactivity to the visits, including increased heart rate and blood pressure from the beginning to the end of the visit (Kleman et al., 1993).

Observing the family at the patient's bedside can provide information about the nature of the patient–family relationship as well as clues to family needs. The more acutely ill the patient, the more urgent it becomes for family members to see the patient. It is not necessary to "clean the patient up"; rather, signs of illness and injury can help the family to accept reality (Hopkins, 1994; Leske & Jiricka, 1998).

Children of critically ill parents experience disbelief at the hospitalization. The equipment is frightening, and the child fears the parent's death (Craft et al., 1993). The children desire more information about their parent's illness. It is important to most children to visit the parent, and children should be given the choice of visiting. In one study, children who had facilitated visitation with their critically ill parent (i.e., emotional support before, during, and after visitation) experienced fewer behavioral and emotional changes than those not allowed to visit (Nicholson et al., 1993).

Families may need directions in how to visit. The nurse may discuss with family what the patient looks like prior to the family visit. It is helpful for the family to know to speak to the patient in a normal tone of voice, to be comfortable simply being with the patient and not speaking at all, and to ask questions away from the bedside (Twibell, 1998).

A unit brochure is one way of communicating visitation policies and their rationale while the family is experiencing high anxiety. The brochure should list the primary nurse to facilitate family questions (Hopkins, 1994). Contracts can be developed with the family to facilitate completion of nursing care as well as an uninterrupted visit. Times to avoid visitation should be discussed and agreed on based on the family's and nursing schedule.

In summary, critically ill patients as well as nurses differ in their opinion regarding the value and nature of visitation. Each situation should be examined and uniquely managed. Negotiations between the patient, family, and nurse may be the most effective way of facilitating visitation that is therapeutic to all involved.

SECTION SIX REVIEW

1. Amy Miller, age 6, asks to see her father, who is comatose and being mechanically ventilated. The nurse should
   - **A.** clean Mr. Miller up first
   - **B.** grant Amy's request
   - **C.** explain to Amy that she shouldn't see her father until he gets more energy
   - **D.** adhere to the policy that prohibits visitors under age 16
2. The physiologic effects of visitation are
   - **A.** the same for everyone
   - **B.** detrimental to patient stability
   - **C.** related to patient's preference for visits
   - **D.** positive
3. Contracting visitation policies with the family involves
   - **A.** having the family sign in each time they visit
   - **B.** ensuring that both the family and the nurse agree on mutually acceptable visitation times
   - **C.** arbitration with the charge nurse
   - **D.** developing a brochure

Answers: 1. B, 2. C, 3. B

SECTION SEVEN: Nursing Staffing Issues

At the completion of this section, the learner will be able to identify work design and staffing strategies for the critically ill patient.

Nurses willing to work with critically ill patients are a precious commodity. Hospitals are filled with more acutely ill patients. Decreased Medicare and Medicaid reimbursement has encouraged shorter length of hospital stays and a reduction in professional nursing staff as cost-reducing measures. Ironically, critical care nursing has been associated with a 50 percent reduction in patient mortality. Although critical care is an expensive service, critical care nursing does not count as a major component of that cost (Armstrong et al., 1991).

The early hospital discharge of acutely ill patients encourages employment of critical care nurses outside the hospital environment. New practice areas may include intensive care hospices for terminally ill patients with complex technical needs or special care facilities for the chronically critically ill (such as patients with cardiac and respiratory failure).

Cross-training is a strategy being used to ensure the availability of competent nurses when patient census increases in number and acuity. Cross-training teaches specific skills in an associated clinical area. It differs from orientation in that cross-training focuses on the most frequently encountered patient populations in a new practice setting. Differences between the usual and the new practice setting are stressed (Dirks et al., 1995). Proponents state that cross-training protects nurses' salaries by providing an alternative to mandatory time off. It is also less expensive than hiring registry replacement nurses.

An alternative to cross-training is to prepare nurses in one practice setting to care for acutely ill patients in that setting. An integrated approach allows for patients remaining in one patient care area. During their high-acuity phase, they are assigned a nurse who is competent to care for them during both high and low acuity, thus facilitating the nurse–patient relationship. An example of a patient who may benefit from this type of unit is a patient who receives a bone marrow transplant (high acuity) and does not exhibit rejection (moves into a low-acuity phase). Seminars given by former patients can help both novice and expert nurses gain a better understanding of the needs of critically ill patients.

The reduction in professional nursing staff is encouraging the upgrading of nursing assistant skills. Technical skills are differentiated from cognitive and complex skills such as assessment, planning, and communication (Ackerman & Higgins, 1992). When unlicensed individuals provide direct patient care, they are accountable to and work under the direct supervision of a professional critical care nurse (AACN, 1989b).

In summary, changes in Medicare and Medicaid reimbursement have encouraged hospital administrators to decrease the number of professional nursing staff. The reduction of professional nurses combined with high patient acuity has stimulated work redesign. Three approaches are cross-training, integrating higher-acuity patients into traditionally low-acuity settings, and upgrading nursing assistant roles and responsibilities. There is a need to evaluate the impact of these staffing strategies on patient outcomes.

SECTION SEVEN REVIEW

1. Cross-training involves
   A. teaching nursing assistants to perform technical skills
   B. integrating critically ill patients into low acuity settings
   C. developing special care facilities
   D. teaching specific skills in an associated clinical area to professional nurses

2. Which of the following stimulated a reduction in professional nursing staff?
   A. the registered nurse (RN) shortage
   B. decreased enrollment in nursing schools
   C. decreased patient acuity
   D. changes in Medicaid and Medicare reimbursement

Answers: 1. D, 2. D

SECTION EIGHT: Interface Between Technology and Caring

At the completion of this section, the learner will be able to describe the interface between technology and caring.

A major criticism of nurses who work with critically ill patients is that they are strictly technologically oriented. This criticism was derived historically. The advances in surgery created a need for an area where the patient could undergo an operation and recover from anesthesia. The nurse in this area functioned in a monitoring role by using instruments and equipment that recorded physiologic responses (Levine, 1989). Patients were not aware of their surroundings, so the areas were designed to facilitate work flow, not for esthetics.

Patients, by signing the operative permit, became dependent on the health care provider, and an attitude of trust—the professionals know best—was created. Nurses working in recovery rooms were exposed to constant stress, since the patients required continuous monitoring, and the nurse was unable to leave the bedside. Patients were not encouraged to participate in their care. Eventually, machinery allowed nurses to care for more than one critically ill patient at a time. It has been suggested that nurses focused on the technology in order to cope with the stress and to exclude their personal feelings (Levine, 1989).

There has been much deliberation over what separates medical from nursing practice. Because of the autonomous use of technology in caring for the critically ill patient, nurses working with this patient population have been referred to as "junior physicians" or "minidoctors." Nurses have used the words *technical, curative,* and *prescribing* to describe caring for the critically ill patient (Schultz & Daly, 1989).

There are inherent hazards to using technology. The use of technology can be so intriguing that the primary purpose for using the technology—to support the well-being of the patient—may be lost. Another hazard is that technology creates demands where no demands existed before by fragmenting patients into subpopulations (e.g., bone marrow transplant floor, cardiac surgery unit). Each subpopulation has its own health care staff. Staff begin to compete for the resources within the hospital system.

Several other problems result from current technology. Technologic advances make it easy to provide services to patients who may not benefit from use of the equipment. Machines compete with the patient for nursing surveillance. It is possible that nurses may become so dependent on monitoring devices that they trust the equipment even when the data conflict with their own clinical assessment of the situation. Having responsibility for multiple pieces of equipment can increase the nurse's stress level. Data from monitoring devices can either support or help to incriminate a nurse in legal proceedings. Technical devices present mechanical impediments to touching. Little surface area may be available for physical contact. The lack of physical contact can lead to a feeling of depersonalization. A patient who has felt depersonalized may be more likely to sue a nurse.

Nursing interventions should focus on humanizing the patient and the situation. Interventions may include (1) exchanging names, (2) sharing something about self with the patient, (3) interacting with the patient's family, (4) giving the family permission to touch the patient by lowering side rails and pulling a chair up to the bedside, and (5) developing a personality display board with pictures and information about the patient, to encourage interaction (Halm & Alpen, 1993; Williams, 1993).

Parents of critically ill children experience distress over their loss of the parenting role of a healthy child. As they adjust to becoming the parent of a critically ill child, they relinquish the child to health care providers, assess their strength and resources as a family, and then get involved (Cox, 1992). As parents relinquish their child, it is necessary for the nurse to foster competence and caring and thus trust.

Technology may evoke fear in patients and contribute to their anxiety regarding their ability to recover. Fear and anxiety stimulate the sympathetic nervous system, resulting in myocardial stimulation and bronchoconstriction. These physiologic responses may make ventilator weaning difficult, or may produce ischemia, further increasing the patient's need for technology (Halm & Alpen, 1993). Orienting the patient to the purpose, function, and sounds of a machine may decrease the patient's fear.

Nurses working with critically ill patients must be capable of making critical decisions. Although decision making has been viewed as somewhat artful and intuitive, computers have used a scientific, programmed approach to decision making. Because of the massive amount of patient information available related to the multiple pieces of machinery, nurses may be reaching a saturation point in data processing. Computer software programs are available to help diagnose patient conditions.

The nurse must be proficient in the use of machinery. Proficiency is fostered by having the opportunity to become familiar with the machinery before its use in patient care and by having an available resource person who understands the machine's operation. Once the nurse is proficient, he or she can encourage the questions of patient and family members about the machinery. Explaining machinery can increase patient and family trust in the nurse. Most nurses think that machines provide reassurance because they can alert the nurse to a problem situation before clinical manifestations occur (McConnell, 1990). It is essential, however, that the nurse validate the machine data with nursing assessment data. In addition, nurses must appreciate the techniques that patients have developed to interact with the technology. This may include denial, humor, and a compulsiveness to learn everything about a machine.

Caring has been described differently depending on the context where the nurse practices. In the ICU, caring has been described as technical. On medical–surgical floors, caring has been described as a team effort. Traditionally, caring has been viewed as humanistic behavior involving spiritual and ethical aspects. The modern health care delivery system has created a form of bureaucratic caring that includes economic, legal, and technical aspects (Ray, 1989). The nurse caring for the critically ill patient has to address all views, even though they may be theoretically contradictory in nature.

Nurses working with critically ill patients perform

technologic caring where technologic competence is blended with moral principles (Ray, 1989). Technology in the ICU is designed to be invulnerable and predictable, in contrast to the patient's characteristics of vulnerability and unpredictability. Although nurses may appreciate machines as extensions of the patient, patients view the machines as intrusions that reinforce their powerlessness (Cooper, 1993). Ultimately, caring is protecting the patient from being reduced to the moral status of an object (Mendyka, 1993). Critically ill patients define *caring* as a healing process that involves vigilance, highly skilled practice, going beyond the basics, and nurturing. Caring relieves patients' anxiety and allows them to focus their energy on getting well (Burfitt et al., 1993).

In summary, nurses who care for critically ill patients must be able to use technology in the caring process and still recognize the limitations of technology. Equipment and technologic advances cannot be substituted for the nurse's personal knowledge, observation skills, and senses. The nurse must be able to integrate complex technology with individualized, humanistic care (Cooper, 1993).

SECTION EIGHT REVIEW

1. The referral to nurses who work with critically ill patients as junior physicians was derived from
   A. the close collaborative relationship between nurse and physician
   B. increased use of advanced technology
   C. the constant stress of continuous monitoring
   D. the decreased nurse–patient ratio
2. The implications of advanced technology for nursing include
   A. decreased likelihood of malpractice and negligence
   B. provision of data to incriminate or support nurses in court proceedings
   C. allowing greater time for patient contact
   D. encouraging greater use of nursing assessment skills
3. The hazards of technology include all of the following EXCEPT
   A. creates demands for new services
   B. decreases demands for nursing staff
   C. fosters depersonalization of the patient
   D. creates machine competition with patient for nursing time
4. An intervention that helps to humanize the patient is
   A. developing a personality display board
   B. leaving machine alarms volume low
   C. wearing a name badge
   D. viewing the machine as an extension of the patient

Answers: 1. B, 2. B, 3. B, 4. A

SECTION NINE: Nursing Critically Ill Patients

At the completion of this section, the learner will be able to discuss the stressful and satisfying aspects to caring for critically ill patients.

The term **burnout** has been used to describe a crisis state evolving from stress. It has been defined as "to fail, wear out, or become exhausted by making excessive demands on energy, strength, or resource" (Freudenberg, 1974). Burnout is an automatic response that protects the nurse from pain and conflict. In a classic study conducted by Claus and Bailey (1980), 1,794 nurses who work with critically ill patients were surveyed to identify sources of stress. The major sources of stress were (1) interpersonal conflict, (2) management of the patient care area, (3) nature of the direct patient care, and (4) inadequate knowledge. In a more recent study, family demands, health difficulties, supervision, pay, job security, and situational stress were major sources of stress (Stechmiller & Yarandi, 1993). There are several symptoms that indicate burnout (Table 1–4). Although basic nursing programs usually offer structured coursework in meeting the psychosocial needs of patients, few programs offer instruction in meeting the psychosocial needs of nurses (Continenza, 1989).

Posttraumatic stress disorder (PTSD) occurs from stress associated with dramatic, emotionally overwhelming situations, outside the range of usual human experience, that overcomes normal coping mechanisms (Spitzer & Burke, 1993; Acker, 1993). Incident stress may manifest the same symptoms as burnout. Table 1–4 includes additional symptoms that may occur in PTSD. Critical care nurses may experience PTSD from an accumulation of environmental stress and having to inflict pain (Acker, 1993).

Primary nursing may be a source of burnout. Nurses who work with critically ill patients usually have responsibility for one or two patients. Primary nursing, although once regarded as the ultimate method of nursing assignment, can be a stressor because of the intensity and intimacy of the nurse–patient relationship. There is a constant threat that the patient may die. The nurse may experience repetitive losses but still has to reinvest energy into a new patient before adequately mourning the loss of the previous patient.

TABLE 1–4. SYMPTOMS OF BURNOUT AND POSTTRAUMATIC STRESS DISORDER (PTSD)

BURNOUT	PTSD
Behavioral	
Withdrawal	Excessive silence
Risk taking and impulsiveness	Feeling hopeless
Ambivalence	Feeling guilty
Decreased productivity	
Contemplating career change	
Increased use of caffeine, alcohol, and nicotine	
Physiologic	
Chronic fatigue	Tremors
Frequent minor ailments	Diarrhea
Sleep changes	Tachycardia
Appetite change	
Sexual difficulty	
Psychological	
Attempt to blame others	Grief
Stereotype patients	Anger
Nightmares	Fear
Depression	
Hostility and negativism	
Loss of tolerance	
Cognitive	
Decreased ability to make decisions	Confusion
Poor judgment	Calculation difficulties
Lack of initiative	
Forgetfulness	

Another source of burnout is the patient's changing condition. Frequently, the aims of the patient's treatment will change drastically within the course of a shift, requiring the nurse to be philosophically flexible. A patient with a presumably poor prognosis may have a prolonged stay that involves the use of all available technology, and in the middle of the shift, a decision to cease extraordinary efforts may be made. The patient may then begin to improve, requiring reevaluation and escalation of care. Conversely, the patient may be pronounced brain dead, and the individual becomes a cadaveric donor. The nursing care for the cadaveric donor may detract from the nursing care of other viable patients, producing a nursing conflict (Fitzgerald, 1989). A significant degree of uncertainty is confronted on a daily basis. In addition, the nurse must view the worst of humanity (gunshot wounds and stabbings) and deal with injury in the prime of life.

Noise-induced stress and burnout may be related. Just as the patient may experience problems from the stimulation in the patient care area, nurses also may be affected. The top three disturbing noises identified by nurses were beeping monitors, equipment alarms, and telephones (Topf & Dillon, 1988).

Burnout may be prevented if the nurse exhibits hardiness. Hardiness comprises three components: a sense of commitment, a perception of life changes as challenges, and a sense of control over life. Of the three components, less commitment to work has been linked with greater work stress (Topf, 1989). Thus, commitment to career, dealing with others at work, and job satisfaction protect against burnout (Stechmiller & Yarandi, 1993).

Nurses must enhance self-awareness of personal sources of tension. Fatigue, frustration, and anxiety have been listed as nurses' most frequent responses to stress (Robinson & Lewis, 1990). Once these sources of tension are identified, strategies for alleviating the stressors can be developed. The use of written protocols to assist in defining practice and clarifying boundaries, regular assessment of staff goals and achievements, and continuing education programs for personal growth are stress-relieving factors. Discussing problems with coworkers and watching television or reading are strategies listed by nurses for coping with work-related stress. The presence of social support has demonstrated a buffering effect on stress in nurses working with critically ill patients.

Establishing critical incident stress debriefings (CISDs) may facilitate coping with specific situations. Informal defusings are held within 4 hours of a traumatic event to stabilize the health care professionals involved and allow their reentry into the situation. Formal debriefings are held with larger groups to promote team building (Spitzer & Burke, 1993). In essence, CISDs are a formal way of managing stress before it becomes debilitating or fosters burnout.

There are advantages to working with critically ill patients. Generally, nurses and physicians have better collaboration because the nature of the patient situation requires close communication. Nurses may have greater freedom in implementing medical guidelines, since there is less emphasis on nonclinical maintenance activities (e.g., ordering supplies). Research findings suggest that nurses who work with critically ill patients are more satisfied in their role than nurses who work with less acute patients (Boumans & Landeweerd, 1994). Nurses who experience psychological stress usually are younger and have less experience and less education (Harris, 1989).

Some of the stressors associated with caring for critically ill patients also can produce satisfaction. The fast-paced environment is stimulating to some nurses. The ability to interact with patients and families during crisis can be satisfying. Claus and Bailey (1980) discovered that intellectual challenge, opportunities for learning, smaller nurse–patient ratio, and proficient use of skills were the most frequently mentioned motivators for working with critically ill patients.

In summary, nurses who work with critically ill patients do not appear to have greater degrees of work-related stress than nurses working with less acute patient populations. However, nurses working with the critically ill are still susceptible to burnout. The symptoms of burnout and PTSD are cognitive, psychological, physiologic, and behavioral in nature (Table 1–4). Strategies useful in limiting or buffering job-related stressors are an available social support system, developing guidelines to delineate practice boundaries, periodic assessment of personal and unit goals, comprehensive unit orientation, and continuing education for stress reduction. Establishment of CISDs accelerates recovery of health professionals who are suffering painful reactions to abnormal events.

SECTION NINE REVIEW

1. Primary nursing
   A. produces stress because of the intensity of the nurse–patient relationship
   B. discourages collaboration among health team members
   C. prevents the nurse from reinvesting energy into a new patient after a previous patient is discharged
   D. is the preferred method of patient assignment
2. Nurses who work with critically ill patients as opposed to nurses who work with less acute patients
   A. experience greater stress
   B. have a stronger support system
   C. are more satisfied in their role
   D. are more susceptible to burnout
3. Which of the following components of hardiness has been linked to burnout?
   A. a sense of control over the patient care area
   B. less commitment to work
   C. perception of change as a challenge
   D. sense of control over life

Answers: 1. A, 2. C, 3. B

SECTION TEN: Resource Allocation

At the completion of this section, the learner will be able to discuss resource allocation issues as they relate to critically ill patients.

Allocation of resources within critical care occurs when ICU beds are filled and the demand for the existing beds increases, forcing premature transfer of patients and acceleration of the process of withdrawing life-sustaining treatment (Marsden, 1992). It is difficult for the nurse to reconcile the dual roles of patient advocate and resource allocater. Advocacy means to act to safeguard and advance the interests of others (Rushton, 1994). If acting as an advocate requires supporting the patient's basic values, rights, and beliefs, then controversy may occur when the patient's beliefs conflict with the nurse's beliefs. Section Ten addresses personal values. Many view supporting the patient's beliefs as functioning ethically.

Who is in need of the greatest health care resources when they are critically ill? The criteria for resources may be based on age, diagnosis, physician preference, and bed and nursing staff availability, as well as community and hospital standards. One could argue that resources should be used for patients who want to receive extraordinary support, have a better probability of surviving, or have a higher quality of life (Carlon, 1988). If resource allocation were based on these principles, the actual precipitating event that created the need for resources would be irrelevant. Therefore, oncology patients, trauma patients, the young, and the old should be considered equally. It has been suggested that futility of treatment and informed refusal by the patient are acceptable reasons for physicians to limit treatment. However, only the patient or society, through the legal system, can make decisions to withhold treatment based on quality of life or cost considerations (Lo & Jonsen, 1980).

Several patient populations are vulnerable with regard to the resource allocation issues frequently encountered by nurses who work with critically ill patients. Critically ill neonates are considered a vulnerable population. Almost all infants are born in a hospital. Each hospital has policies regarding resuscitation of the newborn. It is almost impossible to differentiate at birth infants who may benefit from lifesaving interventions from those with poor prognoses. Therefore, all neonates usually are resuscitated (Kohrmann, 1985). Issues arise when cessation of life support is considered later in the infant's hospitalization.

Oncology patients often are stereotyped as not being candidates for aggressive treatment. This can result in a self-fulfilling prophecy, because critically ill patients who are denied technical life support eventually will die (Carlon, 1988). However, oncology patients frequently become critically ill from interventions administered by health care providers. Should these patients be denied access to resources when their condition has been induced? Conversely, oncology patients may be kept alive for research purposes to determine the ultimate effects of certain interventions.

Age has been used to justify the withholding of resources from the elderly. Interestingly, age has not been solely related to mortality. The severity of the illness episode, admitting diagnosis, and the patient's previous health status have been positively related to health outcomes (Chelluri et al., 1993). The Medicare and Diagnostic-Related Grouping systems send strong signals to hospitals to limit resources provided to the elderly. Financial reimbursement is less than the hospital's cost for providing the resources.

It is difficult to predict who will benefit from intensive care. Severity of illness scales and probability models have been developed for this purpose. The APACHE III (Knaus et al., 1991) is an example. However, these indices have not predicted mortality consistently in cases of middle severity (Snider, 1994). The functional capacity of the patient prior to illness has been associated with outcome (Rockwood et al., 1993). Individual factors have been highly correlated with mortality: presence of coma at time of ICU admission (Snyder & Colantonio, 1994) and arterial lactate levels (Tuchschmidt & Mecher, 1994) are two of these factors. Mortality is best predicted at admission and at 24 hours postadmission (Teres & Lemeshow, 1994). Mortality is usually the outcome studied in relation to ICU care. However, outcomes may include patient comfort, well-being, functional status, and other variables in addition to living or dying (Jones, 1993). Patients and their families consider multiple outcomes when deciding to withdraw life support.

Because of the nature of critical illness, it is difficult to remember that the patient's freedom of choice should still be placed above every other value. Patient situations change rapidly, often preventing discussion with the patient about treatment decisions. Health care providers, including nurses, have a tendency to believe that what they think is good for the patient is indeed good for the patient. The underlying reason for this belief may be to rationalize interventions that produce patient pain. The nurse has the responsibility to act as patient advocate because of the vulnerable nature of the critically ill patient.

Intensive care units account for 7.5 percent of all hospital beds, yet charges for ICU comprise 28 percent of total hospital charges (Snider, 1994). Technology forces health care providers to make choices about who receives costly resources. Nurses are encouraged to be more cost conscious and frequently are asked what is a reasonable reduction below ideal care for their patients. Making decisions about allocation of resources is a real but usually unspecified aspect of the nursing role with critically ill patients. These decisions force health care providers to make comparisons based on personal beliefs. Technology alone cannot provide information about who may live and die. A patient's intangibles, such as their family support systems, personal value system, and purpose in life, also may contribute to a patient's ability to recover even when technologic data provide no hope (Van Ora, 1989).

Technology is used not only for its original intention—to resuscitate patients who can benefit—but also for patients who have virtually no possibility of recovering. Patients whose outcome is opposite to what is expected on ICU admission generate the most cost. These are patients who are expected to die but who survive, and those who are expected to survive but who die (Snider, 1994). Health care reform is supporting the transition from a "rule of rescue" to a "rule of reason" (Luce, 1994). Health care providers appear more comfortable with stopping life support measures than with not starting life support measures, although there is no moral difference between the two (Cassell, 1986). Because the patient may be distracted by pain or unable to communicate verbally because of intubation or altered mental status, each situation is unique. In some situations, however, nurses working with critically ill patients can be proactive in identifying the wishes of the patient before the moment of need, so that patients and families can express coherent desires. Permission for resuscitation can be obtained as an informed consent, like other invasive procedures. As the patient's clinical condition changes, patients and families need to be informed to ensure that consent for resuscitation is still valid.

Cardiopulmonary resuscitation (CPR) is an example of a technique that has been misused. Guidelines for using the technique originally stated that it was not to be used in cases of terminal irreversible illness in which death is expected. Ironically, hospitals now require that every patient be a candidate to receive CPR unless an order is written to withhold it (Bellamy & Oye, 1987). Failed CPR is a major cause of inappropriate ICU admissions (Snider, 1994). It may also indicate a failure to obtain the patient's wishes regarding resuscitation. Technology encourages death to be viewed as a symptom to be treated, not as a life event.

Do Not Resuscitate (DNR) orders were developed to prevent the use of CPR and advanced cardiac life support measures, not to prevent other forms of treatment for the patient, including the use of critical care resources (Edwards, 1990). However, DNR patients consume more resources and have a higher mortality rate than non-DNR patients. DNR orders may be written for reasons other than terminal illness, such as patient request; chronic, irreversible illness; and poor quality of life. Since DNR patients may be able to benefit from receiving care from nurses skilled in working with critically ill patients, is it fair to withhold these resources? Some argue that scarce resources would be redistributed to non-DNR patients and costs would be reduced if resources were not provided to the DNR patient (Edwards, 1990). The immediate needs of the person may be in conflict with the interests of society. Because of limited resources, patients who can be treated successfully may be denied resources because available resources are being used by patients with questionable survival capability.

Health care providers justify not providing services to the critically ill by stating that they are relieving suffering. However, in some situations, it cannot be verified that suffering is being relieved (Levine, 1989). It is not a nursing responsibility to evaluate the social worth of a patient. Whenever possible, decisions to use or not to use technology to sustain life should be made in advance by the patient. In cases in which advanced decision making has not taken place, family members and other individuals requested by the patient should be included in decision making. An ethical review committee may be used in some circumstances. It has been stated that it is impossible for caregivers whose philosophy is to protect life and relieve suffering to make these decisions (Levine, 1989). Historically, the public has not wanted to know that there are times when health care providers do not know which action is best. Added to this is the fact that health care providers have not wanted public scrutiny of their actions. The development of ethical review committees can be viewed as both a curse and a blessing. They can diminish individual consideration of cases in favor of implementing general standards of treatment based on criteria. The positive aspect of these committees is that a decision is made by a group instead of by an individual health care provider.

Other ethical decision making strategies include (1) establishing a nursing ethics council that addresses broad issues, such as allocation of resources, rather than specific patient cases; (2) identifying a consistent process to use when considering ethical issues for the institution; and (3) developing unit-based ethics rounds (Holly & Lyons, 1993). Critical paths can be developed for terminally ill patients to ensure that family and patient needs are met (Henneman, 1993).

In summary, technology has produced ethical dilemmas for nurses working with critically ill patients. Recent dilemmas have focused on the use of valuable critical care resources by infants with congenital abnormalities, oncology patients, the elderly, and DNR patients. It is not the nurse's role to solve these dilemmas alone. Rather, the nurse's responsibility is to become involved in establishing guidelines for resource allocation and to represent nursing's viewpoint on ethical review committees and in hospital policy.

SECTION TEN REVIEW

1. CPR was developed to be used
   A. for those who experience sudden unexpected death
   B. for every witnessed arrest
   C. for every arrest situation (witnessed or not)
   D. only in the hospital
2. The DNR order was developed to
   A. provide only custodial care to terminal patients
   B. prevent use of CPR
   C. provide greater resources for non-DNR patients
   D. decrease health costs
3. Resource allocation for critically ill patients may be based on all of the following EXCEPT
   A. admitting diagnosis
   B. bed availability
   C. hospital standards
   D. gender of the patient

Answers: 1. A, 2. B, 3. D

SECTION ELEVEN: Personal Values

At the completion of this section, the learner will be able to examine personal values as they relate to the nurse's role in working with critically ill patients and discuss end-of-life issues to be considered in caring for critically ill patients.

The American Nurses Association (ANA) (1995) states that essential components of professional nursing practice include care, cure, and coordination. The AACN (1994) believes that nurses who work with critically ill patients should base their practice on individual professional accountability; thorough knowledge of the interrelatedness of body systems; recognition and appreciation of a person's wholeness, uniqueness, and significant social–environmental relationships; and appreciation of the collaborative role of all health care team members.

Nurses can improve assessment and technical skills by providing nursing care for critically ill patients. The nurse must be able to interpret and anticipate health outcomes that may result from applying patient care protocols. Verbal and nonverbal communication skills can be refined because communication must be precise and perceptive in these settings. The exposure to death and the saving of human life can strengthen one's integrity. Personal values can be identified and clarified by examining bioethical issues encountered when working with critically ill patients.

The value clarification exercise shown in Table 1–5 is designed to help the learner explore personal values in relation to the profession of nursing and bioethical issues. By reflecting on personal values, one gains a better understanding of what factors may limit one's ability to reason clearly and when one may not be suitable for being a patient advocate (Bertolini, 1994).

There may be circumstances in which conflicts occur between the nurse's world view and that of the patient, such as in decisions regarding withholding or withdrawing life-sustaining treatment. In these circumstances, the nurse should transfer the care of the patient to another qualified critical care nurse (AACN, 1991).

TABLE 1–5. VALUE CLARIFICATION EXERCISE

To the left of each statement, place the number that best explains your position: 1 = mostly agree, 2 = somewhat agree, 3 = neutral, 4 = somewhat disagree, 5 = mostly disagree

___ 1. Infants with severe handicaps ought to be left to die.
___ 2. Extraordinary medical treatment is always indicated.
___ 3. My role as a nurse is to always resuscitate patients who could benefit from it, no matter what has been decided previously.
___ 4. I must follow physician's orders.
___ 5. Older patients should be allowed to die with dignity.
___ 6. Medical technology has advanced the quality of life.
___ 7. Children should not be involved in giving consent for treatments.
___ 8. Families ought to make decisions about life or death situations without involving the patient.
___ 9. Children should participate in human experimentation that is not harmful even if it has no benefit to them.
___ 10. Prisoners should participate in scientific experiments to repay society for their wrongdoings.
___ 11. Women should seek medical care from female physicians to avoid potential discrimination.
___ 12. Children whose parents refuse to have them receive medical care should be removed from their families through court action.
___ 13. Research using fetuses should be pursued vigorously.
___ 14. Life support systems should be discontinued after several days of flat electroencephalogram.
___ 15. Health professionals are a scarce resource in many parts of the country.
___ 16. Nursing is a subservient profession, especially to the medical profession.
___ 17. As a nurse, I must relinquish my personal philosophy to support the philosophies of others.
___ 18. All patients, regardless of differences, should be treated in a humanistic way.
___ 19. I should give mouth-to-mouth resuscitation to a derelict if he needs it.
___ 20. A child who is disabled has value.
___ 21. All forms of human life have value.
___ 22. I should be involved in decision making regarding ethical issues in practice.
___ 23. Committees should decide who receives scarce resources, such as kidneys.
___ 24. Patients' individual rights should be more important than the rights of society at large.
___ 25. A person has the right to make a living will.
___ 26. Underdeveloped countries should be given health and financial support from developed countries.
___ 27. I should support all the positions taken on ethical issues taken by my professional association.
___ 28. The care component of nursing practice is not as important as the cure component of medical practice.
___ 29. The nurse's primary role in decision making on ethical issues is to implement the selected alternative.
___ 30. I feel afraid when caring for a patient who is dying.
___ 31. Children who have disabilities should be institutionalized.
___ 32. Patients in mental health institutions and prisons should be given behavior modification therapy to make them conform to society.
___ 33. Personal possessions of patients should be removed to guarantee safekeeping during hospitalization.
___ 34. Patients should have access to their own health information.
___ 35. Withholding health information fosters the patient's recovery.
___ 36. A patient with kidney failure is always able to get kidney dialysis when needed.
___ 37. Society should bear the cost of extraordinary medical interventions.
___ 38. Confidentiality is an important part of the nurse's role.
___ 39. As a nurse, I should value responsibility.
___ 40. Nurses have a right to withhold information to facilitate nursing research on human subjects.
___ 41. The patient who refuses treatment should be dropped from the health supervision of an agency or professional.
___ 42. Transplantations should be done whenever needed.

Personal Application

1. Add the number of 1s, 2s, 3s, 4s, and 5s that you have.
2. How many statements do you have clear ideas (1s and 5s) about?
3. Do these outweigh the number of ambivalent (neutral) statements you listed?
4. Look at the statements that you agree with (1s and 2s). Is there a relationship between the statements that influenced your responses (e.g., age of patient, patient acuity)?
5. Look at the statements that you disagree with (4s and 5s). Is there a relationship between these statements that influenced your responses?
6. Analyze the cluster of statements below. Is there any consistency in the way that you rated these statements? What variables influenced your decision?

Cluster 5, 8, 14, 25, and 30: Relates to issues pertaining to death
Cluster 3, 4, 16, 17, 22, 27, 28, 29, and 38: Relates to the profession of nursing
Cluster 2, 6, 14, 36, 37, and 42: Relates to issues raised by advanced technology
Cluster 1, 7, 9, 12, 20, and 31: Relates to children
Cluster 9, 10, 13, and 40: Relates to human experimentation
Cluster 3, 7, 8, 11, 12, 18, 19, 21, 24, 25, 33, 34, 35, 38, and 41: Relates to patients' rights
Cluster 9, 10, 24, 26, 32, and 37: Relates to society's rights
Cluster 15, 23, and 36: Relates to allocation of resources
Cluster 3, 4, 17, 18, 19, 22, 27, 29, and 39: Relates to perceptions of obligations

Adapted from Steele, S., and Harmon, V. (1979). Value Clarification in Nursing. *New York: Appleton-Century-Crofts.*

The Patient Self Determination Act, passed as part of the Omnibus Budget Reconciliation Act of 1990, requires that all patients be given information about their right to formulate advanced directives of two types: treatment directives (living wills) and appointment directives (power of attorney for health care). This has increased the role of the patient and family in making end-of-life decisions. Nurses have a primary role in ensuring that the patient makes informed decisions regarding end-of-life care (ANA, 1991). The nurse working in critical care serves as patient advocate and intercedes for patients who cannot speak for themselves and supports the decisions of the patient or the patient's designated surrogate (AACN, 1989a). Nurses are also directed to uphold the choices and values of the patient even when these wishes conflict with those of health care providers and families (ANA, 1992).

In summary, the nurse has several different roles when caring for the critically ill patient. These roles include but are not limited to prevention of illness, counselor, teacher, and patient advocate. The ability to interpret multiple clinical data and anticipate events based on knowledge of physiology is an inherent requirement. As technology advances, patient care has the tendency to become fragmented. The nurse glues the pieces together. Nurses need to be aware of the personal fears and feelings they experienced when they first began to work with critically ill patients. Once one becomes a native, it is easy to forget and not appreciate or overlook these same feelings and fears in the critically ill patient.

There are many similarities in nursing regardless of practice setting and patient population. Evaluation of one's personal philosophy can improve one's satisfaction in working with critically ill patients. Clarification of one's values helps to anticipate problems that may be encountered in the practice setting and supports development of positive coping strategies. This knowledge can be transferred for use in other health care settings with less acutely ill patients.

SECTION ELEVEN REVIEW

1. Nurses who work with critically ill patients should base their practice on all of the following EXCEPT
   A. delegated responsibility
   B. thorough knowledge of the interrelatedness of body systems
   C. recognition and appreciation of a person's uniqueness and social–environmental relationships
   D. appreciation of the collaborative role of all health team members
2. Common aspects of the critical care nursing role include
   A. community referral
   B. teacher
   C. disaster management
   D. staff liaison

Answers: 1. A, 2. B

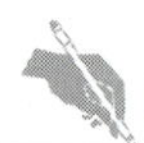

POSTTEST

1. A patient is crying about a below-knee amputation (BKA) sustained as a pedestrian in a pedestrian–vehicle crash. She expresses fears about ambulating in physical therapy. This behavior is a sign of which stage of illness?
   A. denial
   B. awareness
   C. restitution
   D. resolution
2. Which of the following groups of critically ill patients is at greatest risk for experiencing sensory problems?
   A. middle-aged adults
   B. renal transplant patients
   C. patients in windowless patient care areas
   D. patients who have been hospitalized previously
3. Mrs. Baker states she has heard her dead mother calling her. The nurse recognizes this as a symptom of
   A. sensory shutdown
   B. sensory deprivation
   C. auditory damage
   D. antibiotic toxicity
4. One of the most disturbing noises listed by nurses working with critically ill patients is
   A. physician yelling
   B. equipment alarms
   C. ventilator cycling
   D. suction equipment
5. The more acutely ill the patient, the greater the need of families to
   A. visit the patient
   B. understand the technology used in caring for the patient
   C. have a detailed explanation of procedures
   D. have a unit brochure explaining unit policies
6. Extended orientation programs for new graduates to prepare them to work with critically ill patients
   A. are more successful
   B. promote nurse retention
   C. decrease the number of incident reports
   D. are expensive
7. The primary purpose of using technology is to
   A. support the patient's well-being
   B. decrease the patient's length of hospitalization
   C. anticipate complications of therapy
   D. decentralize patient care into specialized units

8. A hazard of technology is
   A. not trusting nursing assessment data
   B. too much touching of the patient
   C. increased nursing surveillance of the patient
   D. the demise of nursing specialty practice

9. Which of the following has been identified by nurses who work with critically ill patients as a primary stressor?
   A. lack of pay
   B. interpersonal conflict
   C. overtime
   D. performing complex skills

10. To relieve stress associated with nursing critically ill patients, the nurse should
   A. request a transfer
   B. drink more decaffeinated beverages
   C. work with fewer protocols
   D. attend a continuing education program for personal growth

11. Burnout is
   A. the result of sensory overload
   B. associated with ICU psychosis
   C. an automatic protective response
   D. associated with tenure as a nurse

12. Commitment to work
   A. is associated with less burnout
   B. produces greater work stress
   C. results from extensive orientation to the work area
   D. is associated with the number of years the nurse has worked in the area

13. Burnout may be manifested by all of the following EXCEPT
   A. pessimism
   B. forgetfulness
   C. tolerance
   D. nightmares

14. The decision not to use technology to sustain life should be made
   A. by the health care provider
   B. before an emergency situation
   C. by community standards
   D. when the patient is transferred to the ICU

15. Informed refusal by the patient
   A. is an acceptable reason for limiting treatment
   B. jeopardizes the health care provider's legal status
   C. indicates that the patient did not receive adequate explanation of treatment
   D. indicates that the patient is angry

16. All of the following variables have been associated with health outcomes EXCEPT
   A. severity of illness
   B. age
   C. patient's previous health status
   D. admission diagnosis

17. Do Not Resuscitate orders were developed to prevent
   A. treatment for the patient
   B. use of CPR
   C. use of critical care resources
   D. patient transfer

18. An ethical review committee may
   A. decrease public scrutiny of health care providers' actions
   B. promote implementation of general standards
   C. enhance health care providers' liability
   D. increase individual responsibility for decision making

19. The essential components of professional nursing practice are all of the following EXCEPT
   A. care
   B. cure
   C. coordination
   D. culture

20. Clarification of one's values as a nurse may
   A. decrease the nurse's liability
   B. help the nurse anticipate patient care problems
   C. promote burnout
   D. decrease sensory overload

POSTTEST ANSWERS

Question	Answer	Section	Question	Answer	Section
1	C	Two	11	C	Nine
2	C	Four	12	A	Nine
3	B	Four	13	C	Nine
4	B	Four	14	B	Ten
5	A	Six	15	A	Ten
6	D	Seven	16	B	Ten
7	A	Eight	17	B	Ten
8	A	Eight	18	B	Ten
9	B	Nine	19	D	Eleven
10	D	Nine	20	B	Eleven

REFERENCES

Acker, K. (1993). Do critical care nurses face burnout, PTSD, or is it something else?: Getting help for the helpers. *AACN Clin Issues* 4:558–565.

Ackerman, N., & Higgins, V. (1992). Upgrading critical care nursing assistant skills. *Nursing Management* 23:80A–80H.

American Association of Critical Care Nurses. (1989a). Position statement: Role of the critical care nurse as patient advocate. Laguna Niguel, CA: Author.

American Association of Critical Care Nurses. (1989b). Use of nursing support personnel in critical care units. *Focus Crit Care* 16:327–328.

American Association of Critical Care Nurses. (1991). Position statement: Withholding or withdrawing life-sustaining treatment. Laguna Niguel, CA: Author.

American Association of Critical Care Nurses. (1994). Definition of critical care nursing. Newport Beach, CA: Author.

American Nurses Association. (1991). Position statement on nursing and the patient self-determination act. Kansas City, MO: Author.

American Nurses Association. (1992). Position statement on nursing care and do-not-resuscitate decisions. Kansas City, MO: Author.

American Nurses Association. (1995). Nursing: A social policy statement. Kansas City, MO: Author.

Armstrong, S., Simpson, T., Nield, M., Lentz, M., & Mitchell, P. (1991). The cost of nursing excellence in critical care. *J Nursing Admin* 21(2):27–34.

Aultschuler, J. (1997). Family relationships during serious illness. *Nursing Times* 93(7):48–49.

Baggs, J. (1989). Intensive care unit use and collaboration between nurses and physicians. *Heart Lung* 18:332–338.

Baker, C. (1993). Annoyance to ICU noise: A model of patient discomfort. *Crit Care Nursing Q* 16(2):83–90.

Bartz, B. (1993). Fostering comforting touch in caring for critically ill patients. In M. Harvey et al. (eds.). Results of the consensus conference on fostering more humane critical care: Creating a healing environment. *AACN Clin Issues* 4:509.

Bellamy, P., & Oye, R. (1987). Admitting elderly patients into the ICU: Dilemmas and solutions. *Geriatrics* 42(3):61–68.

Bertolini, C. (1994). Ethical decision making in intensive care: A nurse's perspective. *Intensive Crit Care Nursing* 10:58–63.

Bouley, G., von Hofe, K., and Blatt, L. (1994). Holistic care of the critically ill: Meeting both patient and family needs. *Dimensions Crit Care Nursing* 13(4):218–223.

Bouman, C. (1984). Identifying priority concerns of families of ill patients. *Dimensions Crit Care Nursing* 3:313–319.

Boumans, N., & Landeweerd, J. (1994). Working in an intensive or non-intensive care unit: Does it make any difference? *Heart Lung* 23:71–79.

Burfitt, S., Greiner, D., Miers, L., Kinney, M., & Branyon, M. (1993). Professional nurse caring as perceived by critically ill patients: A phenomenologic study. *Am J Crit Care* 2:489–499.

Carlon, G. (1988). Admitting cancer patients to the ICU. *Crit Care Clin* 4:183–192.

Cassell, E. (1986). Autonomy in the ICU: Refusal of treatment. *Crit Care Clin* 2:27–40.

Chelluri, L., Pinsky, M., Donahoe, M., & Grenvik, A. (1993). Long term outcome of critically ill elderly patients requiring intensive care. *JAMA* 269:3119–3123.

Clark, S. (1993, August). Challenges in critical care nursing: Helping patients and families cope. *Crit Care Nursing* (Suppl) 14–20.

Claus, K., & Bailey, J. (1980). Living with stress and promoting well-being. St. Louis: C.V. Mosby.

Clement, J. (1986). Caring and touching as nursing interventions. In C. Hudak, B. Gallo, & T. Lohr (eds.). *Critical care nursing: A holistic approach* (p. 36). Philadelphia: J.B. Lippincott.

Clement, J. (1988). The need for and effects of touch in intensive care patients. In B. Heater & B. AuBuchon (eds.). *Controversies in critical care nursing* (p. 81). Rockville, MD: Aspen.

Cleveland, A. (1994). ICU visitation policies. *Nursing Management* 25:80A–80D.

Continenza, K. (1989). Who cares for the care givers? *Focus Crit Care* 16:435–436.

Cooper, M. (1993). The intersection of technology and care in the ICU. *Adv Nursing Sci* 15(3):23–32.

Cox, P. (1992). Children in critical care: How parents cope. *Br J Nursing* 1:764–768.

Craft, M., Cohen, M., Titler, M., & DeHamer, M. (1993). Experiences in children of critically ill patients: A time of emotional disruption and need for support. *Crit Care Nursing Q* 16(3):64–71.

Davis-Martin, S. (1994). Perceived needs of families of long term critical care patients: A brief report. *Heart Lung* 23:515–518.

Dirks, J., Lough, M., & Moungey, S. (1995). Cross training across acuity levels. *Crit Care Nurse* 15(1):68–74.

Dominion, J. (1971). The psychological significance of touch. *Nursing Times* 67:163–171.

Dossey, B. (1990). Psychophysiologic self-regulation interventions. In B. Dossey, C. Guzzetta, & C. Kenner (eds). *Essentials of critical care nursing: body, mind, spirit* (Chap. 5). Philadelphia: J.B. Lippincott.

Easton, C., & MacKenzie, F. (1988). Sensory-perceptual alterations: Delirium in the ICU. *Heart Lung* 17:229–235.

Edwards, B.S. (1990). Does the DNR patient belong in the ICU? *Crit Care Clin North Am* 2:473–480.

Farrimond, P. (1984). Post-cardiotomy delirium. *Nursing Times* 80(30):39–41.

Fitzgerald, K. (1989). Trauma. In B. Riegel & D. Ehrenreich (eds.). *Psychological aspects of critical care nursing* (pp. 210–233). Rockville, MD: Aspen.

Foss, K., & Tenholder, M. (1993). Expectations and needs of persons with family members in an intensive care unit as opposed to a general ward. *South Med J* 86:380–384.

Freudenberg, H. (1974). Staff burnout. *J Social Issues* 30:159–165.

Guzetta, C., Kessler, C., Dossey, B., & Moser, D. (1998). Alternative/Complimentary Therapies. In M. Kinney, S. Dunbar, J. Brooks-Brunn, N. Molter, & J. Vitello-Cicciu (eds.). *AACN's clinical reference for critical care nursing* (4th ed). St. Louis: C.V. Mosby.

Halm, M., & Alpen, M. (1993). The impact of technology on patients and families. *Nursing Clin North Am* 28:443–457.

Hansell, H. (1984). The behavioral effects of noise on man: The patient with "ICU psychosis." *Heart Lung* 13:59–65.

Harris, R. (1989). Reviewing nursing stress according to a proposed coping-adaptation framework. *Adv Nursing Sci* 11:12–28.

Harvey, M., et al. (1993). Results of the consensus conference on fostering more humane critical care: Creating a healing environment. *AACN Clin Issues* 4:484–507.

Henneman, E. (1993). Multidisciplinary care plan for the dying patient: A strategy to promote humane caring in ICU. In M. Harvey et al. (eds). Results of the consensus conference on fostering more humane critical care: creating a healing environment. *AACN Clin Issues* 4:527.

Hickey, M. (1990). What are the needs of families of critically ill patients? A review of the literature since 1976. *Heart Lung* 19:401–415.

Hoekstra, L. (1994). Exploring the scientific bases of holistic nursing. *Nursing Connections* 7:5–14.

Holly, C., & Lyons, M. (1993). Increasing your decision making role in ethical situations. *Dimensions Crit Care Nursing* 12:264–270.

Hopkins, A. (1994). The trauma nurse's role with families in crisis. *Crit Care Nurse* 14:35–43.

Jones, K. (1993). Outcomes analysis: Methods and issues. *Nursing Economics* 11:145–152.

Kirchhoff, K., Hansen, C., & Fullmer, N. (1985). Open visiting in the intensive care unit: A debate. *Dimensions Crit Care Nursing* 4:296–304.

Kirchhoff, K., Pugh, E., Calame, R., & Reynolds, N. (1993). Nurses' beliefs and attitudes toward visiting in adult critical care settings. *Am J Crit Care* 2:238–245.

Kleman, M., et al. (1993). Physiologic responses of coronary care patients to visiting. *J Cardiovasc Nursing* 7:(3):52–62.

Kohrmann, A. (1985). Selective non-treatment of handicapped newborns: A critical essay. *Social Sci Med* 20:1091–1095.

Knaus, W.A., Wagner D.P., Draper E.A., Zimmerman J.E., et al. (1991). The Apache III prognostic system. Risk prediction of hospital mortality for critically ill hospitalized adults. *Chest* 100(6):1619–1636.

Krachman, S.L. (1995). Sleep in the intensive care unit. *Chest* 107:1713–1720.

Leske, J.S., & Jiricka, M.K. (1998). Impact of family demands and family strengths and capabilities on family well being and adaptation after critical injury. *Am J Crit Care* 7:383–389.

Levine, M. (1989). Ration or rescue: The elderly patient in critical care. *Crit Care Nursing Q* 12:82–89.

Lo, B., & Jonsen, A. (1980). Clinical decisions to limit treatment. *Ann Intern Med* 93:764–768.

Luce, J. (1994). The changing physician-patient relationship in critical care medicine under health care reform. *Am J Resp Crit Care Med* 150:266–270.

Marsden, C. (1992). An ethical assessment of intensive care. *Int J Technol Assess Health Care* 8:408–418.

Maslow, A. (1970). *Motivation and personality*. New York: Harper & Row.

McConnell, E. (1990). The impact of machines on the work of critical care nurses. *Crit Care Nursing Q* 12:45–52.

Mendyka, B. (1993). The dying patient in the intensive care unit: Assisting the family in crisis. *AACN Clin Issues* 4:550–557.

Miller, J. (1989). Hope-inspiring strategies of the critically ill. *Appl Nursing Res* 2:23–29.

Miracle, V., & Hovekamp, G. (1994). Needs of families of patients undergoing invasive cardiac procedures. *Am J Crit Care* 3:155–157.

Nicholson, A., et al. (1993). Effects of child visitation in adult critical care units: A pilot study. *Heart Lung* 22:36–45.

Patel, C.T. (1996). Hope-inspiring strategies of spouses of critically ill patients. *J Holistic Nursing* 14(1):44–65.

Pelletier, M. (1993). The needs of family members of organ and tissue donors. *Heart Lung* 22:151–157.

Quinn, J. (1993). Psychoimmunologic effects of therapeutic touch on practitioners and recently bereaved recipients: A pilot study. *Adv Nursing Sci* 15(4):13–26.

Ray, M. (1989). The theory of bureaucratic caring for nursing practice in the organizational culture. *Nursing Admin Q* 13:31–42.

Robinson, J., & Lewis, D. (1990). Coping with ICU work-related stressors: A study. *Crit Care Nurse* 10:80–88.

Rockwood, K., et al. (1993). One-year outcome of elderly and young patients admitted to intensive care units. *Crit Care Med* 21:687–691.

Rose, P.A. (1995). The meaning of critical illness to families. *Can J Nursing Res* 27(4):83–87.

Rushton, C. (1994). The critical care nurse as patient advocate. *Crit Care Nurse* 14:102–106.

Schnaper, N., & Cowley, R. (1976). Overview: Psychological sequelae to multiple trauma. *Am J Psychiatry* 133:883–890.

Schultz, M., & Daly, B. (1989). Differences and similarities in nurses' perceptions of intensive care nursing and non-intensive care nursing. *Focus Crit Care* 16:465–471.

Simpson, T. (1993). Visit preferences of middle aged versus older critically ill patients. *Am J Crit Care* 2:339–345.

Smith, J. (1994). Psychosocial concepts and the patient's experience with critical illness. In C. Hudak & B. Gallo (eds.). *Critical care nursing: A holistic approach*. Philadelphia: J.B. Lippincott.

Snider, G. (1994). Allocation of intensive care: The physician's role. *Am J Resp Crit Care Med* 150:575–580.

Snyder, J., & Colantonio, A. (1994). Outcome from central nervous system injury. *Crit Care Clin* 10:217–228.

Spitzer, W., & Burke, L. (1993). A critical incident stress debriefing program for hospital based health care personnel. *Health Social Work* 18:149–156.

Stechmiller, J., & Yarandi, H. (1993). Predictors of burnout in critical care nurses. *Heart Lung* 13:534–541.

Suchman, E. (1965). Stages of illness and medical care. *J Health Hum Behav* 6:114.

Teres, D., & Lemeshow, S. (1994). Why severity models should be used with caution. *Crit Care Clin* 10:93–115.

Topf, M. (1989). Personality hardiness, occupational stress, and burnout in critical care nurses. *Res Nursing Health* 12:179–186.

Topf, M. (1992). Stress effects of personal control over hospital noise. *Behav Med* 18:84–94.

Topf, M., & Davis, J. (1993). Critical care unit noise and rapid eye movement (REM) sleep. *Heart Lung* 22:252–258.

Topf, M., & Dillon, E. (1988). Noise-induced stress as a predictor of burnout in critical care nurses. *Heart Lung* 17:567–574.

Tuchschmidt, J., & Mecher, C. (1994). Predictors of outcome from critical illness. *Crit Care Clin* 10:179–195.

Twibell, R.S. (1998). Family coping during critical illness. *Dimensions Crit Care Nursing* 17(2):100–112.

Urban, N. (1998). Patient and family responses to the critical care environment. In M. Kinney, S. Dunbar, J. Brooks-Brunn, N. Molter, & J. Vitello-Cicciu (eds.). *AACN's clinical reference for critical care nursing* (4th ed). St. Louis: C.V. Mosby.

Van Ora, L. (1989). Terminal is a relative term. *Nursing Health Care* 18:97–100.

Williams, M. (1989). Physical environment of the intensive care unit: Elderly patients. *Crit Care Nursing Q* 12:39–54.

Williams, M. (1993). Re-establishment of personalities in the ICU: Use of the personality display board to minimize depersonalization. In M. Harvey et al. (eds.). Results of the consensus conference on fostering more humane critical care: Creating a healing environment. *AACN Clin Issues* 4:546.

Wilson, L. (1993). Sensory perceptual alteration: Diagnosis, prediction, and intervention in the hospitalized adult. *Nurs Clin North Am* 28:747–765.

Wlody, G.S. (1998). Ethics and advocacy in critical care nursing. In M. Kinney, S. Dunbar, J. Brooks-Brunn, N. Molter, & J. Vitello-Cicciu (eds.). *AACN's clinical reference for critical care nursing* (4th ed). St. Louis: C.V. Mosby.

Wood, A. (1993). A review of the literature relating to sleep in hospital with emphasis on the sleep of the ICU patient. *Intensive Crit Care Nursing* 9:129–136.

Module 2

Acute Pain in the High-Acuity Patient

Kathleen Dorman Wagner, Barbara Vanderveer, Susan K. Seely

The focus of this module is on the concept of acute pain rather than chronic pain. The module is composed of seven sections. Section One provides a brief discussion of the physiology involved in the transmission of pain. Section Two defines acute pain and presents a multifaceted model of pain. Section Three discusses potential sources of pain and the effects of pain on the body. Section Four presents a variety of pain assessment tools, including unidimensional and multidimensional assessment tools. Sections Five, Six, and Seven focus on the management of pain. Information covered in these sections includes pharmacologic and nonpharmacologic approaches to pain management, reasons for undertreatment of acute pain, and special considerations regarding pain management in specific patient populations. Each section includes a set of review questions to help the learner evaluate his or her understanding of the section's content before moving on to the next section. All Section Reviews, and the module Pretest and Posttest include answers. It is suggested that the learner review those concepts answered incorrectly in the review questions before proceeding to the next section.

Objectives

Following completion of this module, the learner will be able to

1. Identify the basic physiology involved in the transmission of pain.
2. Explain the multifaceted nature of pain.
3. Describe potential sources and effects of pain.
4. Discuss pain assessment.
5. Describe effective management of pain for the high-acuity patient.
6. Discuss issues related to the undertreatment of pain.
7. Identify considerations associated with pain management in special populations.

Pretest

1. The five types of sensory receptors include all of the following EXCEPT
   A. chemoreceptors
   B. nociceptors
   C. thermoreceptors
   D. odoreceptors

2. The A nerve fibers have which of the following characteristics?
   A. myelinated
   B. primitive
   C. transmit slowly
   D. transmit aching sensations

3. Acute persistent pain is associated with
   A. a short duration
   B. a rapid healing process
   C. chronic pain conditions
   D. a distinct organic pathology
4. A second-degree burn on the arm is an example of what type of noxious stimulus?
   A. thermal
   B. physiologic
   C. chemical
   D. mechanical
5. When the stress response becomes too high, it is associated with all of the following physiologic changes EXCEPT
   A. organ hypoperfusion
   B. elevated blood endorphin levels
   C. increased vascular shunting
   D. enhanced hormone function
6. The clinician would anticipate a masking of the sympathetic symptoms of pain by increased parasympathetic response under which of the following circumstances?
   A. fractured ribs
   B. leg amputation
   C. injury to the bowel
   D. severe pneumonia
7. If a patient is mildly confused, the nurse should initially try to assess pain using
   A. vital signs
   B. self-report
   C. facial expression
   D. body posturing
8. A major weakness of multidimensional tools is that
   A. the nurse performs the assessment
   B. they measure only pain intensity
   C. the patient must comprehend the vocabulary
   D. they are unable to measure degree of anxiety
9. Which of the following statements is correct regarding nonopioid therapy?
   A. nonopioids have more severe side effects than opioids
   B. nonopioids are harder to access than opioids
   C. nonopioids can manage pain as effectively as opioids
   D. combining opioids with nonopioids enhances analgesia effectiveness
10. The most common route used for patient-controlled analgesia (PCA) is
    A. intramuscular
    B. intravenous
    C. subcutaneous
    D. epidural
11. Which of the following statements is correct regarding opioid use and respiratory depression?
    A. respiratory depression precedes onset of sedation
    B. respiratory depression worsens as tolerance develops
    C. sedation occurs before respiratory depression
    D. respiratory depression is a common problem in hospitalized patients
12. Accumulation of morphine metabolites in the blood secondary to renal dysfunction can cause
    A. seizures
    B. tachycardia
    C. central nervous system (CNS) stimulation
    D. severe respiratory depression
13. Elderly patients have fewer endogenous receptors and neural transmitters than younger patients. The primary clinical significance of this statement is
    A. pain relief using opioids is less effective
    B. pain relief using opioids is more unpredictable
    C. smaller doses of opioids are required to achieve pain relief
    D. larger doses of opioids are required to achieve pain relief

Answers: 1. D, 2. A, 3. D, 4. A, 5. D, 6. C, 7. B, 8. C, 9. D, 10. B, 11. C, 12. D, 13. C

GLOSSARY

Acute pain. Pain that is continually changing and transient; onset is rapid and pain is of brief duration (≤ 6 months)

Addiction. See Psychological dependence

Epidural. Situated within the spinal canal, on or outside the dura mater (tough membrane surrounding the spinal cord); synonyms are *extradural* and *peridural* (AHCPR, 1992)

Intrathecal. Within a sheath (e.g., cerebrospinal fluid that is contained within the dura mater) (AHCPR, 1992)

Nociception. The activation of pain receptors and the pain pathway by a noxious stimulus of sufficient strength to threaten tissue integrity

Nociceptors. Pain receptors

Opioid agonist. Any morphine-like compound that produces bodily effects including pain relief, sedation, constipation, and respiratory depression (AHCPR, 1992)

Opiophobia. The fear of prescribing (or consuming) adequate amounts of opiates for therapeutic results

Opioid pseudoaddiction. A term that has been applied to patient behaviors that mimic those associated with addiction; the behaviors result from inadequate pain management rather than psychological dependence

Pain. An unpleasant sensory and emotional experience associated with actual or potential tissue damage or described in terms of such damage (AHCPR, 1992, p. 95)

Pain. An unpleasant phenomenon that is uniquely experienced by each individual; it cannot be adequately defined, identified, or measured by an observer (Ludwig-Beymer & Huether, 1996, pp. 319–320)

Pain. Whatever the experiencing person says it is, existing whenever the experiencing person says it does (McCaffery & Pasero, 1999, p. 17)

Pain behavior. A person's physical reaction to the conscious perception of pain

Physical dependence. A physical adaptation of the body to the presence of opioids, existing when rapid drug withdrawal produces signs and symptoms

Psychological dependence (addiction). A pattern of compulsive drug use characterized by a continued craving for an opioid and the need to use the opioid for effects other than pain relief (or other medical indications) (AHCPR, 1994)

Sedation. A state of drowsiness and clouding of mental activity that may be accompanied by impaired reasoning ability (Way et al., 1998)

Tolerance. A common physiologic result of chronic opioid use; it means that a larger dose of opioid is required to maintain the same level of analgesia

ABBREVIATIONS

AHCPR. Agency for Health Care Policy and Research

CSF. Cerebrospinal fluid

ICU. Intensive care unit

MPQ. McGill Pain Questionnaire

NRS. Numeric rating scale

NSAID. Nonsteroidal anti-inflammatory drug

PCA. Patient-controlled analgesia

SF-MPQ. Short-Form McGill Pain Questionnaire

VAS. Visual analog scale

WHO. World Health Organization

SECTION ONE: Pain Physiology—A Review

At the completion of this section, the learner will be able to identify the physiology involved in the transmission of pain.

A review of pain sensory receptors and their pathways is presented to provide a basic understanding of the assessment and management of the patient in acute pain. A description of the transmission of pain impulses is presented to provide a foundation for understanding the numerous problems involved in the effective management of pain.

The two major types of **pain** are *somatic pain*, which arises from stimulation of receptors in the skin, muscle, joints, and tendons; and *visceral pain*, which arises from stimulation of receptors in the viscera. Sensory stimuli, such as cold, heat, touch, and pain, are communicated to the nervous system through sensory receptors. There are five types of sensory receptors, each one with the ability to detect changes in a specific type of sensory input (Table 2–1). Sensory receptors require a certain level of excitation (called the *threshold*) before they will transmit input. Once the sensory threshold has been achieved, the nerve fiber is stimulated and the impulse travels the length of the associated sensory nerve (Guyton & Hall, 1997a).

Pain Nerve Fibers

The nerves that carry pain impulses are categorized in terms of their size and whether or not a myelin sheath is present. Nerves termed *A beta fibers* are large in diameter and have a myelin sheath. *A delta fibers* are small in diameter and are also myelinated. *C fibers* are small in diameter and are usually unmyelinated. Impulses are conducted more quickly over large, myelinated nerves in comparison to small or unmyelinated nerves (Guyton & Hall, 1997a). For example, A delta fibers conduct impulses rapidly. Sharp, pinprick-like pain is conducted along these fibers. C fibers, on the other hand, have a slow conduction rate, and transmit aching, throbbing sensations (Guyton & Hall, 1997b).

TABLE 2–1. SENSORY RECEPTORS

RECEPTOR	FUNCTION
Pain receptors (nociceptors)	Detection of tissue damage
Thermoreceptors	Detection of temperature changes
Electromagnetic receptors	Detection of light on eye retina
Chemoreceptors	Detection of smell, taste, concentration of arterial blood oxygen and carbon dioxide, and others
Mechanoreceptors	Detection of mechanical changes in cells adjacent to receptors (e.g., position and tactile senses)

Pain Transmission

Pain impulses initiated at receptor sites are transmitted to the brain along multiple pathways. A major dual pathway consists of the neospinothalamic tract and paleospinothalamic tract. An example of this dual pathway is as follows: A delta pain fibers primarily transmit thermal and mechanical pain through the neospinothalamic tract. The theory underlying the A delta route of transmission is that pain impulses travel along first-order neurons to the dorsal horn of the spinal cord, terminating primarily in the lamina marginalis. Upon reaching the lamina marginalis in the dorsal horn, the impulse excites second-order neurons and immediately crosses to the opposite side of the spinal cord. The impulse then ascends through the brain stem to the thalamus, where it is consciously acknowledged. From the thalamus it travels to the cerebral cortex, where analysis of pain quality takes place. The slower-transmitting C fibers travel along a cruder, more primitive pain pathway, the paleospinothalamic tract, which primarily terminates in a broad area of the brain stem, with less than a quarter of the fibers passing on through to the thalamus (Guyton & Hall, 1997b).

Endogenous Analgesia System

Although the transmission of the impulse along the spinothalamic pathways appears relatively simple and straightforward, the process is complex. Guyton & Hall (1997b) explain that the body has its own analgesia system that significantly influences how each person reacts to pain. There are three components to this system (in order of their location in the CNS): (1) the periventricular and periaqueductal gray (PAG) areas, located in the third ventricle, hypothalamus, and upper brain stem; (2) the raphe magnus nucleus, located in the brain stem; and (3) the pain inhibitory complex, located in the spinal cord's dorsal horns. Stimulation of the PAG or raphe magnus nucleus causes significant suppression of extremely strong pain signals that are coming in through the dorsal spinal roots. Pain signals that primarily stimulate the periventricular and PAG areas are suppressed but to a lesser degree. Pain signals that are blocked by the pain inhibitory complex in the spinal cord are suppressed at that level and may not be transmitted on to the brain.

The analgesia system secretes special pain modulating neurotransmitters that influence pain impulses at various stages of transmission. These endogenously produced analgesic substances are called *endogenous opioid peptides*. When these substances are released, they bind to special receptor sites along the ascending pain pathway and modify the pain transmission. Three types of endogenous opioid peptides have been identified: enkephalins, beta-endorphins, and dynorphins. These substances modulate pain transmission in response to specific physiologic events, such as pain and stress (Curtis, Kolotylo, & Broome, 1998; Guyton & Hall, 1997b; Hawthorn & Redmond, 1998; Way, Fields, & Way, 1998). Table 2–2 provides a brief summary of the endogenous opioid peptides.

In addition, theorists Melzack and Wall (1965), in their classic work on pain mechanisms, contended that the substantia gelatinosa acts as a gate for pain impulses. Whether the gate is open (allowing impulses to continue along the pain pathway) or closed depends on whether large-fiber firing or small-fiber firing predominates. Large-fiber firing causes the gate to close, whereas small-fiber firing opens the gate.

In summary, the transmission and eventual response to pain impulses is a complex process that is not as yet fully understood. Multiple pain pathways are thought to exist, including a dual pathway, consisting of the neospinothalamic tract and paleospinothalamic tract. The precise mechanisms of pain transmission cannot be described with certainty. The complexity of the process is due, in part, to known and suspected influences on the impulse as it travels along the pain pathway.

TABLE 2–2. ENDOGENOUS OPIATES

GROUP	PRIMARY LOCATION	COMMENTS
Enkephalins	Periaqueductal gray (PAG) in midbrain and brain stem	Most widely distributed in body Effects last minutes to hours Serotonin causes enkephalin release at dorsal horn
Beta-endorphin	Hypothalamus and pituitary gland	Hypothalamus and pituitary gland Most like morphine
Dynorphins	PAG and spinal cord	Present in minute quantities Extremely powerful (perhaps 200 times more powerful than morphine)

From Hawthorn, J., & Redmond, K. (1998). Pain: Causes and management. *Malden, MA: Blackwell Science; Guyton, A.C., & Hall, J.E. (1997). Pain, headache, and thermal sensations. In A.C. Guyton & J.E. Hall (eds.).* Human physiology and mechanisms of disease *(6th ed.). Philadelphia: W.B. Saunders; and Thelan, L.A., Urden, L.D., Lough, M.E., & Stacy, K.M. (eds.).* Critical care nursing: Diagnosis and management *(3rd ed.). St. Louis: C.V. Mosby.*

SECTION ONE REVIEW

1. The five types of sensory receptors include all of the following EXCEPT
   A. chemoreceptors
   B. nociceptors
   C. thermoreceptors
   D. odoreceptors
2. Type A nerve fibers have which of the following characteristics?
   A. myelinated
   B. primitive
   C. transmit slowly
   D. transmit aching sensations
3. Pain is analyzed in which part of the brain?
   A. cerebellum
   B. thalamus
   C. cerebral cortex
   D. brain stem
4. When pain is suppressed at the pain inhibitory complex it
   A. moves on to the PAG
   B. is blocked at the spinal cord level
   C. transfers to the raphe magnus nucleus
   D. is ultimately suppressed in the hypothalamus
5. The neospinothalamic pain pathway terminates in the
   A. cerebral cortex
   B. brain stem
   C. dorsal horns
   D. substantia gelatinosa
6. The paleospinothalamic tract
   A. is the primary pain pathway
   B. terminates throughout the brain stem
   C. transmits signals to specific sensory areas
   D. transmits signals identically to the fast pathway

Answers: 1. D, 2. A, 3. C, 4. B, 5. A, 6. B

SECTION TWO: The Multifaceted Nature of Pain

At the completion of this section, the learner will be able to explain the multiple facets of pain.

A Working Definition of Acute Pain

McCaffery has defined pain as "whatever the experiencing person says it is, existing whenever the experiencing person says it does" (McCaffery & Pasero, 1999). The AHCPR Guidelines (1992) state that pain is "an unpleasant sensory and emotional experience associated with actual or potential tissue damage or described in terms of such damage."

Acute pain has been defined as pain that is continually changing and transient. It is accompanied by a high level of emotional and autonomic nervous system arousal and is usually associated with tissue pathology or surgery. It can be further divided into two types—brief acute pain (short duration, minutes to days) and acute persistent pain (longer duration, weeks to months). Acute persistent pain is primarily associated with a distinct organic pathology and a slow healing process (Chapman & Syrjala, 1990). Acute pain serves a major protective function by acting as an early warning system of impending or actual tissue injury and typically diminishes as the injury heals (Curtis, Kolotylo, & Broome, 1998).

A Multifaceted Model of Pain

Loeser and Cousins (1990) propose that pain is multifaceted and composed of nociception, pain, suffering, and pain behaviors (Fig. 2–1). Only the outermost facet, pain behaviors, can be observed by someone other than the person experiencing the pain. The other three facets are completely personal and can only be inferred. The relative contribution of each of the four facets to the pain experience is variable. Each facet is present to some degree in any pain experience. In general, the noxious stimulus and the process of nociception predominate during acute pain.

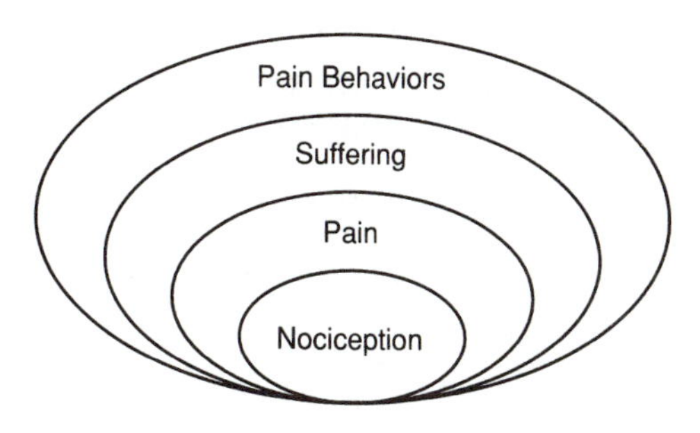

Figure 2–1. A multifaceted conceptual approach to the pain experience. *(Adapted from Loeser, J.D., & Cousins, M.J. [1990]. Contemporary pain management.* Med J Aust *153:208–212, 216.)*

Noxious Stimulus

Noxious stimuli may be mechanical, thermal, or chemical, and they have the potential to excite pain receptors. These stimuli must exist in sufficient quantities to trigger the release of biochemical mediators that activate the pain response (nociception). Activation of the pain response may also be triggered:

- In response to what would typically be defined as non-noxious stimuli
- In response to sympathetic discharge (sympathetically maintained pain)
- Spontaneously

The First Facet: Nociception

Nociception refers to the activation of pain receptors (nociceptors) and the pain pathway by a noxious stimulus of sufficient strength to threaten tissue integrity. Under normal circumstances it leads to the sensation of pain. Acute pain is primarily of nociceptive origin. Nociception does not, however, always lead to pain. Certain factors or conditions can alter or eliminate the sensation of pain even when the person is subjected to extremely noxious stimuli. Such factors include severe nerve damage (spinal cord injury, peripheral neuropathy), anesthesia, and strong analgesia therapy. Pain can also occur without nociception, such as may be found in patients with neuropathic pain and other chronic pain conditions (Loeser & Cousins, 1990).

The Second Facet: Pain

According to Loeser and Cousins (1990), pain "is the perception of a noxious stimulus dependent upon events in the neurones of the spinal cord and brain stem" (p. 179). A person can perceive pain only when transmission of the noxious stimulus terminates within the brain. It is unknown whether the patient's ability to perceive pain remains intact when cortical function is compromised or when cortical function has been chemically altered by sedative–hypnotics.

The Third Facet: Suffering

The multifaceted model describes the term *suffering* as a negative affective response that is generated in the higher nervous centers of the brain. It further states that suffering can be caused by pain or a variety of situations such as stress, anxiety, fear, loss of a loved one, and depression. The concept of suffering seems closely connected to the personal meaning of the pain. The clinician's objective assessment of suffering is restricted to observing for the presence or absence of pain behaviors. According to Loeser and Cousins (1990), suffering is particularly associated with chronic pain. The complex concept of suffering has received increased attention over the past decade and there is a growing body of literature in this area. The reader is referred to suggested additional readings in the reference section of this module.

The Fourth Facet: Pain Behaviors

It is not coincidental that the outside circle of the multifaceted model of pain is pain behavior. **Pain behavior** refers to a person's physical reaction to the conscious perception of pain; it is what leads the observer to conclude that pain is being experienced. There are two types of pain behaviors: those that are intended to communicate pain (pain-expressing behaviors), and those that are intended to lessen or control the pain (pain-controlling behaviors). Common pain-expressing behaviors include groaning, rubbing the painful part, or lying motionless. It is often difficult for the observer to differentiate pain-controlling from pain-expressing behaviors. For example, rubbing or massaging the painful part may be a means of moderating the sensory input (pain-controlling behavior) rather than a means of communicating (expressing) the pain to others. Pain behaviors are discussed further in Section Four: Pain Assessment.

In summary, pain can be defined in a variety of ways but is consistently viewed as a very personal, subjective experience. A multifaceted model of pain illustrates the complex nature of the pain experience. The model proposes that there are four facets of pain, including nociception, pain, suffering, and pain behaviors. The first three facets can only be inferred by anyone other than the person experiencing the pain. Only the fourth facet, pain behaviors, can be observed. Pain behaviors may be either pain expressing or pain controlling.

SECTION TWO REVIEW

1. Acute persistent pain is associated with
   A. a short duration
   B. a rapid healing process
   C. chronic pain conditions
   D. a distinct organic pathology
2. A second-degree burn on the arm is an example of what type of noxious stimulus?
   A. thermal
   B. physiologic
   C. chemical
   D. mechanical
3. The activation of pain receptors and the pain pathway by a noxious stimulus of sufficient strength to threaten tissue integrity is known as
   A. acute pain
   B. suffering
   C. nociception
   D. neuropathy

4. Suffering is most commonly associated with which type of pain?
   A. acute
   B. persistent acute
   C. slow chronic
   D. intermittent
5. Behaviors that are intended to communicate pain are called what type of pain behaviors?
   A. expressing
   B. heralding
   C. controlling
   D. communicating

Answers: 1. D, 2. A, 3. C, 4. C, 5. A

SECTION THREE: Acute Pain in the High-Acuity Patient

At the completion of this section, the learner will be able to discuss potential sources and effects of pain.

Potential Sources of Pain

High-acuity patients are at risk for brief acute as well as acute persistent types of pain. The initial insult requiring admission to the hospital is often linked to acute pain (e.g., traumatic injury, organ ischemia, surgical manipulation). In addition, high-acuity patients commonly have invasive lines and tubes inserted (e.g., chest tubes, intravenous lines, endotracheal and tracheostomy tubes), all of which irritate delicate tissues and cause varying degrees of pain. The patient may also be required to undergo painful procedures such as lumbar puncture or endoscopic examinations. Forced immobility owing to the serious or critical nature of an illness, and attachment to multiple tubes, may exacerbate more chronic conditions, such as back or arthritic pain.

Acute pain is usually accompanied by some degree of anxiety, which may be further aggravated by the stress and anxiety associated with the hospital or critical care environment. High-anxiety states are associated with an increase in pain perception and may decrease pain tolerance. Pain may also be a contributor to patient confusion and inadequate sleep.

The Effects of Stress and Pain on the Body

In the high-acuity patient, pain can result from a variety of sources such as tissue injury, ischemia, metabolic or chemical mediators, inflammation, or muscle spasm. Pain is also affected by stress. The stress response is a crucial part of self-preservation. It initiates events that increase the body's chances of survival through a life-threatening event. When the body experiences a massive insult, however, the stress response can become too high, which can cause physiological changes that are associated with poor patient outcomes. A high-stress response increases vascular shunting, resulting in hypoperfusion of vital organs. It also increases serum levels of endogenous opioid peptides, which may result in counterregulation of hormonal responses. Tissue injury is a strong stress response stimulus. The acute pain created by injured tissue initially increases both hormonal and sympathetic nervous system responses. However, if the pain becomes prolonged, the sympathetic response to pain diminishes due to a parasympathetic rebound effect, which results in the vital signs returning more toward normal. This is an important consideration when assessing pain in the high-acuity patient. Although the sympathetic response is important to assess, reliance on it as the sole indicator of acute pain may significantly misrepresent the intensity of pain.

Patients who are experiencing moderate to high levels of pain are often at increased risk for developing stasis-related complications due to immobility. Pain is associated with a natural limiting of activity that encourages a person to rest and, therefore, aids the healing process. This decrease in activity, however, is also associated with negative outcomes, such as pulmonary complications and deep vein thrombosis. Pulmonary complications, such as atelectasis and stasis pneumonia, result from splinting that decreases spontaneous ventilatory movement and oxygenation. For example, pulmonary complications are frequently noted in patients who have had thoracic surgery, abdominal surgery, or trauma, and prolonged bedrest is a significant risk factor in development of deep vein thrombosis. By decreasing the level of pain, patients may become more active earlier in their recovery period, thus significantly decreasing the risk of developing stasis complications.

In summary, pain is a major life-protecting sensation that is frequently accompanied by varying levels of stress and anxiety. When pain is prolonged or severe, it can have a negative physiologic impact. There are many potential sources of pain for the high-acuity patient, including those associated with the patient's admission and those associated with painful procedures, invasive lines, insertion of tubes, and imposed immobility.

SECTION THREE REVIEW

1. Which of the following statements reflects the relationship between pain, stress, and anxiety?
   A. increased levels of stress and anxiety worsen pain
   B. increased levels of stress worsen pain but anxiety has no significant effect
   C. increased levels of anxiety worsen pain but stress has no significant effect
   D. there is no significant relationship between pain, stress, and anxiety
2. The stress response is
   A. an avoidable reaction
   B. a maladaptive response to crises
   C. a crucial part of self-preservation
   D. an unpredictable reaction to pain
3. When the stress response becomes too great, it is associated with all of the following physiologic changes EXCEPT
   A. organ hypoperfusion
   B. elevated blood endorphin levels
   C. increased vascular shunting
   D. enhanced hormone function
4. If acute pain is sustained for a prolonged period of time, the
   A. sympathetic response diminishes
   B. parasympathetic response diminishes
   C. pain threshold increases
   D. pain tolerance decreases

Answers: 1. A, 2. C, 3. D, 4. A

SECTION FOUR: Pain Assessment

At the completion of this section, the learner will be able to discuss pain assessment in the high-acuity patient.

Pain is a complex, subjective response that is multidimensional in nature. The patient's self-report is the most reliable indicator of the existence and intensity of adult pain, and yet it has been shown that nurses' attitudes frequently alter the assessment by subjectively interpreting the patient's self-report of pain (AHCPR, 1992; McCaffery & Pasero, 1999; Stephenson, 1994). Strict attention to applying the nursing process is crucial if acute pain is to be managed effectively, since pain is an ongoing process that requires continual reassessment and reevaluation.

Pain levels vary in each individual primarily because of the biopsychological nature of pain. To manage pain effectively, it is essential to use self-report pain assessment tools whenever possible. These assessment tools help clinicians establish baseline criteria for evaluating pain and facilitate the development of appropriate comfort interventions. The ongoing challenge for caregivers and researchers is to find an effective alternative means of assessment for unconscious patients and other patients who for some reason cannot self-report their levels of pain (e.g., very confused).

Numerous studies over the past decade have described the lack of pain assessments by nurses; yet nurses are consistent in obtaining vital signs. For this reason, the American Pain Society (APS) has suggested making pain the fifth vital sign. The APS believes that by keeping the assessment of pain highly visible, it is more likely to be treated effectively (American Pain Society Quality of Care Committee, 1995).

Pain History

The pain history provides valuable information regarding the patient's preexisting pain experiences, treatment modalities, and medication history. In addition, it may also be used for obtaining information regarding the patient's usual pain behaviors and relief methods at home. Having knowledge of an individual's usual pain behaviors would be of particular value if the patient should lose the ability to communicate with the health care team during hospitalization. Table 2–3 lists important information that can be obtained through a pain history.

The Acute Pain Assessment

Unidimensional and Multidimensional Assessment

Unidimensional pain assessment tools provide the patient with a means to rate a single pain dimension, such as pain

TABLE 2–3. PAIN HISTORY

Drug allergies
Prior acute pain experiences
Chronic pain problems—location? Description of pain? How often? For how long?
Activity level maintained during pain?
Any recent changes in usual pain/discomfort pattern?
How does patient express pain at home? (e.g., paces, lies motionless, cries, distraction, etc.)
How does the pain make the person feel? (e.g., sad, angry, frustrated, etc.)
Usual relief measures:
- Drug therapy—what? How much? How often? Level of relief?
- Nonpharmacologic—what? (e.g., hot water bottle, ice, heating pad, etc.) Level of relief?

intensity, affective distress, or the subjective meaning of the pain. When the specific cause of pain is apparent (e.g., postsurgical incisional pain), a unidimensional pain assessment tool is often considered sufficient. Unidimensional tools are especially useful in evaluating the effectiveness of the interventions used to decrease the pain. These tools are simple to use and take little time to administer. Examples of unidimensional pain assessment tools include the Visual Analog Scale (VAS), the Numeric Rating Scale (NRS), and verbal descriptor scales such as the Adjective Rating Scale (ARS). Unidimensional tools can also be used as part of a multidimensional pain assessment.

Multidimensional pain assessment tools provide the patient with a means to express the affective and evaluative aspects of the pain experience in addition to the sensory aspect. These tools work best for patients with more complex pain such as pain of unknown origin or chronic pain. Examples of multidimensional tools include the McGill Pain Questionnaire (MPQ) and the short-form McGill Pain Questionnaire (SF-MPQ) (Wall & Melzack, 1994).

Unidimensional Pain Assessment

VISUAL ANALOG SCALE (VAS). The VAS has been shown to be an effective measurement of pain intensity. There are several variations of the VAS. The most common is a horizontal or vertical line with one end labeled "no pain" and the opposite end labeled "worst pain imaginable." The patient self-reports where the pain is along this line. The line is usually 10 cm in length. Once the patient has indicated the point on the scale that best represents the current level of pain, a centimeter ruler is placed on the scale and a numeric rating of 0 to 10 is given. On some VAS variations, a numeric scale is present on the reverse side, with a slide rule type of device for converting the VAS to a numeric score. Figure 2–2 illustrates an example of a VAS.

THE NUMERIC RATING SCALE (NRS). The NRS (see Fig. 2–2) is a variation of the VAS. It uses a sequence of numbers from which the patient chooses. The most common use of the NRS is measurement of pain intensity based on a continuum of pain, with 0 being "no pain" and the extreme opposite number (5, 10, or 100) being the "worst pain imaginable." The most common and clinically proven NRS is the 0 to 10 scale. The NRS has also been used to rate numerically other dimensions of pain. An advantage of using the NRS is that the directions for using it have been translated into a variety of languages (McCaffery & Pasero, 1999).

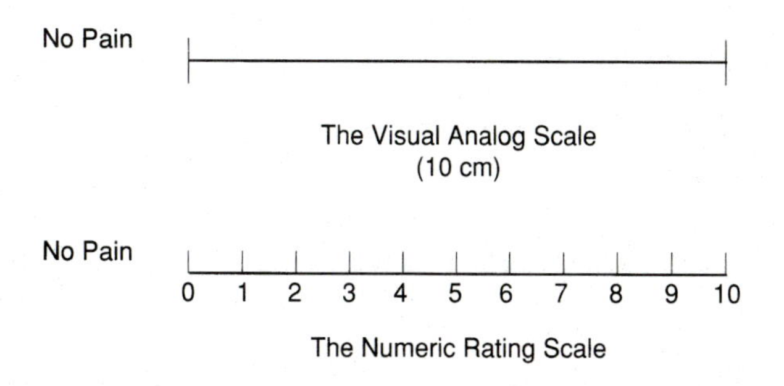

Figure 2–2. Examples of unidimensional pain assessment tools.

VERBAL DESCRIPTOR SCALES. As a unidimensional assessment tool, a verbal descriptor scale, such as the ARS, may be used to measure any of the pain dimensions. For example, as a sensory dimension measure, the scale might include a listing of adjectives, such as flickering, quivering, pulsing, throbbing, beating, pounding (from the MPQ, in Chapman & Syrjala, 1990). Using this list of words, the patient is asked to choose the adjective that best describes his or her current pain. The words should reflect different levels of the dimension being measured. Using this type of tool has several potential disadvantages. First, careful choice of descriptor words is necessary if this type of scale is to be a useful pain assessment tool. Second, patients have a tendency to choose words from the middle of the scale rather than choosing from either end (Chapman & Syrjala, 1990).

WONG–BAKER FACES SCALE (FACES). The Faces Scale has been shown to be popular with both children and adults (Carey et al., 1997). It consists of six facial drawings ranging from smiling to crying. Each face is assigned a number from 0 to 5 or 0 to 10. The patient simply points to the face that represents his or her current level of pain. Directions for the Wong–Baker Faces Scale have also been translated into a variety of languages (McCaffery & Pasero, 1999).

Adapting the Unidimensional Pain Assessment Tool for the Severely Ill Patient

A patient who is extremely ill or weak may be able to use unidimensional tools with the nurse's assistance. For example, the nurse can run a pencil along a VAS and have the patient nod or indicate in some way where the "point" of pain is on the scale. Sometimes, the patient may be able to point to the number on an NRS or to the location on the line of a VAS that best indicates the intensity of pain. As an alternative, the patient may be able to raise up the number of fingers that indicate the level of pain, with no fingers raised being "no pain" and 5 or 10 fingers raised being the "worst pain imaginable."

Nurses frequently assume that extreme illness, weakness, or mild confusion prevents the patient from being able to self-report pain. This is not necessarily true. Self-report methods should be attempted in this patient group even though it may require patience and flexibility on the part of the nurse. If the nurse is to have success using these methods, brief but clear directions must be given and repeated as needed during the assessment procedure.

It has been shown that even when nurses use self-report tools, they rely more on their own nursing observations of behavioral cues in determining whether or not the patient is in pain (Ferrell, McCaffery, & Grant, 1991). This may result in the nurse's applying a numeric value based on nursing observation and estimation of the patient's level of pain intensity (i.e., documenting a patient as a 5/10 based strictly on nursing observation). This is an inappropriate use of the unidimensional self-report tools.

Both types of tools have strengths and limitations associated with their use. Table 2–4 summarizes the advantages and disadvantages of using unidimensional and multidimensional pain assessment tools. The clinician also should be aware that discrepancies may exist between the patient's self-reported level of pain and nurse-observed pain behaviors. For example, a patient may describe pain intensity as a 7 out of 10 while watching television or talking on the phone. This individual may be using coping skills that subjectively do not reflect high pain scores. A patient's use of distraction and relaxation techniques can be misinterpreted as stoicism or exaggeration of self-reported pain levels (AHCPR, 1992).

Multidimensional Pain Assessment

The most frequently used measurement of sensory and affective pain is the MPQ. This questionnaire measures four aspects (categories) of the pain experience: sensory, affective, evaluative, and miscellaneous. Each pain category is measured using a cluster of descriptive words. The patient's choice of words assists the clinician in determining which category the pain is originating from and aids the clinician in choosing a therapeutic pain regimen that is individualized to the patient's needs. The SF-MPQ is recommended for conscious patients in the critical care area. The SF-MPQ takes 2 to 5 minutes to administer. It is more practical for many high-acuity patients, assuming that vocabulary is not a problem and that the patient is functioning at a sufficiently high cognitive level. The words are simple and are understood by most patients. Administration of SF-MPQ can be adjusted for patients who cannot communicate verbally (e.g., intubated patients) by having them either point to desired descriptive words or, if they are too weak, use a head nod when the nurse reads the desired descriptive word. In addition to the McGill tools, the clinician can develop a simple word list using words describing emotions and sensations that would be appropriate for a particular patient or patient population.

Alternative Pain Assessment

High-acuity patients have many reasons for experiencing acute pain, and a significant number are at risk for undertreatment owing to their inability to self-report pain. Many high-acuity patients have altered communication abilities for a variety of reasons, such as altered level of consciousness and extreme weakness. Nurses must be flexible in how they assess pain in this patient population, first trying self-report whenever possible. When self-report cannot be used, the clinician can use additional data-gathering sources, such as obtaining information from the family regarding usual expressions of pain and relief measures, and by direct nursing observations to make the determination of the presence of pain rather than trying to quantify pain intensity. Figure 2–3 is an example of an alternative pain assessment tool that has been developed by nurses in a medical intensive care unit (ICU) to better assess vulnerable patient populations.

Patient behaviors (cues) that may indicate the presence of pain can be divided into four groups: vocal, facial, body posturing, and sympathetic nervous system response. Vocal behaviors are sounds such as crying, moaning, or

TABLE 2–4. ADVANTAGES AND DISADVANTAGES OF PAIN ASSESSMENT TOOLS

UNIDIMENSIONAL TOOLS	
Advantages	**Disadvantages**
Provide baseline data	Measure only one dimension of the pain experience
Provide a means of comparing pre- and postintervention pain intensity	Unable to measure degree of anxiety or stress accompanying the pain
Provide a standardized method for assessment of pain intensity	Require relatively high cognitive level
Can be clearly documented and reported	Require some means of communication
Adaptable for patients who cannot verbalize	
Easy to perform	
Short assessment time	
MULTIDIMENSIONAL TOOLS	
Advantages	**Disadvantages**
Provide baseline data	Valid only if patient understands vocabulary
Provide a standardized method for assessment of pain	Long length of completion time (McGill Pain Questionnaire)
Can be clearly documented and reported	Require a high cognitive level
Assess multiple aspects of the pain experience	
Provide data for choosing nonpharmacologic interventions	
Adaptable for patients who cannot verbalize	

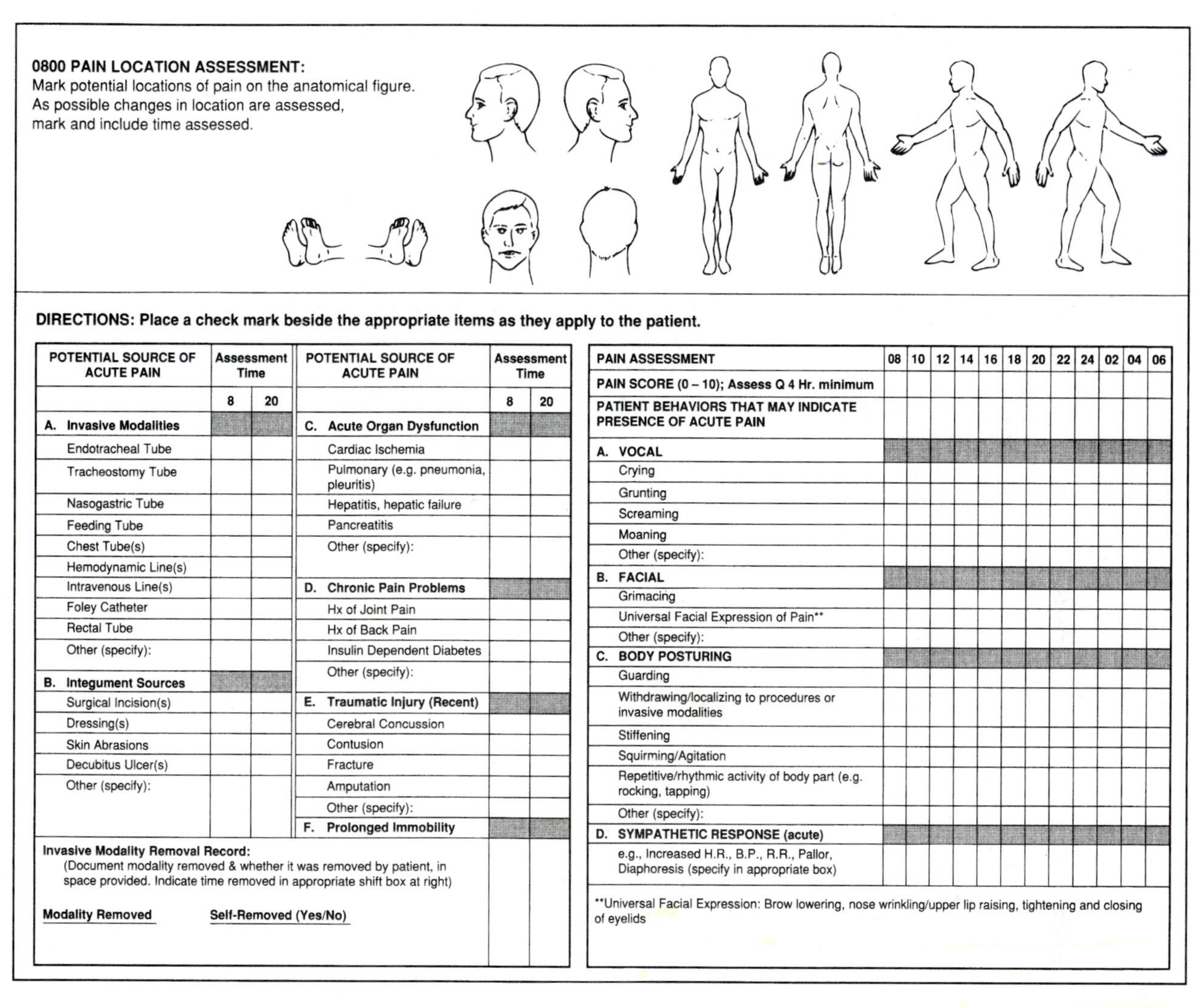

0800 PAIN LOCATION ASSESSMENT:
Mark potential locations of pain on the anatomical figure.
As possible changes in location are assessed,
mark and include time assessed.

DIRECTIONS: Place a check mark beside the appropriate items as they apply to the patient.

POTENTIAL SOURCE OF ACUTE PAIN	Assessment Time	
	8	20
A. Invasive Modalities		
Endotracheal Tube		
Tracheostomy Tube		
Nasogastric Tube		
Feeding Tube		
Chest Tube(s)		
Hemodynamic Line(s)		
Intravenous Line(s)		
Foley Catheter		
Rectal Tube		
Other (specify):		
B. Integument Sources		
Surgical Incision(s)		
Dressing(s)		
Skin Abrasions		
Decubitus Ulcer(s)		
Other (specify):		

POTENTIAL SOURCE OF ACUTE PAIN	Assessment Time	
	8	20
C. Acute Organ Dysfunction		
Cardiac Ischemia		
Pulmonary (e.g. pneumonia, pleuritis)		
Hepatitis, hepatic failure		
Pancreatitis		
Other (specify):		
D. Chronic Pain Problems		
Hx of Joint Pain		
Hx of Back Pain		
Insulin Dependent Diabetes		
Other (specify):		
E. Traumatic Injury (Recent)		
Cerebral Concussion		
Contusion		
Fracture		
Amputation		
Other (specify):		
F. Prolonged Immobility		

Invasive Modality Removal Record:
(Document modality removed & whether it was removed by patient, in space provided. Indicate time removed in appropriate shift box at right)

Modality Removed **Self-Removed (Yes/No)**

PAIN ASSESSMENT	08	10	12	14	16	18	20	22	24	02	04	06
PAIN SCORE (0 – 10); Assess Q 4 Hr. minimum												
PATIENT BEHAVIORS THAT MAY INDICATE PRESENCE OF ACUTE PAIN												
A. VOCAL												
Crying												
Grunting												
Screaming												
Moaning												
Other (specify):												
B. FACIAL												
Grimacing												
Universal Facial Expression of Pain**												
Other (specify):												
C. BODY POSTURING												
Guarding												
Withdrawing/localizing to procedures or invasive modalities												
Stiffening												
Squirming/Agitation												
Repetitive/rhythmic activity of body part (e.g. rocking, tapping)												
Other (specify):												
D. SYMPATHETIC RESPONSE (acute)												
e.g., Increased H.R., B.P., R.R., Pallor, Diaphoresis (specify in appropriate box)												

**Universal Facial Expression: Brow lowering, nose wrinkling/upper lip raising, tightening and closing of eyelids

Figure 2–3. Alternative pain assessment tool. *(Developed by Medical ICU, University of Kentucky Hospital.)*

grunting. The primary facial cues that suggest pain are facial grimacing and a crying expression (tears may be noted). Certain body posturing behaviors are associated with the presence of pain. Typical observations include agitation or lying completely still, guarding, splinting respirations, withdrawing or localizing to invasive modalities and procedures, stiffening, and repetitive/rhythmic activity of a body part (such as rocking or tapping). Acute pain is associated with stimulation of the sympathetic nervous system response, which causes elevation of heart rate, blood pressure, and respiratory rate, and increased pallor and diaphoresis. While of value in assessing short-term acute pain, use of the sympathetic response criteria for the presence of pain loses validity over time. The sympathetic response is known to adapt rapidly, within 24 hours, even in the patient experiencing severe pain.

In summary, acute pain is a subjective, multidimensional experience. The patient's self-report is the single most reliable indicator of the existence and intensity of acute pain. An effective pain manager uses patient self-report as the major pain indicator and uses nursing observations to gather additional data. Use of self-report tools provides an effective means for measurement and documentation of pain. When patients cannot self-report their pain levels, it is necessary for the nurse to rely on observing for behaviors typically associated with the presence of pain and on prior history ascertained from family members and significant others. When the patient is not able to self-report, the nurse should not prematurely judge the quantity and quality of pain until appropriate pain assessment data have been collected and analyzed. Patients who cannot self-report are particularly vulnerable to inadequate pain management by nurses who either do not use alternative pain assessment methods or misinterpret patient behaviors. Therefore, it is imperative that nurses carefully assess pain when patients cannot actively participate in the assessment process.

SECTION FOUR REVIEW

1. The Numeric Rating Scale is most commonly used to measure what part of the pain experience?
   A. affective
   B. evaluative
   C. intensity
   D. coping
2. If a patient is mildly confused, the nurse should initially try to assess pain using
   A. vital signs
   B. self-report
   C. facial expression
   D. body posturing
3. A major weakness of multidimensional tools is that
   A. the patient must comprehend the vocabulary
   B. they measure only pain intensity
   C. the nurse performs the assessment
   D. they are unable to measure degree of anxiety
4. All of the following are examples of vocal pain behaviors EXCEPT
   A. grunting
   B. moaning
   C. crying
   D. guarding

Answers: 1. C, 2. B, 3. A, 4. D

SECTION FIVE: Management of Acute Pain

At the completion of this section, the learner will be able to describe effective pain management for the high-acuity patient.

Organized Approach to Pain Management

Effective pain management is facilitated by use of an organized, systematic approach. The WHO Analgesic Ladder provides an example of such an approach. The ladder (Fig. 2–4) suggests general pain management choices based on the level of pain (i.e., mild, mild to moderate, or moderate to severe). In addition, it provides a step-by-step approach to adjusting the pharmacologic choices if the patient's pain is persistent or increases.

The high-acuity patient is particularly at risk for moderate to severe pain; thus, discussion will focus on management at this level of the ladder. Opioids are generally the drugs of choice for pain management at this level. In addition, the ladder recommends consideration of nonopioid and adjuvant therapies to further enhance the effects of opioid therapy.

Pharmacologic Pain Management

The pharmacologic management of pain involves modulation of pain transmission at different levels of the nervous system. For example, opioids bind with opioid receptors in such areas as the spinal cord, peripheral nervous system, and central nervous system. Nonsteroidal anti-inflammatory drugs (NSAIDs) may relieve pain by working peripherally at the site of injury, by inhibiting the formation of prostaglandins, proteolytic enzymes, and bradykinins. They may also have a CNS effect.

Nonopioid Therapy

Effective pain management can be enhanced by a combination of opioid and nonopioid therapy. A better level of analgesia is often achieved in combination than when either is administered alone. Nonopioids include such drugs as acetaminophen, aspirin, and, in particular, NSAIDs. Nonopioids are associated with fewer side effects than opioids.

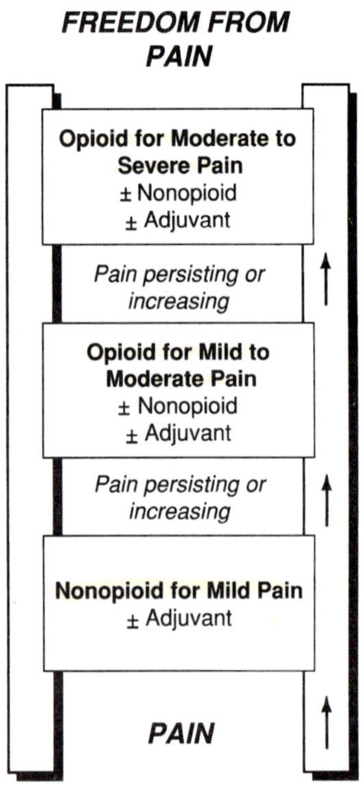

Figure 2–4. The WHO Ladder. *(Adapted from WHO. [1996].* Cancer pain relief, *2nd ed. Geneva, Switzerland: World Health Organization.)*

Adjuvant Therapy

Adjuvant therapy includes drugs that can assist in reducing certain types of pain. Their assistance may be indirect (by decreasing other symptoms associated with the underlying condition) or direct, as a co-analgesic. These drugs are generally used in addition to opioid and nonopioid analgesics. Several specific examples of adjuvant drugs include corticosteroids for cancer-related pain, and antidepressants or anticonvulsants for treatment of neuropathic pain (Hawthorn & Redmond, 1998; McCaffery & Pasero, 1999).

Opioid Therapy

Therapeutic use of opioids begins with the selection of a specific opioid drug and route of administration. Once the choice of drug and route are determined, decisions are made regarding the suitable initial dose; frequency of administration; optimal doses of nonopioid analgesics, if these are to be given; and incidence and severity of side effects. The importance of careful adjustment of these medications for therapeutic effects cannot be overemphasized, as dosing needs and analgesic responses vary greatly among individual patients (AHCPR, 1992).

Routes of Administration

There are many routes available for administration of analgesia. The oral, subcutaneous, intramuscular, and intravenous routes can be accessed by the nurse. Most other routes, however, require initial access by an anesthesiologist.

The oral route is most commonly used for opioids. This route is also the most inexpensive and convenient. For the high-acuity patient, however, the oral route may not be available due to a nothing-by-mouth status. While these individuals are not able to take medications orally, many have feeding tubes that act as an alternate medication route.

AHCPR guidelines state that when IV access is not possible, the rectal or sublingual routes should be considered in preference to the traditional use of subcutaneous and intramuscular routes. Repeated use of the subcutaneous and intramuscular routes are painful to the patient and may cause tissue trauma. In addition, the lag time between injection and absorption into the circulation makes these injection routes less desirable alternatives (AHCPR, 1992).

The intravenous route can be used by the nurse or self-administered by the patient using intravenous patient-controlled analgesia (PCA). The most common method of PCA allows the patient to self-dose intravenously by pushing a button that is attached via a cord to an infusion device. The infusion device can be programmed for the patient to self-administer doses of opioid without becoming overly sedated (AHCPR, 1992). Other forms of PCA are subcutaneous, intramuscular, and epidural.

Intraspinal opioids can be administered in a variety of ways:

- Single-dose epidural or intrathecal
- Intermittent scheduled dose epidural or intrathecal
- Intermittent patient-controlled epidural (PCEA) or intrathecal
- Continuous infusion of opioid alone or in combination with local anesthetic epidural or intrathecal
- Continuous infusion plus patient-controlled opioid alone or in combination with local anesthetic (American Pain Society, 1999)

The **epidural** route requires insertion of a small catheter into the space located just before the dura mater. Opioid, or a combination of opioid and local anesthetic, is delivered using an infusion device. The opioids diffuse across the dura mater and bind at opioid receptors. The local anesthetic selectively blocks sensory nerve fibers that make up the spinal nerve roots, acting as a neural blockade. The spinal nerve roots pass through the epidural space to the spinal cord, thus making the epidural space a convenient place to infuse drugs. Combinations of opioid and local anesthetic agents are used to modulate the transmission of pain at different sites. This route requires low doses of analgesic, whether administered alone or in combination. This route also minimizes the potential for side effects. Neural blockade provides analgesia without the central nervous system effects of sedation, drowsiness, and respiratory depression that can occur when analgesics are given systemically (PO, IV, or IM).

The **intrathecal** route for analgesia requires the passage of a small catheter into the cerebrospinal fluid (CSF) space. Opioid flows through the CSF and rapidly binds to opioid receptors in the spinal cord. Smaller amounts of intrathecally administered drug are required to achieve the same effects as epidural administration. This method places the spinal cord at some degree of risk, however, owing to the potential for mechanical or chemical irritation and/or damage. There is also a higher risk of infection than with the epidural route. Many methods are available to deliver intrathecal medications, including percutaneous catheters, implanted ports, and implanted pumps. Use of the epidural or intrathecal routes requires close communication between anesthesiology and nursing staffs and careful monitoring of the patient.

Peripheral nerve blocks and pleural infusion routes also require an anesthesiologist. When a peripheral nerve block is performed, the peripheral nerve path that is transmitting the pain is located, and local anesthetic is injected medial to the point of pain origin. The sites most frequently used for peripheral nerve blocking are the intercostal nerves medial to the insertion site of chest tubes. The duration of the analgesia depends on the half-life of the local anesthetic that has been injected.

The pleural infusion route primarily is used when multiple rib fractures are present. A small catheter is placed into the pleural space (between the visceral and parietal pleura) and local anesthetic is injected. By administering a local anesthetic via this route, multiple intercostal nerves can be blocked at one time without repeated needle sticks to the skin.

Whenever local anesthetics are administered, it is important for the health care provider to monitor the patient for systemic anesthetic toxicity. Signs and symptoms of this complication include a 25 percent drop in baseline heart rate, tinnitus, slurred speech or thick tongue, and mental confusion. Table 2–5 provides a comparison of pharmacologic pain interventions.

Nonpharmacologic Interventions

Nonpharmacologic therapies can be used concurrently with medications to manage pain. The role of the clinician is to assist the patient in identifying effective alternative interventions to be systematically incorporated into the care plan. All clinicians involved in the patient's care have a role in providing the necessary support for utilization of these therapies as outlined in the care plan. Guidelines for choice of nonpharmacologic interventions include pain problem identification, effectiveness for a specific patient, and the skill of the clinician. Table 2–6 lists examples of nonpharmacologic interventions for the management of pain.

The AHCPR (1992) guidelines support use of nonpharmacologic interventions in patients who:

- Find such an intervention appealing
- May benefit from avoiding or reducing drug therapy (e.g., history of adverse reactions, fear of or physiologic reason to avoid, oversedation)
- Have incomplete pain relief following appropriate pharmacologic intervention
- Are likely to experience and need to cope with a prolonged period of postoperative pain, particularly if punctuated by recurrent episodes of intense treatment or procedure-related pain
- Express anxiety or fear, as long as the anxiety is not incapacitating or secondary to a medical or psychiatric condition that has a more specific treatment

The last three guidelines could apply to many high-acuity patients; thus, nonpharmacologic interventions should be seriously considered in this patient population.

TABLE 2–5. PHARMACOLOGIC INTERVENTIONS

INTERVENTION	COMMENTS
Nonsteroidal Anti-inflammatory Drugs (NSAIDs)	
Oral (alone)	Effective for mild-to-moderate pain. Begin preoperatively. Relatively contraindicated in patients with renal disease and risk of or actual coagulopathy. May mask fever.
Oral (adjunct to opioid)	Potentiating effect resulting in opioid sparing. Begin preop. Cautions as above.
Parenteral (ketoralac)	Effective for moderate to severe pain. Expensive. Useful where opioids contraindicated, especially to avoid respiratory depression and sedation. Advance to opioid.
Opioids	
Oral	As effective as parenteral in appropriate doses. Use as soon as oral medication tolerated. Route of choice.
Intramuscular	Has been the standard parenteral route, but injections painful and absorption unreliable. Hence, avoid this route when possible.
Subcutaneous	Preferable to intramuscular when a low-volume continuous infusion is needed and intravenous access is difficult to maintain. Injections painful and absorption unreliable. Avoid this route for long-term repetitive dosing.
Intravenous	Parenteral route of choice after major surgery. Suitable for titrated bolus or continuous administration (including PCA), but requires monitoring. Significant risk of respiratory depression with inappropriate dosing.
PCA (systemic)	Can be used for intravenous, subcutaneous, and epidural routes. Good steady level of analgesia. Popular with patients but requires special infusion pumps and staff education.
Epidural and intrathecal	When suitable, provides good analgesia. Requires careful monitoring. Use of infusion pumps requires additional equipment and staff education.
Local Anesthetics	
Epidural and intrathecal	Effective regional analgesia. Opioid sparing. Addition of opioid to local anesthetic may improve analgesia. Risks of hypotension, weakness, numbness. Requires careful monitoring. Use of infusion pump requires additional equipment and staff education.
Peripheral nerve block	Limited indications and duration of action. Effective regional analgesia. Opioid sparing. May be used as a one-time injection or with a continuous infusion through a catheter.

Adapted from AHCPR. (1992). Acute pain management: Operative or medical procedures and trauma clinical practice guideline. *Rockville, MD: Agency for Health Care Policy and Research, Public Health Service, U.S. Department of Health and Human Services. ACHPR Pub. No. 92–0032.*

TABLE 2–6. NONPHARMACOLOGIC INTERVENTIONS

Simple Relaxation (begin preoperatively)	
Interventions:	Jaw relaxation, progressive muscle relaxation, and simple imagery
Comments:	Effective in reducing mild to moderate pain and as an adjunct to analgesic drugs for severe pain. Use when patients express an interest in relaxation. Requires 3 to 5 minutes of staff time for instructions.
Intervention:	Music
Comments:	Effective for reduction of mild to moderate pain. Requires skilled personnel.
Complex Relaxation (begin postoperatively)	
Intervention:	Biofeedback
Comments:	Effective in reducing mild to moderate pain and operative site muscle tension. Requires skilled personnel and special equipment.
Intervention:	Imagery
Comments:	Effective for reduction of mild to moderate pain. Requires skilled personnel.
Education/Instruction (begin preoperatively)	
Comments:	Effective for reduction of pain. Should include sensory and procedural information and instruction aimed at reducing activity-related pain. Requires 5 to 15 minutes of staff time.
TENS (transcutaneous electrical nerve stimulation)	
Comments:	Effective in reducing pain and improving physical function. Requires skilled personnel and special equipment. May be useful as an adjunct to drug therapy.

Adapted from AHCPR. (1992). Acute pain management: Operative or medical procedures and trauma clinical practice guideline. *Rockville, MD: Agency for Health Care Policy and Research, Public Health Service, U.S. Department of Health and Human Services. ACHPR Pub. No. 92–0032.*

In summary, effective pain management requires the use of pharmacologic as well as nonpharmacologic interventions. To increase effectiveness of the analgesic response, medications can be given by a variety of routes and in combination with other medications. The use of nonpharmacologic interventions can also modulate the analgesic response. Health care providers are encouraged to explore which interventions (both pharmacologic and nonpharmacologic) have been used by the patient in the past when formulating a plan of care for decreasing pain.

Section Five Review

1. The World Health Organization (WHO) Analgesic Ladder provides the clinician with
   - **A.** general pain management choices based on level of pain
   - **B.** nonpharmacologic interventions based on level of pain
   - **C.** specific pain management choices based on severity of pain
   - **D.** pharmacologic and nonpharmacologic pain management choices
2. Which of the following statements is correct regarding nonopioid therapy?
   - **A.** nonopioids have more severe side effects than opioids
   - **B.** nonopioids are harder to access than opioids
   - **C.** nonopioids can manage pain as effectively as opioids
   - **D.** combining opioids and nonopioids enhances analgesia effectiveness
3. The most common route used for PCA is
   - **A.** intramuscular
   - **B.** intravenous
   - **C.** subcutaneous
   - **D.** epidural
4. A major advantage of using the epidural route for analgesia is that it
   - **A.** can be accessed by the nurse
   - **B.** uses only nonopioid analgesics
   - **C.** blocks a specific peripheral nerve path
   - **D.** provides analgesia without CNS side effects
5. The guidelines for choosing appropriate nonpharmacologic interventions include all of the following EXCEPT
   - **A.** skill of clinician
   - **B.** effectiveness for patient
   - **C.** type of opioid being used
   - **D.** pain problem identification

Answers: 1. A, 2. D, 3. B, 4. D, 5. C

SECTION SIX: Issues in Inadequate Treatment of Acute Pain

At the completion of this section, the learner will be able to discuss issues related to the undertreatment of pain.

Definitions

It is important to differentiate between *tolerance*, *dependence*, and *addiction*, terms that are misused and have potentially negative connotations. These terms are defined as follows:

- **Tolerance:** A common physiologic result of chronic opioid use; it means that a larger dose of opioid is required to maintain the same level of analgesia (AHCPR, 1994)
- **Physical dependence:** A physical adaptation of the body to the presence of opioids, existing when rapid drug withdrawal produces signs and symptoms (Hawthorn & Redmond, 1998)
- **Psychological dependence (addiction):** A pattern of compulsive drug use characterized by a continued craving for an opioid and the need to use the opioid for effects other than pain relief (or other medical indications) (AHCPR, 1994)
- **Opioid pseudoaddiction:** A term applied to patients who develop behaviors that mimic those associated with addiction. The individual may be labeled as drug craving or drug seeking. Pseudoaddiction, however, results from inadequate pain management, not psychological dependence (Hudak, Gallo, & Morton, 1998). A variety of responses are noted in patients who experience unrelieved pain, from acceptable drug seeking to pathologic behaviors. Pain relief usually eliminates the aberrant behaviors in this patient population.

Reasons for Opioid Undertreatment of Pain

Inadequate treatment of pain is a complex problem that is based on misconceptions widely held by physicians, nurses, and patients. Physicians underprescribe opioids by two methods: prescribing subtherapeutic doses, and prescribing time intervals for drug doses that are less than the pharmacologic duration of action. Nurses undertreat pain by administering less than what the patient can receive per physician orders, and administering opioids at longer intervals than prescribed. Patients often contribute to their own undertreatment of pain by not requesting PRN pain medications, taking medication at longer-than-ordered intervals, taking less than the amount prescribed, or refusing to take the drug at all (McCaffery & Pasero, 1999).

There are four common misconceptions regarding opioid use that contribute to inadequate treatment: fear of addiction, physical dependence, tolerance, and respiratory depression.

Fear of Addiction (Psychological Dependence)

Fear of addiction is probably the major cause of undertreatment of pain. The term **opiophobia** has been used to describe the irrational fear of prescribing (or consuming) adequate amounts of opiates for therapeutic results. In fact, very few hospitalized patients who receive opioids become addicted; as the pain subsides, so does use of opioids. The term **addiction** should be used with extreme caution. The indiscriminate labeling of a person who uses drugs as being an addict carries a strong social stigma that may label an individual negatively (McCaffery & Pasero, 1999).

Fear of Physical Dependence

Some of the fear associated with physical dependence is generated from the belief that opioid withdrawal is life threatening, the symptoms associated with physical dependence are difficult to control, and the presence of symptoms of physical dependence prevent decreases in opioid doses as the pain decreases. In addition, many people believe that addiction is the natural progression of physical dependence. It is true that any patient who receives repeated doses of opioids is at risk for some degree of withdrawal symptoms if the opioid is suddenly stopped. These symptoms, however, can be effectively managed by gradual reduction in opioid dosage as the patient's pain subsides (McCaffery & Pasero, 1999).

Fear of Tolerance

Fear of tolerance is usually seen in patients with long-term pain associated with either a disease process or painful treatments (e.g., patients with burns, cancer, or life-threatening illnesses). Patients, physicians, and nurses have expressed fear that opioids lose their effectiveness over time and may not work when really needed. A part of this fear is the belief in an imaginary dose ceiling, beyond which the patient cannot be taken. In fact, this feared dose ceiling does not seem to exist. As tolerance to an opioid develops, so does the patient's tolerance to the side effects of sedation and respiratory depression. Tolerance is treated by decreasing the dose interval or increasing the dose. Nursing management should focus on patient education about the concept of tolerance, and monitoring for the therapeutic and nontherapeutic effects of the adjusted dosage (McCaffery & Pasero, 1999).

Fear of Respiratory Depression

Physicians and nurses are particularly sensitive to the fear of respiratory depression. All opioids have the capability of causing respiratory depression, yet it need not be a life-threatening problem and should not prevent therapeutic opioid use. In the majority of hospitalized patients, respiratory depression has not been shown to be a significant problem. Nursing management should focus on close observation of the patient's response. **Sedation** develops before respiratory depression; therefore, the nurse should observe and document the patient's sedation level (e.g., wide awake, drowsy, dozing intermittently, mostly sleeping, or awakens only when aroused). Respiratory depression is dose related, and low doses are generally considered safe. It is impossible, however, to know what dose of an opioid will cause respiratory depression in any given patient. It is more important to watch the individual's response, especially to the first dose (McCaffery & Pasero, 1999).

Nursing Approach in Acute Pain Management

McCaffery and Pasero (1999) state that the way in which an analgesic is used is probably more important than which drug is used. In the acute care setting, the nurse maintains significant control over how analgesics are used. Nursing activities that have an impact on therapeutic pain management include:

- Selecting an appropriate opioid or nonopioid from the analgesics ordered
- Evaluating when to administer the analgesic
- Evaluating how much analgesic to administer
- Obtaining a change in prescription when required

Effective pain management requires objective assessment skills and specific knowledge of opioids and nonopioids. In addition, the nurse must individualize the care plan to best meet the patient's individual comfort needs.

There are two major approaches to effective pain management: the preventive and the titration approaches.

Preventive

Using the preventive approach, analgesics are administered before the patient complains of pain. For example, when pain is occurring consistently over a 24-hour period, administering analgesics on a regular schedule (around the clock) is more effective than administering them PRN. This method helps to maintain a consistent therapeutic level of analgesic in the bloodstream.

Administering pain medication on a PRN basis can cause prolonged delays in treating the patient's pain. If PRN analgesia is to be used, it is important for the clinician to know the half-life and effectiveness of the medication being administered, to be able to predict when the patient is likely to need another dose. Staying on top of pain by offering pain medication on a routine basis is more effective for pain control than requiring the patient to ask for medication (PRN). The patient may wait for the pain to become severe before requesting analgesia, or the clinician may be delayed in getting the drug to the patient. Either situation makes adequate pain relief more difficult to obtain. There are times when PRN administration is an acceptable option, such as changing to PRN late in the postoperative course to help decrease side effects; or when the pain is incidental, intermittent, or unpredictable (AHCPR, 1992; McCaffery & Pasero, 1999). In addition, PRN analgesics may be used as supplemental doses to regularly scheduled analgesics, primarily when a certain known activity causes pain (i.e., ambulation, sitting up in a chair, coughing, and deep breathing).

Titration

The titration approach calls for adjusting and individualizing therapy based on the effects the drug is having on the patient rather than the milligrams being administered. The goal is to gain the desired level of pain relief with minimum side effects. When using this approach, the clinician should consider:

- *Dose*—Analgesic potency helps provide a rational basis for choosing the appropriate starting dose (AHCPR, 1992).
- *Interval between doses*—Assess the patient regarding the amount of time it takes for the pain to increase. For example, if the nurse is administering an analgesic every 4 hours and the patient notices that the pain increases quickly after 3 hours, the interval should be changed to 3 hours.
- *Route of administration*—Use a conversion chart for equal analgesic dosing when switching from one route to another (Table 2–7). Dosing conversion factors based on relative potency estimates may differ between patients (AHCPR, 1992).
- *Choice of drug*—Opioids are classified as full (pure) **opioid agonists,** partial agonists, or mixed agonist–antagonists. Full agonists are more potent than partial agonists. Agonist–antagonists activate one type of opioid receptor and at the same time block another type (AHCPR, 1992). Withdrawal-like symptoms can occur when switching a patient from a pure agonist to an agonist–antagonist.

In summary, undertreatment of pain results from misconceptions regarding addiction, physical dependence, tolerance, and respiratory depression. These misconceptions may be held by physicians and nurses, as well as by patients. Effective pain management can be approached using two methods, called the preventive and titration approaches. The preventive approach focuses on "staying on top" of the pain, while the titration approach emphasizes the patient's response to therapy rather than dose and interval between doses. The PRN approach for pain management is not recommended except in specific situations.

TABLE 2–7. EQUIANALGESIC DOSES OF SELECTE OPIOIDS

DRUG	TRADE NAME	ROUTES	EQUIANALGESIC DOSE (MG)	DURATION (HOURS)
Morphine	Generic	IM/IV	10	4–6 (IM)
		PO/R	60	4–7
Hydromorphone	Generic; Dilaudid	IM/IV	1.5	4–5 (IM)
		PO/R	7.5	4–6
Codeine	Generic; 2 APAP; Tylenol #3, etc	IM/IV	130	4–6 (IM)
		PO	200[a]	4–6
Oxycodone	Generic; w/APA; Percocet w/ASA; Percodan	PO	30	3–5
Fentanyl	Generic; Sublimaze; Duragesic	IM/IV	0.1	1–2
		Topical		
Oxymorphone	Numorphan	IM	1	4–6
		R	10	4–6
Meperidine[b]	Generic; Demerol	IM/IV	75	4–5 (IM)
		PO	300	4–6

[a]The dose of codeine may be lowered when administered as a combination product containing aspirin or acetaminophen, which work synergistically.
[b]Meperidine has very limited use in cancer pain, as the toxic metabolite, normeperidine, builds to unacceptable levels in the CNS.

SECTION SIX REVIEW

1. A common physiologic consequence of chronic opioid use that results in a person's requiring an increasing dose of opioids to maintain the same level of analgesia is the definition of
   A. pseudoaddiction
   B. tolerance
   C. psychologic dependence
   D. physical dependence
2. Which of the following statements is correct regarding opioid use and respiratory depression?
   A. respiratory depression precedes the onset of sedation
   B. respiratory depression worsens as tolerance develops
   C. sedation occurs before respiratory depression
   D. respiratory depression is a common problem in hospitalized patients
3. PRN analgesics are appropriately used in all of the following situations EXCEPT
   A. when pain is intermittent
   B. when pain is consistent
   C. when pain is unpredictable
   D. when used as a supplement to scheduled doses
4. When the titration approach to pain management is used, the emphasis is on
   A. patient's analgesic response
   B. total milligrams per day
   C. physical dependence
   D. psychological dependence

Answers: 1. B, 2. C, 3. B, 4. A

SECTION SEVEN: Pain Management in Specific Patient Populations

At the completion of this section, the learner will be able to identify considerations associated with pain management in special populations.

Several important patient-focused factors influence acute pain management. These factors include age, concurrent medical disorders, and history of substance abuse. A basic understanding of these factors helps to facilitate effective pain management.

Elderly Patients

According to Katzung (1998), opioid use in the elderly is associated with variable alterations in pharmacokinetics. This patient population is particularly at risk for respiratory depression; thus opioids should be initiated with caution until sensitivity is determined. Studies have shown that opioids are underutilized in elderly patients who could significantly benefit from their use. Katzung suggests that there is no justification for this underutilization if opioids are administered according to an appropriate pain management plan.

Pediatric Patients

Historically, many misconceptions have evolved regarding pain management in children, including that children do not feel as much pain as adults do, children do not remember pain, children become addicted to opioids, opioids are not safe for children, and if a child does not display overt pain behaviors, she or he is not in pain (Pounder & Steward, 1992). Research does not support these misconceptions. The clinician should assume that the child's pain perception is accurate, and analgesia should be administered as appropriate. Opioids continue to be the mainstay of postoperative pain relief, and careful titration of dosage based on weight and desired effect is necessary. Respiratory depression is not commonly noted when age-appropriate doses of opioids are administered (Thelan et al., 1998). Children can receive opioids by many different routes; however, alternatives to administration by painful intramuscular injection should be used whenever possible (AHCPR, 1992). Thelan et al. suggest intravenous (continuous or intermittent), epidural, or caudal as possible alternative routes.

Patients with Concurrent Medical Disorders

High-acuity patients frequently have more than one dysfunctioning organ at any single time. Impaired function of the liver and kidneys has serious implications for analgesic therapy. Analgesics are primarily metabolized in the liver, with a small percentage being excreted unchanged. The kidneys have the major responsibility for opioid excretion. When either of these organs has decreased functioning, serum drug levels increase, placing the patient at increasing risk for the development of adverse effects.

Certain opioids (e.g., morphine) are converted into polar glucuronidated metabolites in the liver and then excreted through the kidneys. The glucuronidated metabolites maintain analgesic capabilities that may be stronger than the actual opioid. If kidney function is significantly impaired, these metabolites may accumulate in the blood, resulting in prolonged and deeper analgesia. This can compromise the patient by precipitating severe respiratory depression, deep sedation or intractable nausea. Meperidine, a synthetic opioid, may also accumulate in the presence of renal dysfunction or when high doses are used. Normeperidine, the metabolite of meperidine, is associated with CNS stimulation, which can precipitate tachycardia and seizure activity. The risk of seizures increases as normeperidine levels increase (Way et al., 1998). The half-life of normeperidine is 15 to 20 hours, which is significantly longer than that of the parent compound meperidine (3 to 8 hours); thus, adverse effects caused by elevated levels of normeperidine can remain for a prolonged period in patients with liver or kidney dysfunction (Deglin & Vallerand, 1998). When kidney or liver impairment is present, doses of most opioids must be reduced and the patient monitored closely for the development of accumulative effects.

Patients who have been receiving long-term opioid therapy for chronic pain are at risk for undertreatment of acute pain owing to the presence of opioid drug tolerance. In such cases, the opioid dose requirements may be significantly higher than what is usually recommended (or needed) to reach a satisfactory level of analgesia. A thorough pain history provides valuable information regarding the potentially altered dose requirements of this patient population.

The Known Substance Abuser as Patient

Pain management in the substance abuser is becoming increasingly common. Substance abusers experience traumatic injuries and a variety of health problems more often than the general population (AHCPR, 1992). During the postoperative period, the issue of opioid withdrawal becomes apparent when sympathetic symptoms such as restlessness, tachycardia, and sleeplessness impair progress toward a typical convalescence period.

The AHCPR (1992) offers the following guidelines for pain management in the known substance abuser:

- Define the origin of the pain.
- Past history of drug abuse may influence drug abuse behaviors. More recent drug abuse may require higher initial opioid doses than the opioid-naive patient.
- The use of an antagonist–agonist pain medication may precipitate withdrawal symptoms.
- Adjunctive pain-relieving methods should be used concurrently with opioids.
- Deal firmly and frankly with negative behaviors such as tampering with the PCA delivery device.
- Set limits to avoid excessive negotiation about drug selections or choices.

These guidelines can aid the clinician in determining whether the patient is exhibiting "drug-seeking" or "pain-avoidance" behaviors.

In summary, certain patient populations need special consideration when managing the analgesic response. To manage pain effectively in the elderly, the clinician must consider the physiologic changes associated with aging. Medication doses must be adjusted on the basis of metabolic and analgesic responses. Misconceptions must be clarified, especially when managing children's analgesic responses. Concurrent medical problems complicate pain management, particularly the presence of impaired liver or kidney function. Finally, treatment of pain in the known substance abuser requires special consideration to be able to differentiate between drug-seeking and pain-avoidance behaviors.

Section Seven Review

1. Elderly patients have fewer endogenous receptors and neurotransmitters than younger patients. The primary clinical significance of this statement is
   - **A.** larger doses of opioids are required to achieve pain relief
   - **B.** pain relief using opioids is more unpredictable
   - **C.** smaller doses of opioids are required to achieve pain relief
   - **D.** pain relief using opiates is less effective
2. In pediatric patients, it is suggested that what route be avoided?
   - **A.** oral
   - **B.** intramuscular
   - **C.** rectal
   - **D.** subcutaneous
3. Accumulation of morphine metabolites in the blood owing to renal dysfunction can cause
   - **A.** severe respiratory depression
   - **B.** seizures
   - **C.** tachycardia
   - **D.** CNS stimulation
4. Accumulation of the metabolite of meperidine (normeperidine) in the blood can result in
   - **A.** severe sedation
   - **B.** bradycardia
   - **C.** severe respiratory depression
   - **D.** seizures
5. The known substance abuser who is hospitalized
   - **A.** should receive no opioids
   - **B.** may require higher-than-usual opioid dose ranges
   - **C.** should receive only one type of opioid
   - **D.** may require lower-than-usual opioid dose ranges

Answers: 1. C, 2. B, 3. A, 4. D, 5. B

Posttest

The following Posttest is constructed in a case study format. A patient is presented, and questions are asked based on available data. New data are presented as the case study progresses.

Marcos M, 32 years old, was involved in a pedestrian–car crash in which he sustained multiple injuries. It is now 4 days after open reduction of his left femur and left humerus; a splenectomy was also necessary. He is complaining of severe sharp pain at his abdominal incision site.

1. His sharp pain is transmitted through
   - **A.** A fibers
   - **B.** B fibers
   - **C.** C fibers
   - **D.** D fibers
2. Marcos's acute pain sensation is transmitted up the spinal cord and terminates in the
   - **A.** thalamus
   - **B.** substantial gelatinosa
   - **C.** cerebral cortex
   - **D.** brain stem

It is now 1 week postinjury. Marcos's wounds are healing well but he continues to require pain management.

3. The type of pain that Marcos is most likely experiencing at this time is
   - **A.** brief acute
   - **B.** acute persistent
   - **C.** chronic
   - **D.** chronic intermittent
4. Which of the following statements is correct regarding suffering?
   - **A.** it is related to the personal meaning of pain
   - **B.** it is measurable
   - **C.** it is associated with acute pain
   - **D.** it bears no relationship to stress and anxiety

The nurse notes that Marcos continues to be in a high-anxiety state and continues to require analgesia at regular intervals.

5. The relationship between pain and anxiety is
   - **A.** anxiety increases pain tolerance
   - **B.** anxiety decreases pain complaints
   - **C.** anxiety decreases pain-related stress
   - **D.** anxiety increases pain perception
6. If Marcos's stress response becomes too high, it can result in all of the following EXCEPT
   - **A.** counterregulation of hormone responses
   - **B.** decreased vascular shunting
   - **C.** hypoperfusion of vital organs
   - **D.** elevated levels of blood endorphins

The nurse notes that Marcos is becoming increasingly agitated and he has begun rhythmically hitting his right foot on the rail of the bed.

7. The nurse's initial intervention should consist of
   - **A.** administering his ordered analgesic
   - **B.** contacting the physician

C. having him indicate his pain level on a VAS
D. documenting his new behaviors

8. The best method of assessing Marcos for pain is to assess by
A. self-report
B. facial cues
C. vital sign changes
D. body posturing behaviors

Marcos is bilingual, with Spanish as his first language. His understanding of spoken English is only fair and he states that he does not read English well.

9. Based on Marcos's language status, which of the following assessment approaches would be most valid (assuming all assessments are written in English)?
A. Short-Form McGill
B. VAS/NRS
C. McGill Pain Questionnaire
D. nurse observation

10. Marcos describes his pain as being severe and sharp. He is grimacing and continues to tap his foot on the bed rail. The nurse assigns him a pain intensity score of 8/10 (8 out of a possible 10). This method of assigning a score is
A. probably accurate in reflecting his pain level
B. an acceptable alternative pain assessment tool
C. acceptable only under special circumstances
D. an inappropriate use of a unidimensional tool

Marcos is complaining of pain at a level of 7/10. The nurse notes that his vital signs are normal and he is watching television. He is requesting pain medication.

11. Based on this new information, the nurse should
A. contact the physician
B. wait for 1 hour and recheck his vital signs
C. administer his ordered analgesic
D. suspect that he is exaggerating

Marcos has the following pain management orders:

Morphine 10 mg (IM) every 3 to 4 hours PRN
Ibuprofen 400 mg (PO) every 6 hours

12. Marcos's combination pain therapy is ordered for which primary purpose?
A. to enhance the level of analgesia
B. to increase sedation effects
C. to decrease respiratory depressive effects
D. to significantly reduce opioid dose

Marcos is switched to intravenous PCA.

13. The primary advantage for switching Marcos from injections to intravenous PCA is that PCA
A. decreases the number of painful injections
B. allows Marcos to gain some control over his analgesia
C. decreases the frequency of patient assessment
D. reduces the risk of severe respiratory depression

14. If the epidural route for analgesia had been chosen, the nurse would focus the pain assessment on the degree of
A. sedation
B. respiratory depression
C. pulse decrease
D. pain relief

Marcos indicates that he is interested in trying some nonpharmacologic interventions.

15. The AHCPR guidelines support use of nonpharmacologic interventions in all of the following patient situations, EXCEPT for patients who
A. are comatose
B. have prolonged pain
C. express anxiety or fear
D. would benefit from reducing drug therapy

Marcos has been receiving morphine on a regular basis for several weeks. He is now complaining that the usual dose he has been receiving is no longer relieving his pain as effectively.

16. Assuming nothing has changed in Marcos's condition, the nurse would suspect that Marcos is
A. exaggerating his level of pain
B. becoming psychologically dependent
C. developing tolerance to the morphine
D. needing to have the morphine discontinued

17. The term *pseudoaddiction* refers to behaviors that mimic those associated with addiction but are motivated by
A. drug craving
B. drug tolerance
C. PRN drug administration
D. pain undertreatment

18. Marcos is refusing to take any more morphine because he is afraid he will stop breathing. The nurse teaches Marcos about opioid therapy based on all of the following facts EXCEPT
A. opioid use places him at high risk for respiratory depression
B. sedation occurs before respiratory depression
C. respiratory depression is dose related
D. his level of sedation and respiratory rate will be closely monitored

19. If Marcos develops renal function impairment while receiving morphine, he will need to be monitored closely for
A. tachycardia
B. severe tachypnea
C. seizure activities
D. severe respiratory depression

POSTTEST ANSWERS

Question	Answer	Section	Question	Answer	Section
1	A	One	11	C	Four
2	C	One	12	A	Five
3	B	Two	13	B	Five
4	A	Two	14	D	Five
5	D	Three	15	A	Five
6	B	Three	16	C	Six
7	C	Four	17	D	Six
8	A	Four	18	A	Six
9	B	Four	19	D	Seven
10	D	Four			

REFERENCES

AHCPR. (1994). *Management of cancer pain.* Clinical Practice Guideline No. 9. Rockville, MD: U.S. Department of Health and Human Services. [AHCPR Publication No. 94-0592.]

AHCPR. (1992). *Acute pain management: Operative or medical procedures and trauma.* Clinical Practice Guideline No. 1. Rockville, MD: U.S. Department of Health and Human Services. [AHCPR Publication No. 92-0032.]

American Pain Society. (1999). *Principles of analgesic use in the treatment of acute pain and cancer pain* (4th ed.). Glenview, IL: Author.

American Pain Society Quality of Care Committee. (1995). Quality improvement guidelines for treatment of acute pain and cancer pain. *JAMA* 274(23):1874–1880.

Carey, S.J., Turpin, C., Smith, J., et al. (1997). Improving pain management in an acute care setting. *Orthop Nurs* 16(4): 29–36.

Chapman, C.R., & Syrjala, K.L. (1990). Measurement of pain. In J.J. Bonica (ed.). *The management of pain,* Vol. 1 (2nd ed.) (pp. 480–594). Philadelphia: Lea & Febiger.

Curtis, S., Kolotylo, C., & Broome, M.E. (1998). Somatosensory function and pain. In C.M. Porth (ed.). *Pathophysiology: Concepts of altered health states* (5th ed.) (pp. 959–992). Philadelphia: J.B. Lippincott.

Deglin, J.H., & Vallerand, A.H. (1998). *Davis's drug guide for nurses* (6th ed.). Philadelphia: F.A. Davis.

Ferrell, B.R., McCaffery, M., & Grant, M. (1991). Clinical decision making and pain. *Behav Res Ther* 30(1):71–73.

Guyton, A.C., & Hall, J.E. (1997a). Sensory receptors; neuronal circuits for processing information; tactile and position senses. In A.C. Guyton & J.E. Hall (eds.). *Human physiology and mechanisms of disease* (6th ed.) (pp. 376–391). Philadelphia: W.B. Saunders.

Guyton, A.C., & Hall, J.E. (1997b). Pain, headache, and thermal sensations. In A.C. Guyton & J.E. Hall (eds.). *Human physiology and mechanisms of disease* (6th ed.) (pp. 392–399). Philadelphia: W.B. Saunders.

Hawthorn, J., & Redmond, K. (1998). *Pain: Causes and management.* Malden, MA: Blackwell Science.

Hudak, C.M., Gallo, B.M., & Morton, P.G. (eds.). (1998). *Critical care nursing: A holistic approach* (7th ed.) (p. 49). Philadelphia: J.B. Lippincott.

Loeser, J.D., & Cousins, M.J. (1990). Contemporary pain management. *Med J Aust* 153:208–212, 216.

Katzung, B.G. (1998). Special aspects of geriatric pharmacology. In B.G. Katzung (ed.). *Basic & clinical pharmacology* (7th ed.) (pp. 989–998). Stamford, CT: Appleton & Lange.

McCaffery, M., & Pasero, C. (1999). *Pain: Clinical manual for nursing practice* (2nd ed.). St. Louis: C.V. Mosby.

Melzack, R., & Wall, P. (1965). Pain mechanisms: A new theory. *Science* 150(699):971–979.

Pounder, D.R., & Steward, D.J. (1992). Postoperative analgesia: Opioid infusions in infants and children. *Can J Anaesth* 39(9):969–974.

Stephenson, N.A. (1994, September/October). A comparison of nurse and patient perceptions of postsurgical pain. *J Intravenous Nurs* 17:235–239.

Thelan, L.A., Urden, L.D., Lough, M.E., & Stacy, K.M. (1998). Pain and sensation. In L.A. Thelan, L.D. Urden, M.E. Lough, & K.M. Stacy (eds.). *Critical care nursing: Diagnosis and management* (3rd ed.) (pp. 169–201). St. Louis: C.V. Mosby.

Wall, P.D., & Melzack, R. (eds.). (1994). *Textbook of pain* (3rd ed.). New York: Churchill Livingstone.

Way, W.L., Fields, H.L., & Way, E.L. (1998). Opioid analgesics and antagonists. In B.G. Katzung (ed.). *Basic and clinical pharmacology* (7th ed.) (pp. 496–515). Stamford, CT: Appleton & Lange.

World Health Organization. (1996). *Cancer pain relief* (2nd ed.). Geneva, Switzerland: Author.

ADDITIONAL READINGS

Brand, P., & Yancy, P. (1993). *Pain: The gift nobody wants.* New York: HarperCollins Publishers.

Cassell, E.J. (1991). *The nature of suffering.* New York: Oxford University Press.

Duffy, M.E. (1992). A theoretical and empirical review of the concept of suffering. In P. Stark & J. McGovern (eds.). *The hidden dimension of illness: Human suffering.* New York: NLN Press.

Kahn, D.L., & Steeves, R.H. (1986). The experience of suffering: Conceptual clarifications and theoretical definition. *J Adv Nursing* 11:623–631.

MODULE 3

Fluid and Electrolyte Balance in the High-Acuity Patient

Kathleen D. Wagner

The focus of this module is on the physiologic and pathologic processes involved in fluid and electrolyte balance. Maintenance of fluid and electrolyte balance is a major goal in improving the outcomes of patients with diverse health problems. Therefore, in many of the text's modules, fluid and electrolyte balance is addressed as it applies to specific module topics.

This module is composed of 10 distinct sections. Sections One and Two present the concepts of body fluid distribution and fluid balance regulation. Section Three focuses on fluid imbalances, including edema, third spacing, and fluid volume deficit and excess. Section Four describes nursing implications associated with fluid imbalance problems. In Sections Five through Seven, specific extracellular electrolytes are discussed: sodium, chloride, and calcium. Sections Eight through Ten address three major intracellular electrolytes: potassium, magnesium, and phosphorus. Discussion of each electrolyte includes major functions, causes, and clinical manifestations of imbalances.

Each section includes a set of review questions to assist the learner evaluate his or her understanding of the section's content before moving on to the next section. All Section Reviews and the Module Pretest and Posttest include answers. It is suggested that the learner review those concepts answered incorrectly in the review questions before proceeding to the next section.

OBJECTIVES

At the completion of this module, the learner will be able to

1. Discuss the distribution of body fluids.
2. Describe the regulation of fluid balance.
3. Discuss fluid imbalance, including edema, third spacing, fluid volume deficit, and fluid volume excess.
4. Discuss the nursing implications associated with fluid imbalances.
5. Discuss the extracellular compartment electrolyte, sodium.
6. Describe the extracellular compartment electrolyte, chloride.
7. Discuss the extracellular compartment electrolyte, calcium.
8. Discuss the intracellular compartment electrolyte, potassium.
9. Describe the intracellular compartment electrolyte, magnesium.
10. Discuss the intracellular compartment electrolyte, phosphorus (phosphate).

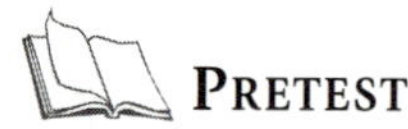

PRETEST

1. Two thirds of total body fluid is in which of the following compartments?
   A. intracellular
   B. extracellular
   C. intravascular
   D. interstitial
2. The elderly patient is at increased risk for developing a fluid volume problem related to
   A. high metabolic rate
   B. diminished renal function
   C. inability to concentrate urine
   D. greater ratio of surface area to volume
3. Which of the following electrolytes are found predominantly in the extracellular fluid?
   A. potassium
   B. magnesium
   C. phosphate
   D. sodium
4. Which of the following is the primary regulator of water intake?
   A. nervous system
   B. endocrine system
   C. renal system
   D. hypothalamus
5. The sympathetic nervous system responds to decreased volume by producing
   A. antidiuretic hormone (ADH)
   B. adrenocorticotropic hormone (ACTH)
   C. vasoconstriction
   D. aldosterone
6. When the hypothalamus senses a decrease in serum sodium or potassium, it responds by stimulating the pituitary to release
   A. renin
   B. aldosterone
   C. ADH
   D. ACTH
7. A low serum osmolality may suggest
   A. fluid volume deficit
   B. fluid volume overload
   C. dehydration
   D. isotonic balance
8. The most common cause of edema resulting from increased capillary hydrostatic pressure is
   A. liver failure
   B. congestive heart failure
   C. immune reactions
   D. burn injury
9. Nursing assessment data found in the patient with fluid volume excess would include
   A. low pulmonary artery wedge pressure (PAWP)
   B. increased hematocrit
   C. moist crackles
   D. decreased blood pressure
10. Which of the following intravenous solutions closely approximates serum osmolality?
    A. 0.45 percent normal saline
    B. 5 percent dextrose in normal saline
    C. lactated Ringer's
    D. 3 percent normal saline
11. Signs and symptoms of hypernatremia include
    A. diarrhea
    B. muscle twitching
    C. stomach cramps
    D. decreased muscle tone
12. Hyponatremia is associated with which of the following symptoms?
    A. edema
    B. hyperreflexia
    C. lethargy
    D. restlessness
13. Chloride levels closely follow the levels of which of the following electrolytes?
    A. potassium
    B. sodium
    C. calcium
    D. magnesium
14. Calcium is absorbed in the intestines under the influence of
    A. phosphorus
    B. vitamin D
    C. sodium
    D. vitamin C
15. Hypocalcemia is associated with which of the following clinical findings?
    A. tingling and numbness
    B. constipation
    C. lethargy
    D. shortened QT interval
16. The presence of hypokalemia alters renal excretion of potassium in which of the following ways?
    A. urine output increases
    B. potassium excretion increases
    C. potassium is reabsorbed
    D. potassium excretion does not change
17. The normal range of serum magnesium is
    A. 1.5 to 2.5 mEq/L
    B. 3.5 to 5.3 mEq/L
    C. 4.5 to 5.5 mEq/L
    D. 135 to 145 mEq/L
18. The symptoms of hypomagnesemia reflect
    A. central nervous system (CNS) hypoactivity
    B. fluid compartment shifts
    C. cardiac depressant effects
    D. neuromuscular and CNS hyperactivity
19. Hypophosphatemia is associated with which of the following conditions?

A. malnourished state
B. metabolic alkalosis
C. hypocalcemia
D. hyperthyroidism

20. Severe hypophosphatemia is associated with which of the following symptoms?
A. joint pain
B. muscle cramping
C. respiratory arrest
D. peptic ulcer disease

Answers: 1. A, 2. B, 3. D, 4. D, 5. C, 6. D, 7. B, 8. B, 9. C, 10. C, 11. B, 12. C, 13. B, 14. B, 15. A, 16. D, 17. A, 18. D, 19. A, 20. C

GLOSSARY

Anions. Negatively charged ions

Baroreceptors. Pressure receptors located in the arch of the aorta and carotid sinus that detect arterial pressure changes

Cations. Positively charged ions

Dilutional effect. Net gain of water in the extracellular spaces

Electrolytes. Electrically charged microsolutes found in body fluids

Extracellular. Fluid compartment within the body composed of plasma and interstitial fluid

Hypertonic. A high-osmolality state in which the concentration of particles is greater on one side of a membrane than the other side of the membrane; in the body, the solution has a higher osmolarity than exists inside of the cells

Hypervolemia. Excess volume of circulating fluids

Hypotonic. A low-osmolarity state in which the concentration of particles in a solution is greater on one side of a membrane than the other side of the membrane; in the body, the solution has a lower osmolality than exists inside of the cells

Hypovolemia. Decreased volume of circulating fluids

Intracellular. Fluid compartment within the body's cells; composes approximately two thirds of the total body water

Intravascular. Fluid compartment in the blood vessels; fluid is available for exchange of nutrients and oxygen

Isotonic. The concentration of particles in a solution on one side of a membrane is the same as it is on the other side of the membrane; in the body, it closely approximates normal serum plasma osmolality

Osmosis. The net diffusion of water from an area of greater concentration to an area of lesser concentration across the cell membrane; occurs as the result of osmotic pressure

Osmolality. The solute concentration per volume of a solution (refers to body fluids)

Osmolarity. The solute concentration per volume of a solution (refers to outside of body)

Serous cavity. A body cavity that is lined with serous membrane (e.g., pericardial sac, pleural, peritoneal)

Tonicity. Osmolarity of an intravenous fluid

ABBREVIATIONS

ACTH. Adrenocorticotropic hormone

ADH. Antidiuretic hormone

ATN. Acute tubular necrosis

BUN. Blood urea nitrogen

Ca. Calcium

Cl. Chloride

CNS. Central nervous system

CVP. Central venous pressure

DKA. Diabetic ketoacidosis

ECF. Extracellular fluid

HHNS. Hyperglycemic hyperosmolar nonketotic syndrome

ICF. Intracellular fluid

IV. Intravenous

K. Potassium

Mg. Magnesium

mOsm. Milliosmole

Na. Sodium

PAWP. Pulmonary artery wedge pressure

PO_4. Phosphate

PTH. Parathyroid hormone

SIADH. Syndrome of inappropriate antidiuretic hormone

TPN. Total parenteral nutrition

SECTION ONE: Body Fluid Distribution

At the completion of this section, the learner will be able to discuss the distribution of body fluid.

Body fluids compose about 60 percent of the body weight in the average adult male. The composition of body fluids is primarily water with various electrolytes and glucose, urea, and creatinine. These fluids provide both an internal and external environment for the cells, playing crucial roles as a medium for metabolic reactions, a cushion to protect body parts from injury, and an influence on regulation of body heat.

Age as a Variable Affecting Body Fluid Content

The percentage of body water diminishes as one grows older. Greater percentages of body fluids are found in individuals with a small body surface area; thus, infants have a larger fluid reserve. Infants, however, are predisposed to serious, rapid fluid volume deficit due to their limited ability to concentrate urine, their proportionately greater ratio of surface area to volume, and their higher metabolic rate. Individuals over the age of 65 have a reduction in total fluid body weight. The elderly patient's fluid balance is affected by alterations in thirst and nutritional intake, diminished renal function, chronic illness, and medications. The elderly are predisposed to developing fluid volume deficit related to decreased muscle mass, smaller fat stores, and a reduction in percentage of body fluids.

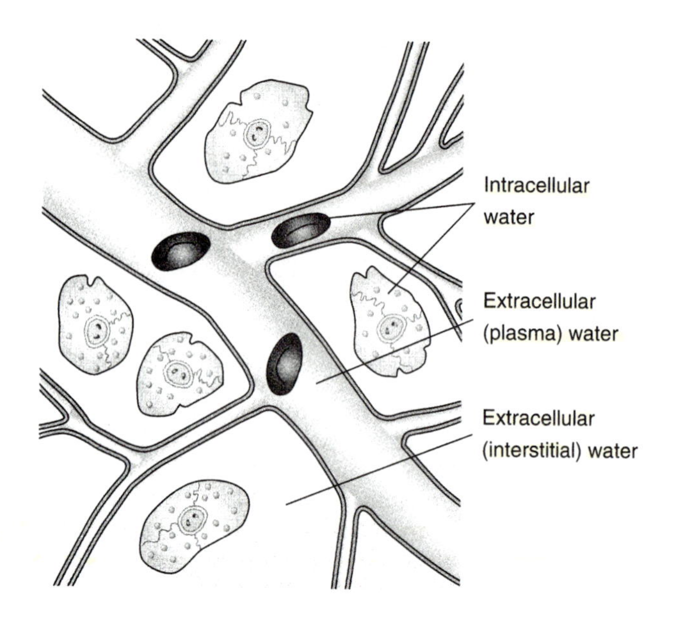

Figure 3–1. Distribution of body water. The extracellular space includes the vascular compartment and the interstitial spaces. *(From Porth, C.M. [1998]. Pathophysiology: Concepts of altered health states, 5th ed. [p. 586]. Philadelphia: J.B. Lippincott.)*

Fluid Compartments

Body fluids are primarily found in two compartments: the **intracellular** compartment (within the cells) and the **extracellular** compartment (all other body fluids) (Fig. 3–1). About two thirds of total body fluid is intracellular and the remaining one third is extracellular. Table 3–1 summarizes water distribution in the adult.

Intracellular Compartment

The intracellular fluids (ICFs) are rich in potassium, phosphate, and protein and contain moderate amounts of magnesium and sulfate ions. Intracellular fluids provide the cells with nutrients and assist in cellular metabolism. Porth (1998) explains that ICF volume is regulated by several important mechanisms. First, the presence of nondiffusible intracellular protein attracts fluid into the cells. Second, negatively charged ions within the cells attract positively charged ions such as sodium and potassium. These two activities draw fluid into the cells, causing cellular expansion. Without the counterregulating forces provided by the Na^+/K^+ pump, the cells would rupture and die. The Na^+/K^+ pump is an active transport mechanism that exchanges Na^+ ions for K^+ ions at a ratio of 3:2; thus, more Na^+ ions are moved out of the cells than K^+ ions. Since water is attracted to Na^+ ions, more water accumulates in the extracellular compartment and ICF balance is maintained. Certain pathologic situations harm the Na^+/K^+ pump, including hypoxia and cell expansion associated with excess Na^+ ions within the cells (e.g., overload of a hypotonic saline IV fluid).

Extracellular Compartment

All body fluid outside of the cells exists in the extracellular compartment and is referred to as extracellular fluid (ECF). The major components of the ECF are plasma (intravascular compartment) and interstitial fluid (interstitial compartment). A minor but potentially significant ECF component is transcellular fluid (transcellular compartment). Plasma is the fluid portion of the blood and is composed of water (about 90 percent), plasma proteins (about 7 percent), and other substances (Gaspard, 1998). According to Porth (1998), interstitial fluid functions as

TABLE 3–1. WATER DISTRIBUTION IN THE BODY (ADULT)*

COMPARTMENTS/ SUBCOMPARTMENTS	% BODY WEIGHT	VOLUME
Intracellular	40	25
Extracellular		
Interstitial	15	11
Plasma	4	3
Transcellular	1	2
TOTAL	60	41

*Approximate

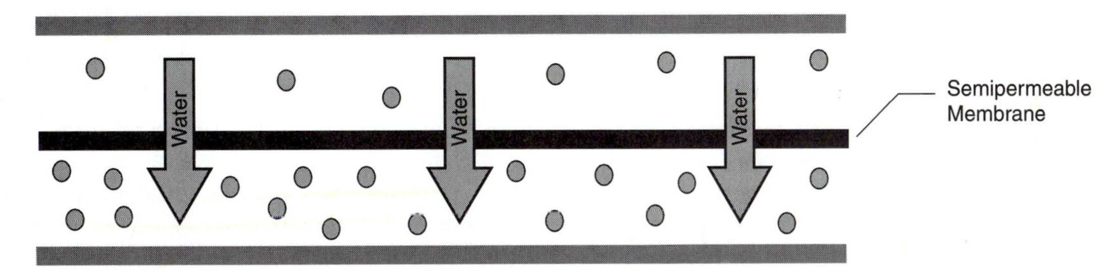

Figure 3–2. Osmosis. Fluid moves across a semipermeable membrane from an area of low concentration to an area of higher concentration.

a transport medium for shuttling nutrients, gases, waste products, and other substances between the blood and the body cells. It also acts as a back-up fluid reservoir that can rapidly provide fluid during situations in which there is vascular fluid loss (e.g., hemorrhage). The interstitial compartment contains a spongelike substance called *tissue gel* that helps distribute interstitial fluid evenly. The gel is held together with collagen fibers. Tissue gel exerts force against the capillaries, which helps maintain fluids inside of the capillaries. It also keeps free water from accumulating in the interstitial spaces. *Transcellular fluid* normally comprises about 1 percent of total ECF. It is located in joints, connective tissue, bones, body cavities, cerebrospinal fluid (CSF), and other tissues (Porth, 1998; Woods, 1998). Transcellular fluid has the potential to increase significantly when fluids become abnormally sequestered in body cavities and tissues, as occurs with third spacing.

Intercompartmental Movement of Fluids

To understand intercompartmental fluid movement, it is crucial to first understand the concepts of osmosis and osmolality. The principle of **osmosis** explains the net diffusion or movement of water across the cell membrane (Fig. 3–2). Water moves across a semipermeable (or selectively permeable) cell membrane from an area of lesser concentration of solutes to an area of greater concentration of solutes. Osmosis is a passive process, requiring no expenditure of energy. Its purpose is to maintain fluid equilibrium between the fluid compartments. Water moves freely between the various fluid compartments; therefore, an alteration in one compartment produces a shift in body fluids in another compartment.

Osmolality refers to the concentration of solute in body water and reflects a patient's hydration status. The osmolarity of a solution is the solute (or particle) concentration per volume of water. Measurement of the *serum* osmolality can be used as an approximation of the extracellular fluid volume. According to Kee (1999), osmolality is expressed in milliosmoles (mOsm), with normal serum osmolality in an adult being 280 to 300 mOsm/kg. Serum values of less than 240 mOsm/kg or above 320 mOsm/kg are considered critically abnormal. A low serum osmolality suggests fluid volume excess or hemodilution, meaning there is more fluid than solute in the serum. A high serum osmolality suggests fluid volume deficit or hemoconcentration, meaning there is less fluid than solute in the serum. Kee (1999) suggests the following formula for determining serum osmolality:

$$\text{Serum Osm/L} = (\text{serum Na} \times 2) + \frac{\text{BUN}}{3} + \frac{\text{Glucose}}{18}$$

[For example: Given that a patient's Na is 140 mEq/L, BUN 20 mg/dL, glucose 250 mg/dL; using the above formula, it can be calculated that the serum osmolality is 301 Osm/L. This indicates that there are more particles than fluid in this patient's serum. This osmolality is slightly high, which suggests fluid volume deficit.]

Clinically, serum osmolality can be used to determine the need for fluid replacement in the high-acuity patient.

Serum osmolality may be increased or decreased in various diseases. Hyperglycemia, diabetes insipidus, and hypernatremia produce an increased serum osmolality, while syndrome of inappropriate antidiuretic hormone (SIADH) and certain ADH-secreting carcinomas of the lung can produce a low serum osmolality. The clinical manifestations of decreased serum osmolality (fluid volume excess) are similar to those of hyponatremia and those of increased serum osmolality (fluid volume deficit) are similar to those of hypernatremia.

Through the processes of osmosis and diffusion, body fluids move freely between the interstitial and intravascular compartments. According to Porth (1998), there are four forces, called *Starling forces*, that control this movement (Fig. 3–3). The forces include capillary hydrostatic pressure, capillary colloidal osmotic pressure, tissue hydrostatic pressure, and tissue colloid osmotic pressure. *Capillary hydrostatic pressure* is the pressure exerted by fluid moving through the capillaries to push fluid out of the capillary into the interstitial space. The majority of this movement occurs at the arterial end of the capillary, where the pressure is greatest (30 to 40 mm Hg). The venous end of the capillary has a much lower pressure (10 to 15 mm Hg) and fluid is reabsorbed back into the capillary at this end. *Capillary colloidal osmotic pressure* is the

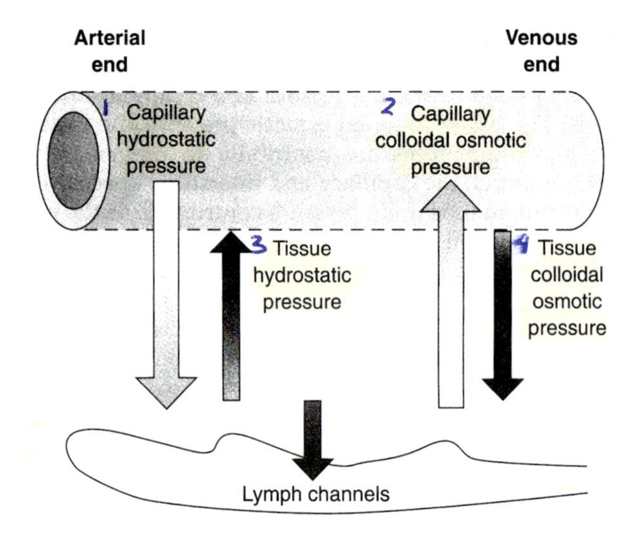

Figure 3–3. Exchange of fluid at the capillary level. *(From Porth, C.M. [1998].* Pathophysiology: Concepts of altered states, *5th ed. [p. 589]. Philadelphia: J.B. Lippincott.)*

pressure exerted by plasma proteins as they flow through the capillary to draw fluid into the capillary. *Tissue hydrostatic pressure* is the pressure exerted by fluid in the interstitial space that pushes against the capillaries, opposing shifts of fluid out of the capillaries. *Tissue colloidal pressure* is pressure exerted by the small amount of proteins located in the interstitial space, which attracts fluid out of the capillaries and into the interstitium. As can be seen, the opposing forces found in the capillaries and the interstitial spaces cause fluids to shift in and out of the capillaries, maintaining fluid balance between compartments and preventing excess fluid buildup in the interstitial spaces. In high-acuity patients, these forces can become unbalanced; causing abnormal fluid shifts such as seen with the occurrence of third spacing.

In summary, body fluids compose more than 60 percent of total body weight. Age can influence total fluid volume. Infants and the elderly are both at increased risk for imbalances in fluid volume. Two thirds of the body's fluids are found in the intracellular fluid and one third exists in the extracellular fluid compartments. Each compartment has its own functions and major electrolytes. The processes of osmosis and diffusion allow intercompartmental shifting of fluids. Fluid shifts alter serum osmolality, which is a measure of the solute concentration in body water. There are two major fluid compartments—intracellular and extracellular. The extracellular compartment can be further divided into the interstitial and intravascular compartments. The transcellular compartment is a small part of the extracellular compartment and is normally an insignificant volume of fluid but has the potential to expand under pathologic circumstances. Fluid shifts out of the intravascular compartment can disrupt homeostasis, resulting in decreased circulating volume.

SECTION ONE REVIEW

1. Two thirds of total body fluid is in which of the following compartments?
   A. intracellular
   B. extracellular
   C. intravascular
   D. interstitial
2. The elderly patient is at increased risk for developing a fluid volume problem related to
   A. high metabolic rate
   B. diminished renal function
   C. inability to concentrate urine
   D. greater ratio of surface area to volume
3. Which of the following electrolytes are found predominantly in the extracellular fluid?
   A. potassium
   B. magnesium
   C. phosphate
   D. sodium
4. The major function of tissue gel in the interstitial compartment is to
   A. shift fluid out of capillaries
   B. provide a source of electrolytes
   C. distribute fluid evenly
   D. dispose of cellular waste products
5. Which of the following statements is correct regarding a low serum osmolality?
   A. it reflects fluid volume deficit
   B. it reflects fluid volume excess
   C. it is associated with dehydration
   D. it is associated with hypernatremia
6. Capillary hydrostatic pressure is the pressure exerted by
   A. plasma proteins in the capillaries
   B. fluid in the interstitial spaces
   C. plasma proteins in the interstitial spaces
   D. fluid moving through the capillaries

Answers: 1. A, 2. B, 3. D, 4. C, 5. B, 6. D

SECTION TWO: Regulation of Fluid Balance

At the completion of this section, the learner will be able to describe the regulation of fluid balance.

Nervous System Regulation

Hypothalamus

According to Guyton and Hall (1997a), the lateral area of the hypothalamus regulates body water, especially thirst and renal excretion of excess water. Cells located in the hypothalamus are sensitive to body fluid concentration (serum osmolality). Thirst is activated by an increase in serum osmolality, decreased arterial blood pressure or circulating blood volume, increased secretion of angiotensin II, and mouth dryness. Thirst is decreased by a lower-than-normal serum osmolality, decreased angiotensin II, increased circulating blood volume or arterial blood pressure, and distention of the stomach. When thirst is triggered, the conscious person responds by drinking fluids. Clinical conditions that decrease the sense of thirst or the individual's ability to respond to thirst can decrease the circulating extracellular volume. The unconscious and/or high-acuity patient often cannot respond to the thirst signals. For this reason, in the clinical setting, the nurse needs to closely evaluate the patient's fluid status using objective data obtained through physical assessment, and urine and serum lab analysis data.

Arterial Baroreceptors

Arterial **baroreceptors** (pressure receptors) located in the arch of the aorta and carotid sinus detect arterial pressure changes. When baroreceptors sense a decrease in arterial blood pressure, they send a message to the autonomic nervous system. The sympathetic nervous system responds to this message by causing peripheral vasoconstriction. Vasoconstriction of renal arteries decreases glomerular filtration, which reduces urine output in an attempt to increase circulating blood volume. The baroreceptors trigger opposite actions if they detect increased arterial blood pressure, causing vasodilation.

Renal and Endocrine Regulation

Adrenocorticotropic Hormone

The renal and endocrine systems work synergistically to regulate blood volume. When the hypothalamus senses a decrease in serum sodium or an increase in serum potassium, it sends a message to the pituitary to release adrenocorticotropic hormone (ACTH). In response, the ACTH stimulates the adrenal cortex to release aldosterone. Aldosterone is the most potent of the mineralocorticoids and is sometimes referred to as the *salt-regulating hormone*. It regulates water balance by facilitating sodium reabsorption in the renal distal tubules, the collecting tubules, and collecting duct (Guyton & Hall, 1997b). As sodium is reabsorbed, potassium is excreted by the kidneys. The sodium reabsorption increases circulating blood volume by increasing water reabsorption. In this way, circulating blood volume and arterial blood pressure increase.

Antidiuretic Hormone

When the hypothalamus detects a change in the concentration of body fluid, it also sends a message to the posterior pituitary to either decrease or increase the release of antidiuretic hormone (ADH), which is also called *vasopressin*. For example, when serum osmolality increases, ADH increases permeability of the renal distal tubules and collecting ducts, which allows a large volume of water to be reabsorbed. This results in expansion of the ECF, decreases serum osmolality, and improves arterial blood pressure and perfusion. (The ADH-regulating mechanism is further described in Module 10.)

Renin–Angiotensin System

When sodium concentration in the ECF is decreased or blood flow through the kidneys is diminished, the kidneys release renin, a protein enzyme. In response to a drop in arterial blood pressure, renin acts on a plasma protein (renin substrate) to release angiotensin I. Angiotensin I ultimately converts to angiotensin II, a powerful vasoconstrictor. Angiotensin II also causes retention of sodium and water by the kidneys. The combination of actions results in a rapid increase in blood pressure, which improves perfusion. The renin, aldosterone, and ADH mechanisms are three endocrine responses to decreased circulating blood volume. (For further discussion of the renin–angiotensin system, refer to Module 26 and Module 10.)

In summary, the nervous, renal, and endocrine systems work synergistically to maintain fluid balance. Aldosterone, ADH, and the renin–angiotensin–aldosterone cycle regulate fluid balance. When these physiologic mechanisms fail or when conditions exist that affect fluid elimination, a fluid volume imbalance occurs.

SECTION TWO REVIEW

1. Which of the following is the primary regulator of water intake?

A. nervous system
B. endocrine system
C. renal system
D. hypothalamus

2. The sympathetic nervous system responds to decreased volume by producing
   A. ADH
   B. ACTH
   C. vasoconstriction
   D. aldosterone
3. When the hypothalamus senses a decrease in serum sodium or potassium, it responds by stimulating the pituitary to release
   A. ACTH
   B. ADH
   C. aldosterone
   D. renin
4. When the hypothalamus senses a change in serum osmolality, it stimulates the posterior pituitary to release
   A. renin
   B. aldosterone
   C. ADH
   D. ACTH
5. Angiotensin II is a powerful
   A. diuretic
   B. vasoconstrictor
   C. thirst trigger
   D. sodium waster

Answers: 1. D, 2. C, 3. A, 4. C, 5. B

SECTION THREE: Fluid Imbalance

At the completion of this section, the learner will be able to discuss fluid imbalance, including edema, third spacing, fluid volume deficit, and fluid volume excess.

Edema

Edema refers to an accumulation of fluid in the interstitial tissues. It most commonly occurs in the extracellular compartment but can occur intracellularly if the active transport Na^+/K^+ pump fails. Edema is not a disease; rather, it is an important manifestation of some underlying problem. The mechanisms that lead to edema are interrelated and include (1) an imbalance in one or more of Starling forces and/or (2) an obstruction in the lymphatic system.

Problems of Starling Forces

INCREASED CAPILLARY HYDROSTATIC PRESSURE. As described in Section One, capillary hydrostatic pressure exerts force against the capillary walls, which shifts fluid out of the capillaries and into the interstitium at the arterial end of the capillary. The fluid is then reabsorbed at the venous end of the capillary (low capillary hydrostatic pressure) or is taken up by the lymphatic system. Under normal conditions, these activities maintain fluid balance. With certain pathologic conditions, the capillary hydrostatic pressure becomes abnormally increased and the fluid cannot be reabsorbed back into the capillaries at the venous end. This usually results in a localized form of edema. The most common cause of increased capillary hydrostatic pressure is congestive heart failure (CHF), due to increased blood volume and increased systemic venous pressure. Other causes include renal failure, prolonged standing, hepatic obstruction (portal hypertension), and decreased venous circulation (e.g., phlebothrombosis) (Mulvey & Bullock, 2000).

DECREASED CAPILLARY COLLOIDAL OSMOTIC PRESSURE. Plasma proteins (primarily albumin) within the capillaries exert a force that draws fluid into the capillaries, counterbalancing the outward fluid movement caused by capillary hydrostatic forces. When plasma proteins are decreased, the capillary hydrostatic pressure pushes fluid out of the capillaries faster than it can be drawn in, causing generalized edema and decreased intravascular fluid volume. Examples of pathologic conditions associated with decreased plasma proteins include liver failure, starvation and protein malnutrition, and burn injury (Mulvey & Bullock, 2000).

INCREASED CAPILLARY PERMEABILITY. Under certain circumstances, the capillaries develop increased permeability, which allows more fluid, plasma proteins, and other active particles to escape into the interstitial spaces (Mulvey & Bullock, 2000; Porth, 1998). This can result from loss of capillary wall integrity through injury or enlargement of capillary pores (e.g., problems causing vasodilatation) (Porth, 1998). The edema resulting from increased capillary permeability can be either localized or generalized, depending on how widespread the underlying problem is. Edema is further increased as plasma proteins escape into the interstitial spaces and begin exerting an increased tissue colloidal osmotic pressure, which attracts more fluid into the area. Examples of conditions associated with increased capillary permeability include burns, inflammation, direct trauma, immune reactions, bacterial infections, and certain toxins (Guyton & Hall, 1997b; Mulvey & Bullock, 2000).

Lymphatic Obstruction

Normally, the lymphatics pick up excess fluid and plasma proteins that have leaked out of the capillaries and return them to the circulation. If the lymphatics become obstructed, however, fluid and plasma proteins accumulate in the affected interstitial spaces. According to Mulvey and Bullock (2000), the most common cause of lymphatic obstruction is the surgical removal of lymph nodes as part of cancer treatment. Other pathologic conditions associated with lymphatic obstruction include cancer (involving lymphatic structures), and a rare parasitic disorder of the lymph vessels called *filariasis* (filaria nematodes) (Guyton & Hall, 1997; Mulvey & Bullock, 2000).

Regardless of the mechanism that precipitates the development of edema, fluid accumulates in the interstitial spaces in the body. As fluid shifts out of the **intravascular** compartment, the intravascular volume becomes depleted, causing a decrease in arterial blood pressure. When the blood pressure drops significantly, the renin–angiotensin system is activated. Sodium and water are conserved and arterioles vasoconstrict, resulting in an increase in the arterial blood pressure. In addition to accumulating in the interstitial spaces, fluid can also accumulate in the transcellular spaces, causing third spacing.

Third Spacing

According to Porth (1998), third spacing is the shift of fluid from the intravascular compartment into a "third" (transcellular) space—usually a **serous cavity.** Normally, there is no accumulation of serosal fluid in a serous cavity. The cavities usually remain empty because of balanced Starling forces and the presence of a rich lymphatic network. If, however, any of the Starling forces become imbalanced or lymphatic drainage becomes obstructed or inadequate, a significant volume of serous fluid or exudate can rapidly accumulate. As fluid fills the cavity, pressure is exerted on the soft structures in the cavity, which can result in compression of those structures (e.g., cardiac tamponade). Fluids that are sequestered in a third space are unavailable for physiologic use by the body and may accumulate rapidly due to protein-rich contents, which causes increased tissue colloidal osmotic pressure, attracting more fluids. Third spacing may occur in the peritoneal cavity, pleural cavity, and pericardial sac and is associated with underlying problems such as intestinal obstruction, liver or renal failure, and peritonitis. Clinically, third spacing manifests itself as ascites, pericardial and pleural effusions, and other conditions.

Fluid Volume Deficit

Extracellular fluid volume deficit exists when there is an abnormally low volume of body fluid in the intravascular and/or interstitial compartments. It produces a state of extracellular dehydration associated with serum hyperosmolality that can lead to intracellular dehydration as fluid shifts out of the cells to increase extracellular volume. It is a common and potentially serious problem in the high-acuity patient. Many factors can cause or contribute to development of fluid volume deficit. These factors are summarized in Table 3–2. The clinical manifestations of ECF volume deficit are presented in Section Four.

TABLE 3–2. FACTORS THAT PRODUCE FLUID VOLUME DEFICIT

SOURCE OF FLUID LOSS	RELATED FACTORS
Gastrointestinal	Diarrhea, vomiting, nasogastric suction, fistulas
Urinary	Uncontrolled diabetes, diabetes insipidus, diuretic phase of acute tubular necrosis
Integumentary	Burns, diaphoresis, increased capillary permeability
Insensible	Hyperventilation, fever, hypermetabolism, tachypnea, mechanical ventilation
Other	Wound drainage

Fluid Volume Excess

Extracellular fluid volume excess, also called fluid overload, produces a state of overhydration in the intravascular, interstitial, and/or transcellular compartments. It is associated with fewer contributing factors than are seen with fluid volume deficit. These factors are summarized in Table 3–3. The clinical manifestations associated with ECF volume excess are presented in Section Four.

In summary, edema is an accumulation of fluid in the interstitial spaces. It is caused by imbalances in Starling forces or lymphatic obstruction. Third spacing of fluids occurs when intravascular fluids shift into the transcellular compartment, usually a serous body cavity. Third spacing results in development of ascites and pleural or pericardial effusions. Third spacing can occur in the presence of edema. *ECF volume deficit* is a term used to describe dehydration in the interstitial and/or intravascular compartments. It is associated with conditions in which there is a

TABLE 3–3. FACTORS THAT PRODUCE FLUID VOLUME EXCESS

SOURCE OF FLUID GAIN	RELATED FACTORS
Cardiovascular	Heart failure
Urinary	Renal failure (acute or chronic)
Hepatic	Cirrhosis
	Liver failure
Other	Cancer
	Thrombus
	Peripheral vascular disease
	Drug therapy (e.g., corticosteroids)
	High sodium intake
	Protein malnutrition

fluid loss in excess of fluid gain. ECF volume deficit can eventually lead to intracellular dehydration. ECF volume excess (fluid overload) describes a state of overhydration in the intravascular, interstitial, and, possibly, the transcellular compartments. It commonly results in edema or third spacing. Fluid volume excess is associated with pathologic conditions in which there is a net fluid gain in relation to fluid loss.

SECTION THREE REVIEW

1. The most common cause of edema resulting from increased capillary hydrostatic pressure is
   - A. liver failure
   - B. burn injury
   - C. immune reactions
   - D. congestive heart failure
2. When capillary plasma protein levels are lower than normal, it results in
   - A. increased intracellular fluid volume
   - B. decreased intravascular fluid volume
   - C. increased intravascular fluid volume
   - D. decreased interstitial fluid volume
3. Edema resulting from escape of fluid and plasma proteins through enlarged pores in the capillary walls is caused by
   - A. increased capillary permeability
   - B. decreased capillary permeability
   - C. increased colloidal osmotic pressure
   - D. decreased tissue colloidal osmotic pressure
4. The most common cause of edema due to lymphatic obstruction is
   - A. lymphatic cancer
   - B. filariasis parasitic infection
   - C. surgical removal of lymph nodes
   - D. tumor compression on lymph nodes
5. Which of the following is an example of third-spaced fluids?
   - A. pericardial effusion
   - B. wound swelling
   - C. dependent edema
   - D. peripheral edema
6. Third spacing of fluids is most commonly located in
   - A. joints
   - B. a serous cavity
   - C. the cranial vault
   - D. interstitial fluid
7. Which of the following statements is correct regarding ECF volume deficit?
   - A. In can lead to transcellular expansion
   - B. It can lead to intracellular expansion
   - C. It is associated with low serum osmolality
   - D. It is associated with high serum osmolality

Answers: 1. D, 2. B, 3. A, 4. C, 5. A, 6. B, 7. D

SECTION FOUR: Nursing Implications

At the completion of this section, the learner will be able to describe the nursing implications associated with fluid imbalances.

Clinical Manifestations of Edema and Third Spacing

If a hemodynamically significant volume of fluid escapes from the intravascular compartment into the interstitial and/or transcellular spaces, the high-acuity patient is at high risk for developing clinical manifestations consistent with **hypovolemia** or hypovolemic shock. (Hypovolemia and hypovolemic shock are discussed in detail in Module 10.)

Edema and third spacing can be described in terms of certain characteristics, including location, whether it is pitting or nonpitting, and amount of fluid weight gain.

Location

Determining whether the edema is localized or generalized gives important clues as to its possible origin since pathologic conditions are usually associated with one or the other. Generalized edema is present all over the body and is primarily seen in the presence of decreased plasma proteins resulting from severe protein malnutrition. Localized edema results from a more localized pathologic condition, for example, local inflammation and infection. Sometimes, however, generalized edema develops secondary to a localized process that has expanded, causing widespread damage to the capillary endothelium and generalized edema. Examples of severe conditions in which this form of secondary generalized edema can occur are septic and anaphylactoid shock.

Localized edema is confined to areas in which the causative condition is affecting the capillaries or lymph tissues (e.g., the area of inflammation, obstruction, or high capillary hydrostatic pressure). The edema associated with congestive heart failure is considered localized since it is confined to the gravity-dependent body areas (e.g., feet, lower legs, and sacrum). Pulmonary edema caused by left-sided heart failure is localized edema created by increased capillary hydrostatic pressure in the lungs due to elevated left heart pressures.

The exact clinical manifestations associated with edema and third spacing depend on their location. For example, a patient with pulmonary edema or pleural effusion is at risk for developing pulmonary gas exchange problems, usually hypoxemia. A patient with cerebral edema is at risk for cerebral herniation, which is a life-threatening complication that clinically presents as a rapid deterioration of the patient's level of consciousness, visual, motor, and respiratory status. Edema around a joint immobilizes the joint. Severe edema can compress capillary blood flow, causing tissue ischemia and pain. A patient with ascites may develop problems with gas exchange as fluid in the peritoneal cavity begins to displace the diaphragm upward or impede diaphragmatic movement. A patient with pericardial effusion may develop signs of circulatory shock in the presence of cardiac tamponade.

Pitting or Nonpitting Edema

Porth (1998) suggests that pitting edema develops when the accumulation of fluid exceeds what can be absorbed by the interstitial tissue gel. Firm pressure applied to the edematous area displaces the interstitial fluid, causing a temporary pitting. It can be measured on a scale of +1 to +4 based on the depth and the length of time it takes for the indentation to disappear.

- **+1:** 0- to ¼-inch (< 6.4-mm) indentation; disappears rapidly
- **+2:** ¼- to ½-inch (6.4-mm to 12.8-mm) indentation; disappears in 10 to 15 seconds
- **+3:** ½- to 1-inch (12.8-mm to 2.5-cm) indentation; disappears in 1 to 2 minutes
- **+4:** > 1-inch (> 2.5-cm) indentation; disappears in 2 to 5 minutes (Porth, 1998)

Body Weight

In the adult, peripheral edema develops when ≥ 5 L of fluid have accumulated in the interstitial spaces and pitting edema develops with an accumulation of ≥ 10 L of interstitial fluid. Clinically, a weight gain or loss of 1 kg (2.2 pounds) represents a fluid gain or loss of about 1 L (Larocca & Otto, 1997). Evaluating daily weight trends provides valuable information on fluid status (Whalen & Kelleher, 1998).

Assessment of third-spaced fluids is more difficult since the serous cavities are deep structures, particularly the pericardial sac and pleural cavity. A thorough evaluation is necessary, and may include auscultation, chest or abdominal radiology, electrocardiogram, echocardiogram, and others. Ascites can involve fluid shifts that are hemodynamically significant. For this reason, close evaluation of arterial blood pressure and serum albumin is important. In addition, daily weights and abdominal girth measurements provide valuable trending data.

Assessment of Fluid Volume Deficit

Assessing the high-acuity patient for the presence of fluid volume deficit is an important part of the daily nursing assessment. Table 3–4 summarizes common clinical assessments. High-acuity patients with fluid volume deficit require close monitoring and additional fluids to achieve and maintain a balanced intake and output.

Nursing interventions may include measures to decrease vomiting, diarrhea, and/or fever; increasing oral fluid intake or administration of intravenous solutions; and monitoring of fluid and electrolyte status. Desired patient outcomes include: pulse, blood pressure, central venous pressure (CVP), and pulmonary artery wedge pressure (PAWP) within acceptable ranges for the patient; normal serum osmolality; increased urine output with normal specific gravity; improved skin turgor; balanced intake and output; stable weight; moist mucous membranes; hematocrit and blood urea nitrogen (BUN) within acceptable limits; and absence of other dehydration manifestations.

Assessment of Fluid Volume Excess

ECF volume excess can be generalized or localized. The assessment procedures are essentially the same as those used for assessing for fluid volume deficit. The findings, however, are almost in complete opposition, with the exception of urinary output. A low urine output can be in-

TABLE 3–4. NURSING ASSESSMENT OF A PATIENT WITH FLUID VOLUME DEFICIT

ASSESSMENT	DATA
Physical assessment	Weight loss Poor skin turgor Dry mucous membranes Flattened neck veins Mental status changes
Vital signs	Orthostatic changes Decreased blood pressure Rapid, weak, thready pulse Rapid, shallow respirations Temperature may be elevated Low CVP and PAWP Decreased cardiac output
Laboratory data	Elevated hematocrit Elevated BUN (normal creatinine) High serum osmolality
Urine	Increased osmolality Increased specific gravity Decreased volume

dicative of either a deficit or an excess. For example, a low urine output (< 30 mL/hr) may be indicative of dehydration or renal failure. Decreased urinary output in the patient with dehydration is actually a protective mechanism for the body to reserve volume. Decreased urinary output in the patient with renal failure, however, causes fluid volume excess. Nursing assessment of the patient for fluid volume excess is summarized in Table 3–5.

Nursing interventions may include fluid and/or salt restrictions; administration of diuretics; or dialysis. The desired patient outcomes for intravascular fluid excess include pulse, blood pressure, CVP, and PAWP within acceptable ranges for the patient; lung sounds clear to auscultation; balanced intake and output; weight loss and resolution of edema; and hematocrit and BUN within acceptable limits.

Use of Intravenous Fluids to Manage Fluid Volume Imbalances

High-acuity patients frequently require fluid and/or electrolyte support through use of intravenous (IV) fluid administration. IV fluids are classified according to their **osmolarity** or tonicity. **Tonicity** refers to the effect the solution has on the ECF and ICF compartments. Intravenous solutions are classified as isotonic, hypotonic, or hypertonic. (See Fig. 3–4.)

Isotonic Solutions

The term **isotonic** means that the osmolarity of the solution on one side of a membrane is the same as the osmolarity on the other side of the membrane. The osmolarity of isotonic fluid closely approximates normal serum plasma osmolality (280 to 300 mOsm/L) (Kee, 1999). For this reason, a steady osmolar state is maintained between the ICF and ECF. Isotonic fluids are used when rapid ECF expansion is needed (Halperin & Goldstein, 1999). The most common reason for administration of isotonic solutions is intravascular dehydration (intravascular fluid volume deficit). In the high-acuity patient, intravascular dehydration can result from hemorrhage, massive gastrointestinal bleed, or dehydration. See Table 3–6 for examples of commonly used isotonic solutions.

TABLE 3–5. NURSING ASSESSMENT OF THE PATIENT WITH FLUID VOLUME EXCESS

ASSESSMENT	DATA
Physical assessment	Weight gain Distended neck veins Periorbital edema, pitting edema over body processes Adventitious lung sounds, moist crackles Shortness of breath Mental status changes Generalized or dependent edema
Vital signs	Elevated blood pressure High CVP/PAWP Increased cardiac output
Laboratory data	Decreased hematocrit (dilutional) Low serum osmolality Radiography: pulmonary vascular congestion, pleural effusion, pericardial effusion, ascites Low urine-specific gravity

Hypotonic Solutions

Hypotonic solutions contain a lower concentration of particles than exists in the ICF and ECF, giving them a low osmolarity. The low osmolarity shifts fluid from the intravascular compartment into the intracellular compartments. Hypotonic fluids are primarily used for treatment of cellular dehydration since they expand the intracellular volume. Hypotonic solutions are useful for prevention of dehydration or for hydration. Hypotonic solutions are used with caution, however, since their overuse causes cells (including blood cells) to expand and burst, resulting in cellular destruction (Thelan et al., 1998). See Table 3–6 for examples of commonly used hy-

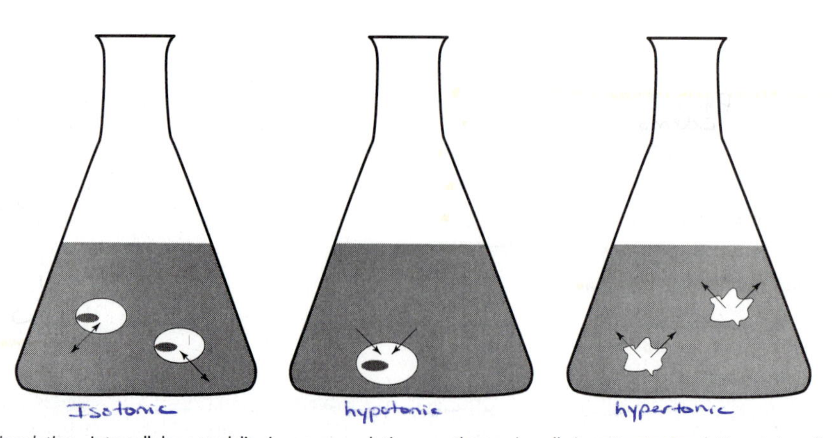

Figure 3–4. Tonicity. *Isotonic solution*—Intracellular osmolality is same as solution; no change in cell size. *Hypotonic solution*—Intracellular osmolality is lower than solution. Fluid moves into cells, enlarging them. *Hypertonic solution*—Intracellular osmolality is higher than solution. Fluid moves out of cells, shrinking them.

TABLE 3–6. COMMON INTRAVENOUS SOLUTIONS CLASSIFIED BY TONICITY

SOLUTION TYPE	SOLUTION EXAMPLES	COMMENTS
Isotonic	5% dextrose in water 0.9% normal saline (NS) Lactated Ringer's	Solution osmolarity approximates serum osmolality Expands intravascular volume Used for dehydration, shock states
Hypotonic	0.45% normal saline 0.2% normal saline 2.5% dextrose	Low solution osmolarity in relation to serum osmolality Fluid shifts into intracellular compartment Used for replacement of hypotonic fluid deficit (e.g., intracellular dehydration)
Hypertonic	5% dextrose in 0.45% normal saline 10% dextrose in water 3% normal saline	High solution osmolarity in relation to serum osmolality Fluid shifts from intracellular to extracellular compartments Used for treatment of water intoxication, symptomatic hyponatremia

potonic solutions. (Refer to Module 10 for further discussion of hypotonic solutions.)

Hypertonic Solutions

Hypertonic solutions have a high osmolarity because they contain a higher concentration of particles than exists in the ICF and ECF. The high osmolarity of the hypertonic solutions shifts fluids from the ICF and ECF into the intravascular compartment, expanding blood volume. Kee and Paulanka (1999), explain that hypertonic solutions are used in the treatment of water intoxication (intracellular fluid volume excess). In the high-acuity patient, water intoxication can be caused by administration of large amounts of electrolyte-free water, overuse of hypotonic solutions (e.g., 0.45 percent sodium chloride), elevated ADH secretion, or renal failure. In addition, overuse of 5 percent dextrose and water (an isotonic solution) can result in water intoxication owing to the rapid metabolizing of glucose, which then leaves a hypotonic water solution remaining in the intravascular compartment. See Table 3–6 for examples of commonly used hypertonic solutions.

In summary, assessment of the patient with fluid imbalances should include a physical assessment, vital signs, and laboratory data. Clinical assessment of edema and third-spaced fluids includes evaluation based on the specific location. Edema is further evaluated as to whether it is pitting or nonpitting. Body weight changes can provide important clues regarding net fluid gain or loss. Evaluation of third-spaced fluid is more difficult, owing to the deep locations of some of the serous cavities, and usually requires an evaluation that is more complex. Nursing diagnoses for alterations in fluid balance may include fluid volume deficit or fluid volume excess. The assessment procedures of these two diagnoses are similar, but the findings are opposite.

Section Four Review

1. A weight gain of 10 kg, indicates what volume of fluid volume excess?
   A. 5 L
   B. 10 L
   C. 15 L
   D. 20 L
2. An example of a patient problem in which the patient develops generalized edema stemming from a problem that usually causes localized edema is
   A. sepsis
   B. congestive heart failure
   C. pulmonary edema
   D. burns
3. Which of the following complications is specifically associated with third spacing of fluid into the pericardial sac?
   A. pulmonary edema
   B. peripheral edema
   C. right heart failure
   D. cardiac tamponade
4. The nurse charts that a patient has "+3 pitting edema." Which of the following assessments best fits this notation?
   A. indentation was ⅛ inch and disappeared within 20 to 30 seconds
   B. indentation was ¼ inch and disappeared rapidly

C. indentation was ½ inch and disappeared within 10 to 15 seconds
D. indentation was ¾ inch and disappeared within 1 to 2 minutes

5. Nursing assessment data found in the patient with fluid volume excess would include
A. low PAWP
B. increased hematocrit
C. moist crackles
D. decreased blood pressure

6. Which of the following intravenous solutions closely approximates serum osmolality?
A. 0.45 percent normal saline
B. 5 percent dextrose in normal saline
C. lactated Ringer's
D. 3 percent normal saline

Answers: 1. B, 2. A, 3. D, 4. D, 5. C, 6. C

SECTION FIVE: Sodium

At the completion of this section, the learner will be able to discuss the extracellular compartment electrolyte, sodium.

Electrolytes are electrically charged microsolutes found in body fluids. There are two types of electrolytes: **cations** (positively charged ions) and **anions** (negatively charged ions). Electrolytes play a vital role in many physiologic activities, including enzyme activities, muscle contraction, and metabolism. There are three major extracellular electrolytes—sodium, chloride, and calcium—and three major intracellular electrolytes—potassium, magnesium, and phosphorus. Sections Five through Ten present an overview of these six major electrolytes. Table 3–7 lists the normal serum electrolytes ranges as well as the panic, or life-threatening, levels.

Normal serum sodium is 135 to 145 mEq/L (Kee, 1999). It is the most abundant cation in the extracellular fluid. Sodium is responsible for shifts in body water and the amount of water retained or excreted by the kidneys. It is required for normal transmission of impulses across muscle and nerve cells, through the sodium pump mechanism. It helps maintain acid–base balance by combining with chloride or bicarbonate to increase or decrease serum pH.

Sodium and Water Balance

Changes in sodium levels alter water balance; thus, the clinical manifestations of sodium alterations also reflect symptoms of water imbalance. Since water is drawn to sodium, an excess sodium level in the extracellular fluid pulls water from the intracellular spaces. This results in shrinking of the intracellular fluid compartment and expansion of the extracellular compartment. Such expansion may precipitate congestive heart failure and pulmonary edema in patients whose renal or cardiovascular system cannot tolerate such fluid shifts.

When serum levels of sodium are low, water moves from an area of low sodium concentration (extracellular) to an area of high sodium concentration (intracellular). This causes excess volume in the intracellular compartment and fluid volume deficit in the extracellular compartment.

The amount of sodium in the diet varies widely,

TABLE 3–7. SERUM ELECTROLYTES AND OSMOLALITY NORMAL RANGES AND CRITICAL ABNORMAL VALUES

ELECTROLYTE	NORMAL RANGE	CRITICAL ABNORMALS
Sodium (Na^+)	135–145 mEq/L (or mmol/L)	
Chloride (Cl^-)	95–105 mEq/L (or mmol/L)	
Calcium (Ca^{++})	4.5–5.5 mEq/L (9–11 mg/dL)	> 14 mg/dL
Potassium (K^+)	3.5–5.3 mEq/L (or mmol/L)	< 2.5 mEq/L or > 7 mEq/L
Magnesium (Mg^{++})	1.5–2.5 mEq/L (1.8–3.0 mg/dL)	< 1.0 mEq/L or > 10 mEq/L
Phosphate (PO_4^-)	1.7–2.6 mEq/L (2.5–4.5 mg/dL)	< 0.5 mEq/L
Serum osmolality	280–300 mOsm/kg	< 240 or > 320

Values from Kee, J.L. (1999). Laboratory diagnostic tests with nursing implications, *5th ed. Stamford, CT: Appleton & Lange; Kee, J.L., & Paulanka, B.J. (1999).* Handbook of fluid, electrolyte and acid–base imbalances. *Albany, NY: Delmar Publishers.*

since the supply is abundant in many (particularly processed) foods. When sodium intake is excessive, fluid volume in the intravascular compartment increases. In response, the kidneys increase urinary excretion of sodium through enhanced filtering from the blood; inhibition of ADH prevents reabsorption of sodium by the kidneys; and aldosterone release is suppressed, enhancing urinary excretion of sodium. When sodium intake is excessively low, plasma volume is decreased. The kidneys sense the decreased volume, triggering the renin–angiotensin–aldosterone system, which causes increased sodium reabsorption; thus, decreasing urine output and increasing fluid volume.

Hypernatremia

Serum sodium levels above 145 mEq/L can result from excessive sodium intake or excess water loss. In the high-acuity patient, excessive sodium intake can occur from the overadministration of hypertonic intravenous fluid or sodium bicarbonate, or overconsumption of dietary sodium. High serum sodium pulls water from the ICF compartment into the intravascular compartment. The cells shrink and shrivel owing to cellular dehydration while the ECF becomes overloaded with water.

Hypernatremia caused by excess water loss can result from renal dysfunction, profuse diaphoresis, or increased ACTH secretion (Cushing's syndrome) (Kee & Paulanka, 1999). Excess fluid loss can also develop from gastrointestinal loss if fluid loss exceeds electrolyte loss (e.g., severe vomiting and/or diarrhea and nasogastric suction drainage). Diabetes insipidus and administration of osmotic diuretics can cause a significant loss of body water without equivalent loss of sodium, which drives up the serum sodium concentration.

Hyponatremia

Hyponatremia occurs when the serum sodium levels fall below 135 mEq/L. It can result from excessive sodium loss, or water gain, which produces a **dilutional effect.**

Excessive Sodium Loss

In high-acuity patients, major sources of sodium loss are through the gastrointestinal tract and kidneys. Gastrointestinal-related losses occur when electrolyte loss is in excess of fluid loss and may result from severe diarrhea, vomiting, or nasogastric suction. Renal loss of sodium is usually due to diuretic therapy or severe renal dysfunction. Severe diaphoresis can also lead to significant loss of sodium through the skin. Excessive sodium loss also results from hyperglycemic osmotic diuresis, as seen with diabetic ketoacidosis (DKA). Persistent sodium excretion can occur with consistent release of ADH from the pituitary or ectopic production of ADH. This unregulated production of ADH is associated with SIADH, which is associated with cerebral trauma, narcotic use, lung cancer, and certain drugs.

Dilutional Effect

Hyponatremia can result from a net gain of water in the ECF compartment. This occurs when water moves into an area without an equivalent increase in sodium. For example, when a patient develops DKA, excessively high serum glucose levels cause a shift of water from the ICF and other compartments into the intravascular compartment to dilute the glucose and regain equilibrium.

Clinical Manifestations of Sodium Imbalances

The clinical manifestations of hypernatremia are predominantly neurologic because brain cells are especially sensitive to sodium levels. If hypernatremia develops rapidly, cellular shrinkage also contributes to the neurologic symptoms. Hyponatremia is associated with early changes in muscle tone since sodium plays a role in transmission of neuromuscular impulses. If sodium levels continue to fall (< 120 mEq) intracellular edema occurs, producing further neurologic deterioration. The clinical manifestations of hypernatremia and hyponatremia are summarized in Table 3–8.

In summary, sodium is the major extracellular cation. It is crucial to regulation of body fluids. It also plays an important role in nerve impulse transmission. Hypernatremia primarily results from excessive sodium intake or excess water loss. Hyponatremia usually results from excessive sodium loss or the dilutional effect. The clinical manifestations of sodium imbalances are predominantly neurologic, due to the sodium sensitivity of brain cells.

TABLE 3–8. CLINICAL MANIFESTATIONS OF SODIUM IMBALANCES

Hypernatremia (> 145 mEq/L)	*Moderate:* Confusion, thirst
	Severe: Cardiovascular: hypertension, tachycardia Neurologic: restlessness, seizures, coma Neuromuscular: hyperreflexia, muscle twitching Gastrointestinal: nausea and vomiting
Hyponatremia (< 135 mEq/L)	Cardiovascular: hypotension Neurologic: confusion, headache, lethargy, seizures Neuromuscular: decreased muscle tone, muscle twitching, tremors Gastrointestinal: vomiting, diarrhea, cramping

SECTION FIVE REVIEW

1. The normal range of serum sodium is
   A. 1.5 to 2.2 mEq/L
   B. 3.5 to 5.5 mEq/L
   C. 8.5 to 10.5 mg/dL
   D. 135 to 145 mEq/L
2. Hypernatremia can be caused by which of the following?
   A. diabetes insipidus
   B. hyperglycemia
   C. SIADH
   D. DKA
3. Signs and symptoms of hypernatremia include
   A. diarrhea
   B. muscle twitching
   C. stomach cramps
   D. decreased muscle tone
4. Hyponatremia is associated with which of the following symptoms?
   A. edema
   B. hyperreflexia
   C. lethargy
   D. restlessness
5. The major function of sodium is
   A. carbohydrate metabolism
   B. tissue oxygenation
   C. blood coagulation
   D. fluid balance

Answers: 1. D, 2. A, 3. B, 4. C, 5. D

SECTION SIX: Chloride

At the completion of this section, the learner will be able to describe the extracellular compartment electrolyte, chloride.

Chloride is the most abundant anion in the ECF. The normal serum chloride range is 95 to 105 mEq/L (Kee, 1999). Chloride works with sodium in regulation of body fluids by its influence on osmotic pressures within the interstitial and intravascular compartments. Serum chloride levels tend to closely follow sodium levels, as chloride normally follows sodium in the body. Aldosterone regulates chloride levels indirectly by stimulating reabsorption of sodium in the kidney. Chloride assists in maintaining the resting membrane potential of cells and, with sodium, maintains osmolality of the extracellular fluid space.

The extracellular fluid acid–base status requires a balance between the total number of anions and cations within the fluid. Thus, the major cation (sodium) must be in balance with the two major extracellular anions (chloride and bicarbonate). To regulate this balance, chloride and bicarbonate maintain an inverse relationship, competing for sodium ions. For example, if a patient receives an excessive dose of sodium bicarbonate to treat metabolic acidosis, the presence of excess bicarbonate ions in the serum results in the excretion of chloride ions, precipitating hypochloremia.

Hyperchloremia

Hyperchloremia is defined as a serum chloride of more than 105 mEq/L. Hyperchloremia is associated with excessive loss of bicarbonate and normal anion gap metabolic acidosis (refer to Module 25). Normal anion gap metabolic acidosis is most commonly caused by loss of bicarbonate ions through either renal or gastrointestinal loss (e.g., diarrhea). As bicarbonate is lost, chloride is reabsorbed to maintain acid–base balance.

Hypochloremia

Hypochloremia is defined as a serum chloride of < 95 mEq/L. Hypochloremia can result from metabolic alkalosis or hypokalemia. Excessive use of loop diuretics, such as furosemide, enhances the loss of chloride and sodium in the urine. When chloride levels are low, the kidneys sense the need for more anions to maintain electrical neutrality and bicarbonate is reabsorbed.

Clinical Manifestations of Chloride Imbalances

The signs and symptoms of chloride imbalance reflect the manifestations of the associated acid–base imbalance. Neurologic, musculoskeletal, respiratory dysfunction, and the symptoms of a concurrent sodium imbalance are also associated with chloride imbalances. The clinical manifestations of chloride imbalances are listed in Table 3–9.

TABLE 3–9. CLINICAL MANIFESTATIONS OF CHLORIDE IMBALANCES

Hyperchloremia (> 105 mEq/L)	Musculoskeletal: muscle weakness Respiratory: rapid, deep respirations Neurologic: headache, lethargy, decreasing level of consciousness Symptoms of hypernatremia and fluid volume deficit
Hypochloremia (< 95 mEq/L)	Neurologic: irritability, tetany, agitation Respiratory: shallow breathing, bradypnea Musculoskeletal: muscle weakness Symptoms of hyponatremia

In summary, chloride is the major extracellular anion. It maintains a direct relationship with sodium and an inverse relationship with bicarbonate. Chloride is important in fluid regulation and acid–base balance. Hyperchloremia is associated with loss of bicarbonate ions and metabolic acidosis (normal anion gap). Hypochloremia is associated with loss of sodium or potassium ions and metabolic alkalosis.

SECTION SIX REVIEW

1. Chloride levels closely follow the levels of which of the following electrolytes?
   A. potassium
   B. sodium
   C. calcium
   D. magnesium
2. Hypochloremia is associated with which of the following symptoms?
   A. tetany
   B. headache
   C. lethargy
   D. rapid, deep respirations
3. The normal serum chloride range is
   A. 3.5 to 5.3 mEq/L
   B. 4.5 to 5.5 mEq/L
   C. 95 to 105 mEq/L
   D. 135 to 145 mEq/L
4. Hyperchloremia is associated with which of the following problems?
   A. metabolic acidosis (normal anion gap)
   B. metabolic acidosis (high anion gap)
   C. metabolic alkalosis (normal anion gap)
   D. metabolic alkalosis (high anion gap)
5. Which of the following substances indirectly regulates serum chloride levels?
   A. parathyroid hormone
   B. calcitonin
   C. renin
   D. aldosterone

Answers: 1. B, 2. A, 3. C, 4. A, 5. D

SECTION SEVEN: Calcium

At the completion of this section, the learner will be able to discuss the extracellular compartment electrolyte, calcium.

The normal serum calcium level is 4.5 to 5.5 mEq/L (Kee, 1999). Almost all of the body's calcium is located within bone, with a small amount existing in the ECF and soft tissues. Calcium is required for blood coagulation, neuromuscular contraction, enzymatic activities, and for intact bones.

Calcium regulation is under the influence of parathyroid hormone (PTH), calcitonin, and calcitriol. Serum calcium levels are maintained by calcium excretion from the kidneys, absorption of calcium from the gastrointestinal tract, and mobilization of calcium from the bone. Calcium is absorbed in the intestines only under the influence of vitamin D, which is activated in the kidneys. It is reabsorbed in the proximal renal tubules after being filtered by the glomerulus and is excreted by the kidneys. Renal disease prevents activation of vitamin D, thus reducing the body's ability to absorb calcium.

Calcitonin and parathyroid hormone work in opposition to regulate calcium levels. When calcium levels are low, PTH is released by the parathyroid gland, stimulating the conversion of calcitriol (the active form of vitamin D), which causes the small intestines to absorb more calcium. PTH also stimulates release of calcium from bony tissues into the blood. When calcium levels are high, PTH secretion is suppressed and calcitonin is secreted by the thyroid, inhibiting the release of calcium from bone into the blood.

Serum calcium can be measured in two different ways: as total calcium and as ionized calcium. These two measurements evaluate body calcium in two different states:

- *Total calcium*—Normal levels: 4.5 to 5.5 mEq/L or 9 to 11 mg/dL (Kee, 1999). Total calcium reflects calcium that is bound to proteins (primarily albumin) in the serum. Total calcium levels are influenced by the patient's nutritional state.
- *Ionized calcium*—Normal levels: 2.2 to 2.5 mEq/L or 4.25 to 5.25 mg/dL (Kee, 1999). Approximately 50 percent of serum calcium exists in an ionized state. Ionized calcium represents the calcium that is used in the physiologic activities and is crucial for neuromuscular activity. Ionized calcium levels may remain normal even when total calcium levels are low.

Hypercalcemia

Hypercalcemia is defined as a serum calcium level above 5.5 mEq/L (11 mg/dL). Hypercalcemia results from mobilization of calcium from bone. Malignancy is a common cause of hypercalcemia, usually through destruction of bone (from bone metastasis). Another malignancy-

TABLE 3–10. CLINICAL MANIFESTATION OF CALCIUM IMBALANCES

Hypercalcemia (> 5.5 mEq/L or 9–11 mg/dL) (Severe = > 14 mg/dL)	Gastrointestinal: anorexia, constipation, peptic ulcer disease Neurologic: lethargy, depression, fatigue; if severe: confusion, coma Cardiovascular: cardiac dysrhythmias, heart block, shortened QT interval, decreased ST segment Skeletal: pathologic bone fractures, bone thinning Other: renal stones
Hypocalcemia (< 4.5 mEq/L or 9 mg/dL)	Musculoskeletal: cramps: abdominal, extremities; tingling, and numbness; severe: positive Chvostek's or Trousseau's sign, tetany Neurologic: irritability, reduced cognitive ability, seizures Cardiovascular: electrocardiographic changes: prolonged QT interval, long ST segment, decreased blood pressure, and myocardial contractility Skeletal: bone fractures possible Hematologic: abnormal clotting

related mechanism for hypercalcemia is the presence of PTH-secreting tumors. Malignancies that are most commonly associated with development of hypercalcemia include pulmonary, breast, ovarian, and others (Kee & Paulanka, 1999). Hypercalcemia also develops from prolonged immobility, hyperparathyroidism, thyrotoxicosis, and thiazide diuretics. Excessive ingestion of vitamin D or calcium and altered renal tubular absorption of calcium also elevates serum calcium levels. Gastrointestinal and renal absorption of calcium decreases the reabsorption of phosphorus; therefore, hypercalcemia accompanies hypophosphatemia, as calcium and phosphorus levels shift in opposite directions.

Hypocalcemia

Hypocalcemia is defined as a serum level below 4.5 mEq/L (9 mg/dL). In the high-acuity patient, the most common cause of hypocalcemia is depressed function or surgical removal of the parathyroid gland. It is also associated with hypomagnesemia and hyperphosphatemia, which can cause diminished vitamin D synthesis by the kidneys. Hypocalcemia can be induced by the administration of large amounts of stored blood because stored blood is preserved with citrate. When citrate is administered, it binds with calcium, which lowers serum calcium.

Clinical Manifestations of Calcium Imbalances

The signs and symptoms of hypercalcemia primarily reflect dysfunction of the gastrointestinal and musculoskeletal systems. The signs and symptoms of hypophosphatemia can accompany hypercalcemia. Hypocalcemia becomes symptomatic when ionized calcium levels fall to below normal limits. Symptomatic hypocalcemia affects the musculoskeletal, neurologic, and cardiovascular systems. The clinical manifestations associated with hypercalcemia and hypocalcemia are presented in Table 3–10.

In summary, calcium plays an important part in blood coagulation and is the major component of bone tissue. It is regulated by PTH, calcitonin, and calcitriol. Calcium is measured in its protein bound state (total calcium) and its ionized state (ionized calcium). Hypercalcemia results from movement of calcium from the bone. Hypocalcemia is associated with depressed parathyroid function. Calcium imbalances are particularly associated with neuromuscular and cardiac dysfunction.

SECTION SEVEN REVIEW

1. The normal range of total serum calcium is
   A. 1.5 to 2.5 mEq/L
   B. 3.5 to 5.3 mEq/L
   C. 4.5 to 5.5 mEq/L
   D. 135 to 145 mEq/L
2. Calcium is absorbed in the intestines under the influence of
   A. phosphorus
   B. vitamin D
   C. sodium
   D. vitamin C
3. Hypocalcemia is associated with which of the following?
   A. tingling and numbness
   B. constipation
   C. lethargy
   D. shortened QT interval
4. Calcium regulation is under the influence of all of the following EXCEPT
   A. calcitriol
   B. calcitonin
   C. PTH
   D. aldosterone

5. Which of the following statements is correct regarding serum total calcium?
   - A. it may remain normal even if ionized calcium is abnormal
   - B. it represents calcium that is physiologically active
   - C. it is influenced by the patient's nutritional state
   - D. it measures calcium that is not bound to protein

Answers: 1. C, 2. B, 3. A, 4. D, 5. C

SECTION EIGHT: Potassium

At the completion of this section, the learner will be able to discuss the intracellular compartment electrolyte, potassium.

The normal serum potassium level is 3.5 to 5.3 mEq/L (Kee, 1999). Potassium is the major intracellular cation, with almost all potassium being located within the cells. Although the concentration in the plasma is small, monitoring serum potassium is very important because the body is intolerant of abnormal serum levels. Potassium is readily found in many foods; thus, we normally consume sufficient quantities of potassium to meet daily requirements. Excess potassium is eliminated in the urine by the kidneys, and about 40 mEq/L of potassium is excreted daily in the urine (Kee, 1999).

Potassium is vital in maintaining normal cardiac and neuromuscular function because it affects muscle contraction. Potassium also influences nerve impulse conduction; therefore, abnormal serum potassium levels can produce potentially lethal cardiac conduction abnormalities, which could result in cardiac arrest. Potassium is vital to carbohydrate metabolism and plays an important role in normal cell membrane function. It is important in maintaining acid–base balance because hydrogen ions exchange with potassium ions.

Hyperkalemia

Hyperkalemia is defined as a potassium level above 5.3 mEq/L. Hyperkalemia can result from a variety of situations. In the high-acuity patient, administration of potassium supplements, either oral or IV can cause hyperkalemia, particularly in the presence of reduced urinary output (e.g., renal dysfunction). Significant quantities of intracellular potassium are released into the extracellular space in response to injury, stress, acidosis, or a catabolic state. Acidosis contributes to hyperkalemia since excess hydrogen ions shift into the cells, forcing potassium out into the serum (Kee & Paulanka, 1999). Additionally, sodium depletion results in hyperkalemia as potassium is exchanged for sodium across the proximal renal tubule.

Hypokalemia

Hypokalemia is defined as a serum potassium below 3.5 mEq/L. Hypokalemia can result from:

- A loss of gastrointestinal secretions (e.g., vomiting, diarrhea, excessive nasogastric loss, and fistulas)
- Excessive renal excretion of potassium
- Movement of potassium into the cells (e.g., diabetic ketoacidosis)
- Prolonged fluid administration without potassium supplementation
- Excessive use of potassium-wasting diuretics without adequate potassium supplementation

When hypokalemia occurs, the body does not attempt to retain or reabsorb potassium. The kidneys continue to excrete it regardless of the existing potassium state. If allowed to continue, the hypokalemia becomes increasingly severe, causing a steady deterioration in the patient's condition. Because the body does not compensate for potassium loss, it is essential that hypokalemia be rapidly detected and corrected through appropriate potassium supplementation. The body is intolerant of abnormal serum potassium levels. According to Kee and Paulanka (1999), potassium levels that are < 2.5 mEq/L or > 7 mEq/L are critically deranged and can result in cardiac arrest.

Clinical Manifestations of Potassium Imbalances

Since potassium is important in nerve impulse conduction, muscle contraction, and cell membrane function, the signs and symptoms of imbalances reflect interference with these activities. The clinical manifestations of potassium imbalances are summarized in Table 3–11.

In summary, potassium is the major intracellular cation. It is vital in maintaining normal cardiac and neuromuscular function. Hyperkalemia results from excessive potassium intake, renal failure, or use of potassium-sparing diuretics. Hypokalemia results from excessive loss of potassium through the gastrointestinal tract or urine, shifting of potassium into the cells, or excessive administration of potassium-free intravenous fluids. The clinical manifestations of potassium imbalances reflect dysfunctions in nerve impulse conduction, muscle contraction, and cell membrane activities.

TABLE 3–11. CLINICAL MANIFESTATIONS OF POTASSIUM IMBALANCES

Hyperkalemia (> 5.3 mEq/L)	Musculoskeletal: weakness, muscle cramps Gastrointestinal: nausea, vomiting, abdominal cramping, diarrhea Cardiovascular: electrocardiographic changes: progression from tachycardia to bradycardia to cardiac arrest is possible; prolonged P-R interval; flat or absent P wave; slurring of QRS; tall peaked T wave; ST segment depression Acid–base effect: metabolic acidosis
Hypokalemia (< 3.5 mEq/L)	Musculoskeletal: skeletal muscle weakness; decreased smooth muscle function; decreased deep tendon reflexes Cardiovascular: hypotension, electrocardiogram: ST segment depression; U waves; T wave inversion, flattening, or depression; cardiac arrest if severe Gastrointestinal: nausea and vomiting, paralytic ileus, diarrhea Acid–base effect: metabolic alkalosis Neurologic: depression, confusion

SECTION EIGHT REVIEW

1. The normal range of serum potassium is
   A. 1.5 to 2.2 mEq/L
   B. 3.5 to 5.3 mEq/L
   C. 4.5 to 5.5 mEq/L
   D. 135 to 145 mEq/L
2. Hyperkalemia can be caused by which of the following?
   A. renal failure
   B. potassium-wasting diuretics
   C. metabolic alkalosis
   D. severe diarrhea
3. Signs and symptoms of hyperkalemia include
   A. muscle weakness, T wave inversion
   B. muscle twitching, ST segment depression
   C. vomiting, peaked T wave
   D. diarrhea, presence of U wave
4. The presence of hypokalemia alters renal excretion of potassium in which of the following ways?
   A. urine output increases
   B. potassium excretion increases
   C. potassium is reabsorbed
   D. potassium excretion does not change

Answers: 1. B, 2. A, 3. C, 4. D

SECTION NINE: Magnesium

At the completion of this section, the learner will be able to describe the intracellular compartment electrolyte, magnesium.

Magnesium is an intracellular electrolyte with a distribution similar to potassium. The normal serum magnesium level is 1.5 to 2.5 mEq/L (Kee, 1999). Magnesium ensures sodium and potassium transportation across cell membranes. It is needed for activation of certain enzymes required for normal protein and carbohydrate metabolism (Kee, 1999). Magnesium is crucial to many biochemical reactions and plays a significant role in nerve cell conduction. It is important in transmitting CNS messages and maintaining neuromuscular activity.

Magnesium is predominantly excreted in feces, but a small amount is excreted in the urine. The kidneys, however, have a remarkable ability to conserve magnesium. Magnesium balance is closely related to potassium and calcium balance.

Hypermagnesemia

Hypermagnesemia results when magnesium levels rise above 2.5 mEq/L. This abnormality is rare, but can occur with diminished renal excretion as seen in renal dysfunction, or excessive magnesium intake. Consumption of large quantities of magnesium-containing antacids or laxatives can be a source of excessive intake.

Hypomagnesemia

Hypomagnesemia is defined as a serum magnesium of < 1.5 mEq/L. It can result from decreased intake or decreased absorption of magnesium, or excessive loss through urinary or bowel elimination. Magnesium deficiency can be caused by many disorders, including acute pancreatitis, starvation, malabsorption syndrome, chronic alcoholism, burns, and prolonged hyperalimentation without adequate magnesium replacement. Hypoparathyroidism, with resultant hypocalcemia, can also cause hypomagnesemia since the regulatory mechanisms of magnesium and calcium are closely related.

Clinical Manifestations of Magnesium Imbalances

The signs and symptoms of magnesium and calcium imbalances are similar. Since magnesium is important in maintaining normal CNS and neuromuscular function, magnesium imbalances can cause dysfunction of these ac-

TABLE 3–12. CLINICAL MANIFESTATIONS OF MAGNESIUM IMBALANCES

Hypermagnesemia (> 2.5 mEq/L or 3.0 mg/dL)	Neuromuscular: absent deep tendon reflexes, lethargy, drowsiness Cardiovascular: hypotension, bradycardia, cardiac arrest; electrocardiogram: prolonged P-R intervals, complete heart block, wide QR complex Respiratory: depression
Hypomagnesemia (< 1.5 mEq/L or 1.8 mg/dL)	Neuromuscular: tremors, tetany, positive Chvostek's and Trousseau's signs Cardiovascular: premature ventricular contractions, ventricular tachycardia and/or fibrillation; T wave flattening, decreased ST segment

tivities. Hypermagnesemia has a depressant effect, and hypomagnesemia is associated with hyperactivity. The clinical manifestations associated with hypermagnesemia and hypomagnesemia are presented in Table 3–12.

In summary, magnesium is primarily an intracellular cation with a distribution similar to potassium. Magnesium has many functions, including assisting in transport of sodium and potassium across the cell membrane, and transference of energy. Hypermagnesemia is rare and is primarily caused by either excessive intake of magnesium-containing drugs, or renal failure. Hypomagnesemia can result from decreased intake or excessive loss of magnesium. The clinical manifestations of magnesium imbalances primarily reflect CNS and neuromuscular dysfunction.

Section Nine Review

1. The normal range of serum magnesium is
   A. 1.5 to 2.5 mEq/L
   B. 3.5 to 5.3 mEq/L
   C. 4.5 to 5.5 mEq/L
   D. 135 to 145 mEq/L
2. Magnesium balance is closely related to which other two electrolytes?
   A. potassium and phosphorus
   B. calcium and sodium
   C. sodium and phosphorus
   D. calcium and potassium
3. The symptoms of hypomagnesemia reflect
   A. CNS hypoactivity
   B. fluid compartment shifts
   C. cardiac depressant effects
   D. neuromuscular and CNS hyperactivity
4. Hypermagnesemia is associated with which of the following symptoms?
   A. tetany
   B. lethargy
   C. tremors
   D. positive Chvostek's sign
5. Magnesium plays an active part in all of the following physiologic functions EXCEPT
   A. sodium and potassium transport
   B. nerve cell conduction
   C. fluid regulation
   D. transference of energy

Answers: 1. A, 2. D, 3. D, 4. B, 5. C

SECTION TEN: Phosphorus/Phosphate

At the completion of this section, the learner will be able to discuss the intracellular compartment electrolyte, phosphorus/phosphate.

Phosphorus is an intracellular mineral commonly found in many foods. According to Kee and Paulanka (1999), the normal serum level of inorganic phosphorus is 1.7 to 2.6 mEq/L or 2.5 to 4.5 mg/dL. In the body, it predominantly exists as phosphate (PO_4). Phosphorus plays an essential part in development of teeth and bones. It is vital for normal neuromuscular function and is required for energy in the production of adenosine triphosphate (ATP). It also contributes to protein, fat, and carbohydrate metabolism and assists in the maintenance of acid–base balance.

The serum phosphate level is under the influence of PTH and maintains an inverse relationship to calcium. The kidneys are essential to phosphorus regulation through reabsorption and excretion. When glomerular filtration is decreased, phosphorus reabsorption increases, causing an elevation in serum levels. As glomerular filtration increases, phosphorus reabsorption diminishes and more phosphorus is excreted by the kidneys, reducing the serum phosphate level.

TABLE 3–13. CLINICAL MANIFESTATIONS FOR PHOSPHATE IMBALANCES

Hyperphosphatemia (> 2.6 mEq/L or 4.5 mg/dL)	Musculoskeletal: muscle cramping and weakness Cardiac: tachycardia Gastrointestinal: diarrhea, nausea, abdominal cramping *Note:* Many other symptoms are those of hypocalcemia
Hypophosphatemia (< 1.7 mEq/L or 2.5 mg/dL)	Musculoskeletal: weakness, numbness, and tingling; pathologic fractures Cardiac: diminished myocardial function Gastrointestinal: nausea and vomiting, anorexia Neurologic: disorientation, irritability, seizures, coma *Severe hypophosphatemia:* severe myocardial, respiratory, and nervous system dysfunction; hemolysis, WBC and platelet dysfunction

Hyperphosphatemia

Hyperphosphatemia is defined as a serum level above 2.6 mEq/L (4.5 mg/dL). Hyperphosphatemia is not as common in the high-acuity patient as hypophosphatemia. It is predominantly associated with chronic renal failure. Other causes include hyperthyroidism, hypoparathyroidism, severe catabolic states, and conditions causing hypocalcemia.

Hypophosphatemia

Hypophosphatemia is defined as a serum phosphorus level below 1.7 mEq/L (2.5 mg/dL). This condition is associated with malnourished states, and is a relatively common imbalance in the high-acuity patient. Other conditions that can cause hypophosphatemia include hyperparathyroidism, certain renal tubular defects, metabolic acidosis (including DKA), and disorders that cause hypercalcemia.

Clinical Manifestations of Phosphate Imbalances

Hypophosphatemia depresses cellular function, particularly of the hematologic and cardiovascular systems. This results in symptoms of impaired heart function and poor tissue oxygenation. Because phosphorus is essential in providing energy for ATP, muscle fatigue develops. The clinical manifestations associated with hyperphosphatemia and hypophosphatemia are presented in Table 3–13.

In summary, phosphorus, which exists in the serum as phosphate, works closely with calcium and is important in tissue oxygenation and energy production. Hyperphosphatemia is most commonly associated with chronic renal failure. Hypophosphatemia most commonly results from malnourished states. The clinical manifestations of phosphate imbalances primarily reflect dysfunction of the hematologic, cardiovascular, and neuromuscular systems.

SECTION TEN REVIEW

1. The normal range of serum phosphorus is
   - **A.** 1.7 to 2.6 mEq/L
   - **B.** 3.5 to 5.3 mEq/L
   - **C.** 4.5 to 5.5 mEq/L
   - **D.** 135 to 145 mEq/L
2. Hypophosphatemia is associated with which of the following conditions?
   - **A.** malnourished state
   - **B.** metabolic alkalosis
   - **C.** hypocalcemia
   - **D.** hyperthyroidism
3. Severe hypophosphatemia is associated with which of the following symptoms?
   - **A.** joint pain
   - **B.** muscle cramping
   - **C.** respiratory arrest
   - **D.** peptic ulcer disease
4. Phosphorus is important for all of the following functions EXCEPT
   - **A.** tissue oxygenation
   - **B.** sodium transport
   - **C.** calcium regulation
   - **D.** production of ATP
5. The clinical picture of hyperphosphatemia frequently reflects which other electrolyte abnormality?
   - **A.** hypercalcemia
   - **B.** hypochloremia
   - **C.** hypernatremia
   - **D.** hypocalcemia

Answers: 1. A, 2. A, 3. C, 4. B, 5. D

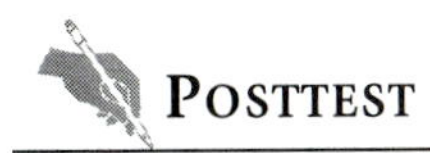

POSTTEST

The following Posttest is constructed in a case study format. A patient is presented, and questions are asked based on available data. New data are presented as the case study progresses.

Donald R, 75 years old, was admitted to the hospital with severe dyspnea. He has a history of chronic alcohol abuse and cirrhosis. On admission, the nurse assesses the following: Thin, chronically ill-appearing male. Blood pressure, 108/62; pulse, 118/min; RR, 26/min; temperature, 97.8°F., +3 pitting generalized edema is noted. His abdomen is distended and tight. He is orthopneic and complains of shortness of breath. Mr. R states that he has been confined to his chair or couch for the past two weeks due to his breathing difficulty and general weakness.

1. Mr. R's age and poor physical condition place him at risk for development of
   - **A.** hypertension
   - **B.** dehydration
   - **C.** acute renal failure
   - **D.** congestive heart failure
2. Mr. R's edema is an example of fluid located in which space?
   - **A.** intracellular
   - **B.** intravascular
   - **C.** interstitial
   - **D.** transcellular
3. Assuming Mr. R's abdominal distention is ascites, the shift of intravascular fluid into his peritoneal cavity is referred to as
   - **A.** third spacing
   - **B.** congestive failure
   - **C.** edema
   - **D.** peritonitis
4. As Mr R's blood pressure decreases, the baroreceptors will trigger
   - **A.** renal vasodilation
   - **B.** increased heart rate
   - **C.** suppression of ACTH release
   - **D.** peripheral vasoconstriction

Mr. R's urine output has been 25 mL/hr for the past 2 hours. His most current serum osmolality is 315 mOsm/L. He is complaining of extreme thirst.

5. Based on the available data, his urine output and serum osmolality are most likely due to
   - **A.** renal failure
   - **B.** peripheral edema
   - **C.** suppressed ADH release
   - **D.** intravascular fluid deficit
6. His thirst is activated by
   - **A.** hemodilution
   - **B.** release of aldosterone
   - **C.** increased osmolality
   - **D.** ADH release

Mr. R has a serum albumin drawn. The results show a significantly low albumin level.

7. A low serum albumin directly alters the Starling forces in which of the following ways?
   - **A.** fluids escape out of the capillaries
   - **B.** fluids are drawn into the capillaries
   - **C.** fluids escape out of the interstitial spaces
   - **D.** fluids are drawn into the interstitial spaces

It is decided that Mr. R requires intravenous fluids.

8. The decision of which type of IV fluid is best for Mr. R is based on osmolarity. A solution's osmolarity refers to its __________ concentration in relation to the ICF and ECF.
   - **A.** particle
   - **B.** protein
   - **C.** glucose
   - **D.** anion
9. Which type of IV solution would be best for treating intravascular fluid deficit?
   - **A.** hypertonic solutions
   - **B.** isotonic solutions
   - **C.** hypotonic solutions
   - **D.** colloid solutions
10. Mr. R receives an IV fluid to increase his intravascular volume and increase his arterial blood pressure. The best IV fluid to accomplish this goal is
    - **A.** 5 percent dextrose in normal saline
    - **B.** 0.45 percent normal saline
    - **C.** 5 percent dextrose in water
    - **D.** 0.2 percent normal saline

Mr. R has received a large volume of IV fluids. His serum electrolytes are drawn. The results are

Sodium: 128 mEq/L
Chloride: 90 mEq/L
Total calcium: 5.8 mEq/L
Potassium: 5.2 mEq/L
Magnesium: 2.7 mEq/L
Phosphate: 1.5 mEq/L

11. Mr. R's serum sodium can cause body water to shift from the
    - **A.** extracellular into intravascular compartment
    - **B.** interstitial into intravascular compartment
    - **C.** extracellular into intracellular compartment
    - **D.** intracellular into extracellular compartment

12. If Mr. R's chloride level continues to fall, he will need to be assessed for
    A. rapid, deep respirations
    B. muscle weakness
    C. depressed breathing
    D. lethargy
13. Mr. R's total calcium level is 4.0 mEq/L. This level is most likely caused by his
    A. renal status
    B. nutritional status
    C. chloride status
    D. immobilized status
14. Should Mr. R's serum potassium level approach 7 mEq/L, the nurse would be MOST concerned about changes in which body system?
    A. cardiovascular
    B. respiratory
    C. neurologic
    D. renal
15. If Mr. R's chloride level dropped significantly, the nurse would need to monitor him for development of which of the following primary acid–base problems?
    A. metabolic acidosis
    B. metabolic alkalosis
    C. respiratory acidosis
    D. respiratory alkalosis
16. Hypomagnesemia, such as Mr. R has, can be caused by all of the following problems EXCEPT
    A. hypercalcemia
    B. chronic alcoholism
    C. starvation
    D. acute pancreatitis
17. Mr. R's hypophosphatemia can affect his musculoskeletal system in which of the following ways?
    A. muscle spasm
    B. joint pain
    C. muscle weakness
    D. muscle cramping

POSTTEST ANSWERS

Question	Answer	Section
1	B	One
2	C	One
3	A	Three
4	D	Two
5	D	One
6	C	One
7	A	One, Three
8	A	Four
9	B	Four
10	C	Four
11	C	Five
12	C	Six
13	B	Seven
14	A	Eight
15	B	Six
16	A	Nine
17	C	Ten

REFERENCES

Gaspard, K.J. (1998). Blood cells and the hematopoietic system. In C.M. Porth (ed.). *Pathophysiology: Concepts of altered health states* (5th ed.) (pp. 113–119). Philadelphia: J.B. Lippincott.

Guyton, A.C., & Hall, J.E. (1997a). Activation of the brain; wakefulness and sleep; behavioral function of the brain. In A.C. Guyton & J.E. Hall (eds.). *Human physiology and mechanisms of disease* (6th ed.) (pp. 482–494). Philadelphia: W.B. Saunders.

Guyton, A.C, & Hall, J.E. (1997b). The body fluid compartments: Extracellular and intracellular fluids. In A.C. Guyton & J.E. Hall (eds.). *Human physiology and mechanisms of disease*, (6th ed.) (pp. 201–211). Philadelphia: W.B. Saunders.

Halperin, M.L., & Goldstein, M.B. (1999). *Fluid, electrolyte, and acid–base physiology: A problem-based approach* (3rd ed.). Philadelphia: W.B. Saunders.

Kee, J.L. (1999). *Laboratory diagnostic tests with nursing implications* (5th ed.). Stamford, CT: Appleton & Lange.

Kee, J.L. & Paulanka, B.J. (1999). *Handbook of fluid, electrolyte and acid–base imbalances*. Albany, NY: Delmar Publishers.

Larocca, J.C., & Otto, S.E. (eds.). (1997). *Pocket guide series: Intravenous therapy* (3rd ed.). St. Louis: C.V. Mosby.

Mulvey, M., & Bullock, B.L. (2000). Fluid, electrolyte, and acid–base balance. In B.L. Bullock, & R.L. Henze (eds.). *Focus on pathophysiology*. Philadelphia: J.B. Lippincott.

Porth, C.M. (1998). Alteration in fluid and electrolytes. In C.M. Porth (ed.). *Pathophysiology: Concepts of altered health states* (5th ed.) (pp. 585–624). Philadelphia: J.B. Lippincott.

Thelan, L.A., Urden, L.D., Lough, M.E., & Stacy, K.M. (1998). Renal anatomy and physiology. In L.A. Thelan et al. (eds.). *Critical care nursing: Diagnosis and management* (3rd ed.) (pp. 849–864). St. Louis: C.V. Mosby.

Whalen, D.A., & Kelleher, R.M. (1998). Cardiovascular patient assessment. In M.R. Kinney, S.B. Dunbar, J.A. Brooks-Brunn, N. Molter, & J.M. Vitello-Cicciu (eds.). *AACN's clinical reference for critical care nursing* (4th ed.) (pp. 277–318). St. Louis: C.V. Mosby.

Woods, S. (1998). Fluid and electrolyte homeostasis. In M.R. Kinney, S.B. Dunbar, J.A. Brooks-Brunn, N. Molter, & J.M. Vitello-Cicciu (eds.). *AACN's clinical reference for critical care nursing* (4th ed.) (pp. 113–133). St. Louis: C.V. Mosby.

MODULE 4

Organ Transplantation

Kathleen D. Wagner, Diana Thacker

This self-study module provides the learner with a broad picture of solid organ transplantation. The module is organized into two parts. As an introduction, Section One presents a brief history of solid organ transplantation.

Part I, which is composed of Sections Two through Four, focuses on the donor. Section Two differentiates between the various types of grafts and donors. It also includes a brief summary of some of the major laws intended to protect the donor and establish procurement protocols. Section Three explains organ procurement and includes establishing brain death, obtaining consent, and working with the family to obtain consent. It concludes with the typical sequence of events involved in the procurement process. Section Four discusses management of the donor prior to organ removal and organ preservation.

Part II focuses on the organ recipient. Sections Five through Eight present specific recipient topics. Section Five explains immunologic considerations such as histocompatibility and donor–recipient compatibility testing. Section Six describes how the need for an organ transplant is determined. Key concepts include determination of need and transplant recipient evaluation. Section Seven discusses posttransplantation complications, dividing them into three categories: technical, organ rejection, and immunosuppressant related. Section Eight describes some of the major immunosuppressants currently in use. Section Nine paints a broad picture of selected organ transplants, including kidney; heart, lung, and heart–lung; and liver. The discussion of each type of organ transplant includes major indications for transplantation, preparation of the recipient, postoperative management, and evaluation of organ function. Each section includes a set of review questions to help the learner evaluate his or her understanding of the section's content before moving on to the next section. All Section Reviews and the module Pretest and Posttest include answers. It is suggested that the learner review those concepts answered incorrectly in the review questions before proceeding to the next section.

OBJECTIVES

Following completion of this module, the learner will be able to

1. Discuss the history of organ transplantation.
2. Describe types of grafts and donors.
3. Explain the general organ procurement process.
4. Discuss donor and organ management.
5. Explain the immunologic considerations of organ transplantation.
6. Describe the determination of transplant need.
7. Discuss the major complications associated with organ transplantation.
8. Describe the immunosuppressant therapy.
9. Discuss the general concepts related to transplantation of selected organs, including postprocedure management implications.

GLOSSARY

Acute rejection. A cell-mediated immune response in which the T lymphocytes and macrophages of the host attack and destroy the graft tissue; it occurs within days or months following the transplant

Allograft. Tissue that is transplanted between members of the same species

Anastomosis. Site at which a graft is sutured into a recipient

Antigens. Substances that are capable of eliciting the immune response

Autograft. Transplantation of tissue from one part of a person's body to another part

Cadaver donor. A donor from whom a tissue or organ is recovered after death

Chronic rejection. A humoral immune response in which antibodies slowly attack the graft

Cytokine-release syndrome. A group of clinical manifestations associated with the initial dose of monoclonal antibody therapy

Cytotoxic agents. Drugs that have the capability of destroying target cells

Donor. One who donates an organ or tissue

Graft. The transfer of tissue or organ from one part of the body to a different part, or from another donor source

Heterograft. Transplantation of tissue between two different species

Histocompatibility. The ability of cells and tissues to live without interference from the immune system

HLA antigens. Human leukocyte antigens—proteins found on the sixth chromosome (also called histocompatibility antigens)

Hyperacute rejection. A humoral immune response in which the B lymphocytes are activated to produce antibodies against the donor organ; it occurs within minutes to hours following transplantation

Immunosuppressant. A drug that suppresses the immune response

Isograft. Transplantation of tissues between identical twins

Monoclonal antibodies. Antibodies that are pure clones of specific B lymphocytes

Polyclonal antibodies. Antibodies produced by immunizing animals with human lymphocytes

Recipient. One who receives an organ or tissue

Rejection. The activation of the immune response against a transplanted tissue or organ

Syngraft. See **isograft**

Tissue typing. Identification of the HLA antigens of both the donor and the recipient

Vascular thrombosis. A blood clot in the vasculature of the graft

Xenograft. See **heterograft**

ABBREVIATIONS

ALG. Antilymphocyte globulin

ALT. Alanine aminotransferase (SGPT)

AST. Aspartate aminotransferase (SGOT)

ATG. Antithymocyte globulin

CMV. Cytomegalovirus

CPB. Cardiopulmonary bypass

CRS. Cytokine-release syndrome

CyA. Cyclosporine

EBV. Epstein–Barr virus

ESRD. End-stage renal disease

HBV. Hepatitis B virus

HCV. Hepatitis C virus

HIV. Human immunodeficiency virus

HLA. Human leukocyte antigen

IDDM. Insulin-dependent diabetes mellitus

KODA. Kentucky Organ Donor Affiliates

MAb. Monoclonal antibody

OPO. Organ Procurement Organization

OPTN. National Organ Procurement and Transplantation Network

PEEP. Positive end-expiratory pressure

UAGA. Uniform Anatomical Gift Act

UNOS. United Network for Organ Sharing

PRETEST

1. The early focal point of interest for organ transplantation was the
   A. lungs
   B. kidney
   C. heart
   D. liver
2. Skin grafts were first experimented with as a treatment for
   A. leg ulcers
   B. traumatic injury
   C. skin cancer
   D. burn injury
3. The specific term referring to transplantation between identical twins is
   A. isograft
   B. autograft
   C. heterograft
   D. allograft
4. Segmental (partial) live-organ donations are usually between
   A. identical twins
   B. husband and wife
   C. parent and child
   D. human and ape
5. All of the following are major criteria for brain death EXCEPT no
   A. hyperthermia
   B. response to pain
   C. body movement
   D. cranial nerve reflexes
6. The major advantage of early notification of the Organ Procurement Coordinator when a potential donor has been identified is that __________ can be initiated.
   A. family counseling
   B. life-support measures
   C. signing of the consent form
   D. preliminary evaluation for suitability
7. Major management goals for caring for the donor patient include all of the following EXCEPT maintaining
   A. stable hemodynamic status
   B. infections at minimum level
   C. fluid and electrolyte balance
   D. optimal oxygenation status
8. The most common underlying cause of hypotension in the donor is
   A. dehydration
   B. cardiac failure
   C. fluid overload
   D. increased systemic vascular resistance
9. Histocompatibility antigens are also known as
   A. monocytes
   B. macrophages
   C. human leukocyte antigens
   D. polymorphonuclear lymphocytes
10. Human leukocyte antigen (HLA) are important because they
    A. are the source of donor organ rejection
    B. indicate the degree of organ failure
    C. are identical only within same species
    D. reflect the need for transplantation
11. General guidelines for determination of organ transplant need include all of the following EXCEPT
    A. severe function disability
    B. end-stage organ failure
    C. psychological readiness
    D. additional serious health problems
12. The decision of whether or not a person is placed on the organ transplant waiting list as a potential recipient is usually made by
    A. the patient/family
    B. a multidisciplinary committee
    C. the organ procurement team
    D. the potential recipient's physician
13. All of the following are examples of technical complications of organ transplantation EXCEPT
    A. bleeding
    B. infection
    C. anastomosis leakage
    D. vascular thrombosis
14. Organ rejection that takes place within minutes to hours following transplantation and results from the presence of preformed graft-specific cytotoxic antibodies is called __________ rejection.
    A. subacute
    B. acute
    C. hyperacute
    D. chronic
15. The immunosuppressant that selectively acts against the helper T cells without affecting other types of immune cells is
    A. corticosteroids
    B. azathioprine
    C. cyclosporine
    D. OKT3
16. Long-term posttransplantation steroid therapy is particularly associated with potentially severe __________ disorders.
    A. bone
    B. heart
    C. liver
    D. blood

17. The major indication for kidney transplantation is end-stage renal disease, which most commonly results from all of the following problems EXCEPT
    A. diabetes mellitus
    B. hypertension
    C. glomerular nephritis
    D. nephrotoxicity
18. Dysfunction of a renal graft is most commonly associated with the
    A. preoperative condition of the donor
    B. preoperative condition of the recipient
    C. length of time the organ was preserved
    D. length of time required to perform the transplant
19. Major conditions that are associated with the need for heart transplantation include all of the following EXCEPT
    A. myocardial infarction
    B. congenital malformations
    C. ventricular aneurysm
    D. cardiomyopathy
20. Major indications for liver transplantation include all of the following EXCEPT
    A. fulminant hepatic failure
    B. acute hepatotoxicity
    C. malignant hepatic tumors
    D. irreversible chronic liver disease
21. Liver transplant patients are at particularly high risk for development of which early complication?
    A. hemorrhage
    B. rejection
    C. infection
    D. obstruction

Pretest answers: 1. B, 2. D, 3. A, 4. C, 5. A, 6. D, 7. B, 8. A, 9. C, 10. A, 11. D, 12. B, 13. B, 14 C, 15. C, 16. A, 17. D, 18. C, 19. A, 20. B, 21. A

SECTION ONE: Brief History of Organ Transplantation

At the completion of this section, the learner will be able to discuss the history of organ transplantation.

Organ transplantation is not a new concept. For centuries there have been attempts to replace various body tissues. It was not until the dawn of the twentieth century, however, that surgical skills and knowledge of immunology and immunosuppression became advanced enough to facilitate tissue survival following transplantation. This section highlights strategic events in the development of modern organ transplantation as described by Dr. Joseph Murray, a pioneer in transplantation (Murray, 1991).

1910 to 1930: The Beginnings

The kidney was the early focal point of interest for organ transplantation. Surgeons had struggled with young patients who, while otherwise healthy, were dying of end-stage renal failure. Prior to 1912, although there was interest in performing such transplants, surgeons had not yet developed a successful method of reconnecting the organ vasculature to make transplantation a feasible option. It was in 1912 that the Nobel Prize winner Dr. A. Carrel developed a landmark method of successfully suturing and transplanting blood vessels and organs. It was also during this period that animal research began exploring tissue survival following autografts and allografts.

1930 to 1950: In Search of Long-Term Success

In the early 1930s, experimentation in skin grafting as a treatment for burns contributed greatly to the advancement of transplantation knowledge. It was noted that, although no skin grafts survived for long, skin grafts from family members survived longer than those from nonfamily members. In 1937, it was discovered that skin grafting between identical twins could provide permanent graft survival. This discovery rekindled interest in organ and tissue replacement, although the reasons for tissue acceptance or rejection were still unknown.

It was in the late 1940s that renal transplantation programs began to develop in earnest. Following World War II, research began to focus on allograft rejection. A common antigen was discovered between kidney and skin allografts that would cause sensitization of a recipient for subsequent graftings. Scientists knew that, if renal transplantation was to be a feasible option, they must find a way to get around the immunologic problems experienced thus far. By the end of the 1940s, transplanted kidneys were surviving for up to 6 months. Long-term organ transplant survival remained just out of reach.

1950 to 1960: The Isograft and Immunosuppressant Discovery Years

In 1954, the first renal transplants between identical human twins took place. Tissue matching was performed by cross skin grafting between two twin brothers. The success of the isograft demonstrated that identical twins provided a method of bypassing the tissue incompatibility problem.

Research continued toward solving the problem of tissue incompatibility. Total body x-ray was performed experimentally, as a means to depress the immune system. After the x-ray treatments were completed, bone marrow infusions were performed and the renal allograft transplant was completed. This method, however, had only marginal success in the short term and little success in the long term.

During this decade, research also focused on pharmacologic immunosuppression. In 1959, animal experimentation began using 6-mercaptopurine, an antimetabolite, with encouraging success. It was during the next year that azathioprine (Imuran) was introduced. Early use of azathioprine was associated with patient death from high-dose–related complications. Once the correct dose was established, however, azathioprine was very successful during human clinical trials, and it continues to be a major form of immunosuppression therapy. Not long after initiating the use of azathioprine, corticosteroids were introduced as adjunctive therapy.

1961 to the Present

The 1960s saw a rapid increase in transplant knowledge. Renal transplant survival rates increased dramatically. New forms of immunosuppressive therapy were discovered. Organ procurement programs were initiated both regionally and nationally. There was great enthusiasm to take what was learned from the renal transplantation programs and expand it to transplantation of other organs.

In the late 1960s, liver transplantation was initiated, followed by heart transplantation. Early attempts at heart transplantation were not very successful. The poor success rate associated with heart transplantation "between 1968 and 1970 was undoubtedly transplantation's darkest hour" (Murray, 1991). Today, however, cardiac transplantation is successful, in part due to improved immunosuppressant therapy, particularly cyclosporine. Following the attainment of a successful cardiac transplant program, surgeons turned to perfecting the heart–lung, single-lung, and double-lung transplants.

In summary, the history of organ transplantation is relatively short. Most dysfunctional organs can now be replaced by healthy ones. The problems associated with histocompatibility and organ rejection required years of research to overcome. This section presented an overview of events that led to present-day organ transplant programs.

SECTION ONE REVIEW

1. The early focal point of interest for organ transplantation was the
   A. kidney
   B. lungs
   C. heart
   D. liver
2. Skin grafts were first experimented with as a treatment for
   A. leg ulcers
   B. traumatic injury
   C. skin cancer
   D. burn injury
3. One of the earliest immunosuppressants to be successfully used on transplant patients was
   A. cyclosporine
   B. azathioprine
   C. corticosteroids
   D. 6-mercaptopurine

Answers: 1. A, 2. D, 3. B

THE ORGAN DONOR

SECTION TWO: The Graft and Donor

At the completion of this section, the learner will be able to describe types of grafts and donors.

The term **graft** refers to the transfer of tissue from one part of the body to a different part or from another donor source. There are three major types of grafts: the autograft, the heterograft, and the allograft.

The Autograft

The **autograft** is the transplantation of tissue from one part of a person's body to another part. It is the ideal situation for tissue compatibility and graft survival. A common example of autografting is the skin graft. For example, when a person receives severe burns, healthy tissue can be removed from an undamaged body area and transplanted over the burned area to promote healing and recovery. Autografting is not used for organ transplantation and thus will not be discussed further in this section. (See Module 33 for more information.)

The Heterograft

The **heterograft**, also called a **xenograft**, refers to transplantation of tissue between two different species. Examples of heterografts are porcine skin grafts and experimental baboon heart transplants. At this time, heterografts are primarily used as temporary transplantations until a permanent homograft becomes available. Tissue rejection occurs rapidly due to the dissimilarities of tissues between species.

The Allograft

The **allograft** (homograft) refers to tissue that is transplanted between members of the same species. One form of allograft, the **isograft (syngraft)**, refers to transplantation between identical twins. The allograft is the most common type of organ transplantation. Allografts, with the exception of isografts, trigger an immune reaction that will cause rejection of the graft. Allografts are obtained either from live or cadaver donors.

The Live Donor

The kidney is the primary solid organ that is recovered, en total, from a live **donor**. Ideally, the live donor is related to the recipient as part of the immediate family (e.g., parents, siblings). When a related donor is not available, a nonrelated live donor is used. Related donors are preferred because of increased histocompatibility and, therefore, longer graft life. If an isograft is used, no rejection is expected since the two tissues are completely histocompatible. Segmental (partial) organ donation such as one lobe of a liver or lung, or part of the pancreas, may be performed using a live donor. Segmental organ donation is usually provided by the parents of a recipient child.

The Cadaver Donor

The **cadaver donor** is one who has an organ or tissue recovered after death. Cadaver donors are most commonly healthy individuals who die as the result of a traumatic event or a sudden death. Cadaver donors comprise the majority of solid organ donors. Potential cadaver donors are initially evaluated for suitability.

There are two types of potential cadaver donors: those who die of cardiac death and those who die of brain death.

DONORS WHO DIE OF CARDIAC DEATH. Cardiac death refers to death by termination of cardiac and respiratory function. Transplantable tissues may be limited to heart valves, corneas, eyes, saphenous veins, skin, and bones. These tissues are to be recovered within 12 to 24 hours post declaration of death (KODA, 1994). On occasion, organs may be recovered following cardiac death. This must be initiated within minutes of cardiac arrest with the appropriate personnel available to complete the organ recovery.

DONORS WHO DIE OF BRAIN DEATH. Brain death refers to the cessation of the entire brain and brain stem function. Loss of brain stem function destroys the vital centers for blood pressure, temperature, and respiratory control, making cardiopulmonary death imminent. Organ donations resulting from brain death comprise the majority of cadaver organs. Transplantable tissues from this group of donors include soft tissues as well as solid organs such as the kidneys, lungs, heart, liver, pancreas, and small bowel (Thacker, 1999).

Strict laws and formal procurement protocols have been established to protect the potential donor's rights.

Legal Aspects of Donation and Transplantation

Many laws are in place at both the national and state levels to protect the potential organ donor and to organize and facilitate organ procurement and distribution. The following are examples of some of this legislation.

Uniform Anatomical Gift Act (UAGA)

The UAGA authorizes the donation of all or part of the human body following death for a variety of uses (research, transplantation, and education). The act also includes guidelines regarding who can donate, how donation is to be carried out, and who can receive the organ donation. The act provides for the donor card as a means for individuals to convey their desire to be donors. The act also includes liability protection for health care providers. All states have passed the Uniform Anatomical Gift Act.

Required-Request Legislation

A section of the Uniform Anatomical Gift Act, called the "Routine Inquiry and Required Request; Search and Notification," stipulates hospital responsibilities toward identifying potential donors and providing donor information to families to make them aware of their opportunities to donate. Hospitals that do not comply with the required-request stipulations may be open to penalties or administrative actions.

National Organ Transplant Act

The National Organ Transplant Act sets up the National Organ Procurement and Transplantation Network (OPTN). The OPTN establishes national registries to track potential recipients and posttransplantation organ recipients. It also provides for a national system to match organs and potential recipients. In addition, the act prohibits selling of human organs and tissues. This act has been adopted in all 50 states.

Uniform Determination of Death Act

The Uniform Determination of Death Act has been enacted as a guideline for states to establish a legal definition of death. Most states have adopted some form of this act. For example, in Kentucky, KRS 446.400: Determination of death; minimal conditions to be met, states:

> For all legal purposes, the occurrence of human death shall be determined in accordance with the usual and customary standards of medical practice, provided that death shall not be determined to have occurred unless the following minimal conditions have been met: (1) When respiration and circulation are not artificially maintained, and there is a total and irreversible cessation of spontaneous respiration and circulation; or (2) When respiration and circulation are arti-

ficially maintained, and there is a total and irreversible cessation of all brain function, including the brain stem and that such determination is made by two (2) licensed physicians.

Hospital Conditions of Participation

Enacted in 1998, these guidelines directed at hospitals stipulate Medicare conditions of participation. The guidelines specifically indicate the responsibilities of hospitals toward notifying and working with their organ procurement organization (OPO). They also require personnel, who will be working with families of potential donors, to have special training by the OPO. In addition, hospitals are required to provide transplant related data as requested by their OPO or the OPTN.

In summary, there are three major types of grafts, including the autograft, the heterograft, and the allograft. One type of allograft, the isograft, is a graft between identical twins. Allografts comprise the majority of grafts. Allografts can be obtained from live or cadaver donors. The majority of grafts are of cadaver origin. Cadaver organs and tissues come from two sources: donors who die of cardiac death and those who die of brain death. Strict laws and formal procurement protocols protect the potential donor's rights. Examples of some of the major laws include the Uniform Anatomical Gift Act, required-request legislation, the National Organ Transplant Act, the Uniform Determination of Death Act, and the Hospital Conditions of Participation.

SECTION TWO REVIEW

1. Tissue that is transplanted between members of the same species is the definition of
   A. autograft
   B. heterograft
   C. xenograft
   D. allograft
2. The specific term referring to transplantation between identical twins is
   A. isograft
   B. autograft
   C. heterograft
   D. allograft
3. Segmental (partial) live-organ donations are usually between
   A. identical twins
   B. husband and wife
   C. parent and child
   D. human and ape
4. The major legislation that authorizes the donation of all or part of the human body following death is called the
   A. National Organ Transplant Act
   B. Uniform Anatomical Gift Act
   C. Uniform Determination of Death Act
   D. Omnibus Reconciliation Act

Answers: 1. D, 2. A, 3. C, 4. B

SECTION THREE: Organ Procurement

At the completion of this section, the learner will be able to explain the general organ procurement process.

The specific procedures used to procure and distribute organs differ among transplant programs and organizations. This section will provide information regarding the procurement process in general.

Establishing Brain Death

The initial step in obtaining an organ is the evaluation of a patient for brain death. Brain death is often a difficult concept for family members and health care providers. The physical appearance of a brain-dead person does not fit the typical visual image associated with cardiac death. The brain-dead patient often has a regular heartbeat and may have normal skin temperature and coloring. The patient's chest is rising and falling with respirations, the motion appearing relatively normal even though breathing is being completely controlled by a mechanical ventilator.

The Uniform Determination of Death Act is stated in very broad terms. The broad terms allow hospitals to use the equipment and personnel available in their facilities, as well as implement new technology as it becomes available to make a death pronouncement. As an example, death is defined by Kentucky Statute (KRS 446.400) as:

- **Cardiac standstill death**—when artificial respiration and circulation are not maintained and there is an irreversible cessation of spontaneous respiration and circulation

- **Brain death**—when respiration and circulation are artificially maintained and there is total and irreversible cessation of all brain function including the brain stem

Patients who die from a cardiac standstill death (i.e., myocardial infarction, cancer, or gastrointestinal hemorrhage) are eligible to donate tissues only. Tissues that can be donated include eyes; corneas; heart valves; skin grafts from the abdomen, back, buttocks, and thighs; bone and connective tissue; and saphenous veins. The donor program has up to 24 hours to complete a tissue recovery after the patient's heart stops.

Patients pronounced brain dead can donate both organs and tissues. Recoverable organs include the heart, lungs, liver, pancreas, kidneys, and small intestine. Brain death most often occurs within five categories:

- **Traumatic brain injury.** *Examples:* motor vehicle crashes, blows to the head, shaken child syndrome, falls, closed head injuries, gunshot wounds to the head, and skull fractures
- **Bleeding in the brain.** *Examples:* stroke, intracerebral bleeds, subdural hematomas, and subarachnoid hemorrhage
- **Anoxia.** *Examples:* near drowning, post–cardiopulmonary resuscitation, drug overdoses, and hypoxia
- **Primary central nervous system (CNS) brain tumors.** *Examples:* astrocytomas and glioblastoma (metastatic brain tumors are not candidates for donation)
- **Others.** *Examples:* meningitis and encephalitis

By necessity, specific accepted medical standards are used for establishing death. Some of the brain-death criteria are required and some are optional. Legislation does not specify particular criteria to determine brain death; however, they do recommend guidelines specified in the President's Commission for the Study of Ethical Problems in Medicine and Biomedical and Behavioral Research of 1980.

When brain death testing is being considered, three factors must be determined: (1) known cause of patient's unresponsiveness; (2) absence of toxic CNS depression (such as sedative drugs, ETOH, neuromuscular blockades); and (3) absence of metabolic CNS depression (such as hypothermia, hypotension, severe acid–base imbalance). Brain-death determination must be made by one of three tests, including clinical examination, cerebral blood flow test, or electroencephalogram (EEG). The type of testing to be used is determined by the extent of the patient's injuries, hemodynamic stability, and toxic or metabolic CNS depressive status. Table 4–1 summarizes specific criteria for establishing brain death.

Clinical Examination

Clinical examination is the most cost-effective type of testing and can be completed at the bedside. This exam can be done only if no toxic or metabolic CNS depression exists. Clinical exams cannot be utilized in a patient where respiration cannot be maintained by the patient with injuries that would prevent a respiratory effort in the presence of brain activity (i.e., C1–2 fracture). The following criteria must be found on a clinical exam:

- No response to painful or verbal stimuli. Glasgow Coma Scale score = 3
- No pupillary reflex

TABLE 4–1. CRITERIA FOR ESTABLISHING BRAIN DEATH

CRITERION	CRITICAL ASSESSMENTS	REQUIRED/OPTIONAL TEST
Absence of Reflexes		
Corneal	No blink reflex	Required
Oculovestibular	Negative ice calorics (no eye movement or nystagmus) as a result of procedure	Required
Oculocephalic	No eye movement away from midline; no doll's eye reflex	Required
Other cranial reflexes	No gag, yawning, vocalization, swallowing, coughing	Required
Absence of Other		
Respirations	No spontaneous respirations when removed from mechanical ventilation[a]	Required
Pupillary response	Fixed & fully dilated with direct light	Required
Hypothermia	Temperature > 90°F	Required
Drug screening	No CNS depressants or neuromuscular blockades (if present, blood flow must be determined)	Required
External stimuli	No response to noise, pain, the environment	Required
Spontaneous movement	No response to painful stimuli (spinal reflexes may be present)	Required
Cause of coma	Known	Required
Study Results:	*The following tests confirm brain death but are not required if the other criteria are present*	
Electroencephalogram	Flat; electrocerebral silence	Optional
Radionuclide blood flow scans	Absent	Optional
Carotid arteriography	Absent	Optional
Transcranial Dopplers	Absent	Optional

[a]See Apnea Testing in Clinical Examination for further explanation.

- No doll's eye response
- No response to iced water calorics
- No corneal reflex
- No gag reflex
- No cough reflex
- Apnea (see explanation of apnea testing)

Apnea testing is performed to determine if the patient has the ability to initiate respirations by increasing the patient's PCO_2 level. This testing should be approached with caution; thus, monitoring the patient's stability throughout the testing period is necessary. Prior to starting apnea testing the patient should be preoxygenated and the PCO_2 level normalized. Apnea testing includes the following procedure:

- Disconnect the ventilator and place the patient on passive O_2 via a cannula inserted down the endotracheal tube **or** by placing the patient's ventilator on continuous positive airway pressure (CPAP) mode to supply passive O_2 without giving the patient ventilatory support.
- Observe the patient for spontaneous breathing and monitor vital signs.
- After approximately 10 minutes, draw an arterial blood gas (ABG) and reconnect the ventilator **or** return ventilator mode to the previous settings.
- The patient is considered apneic if the PCO_2 is ≥ 60 mm Hg and there is no evidence of respiratory effort.
- If the patient becomes hypotensive and/or ventricular arrhythmias develop, immediately draw an ABG and place the patient back on the ventilator. If the PCO_2 is ≤ 60 mm Hg, consider other tests to confirm brain death.

Each institution's policy should outline perimeters of time requirements for clinical testing and if repetitious testing is required (i.e., two exams with a 12-hour period of observation between tests). All of the reflexes listed in the clinical exam must be absent; however spinal reflexes such as a Babinski reflex may be present. When spinal reflexes are present, it is important to distinguish these movements from reflex movement coming from the brain.

Cerebral Blood Flow

A cerebral blood flow study, such as a cerebral angiogram, cerebral nuclear flow study, or transcranial Doppler study, is required if the clinical exam cannot be performed, toxic CNS depression exists, or to expedite brain-death testing. An absence of cerebral blood flow confirms brain death. When this is found, no other testing or observation period needs to be utilized or determined.

Electroencephalogram

The EEG measures the electrical activity of the brain. There are two complicating factors in using the EEG for diagnosing brain death. First, it is unable to measure brain stem electrical activity; second, there is a potential problem with the EEG's picking up electrical activity from the machinery connected to the patient (i.e., IV pumps, ventilator, electrocardiographic [ECG] monitor). To assess for presence of brain stem activity, a clinical exam must also be performed.

Obtaining Consent

The UAGA outlines who can give consent for organ donation. The order of priority is spouse, adult child, either parent, adult sibling, either grandparent, guardian, or other. Many states recognize consent given if an organ donor card or driver's license is signed by the patient and legally witnessed by two individuals. However, due to public scrutiny many organ procurement organizations prefer to obtain consent from the legal next of kin.

When caring for a severely brain-injured patient, notification of the patient should be made to the OPO. Most OPOs request that a referral be made to them while the patient has minimal brain function remaining (i.e., Glasgow Coma Scale score ≤ 4). The major advantage of early notification is that the OPO can perform a preliminary evaluation to determine if the patient meets the criteria for donation. By allowing a preliminary evaluation, unsuitable patients can be identified and approaching the family about donation need not occur. It also allows the OPO coordinator to be present at the hospital when brain death is pronounced. This facilitates the coordinator's ability to be able to offer information to the family about their donation options.

It is often the critical care nurse who first identifies the patient as a potential donor, since the nature of the illnesses that proceed rapid deterioration requires management in the critical care environment. To facilitate evaluation of suitability, there are certain data that the nurse can obtain and have ready for the OPO to help them determine the patient's suitability (see Table 4–2).

TABLE 4-2. DONOR REFERRAL INITIAL NURSING DATABASE

- Age, gender
- Attending physician
- Cause of death
- Brain death declaration: Whether or not it has been established (if has been declared, give date and time)
- Height and weight
- Past medical, social, and surgical history
- Laboratory data (current)
  - Serum electrolytes, BUN and creatinine, creatinine clearance, osmolality, glucose
- Vital signs and functions (highest, lowest, average)
  - Heart rate; arterial blood pressure; mean arterial pressure
  - Temperature
  - Urine output (mL/hr)
- Current medications (drug names and doses)
- Whether or not consent has already been given and by whom

Determination of a Patient's Suitability for Donation

To be an organ donor several things must be considered to determine eligibility. Some of these factors are past medical history, past social history, and current hemodynamic stability/instability.

Past Medical /Social History

Illnesses and social behaviors affect the body's functions and influence the transmission of diseases. It is important for the transplant society to become aware of such diseases and/or behaviors in potential donors, to determine the risks posed to their recipients. Factors that will prevent a patient from becoming a donor include being positive for human immunodeficiency virus (HIV), acquired immune deficiency syndrome (AIDS), or active hepatitis B. Other factors that do not preclude donation but are approached with caution are sepsis, high-risk behavior for disease transmission (IV drug abuse, male-to-male sex, extended jail terms, hemophilia, and others), and a noncompliant health history. If the extent of a patient's medical and social history is not known, he or she should still be considered a potential donor. The donor program will always obtain a thorough medical/social history and review the patient's medical records if he or she desires donation.

Hemodynamic Stability/Instability

The donor organs must be well oxygenated and perfused to maintain adequate function in order to be transplanted. Common hemodynamic sequelae that occur in the brain-dead patient are diabetes insipidus, inability to control body temperature, neurogenic pulmonary edema, and initial hypertension (from catecholamine release) followed by hypotension (from inadequate catecholamine production). The goals of management are to maintain the potential donor within certain hemodynamic parameters to assure organ viability. However, failing to meet these parameters does not mean donation cannot occur. In addition, previous cardiac and respiratory arrest does not preclude donation.

Signing the Consent Form

Consent from the next of kin is sought even if the decedent has already indicated consent on a donor card. This is done to avoid any conflicts with the family who might disagree with the decedent's desire to donate. According to the UAGA, to be considered legal, the consent form must be signed by the next of kin and witnessed. If the next of kin cannot be present to sign for consent, a recorded consent can be obtained by the organ procurement coordinator. The determination of who must give consent is prioritized as specified earlier in this section.

Working with the Family

As outlined in the 1998 Medicare Conditions of Participation, only an OPO coordinator or an individual trained by the OPO should discuss donation with the family. Making an early referral to the OPO allows the coordinator an opportunity to be present at the hospital when the family is informed of the patient's death. According to the UAGA, the consent form must be signed by the legal next of kin along with the signature of two witnesses.

The UAGA stipulates that consent must be obtained from the legal next of kin during a very emotional event, the death of a loved one. A crucial part of the interaction with the family at this time is to first ensure that they understand and acknowledge the patient's death. If the family is not able to understand the patient's death, they may be unable to make rational decisions regarding donation. The OPO coordinator has extensive training on how to approach the family with sensitivity and care. When a potential brain-death patient is admitted to the hospital, family teaching must begin immediately. Families desire honest information that helps them understand their loved one's condition. When describing brain death, it is crucial for the family to hear that brain death means the patient is dead. When describing brain death to a family, it is important not to use conflicting terms (e.g., referring to the ventilator as "life-support" rather than "artifical support").

It is imperative that donation *not* be discussed with the family until they have heard and acknowledged the patient's death (decoupling). If donation is brought up early with a family, their perception of the care being given to their loved one seems focused on society's needs and not the needs of the patient or family. This can cause the family to be mistrustful of the nurses and medical team. Therefore, it is important not to talk about donation with the family prior to the patient's death being confirmed. Research has shown that correct timing in approaching the family about donation is crucial. A 1991 retrospective study examined the effects of decoupling on families being approached about organ donation (Garrison et al., 1991). Of 143 families studied, 65 percent approached after decoupling occurred consented to organ donation, whereas only 18 percent of those approached prior to decoupling consented.

The Sequence of Events

Once consent has been obtained, a process of extended evaluation takes place with each organ prior to matching the organ to a recipient. The OPO coordinator first ensures that the patient is hemodynamically stable. Blood samples are drawn for blood typing and serological testing for the presence of transmittable diseases. Food and Drug Administration (FDA) guidelines regulate that all donors be tested for the presence of HIV I and II, human T-lymphotropic virus (HTLV) I and II, hepatitis B antigen, hepatitis B core antibody, hepatitis C antibody, cytomegalovirus (CMV), and syphilis. If testing reveals a positive HIV, HTLV, or hepatitis B surface antigen (HBsAg), the donation must be terminated.

If the patient is hemodynamically stable, further evaluation continues. The heart is evaluated by echocardiogram, chest x-ray, and a 12-lead ECG. If the patient has risk for coronary artery disease or is 50 years of age or older, a cardiac catheterization may be performed. The lungs are evaluated by chest x-ray, sputum Gram stains, and a PO_2 level is drawn after administration of 100 percent O_2 for 15 minutes. If these findings indicate that the lungs are suitable for transplant, a bronchoscopy may be performed. The liver is evaluated by measuring liver enzymes and electrolytes. The kidneys are evaluated by monitoring blood urea nitrogen (BUN), serum creatinine, and urine output. The pancreas is evaluated by monitoring the glucose, amylase, and lipase.

Once blood typing is known, a list of recipients can be matched through the national computer center in Richmond, Virginia, at the United Network of Organ Sharing (UNOS). A computer-printed list of potential recipients is given to the coordinator to begin the search for an appropriate recipient. The recipient lists are matched to the donor through algorithms established by the transplant community. Each organ has a different algorithm designed to find the best recipient to the organ. The heart, lungs, and liver must match by blood type compatibility as well as be an appropriate size match. The kidney and pancreas matching includes blood type compatibility and human leukocyte antigen (HLA) matching.

In most cases, the designation of organs to a matching recipient takes place prior to taking the donor to the operating room. This allows the recipient time to arrive at his or her transplant hospital and be prepared for the transplant before the organ is removed from the donor. This decreases the amount of time the organ is outside of a body—the shorter the time the organ is outside of a body (cold ischemic time), the better the function of the organ after transplantation.

If the patient is hemodynamically unstable when consent is obtained, and cardiopulmonary arrest is imminent, the patient will immediately be taken to the OR for recovery of abdominal organs. Long-term hypotension and hemodynamic instability causes ischemic damage to the organs, making them unsuitable for transplant. This results in the need for immediate removal of the organs to maintain suitability. In the instance of rapid organ removal, thoracic organs can rarely be considered for transplant.

Once the organ–recipient matches have been found, a computer list is generated. The more urgent the need, the higher on the priority list the name will be. As soon as the decision is made as to who the organ recipient(s) will be, operating room times are coordinated by all teams involved. Transportation of the organ(s) from one location to another must be carefully planned. Organs will be transported by air if the recipient is out of state.

Non–Heart-Beating Organ Donation

When organ donation was first being attempted, artificial respiratory support by mechanical ventilators was not known. It was not until the 1980s that brain death was recognized as a type of death. With the advent of brain death, there was a shift in the transplant community to pursue organ donation only in the brain-dead patient, since organ perfusion could be maintained until the time of recovery. As the waiting list has continued to increase at a rate of 20 to 30 percent each year, and organ donation has remained constant, there is an increasing gap between the supply and demand of organs. Because of this widening gap, there has been a recent resurgence in pursuing non–heart-beating organ donation. For non–heart-beating organ donation to occur, an organ procurement coordinator or a trained hospital designee must be present when cardiac cessation occurs. The organs must undergo in situ cooling soon after cardiac death is pronounced, and organ recovery should occur in a short time period. Patient criteria vary in each institution and OPO regarding non–heart-beating organ donation.

In summary, organ procurement requires a carefully executed series of events. Identification of the potential brain-death patient and notification of the organ procurement agency is a crucial first step. This is followed by establishing the diagnosis of brain death in the potential donor. There are accepted medical standards for brain death, which are specific to each institutional policy and state law. Consent for organ donation is sought from the next of kin. The manner in which the family is approached in seeking permission is very important.

SECTION THREE REVIEW

1. A major advantage of early notification of the Organ Procurement Coordinator when a potential donor has been identified is that __________ can be initiated.

   A. family counseling
   B. life-support measures
   C. signing of the consent form
   D. preliminary evaluation for suitability

2. The topic of organ donation should not be initiated with the family until the
   A. patient has died
   B. family signs the consent form
   C. family acknowledges the patient's death
   D. family asks about possible donation
3. Assuming the potential donor has signed an organ donor card, which of the following statements is correct regarding obtaining consent?
   A. consent is usually obtained from the legal next of kin
   B. consent is not usually obtained from the legal next of kin
   C. consent cannot legally be obtained from the next of kin
   D. decedent's organ donor card takes precedence over next of kin's wishes
4. When apnea testing is performed on the patient, he or she is considered apneic if the PCO_2 is ______ mm Hg after _____ minutes.
   A. 50, 5
   B. 50, 10
   C. 60, 5
   D. 60, 10
5. Non–heart-beating organ donation has made a resurgence primarily due to
   A. improved evaluation criteria
   B. scarcity of resources
   C. better transplantation results
   D. family's wishes

Answers: 1. D, 2. C, 3. A, 4. D, 5. B

SECTION FOUR: Donor Management and Organ Preservation

At the completion of this section, the learner will be able to discuss donor and organ management.

Donor Management

There are five major management goals when caring for the donor patient who is awaiting organ removal (Thacker, 1999a).

Maintain Hemodynamic Stability

Adequate organ perfusion is crucial if the organs are to be successfully transplanted. The goals of hemodynamic management are to maintain a systolic blood pressure of 90 to 100 mm Hg with a urine output of 50 to 100 mL/hr. Most often, hypotension is caused by dehydration. Intake and output balance is essential. Dopamine or dobutamine, which are usually considered drugs of choice, may be ordered in small doses to maintain adequate blood pressure. Vasoconstrictive drugs, such as epinephrine and norepinephrine, should be avoided; however, they cause less damage to organs than is seen with long-term hypotension.

Maintain Optimal Oxygenation

The donor should be maintained on an oxygen concentration via the mechanical ventilator sufficient to maintain the PO_2 at > 100 mm Hg. The donor may be placed on 5 cm H_2O of positive end-expiratory pressure (PEEP) to further facilitate oxygenation. Normal pulmonary toilet procedures are continued, such as suctioning and turning every two hours.

Maintain Normothermia

The donor's temperature should be maintained between 96 and 100°F. If the temperature drops, a warming blanket should be used under the patient. To rewarm a patient whose temperature has dropped to less than 94°F, rewarming alternatives such as increasing the ventilator heater, covering the head, warm nasogastric lavage, and/or increasing the temperature in the room need to be considered.

Maintain Fluid and Electrolyte Balance

Fluids should be replaced as needed to prevent volume depletion. Routine monitoring of electrolytes is continued (every six hours and PRN) and depletions are replaced to maintain electrolyte balance. Urine output should be maintained above 50 mL/hr or a minimum of 1 mL/kg/hr. If the patient develops diabetes insipidus, vasopressin may be ordered to maintain the urine output between 100 and 200 mL/hr. The donor's urine output may be replaced mL/mL with IV fluids.

Prevent Infections

Sterile technique must be judiciously maintained. Potential sources of infection include the lungs via the endotracheal tube, and invasive treatments involving central lines and catheters.

Preservation of Organs

A single donor may provide one or multiple organs and tissues. At a prearranged time agreed on by all the transplant teams involved, the donor is taken to the operating room and prepared for surgery. When the donor is brought to the OR, he or she must have the correct documentation present: date and time of the death declaration and the signed or recorded consent form. In addition, the hospital may require a signed death certificate or other documentation. The procedures followed in the OR are similar to any other surgery. The anesthesiologist monitors and maintains the donor's cardiopulmonary and renal status and the fluid and electrolyte balance throughout the organ recovery period. There may be more than one organ recovery team in the OR, each team being responsible for recovering a particular organ or organ set. The donor's attending physician cannot be part of the recovery teams.

During the organ recovery surgery, the transplant surgeon(s) makes one incision from the suprasternal notch to the symphysis pubis. The surgeon inspects the donor for the presence of any unexpected disease such as an undiagnosed cancer, then begins the process of dissecting each organ from its surrounding anatomical structures. Once all of the organs are ready to be removed, cannulas are placed in the thoracic aorta, pulmonary artery, portal vein, and the abdominal aorta. A clamp is placed on the aorta and perfusion of the organs begins with a cold preservation solution. The solution runs through each organ, removing the blood from the organ. This procedure slows the organ metabolic rate and preserves it until the organ is transplanted. Once removed from the donor, the organ is packaged in the preservative solution and sterile triple bagged. It is then placed on ice and transported to the recipient's hospital. Table 4–3 lists the allowed cold ischemic time for each organ.

TABLE 4–3. COMMON ORGAN PRESERVATION TIMES

DONOR ORGAN	TIME OF PRESERVATION (HOURS)
Lung	4–6
Heart	4–6
Liver	12–24
Pancreas	12–24
Kidneys	24–60

Once the organs have been recovered, the transplant surgeon may elect to do further evaluative studies if a disease process is suspected in an organ (i.e., long-standing hypertension can lead to nondiagnosed renal insufficiency or impending renal failure). This is determined by biopsy of the organ.

In summary, management of the donor prior to organ recovery focuses on maintenance of a stable hemodynamic status, optimal oxygenation state, normothermia, fluid and electrolyte balance, and prevention of infection. An organ donor may donate one or multiple organs. Organ recovery is performed by surgical teams in an operating room. Organs require careful handling and special preservation techniques; and they are cooled to decrease metabolic processes.

SECTION FOUR REVIEW

1. Major management goals for caring for the donor patient include all of the following EXCEPT maintain
   A. stable hemodynamic status
   B. fluid and electrolyte balance
   C. infections at minimum level
   D. optimal oxygenation status
2. The most common underlying cause of hypotension in the donor is
   A. dehydration
   B. cardiac failure
   C. fluid overload
   D. increased systemic vascular resistance
3. Which of the following statements best reflects procedures related to organ recovery in the operating room?
   A. an anesthesiologist is not necessary
   B. the recipient's physician must be part of the recovery team
   C. only one organ recovery team can be present in the operating room
   D. the donor's physician is not part of the recovery team
4. The organ preservation method that is common to all organs is
   A. hypothermia
   B. concentration of electrolytes
   C. type of diuretic
   D. preservation formula

Answers: 1. C, 2. A, 3. D, 4. A

THE ORGAN RECIPIENT

SECTION FIVE: Immunologic Considerations

At the completion of this section, the learner will be able to explain the immunologic considerations of organ transplantation.

Histocompatibility

The term **histocompatibility** comes from the Greek word *histos*, meaning tissue, and the Latin word *compati*, meaning to sympathize with. Histocompatibility, then, refers to the ability of cells and tissues to live without interference from the immune system. In Section One, it was noted that historically, histocompatibility problems lead to rapid tissue or organ rejection, thereby limiting successful long-term transplant results to those performed between identical twins. Why is histocompatibility so important in transplantation?

Sommers (1998) explains that major histocompatibility complexes (MHC) are special key molecules that allow the body to be able to distinguish self from nonself. In humans, MHC molecules are known as *human leukocyte antigens* (HLA). **Antigens** are defined as substances that are capable of eliciting the immune response. Antigens can be composed of foreign materials or they can exist as normal cellular components (such as MHC). HLA antigens are proteins found on chromosome six. They exist in pairs (called *haplotypes*) on the surface of cells and are genetically determined. MHC molecules that are involved in intracellular communication for self-recognition are classified into two groups, called MHC I (or class I antigens) and MCH II (or class II antigens).

MHC I (Class I Antigens)

The MHC I proteins have been labeled HLA-A, HLA-B, and HLA-C. They are found on the surface of essentially all nucleated cells (Sommers, 1998).

MHC (Class II Antigens)

The MHC II proteins have been labeled HLA-DR, HLA-DP, and HLA-DQ. They are primarily found on the cell surfaces of macrophages, and B lymphocytes (Sommers, 1998).

The HLA antigens in the MHC I and II classes help the immune system distinguish self from nonself, functioning somewhat like "fingerprints" that are unique to the individual. Normally, the immune system is able to recognize its own HLA "fingerprint" as self, and the immune response is not triggered. HLA antigens are inherited; thus, each full sibling in a family will have some combination of HLA inherited from both biologic parents. The closer the HLA antigen combination matches between two people, the more the "fingerprint" is recognized as self.

A multitude of combinations of pairings can occur; thus, complete HLA matching is virtually impossible with the exception of identical twins. Since full siblings share the same biologic parents, they often have some degree of HLA matching. In contrast, cadaver organs are completely unmatched when chosen randomly for a **recipient.** For this reason, immediate family members most often make the best kidney transplant donors since they are more likely to have a better matched tissue type. Identical twins, however, have the same histocompatibility pairings and are, therefore, perfect HLA matches. In the case of identical twins, a transplanted tissue or organ is recognized as having a self-HLA fingerprint and is accepted into the recipient without an immune assault. (For more detailed information on histocompatibility antigens, the reader is referred to Module 22.)

Donor–Recipient Compatibility Testing

Three common tests used to evaluate the compatibility of the donor's tissues to the recipient's are tissue typing, crossmatching, and ABO typing.

Tissue Typing

Tissue typing refers to the identification of the HLA (histocompatibility) antigens of both the donor and the recipient. It evaluates the degree to which the two sets of tissues are HLA matched. The closer the HLA match is between the donor and the recipient, the better chance for long-term transplant success. The opposite is true, as well.

Crossmatching

Crossmatching tests the potential recipient for antidonor (preformed) antibodies. When such preformed antibodies are present, the patient is referred to as presensitized. Histocompatibility can be tested by evaluating the degree of reactivity of the immune response to crossmatch testing of donor and recipient cells and serum. When a serum crossmatching is performed, a sample of the recipient's serum is subjected to the serum of a sample of the prospective donor's blood. The serum is analyzed for the formation of antidonor antibodies. A recipient can become sensitized to foreign HLA antigens through prior organ transplantation, blood transfusions, or pregnancy. In such cases, the reintroduction of a new organ containing the sensitized HLA antigens can cause rapid organ rejection and possibly death.

ABO Typing

ABO typing identifies the blood group of the donor and the recipient. ABO compatibility is an initial criteria for transplantation. The rules for blood type matching are the same as for transfusions: Unmatched protein types will cause a rapid immune reaction. The type O allograft is considered the universal transplant donor type since it can be safely transplanted into a recipient with any blood type. Type AB is considered to be the universal organ recipient since it can receive an allograft from all blood types. Types A and B can only receive an allograft from their own blood type or type O donors. Table 4–4 summarizes ABO compatibility.

TABLE 4–4. ORGAN DONOR AND RECIPIENT ABO COMPATIBILITY

RECIPIENT'S BLOOD TYPE	COMPATIBLE POTENTIAL DONOR'S BLOOD TYPE
A	A or O
B	B or O
AB (universal recipient)	A, B, or O
O	O only

In summary, histocompatibility is the ability of cells and tissues to live without interference from the immune system. HLA antigens are histocompatibility antigens found on the sixth chromosome. There are two classes of HLA antigens that are involved in self-recognition, and therefore of interest to organ transplantation. HLA antigens are inherited, with a multitude of possible pairing combinations. Identical twins have the same HLA pairings; thus, they can donate and receive each other's organs without rejection problems. To assure the best histocompatible match, donor–recipient compatibility testing is performed. Three tests are usually performed, including tissue typing, crossmatching, and ABO typing.

SECTION FIVE REVIEW

1. Histocompatibility antigens are also known as
   A. monocytes
   B. macrophages
   C. human leukocyte antigens
   D. polymorphonuclear lymphocytes
2. HLA antigens are located on (in) the cell
   A. surfaces
   B. nucleus
   C. cytoplasm
   D. mitochondria
3. The best histocompatibility matching is found between
   A. siblings
   B. identical twins
   C. parent and child
   D. fraternal twins
4. The identification of the histocompatibility antigens of both the donor and the recipient is called
   A. crossmatching
   B. ABO typing
   C. antigen classifying
   D. tissue typing
5. A recipient can become sensitized to foreign HLA antigens through all of the following ways EXCEPT
   A. pregnancy
   B. donating blood
   C. prior organ transplantation
   D. receiving blood transfusions

Answers: 1. C, 2. A, 3. B, 4. D, 5. B

SECTION SIX: Determination of Transplant Need

At the completion of this section, the learner will be able to describe the determination of transplant need.

Scarcity of organ resources and the physical and financial costs involved make determination of transplant need a major issue. In January 2000, there were almost 67,000 patients on the waiting list for transplants (UNOS, 2000a). Transplant surgery can cost between $60,000 and $250,000 or more. The cost of antirejection and other necessary drugs can exceed $8,500 per year (UNOS, 2000a). The choice of who will receive an organ is not a simple one. Hundreds or possibly thousands of patients are on the national waiting list for the same organ at any one time. Organs are allocated to recipients based on a point system established by UNOS.

Determination of Need

The criteria used for determination of need are multifocused. Specific guidelines vary between transplant programs but the general guidelines are fairly consistent and include end-stage organ failure, short life expectancy, severe functional disability, no additional serious health problems, and psychological readiness.

End-stage organ disease is the primary indicator for transplantation need and is established by evaluation of organ function. The short life expectancy criterion is generally considered 6 to 12 months. Measurement of functional disability evaluates the potential recipient's ability to lead a reasonable lifestyle (e.g., ability to work or perform activities of daily living). This can be evaluated through interviewing the patient and family, observation, and cardiopulmonary exercise testing. Psychological readiness is established through interviewing, known history, and possible psychological testing. Due to the highly stressful nature of transplantation, the presence of additional serious medical problems increases the risk of postoperative complications and is associated with a higher mortality rate.

Transplant Recipient Evaluation

The patient is considered as a potential transplant candidate only after maximum medical therapy has become ineffective, leaving transplantation as the final option. Evaluation of the potential recipient is an extensive process. Many factors must be thoroughly evaluated prior to placing the patient on the UNOS national patient waiting list for organ transplantation. These factors usually include the potential recipient's clinical, psychological, and financial status.

Clinical Status

Organ-specific diagnostic studies and laboratory testing are conducted; preexisting or concurrent medical problems (risk factors for transplantation) are closely scrutinized and discussed with the patient and family. Table 4–5 summarizes the common major studies and tests for organ transplantation preparation.

Psychological Status

Chronic illness and its treatment are known to have profound long-term psychological effects on the patient and family. These psychological effects may have an impact on the long-term success of the transplant. In addition, the stresses associated with organ transplantation can further strain the coping abilities of this population. For these reasons, the potential organ recipient, and possibly the family, will undergo a psychological evaluation. If problems are assessed, appropriate counseling is initiated.

Financial Status

The total cost of organ transplantation varies with the organ being grafted. Costs that are factored in include pretransplantation evaluation, interim transplantation, and posttransplantation care. Medicare, state medical programs, and private health insurance coverage vary widely. Coverage is often differentiated by the type of organ being transplanted. If financial resources are questionable, financial options are explored.

Once the decision is made to accept a patient as a suitable recipient, the patient's name and vital information are entered into the computer bank at the United Network for Organ Sharing (UNOS, 2000a). This organization is charged with distributing organs in an equitable and nondiscriminatory manner. The potential recipient remains on the UNOS organ waiting list until an organ becomes available.

In summary, scarcity of donor organs and the transplantation costs make determination of transplantation need a crucial issue. General guidelines to establish need include end-stage organ disease, short life expectancy, and functional disability. A person is considered for organ transplantation only after receiving maximum medical therapy. A potential recipient is evaluated in regard to clinical, psychological, and financial status. Once need and eligibility have been established, the potential recipient's vital information is entered onto the UNOS national organ transplant waiting list.

TABLE 4–5. COMMON ORGAN EVALUATION STUDIES AND TESTS

ORGAN	STUDIES/TESTS
All organs	**Immune Specific**
	ABO, HLA tissue typing, presensitization, crossmatching, HIV profile
	General
	Complete blood count with differential, blood chemistries, coagulation studies, urinalysis
	Cardiovascular
	ECG, echocardiogram
	Radiographic
	Chest x-ray
	Other
	Blood typing and crossmatching, examination and testing for infection (e.g., culturing of blood, urine, etc.); viral titers; possible multiple organ function studies
Kidneys	**Radiographic**
	Gastrointestinal x-rays, abdominal ultrasound, voiding cystourethrogram
Heart, heart–lung, and lung	**Cardiovascular**
	Endomyocardial biopsy (to rule out myocarditis and sarcoidosis)
	Pulmonary
	Arterial blood gas, chest x-ray, pulmonary function testing, ventilation/perfusion scan, computed tomographic (CT) scan of chest, exercise testing
	Other
	Echocardiogram; Doppler study; legs duplex scan; cardiac catheterization
Liver	**Laboratory Tests**
	Liver function tests
	Other
	Portal vein sonogram and Doppler, abdominal CT scan, liver biopsy

Data from Blanford, N.L. (1993). Renal transplantation: A case study of the ideal. Crit Care Nurse *13(1):46–57; Williams, B.A., & Sandiford-Guttenbeil, D.M. (1991). In B.A. Williams, K.L. Grady, D.M. Sandiford-Guttenbeil (eds.),* Organ transplantation: A manual for nurses *(pp. 129–164), New York: Springer Publishing Co.; Staschak, S., & Zamberlan K. (1990). Liver transplantation: Nursing diagnoses and management. In K.M. Sigardson-Poor & L.M. Haggerty (eds.).* Nursing care of the transplant recipient *(pp. 140–179). Philadelphia: W.B. Saunders; Haggerty, L.M., & Sigardson-Poor, K.M. (1990). Kidney transplantation. In K.M. Sigardson-Poor & L.M. Haggerty (eds.),* Nursing care of the transplant recipient *(pp. 114–139). Philadelphia: W.B. Saunders; and Augustine, S.M., & Masiello-Miller, M. (1995). Heart transplantation. In M.T. Nolan & S.M. Augustine (eds.).* Transplantation nursing: Acute and long-term management *(pp. 109–140). Norwalk, CT: Appleton & Lange.*

Section Six Review

1. General guidelines for determination of organ transplant need include all of the following EXCEPT
   A. severe functional disability
   B. end-stage organ failure
   C. psychological readiness
   D. additional serious health problems
2. The decision of whether or not a person is placed on the organ transplant waiting list as a potential recipient is usually made by
   A. the patient/family
   B. a multidisciplinary committee
   C. the organ procurement team
   D. the potential recipient's physician
3. The determination of end-stage organ disease is primarily based on which of the following criteria?
   A. tissue biopsy
   B. patient history
   C. functional disability
   D. age/gender
4. A potential transplant recipient has his or her psychological status thoroughly assessed because
   A. there is a risk of posttransplant psychosis
   B. a depressed state is a major contraindication for transplantation
   C. there is a higher mortality associated with psychological distress
   D. stress associated with transplantation strains coping abilities

Answers: 1. D, 2. B, 3. A, 4. D

SECTION SEVEN: Posttransplantation Complications

At the completion of this section, the learner will be able to discuss the major complications associated with organ transplantation.

Although each type of organ transplant has many unique features, certain aspects have commonalities; this is true also of organ transplant complications. Three major types of complications are associated with transplantation:

- Technical
- Graft rejection
- Immunosuppressant related

Technical Complications

The technical procedures involved in performing the transplantation are not without risks. Three major groups of technical complications are associated with the surgical procedure: vascular thrombosis, bleeding, and anastomosis leakage.

Vascular Thrombosis

Vascular thrombosis is a fairly rare complication that usually develops during the early postoperative period. It refers to the development of a blood clot in the vascular system. As a complication of organ transplantation, it refers to a blood clot in the vasculature of the graft, often the major artery. The presence of a thrombosis may not be detected initially, as the patient is frequently asymptomatic. Diagnostic tests may be performed soon after surgery (e.g., duplex ultrasonography) to assure arterial patency. Early detection and immediate thrombectomy are essential if the graft is to survive. Even then, the graft is at high risk for failure. Any delay in detection of thrombosis frequently leads to loss of the graft.

Bleeding

Postoperative transplantation bleeding is managed in a fashion similar to other postsurgery patients, with the exception of liver transplants. In the liver transplant patient, it is often difficult to differentiate bleeding that is secondary to coagulopathy associated with a dysfunctional liver from bleeding that has resulted from a surgical (technical) problem. Postoperatively, a transplanted liver may have some degree of coagulopathy present, which makes control of otherwise normal postoperative bleeding extremely difficult. The decision must be made as to whether to allow bleeding to continue until the coagulopathy resolves as liver function returns, or whether to take the patient for exploratory surgery immediately under the assumption that the cause is surgical.

Anastomosis Leakage

The term **anastomosis** refers to the site at which the graft is sutured into the recipient. Problems at the anastomosis site usually occur one to three weeks following transplantation. The problem may be failure of the anastomosis to seal completely, usually at the epithelial layer, which results in leakage of fluids (e.g., urine following a postrenal graft, or air as in bronchial dehiscence). The leak results from inadequate healing, possibly due to a deficient blood supply or steroid therapy. Anastomosis leaks usually require surgical exploration and repair.

Graft Rejection

Graft rejection refers to the activation of the immune response against a transplanted tissue or organ. It is the result of the body recognizing the new tissue as nonself, which then triggers an immune system attack to eliminate the invader. Graft rejection is primarily due to T lymphocyte and B lymphocyte activities. There are three types of graft rejection.

Acute Rejection

Acute rejection is characterized by a sudden onset and usually occurs within days or months following the transplant. Acute rejection begins as a type IV hypersensitivity response; that is, it is a cell-mediated immune response in which the T lymphocytes and macrophages of the host attack and destroy the graft tissue. The graft's HLA antigens are recognized as foreign (nonself), thereby triggering T lymphocyte proliferation and attack. As the acute rejection continues, graft-specific cytotoxic antibodies are produced, which further aggravate the acute rejection process.

Hyperacute Rejection

Hyperacute rejection is a type III (Arthus) hypersensitivity response; that is, it is a humoral response in which the B lymphocytes are activated to produce antibodies. It occurs within minutes to hours following transplantation and results from the presence of preformed graft-specific cytotoxic antibodies. Since the antibodies are already formed, as soon as the graft is placed, the immune system recognizes the foreign tissue and increases graft-specific antibody production. In turn, the antibodies accumulate rapidly and trigger agglutination of platelets, activation of the complement system, and phagocytic activities. Fortunately, hyperacute rejection is now rare due to improved donor–recipient screening and matching procedures.

Chronic Rejection

Chronic rejection is a humoral immune response in which antibodies slowly attack the graft. Chronic rejection may begin at any time following transplantation and may take years to render the graft nonfunctional. The antibodies trigger the same immune response as seen with hyperacute rejection but at a very low level. In time, the organ becomes ischemic and dies.

Immunosuppressant-Related Problems

Immunosuppressants are the cornerstone to successful long-term transplantation. This group of drugs, however, is associated with side effects that can cause serious problems, such as infection, organ dysfunction, malignancy, and steroid-induced problems such as hyperglycemia.

Infection

Infection is a major posttransplantation problem since each type of immunosuppressant therapy manipulates the immune system in some way. Infection is a leading cause of death in posttransplantation patients. Common sources of infection include invasive tubes (e.g., indwelling catheters), pneumonia, abscesses, and wound infections. Treatment of the infections with repeated runs of antibiotics may precipitate a superinfection (e.g., *Clostridium difficile* or *Candida*) or development of a resistant strain of bacteria. There is a particular risk for development of cytomegalovirus (CMV) infection (Thelan et al., 1998). The CMV may have already been present in the recipient or it may have been introduced in conjunction with the transplant. CMV-seropositive patients may develop reactivation of the virus owing to their immunosuppressed state. CMV infections may be mild or severe. A severe CMV infection can potentially cause dysfunction of multiple organs. This is especially a problem in seronegative recipients who received a seropositive organ or CMV-positive blood products. In addition, the recipient is at increased risk for development of opportunistic infections such as fungus (e.g., *Aspergillus*).

The immunosuppressed patient is unable to muster the same response to acute infection as a person who is immunocompetent; therefore, infection presents itself in more subtle ways. The primary symptom of infection is a fever greater than 38°C (100.4°F) (Thelan et al., 1998). Other assessments may include tachypnea, fatigue, tachycardia, and pain. Development of a fever requires a rapid but thorough search for the source of the infection and aggressive treatment. The lungs and urinary tract are the most common sources of nosocomial infection.

Organ Dysfunction

Almost all solid organ transplant patients receive a similar regimen of immunosuppressant therapy. Immunosuppressants are associated with multiple side effects, many of which target specific organs. Some degree of graft dysfunction is common immediately following organ transplantation. Development of nephrotoxicity and hepatotoxicity can occur with any organ transplant but are considered especially serious in kidney and liver transplants, respectively. The combination of the adverse effects of the drug and postgraft dysfunction may precipitate a severe graft crisis. Immunosuppressant therapy is discussed in Section Eight.

Malignancy

Patients on long-term immunosuppressant therapy are at increased risk for development of some form of malignancy. Malignancies that have been associated with organ transplantation include non-Hodgkin and other lymphomas, Kaposi's sarcoma, hepatobiliary and renal malignancies, skin tumors, and others. For example, Bartucci (1999) states that about 5 percent of renal transplant patients develop a malignant disease, which is about 100 times higher than is found in the general population.

Steroid-Induced Problems
Long-term steroid therapy carries with it multiple potentially serious side effects. For example, steroid-induced hyperglycemia and significant weight gain are both common problems. Steroid therapy is discussed further in Section Eight.

In summary, three general types of complications are associated with solid organ transplantation; technical, organ rejection, and immunosuppressant-related problems. Technical complications include vascular thrombosis, bleeding, and anastomosis leakage. Organ rejection is due to T and B lymphocyte activities acting against the graft. There are three types of rejection: acute, hyperacute, and chronic. Immunosuppressant-related problems include infection, organ dysfunction, malignancy, and steroid-induced problems. Certain immunosuppressive agents have the potential of exacerbating organ dysfunction.

Section Seven Review

1. All of the following are examples of technical complications of organ transplantation EXCEPT
   A. bleeding
   B. infection
   C. anastomosis leakage
   D. vascular thrombosis
2. Organ rejection that takes place within minutes to hours following transplantation and results from the presence of preformed graft-specific cytotoxic antibodies is called _________ rejection.
   A. subacute
   B. acute
   C. hyperacute
   D. chronic
3. Posttransplantation patients are at particular risk for developing a(n) _________ infection either from being seropositive prior to the transplant or by receiving a seropositive organ or blood transfusion.
   A. hepatitis A
   B. pneumonia
   C. cytomegalovirus
   D. wound
4. Posttransplant patients are at increased risk for development of malignancies secondary to _________.
   A. organ toxicity
   B. preexisting conditions
   C. underlying tissue incompatibility
   D. prolonged immunosuppressant therapy

Answers: 1. B, 2. C, 3. C, 4. D

SECTION EIGHT: Immunosuppressant Therapy

At the completion of this section, the learner will be able to describe immunosuppressant therapy.

The long-term success of organ transplantation has been made possible by use of immunosuppressant therapy. Prior to the discovery and refinement of immunosuppressant therapy, tissue transplantation was considered only a very short-term therapy with the exception of identical twin grafts. This section presents an overview of some of the major drugs or drug groups that are administered for their ability to alter immune function.

Cyclosporine

Cyclosporine (CyA or CsA), a unique drug of fungal origin, is the major immunosuppressant agent for prevention of allograft rejection. Cyclosporine's powerful immunosuppressant activities are directed against the helper T cells without affecting other types of immune cells such as macrophages, B cells, granulocytes, and suppressor T cells. The high degree of specificity of cyclosporine allows the immune system to maintain some degree of protection from infection, especially bacterial infections. According to Barbuto, Akporiaye, and Hersh (1998), cyclosporine may be used as sole or combination therapy in prevention of rejection. It is also an effective agent in treating graft-versus-host syndrome. Cyclosporine acts, in part, by blocking the production of interleukin-2 and -3 (IL-2, IL-3). It is associated with multiple serious side effects, including hepatotoxicity, nephrotoxicity, neurotoxicity, hyperglycemia, hirsutism, and gingival hyperplasia (Bush, 1999). Two formulations of cyclosporine are Sandimmune and Neoral.

Corticosteroids

Corticosteroids are steroid hormones. Prednisone is a synthetic corticosteroid that is commonly used as adjunct immunosuppressant therapy following organ transplantation. Corticosteroids have both anti-inflammatory and immunosuppressant capabilities. In the posttransplant patient, corticosteroids are administered primarily for their immunosuppressant activities. They significantly decrease the number of lymphocytes, particularly T lymphocytes, by interfering with the production and secretion of interleukin-2. In addition, large doses of corticosteroids suppress B lymphocyte production, particularly immunoglobulin G (IgG) and IgA, and significantly impair monocyte–macrophage function. Steroid therapy is useful for prevention of rejection and is used in rescue therapy for organ rejection; however, long-term use is associated with severe bone disorders.

Antimetabolites

Antimetabolites, or **cytotoxic agents**, are drugs that have the capability of destroying target cells. Certain drugs target immunocompetent cells and thus are of use as immunosuppressants. Two commonly used cell cycle-specific cytotoxic agents are azathioprine and mycophenolate.

Azathioprine

Before the introduction of cyclosporine, azathioprine (AZA) was the drug of choice for prevention of graft rejection. Now, it is frequently used as part of combination immunosuppressant therapy, or it is sometimes used as a back-up immunosuppressant when a patient becomes toxic on cyclosporine. Azathioprine is a derivative of 6-mercaptopurine. It inhibits DNA and RNA synthesis, which ultimately causes suppression of cell-mediated immunity. Azathioprine primarily targets T lymphocytes but has some effect on B cells and therefore exerts a degree of inhibition on the humoral immune response. Its action is not specific to lymphocytes and can also inhibit proliferation of all blood cell lines; therefore, the patient can develop anemia and thrombocytopenia, as well as leukopenia. A common product name for azathioprine is Imuran.

Mycophenolate Mofetil

A newer drug than azathioprine, mycophenolate (MMF) is a less toxic alternative to AZA therapy. According to Bush (1999), MMF is produced from penicillin mold. It interferes with cell proliferation by inhibiting DNA and RNA synthesis. B and T cell lymphocytes are targeted. MMF has been shown to be more effective than azathioprine in preventing acute rejection and is effective in rejection rescue therapy. The primary side effects of MMF are gastrointestinal, such as nausea and diarrhea. It also causes inhibition of all blood cell lines, causing anemia, thrombocytopenia, and leukopenia. A common product name for mycophenolate is CellCept.

Antibodies

Several preparations have been produced specifically as antilymphocyte antibodies. There are two major antibody preparations: monoclonal and polyclonal antibodies. Both types of antibodies are formed from foreign proteins that may cause antibodies to form against them, resulting in sensitization of the patient and possible development of serum sickness or anaphylactic reactions (Barbuto, Akporiaye, & Hersh, 1999). Monoclonal and polyclonal antibodies cannot be used as repeated therapy in sensitive individuals (Thelan et al., 1998).

Monoclonal Antibodies

Monoclonal antibodies were developed, in part, to increase the specificity of attack by targeting the lymphocyte subsets responsible for the immune rejection reaction. Ideally, this would allow the majority of the immune system to remain intact. Muromonab-CD3 (OKT3), a murine antihuman-CD3 monoclonal antibody, is the primary agent currently in use. It specifically targets a surface antigen (T3) located on mature T lymphocytes. OKT3 forms antibody–antigen complexes, which renders the T3 nonfunctioning. OKT3 is primarily used to treat a severe graft rejection episode but may be used to induce immunosuppressive therapy following the transplant (Bush, 1999).

Polyclonal Antibodies

Polyclonal antibodies, such as antithymocyte globulin (ATG) or antilymphocyte globulin (ALG), are usually produced by immunizing animals with human lymphocytes or thymocytes. If cells from the thymus gland are used, the resulting preparation is called "antithymocyte serum," which is used to produce ATG. If cells from human lymphocytes are used, the resulting serum preparation is called "antilymphocyte serum" and the antibody is ALG. Polyclonal antibodies particularly target T lymphocytes and are used primarily for treatment of graft rejection, but can be used prophylactically in the immediate posttransplant period.

Cytokine-Release Syndrome (CRS)

Cytokine-release syndrome (CRS) is a reaction that is particularly associated with initiation of monoclonal antibody therapy. When first described, it was called "first-dose response" since it typically develops within the first hour following the initial dose of OKT3. CRS is caused by the release of cytokines following an initial activation of T lymphocytes (Bush, 1999). Cytokines are cell mediators that are responsible for cell function and growth regulation.

CRS can be mild or life threatening. Severe flulike symptoms are the most common, such as chills, fever, and headache (Bush, 1999). Additional symptoms may include nausea, vomiting, and diarrhea. CRS symptoms usually diminish with each day of treatment. Severe symptoms are rare and may include pulmonary edema, hypotension, neurotoxicity, nephrotoxicity, and thrombosis. Premedication with diphenhydramine, methylprednisolone, and acetaminophen is usually given 30 minutes prior to OKT3 administration. Symptoms typically disappear after two to three days of therapy.

Tacrolimus (FK 506)

Tacrolimus is classified as an immunosuppressive antibiotic. Although it is unrelated to cyclosporine, it acts in a similar fashion in its attack on helper T lymphocytes. Tacrolimus has a potency that is up to 100 times stronger than cyclosporine in its immunosuppressant capabilities (Barbuto, Akporiaye, & Hersh, 1999). It has been used in human trials since 1989 and evidence is increasing that it is an effective immunosuppressant for a variety of organ transplants.

In summary, immunosuppressant therapy is the major reason for long-term graft success. Immunosuppressants may inhibit T cell or B cell function, or both. A newer group of drugs, monoclonal antibodies, exerts their immunosuppressant attack very specifically, thus leaving more of the immune system intact. Currently, monoclonal antibodies are used for short-term therapy. CRS is a potentially serious phenomenon that is particularly associated with monoclonal antibody therapy. Symptoms usually disappear within several days of therapy. Tacrolimus, a relatively new antibiotic, shows promise as a major powerful immunosuppressant with actions similar to cyclosporine.

Section Eight Review

1. The immunosuppressant that selectively acts against the helper T cells without affecting other types of immune cells is
   A. corticosteroids
   B. azathioprine
   C. cyclosporine
   D. OKT3
2. Long-term posttransplantation steroid therapy is particularly associated with potentially severe _________ disorders.
   A. heart
   B. bone
   C. liver
   D. blood
3. The major gastrointestinal side effect common to almost all immunosuppressant drugs is
   A. nausea and vomiting
   B. heartburn
   C. abdominal cramping
   D. constipation
4. Monoclonal antibodies are unique in that they target
   A. B cells
   B. helper T lymphocytes
   C. suppressor T lymphocytes
   D. specific lymphocyte subsets
5. The MOST common symptoms associated with CRS include which of the following?
   A. chills
   B. vomiting
   C. diarrhea
   D. hypotension

Answers: 1. C, 2. B, 3. A, 4. D, 5. A

SECTION NINE: Overview of Selected Organ Transplantation

At the completion of this section, the learner will be able to discuss the general concepts related to transplantation of selected organs, including postprocedure management implications.

This section presents a brief overview of selected solid organ transplants, including kidney, heart (heart–lung), lung, and liver. Postprocedure management and evaluation of organ function are also discussed.

Kidney Transplantation

Kidney transplants have been in the literature since the early 1930s, when a kidney was transplanted into the thigh of a young woman in Russia. Today, kidney transplants are a highly successful mode of therapy. A diagnosis of end-stage renal disease (ESRD) does not necessitate renal transplantation since dialysis can be used as an alternative therapy for ESRD. A patient who is being considered for transplantation is carefully screened to determine whether the probability of a successful transplant is sufficient to warrant transplantation rather than continuing use of dialysis. When a renal transplant is successful, it is significantly less costly than long-term dialysis therapy.

Major Indications for Transplantation

ESRD is the primary indicator for a renal transplant. ESRD can result from many problems, of which hypertension, diabetes mellitus, and glomerulonephritis are the three most common (Bartucci, 1999). These three conditions comprise more than half of all causes of ESRD. As of January 2000, there were nearly 44,000 patients on the national waiting list for renal transplants (UNOS, 2000a).

Preparation of the Recipient

When a kidney becomes available, the recipient is admitted to the hospital and pretransplant orders are initiated. Admission may be the day before a scheduled surgery if there is a living donor. If a cadaver donor is made available, preparatory time is much shorter. Upon notification, the patient is admitted to the transplant center, with surgery rapidly following the admission. Preoperative hemodialysis is often performed to normalize fluid and electrolyte balance. Before the patient goes to surgery, crossmatching is performed. If the results are negative, an initial dose of an immunosuppressant and prophylactic antibiotics are administered either before or after the patient is transferred to the operating room. Figure 4–1 provides an illustration of a renal transplant

Postoperative Management

Following transplantation, the patient is monitored closely for the first 24 hours, often in an intensive care setting. Medical and nursing priorities depend on the level of graft function and development of any complications. Typical postoperative orders for the first 24 hours include:

- IV fluids at a rate sufficient to keep urine output over 100 mL/hr; rate may also be titrated based on hourly urine outputs
- Diuretic therapy
- Careful monitoring of intake and output balance with hourly urine output
- Close monitoring for blood clots, which can obstruct the urinary catheter
- Daily weights
- Vital signs and central venous pressure readings
- Monitoring for signs and symptoms of fluid volume excess
- Close monitoring of laboratory values: serum creatinine trends, electrolytes (particularly potassium, sodium, bicarbonate, calcium, and phosphorous), hemoglobin and hematocrit, serum glucose, and blood urea nitrogen (BUN)
- Prophylactic antibiotic therapy
- Monitoring for signs and symptoms of acute infection

Graft dysfunction is more commonly noted in cadaver grafts than in live ones. In the cadaver transplant, organ ischemia is more likely due to the increased length of time the organ was preserved. Renal ischemia may lead to acute tubular necrosis, which causes oliguria or anuria. If the dysfunction lasts more than 48 hours, hemodialysis may be necessary until the graft begins functioning sufficiently. Recovery of the graft takes approximately two weeks.

Hypertension is a common problem in the kidney transplant patient (about 70 percent) (Bartucci, 1999). This condition can be exacerbated during the postoperative recovery period due to fluid volume imbalances precipitated by the high volume of IV fluids used to maintain a high urine flow. Antihypertensive agents may be ordered preoperatively and postoperatively to maintain the blood pressure within an acceptable range for the patient.

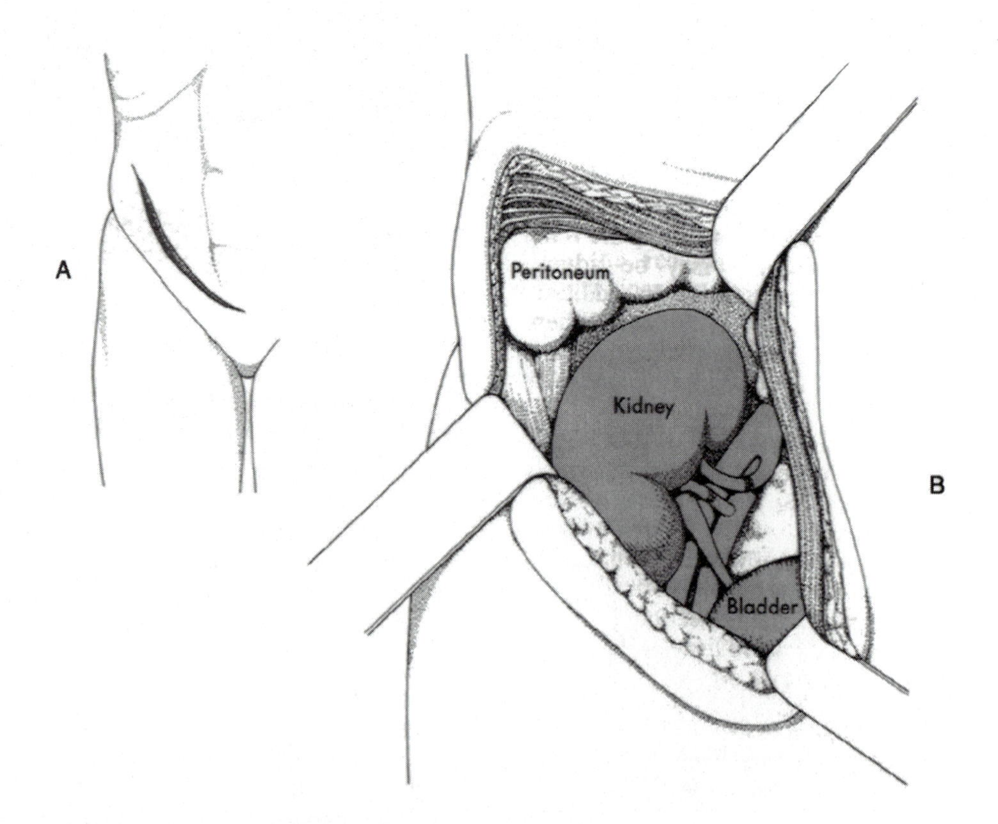

Figure 4–1. Placement of the renal graft into iliac fossa. **A.** The incision is depicted for the right side of the abdomen, representing graft implantation in the right iliac fossa. **B.** The iliac vessels are exposed. *(From Smith, S. L. [1990].* Tissue and organ transplantation: Implications for professional nursing practice *[p. 190]. St. Louis: Mosby Year Book.)*

Evaluation of Renal Function

In addition to laboratory tests, several other procedures can be performed to evaluate function of the renal graft. A needle biopsy using ultrasound is performed to examine renal tissue. This is considered to be the most valuable indicator of renal function. Ultrasound of the kidney may be ordered to look for hydronephrosis, obstruction, or collections of fluid. A renal scan using radioactive isotopes also evaluates renal function.

Post Renal Transplant Complications

General complications associated with organ transplantation are presented in Section Seven. The one-year graft survival rate for cadaver renal transplants is about 83 percent, and for living-donor transplants the graft survival rate is about 97 percent (UNOS, 2000b). The most common long-term complication of renal transplantation is graft rejection.

Heart, Heart–Lung, and Lung Transplantation

Dr. Christiaan Barnard performed the first heart transplant in 1967 in South Africa (Augustine & Masiello-Miller, 1995). The first single-lung transplant was performed by Hardy in 1963, and the first successful heart–lung transplant was performed at Stanford University in 1981 (Owens & Wallop, 1995). The early history of heart, lung, and heart–lung transplants was one of poor graft success rates. Organ rejection, inadequate healing, and infection were major obstacles to success. It was not until the late 1970s (heart) and early 1980s (lung and heart–lung) that technical and immunosuppressant therapy improvements made these transplants a successful surgical option. The introduction of the immunosuppressant cyclosporine played a major role in eventual success of these transplants.

Major Indications for Transplantation

General criteria for determination of transplant need were presented in Section Six. Specific major conditions that are associated with heart, lung, or heart–lung transplantation are listed in Table 4–6. As of January 2000, there were about 4,000 patients on the heart transplant waiting list, about 3,500 patients on the lung transplant waiting list, and about 230 on the heart–lung waiting list (UNOS, 2000a).

Preparation of the Recipient

Once the patient has been found suitable for organ transplantation and he or she has been placed on the transplant waiting list, the major management focus becomes maintaining the patient's cardiac and/or lung status. If the patient lives any distance from the transplant center, he or she may be asked to find lodging close to the transplant center to be readily available. In some cases, the patient may carry a portable communication device to facilitate quick communication and availability.

During the waiting period, the patient may require multiple admissions into the hospital to control cardiac or respiratory failure problems. Health maintenance is promoted through rest; control of cardiac arrhythmias, heart failure, and sodium and fluid intake; and monitoring of drug therapy for therapeutic effects. Lung transplant patients will have pulmonary function closely monitored and controlled through bronchodilators, IV diuretics, oxygen supplementation, and steroid therapy. Some patients may require more aggressive therapy, such as IV inotropic drugs, or the intra-aortic balloon pump. Unfortunately, some patients die before they can receive a transplant due to rapid worsening of heart or lung failure and/or scarcity of organ resources.

When a donor organ is available, the recipient is immediately brought to the hospital and initially prepared with appropriate laboratory tests and a chest x-ray. Preoperative teaching is performed and the patient may receive an initial dose of immunosuppressant therapy and prophylactic antibiotics. Blood is drawn for a retrospective HLA crossmatch with the donor.

As part of the transplant teaching, the patient and family are informed that the surgery will not be performed until the donor organs have been examined and have been determined to be suitable for transplantation. More specifically, the patient is taken to the operating room and intubated but the incision is not made until the procurement team has visualized the organs to be transplanted and they have given the "go-ahead." If the donor organs are determined to be not suitable, the recipient surgery is canceled. Figure 4–2 provides an illustration of a cardiac transplant.

Postoperative Management

Postoperative management of the heart and heart–lung transplant patient is similar to that of all open-heart

TABLE 4–6. MAJOR CONDITIONS ASSOCIATED WITH NEED FOR HEART, LUNG, OR HEART–LUNG TRANSPLANTATION

ORGAN	MAJOR CONDITIONS
Heart	Cardiomyopathy, valvular heart disease, ventricular aneurysm, viral myocarditis, congenital malformations, arteriosclerotic coronary artery disease
Lung	Single lung: End-stage pulmonary fibrosis, chronic obstructive pulmonary disease, pulmonary hypertension secondary to Eisenmenger's syndrome, primary pulmonary hypertension
	Double lung: Cystic fibrosis, bronchiectasis, primary pulmonary hypertension
Heart–lung	Primary pulmonary hypertension (no known cause), congenital heart disease, Eisenmenger's syndrome

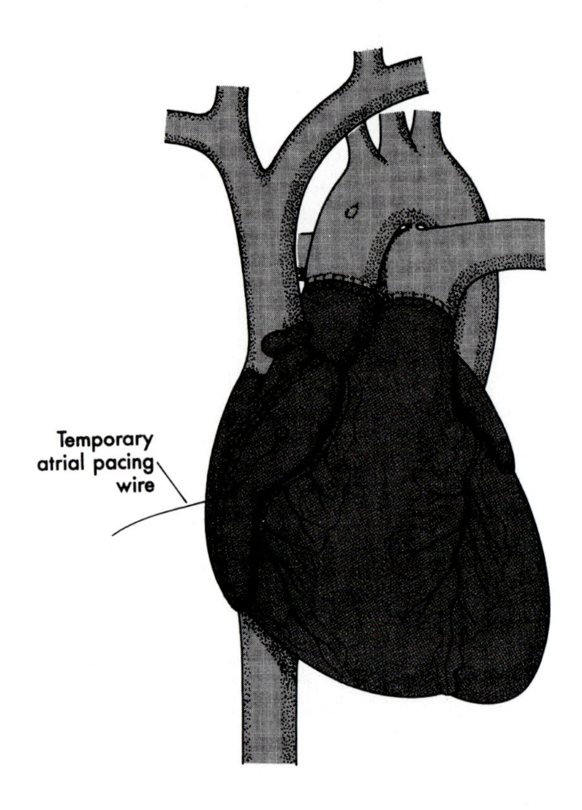

Figure 4–2. Cardiac transplantation. Suture lines connect donor and recipient atria, and then the great vessels are connected. *(From Copeland, J.G. [1984]. Modern techniques in surgery—cardiac thoracic surgery [pp. 66–75]. New York: Futura Publishing.)*

surgery patients. Typical postoperative management includes:

1. Maintaining or correcting problems associated with cardiac function and denervation, including:
   - Hemodynamic and cardiac monitoring for cardiac failure, cardiac dysrhythmias, perioperative myocardial infarction, cardiac tamponade, hemorrhage
   - Pharmacologic therapy based on cardiac status, possibly including diuretics, vasodilators, inotropic agents, and cardiac dysrhythmic agents
2. Maintaining or correcting problems with fluid and electrolyte balance, including:
   - Monitoring intake and output balance and electrolyte trends
   - Intravenous fluid therapy titrated to fluid balance status and cardiac function status
   - Electrolyte replacement as indicated
3. Maintaining and correcting problems with renal function, including:
   - Monitoring patient's urine output and renal laboratory value trends

The heart–lung and lung transplant patients are at risk for development of problems associated with pulmonary dysfunction. The following are management considerations related to the lungs:

Maintaining pulmonary function
- Monitor for signs and symptoms of respiratory insufficiency
  - Administer diuretic therapy
  - Fluid restriction
  - Early weaning from mechanical ventilator with reintubation, if required
  - Monitor fluid balance: intake and output, daily weights
  - Monitor arterial blood gases (ABGs), pulse oximetry, and SvO_2
  - Bronchodilator therapy, as required
  - Early ambulation
  - Incentive spirometry

Preventing infection
- Strict aseptic suctioning technique
- Aggressive postextubation pulmonary toilet
  - Cough and deep-breathing exercises
  - Incentive spirometry
  - Percussion and postural drainage
- Early removal of invasive lines and tubes
- Close monitoring of trends in temperature, chest x-ray, and peak expiratory flow. Although the white blood cell count will be monitored, it is anticipated that it will increase significantly for several days postop secondary to drug therapy

Evaluation for Organ Rejection

Postoperative organ function will be evaluated in a variety of ways, including laboratory tests, electrocardiograms, pulmonary function testing, and tissue biopsies.

The Biopsy

HEART BIOPSY. A biopsy of the right ventricular wall is obtained approximately one week posttransplantation. A special device called an endomyocardial bioptome is inserted into the right ventricle by way of the right jugular vein (Fig. 4–3). The procedure is generally performed in the cardiac catheterization laboratory. The biopsy results can definitively indicate whether rejection is present and to what degree. Immunosuppressant therapy can then be adjusted to halt the rejection process. Biopsies are performed periodically to continue monitoring the graft status.

LUNG BIOPSY. Pulmonary tissue can be obtained by biopsy during a bronchoscopy procedure. In patients who have had a heart–lung transplant, the lung is usually biopsied first because rejection occurs more frequently in the lungs.

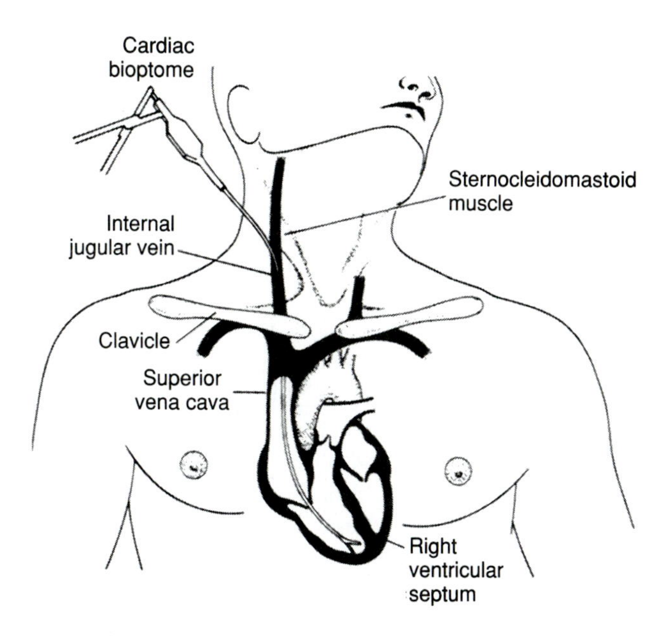

Figure 4–3. Endomyocardial biopsy technique. Transvenous biopsy approach through the right internal jugular vein. *(From Smith, S.L. [1990].* Tissue and organ transplantation: Implications for professional nursing practice *[p. 219]. St. Louis: Mosby Year Book.)*

Liver Transplantation

Liver transplantation was first attempted in a human being in 1963 by Dr. Thomas Starzl. It was not until the early 1980s that the procedure became a long-term option. This change was largely due to the introduction of cyclosporine A, which rapidly increased graft survival rates to approximately 73 percent at one year and 63 percent at four years post-transplantation (UNOS, 2000b). Improvements in immunosuppressant therapy and better surgical and donor organ preservation techniques played important roles in increasing survival rates.

Major Indications for Transplantation

Three major liver problems that are referred for possible liver transplantation include patients with chronic irreversible liver disease, liver and biliary tree primary malignant tumors, and fulminant hepatic failure. Cirrhosis is the most common indicator for liver transplantation in adults. In children, indications include such disorders as biliary atresia, Alagille syndrome, and inborn errors of metabolism.

Preparation of the Recipient

As with other patients on the waiting list for organs, the waiting period is an extremely stressful period. Patients may experience anger, fear, depression, and hopelessness as their condition worsens. The patient and the family members need psychologic support and possibly counseling during this period. When available, patients and their families may be encouraged to join a transplant support group at the transplant medical center.

The patient's hepatic function is monitored intermittently and usually includes laboratory tests. The patient may require admission into the hospital for interim treatment if hepatic function decreases significantly. Preoperative teaching is often initiated during the waiting period since time is short once an organ becomes available for transplantation.

Alternative Transplant Approaches

Not all recipients receive an entire donor liver. Two alternative types of liver grafts may be used: split-liver transplants and living-related donor transplants. The split-liver transplant divides a single donor liver into two pieces to provide a graft for two recipients. Scarcity of resources and the fact that a small child recipient cannot take an entire adult donor liver triggered the original interest in split-liver transplants. The operation is extremely complex and a high morbidity and mortality rate has made this option a limited one at this time. The living-related donor transplant usually involves a donation from a parent to a small child. This procedure is possible because of the liver's great regenerative abilities.

Postoperative Management

Immediate postoperative management in the critical care unit focuses on prevention of complications, particularly those associated with liver dysfunction, abnormalities of fluid and electrolytes, infection, and rejection. Early management also centers on support of the other systems, such as cardiopulmonary, renal, gastrointestinal, and neurologic. The complexity of the liver transplant procedure places the recipient at risk for development of many complications. Nursing care in the intensive care unit setting requires intense multiple system monitoring and rapid analysis of abnormal assessment data.

In addition to the typical postoperative management associated with all transplant patients, the major management goal that is unique to liver transplantation is *maintaining normal liver function*, which includes the following assessments:

- Monitor bile drainage appearance and quantity
- Monitor laboratory tests that reflect liver function:
    - Prothrombin time (PT) and partial thromboplastin time (PTT)
    - Alanine transaminase (ALT) and aspartate transaminase (AST), alkaline phosphatase
    - Bilirubin (total and direct), ammonia levels
    - Glucose
- Monitor neurologic status

Evaluation for Organ Rejection

The general function of the graft is routinely monitored through laboratory testing. **Rejection** often presents itself as a mild elevation in serum transaminase. In addition, the patient may experience general malaise and a mild fever. An ultrasound of the abdomen may be ordered to investigate the general condition of the liver. Liver biopsy, however, is the only means of making the definitive diagnosis of rejection.

In summary, renal transplantation was the first transplant procedure to find widespread acceptance and success. The primary indication for renal transplant is end-stage renal disease. Postoperative management centers on monitoring and enhancement of kidney function and prevention of complications. Graft function can be evaluated by needle biopsy, ultrasound, and renal scan. The early history of heart and lung transplantation was one of frustration and poor success rates. Graft survival rates have increased with improved technical skills and immunosuppressive therapy. During the waiting period, management focuses on maintaining cardiac and/or pulmonary function. Postoperative management focuses on maintenance of cardiac and pulmonary function, detection and correction of rejection, and prevention of infection. Evaluation of posttransplant graft status usually includes biopsy of heart and/or lung tissue. Three major categories of patients undergo liver transplants: those with irreversible chronic liver disease, liver and biliary tree malignant tumors, and fulminant hepatic failure. As an alternative to transplantation of the entire liver, a partial organ transplant may be performed. Two types of partial organ procedures include the split-liver transplant and the living-related donor transplant. Postoperative management focuses on prevention of complications and maintenance of liver function. Organ function is monitored through laboratory testing, and a liver biopsy may be performed to evaluate for rejection.

SECTION NINE REVIEW

1. The major indication for kidney transplantation is end-stage renal disease, which most commonly results from all of the following problems EXCEPT
   A. diabetes mellitus
   B. hypertension
   C. glomerular nephritis
   D. nephrotoxicity
2. Dysfunction of a renal graft is most commonly associated with the
   A. preoperative condition of the donor
   B. preoperative condition of the recipient
   C. length of time the organ was preserved
   D. length of time required to perform the transplant
3. The most common cause of renal graft failure is
   A. rejection
   B. hypoperfusion
   C. hypertension
   D. nephrotoxicity
4. Major conditions that are associated with the need for heart transplantation include all of the following EXCEPT
   A. cardiomyopathy
   B. congenital malformations
   C. ventricular aneurysm
   D. myocardial infarction
5. While the patient is waiting for a lung transplant, health maintenance particularly focuses on the __________ system.
   A. cardiopulmonary
   B. renal
   C. hepatobiliary
   D. neurologic
6. Postoperative management of the patient with a heart transplant includes the goal of preventing infection. Which of the following interventions most directly addresses this goal?
   A. early ambulation
   B. monitor urine output and laboratory trends
   C. monitor ABGs, pulse oximetry, SvO_2
   D. aggressive postextubation pulmonary toilet
7. Approximately one week following a heart transplant, a heart biopsy is performed to evaluate the recipient for
   A. anastomosis leak
   B. rejection
   C. infection
   D. ischemic tissue
8. Major indications for liver transplantation include all of the following EXCEPT
   A. fulminant hepatic failure
   B. acute hepatotoxicity
   C. malignant hepatic tumors
   D. irreversible chronic liver disease
9. Liver transplant patients are at particularly high risk for development of which early complication?
   A. hemorrhage
   B. rejection
   C. infection
   D. obstruction

10. A split-liver type of transplant refers to
    A. a parent-to-small-child liver donation
    B. splitting normal from abnormal parts of liver
    C. dividing the donor liver between several recipients
    D. splitting parts of a live donor liver between several recipients

11. Postoperative monitoring of liver function typically includes all of the following EXCEPT
    A. bilirubin
    B. ammonia
    C. prothrombin time
    D. blood urea nitrogen

Answers: 1. D, 2. C, 3. A, 4. D, 5. A, 6. A, 7. B, 8. B, 9. A, 10. C, 11. D

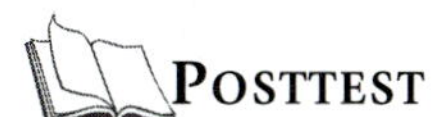

POSTTEST

The following Posttest is constructed in a case study format. A patient is presented. Questions are asked based on available data. New data are presented as the case study progresses.

Kathy S is a critically ill 23-year-old college student who recently sustained multiple trauma in a motor vehicle crash. The health care team is currently initiating evaluation of Kathy for establishing brain death.

1. If it is decided that Kathy may be a potential organ donor, she must be evaluated for suitability as a donor. Common criteria used to determine suitability include all of the following EXCEPT
   A. presence of infection
   B. cardiac arrest resuscitation
   C. preexisting metastatic disease
   D. head trauma
2. Potential donors such as Kathy are protected by law. The legislation that gives specific guidelines regarding how donation is to be carried out is the
   A. National Organ Transplant Act
   B. Uniform Anatomical Gift Act
   C. Uniform Determination of Death Act
   D. required-request legislation
3. Establishing brain death demands careful testing of Kathy. Required brain-death criteria include all of the following EXCEPT
   A. flat electroencephalogram
   B. negative ice calorics
   C. no doll's eye reflex
   D. no CNS depressants
4. The manner in which Kathy's family is approached about organ donation is important. It is suggested that her family not be approached until
   A. Kathy has been declared legally dead
   B. they have asked the physician about possible donation
   C. they have acknowledged that Kathy is brain dead
   D. it is determined whether Kathy has signed a uniform donor card
5. Prior to discussing donation with Kathy's family, she may have a preliminary evaluation performed by the Donor Procurement Coordinator/Team. Initial evaluation is performed primarily to
   A. save time
   B. evaluate for unsuitability
   C. guarantee suitability
   D. meet legal requirements

Kathy has been found suitable as a potential organ donor. Although her family has been in close contact with the physician and nurses, they are unable to be at Kathy's bedside for the next several days. They have expressed an interest in organ donation, but consent has not been given.

6. Kathy meets all of the criteria for brain death. The health care team is anxious to obtain consent to initiate donor supportive measures. Which of the following statements is correct regarding obtaining consent?
   A. any member of Kathy's family can come in to sign a consent form
   B. consent is not mandatory if the family is not available
   C. consent could be obtained over the telephone
   D. because Kathy has signed a uniform donor card, the family does not have to give consent

Kathy is now legally established as a donor.

7. As a donor, maintaining Kathy's fluid and electrolyte balance is a priority. Nursing interventions to accomplish this goal may include all of the following EXCEPT
   A. maintaining urine output at 20 to 25 mL/hr
   B. mL/mL replacement of urine output with IV fluid
   C. monitoring for therapeutic effects of Pitressin
   D. maintaining blood pressure above 90 mm Hg systolic

Kathy is taken to the operating room for organ recovery to be performed.

8. Operating room procedures for donor organ recovery may include all of the following EXCEPT
   A. aseptic procedures are not required
   B. Kathy's physician cannot be present in the operating room
   C. several recovery teams may be in the operating room
   D. anesthesiology department performs usual functions

Juan C, 46 years old, has a long history of chronic renal problems. He has been receiving hemodialysis for the past five years. Mr. C, his family, and his physician have been discussing the possibility of renal transplantation.

9. Mr. C has no siblings. Assuming that he eventually does undergo a renal transplant, he will most likely receive a(n) __________.
   A. autograft
   B. allograft
   C. isograft
   D. heterograft
10. Mr. C and his son (a possible kidney donor) have tissue typing done. Their HLA matching is likely to be
   A. partially matched
   B. identical
   C. totally unmatched
   D. unpredictable
11. Kathy's kidney is being considered for transplantation into Mr. C. He will have a sample of his blood subjected to a sample of Kathy's blood to check for preformed antibodies. This test is called
   A. antigen testing
   B. ABO typing
   C. tissue typing
   D. crossmatching
12. Mr. C has type A blood and Kathy's blood type is O. This combination of donor and recipient blood types is a(n)
   A. unacceptable match
   B. questionable match
   C. acceptable match
   D. ideal match
13. If Mr. C develops a technical type of complication associated with his kidney transplantation, it could include any of the following problems EXCEPT
   A. type III hypersensitivity response
   B. vascular thrombosis of the renal artery
   C. perioperative or postoperative bleeding
   D. urine leakage at the anastomosis site
14. If Mr. C develops a cytomegalovirus infection following the surgery, he would most likely develop it through
   A. incorrect suctioning procedures
   B. reactivation of preexisting CMV
   C. infiltration in wound infections
   D. contamination via invasive tubes
15. Mr. C is currently receiving cyclosporine (CyA). The major advantage of using this drug is that it
   A. affects only helper T cells
   B. directs its action against B cells
   C. is a cell cycle–specific cytotoxic agent
   D. has anti-inflammatory and immunosuppressant capabilities
16. If Mr. C is started on monoclonal antibody therapy, the nurse will need to monitor him closely for the first 48 hours for ______________, in addition to the usual assessments.
   A. infection
   B. renal failure
   C. nausea and vomiting
   D. cytokine-release syndrome

Additional history on Mr. C: History of type 1 diabetes mellitus since age 5. He had several episodes of staphylococcal pneumonia as a child. He is 5 foot 10 and weighs 150 pounds. Several months ago, he was treated for a severe infection with gentamicin. He has a history of hypertension that has been well controlled with antihypertensive therapy.

17. Mr. C's end-stage renal disease most likely resulted from
   A. hypertension
   B. type 1 diabetes mellitus
   C. complications of staphylococcal pneumonia
   D. recent antibiotic therapy
18. If Mr. C develops failure of his transplanted kidney, it is most likely going to be due to
   A. nephrotoxicity
   B. hypertension
   C. hypoperfusion
   D. rejection

POSTTEST ANSWERS

Question	Answer	Section	Question	Answer	Section
1	D	Two	10	A	Five
2	B	Two	11	D	Five
3	A	Three	12	C	Five
4	C	Three	13	A	Seven
5	B	Three	14	B	Seven
6	C	Three	15	A	Eight
7	A	Four	16	D	Eight
8	A	Four	17	B	Nine
9	B	Two	18	D	Nine

REFERENCES

Augustine, S.M., & Masiello-Miller, M. (1995). Heart transplantation. In M.T. Nolan & S.M. Augustine (eds.). *Transplantation nursing: Acute and long-term management* (pp. 109–140). Norwalk, CT: Appleton & Lange.

Barbuto, J.A., Akporiaye, E.T., & Hersh, E.M. (1999). Immunopharmacology. In B.G. Katzung (ed.). *Basic & clinical pharmacology* (7th ed.) (pp. 916–944). Stamford, CT: Appleton & Lange.

Bartucci, M.R. (1999). Kidney transplantation: State of the art. *AACN Clinical Issues* 10(2):153–163.

Bush, W.W. (1999). Overview of transplantation immunology and the pharmacotherapy of adult solid organ transplant recipients: Focus on immunosuppression. *AACN Clinical Issues* 10(2):253–269.

Garrison, R.N., Bentley, F.R., Raque, G.H., et al. (1991). There is an answer to the organ donor shortage. *Surg Gynecol Obstet* 173(5):391–396.

KODA. (1994). Materials provided by Kentucky Organ Donor Affiliates (KODA). Lexington, KY: Author.

Murray, J.E. (1991). Nobel Prize lecture: The first successful organ transplants in man. In P.I. Terasaki (ed.). *History of transplantation: Thirty-five recollections* (pp. 123–138). Los Angeles: UCLA Tissue Typing Laboratory.

Owens, S.G., & Wallop, J.M. (1995). Heart-lung and lung transplantation. In M.T. Nolan & S.M. Augustine (eds.). *Transplantation nursing: Acute and long-term management* (pp. 141–163). Norwalk, CT: Appleton & Lange.

Sommers, C. (1998). Immunity and inflammation. In C.M. Porth (ed.). *Pathophysiology: Concepts of altered health states* (5th ed.) (pp. 189–212). Philadelphia: J.B. Lippincott.

Thacker, D. (1999a). *Organ and tissue donation*. Lexington, KY: Kentucky Organ Donor Affiliates.

Thelan, L.A., Urden, L.D., Lough, M.E., & Stacy, K.M. (eds.). (1998). Transplantation. In L.A. Thelan et al. (eds.). *Critical care nursing: Diagnosis and management* (3rd ed.) (pp. 1171–1220). St. Louis: C.V. Mosby.

UNOS (United Network for Organ Sharing). (1993). *Patients waiting for transplants*. Richmond, VA: Author.

UNOS. (2000a). Critical data. United Network for Organ Sharing. Available online at *http://www.unos.org/Newsroom/critdata_main.htm*.

UNOS. (2000b). Transplants. United Network for Organ Sharing. Available online at *http://www.unos.org/Newsroom/critdata_transplants_survive1.htm*.

PART II

RESPIRATION AND VENTILATION

Module 5

Respiratory Process

Kathleen Dorman Wagner

The focus of this module is on physiologic as well as pathophysiologic processes involved in pulmonary ventilation and respiration. The module is composed of 10 sections. Sections One through Four consider the underlying general principles involved in the respiratory process, including respiration and ventilation, pulmonary diffusion, the relationship between ventilation and perfusion, and pulmonary shunting. Section Five gives a brief overview of evaluation of pulmonary function. Section Six differentiates pulmonary diseases on the basis of restrictive versus obstructive processes. Section Seven describes the pathophysiologic basis of acute respiratory failure. Section Eight presents assessment data frequently used in deriving appropriate nursing diagnoses for a patient with a respiratory problem. Section Nine discusses five calculations that are commonly used for estimating shunt and pulmonary vascular resistance. Section Ten describes respiratory-focused nursing diagnoses and how they apply to patients with restrictive and obstructive pulmonary disorders. Each section includes a set of review questions to help the learner evaluate his or her understanding of the section's content before moving on to the next section. All Section Reviews and the module Pretest and Posttest include answers. It is suggested that the learner review those concepts answered incorrectly in the review questions before proceeding to the next section.

Objectives

Following completion of this module, the learner will be able to

1. Explain the concept of ventilation.
2. Discuss pulmonary diffusion.
3. Explain the relationship between ventilation and perfusion.
4. Describe the physiologic basis of right-to-left shunt.
5. Describe various tests used for evaluation of pulmonary function.
6. Explain the basic difference between restrictive and obstructive pulmonary diseases.
7. Discuss the pathophysiologic basis of respiratory failure.
8. Describe an appropriate database for a patient with a pulmonary disorder.
9. Perform selected respiratory calculations.
10. Develop a plan of care for a patient with altered respiratory function.

Pretest

1. Ventilation is best defined as
   A. movement of gases across the alveolar–capillary membrane
   B. mechanical movement of gases in and out of the lungs
   C. transport of gases through the blood to and from the tissues
   D. movement of gases down a pressure gradient

2. During inspiration, air is drawn into the lungs because intrapulmonary pressure is
   A. above alveolar–capillary pressure
   B. equal to intra-abdominal pressure
   C. below atmospheric pressure
   D. above intrathoracic pressure
3. All of the following factors affect pulmonary diffusion EXCEPT
   A. gradient
   B. thickness
   C. surface area
   D. barometric pressure
4. If the ventilation–perfusion ($\dot{V}/\dot{Q}$) ratio is low, it will affect arterial blood gases in which way?
   A. decreased PaO_2
   B. decreased $PaCO_2$
   C. increased PaO_2
   D. increased pH
5. Physiologic shunt refers to which of the following?
   A. blood that bypasses the heart
   B. blood that bypasses the lungs
   C. blood that does not take part in diffusion
   D. blood that does not release carbon dioxide
6. Normal tidal volume in an average-sized adult male would be how many mL/kg?
   A. 3 to 4
   B. 4 to 5
   C. 5 to 7
   D. 7 to 9
7. The primary ventilatory problem associated with obstructive pulmonary disease is
   A. obstruction to perfusion
   B. decreased diffusion of gases
   C. delay of airflow out of the lungs
   D. inability to achieve normal tidal volumes
8. The major cause of increased pulmonary vascular resistance (PVR) is
   A. hypercarbia
   B. alkalosis
   C. hypoxia
   D. cor pulmonale
9. A patient who has cor pulmonale will have
   A. left heart dilation
   B. right heart hypertrophy
   C. pulmonary fibrosis
   D. left ventricular hyperplasia
10. The nurse would expect a person who has respiratory insufficiency to have which of the following blood gas conditions?
    A. pH below normal
    B. $PaCO_2$ below normal
    C. pH normal
    D. $PaCO_2$ normal
11. Classic symptoms associated with an abnormally high $PaCO_2$ would include
    A. weak, thready pulse
    B. flushed, wet skin
    C. decreased blood pressure
    D. slow, shallow breathing
12. The pulmonary edema associated with ARDS is caused by
    A. capillary microembolism
    B. left ventricular failure
    C. loss of surfactant
    D. increased membrane permeability
13. Chest pain that is typical of pleuritic pain can be best characterized as
    A. sharp
    B. pressurelike
    C. radiating
    D. dull

Pretest answers: 1. B, 2. C, 3. D, 4. A, 5. C, 6. D, 7. C, 8. C, 9. B, 10. C, 11. B, 12. D, 13. A

GLOSSARY

Absolute (true) shunt. The sum of anatomic shunt and capillary shunt; refractory to oxygen therapy (Des Jardins, 1998)

Accessory muscles. Muscles not normally used during quiet breathing that are available for assisting either inspiration or expiration during times of increased work of breathing

Adult respiratory distress syndrome (ARDS). A type of respiratory failure caused by diffuse injury to the alveolar–capillary membrane, resulting in noncardiogenic pulmonary edema

Anatomic shunt. Movement of blood from the right heart and back into the left heart without coming into contact with alveoli

Capillary shunt. Normal flow of blood past completely unventilated alveoli

Chronic bronchitis. A chronic obstructive pulmonary disease of the larger airways that is defined clinically as the presence of chronic productive cough that occurs daily for at least 3 months per year for at least 2 years in succession

Chronic obstructive pulmonary disease (COPD) (chronic airflow limitation diseases). A group of pulmonary diseases that cause obstruction to primarily expiratory airflow

Compliance (CL). Measurement of the relative ease with which the lungs accept a volume of air; reflects relative stiffness of lungs

Cor pulmonale. Right ventricular hypertrophy and dilation secondary to pulmonary disease

Crackles (rales). Adventitious breath sounds associated with fluid or secretions or both in small airways or alveoli

Diffusion. Movement of gases down a pressure gradient from an area of high pressure to an area of low pressure

Dyspnea. Difficulty breathing

Emphysema. A pathologic pulmonary process characterized by enlargement of alveoli and destruction of alveoli and surrounding capillary beds

External respiration. Movement of gases across the alveolar–capillary membrane

Forced expiratory volumes (FEVs). Measure of how rapidly a person can forcefully exhale air after a maximal inhalation; a measurement of dynamic lung function

Hemoptysis. Expectoration of bloody secretions

Internal respiration. Movement of gases across systemic capillary–cell membrane, in the tissues

Minute ventilation ($\dot{V}_E$). The total volume of expired air in 1 minute

Obstructive disorders. Pulmonary disorders that are associated with decreased or delayed airflow during expiration

Oxygenation failure. A respiratory crisis in which the primary problem is one of hypoxemia. Clinically, it is defined as a PaO_2 of ≤ 60 mm Hg

Parietal pleura. The moist membrane that adheres to the thoracic walls, diaphragm, and mediastinum

Paroxysmal nocturnal dyspnea (PND). A symptom usually associated with transient pulmonary edema secondary to heart failure; patient awakens from sleep with severe orthopnea

Physiologic shunt. Movement of blood from the right heart, through the lungs, and on into the left heart without taking part in alveolar–capillary diffusion

Pleurisy (pleuritis). Pain caused by inflammation of the parietal pleura

Pleural rub. Adventitious breath sound caused by inflammation of the pleural membrane

Respiration. The process by which the body's cells are supplied with oxygen and carbon dioxide is eliminated from the body

Respiratory failure. A state of pulmonary decompensation in which the body is no longer able to maintain normal gas exchange. It can be expressed as $PaO_2 < 60$ mm Hg or $PaCO_2 > 50$ mm Hg at pH < 7.30

Respiratory insufficiency. A state of pulmonary compensation in which a normal blood pH is maintained only at the expense of the cardiopulmonary system

Restrictive disorders. Pulmonary disorders associated with a decrease in lung volume

Rhonchi. Adventitious breath sounds associated with an accumulation of fluid or secretions in the larger airways

Sepsis. A pathologic state in which microorganisms, or their toxins, are present in the bloodstream

Shuntlike effect. Effect created by an excess of perfusion in relation to alveolar ventilation

Surfactant. A lipoprotein produced by type II alveolar cells that reduces the surface tension of the alveolar fluid lining

Tidal volume (TV or V_T). The amount of air that moves in and out of the lungs with each normal breath

Total lung capacity (TLC). The amount of gas present in the lungs after maximal inspiration

Venous admixture. The effect that a physiologic shunt has on the oxygen content of the blood as it drains into the left heart

Ventilation. The mechanical movement of airflow to and from the atmosphere and the alveoli

Ventilatory failure. A condition caused by alveolar hypoventilation; clinically it is called *acute respiratory acidosis*

Visceral pleura. The moist membrane that adheres to the lung parenchyma and is adjacent to the parietal pleura

Vital capacity (VC). The maximum amount of air expired after a maximal inspiration; a measurement of lung capacity

$\dot{V}/\dot{Q}$ ratio. A ratio expressing the relationship of ventilation to perfusion

Wheeze. Adventitious breath sound caused by air passing through constricted airways

ABBREVIATIONS

ABG. Arterial blood gas

ARDS. Acute respiratory distress syndrome

C_L. Lung compliance, expressed in cm H_2O/mL

CO_2. Carbon dioxide

COPD. Chronic obstructive pulmonary disease

f. Frequency, rate of breathing, expressed in breaths per minute

FEV. Forced expiratory volume

IPPB. Intermittent positive pressure breathing

NANDA. North American Nursing Diagnosis Association

$\dot{Q}$. Pulmonary capillary perfusion

PCO_2. Partial pressure of carbon dioxide or carbon dioxide tension, expressed in mm Hg; variations:

- **P_ACO_2.** Specifies alveolar carbon dioxide tension
- **$PaCO_2$.** Specifies arterial carbon dioxide tension
- **$P\bar{v}CO_2$.** Specifies mixed venous carbon dioxide tension

PEEP. Positive end expiratory pressure

PO_2. Partial pressure of oxygen or oxygen tension, expressed in mm Hg; variations:

- **PAO_2.** Specifies alveolar oxygen tension
- **PAO_2.** Specifies arterial oxygen tension
- **$P\bar{v}CO_2$.** Specifies mixed venous oxygen tension

$\dot{V}$. Ventilation

VC. Vital capacity

$\dot{V}E$. Minute ventilation

$\dot{V}/\dot{Q}$ ratio. Ventilation-perfusion ratio

VT (TV). Tidal volume, expressed in milliliters (mL) or liters (L)

SECTION ONE: Ventilation

At the completion of this section, the learner will be able to explain the concept of ventilation.

The respiratory process consists of two distinct concepts, **respiration** and **ventilation**. Respiration is the process by which the body's cells are supplied with oxygen and carbon dioxide (cellular waste product) is eliminated from the body. Respiration can be further divided into external and internal respiration. **External respiration** refers to the movement of gases across the alveolar–capillary membrane. **Internal respiration** refers to the movement of gases across systemic capillary–cell membranes in the tissues. External respiration is discussed throughout this module.

Ventilation is defined as the mechanical movement of airflow to and from the atmosphere and the alveoli. Ventilation involves the actual work of breathing and requires adequate functioning of the lungs and conducting airways, thorax, ventilatory muscles, and nervous system control. Decreased functioning of any one of these factors will affect the body's ability to ventilate properly.

Ventilation is accomplished through a bellowslike action. Air is able to move in and out of the lungs as a result of the changing size of the thorax caused by ventilatory muscle activity. When the thorax enlarges, the intrapulmonary pressure drops to below atmospheric pressure. Air then moves from the area of higher pressure to the area of lower pressure, resulting in air flowing into the lungs (inspiration) until the pressure in the lungs becomes slightly higher than atmospheric pressure. At this point, air flows back out of the lungs (expiration) until once again pressures are equalized.

Lung tissue has a constant tendency to collapse due to several important properties. First, the fluid lining of the alveoli has a naturally high surface tension, creating a tendency for the alveolar walls to collapse. To prevent this, special cells in the alveoli secrete a lipoprotein called **surfactant**. Surfactant has a detergentlike action, reducing the surface tension of the fluid lining the alveolar sacs and thereby decreasing the tendency toward collapse. Second, the lungs are composed of elastic fibers. The elastic force of these fibers constantly seeks to return to their resting state, causing a collapsed lung. To maintain the lungs in an inflated state, the elastic forces must constantly be overcome by opposing forces (Fig. 5–1).

The primary opposing force that maintains the lung in an expanded state is the thorax, which, with its associated respiratory muscles, naturally moves outward, thus expanding during inspiration. The thoracic bony structure provides a cagelike framework to maintain the lungs in a baseline inflated state even at rest.

What causes the lungs to adhere to the thoracic walls? An attraction exists between the visceral and parietal pleura. The pleurae are slick-surfaced moist membranes. The parietal pleura adheres to the thoracic walls,

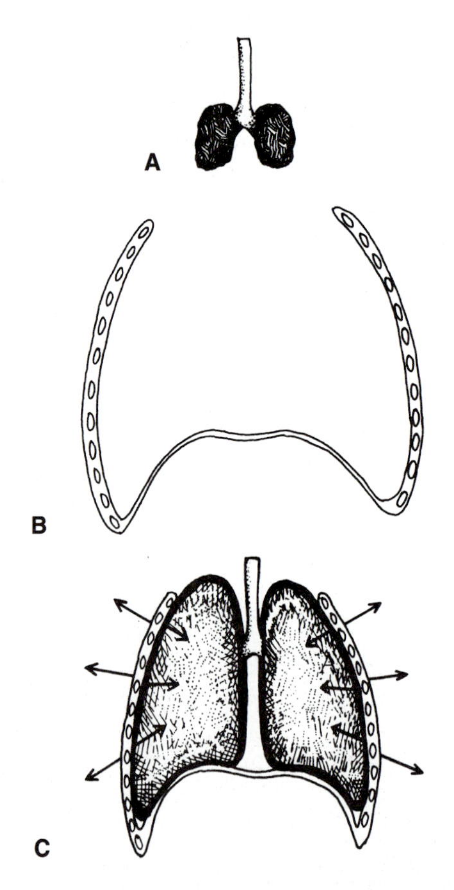

Figure 5–1. Opposing elastic forces of the lungs and thorax. **A.** The resting state of normal lungs when removed from the chest cavity. Elasticity causes total collapse. **B.** Resting state of normal chest wall and diaphragm when apex is open to the atmosphere, and the thoracic contents are removed. **C.** End expiration in the normal, intact thorax. Note that the elastic forces of the lung and chest wall are in opposite directions. The pleural surfaces link these two opposing forces. *(From Shapiro, B.A., et al. [1991].* Clinical application of respiratory care, *4th ed., [p. 22]. St. Louis, MO: Mosby-Year Book.)*

diaphragm, and mediastinum, and the visceral pleura adheres to the lung parenchyma. To understand the pleural attraction, it may help to think of placing two moistened sheets of smooth glass together. Although it would be relatively easy to glide one sheet over the other in a parallel fashion, it would be very difficult to pull them directly apart at a 180-degree angle. The glass sheets represent the two pleurae. Under normal circumstances (a negative intrapleural state), the parietal and visceral pleura act as one membrane. Therefore, as the thorax increases and decreases in volume, so will the lungs.

Compliance

The ease with which the lungs are able to be expanded is measured in terms of lung compliance. For example, it is much more difficult to blow up a small balloon than a large balloon. To inflate the small balloon, you would need to blow harder (exert more pressure force) to obtain the same volume that you would be able to obtain with less force in the large balloon. The small balloon is less compliant than the large balloon. **Compliance (CL)** is defined in terms of lung volume (mL) and pressure (cm H_2O) as

$$C_L = \Delta V / \Delta P$$

where CL is lung compliance, ΔV is change in volume (mL), and ΔP is change in pressure (cm H_2O).

Like a bag of assorted-size balloons, alveoli also come in many sizes. Each size of alveolus has a certain filling capacity beyond which it becomes overexpanded and may even burst. As the alveoli approach their filling capacity, they become less compliant; that is, it takes more force to completely expand the alveoli and even greater force to hyperexpand them. For example, patients with acute respiratory distress syndrome (ARDS) require moderate to high levels of positive end-expiratory pressure (PEEP) to open, expand, or hyperexpand alveoli that have become significantly noncompliant due to the disease process. Use of PEEP ideally increases lung compliance. However, if too much PEEP (measured in cm H_2O pressure) is used, alveoli become so hyperexpanded that compliance decreases dramatically and the alveoli are at risk of rupture, causing pneumothorax. (PEEP is explained in detail in the Mechanical Ventilation Module.)

Many pulmonary and extrapulmonary problems can influence compliance. Compliance is very sensitive to any condition that affects the lung's tissues, particularly if the disorder causes a reduction in pulmonary surfactant, which is crucial to maintenance of functional alveoli. When there is a deficiency of surfactant, compliance is decreased. Decreased compliance is sometimes referred to as "stiff lungs," meaning that it now takes more force (pressure) to increase lung volume. For example, whereas a person with normal lungs can inhale 50 to 100 mL of air for every 1 cm H_2O of pressure exerted, a person with decreased compliance might be able to inhale 30 to 40 mL/cm H_2O of pressure. Decreased compliance increases the work of breathing and causes a decreased tidal volume. Breathing rate increases to compensate for the decreased tidal volume. Pulmonary problems causing decreased compliance are called restrictive pulmonary disorders (Section Six). (Examples of conditions associated with decreased compliance can be found in Table 5–3, p. 121.)

In summary, the respiratory process has two major components: respiration and ventilation. Lung tissue has to constantly overcome the tendency to collapse. The substance surfactant is crucial in maintaining the alveoli in an open state. Lung compliance is decreased by many intrapulmonary and extrapulmonary disorders affecting the volume of air moved in and out of the lungs.

Section One Review

1. The elastic force of lung tissue seeks to
   A. keep lungs expanded
   B. make lungs collapse
   C. flatten the diaphragm
   D. decrease thorax size
2. During expiration, air flows out of the lungs because the intrapulmonary pressure
   A. increases to above atmospheric pressure
   B. is equal to perfusion pressure
   C. drops to below atmospheric pressure
   D. is equal to alveolar pressure
3. The purpose of surfactant is to
   A. decrease lung compliance
   B. increase alveolar surface tension
   C. cleanse the alveoli
   D. decrease alveolar surface tension
4. The lungs adhere to the thoracic walls because of
   A. elastic forces
   B. pulmonary surfactant
   C. hydraulic traction
   D. lung compliance

5. As alveoli near their filling capacity, they become
   A. less compliant
   B. less elastic
   C. more compliant
   D. hyperexpanded

6. External respiration refers to
   A. movement of air from the atmosphere to the alveoli
   B. diffusion of gases across the alevolar–capillary membrane
   C. movement of air from the alveoli to the atmosphere
   D. diffusion of gases across the tissue–capillary membranes

Answers: 1. B, 2. A, 3. D, 4. C, 5. A, 6. B

SECTION TWO: Diffusion

At the completion of this section, the learner will be able to discuss pulmonary diffusion.

Oxygenation of tissues is dependent on the process of diffusion as the vital mechanism for both external and internal respiration. **Diffusion** is the movement of gases down a pressure gradient from an area of high pressure to an area of low pressure. There are four factors that affect diffusion through the alveolar–capillary membrane: gradient, surface area, thickness, and length of exposure.

Gradient

A pressure gradient (difference) exists between the atmosphere and the alveoli and between the alveoli and the pulmonary capillaries. The greater the pressure difference, the more rapid the flow of gases. Several factors that increase the gradient include exercise, positive pressure mechanical ventilation, and intermittent positive pressure breathing (IPPB).

Air enters the alveoli from the atmosphere because the atmospheric air pressure is slightly higher than alveolar pressure. A pressure gradient also exists between the alveoli and the pulmonary capillaries, causing flow of gases across the alveolar–capillary membrane. This process is called **external respiration.** Atmospheric air is composed of molecules of nitrogen, oxygen, carbon dioxide, and water vapor. The combination of all of these gases exerts about 760 mm Hg of pressure at sea level. The respiratory process, however, does not actively involve use of the water vapor or nitrogen. It is concerned with exchange of oxygen and carbon dioxide (Fig. 5–2).

Oxygen and carbon dioxide both exert a certain percentage of the total air pressure. Oxygen in the alveoli exerts approximately 100 mm Hg pressure, and this partial pressure of oxygen is called PO_2, or oxygen tension. When the PO_2 refers to oxygen in the alveoli, it is more precisely referred to as PAO_2. When it refers to arterial blood, it is abbreviated as PaO_2, and when it refers to venous blood, it is specified as PVO_2. Carbon dioxide in the alveoli exerts approximately 40 mm Hg of pressure. This partial pressure is called PCO_2. The abbreviation alterations of A, a, and V used for describing PO_2 also apply to PCO_2.

Venous blood returning to the lungs from the tissues is oxygen poor ($PVO_2 \approx 40$ mm Hg), because the blood has dropped off its load of oxygen for use by the tissues. Venous blood is rich in carbon dioxide ($PVCO_2 \approx 45$ mm Hg) owing to transport of the cellular waste product, carbon dioxide (CO_2), for removal from the lungs.

The alveolar–capillary membrane is very thin. Oxygen and carbon dioxide molecules move easily across the membrane by diffusion. Alveolar oxygen moves into the capillaries, and carbon dioxide moves out of the capillaries into the alveoli. Oxygen and carbon dioxide do not diffuse at the same rate. Carbon dioxide is able to diffuse about 20 times more rapidly than oxygen. Therefore, when a person has diseased lung tissue, severe tissue hy-

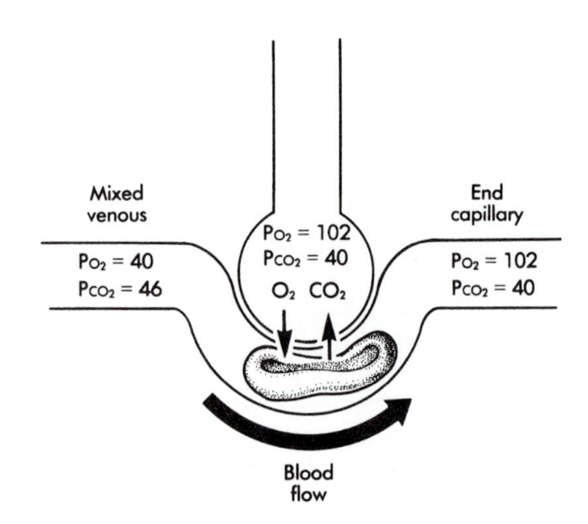

Figure 5–2. Diffusion of oxygen and carbon dioxide. Gas exchange occurs solely by diffusion from a region of relatively high gas pressure to one of relatively low gas pressure. *(From Martin, L. [1987].* Pulmonary physiology in clinical practice: The essentials in clinical practice, *[p. 39]. St. Louis: C.V. Mosby.)*

poxia may exist long before carbon dioxide levels are affected. Figure 5–2 shows the movement of gases during diffusion.

In **internal respiration,** the process is reversed. The arterial blood is rich in oxygen and poor in carbon dioxide, whereas the cells are poor in oxygen and rich in carbon dioxide. The pressure differences between the PaO_2 and $PaCO_2$ in the blood and cells cause oxygen to move from the circulating hemoglobin into the cells. The cells release carbon dioxide into the bloodstream for transport back to the lungs for excretion.

Surface Area

The total surface area of the lung is very large. The greater the available alveolar–capillary membrane surface area, the greater the amount of oxygen and carbon dioxide that can diffuse across it during a specific time period. Emphysema is a major pulmonary disorder that destroys the alveolar–capillary membrane. This greatly reduces surface area and consequently impairs gas exchange. Many pulmonary conditions, including severe pneumonia, lung tumors, pneumothorax, and pneumonectomy, can reduce functioning surface area significantly.

Thickness

The thickness of the alveolar–capillary membrane is of major importance. The thinner the membrane, the more rapid the rate of diffusion of gases. Several conditions can increase membrane thickness, thereby decreasing the rate of diffusion:

- Fluid in the alveoli or interstitial spaces or both (e.g., pulmonary edema)
- An inflammatory process involving the alveoli (e.g., pneumonia)
- Lung conditions that cause fibrosis (e.g., ARDS or pneumoconiosis)

Length of Exposure

During periods of rest, blood flows through the alveolar–capillary system in approximately 0.75 second. Diffusion of oxygen and carbon dioxide requires about 0.25 second to reach equilibrium (the balance between alveolar and capillary gas levels). During the periods of high cardiac output, such as occurs with exercise or stress, blood flow is faster through the alveolar–capillary system. Under these circumstances, diffusion must take place during a shortened exposure time. In healthy lungs, oxygen exchange is usually not impaired with high cardiac output states; however, hypoxemia may result if diffusion abnormalities are present, such as pulmonary edema, alveolar consolidation (e.g., pneumonia), or alveolar fibrosis (Des Jardins, 1998).

In summary, diffusion is the process by which gases are exchanged in the lungs and in the tissues. The factors of gradient, surface area, thickness, and length of exposure all greatly influence the effectiveness of diffusion. Should a pulmonary disorder cause a problem with any one of these factors, gas exchange becomes impaired, which results in an increase in arterial carbon dioxide levels, a decrease in arterial oxygen levels, or both.

SECTION TWO REVIEW

1. Pressure gradient affects diffusion of gases in which of the following ways?
   A. the more rapid the ventilatory rate, the greater the gradient
   B. the greater the difference, the more rapid the gas flow
   C. the less rapid the ventilatory rate, the greater the gradient
   D. the smaller the difference, the more rapid the gas flow
2. Which of the following factors increases the diffusion pressure gradient?
   A. increased exercise
   B. decreased activity
   C. negative pressure ventilation
   D. amount of lung surface area
3. The normal partial pressure of alveolar oxygen is approximately
   A. 60 mm Hg
   B. 80 mm Hg
   C. 100 mm Hg
   D. 110 mm Hg
4. Surface area as a factor affecting diffusion refers to
   A. size of the alveoli
   B. the conducting airways
   C. the functional capillary perfusion
   D. the functional alveoli and surrounding capillaries

5. An example of a disease process that would increase the thickness of the alveolar–capillary membrane is
   A. pneumonia
   B. pneumothorax
   C. lung tumor
   D. pneumonectomy

6. Which of the following statements regarding diffusion is appropriate?
   A. gas flows down a pressure gradient
   B. diffusion refers to alveolar pressure
   C. gas flows up a pressure gradient
   D. diffusion refers to capillary pressure

Answers: 1. B, 2. A, 3. C, 4. D, 5. A, 6. A

SECTION THREE: Ventilation–Perfusion Relationship

At the completion of this section, the learner will be able to explain the relationship between ventilation and perfusion.

Normal diffusion of gases requires a certain balance of alveolar ventilation (movement of gas into the alveoli) and pulmonary perfusion (blood flow through the pulmonary capillaries). Should an imbalance in this relationship develop, normal gas exchange cannot take place in the affected areas. For this reason, it is important to gain a basic understanding of the relationship of ventilation ($\dot{V}$) to perfusion ($\dot{Q}$). This relationship is expressed as a ratio of alveolar ventilation to pulmonary capillary perfusion (**$\dot{V}/\dot{Q}$ ratio**).

For ideal gas exchange to occur, one would expect that for every liter of fresh air coming into the alveoli, 1 L of blood would flow past it, creating a 1:1 ratio of ventilation to perfusion. In reality, for approximately every 4 L of air flowing into the alveoli, about 5 L of blood flows past (an average ratio of 4:5, or 0.8) (Fig. 5–3).

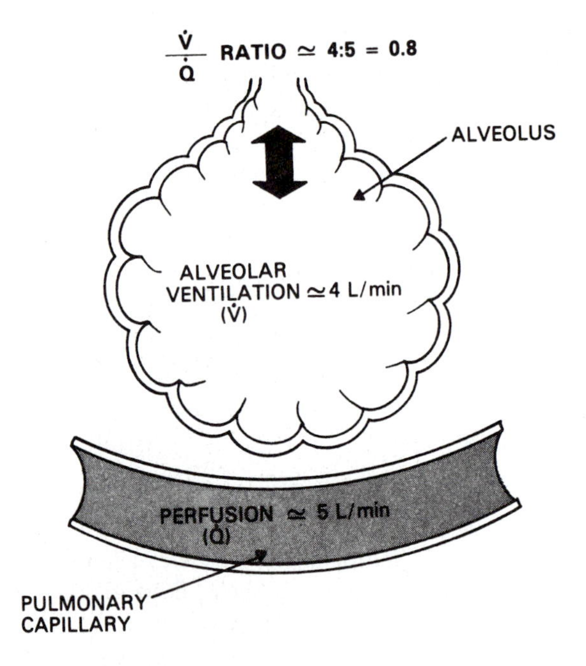

Figure 5–3. The relationship of ventilation to perfusion. The normal ventilation–perfusion ratio ($\dot{V}/\dot{Q}$ ratio) is about 0.8. *(From* Cardiopulmonary Anatomy and Physiology, *2nd ed., by J. R. Des Jardins © 1993. Reprinted with permission of Delmar, a division of Thompson Learning. Fax (800) 730-2215.)*

To facilitate discussion of the $\dot{V}/\dot{Q}$ ratio, the partial pressures of alveolar oxygen and carbon dioxide (PAO_2 and $PACO_2$) must be discussed further. The balance of ventilation to perfusion is greatly affected by the PAO_2 and $PACO_2$. This balance is dependent on adequate diffusion of oxygen and carbon dioxide across the alveolar–capillary membrane, and movement of oxygen into and carbon dioxide out of the alveoli.

Though normal values are given for PAO_2 (100 mm Hg) and $PACO_2$ (40 mm Hg), these numbers only express an average. The actual partial pressures of oxygen and carbon dioxide vary throughout the lungs, since ventilation is not distributed evenly. In an upright person, alveolar ventilation is moderate only in the apices of the lungs because of increased negative pleural pressures in the apices in relation to the lung bases. This makes the alveoli in the lung apices more resistant to airflow during inspiration. When breathing spontaneously, airflow naturally moves toward the diaphragm, which results in more air movement into the bases and peripheral lung during inspiration (airflow follows the path of least resistance). Pulmonary capillary perfusion is gravity dependent. Perfusion is greatest in the dependent areas of the lungs (the bases in an upright person). Consequently, since ventilation and perfusion are both greatest in the bases of the lungs, the greatest amount of gas exchange occurs in this portion of the lung fields.

In the upper lungs, there is moderate alveolar ventilation and very reduced perfusion, making an excess of ventilation to available perfusion. This results in a $\dot{V}/\dot{Q}$ ratio that is higher than the average of 0.8. In the lower lungs, there is a moderate increase in ventilation with a great increase in

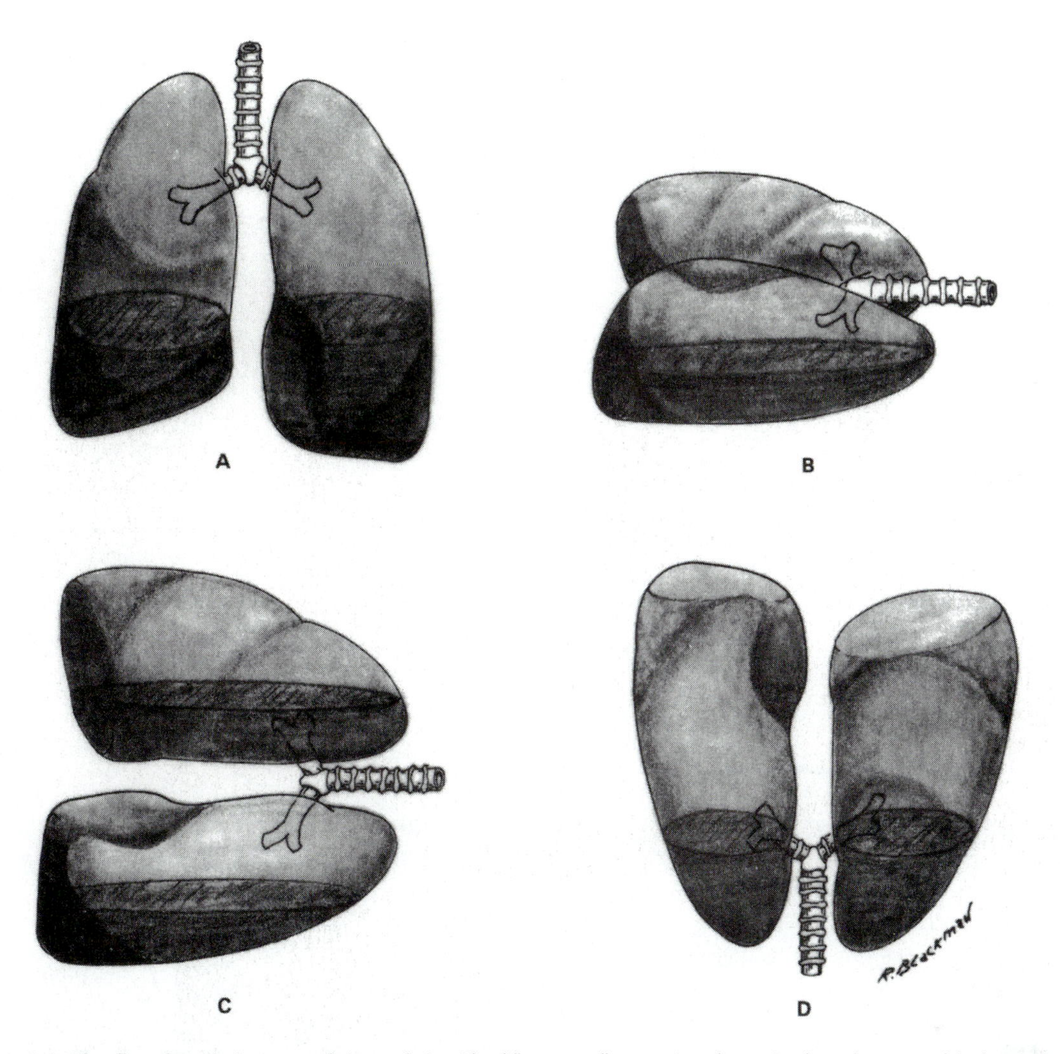

Figure 5–4. The effect of positioning on ventilation-perfusion. Blood flow normally moves into the gravity-dependent areas of the lungs. Thus, body position affects the distribution of the pulmonary blood flow, as illustrated in the erect **(A)**, supine **(B)**, lateral **(C)**, and upside-down **(D)** positions. *(From* Cardiopulmonary Anatomy and Physiology, *2nd ed., by J. R. Des Jardins © 1993. Reprinted with permission of Delmar, a division of Thompson Learning. Fax (800) 730-2215.)*

perfusion. This results in a $\dot{V}/\dot{Q}$ ratio that is lower than the average of 0.8, since there is a relatively moderate increase in ventilation associated with a significant increase in perfusion.

The clinical significance of ventilation–perfusion balance becomes apparent when considering its implications in high-acuity patients. When a high-acuity person is placed in bed, he or she is kept in a relatively horizontal position. Since perfusion is gravity dependent, it will shift from the lung bases to whichever lung area is now in the dependent position (Fig. 5–4).

Keeping the principles of $\dot{V}/\dot{Q}$ ratio in mind, what could happen if a patient is positioned on the right side when there is significant pneumonia in the right lung fields? Since the patient is lying on the right side, maximum pulmonary capillary perfusion will be on the right. Pneumonia is associated with secretions and other factors that cause obstruction to airflow into the affected right lung alveoli. Therefore, since airflow follows the path of least resistance, it will decrease in the diseased right lung area. This combination of significant decrease in ventilation in the presence of normal to increased perfusion causes a mismatching of ventilation to perfusion, creating a low $\dot{V}/\dot{Q}$ ratio. If sufficient mismatching occurs, PaO_2 and oxygen saturation levels could drop significantly. Positioning this patient on the left side would be tolerated better, since $\dot{V}/\dot{Q}$ matching would be improved. This, then, is one reason why some high-acuity patients tolerate being turned on one side more than another. Table 5–1 compares high and low $\dot{V}/\dot{Q}$ ratios.

TABLE 5–1. COMPARISON OF HIGH AND LOW $\dot{V}/\dot{Q}$ RATIOS

HIGH $\dot{V}/\dot{Q}$ RATIO	LOW $\dot{V}/\dot{Q}$ RATIO
Normal to increased alveolar ventilation associated with decreased perfusion	Decreased alveolar ventilation associated with normal to increased perfusion
Alveolar gas effect	**Alveolar gas effect**
Increased cardiac output	Decreased oxygen in alveoli
Decreased alveolar CO_2	Increased carbon dioxide in alveoli
Normally exists in upper lung fields	Normally exists in lower lung fields
Abnormally present with	**Abnormally present with**
Decreased cardiac output	Hypoventilation
Pulmonary emboli	Obstructive lung diseases
Pneumothorax	Restrictive lung diseases
Destruction of pulmonary capillaries	
Arterial blood gas effects	**Arterial blood gas effects**
Increased Pa_{O_2}	Decreased Pa_{O_2}
Decreased Pa_{CO_2}	Increased Pa_{CO_2}
Increased pH	Decreased pH

In summary, the relationship of ventilation to perfusion ($\dot{V}/\dot{Q}$ ratio) varies throughout the lung. An overall balance in this relationship must be maintained to optimize proper diffusion of gases. Pulmonary disorders may create a mismatching of ventilation and perfusion, which creates problems associated either with a high $\dot{V}/\dot{Q}$ ratio or a low $\dot{V}/\dot{Q}$ ratio.

SECTION THREE REVIEW

1. Which of the following statements is true regarding the relationship of ventilation to perfusion in an upright person?
   A. it varies throughout the lung
   B. ventilation is best in the apices
   C. perfusion is best in peripheral lung areas
   D. it maintains a 1:1 relationship
2. During spontaneous breathing, air flows toward
   A. the apices
   B. the diaphragm
   C. higher pressure gradient
   D. higher resistance areas
3. Mr. M has a left lower lobe pneumonia. His remaining lung fields are clear. It is time to reposition Mr. M in bed. Of the following positions, which is most likely to optimize the ventilation–perfusion relationship?
   A. place him on his right side
   B. place him on his back
   C. place him on his left side
   D. place him flat in the bed
4. When ventilation–perfusion mismatching occurs, it can be detected by which of the following parameters?
   A. hemoglobin (Hgb) level
   B. oxygen saturation level (Sa_{O_2})
   C. partial pressure of arterial carbon dioxide (Pa_{CO_2})
   D. arterial sodium bicarbonate level (HCO_3)
5. What causes a decrease of airflow to the apices of the lungs?
   A. increased natural airflow toward lung periphery
   B. increased negative pleural pressure in bases
   C. increased negative pleural pressure in apices
   D. increased positive pleural pressure in apices

Answers: 1. A, 2. B, 3. A, 4. B, 5. C

SECTION FOUR: Right-to-Left Shunt

At the completion of this section, the learner will be able to describe the physiologic basis of right-to-left shunt.

Pulmonary shunting is a major cause of hypoxemia in high-acuity patients. Shunting also helps explain how problems in ventilation and perfusion originate. Not all blood that flows through the lungs participates in gas exchange. **Physiologic shunt** is the term used to describe the blood that moves from the right heart through the lungs and into the left heart without taking part in alveolar–capillary diffusion. Physiologic shunt can be divided into three types: anatomic, capillary, and shuntlike effect (Fig. 5–5). Total physiologic shunting normally ranges

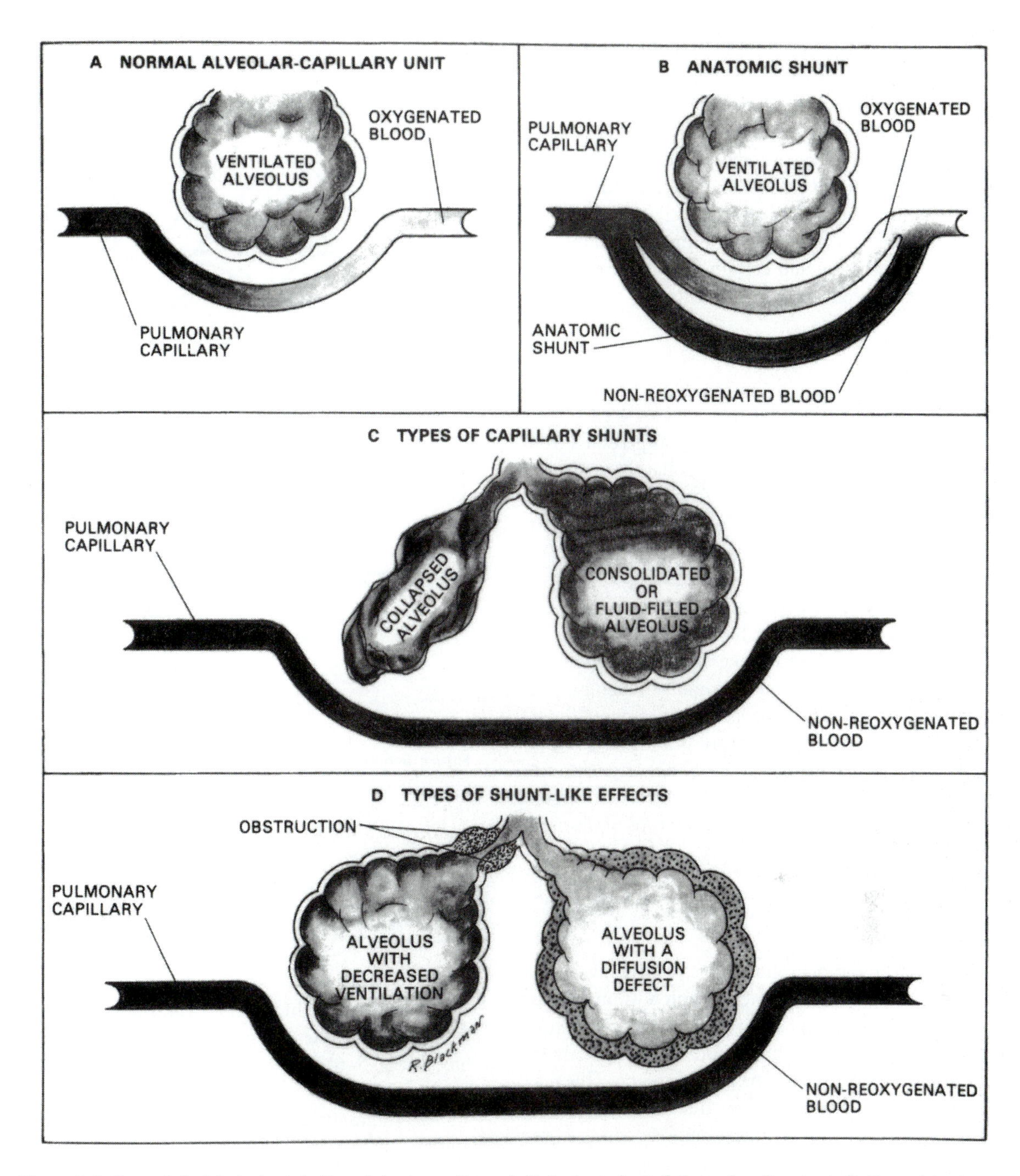

Figure 5–5. Types of physiologic shunt. **A.** Normal alevolar–capillary unit. **B.** Anatomic shunt. **C.** Types of capillary shunts. **D.** Types of shunt-like effects. *(From* Cardiopulmonary Anatomy and Physiology, *2nd ed., by J. R. Des Jardins © 1993. Reprinted with permission of Delmar, a division of Thompson Learning. Fax (800) 730-2215.)*

from 2 percent to 5 percent of cardiac output. Shunting of more than 15 percent of cardiac output can be noted in severe respiratory failure conditions, such as ARDS. Several fairly simple formulas for estimating the degree of shunt are presented in Section Nine.

Anatomic Shunt

Anatomic shunt refers to blood that moves from the right heart and back into the left heart without coming into contact with alveoli. Normally, this is approximately

2 percent to 5 percent of blood flow. Normal anatomic shunting occurs as a result of emptying of the bronchial and several other veins into the lung's own venous system. Abnormal anatomic shunting can occur because of heart or lung problems. For example, a ventricular septal defect, in the presence of pulmonary hypertension, shunts venous blood from the right heart directly into the arterial blood in the left heart. Traumatic injury to pulmonary blood vessels and tissues and certain types of lung tumors also can cause abnormal anatomic shunting.

Capillary Shunt

Capillary shunt is the normal flow of blood past completely unventilated alveoli. Capillary shunt results from such conditions as consolidation or collapse of alveoli, atelectasis, or fluid in the alveoli. Anatomic shunt and capillary shunt together are called **absolute (true) shunt.** The amount of absolute shunt has important clinical implications. Lung tissue that is affected by absolute shunt is unaffected by oxygen therapy, since it involves nonfunctioning alveoli. No matter how much oxygen is administered, diffusion cannot take place if alveoli are completely bypassed or nonfunctioning. For example, patients with ARDS generally have a shunt of over 20 percent of cardiac output. The hallmark of ARDS is refractory hypoxemia (hypoxemia that is not significantly affected by administration of increasing levels of oxygen, which is consistent with the clinical picture of absolute shunt).

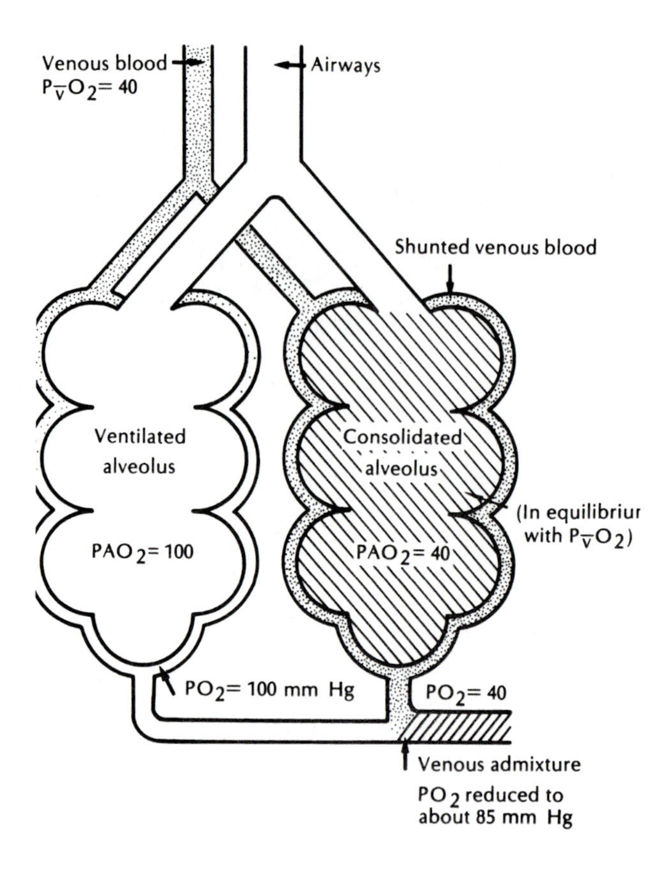

Figure 5–6. Venous admixture. Venous admixture occurs when reoxygenated blood mixes with nonreoxygenated blood distal to the alveoli. *(From Des Jardins, T.R. [1990].* Clinical manifestations of respiratory disease, *2nd ed., [p. 22]. Chicago: Year Book Medical Publishers.)*

Shuntlike Effect

A third type of physiologic shunt is referred to as **shuntlike effect**. Shuntlike effect is not complete shunting but occurs when there is an excess of perfusion in relation to alevolar ventilation. Such a condition exists when alveolar ventilation is reduced but not totally absent. This may be created by pulmonary conditions that cause such problems as bronchospasm, hypoventilation, or pooling of secretions. Fortunately, since the alveoli are still functioning, hypoxemia secondary to shuntlike effect is very responsive to oxygen therapy.

Venous Admixture

Venous admixture refers to the effect that physiologic shunt has on the contents of the blood as it drains into the left heart and out into the system as arterial blood. As the reoxygenated and unoxygenated blood combine in the bloodstream beyond the shunt area, the blood seeks to gain an equilibrium of oxygen molecules. The oxygen molecules remix in the combined blood to establish a new balance. The end resulting PaO_2 is higher than that which existed in the shunted (unoxygenated) blood but lower than what it was in the reoxygenated (nonshunted) blood (Fig. 5–6).

In summary, oxygenation is greatly affected by the amount of blood that does not take part in gas exchange in the lungs. Physiologic shunt helps explain how hypoxemia develops. There are three types of physiologic shunt: anatomic, capillary, and shuntlike effect. The combination of anatomic and capillary shunt is called absolute shunt, which is refractory to oxygen therapy, since it involves nonfunctioning alveoli. Shuntlike effect, however, is correctable using oxygen therapy, since the alveoli are still functioning to some extent. The end result of shunting is called venous admixture, which represents the final oxygen content of the blood as it moves into arterial circulation. It is composed of the blending of the reoxygenated and unoxygenated (shunted) blood. An arterial blood gas (ABG) specimen gives a representative sample of venous admixture blood.

Section Four Review

1. Which of the following best describes the term *physiologic shunt?*
   A. alveoli that have no air flow
   B. alveoli that have air trapped in them
   C. blood that does not take part in pulmonary gas exchange
   D. blood entering the right heart without being oxygenated
2. Normal physiologic shunt ranges from what percentage of cardiac output?
   A. 0 to 5
   B. 2 to 5
   C. 10 to 30
   D. 20 to 40
3. Of the following, anatomic shunt would most likely exist with
   A. pneumonia
   B. pulmonary edema
   C. tuberculosis
   D. ventricular septal defect
4. Normal blood flow past completely unventilated alveoli is the definition of
   A. physiologic shunt
   B. anatomic shunt
   C. capillary shunt
   D. venous admixture
5. Oxygen therapy is most effective in treating which of the following?
   A. shuntlike effect
   B. anatomic shunt
   C. capillary shunt
   D. absolute shunt

Answers: 1. C, 2. B, 3. D, 4. C, 5. A

SECTION FIVE: Pulmonary Function Evaluation

At the completion of this section, the learner will be able to briefly describe various tests used to evaluate pulmonary function.

The medical team generally initiates orders for pulmonary function testing to assist in diagnosing a pulmonary problem or updating or evaluating a patient's pulmonary status. Actual implementation and interpretation of the tests often become an interdisciplinary undertaking.

Pulmonary Function Tests

Ventilation is measured in a variety of ways using pulmonary function tests (PFTs). Pulmonary function tests provide baseline data and also provide a means to monitor the progress of the degree of functional impairment associated with pulmonary diseases. They help differentiate a restrictive pulmonary problem from an obstructive problem. In addition, PFTs are very useful for monitoring the effectiveness of therapeutic interventions.

Total Lung Capacity

Total lung capacity (TLC) is the amount (volume) of gas present in the lungs after maximal inspiration, which is equal to about 6,000 mL in an adult. Total lung capacity is composed of four separate volumes, each of which can be measured separately. These volumes are called inspiratory reserve volume (IRV), tidal volume (TV), expiratory reserve volume (ERV), and residual volume (RV). Volumes also can be measured in combinations called lung capacities. *Lung capacities* include inspiratory capacity (IC), vital capacity (VC), functional residual capacity (FRC), and TLC.

Bedside Pulmonary Function Measurements

High-acuity patients with or without direct pulmonary involvement are at risk of developing pulmonary complications associated with immobility and respiratory muscle fatigue. Pulmonary function may be monitored in patients who are at particular risk for ventilatory decompensation. Of particular interest are tidal volume, vital capacity, and minute ventilation. **Tidal volume (TV or V_T)** is the amount of air that moves in and out of the lungs with each normal breath. Normal TV is approximately 7 to 9 mL/kg (Des Jardins, 1993), about 500 mL in the average-sized man. When TV drops below 4 mL/kg, a state of alveolar hypoventilation develops. If the hypoventilation is severe enough, acute respiratory failure results.

Vital capacity (VC) is the maximum amount of air expired after a maximal inspiration. Normal VC is approximately 4,800 mL in the average-sized man. Both TV and VC help monitor respiratory muscle strength. As the patient experiences respiratory muscle fatigue, these values will decrease. Both of these PFTs can be measured using a respiratory spirometer.

Minute Ventilation

Minute ventilation ($\dot{V}_E$) is the total volume of expired air in 1 minute. It is used as a rapid method of measuring total lung ventilation changes, but it is not considered to be an accurate measure of alveolar ventilation. Minute ventilation is not a direct measurement but a simple calculation,

$$\dot{V}_E = V_T \times f$$

where f = frequency, breaths per minute. Normal minute ventilation is 5 to 10 L/min. When it increases to over 10 L/min, the work of breathing is significantly increased. Minute ventilation below 5 L/min indicates that the patient is at risk for problems associated with hypoventilation.

Forced Expiratory Volumes

Forced expiratory volumes (FEVs) are important diagnostic measurements that help differentiate restrictive pulmonary problems from obstructive problems and measure airway resistance. FEVs measure how rapidly a person can forcefully exhale air after a maximal inhalation, measuring volume (in liters) over time (in seconds). Patients who have a restrictive airway problem will be able to push air forcefully out of their lungs at a normal rate, whereas persons who have an obstructive problem will have a delayed emptying rate (a reduced rate of expiratory air flow).

TABLE 5–2. PULMONARY FUNCTION MEASUREMENTS

MEASUREMENT	NORMAL ADULT RANGE/VALUE
Total lung capacity (TLC)	6,000 mL
Tidal volume (TV, V_T)	7–9 mL/kg
Vital capacity (VC)	4,800 mL (average male)
Minute ventilation ($\dot{V}_E$) ($\dot{V}_E = V_T \times f$)	5–10 mL/min

In summary, there are a wide variety of methods by which pulmonary function can be evaluated. Pulmonary function tests, such as tidal volume, vital capacity, and total lung capacity, help measure the effects of a disease process on ventilation. Table 5–2 lists normal pulmonary function values. Assessment of gas exchange is discussed in depth in Module 6.

SECTION FIVE REVIEW

1. In the acutely ill patient, pulmonary function testing helps monitor for
   - A. impending ventilatory failure
   - B. acute hypoxemia
   - C. acute metabolic acidosis
   - D. impending oxygenation failure
2. Minute ventilation $\dot{V}_E$ is calculated as
   - A. $\dot{V}_E = VC \times f$
   - B. $\dot{V}_E = TV/f$
   - C. $\dot{V}_E = VC \times TV$
   - D. $\dot{V}_E = TV \times f$
3. Patients who have obstructive pulmonary disease will have which of the following patterns of FEVs?
   - A. increased FEVs
   - B. delayed FEVs
   - C. normal FEVs
   - D. variable FEVs
4. Total lung capacity is defined as
   - A. the rate at which air can be forcefully exhaled after a maximal inspiration
   - B. the amount of air that moves in and out of the lungs with each normal breath
   - C. the volume of gas present in the lungs after a maximal inspiration
   - D. the maximum amount of air expired after a maximal inspiration
5. Normal tidal volume in an average-sized adult male would be ______ mL/kg
   - A. 3 to 4
   - B. 4 to 5
   - C. 5 to 7
   - D. 7 to 9

Answers: 1. A, 2. D, 3. B, 4. C, 5. D

SECTION SIX: Restrictive versus Obstructive Pulmonary Disorders

At the completion of this section, the learner will be able to explain the basic differences between restrictive and obstructive pulmonary diseases.

Pulmonary diseases may be divided into acute and chronic problems. Acute problems have a rapid onset and are episodic. Acute pulmonary problems frequently are confined to the lungs. Chronic problems have a slow, often insidious onset. The pulmonary impairment either does not change or slowly worsens over an extended period. Chronic pulmonary problems generally involve other organs as part of the disease process. Patients with chronic pulmonary problems, such as emphysema, may develop an acute problem (e.g., pneumonia) that may further stress their pulmonary status.

Pulmonary diseases may be divided further into problems of inflow of air (restrictive) and problems of outflow of air (obstructive). By being able to differentiate between obstructive and restrictive pulmonary diseases, the nurse can apply appropriate nursing diagnoses regardless of the medical diagnosis of the specific pulmonary disease process.

Restrictive Pulmonary Disorders

Restrictive disorders are associated with decreased lung compliance, and, thus, decreased lung expansion. Restrictive disorders may be caused by a decrease in functioning alveoli, as in pneumonia; by lung tissue loss, as in pneumonectomy or lung tumors; or by external problems, such as chest burns or obesity. (Table 5–3 provides a more complete listing of restrictive disorders.)

Restrictive disorders are problems of volume, not airflow. The term *volume* refers to the amount of air that can be moved in and out of the lung with either normal breathing or maximal breathing. TLC is a measurement of lung volume (see Section Five). TLC is decreased in individuals who have a restrictive disorder. Air cannot move into the alveoli as readily as it should because of limited expansion, which leads to alveolar hypoventilation. Alveolar hypoventilation will lead to hypoxemia if alveolar oxygen is removed (via diffusion) at a rate that is faster than it can be replaced by ventilation. When this occurs, the PaO_2 will fall at approximately the same rate as the $PaCO_2$ rises, assuming that diffusion is normal (Hunt, 1999).

Restrictive disorders do not interfere with airflow (the rate of movement of air into or out of the lungs). The volume of air the person is able to get into the lungs can be exhaled at a normal rate of flow. The relationship of ventilation to perfusion ($\dot{V}/\dot{Q}$ ratio) may be disturbed as a result of restrictive problems. In mild to moderate restrictive disease, the $\dot{V}/\dot{Q}$ ratio may stay normal, since both ventilation and perfusion may be fairly equally disturbed. In many acute restrictive diseases, perfusion can be diminished secondary to edema resulting from the inflammatory process or from reduced or absent blood flow secondary to compression or blockage of capillaries. In severe disease, a low $\dot{V}/\dot{Q}$ ratio may develop because ventilation is greatly diminished, whereas perfusion may be fairly normal or moderately disturbed. A low $\dot{V}/\dot{Q}$ ratio is associated with hypoxemia with a decreasing pH and increasing $PaCO_2$. Table 5–4 lists the typical signs and symptoms associated with restrictive pulmonary disorders.

TABLE 5–3. EXAMPLES OF RESTRICTIVE DISORDERS

EXTERNAL PROBLEMS	INTERNAL (PARENCHYMAL) PROBLEMS
Obesity	Pneumonia
Extensive chest burns	Atelectasis
Flail chest	Congestive heart failure
Neuromuscular diseases	Pulmonary edema
Myasthenia gravis	Pulmonary fibrosis
Muscular dystrophy	Pulmonary tumors
Guillain-Barré syndrome	Pneumothorax
Spinal cord trauma	

TABLE 5–4. SIGNS AND SYMPTOMS OF RESTRICTIVE DISORDERS

Increased respiratory rate
Decreased tidal volume (TV)
Normal to decreased PaO_2
Shortness of breath
Cough
Chest pain or discomfort
Fatigue
History of weight loss

Obstructive Pulmonary Disorders

Chronic obstructive pulmonary disease (COPD) is the term commonly applied in the clinical setting to refer to pulmonary disorders that hinder expiratory airflow. The more accurate and preferred term for these disorders, however, is *chronic airflow limitation.* Currently, these two terms are often used interchangeably. Some of the major **obstructive disorders** include

- Emphysema
- Chronic bronchitis
- Asthma
- Cystic fibrosis

Asthma differs from the other diseases in that it is episodic rather than continuous obstruction. Air is able to flow into the lungs but then becomes trapped, making it very difficult to rid the lungs of the inspired air. The inability to exhale rapidly causes a prolongation of expiratory time. If expiratory time is severely prolonged, the lungs may never be able to empty before the person must inhale again. Expiratory times can be measured using FEV studies (Section Five).

Obstructive problems may be caused by airway narrowing, such as in bronchospasm and bronchoconstriction, or by airway obstruction, such as is seen with pooling of secretions or destruction of bronchioles and alveoli. Obstructive disorders are frequently associated with increased lung compliance accompanied by a loss of elastic recoil; however, a notable exception to this generalization is asthma. The $\dot{V}/\dot{Q}$ ratio also may be disturbed with this group of disorders. In disease processes that do not destroy alveoli **(chronic bronchitis),** a low $\dot{V}/\dot{Q}$ ratio may exist. Ventilation is reduced, whereas perfusion remains normal. If lung tissue is actually destroyed **(emphysema),** the $\dot{V}/\dot{Q}$ ratio may remain normal because both ventilation and perfusion are equally destroyed. A normal $\dot{V}/\dot{Q}$ ratio does not necessarily indicate healthy lungs. It indicates only that a balance exists between ventilation and blood flow. Table 5–5 lists the typical clinical manifestations associated with obstructive pulmonary disorders.

TABLE 5–5. CLINICAL MANIFESTATIONS OF OBSTRUCTIVE PULMONARY DISORDERS

Mucus hypersecretion (except with pure emphysema)
Wheezes, rhonchi
Dyspnea (episodic or progressive)
Diminished breath and heart sounds
Barrel chest (increased AP diameter)
Progressive hypercapnia and respiratory acidosis
Progressive or episodic hypoxemia (particularly in later stages)
Cor pulmonale
Accessory muscle use
Increased expiratory time (E > I)
PFTs: Normal to increased TLC, increased FRC, decreased FEV, decreased VC

Cor Pulmonale

Cor pulmonale refers to right ventricular hypertrophy and dilation secondary to pulmonary disease. It is a complication of both restrictive and obstructive pulmonary diseases. Cor pulmonale can cause right heart failure and is a major cause of death in the COPD patient. To gain a clearer understanding of cor pulmonale, the concept of pulmonary vascular resistance needs to be explained.

Pulmonary Vascular Resistance

Pulmonary vascular resistance (PVR) measures the resistance to blood flow in the pulmonary vascular system, which is a low-resistance system. In effect, it represents right ventricular afterload in much the same way that systemic vascular resistance represents left ventricular afterload (a high-resistance system). The right ventricle pumps oxygen-poor blood into the pulmonary capillaries by way of the pulmonary artery. The amount of right ventricular force required to pump the blood into the lungs depends on the resistance to flow present in the pulmonary vascular system. This resistance to flow is called *pulmonary vascular resistance.* When PVR becomes elevated, the patient is at increased risk for development of a form of right heart failure associated with cor pulmonale.

Three main factors determine the amount of pulmonary resistance: the length and radius of the vessels and the viscosity of the blood. Of these factors, the major determinant of pulmonary vascular resistance is vessel radius (caliber).

VESSEL RADIUS DETERMINANTS. Vessel radius refers to the diameter (caliber) of the vessels. Vessel radius is altered by:

- The volume of blood in the pulmonary vascular system
- The amount of vasoconstriction
- The degree of lung inflation

Factors related to the volume of blood in the pulmonary vascular system include capillary recruitment and distention. Of these factors, recruitment is the most influential. The small pulmonary capillaries open up (are recruited) in response to an increase in blood flow. Under circumstances in which pulmonary blood flow is low (e.g., shock), the smaller capillaries may receive so little blood that they collapse. The concept of pulmonary capillary recruitment is similar to the recruitment and collapse of alveoli based on volume of airflow. The second factor, distention, occurs in response to increased cardiac output or increased intravascular fluid volume. By distending, the capillaries are able to accommodate the increased flow. Distention of the capillaries decreases PVR.

Vasoconstriction occurs in response to hypoxia and acidosis. Vasoconstriction is a major cause of increased PVR in the high-acuity patient, and hypoxia is the strongest stimulant for pulmonary vasoconstriction. When an area of the lung becomes hypoxic, such as is seen in shunt, vasoconstriction is triggered. This response effectively deviates blood flow to more functional areas of the lungs and results in a reduction in the impact of shunt. Unfortunately, in cases involving a generalized pulmonary disease process (e.g., late-stage emphysema), vasoconstriction is also generalized and PVR increases significantly. The elevated PVR requires the right heart to work against elevated pressures. In response to this increased workload, the right heart hypertrophies, and cor pulmonale develops (Des Jardins & Burton, 1995).

The degree of lung inflation also has an impact on the diameter of the pulmonary capillaries. As the lung inflates, capillaries become stretched. In states of high lung inflation, capillaries become very stretched, which decreases their diameter and thus increases PVR. The opposite is also true: Lower lung volumes are associated with decreased PVR.

Calculation of PVR is presented in Section Nine: Respiratory Calculations.

Cor pulmonale is the result of a sequence of events precipitated by pulmonary hypertension. Pulmonary vessels function in a low pressure system. Many pulmonary conditions, both acute and chronic, cause pressures to increase in the vascular bed, creating a state of pulmonary hypertension. When this occurs, PVR increases. Pressure in the pulmonary artery is increased, making it more difficult to push blood out of the right heart during systole. The right heart becomes congested because less blood is moved out with each contraction. Over time, this congestion causes the right heart chambers to dilate. The right heart muscle hypertrophies to compensate for the required increased work of contraction. Figure 5–7 is a diagram showing how the heart is affected by chronic respiratory disorders.

In summary, restrictive diseases are those that interfere with lung expansion. They cause a decrease in lung volumes while expiratory airflow remains normal. They are associated with decreased compliance. Restrictive diseases can be measured by pulmonary function tests, par-

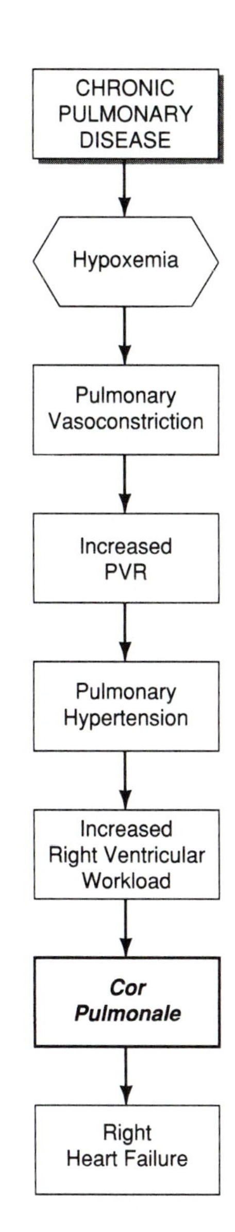

Figure 5–7. Cor pulmonale. Severe chronic pulmonary diseases are associated with a pattern of increasing hypoxemia that causes the lungs to vasoconstrict. The pulmonary vascular vasoconstriction increases PVR, which results in pulmonary hypertension. The right heart is required to work harder to pump blood into the pulmonary vascular system, and, over time, the right ventricle dilates and hypertrophies in response to the increased PVR. The adaptation of the right ventricle is called *cor pulmonale.*

TABLE 5–6. COMPARISON OF RESTRICTIVE AND OBSTRUCTIVE PULMONARY DISEASES

RESTRICTIVE DISORDERS	OBSTRUCTIVE DISORDERS
Characteristics	
Decreased lung expansion	Increased lung expansion
Decreased lung compliance	Increased lung compliance
Normal airflow	Decreased expiratory airflow; prolonged expiratory time
Pulmonary Function Testing	
Decreased TLC	Decreased FEVs
Decreased total volume	
Pathologic Disturbances	
Internal Problems	Bronchoconstriction
Decreased functioning alveoli	Bronchospasm
Loss of pulmonary tissue	Airway obstruction
	Airway collapse
	Pooling of copious secretions
External Problems	
Disorders that decrease lung compliance external to the lungs	
Associated Blood Gas Disturbances	
Decreased Pa_{O_2}	Increased Pa_{CO_2}
Normal to low $\dot{V}/\dot{Q}$ ratio	Decreased pH (if not compensated)
Increased intrapulmonary shunt	
Increased Pa_{CO_2} and decreased pH if ventilatory pump failure is present	Normal to decreased Pa_{O_2} (may stay stable until severe disease state)
Associated Lung Sounds	
Crackles (most common)	Wheezes (most common)
Rhonchi, if secretions build up in large airways	Rhonchi, if secretions build up in large airways
	Crackles (particularly associated with cor pulmonale)

ticularly TLC. Obstructive diseases are those that interfere with expiratory airflow. Airflow is reduced or delayed, whereas lung volume remains normal. Obstructive diseases are associated with increased lung compliance. They can be evaluated by measuring FEV flow rates. Table 5–6 compares these two disease processes. Cor pulmonale is a complication of chronic respiratory diseases. Ultimately, right heart failure develops secondary to increased pulmonary vascular resistance.

SECTION SIX REVIEW

1. Restrictive pulmonary diseases are associated with
   A. increased lung expansion
   B. increased lung compliance
   C. decreased lung expansion
   D. decreased air flow into lungs

2. Which of the following is considered a restrictive disease?
   A. pneumonia
   B. asthma
   C. emphysema
   D. chronic bronchitis
3. Obstructive pulmonary diseases are associated with
   A. decreased lung expansion
   B. decreased lung compliance
   C. decreased air flow into lungs
   D. decreased expiratory airflow
4. An example of an obstructive pulmonary disease is
   A. multiple sclerosis
   B. asthma
   C. tuberculosis
   D. pneumonia
5. Lung compliance is increased with which disorder?
   A. emphysema
   B. pneumonia
   C. pneumothorax
   D. chest burns
6. A patient who has cor pulmonale will have
   A. left heart dilation
   B. right heart hypertrophy
   C. pulmonary fibrosis
   D. left ventricular hyperplasia
7. The major cause of increased PVR is
   A. hypercarbia
   B. alkalosis
   C. hypoxia
   D. cor pulmonale

Answers: 1. C, 2. A, 3. D, 4. B, 5. A, 6. B, 7. C

SECTION SEVEN: Acute Respiratory Failure

At the completion of this section, the learner will be able to discuss the basis of respiratory failure.

Cardiopulmonary System

It is helpful to think of the heart and lungs as a complex integrated cardiopulmonary system. Since the heart and lungs and systemic circulation share a common circuit (Fig. 5–8), whatever affects one part of the system potentially affects the whole. The cardiopulmonary system is very sensitive to pressure changes within it, requiring compensatory adjustments to maintain homeostasis. Problems of cardiac origin can create secondary pulmonary problems. For example, left heart failure can cause cardiogenic pulmonary edema. Pulmonary problems can affect cardiac status, for example, cor pulmonale. If a pulmonary disorder decreases the ability of the lungs to adequately maintain an acid–base balance and oxygenation, the patient's heart will work harder to make more blood available for diffusion, causing a compensatory increase in vital signs (increased blood pressure and pulse). The patient's lungs will work harder by altering the breathing by increasing rate (tachypnea) and depth (hyperventilation).

Insufficiency versus Failure

Respiratory disorders vary greatly in the way in which they affect lung function. The amount of diffusion surface area that becomes impaired is a major factor in altering gas exchange. The extent of impairment coupled with the rate of onset contribute greatly to the ability of the body to cope adequately. The terms *chronic respiratory insufficiency* and *acute respiratory failure* are used to differentiate the level of compensation.

Chronic Respiratory Insufficiency

Respiratory insufficiency is a state in which an acceptable level of gas exchange is maintained only through cardiopulmonary compensatory mechanisms. Chronic pulmonary problems have a slow onset and often are progressive in nature. The body has time to compensate for growing pulmonary deficits, thereby maintaining an adequate level of oxygenation and acid–base balance. A person can lead a relatively normal life in a state of chronic respiratory insufficiency. Arterial blood gases would reflect a normal pH, though the $Pa{CO_2}$ may be abnormal (a compensated respiratory acidosis) with a correspondingly high bicarbonate level, and the $Pa{O_2}$ might reflect some degree of hypoxemia. This compensated state, however, is not normal. A person in chronic respiratory insufficiency is always in a state of impending respiratory failure. Should a new stress overtax the ability of the body to compensate in meeting an even greater demand, the person will develop acute respiratory failure.

Acute Respiratory Failure

Respiratory failure is a life-threatening state in which the cardiopulmonary system is unable to maintain adequate gas exchange. The clinical definition of acute respiratory failure is given in Table 5–7. Acute respiratory failure is caused by an imbalance in supply and demand. Normally, the cardiopulmonary system is able to meet the demands of the body by increasing its work to supply adequate oxygen and ridding the body of carbon dioxide. If

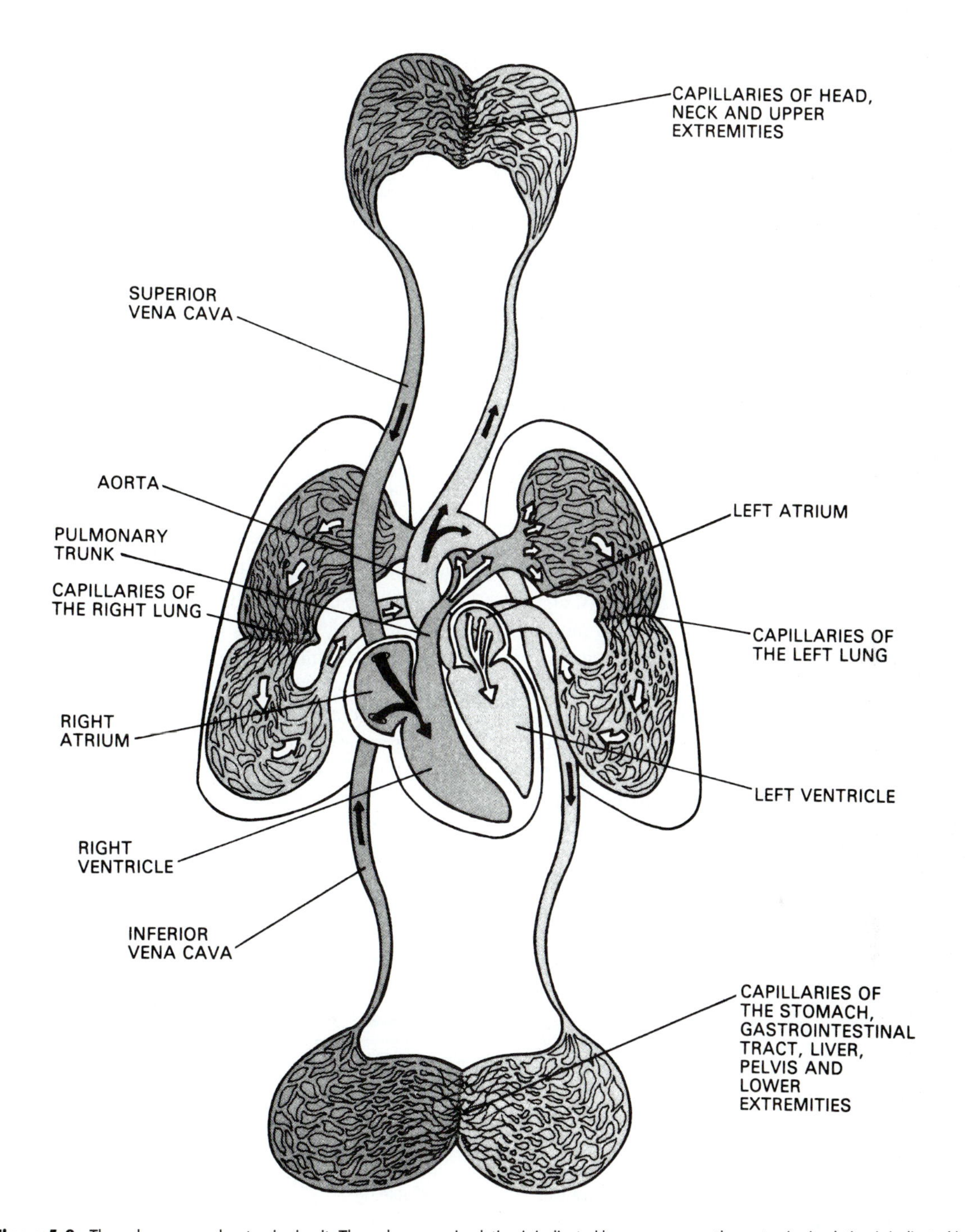

Figure 5–8. The pulmonary and systemic circuit. The pulmonary circulation is indicated by open arrows; the systemic circulation is indicated by solid arrows. *(From* Cardiopulmonary Anatomy and Physiology, *2nd ed., by J. R. Des Jardins © 1993. Reprinted with permission of Delmar, a division of Thompson Learning. Fax (800) 730-2215.)*

the body's demands become higher than the cardiopulmonary system can supply, the system will fail, precipitating acute respiratory failure.

Components of Acute Respiratory Failure

The term **acute respiratory failure** is a general one that pertains to both gas exchange components: oxygen and carbon dioxide. To better understand and clarify respiratory failure, it is helpful to break it down into its two component parts, failure of oxygenation and failure of ventilation. Both components may occur together initially, the patient suffering from both a low PaO_2 and a high $PaCO_2$, with accompanying low pH. At the onset of failure, however, the primary problem is often one or the other rather than both. For this reason, it is important to be able to differentiate the two failure components.

TABLE 5–7. ACUTE RESPIRATORY FAILURE AND ITS COMPONENTS

TYPE OF FAILURE	CLINICAL DEFINITION	CLINICAL MANIFESTATIONS
Acute respiratory failure	$Paco_2 \geq 50$ mm Hg with a pH ≤ 7.30 and/or $Pao_2 \leq 60$ mm Hg	
Oxygenation failure	$Pao_2 \leq 60$ mm Hg	Pulmonary: dyspnea, tachypnea Cardiovascular: increased BP, HR, cardiac dysrhythmias, cyanosis, and increased PVR Central nervous system: altered level of responsiveness; restlessness
Ventilation failure	$Paco_2 \geq 50$ mm Hg with a pH ≤ 7.30 (acute respiratory acidosis)	Pulmonary: tachypnea Vascular: headache; flushed, wet skin Cardiovascular: bounding pulse, increased BP and HR Central nervous system: anesthetic effects of carbon dioxide: lethargy, drowsiness, coma (CO_2 narcosis)

Failure of Oxygenation

When a state of **oxygenation failure** exists, the primary problem is one of hypoxemia. Carbon dioxide (CO_2) is able to diffuse across the alveolar–capillary membrane approximately 20 times more rapidly than is oxygen. For this reason, CO_2 levels may remain normal when diffusion is interfered with, even though the patient is showing signs of moderate to severe hypoxemia. Conditions that can cause oxygenation failure include ARDS, pulmonary embolus, acute asthmatic attack, pneumonia, and others. Should these conditions worsen or should the patient fatigue, the ventilatory component can be initiated.

Shapiro and colleagues (1994) differentiate degrees of hypoxemia, from mild to severe. They also provide guidelines for estimating degree of hypoxemia correction once oxygen therapy is initiated. This information is summarized in Table 5–8. The clinical manifestations and clinical definition of oxygenation failure are presented in Table 5–7.

Failure of Ventilation

Ventilatory failure (acute respiratory acidosis) is caused by alveolar hypoventilation; that is, the inability to move air adequately in and out of the alveoli, allowing a buildup of carbon dioxide. Ventilatory failure can be caused by any problem that interferes with adequate movement of airflow (e.g., neuromuscular disorders, respiratory muscle fatigue, COPD, and many others).

Signs and symptoms of ventilatory failure reflect hypercapnia. The clinical manifestations and clinical definition of ventilatory failure are presented in Table 5–7.

Most of the symptoms associated with hypercapnia are due to the strong vasodilator effect of carbon dioxide. The term CO_2 *narcosis* is sometimes used to describe ventilatory failure based on its anesthetic effects.

Complications of Respiratory Failure

Acute respiratory failure can affect virtually all body systems by causing organ hypoxia. If the respiratory failure is coupled with decreased cardiac output, the patient is at particular risk for development of hypoperfusion/hypoxic organ shock complications, such as those seen with multiple organ dysfunction (MOD). Typical problems triggered by this mechanism include ARDS, acute tubular necrosis (acute renal failure), and many others. (MOD is presented in a separate module.)

As a general rule, ventilation failure is considered to be a more serious problem than oxygenation failure. Acute respiratory acidosis, which is present in ventilatory failure, can quickly deteriorate to systemic acidosis. Cellular function rapidly becomes impaired in acidotic states. Oxygenation failure, on the other hand, is associated with better compensatory mechanisms and, therefore, it is better tolerated.

TABLE 5–8. ASSESSMENT OF HYPOXEMIA

Pao_2 LEVEL[a]	HYPOXEMIA STATUS
On room air	
≥ 80 mm Hg	Normal oxygenation
< 80 mm Hg	Mild hypoxemia
< 60 mm Hg	Moderate hypoxemia[b]
< 40 mm Hg	Severe hypoxemia[b]
On oxygen therapy	
> 100 mm Hg, but less than predicted by[c]	Excessively corrected hypoxemia
60–100 mm Hg	Corrected hypoxemia
< 60 mm Hg	Uncorrected hypoxemia

[a] Minimum acceptable Pao_2 decreases with age: subtract 1 mm Hg from the minimum Pao_2 level for every year of age over 60.

[b] Clinically significant.

[c] Predicted effect of oxygen therapy on Pao_2 in normal lungs:

% O_2	Pao_2
30	> 150 mm Hg
40	> 200 mm Hg
50	> 250 mm Hg
80	> 400 mm Hg
100	> 500 mm Hg

Adapted from Shapiro, B.A. et al. (1994). Clinical application of blood gases, *5th ed, pp. 65, 81. St. Louis: C.V. Mosby.*

Pathogenesis of Respiratory Failure

The sequence of events that leads to the development of respiratory failure is a complicated one. It is initiated by the presence of a respiratory disease (acute or chronic) that interferes with the relationship of ventilation to perfusion ($\dot{V}/\dot{Q}$ ratio) and decreases PaO_2. The body recognizes increased oxygen demand and responds by increasing the rate and depth of respirations to move more air into and out of the alveoli (compensation). This compensatory mechanism increases the PaO_2 and decreases the $PaCO_2$ to regain an adequate level of oxygenation and acid–base balance. Compensatory mechanisms, however, increase the metabolic rate by increasing the work of breathing. When the metabolic rate is increased, more oxygen is consumed by the tissues and more carbon dioxide is produced. The overall effect of the sequence is a progressive increase in arterial carbon dioxide and a decrease in arterial oxygen. A state of acute respiratory failure exists when the patient meets the clinical criteria of $PaCO_2 \geq 50$ mm Hg with a pH of ≤ 7.30 and/or a PaO_2 of ≤ 60 mm Hg.

Should the sequence of events that precipitated the acute respiratory failure not be managed adequately, the level of respiratory failure worsens, causing a further increase in the work of breathing. As the work of breathing increases, the patient develops respiratory muscle fatigue. Once muscle fatigue sets in, the patient will quickly decompensate, worsening both ventilation and oxygenation. If this sequence of events is allowed to continue, arterial blood gas concentrations will steadily worsen, leading to death of the patient.

Acute Lung Injury/Acute Respiratory Distress Syndrome

Acute lung injury (ALI)/Acute respiratory distress syndrome (ARDS) is defined by Curzen and Evans (1998) as "clinically recognizable sequelae of a complex inflammatory reaction to diverse insults" (p. 379). Acute lung injury can be viewed as a continuum of severity from mild, subclinical injury (ALI) to severe injury (ARDS) (see Figure 5–9). In 1992, the American–European Consensus Conference on ARDS defined ALI/ARDS on the basis of clinical criteria as:

- Acute onset
- Bilateral infiltrates on chest x-ray (frontal view)
- Pulmonary artery wedge pressure (PAWP) or ≤ 18 mm Hg and/or no left atrial hypertension (CHF)
- Oxygenation status measured as PaO_2/FIO_2 ratio* (regardless of PEEP)
    - ALI = ≤ 300 mm Hg
    - ARDS = ≤ 200 mm Hg (Vollman and Aulbach, 1998)

Mild ⟵⟶ **Severe**

(Subclinical, no other organs involved) — (ARDS, multiple organ dysfunction)

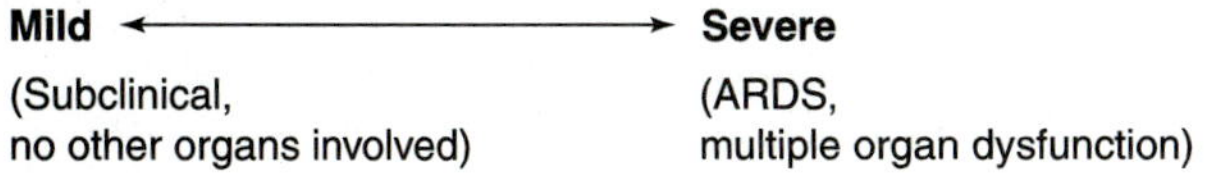

Figure 5–9. ALI/ARDS Continuum of Severity. *(From Curzen, N.P., & Evans, T.W. [1998]. Pulmonary vascular control mechanisms in sepsis and acute lung injury. In E.K. Weir & J.T. Reeves (eds.),* Pulmonary edema: American Heart Association monograph series, *[p. 378]. Armonk, NY: Futura Publishing.)*

In 1995, the Modified Lung Injury Score was developed, which provided a more simple diagnostic approach to diagnosing ARDS that focused only on chest x-ray and PaO_2/FIO_2 ratio findings (Vollman & Aulbach, 1998).

ARDS is a distinct type of acute lung injury resulting in severe respiratory failure. It is caused by diffuse inflammatory injury to the alveolar–capillary membrane, resulting in noncardiogenic pulmonary edema. It is estimated that there are more than 200,000 cases of ARDS per year (Von Rueden, 1998). Acute respiratory distress syndrome is not a disease but a pattern of pathophysiological lung changes resulting in a corresponding pattern of clinical manifestations.

Etiologic Factors. ARDS can be precipitated by direct or indirect pulmonary injury. Patients who are at highest risk for developing ARDS are those experiencing serious infections (particularly **sepsis**), hypovolemic shock, and multiple trauma. A complete list of potential causes of ARDS would be an extensive one. The underlying factor that is common to all precipitating insults is hypoperfusion/hypoxia of lung parenchyma.

Pathogenesis. According to Vollman and Aulbach (1998), ARDS has been associated with systemic inflammatory response syndrome (SIRS). ARDS is the lung's expression of this widespread inflammatory event. No matter what initial direct or indirect insult triggers the onset of ALI/ARDS, the subsequent sequence of events remains relatively predictable. The pathogenesis of ARDS and SIRS is discussed in further detail in Module 11.

Clinical Presentation. There are two patterns of clinical presentation based on the preexisting health state of the individual. In an otherwise healthy person, onset of ARDS usually occurs rapidly, often only a few hours following the triggering insult. The typical early clinical findings are increasing respiratory distress that becomes severe, chest x-ray that is initially normal, acute respiratory alkalosis due to hyperventilation, and either absence of or mild hypoxemia (Vollman & Aulbach, 1998). In persons who have chronic illnesses or comorbid pathologic conditions, the presenting clinical findings are often more insidious, being initially hidden by their other health problems. In this group, ARDS becomes apparent within 24 to 48 hours after the initial insult.

*PaO_2/FIO_2 ratio is easily calculated (see Table 5–14 in Section Nine).

As ARDS progresses, cyanosis and accessory muscle use may be noted. A cough develops, frequently producing sputum that is typical of pulmonary edema. Arterial blood gas findings show a pattern of increasing hypoxemia that is refractory to increasing concentrations of oxygen. The refractory nature of the hypoxemia is largely due to increasing capillary shunt as alveolar units collapse and become dysfunctional. Pulmonary function tests will be consistent with lung restriction, including decreased lung compliance and decreased functional residual capacity (FRC). ARDS can be diagnosed using either the American–European Consensus Conference on ARDS criteria as presented earlier, or the Modified Lung Injury Score. The Modified Lung Injury Score clinically defines ARDS as the presence of bilateral infiltrates by chest x-ray with a decreased PaO_2/FIO_2 ratio of < 175 mm Hg. The Modified Lung Injury Score and the American–European Consensus Conference on ARDS clinical criteria are both considered highly predictive of ARDS (Vollman & Aulbach, 1998).

The mortality rate associated with ARDS varies widely depending on its etiology and comorbidity factors, and ranges from estimates of about 50 percent to over 85 percent mortality. The highest mortality rate is associated with sepsis. Mortality rate highly correlates with the degree of lung injury severity at 72 hours following onset (Vollman & Aulbach, 1998). For those who survive, lung repair occurs slowly and terminates by about six months following the onset of ARDS. Approximately 50 percent will ultimately have no significant permanent lung damage (Vollman & Aulbach). Treatment of ARDS varies widely and is continuously being researched and improved. Nursing emphasis is on supportive measures to maintain the patient until the alveolar–capillary membrane regains its integrity and the syndrome resolves.

In summary, respiratory failure is a potential complication of respiratory insufficiency. Acute respiratory failure can be divided into two components: failure to oxygenate and failure to ventilate. Respiratory failure can cause dysfunction of all organs due to tissue hypoxia, possibly leading to MOD. Adult respiratory distress syndrome is a severe form of acute respiratory failure that is resistant to oxygen therapy.

SECTION SEVEN REVIEW

1. Of the following, which arterial blood gas pH results would be most commonly noted with respiratory insufficiency?
   A. pH within normal limits
   B. pH above normal range
   C. pH below normal range
   D. variable pH
2. Of the following, which arterial blood gas pH results would best reflect acute respiratory failure?
   A. normal pH
   B. pH higher than normal
   C. pH lower than normal
   D. variable pH
3. Failure to oxygenate refers to which of the following primary problems?
   A. ventilation
   B. hypoxemia
   C. arterial pH
   D. carbon dioxide
4. Which of the following symptoms is typical of failure to oxygenate?
   A. bounding pulse
   B. headache
   C. flushed skin
   D. restlessness
5. The primary problem associated with failure to ventilate is
   A. alveolar hypoventilation
   B. capillary hypoperfusion
   C. alveolar hyperventilation
   D. capillary hyperperfusion
6. The symptoms that are typical of ventilatory failure are primarily the result of
   A. vasoconstriction
   B. hypoxemia
   C. vasodilation
   D. acidosis
7. The result of increased metabolic demand is
   A. decreased oxygen consumption
   B. decreased carbon dioxide production
   C. increased oxygen consumption
   D. increased carbon dioxide consumption
8. The pulmonary edema associated with ARDS is caused by
   A. capillary microembolism
   B. left ventricular failure
   C. loss of surfactant
   D. injured alveolar–capillary membrane
9. Which of the following findings are typically present with ARDS?
   A. decreased PaO_2/FIO_2 ratio
   B. increased lung compliance
   C. decreased airway resistance
   D. increased functional residual capacity

10. The refractory (resistant) nature of ARDS to oxygen therapy is based on the amount of
   A. capillary shunt
   B. venous admixture
   C. anatomic shunt
   D. shuntlike effect

Answers: 1. A, 2. C, 3. B, 4. D, 5. A, 6. C, 7. C, 8. D, 9. A, 10. A

SECTION EIGHT: Respiratory Assessment

Nursing History

When a patient is admitted to the hospital in acute distress, the nurse initially assesses airway, breathing, and circulation (ABCs) and immediately takes appropriate action based on those assessments. As soon as is feasible, information regarding the immediate events leading to admission should be obtained. A recent history gives important clues as to the etiology and chain of events related to the current problem.

The presence of severe respiratory distress limits the amount of health history information a patient is able to relate. Minimize questions directed to the patient to reduce the stress on breathing, stating all inquiries in such a way that they require very brief answers.

Historical data of particular importance to assess in the patient with pulmonary problems include the following.

Social History

Assess tobacco and alcohol use. Tobacco use is associated with many pulmonary diseases, and current use may further aggravate acute pulmonary problems. Alcohol use in association with prescribed drug therapy may adversely affect the patient's respiratory condition. Problems with alcohol withdrawal can complicate the cardiopulmonary status should delirium tremens develop.

Nutritional History

The nutritional state of a pulmonary patient is crucial to assess because malnutrition is contributory to the development of respiratory failure. There are several ways in which this can happen. First, a protein–calorie deficit weakens muscles, including the respiratory muscles. Second, malnutrition is associated with a weakened immune system, which increases susceptibility to infection and makes it harder to fight against existing infections. The increased stress associated with an acute infection can precipitate acute respiratory failure. Third, a high-carbohydrate diet increases the overall carbon dioxide load in the body. This may lead to ventilatory complications in certain patients.

Cardiopulmonary History

The lungs, heart, and blood vessels comprise a common circuit. For this reason, factors that alter any part of the circuit can cause a subsequent alteration in other parts. It is often difficult to differentiate between problems of pulmonary and cardiovascular etiology. Because of this, obtaining sufficient data regarding the cardiovascular system will be invaluable in planning the management of the patient. Of particular importance is data concerning preexisting cardiovascular or pulmonary problems and prehospitalization activity tolerance levels.

Elimination History

Urinary elimination is not directly affected by pulmonary function. It can, however, be indirectly affected when the patient experiences a severe hypoxic episode. If the kidneys sustain an acute hypoperfusion/hypoxic episode, acute tubular necrosis and acute renal failure could result.

Bowel elimination can negatively affect pulmonary status when constipation occurs. A full, extended bowel can push abdominal contents against the diaphragm, restricting expansion of the lungs. Oxygen consumption also can be increased when the patient strains to evacuate a hard stool, further compromising oxygen levels in patients with marginal or poor arterial blood gases. Patients with pulmonary disorders often experience constipation related to decreased activity levels and decreased intake of fluids and appropriate foods.

Sleep–Rest History

Pulmonary problems frequently interfere with sleep and rest, for a variety of reasons. If the respiratory problem is severe enough to cause hypoxia, the patient often exhibits restlessness associated with inadequate oxygenation of the brain. Pulmonary disorders often increase the work of breathing, which can interfere with rest and sleep. Patients in respiratory distress may sleep poorly because they fear that they will cease to breathe when they are unaware. Others cannot sleep because of their level of general discomfort. Dyspnea and air hunger are very frightening and threatening experiences for pulmonary patients.

Common Complaints Associated with Pulmonary Disorders

If a respiratory problem is suspected, the nurse should focus on obtaining information concerning the most common respiratory complaints: dyspnea, chest pain, cough, sputum, and hemoptysis. This can be accomplished by interviewing the patient and/or family (subjective data) and by performing a nursing assessment (objective data). Regular assessment of the common respiratory symptoms is also important in monitoring the patient for acute changes in respiratory status.

Dyspnea

SUBJECTIVE DATA. **Dyspnea** is a subjective (patient-based) symptom. It refers to the feeling of difficult breathing or shortness of breath. Physiologically, dyspnea is associated with increased work of breathing—a supply-and-demand imbalance. Increased work of breathing occurs when ventilatory demands go beyond the body's ability to respond. Progressive dyspnea is noted commonly in both restrictive and obstructive pulmonary disorders.

Orthopnea is a type of dyspnea closely associated with cardiac problems or severe pulmonary disease. It refers to a state in which the patient assumes a head-up position to relieve dyspnea. Orthopnea may be mild (the patient may need several pillows to sleep comfortably in bed), or it may be severe (the patient may need to sit upright in a chair or in bed).

One type of dyspnea is of particular interest in differentiating cardiac from pulmonary disorders. **Paroxysmal nocturnal dyspnea (PND)** is associated with left heart failure. The typical patient report is that of waking during the night, after being asleep for several hours, with a sudden onset of severe dyspnea. On sitting up or getting out of bed, the dyspnea is relieved, and the patient is able to resume sleep. Paroxysmal nocturnal dyspnea is a form of transient mild pulmonary edema. It is believed that fluids that have been congested in the lower extremities during the day due to gravity drainage shift to the heart and lungs, causing a fluid volume overload when the person becomes horizontal (as in sleep) for several hours.

OBJECTIVE DATA. Objectively, the nurse may note tachypnea, nasal flaring, use of **accessory muscles,** or abnormal arterial blood gases. The patient may voluntarily assume a high-Fowler sitting position secondary to orthopnea. Severe tachypnea, a respiratory rate of over 30 breaths per minute, significantly increases the work of breathing. If allowed to continue for a prolonged period of time, respiratory muscle fatigue can occur, which may ultimately cause acute respiratory failure.

Chest Pain

SUBJECTIVE DATA. The type of chest pain the patient describes can be helpful in differentiating cardiogenic (originating from the heart) from pleuritic (originating from the pleura) pain. Cardiogenic pain generally is described as dull, pressurelike discomfort often radiating to the jaw, back, or left arm. If asked to point to the painful area, the patient often uses the palm of the hand, indicating a somewhat general area. Cardiogenic pain is unaffected by breathing.

Pleuritic pain frequently is described as sharp and knifelike, and the patient is able to point to the pain focal area with one finger. When the patient is between breaths or the breath is held, pain decreases or ceases. The pain increases with deep breathing. A pleural friction rub may sometimes be auscultated at the focal pain point.

Most pulmonary disorders affecting only the lung parenchyma (lung tissue) are not associated with chest pain as an early symptom because the parenchyma is insensitive to pain. For example, lung cancer frequently goes undetected until a routine chest x-ray is taken or the tumor impinges on innervated thoracic structures, causing deep pain. Like lung tissue, the attached **visceral pleura** is insensitive. The **parietal pleura**, however, is well innervated, and when inflammation (called **pleurisy** or **pleuritis**) occurs, it can trigger the sharp pain as previously described (Fig. 5–10).

OBJECTIVE DATA. Objective data the nurse may note include splinting, shallow respirations, tachypnea, facial changes associated with pain, and increased blood pressure and pulse.

Cough

SUBJECTIVE DATA. Coughing is an important reflex activity that assists the mucociliary escalator in removing secretions and foreign particles from the lower airway. It is triggered by irritation, the presence of foreign particles, or obstruction of the airway. The patient should be asked to provide the following information about cough: frequency, character, duration, triggers, and pattern of occurrence.

OBJECTIVE DATA. The nurse can observe the strength, character, and frequency of the cough.

Sputum

SUBJECTIVE DATA. It is important to obtain a description of sputum production in a pulmonary patient. If the patient has a disease that is associated with chronic production of sputum, he or she should be asked to describe the usual quantity, characteristics, and color. It is important to get the patient to describe any changes in sputum associated with the current pulmonary problem.

OBJECTIVE DATA. Sputum may consist of a variety of substances, such as mucus, pus, bacteria, or blood. Sputum should be monitored on a regular basis for quantity, characteristics (thin, thick, tenacious), color, and odor. Careful attention to sputum changes should be noted and

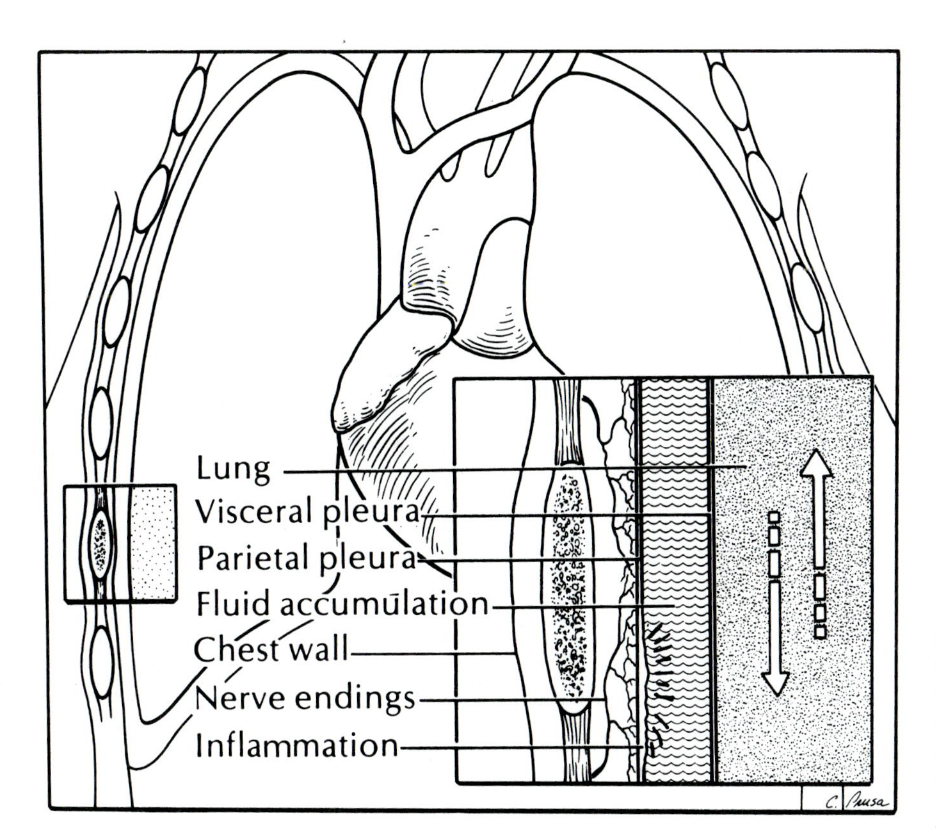

Figure 5–10. The source of pleural pain. When the parietal pleura is irritated and inflamed, the nerve endings located in the parietal pleura send pain signals to the brain. *(From Des Jardins, T.R. [1990].* Clinical manifestations of respiratory disease, *2nd ed., [p. 71]. Chicago: Year Book Medical Publisher.)*

documented, since they may reflect a change in the patient's pulmonary status. Normal secretions are thin and clear. Sputum color varies depending on the underlying problem (Table 5–9).

If a sputum specimen is ordered for laboratory studies, it is best to obtain the specimen in the early morning on awakening because secretions pool during sleep. To ensure that the specimen is not composed of upper airway secretions, instruct the patient to take several large breaths and then cough forcefully from the diaphragm. If the patient's cough is weak and nonproductive, deep tracheal suctioning may be necessary, collecting the specimen in a special suction trap device, such as the Luken tube. The sputum specimen should be obtained before initiation of antibiotic therapy.

Hemoptysis

SUBJECTIVE DATA. **Hemoptysis** refers to expectoration of bloody secretions. It is important to determine the source of the bleeding, which may be from the upper airway (e.g., the oral cavity) or the lower airway (e.g., the lungs). In patients who are experiencing respiratory problems, the presence of hemoptysis can be a significant finding and may be of cardiovascular or pulmonary origin.

Common causes of cardiovascular-related hemoptysis include pulmonary embolism and cardiogenic pulmonary edema secondary to left heart failure. The most common source of hemoptysis, however, is lung disease, particularly as a result of infection and neoplasms. Lung diseases associated with hemoptysis include bronchitis, bronchiectasis, pneumonia, tuberculosis, fungal and parasitic infections, and lung tumors. Information to obtain concerning hemoptysis includes color, consistency and quantity, and frequency and duration.

OBJECTIVE DATA. When hemoptysis is noted, it should be assessed for color, consistency, and quantity. The frequency and duration also should be noted and documented.

TABLE 5–9. SPUTUM COLOR AND CONSISTENCY AND UNDERLYING PROBLEMS

COLOR AND CONSISTENCY	UNDERLYING PROBLEM
Yellow-green	Bacterial infection
White, tenacious, mucoid	Acute asthma
Rust colored/blood-tinged	Trauma of coughing, pneumonia, pulmonary infarction
Frothy, pink-tinged	Pulmonary edema

Respiratory Physical Assessment

The initial general nursing assessment focuses on all body systems in detail. Once the initial assessment is completed and baseline data are documented, the nurse conducts more specific shift assessments. These frequent bedside assessments often are focused on organ systems (or functional patterns) that have the potential for changing rapidly, indicating a status change in actual or potential patient problems.

Vital Signs

Vital signs give important baseline data. They should include at least arterial blood pressure, pulse, respirations, and temperature. They also may include invasive hemodynamic monitoring assessments, such as central venous pressure (CVP), intra-arterial pressure, pulmonary artery pressure, and cardiac output. Hemodynamic monitoring generally is initiated when cardiac involvement is suspected or fluid status is questioned. If the patient's condition is purely pulmonary in nature, data collected from hemodynamic monitoring may be of insufficient use to warrant such an invasive procedure. The presence of pulmonary hypertension can alter hemodynamic measurements.

Inspection and Palpation

Skin coloring should be inspected closely for cyanosis. Observe the lips, earlobes, and beneath the tongue for central cyanosis, which may indicate prolonged hypoxia. In patients with dark skin tones, cyanosis can be observed on the lips and tongue, which will appear ashen-gray. Cyanosis is not a very reliable indicator of hypoxia, since it is dependent on the amount of reduced hemoglobin present. Its value, therefore, is as supportive rather than diagnostic data. Observe chest movement for symmetry of expansion and the rate, depth, and pattern of breathing. If the patient has sustained chest trauma or has chest tubes in place, the chest should be observed for changes in appearance and palpated for subcutaneous emphysema and areas of tenderness.

Percussion

Percussion is an assessment skill that often is not used on a regular shift-by-shift basis in the acute care setting. It can be used to detect the presence of air, fluid, or consolidation under the area being percussed.

Auscultation

Auscultation is one of the most important pulmonary assessments. The diaphragm of the stethoscope is best for hearing most breath sounds, auscultating in a pattern that allows comparison of one lung to the other. One must first be able to recognize normal breath sounds to be able to recognize and differentiate abnormal sounds.

NORMAL BREATH SOUNDS. These are divided into three types: vesicular, bronchial (tubular), and bronchovesicular. Table 5–10 differentiates the various normal sounds.

ABNORMAL BREATH SOUNDS. The chest should be auscultated routinely for diminished or absent sounds in any field. The presence of abnormal breath sounds is associated with a change in lung status, such as partial or complete obstruction of a part of the airway by secretions or fluid.

Adventitious breath sounds are heard on top of other breath sounds. They are never considered normal. Adventitious sounds may be caused by fluid or secretions in the airways or alveoli, by alveoli opening or collapsing, or by bronchoconstriction. Adventitious sounds are classified as crackles, rhonchi, wheeze, and rub.

Crackles (previously called **rales**) are heard as relatively discrete, delicate popping sounds of short duration. They are associated with either fluid or secretions in the small airways or alveoli, or opening of alveoli from a collapsed state. Crackles are heard most commonly during inspiration. Crackles may be described as fine or coarse. Fine crackles are very delicate and high pitched and are of very short duration. Conditions such as atelectasis and pneumonia are associated with fine crackles. Coarse or loud crackles are louder, lower-pitched sounds of longer duration than fine crackles. They are heard in conditions such as bronchitis and pulmonary edema.

Rhonchi are heard as coarse, "bubbly" sounds. They are most commonly present during expiration and are auscultated over the larger airways. Rhonchi are associated with an accumulation of fluid or secretions in the larger airways.

Wheeze is caused by air passing through constricted airways. The constriction may be caused by bronchospasm, fluid, secretions, edema obstructing the airway, or the presence of an obstructing tumor or foreign body. Wheeze has a musical quality that may be high pitched or low pitched. It may be heard on inspiration or expiration and is of long duration.

Pleural rub is caused by an inflammation of the pleural linings (membranes). When inflammation occurs, the linings become resistant to free movement. The characteristic sound is heard during breathing and has been described as sounding like leather rubbing together or creaking.

TABLE 5–10. NORMAL BREATH SOUNDS

BREATH SOUND	NORMAL LOCATION	DESCRIPTION
Vesicular	Peripheral lung fields	Whispering, rustling quality; quiet and low pitched; inspiratory phase is longer than expiratory phase; no distinct pause between inspiration and expiration
Bronchial (tubular)	Over the trachea	High-pitched, loud sound; pause heard between inspiratory and expiratory phases; expiration phase is longer than inspiration (abnormal if heard in peripheral lung; may indicate a consolidation, such as pneumonia)
Bronchovesicular	In all lobes near major airways	Sound is between vesicular and bronchial

Focused Respiratory Assessment

The onset of acute respiratory distress can be rapid and severe. The nurse should be alert to changes from previously assessed baseline data. Rapid respiratory assessment should focus on the following cluster of data that strongly suggest an acute alteration in respiratory function.

- Suddenly increased restlessness and agitation (hypoxia)
- Suddenly decreased level of responsiveness, increased lethargy (hypercapnia)
- Significant change in pattern of breathing:
  - Respiratory rate < 10 or > 30/min
  - Shallow or erratic breathing
- Increased cyanosis or duskiness
- Increased use of accessory muscles
- Increased dyspnea or orthopnea
- Increase in adventitious breath sounds or development of abnormal breath sounds
- Changing trends noted in vital signs (blood pressure, pulse, respirations):
  - Increasing trends indicate that compensation is occurring
  - Decreasing trends indicate that decompensation may be occurring
- Presence of pain

In summary, the most common respiratory-related complaints are dyspnea, chest pain, cough, sputum, and hemoptysis. The nursing history and assessment should include careful data collection focusing on these common complaints. The database can be helpful in differentiating an underlying pulmonary problem from one of cardiac origin. The bedside-focused respiratory assessment includes vital signs, inspection of skin coloring, chest movement and pattern of breathing, and auscultation for the presence of adventitious breath sounds (e.g., crackles, rhonchi, wheeze, or pleural rub).

SECTION EIGHT REVIEW

1. When a patient is admitted in acute respiratory distress, the initial history should focus on which priority?
   A. smoking history
   B. events leading to current admission
   C. nutritional history
   D. events leading to previous admissions
2. The most common complaints associated with pulmonary disease include all of the following EXCEPT
   A. cough
   B. sputum
   C. dyspnea
   D. pneumothorax
3. Chest pain that is typical of pleuritic pain can be best characterized as
   A. sharp
   B. pressurelike
   C. radiating
   D. dull
4. Normal sputum should appear
   A. white and tenacious
   B. yellow-green
   C. clear and thin
   D. frothy and pink-tinged
5. Breath sounds that are auscultated in the peripheral lung fields and have a whispery, rustling quality are
   A. vesicular
   B. bronchovesicular
   C. bronchial
   D. wheezes
6. Crackles are caused by
   A. secretions in the large airways
   B. an inflammation of the pleural linings
   C. air passing through constricted airways
   D. fluid or secretions in the small airways or alveoli

Answers: 1. B, 2. D, 3. A, 4. C, 5. A, 6. D

SECTION NINE: Respiratory Calculations

At the completion of this section, the learner will be able to perform selected respiratory calculations.

A variety of simple calculations can provide significant information regarding the oxygenation status of the high-acuity patient. Increasingly, nurses who take care of this patient population are expected to have a basic understanding of these calculations and their significance. This section presents several of the more uncomplicated but clinically useful equations that can estimate the degree of intrapulmonary shunt (e.g., A–a gradient, a/A ratio, and PaO_2/FIO_2 ratio) and the amount of pulmonary vascular resistance (PVR). Evaluation of PVR has been included because of its clinical relevance in the high-acuity patient population.

Ideal Alveolar Gas Equation

The more simple measurements of shunt require two oxygen-derived variables, PAO_2 and PaO_2. The laws of diffusion state that gases will flow from higher concentration to lower concentration until a state of equilibrium exists. This means that the partial pressure of alveolar oxygen (PAO_2) should approximate the partial pressure of arterial oxygen (PaO_2). As a general clinical guideline, the maximal acceptable range for PaO_2 is 60 to 100 mm Hg, and the maximal acceptable difference between PAO_2 and PaO_2 is 40 mm Hg (Ahrens & Rutherford, 1993). A difference of > 40 mm Hg suggests abnormal intrapulmonary shunt.

Several respiratory calculations (e.g., a/A ratio, and A–a gradient) require an estimate of the PAO_2 level. Unlike its arterial counterpart (PaO_2), alveolar oxygen is not measured directly. It is derived from an equation called the *ideal alveolar gas equation* (or alveolar air equation). At first sight, the equation appears complicated. In fact, it is quite simple to perform because many of the calculation components are constants that are plugged into the equation.

To work the equation, the following bits of data must be obtained: Current $PaCO_2$ and FIO_2 (the concentration of oxygen being breathed). The barometric pressure (PB) should be determined based on the altitude of the local area. This often can be obtained from the respiratory therapy department. Once barometric pressure is determined, it can be used as a constant for your institution. Table 5–11 explains the equation and provides a method for estimating barometric pressure based on the altitude of a general location.

Alveolar–Arterial Pressure Gradient (A–a Gradient)

A–a gradient (also called $P(A\text{–}a)O_2$) is useful for estimating the degree of physiologic shunt and hypoxemia. Although the $PACO_2$ and $PaCO_2$ should approximate each other during gas exchange, in reality, the level of alveolar oxygen is normally slightly higher (about 104 mm Hg) than the level of arterial oxygen (about 95 mm Hg) while breathing room air. The difference between these two levels is called the Alveolar–arterial pressure gradient (A–a gradient) and is attributable to physiologic shunt. Certain factors are associated with a high A–a gradient, including normal aging and of diffusion abnormalities such as shunt and $\dot{V}/\dot{Q}$ mismatch.

TABLE 5–11. IDEAL ALVEOLAR GAS EQUATION

EQUATION	$\mathbf{PAO_2 = [P_B - P_{H_2O}]FIO_2 - PaCO_2(1.25)}$	
Components	$PAO_2 =$	Partial pressure of alveolar oxygen (mm Hg)
	$P_B =$	Barometric pressure (mm Hg)[a] (750 mm Hg is sometimes used as a constant)
	$PH_2O =$	Water vapor constant (mm Hg) (47 mm Hg)
	$FIO_2 =$	Fraction of inspired oxygen (O_2 concentration) (decimal)
	$PACO_2 =$	Partial pressure of arterial carbon dioxide (mm Hg)
	$1.25 =$	A number derived from the respiratory exchange ratio
Example	A patient is receiving oxygen at an FIO_2 of 0.40. Her latest ABG showed a $PaCO_2$ of 45 mm Hg. The barometric pressure (P_B) is 750 mm Hg. $PAO_2 = [750 - 47]0.40 - 45(1.25)$ $PAO_2 = [702]0.40 - 56.25$ $PAO_2 = 280.80 - 56.25$ $\mathbf{PAO_2 = 224.55}$	

[a]Estimating barometric pressure (see examples below)

Near the earth's surface, pressure decreases with altitude at a rate of approximately 2.63 mm Hg for every 100 feet (30 m). To calculate:

$$\frac{\textbf{(Local altitude)}}{\textbf{100 feet}}\ \mathbf{2.63 - 760\ mm\ Hg} = \text{estimated barometric pressure}$$

1. Estimate the altitude of your city (for example, Denver is about 5280 feet above sea level
2. Divide the local altitude by 100 feet
3. Multiply the number derived in Step 2 by 2.63
4. Subtract the number derived in Step 3 from 760 mm Hg

Examples of barometric pressures by altitude:

Sea level = 760 mm Hg
500 feet above sea level = 747 mm Hg estimated P_B
1000 feet above sea level = 734 mm Hg estimated P_B
1500 feet above sea level = 721 mm Hg estimated P_B
2000 feet above sea level = 707 mm Hg estimated P_B

TABLE 5–12. A–a GRADIENT ($P(A–a)O_2$)

EQUATION:[a]	**A–a gradient = P_{AO_2} – Pa_{O_2}**
Components	P_{AO_2} = partial pressure of alveolar oxygen (mm Hg) Pa_{O_2} = partial pressure of arterial oxygen (mm Hg)
Normal values (age dependent)	On room air: 1. Calculate the normal for the person's age: < 4 mm Hg for every decade of life 2. Compare the actual A–a gradient to the answer obtained in Step 1. Normal is any number less than the answer to Step 1. On 100% F_{IO_2}: 1. Estimate 2% shunt for each 50 mm Hg difference in A–a gradient
Examples	On room air: A 40-year-old patient is breathing room air. The patient's P_{AO_2} is 100 mm Hg. An ABG is drawn with the Pa_{O_2} being 89 mm Hg. 100 mm Hg – 89 mm Hg = 11 mm Hg. Normal A–a gradient in a 40 year old would be less than 16 mm Hg. The A–a gradient is less than 16 and therefore is within normal range. On 100% oxygen: A 42-year-old patient is receiving 100% oxygen. She has a P_{AO_2} of 632 mm Hg. Her Pa_{O_2} is 89 mm Hg. A–a gradient = 632 mm Hg – 89 mm Hg A–a gradient = 543 mm Hg Estimating shunt: $\frac{543}{50} = 10.86 = 11$ (rounded) 11 × 2% = 22% estimated shunt is present

Adapted From Chang, D.W. (1998). Respiratory care calculations, *2nd ed. Albany, NY: Delmar Publishing; and Des Jardins, T.R. (1998).* Cardiopulmonary anatomy and physiology: Essentials for respiratory care, *3rd ed. Albany, NY: Delmar Publishing.*

[a]This formula is best used as a rough estimate only. It is not sensitive to changes in oxygen concentration and can give false data regarding the presence and degree of shunt.

Normal Aging

As a person ages, diffusion becomes less efficient. The A–a gradient should be < 4 mm Hg for every decade (10 years) of life (Chang, 1998). For example, in a 50-year-old patient, the A–a gradient should be less than 20 mm Hg (4 mm Hg × 5 decades = 20 mm Hg). When the difference is too high (> 4 mm Hg for every decade) an abnormal process is present that can cause hypoxemia. Caution must be used when interpreting data obtained from evaluation of A–a gradient since it is not sensitive to changing oxygen concentration (F_{IO_2}) levels. As the oxygen concentration is increased, the A–a gradient normally increases and, therefore, does not necessarily reflect intrapulmonary shunt. This measurement then, is of use at the bedside for a quick estimate but should not be relied on as an accurate measurement of shunt. Table 5–12 explains how to calculate A–a gradient.

a/A Ratio and Pa_{O_2}/F_{IO_2} Ratio

Like a–A gradient, arterial/Alveolar (a/A) and Pa_{O_2}/F_{IO_2} ratio are simple equations that can indicate the presence of intrapulmonary shunt, $\dot{V}/\dot{Q}$ mismatch, or a diffusion abnormality. These two measurements are more accurate estimates of intrapulmonary shunt than A–a gradient since they are more sensitive to changes in oxygen concentration.

The a/A ratio is a commonly used measurement. It is a simple calculation, but requires calculation of P_{AO_2} first. The equation takes into consideration changes in F_{IO_2} and Pa_{CO_2}. The a/A ratio is the preferred shunt estimate when the patient's Pa_{CO_2} is unstable. Table 5–13

TABLE 5–13. a/A RATIO

EQUATION[a]	$\frac{Pa_{O_2}}{P_{AO_2}}$
Components	Pa_{O_2} = partial pressure of arterial oxygen P_{AO_2} = partial pressure of alveolar oxygen (derived from Ideal Alveolar Gas Equation)
Normal values	> 0.60—no supplemental oxygen is needed < 0.60—shunt is becoming worse An inverse relationship is present: as the a/A ratio value drops, intrapulmonary shunt worsens
Example	A patient's P_{AO_2} is currently 350 mm Hg. His Pa_{O_2} is 88 mm Hg. $\frac{88}{350} = 0.25$ A significant intrapulmonary shunt is present.

[a]This formula is best used when Pa_{CO_2} is not stable.

Adapted from Chang, D.W. (1998). Respiratory care calculations, *2nd ed. Albany, NY: Delmar Publishing.*

TABLE 5–14. PaO_2/FIO_2 RATIO

EQUATION[a]	$\frac{PaO_2}{FIO_2}$
Components	PaO_2 = partial pressure of arterial oxygen (mm Hg) FIO_2 = fraction of inspired oxygen (O_2 concentration) (decimal)
Normal values	> 350 Minimum clinically acceptable level = 286 Inverse relationship: The lower the ratio value drops below normal, the more intrapulmonary shunt worsens
Example	A patient has a PaO_2 of 92 mm Hg on a FIO_2 of 0.60 $\frac{92}{0.60} = 153$ This is below the minimum acceptable level.

[a]This formula is best used when $PaCO_2$ is stable.

summarizes how to derive the a/A ratio. PaO_2/FIO_2 ratio is the simplest way to estimate intrapulmonary shunt. It is best used when the patient's $PaCO_2$ is stable since it is not sensitive to changes in that value. Table 5–14 provides a summary on calculating PaO_2/FIO_2 ratio.

Pulmonary Vascular Resistance (PVR)

Calculating pulmonary vascular resistance requires the presence of a flow-directed pulmonary artery catheter. The calculation measures resistance, which is a function of pressure and flow. Pressure is determined by the mean pulmonary artery pressure and the pulmonary capillary wedge pressure. Flow is measured as the cardiac output. Table 5–15 summarizes the calculation of pulmonary vascular resistance.

TABLE 5–15. PULMONARY VASCULAR RESISTANCE (PVR)

EQUATION	$PVR = (\overline{PAP} - PCWP) \times \frac{80}{CO}$
Components	$\overline{PAP}$ = mean pulmonary artery pressure PCWP = pulmonary capillary wedge pressure CO = cardiac output 80 = conversion factor
Normal values	50–150 dynes · sec · cm^{-5}
Example	A patient has a $\overline{PAP}$ of 22 mm Hg, a PCWP of 9 mm Hg, and a CO of 4.5 L/min $PVR = 22 - 9 \times \frac{80}{4.5}$ $PVR = 13 \times 17.78$ $PVR = 231.14$
Factors associated with increased PVR	Decreased PAO_2, decreased pH, increased $PaCO_2$; mechanical ventilation, positive end expiratory pressure (PEEP); pulmonary emboli, scleroderma, emphysema, pneumo- and hemothorax; histamine, prostaglandin, angiotensin

Adapted From Des Jardins, T.R. (1998). Cardiopulmonary anatomy and physiology: Essentials for respiratory care, *3rd ed. Albany, NY: Delmar Publishers; and Chang, D.W. (1998).* Respiratory care calculations. *2nd ed. Albany, NY: Delmar Publishers.*

In summary, a variety of respiratory calculations can assist the nurse in determining the oxygenation status of a patient. Several equations were presented that help estimate the degree of intrapulmonary shunt (e.g., A–a gradient, a/A ratio, and PaO_2/FIO_2 ratio). A final equation, pulmonary vascular resistance (PVR), was presented as a common pulmonary problem that can lead to right heart failure. Pulmonary vascular resistance requires readings from a flow-directed pulmonary artery catheter.

SECTION NINE REVIEW

Juan M, 30 years old, is admitted in respiratory distress. His arterial blood gases are as follows: pH = 7.32, $PaCO_2$ = 50 mm Hg, PaO_2 = 79 mm Hg. The barometric pressure is 750 mm Hg. He is currently breathing oxygen at 0.28 FIO_2.

1. Based on the data available regarding Juan, what is his PAO_2?
2. If Juan's PAO_2 is 100 mm Hg and his PaO_2 is 80 mm Hg, what would his A–a gradient be?
   Answer:

   Significance:
3. Given that Juan's PAO_2 is 110 mm Hg and his PaO_2 is 80 mm Hg, what is his a/A ratio?
   Answer:

   Significance:
4. Juan's status has changed. The nurse performs two sequential calculations of his a/A ratio, 1 hour apart. The first is 0.58 and the second is 0.56. What is the significance of this change?
   Significance:

5. The nurse is considering calculating Juan's shunt by using the PaO_2/FIO_2 ratio. This calculation is best used when
A. $PaCO_2$ is unstable
B. PaO_2 is unstable
C. $PaCO_2$ is stable
D. PaO_2 is stable

6. The nurse decides to calculate Juan's PVR. His latest hemodynamic values are $\overline{PAP}$ = 30 mm Hg, PCWP = 15 mm Hg, CO = 5.2 L/min. What is Juan's PVR?
Answer:

Significance:

Answers: 1, 134.34 mm Hg. **2,** 20 mm Hg; significance = abnormally high A–a gradient. **3,** 0.73; significance = > 0.60 suggests no significant shunt. **4,** shunt is worsening. **5,** C. **6,** PVR = 230.7; significance = abnormally high PVR.

SECTION TEN: Developing a Pulmonary Plan of Care

Upon completion of this section, the learner will be able to develop a plan of care for a patient with altered respiratory function.

This section presents a standard respiratory plan of care based on the three NANDA-approved nursing diagnoses that focus on respiratory function. Each nursing diagnosis is defined, major patient outcomes are listed, and some of the major independent nursing interventions are provided.

The Standard Respiratory Plan of Care

The three NANDA-approved respiratory nursing diagnoses are:

- Breathing pattern, ineffective
- Gas exchange, impaired
- Airway clearance, ineffective

All three of the pulmonary-related nursing diagnoses may apply to high-acuity patients during a single illness. For this reason, the nurse may consider using an alternative that joins all three NANDA diagnoses, impaired respiratory function (Ulrich, Canale, & Wendell, 1998).

Breathing Pattern, Ineffective

Ineffective breathing pattern is defined as "a state in which the rate, depth, timing, rhythm, or chest/abdominal wall excursion, or both does not maintain optimum ventilation for the individual" (Ulrich, Canale, & Wendell, 1998, p. 18).

Desired Patient Outcomes

Maintenance of an effective breathing pattern, as evidenced by:

1. Normal respiratory rate, depth, and rhythm
2. ABGs within normal limits for patient
3. No dyspnea

Independent Nursing Interventions

1. Assess for ineffective breathing patterns (report abnormals)
   a. Respirations < 8/min or > 30/min
   b. Increasingly shallow, labored breathing
   c. Increasing dyspnea
   d. Increasingly abnormal ABGs and/or pulse oximetry results
   e. Increasingly irregular breathing pattern
2. Monitor for abdominal or chest pain
3. Reduce level of abdominal or chest pain
   a. Regular administration of pain medication (observe for respiratory depression)
   b. Splint chest or abdomen with pillow or arms for coughing and deep-breathing exercises
4. Implement respiratory muscle strengthening exercises
5. Encourage incentive spirometer use every 1 to 2 hours
6. Encourage slow, deep breaths (as appropriate)
7. Elevate head of bed to 45 degrees or level of comfort
8. Turn (self or assisted) every 2 hours

Gas Exchange, Impaired

Impaired gas exchange is defined as "a state in which an individual experiences an imbalance in oxygenation and/or carbon dioxide elimination at the alveolar–capillary membrane" (Ulrich, Canale, & Wendell, 1998, p. 33).

Desired Patient Outcomes
Maintenance of normal gas exchange, as evidenced by:

1. ABGs within normal limits for patient
2. Usual mental status
3. Breathing unlabored
4. Respiratory rate 12 to 20/min
5. No use (or decreased use) of accessory respiratory muscles

Independent Nursing Interventions

1. Assess for impaired gas exchange (report abnormals)
   a. Change in mental status
      1. increased lethargy
      2. increased restlessness
      3. confusion
   b. Accessory muscle use
   c. Abnormal ABGs
      1. elevated $PaCO_2$ (above acceptable limits)
      2. decreased PaO_2 (below acceptable limits)
   d. Decreasing pulse oximetry readings
2. Turn every 2 hours
3. Encourage incentive spirometer use every 1 to 2 hours
4. Maintain position of comfort, with head of bed elevated > 30 degrees
5. Monitor effects of drug therapy (including oxygen therapy)
6. Encourage early ambulation
7. Assist patient to sit up in chair

Airway Clearance, Ineffective

Ineffective airway clearance is defined as "a state in which an individual is unable to clear secretions or obstructions from the respiratory tract" (Ulrich, Canale, Wendell, 1998, p. 11).

Desired Patient Outcomes
Maintenance of effective airway clearance, as evidenced by:

1. Normal or improved lung sounds
2. No cyanosis
3. Normal respiratory rate and depth
4. No dyspnea

Independent Nursing Interventions

1. Assess for ineffective airway clearance
   a. Adventitious breath sounds
   b. Ineffective cough
   c. Respirations > 24/min
   d. Respiratory depth shallow
   e. Presence of cyanosis
   f. Complaint of dyspnea
2. Assist patient to cough and deep breathe every 1 to 2 hours
3. Encourage fluids to 2 to 2.5 L per 24 hours or 600 to 800 mL per 8-hour shift
4. Perform tracheal suction as necessary
5. Monitor for effects of drug therapy (expectorants, mucolytics)
6. Monitor for and treat acute pain
7. Administer pain medications, as needed
8. Encourage self-care as tolerated
9. Encourage activity and early ambulation

In summary, there are three NANDA-approved respiratory-focused nursing diagnoses. In complex patients in whom all three problems are present, the alternative diagnosis, *impaired respiratory function,* may be used. Many of the expected patient outcomes and independent nursing interventions overlap between the three diagnoses. Regardless of the exact medical diagnosis attached to the patient, a plan of care can be developed if the nurse has an understanding of the underlying pathophysiologic problem. At the end of Part II: Respiration and Ventilation, the entire nursing process is clinically applied (including collaborative interventions) to two case studies, which present a patient with a restrictive disorder and a patient with an obstructive disorder.

SECTION TEN REVIEW

1. Evaluation of the effectiveness of interventions to resolve the nursing diagnosis *ineffective breathing patterns* is best measured by which of the following desired patient outcomes?
   A. usual mental status
   B. normal or improved lung sounds
   C. absent accessory muscle use
   D. normal respiratory rate, depth, and rhythm

2. "The state in which a person experiences decreased passage of oxygen and/or carbon dioxide between the alveoli and the vascular system" is the definition of
   A. impaired gas exchange
   B. ineffective breathing pattern
   C. ineffective airway clearance
   D. altered respiratory function

3. Assessments for impaired gas exchange in the early stage would include all of the following EXCEPT
   A. confusion
   B. increased lethargy
   C. decreased restlessness
   D. change in mental status

4. Nursing interventions that would assist in maintaining effective airway clearance would include
   A. restrict fluids to 1 L/day
   B. cough and deep breathe every 1 to 2 hours
   C. minimize use of opioid analgesics
   D. restrict activities

Answers: 1. D, 2. A, 3. C, 4. B

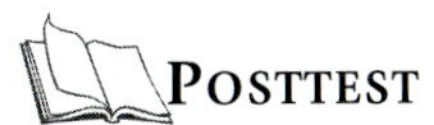

POSTTEST

The following Posttest is constructed in a case study format. A patient is presented, and questions are asked based on available data. New data are presented as the case study progresses.

James Smith is a 55-year-old construction worker. He is active and considers himself fairly healthy. He has a history of smoking one pack of cigarettes per day for 35 years.

1. When Mr. Smith inhales, air moves into his lungs because
   A. intrapulmonary pressure has dropped below atmospheric pressure
   B. intrapleural pressure has dropped below atmospheric pressure
   C. intrapulmonary pressure has risen above atmospheric pressure
   D. intrapleural pressure has risen above atmospheric pressure
2. If his surfactant production would cease, how would it affect the alveoli?
   A. alveoli would hyperinflate
   B. alveoli would be destroyed
   C. alveoli would collapse
   D. alveoli would have decreased surface tension
3. Should Mr. Smith develop a pulmonary problem that decreases his lung compliance, it would
   A. increase his tidal volume
   B. decrease his carbon dioxide level
   C. decrease his oxygen consumption
   D. increase his work of breathing

Mr. Smith becomes ill. He develops a cough and fever and is producing greenish sputum. He is diagnosed as having right middle lobe pneumonia. He also has an underlying chronic obstructive pulmonary disorder.

4. His pneumonia can affect pulmonary diffusion by increasing membrane thickness due to
   A. inflammation
   B. atelectasis
   C. bronchial secretions
   D. surfactant deficiency
5. Ventilation will decrease in the affected lung area because
   A. pressure gradient is increased
   B. gas follows the path of least resistance
   C. decreased perfusion causes decreased ventilation
   D. gas moves from low pressure to high pressure areas
6. Mr. Smith has a low $\dot{V}/\dot{Q}$ ratio. This means that there is
   A. decreased ventilation in relation to perfusion
   B. increased ventilation with decreased perfusion
   C. decreased ventilation with decreased perfusion
   D. increased ventilation in relation to perfusion
7. Mr. Smith has developed a physiologic shunt of 20 percent. As a result, one would anticipate which of the following clinical manifestations?
   A. stupor, bounding pulse
   B. warm, wet skin; cyanosis
   C. headache, flushed appearance
   D. restlessness, cardiac arrhythmias

Mr. Smith's shunt is a capillary shunt. Oxygen therapy has been initiated per Venti-mask.

8. Considering his type of shunt, the nurse can anticipate that his hypoxemia will
   A. remain the same
   B. worsen
   C. be relieved
   D. initially improve and then worsen

Mr. Smith has pulmonary mechanics tests performed. Both his tidal volume and vital capacity are below normal.

9. Inadequate volumes of tidal volume and vital capacity most likely indicate which of the following?
   A. respiratory muscle fatigue
   B. increased atelectasis
   C. loss of pulmonary surfactant
   D. worsening of his pneumonia

10. Based only on available data and considering Mr. Smith's underlying chronic problem, his pneumonia condition would most likely be considered an acute
    A. ventilatory failure
    B. obstructive disease
    C. respiratory failure
    D. restrictive disease
11. Mr. Smith's pneumonia affects expiratory airflow in which way?
    A. increases
    B. no affect
    C. decreases
    D. increases or decreases
12. His obstructive pulmonary disorder is associated with
    A. decreased tidal volumes
    B. increased inspiratory times
    C. decreased inspiratory airflow
    D. increased expiratory times
13. If Mr. Smith develops heart failure secondary to cor pulmonale, he will most likely experience
    A. dependent edema
    B. left ventricular enlargement
    C. low blood pressure
    D. pulmonary edema
14. Based on Mr. Smith's diagnosis of cor pulmonale, the nurse can anticipate that his PVR will be
    A. low
    B. unchanged
    C. high
    D. vacillating
15. PVR increases in response to
    A. hypercapnia
    B. alkalosis
    C. hypoxemia
    D. low lung volumes
16. Assuming Mr. Smith is in a state of chronic respiratory insufficiency, he would most likely exhibit which of the following?
    A. decreased respiratory rate
    B. increased blood pressure
    C. increased temperature
    D. decreased pulse rate
17. If Mr. Smith was to develop acute ventilatory failure, you would anticipate which of the following arterial blood gas findings?
    A. $PaO_2 < 60$ mm Hg
    B. $PaCO_2 > 50$ mm Hg
    C. $PaO_2 > 100$ mm Hg
    D. $PaCO_2 < 35$ mm Hg
18. According to the module, respiratory failure is clinically defined as
    A. $PaCO_2 \geq 50$ mm Hg with a pH ≤ 7.30 and/or $PaO_2 \leq 60$ mm Hg
    B. $PaCO_2 \geq 60$ mm Hg with a pH ≤ 7.30 and $PaO_2 \leq 60$ mm Hg
    C. $PaCO_2 \geq 45$ mm Hg with a pH ≤ 7.35 and/or $PaO_2 \leq 80$ mm Hg
    D. $PaCO_2 \geq 60$ mm Hg with a pH ≤ 7.35 and $PaO_2 \leq 80$ mm Hg
19. ARDS is a pulmonary disorder that initially causes
    A. lung destruction
    B. ventilatory failure
    C. alveolar hypoventilation
    D. oxygenation failure

Una W, a 21-year-old college student, is admitted to the hospital with complaints of severe chest pain and dyspnea. She has an oral temperature of 101°F.

20. When a pulmonary disorder is suspected, obtaining a nutritional history is important for which of the following reasons?
    A. hypoglycemia weakens respiratory muscles
    B. high-carbohydrate diets decrease carbon dioxide levels
    C. high fat intake decreases respiratory rate and depth
    D. poor nutritional status increases susceptibility to infection
21. Una continues to complain of feeling dyspneic. The nurse will need to monitor her closely for other major indicators of respiratory fatigue including all of the following EXCEPT
    A. heart rate of 100
    B. respiratory rate > 30/min
    C. shallow respirations
    D. use of accessory muscles

The nurse has noted the following acute changes in Una's condition: increased restlessness and confusion, respiratory rate 32/min and shallow, increased use of accessory muscles, increased BP and HR.

22. Based only on these changes in Una's status, the nurse would hypothesize that Una is most likely experiencing
    A. a pneumothorax
    B. pneumonia
    C. a pulmonary embolus
    D. an acute alteration in respiratory function

While receiving oxygen at an FIO_2 of 0.40, Una has two ABGs drawn, 1 hour apart. (Assume that barometric pressure is 750 mm Hg.) The results are

#1 @ 10:00 AM: pH = 7.47, $PaCO_2$ = 34 mm Hg, PaO_2 = 90 mm Hg
#2 @ 11:00 AM: pH = 7.49, $PaCO_2$ = 32 mm Hg, PaO_2 = 86 mm Hg

23. The nurse calculates Una's a/A ratios based on ABGs #1 and #2.
    A. a/A ratio on #1 ABG is
    B. a/A ratio on #2 ABG is

24. Based on the a/A ratios calculated in question 23, what can be stated regarding the degree of shunt?

25. The nurse is developing a plan of care for the nursing diagnosis *impaired gas exchange*. Of the following, which expected patient outcome most accurately measures this diagnosis?
   A. ABG within normal limits for patient
   B. SaO_2 = > 95 percent
   C. usual mental status
   D. no cyanosis

26. The nurse writes the nursing diagnosis *ineffective airway clearance* on Una's care plan. All of the following are appropriate interventions to address this diagnosis EXCEPT
   A. administer pain medications, as needed
   B. cough and deep breathe every 1 to 2 hours
   C. limit fluid intake to < 1 L/24 hours
   D. tracheal suction as necessary

POSTTEST ANSWERS

Question	Answer	Section
1	C	One
1	A	One
2	C	One
3	D	One
4	A	Two
5	B	Three
6	A	Three
7	D	Four
8	B	Four
9	A	Five
10	D	Six
11	B	Six
12	D	Six
13	A	Six

Question	Answer	Section
14	C	Six
15	C	Six
16	B	Seven
17	B	Seven
18	A	Seven
19	D	Seven
20	D	Eight
21	A	Eight
22	D	Eight
23	A, 0.38; B, 0.36	Nine
24	shunt is worsening	Nine
25	A	Ten
26	C	Ten

REFERENCES

Ahrens, T., & Rutherford, K. (1993). *Essentials of oxygenation*. Boston: Jones and Bartlett.

Chang, D.W. (1998). *Respiratory care calculations* (2nd ed.). Albany, NY: Delmar Publishers.

Curzen, N.P., & Evans, T.W. (1998). Pulmonary vascular control mechanisms in sepsis and acute lung injury. In E.K. Weir & J.T. Reeves, *Pulmonary edema: American Heart Association Monograph Series*. Armonk, NY: Futura Publishing.

Des Jardins, T.R. (1993). *Cardiopulmonary anatomy and physiology: Essentials for respiratory care* (2nd ed.). Albany, NY: Delmar Publishers.

Des Jardins, T.R., & Burton, G.G. (1995). *Clinical manifestations of respiratory disease* (3rd ed.). Chicago: Year Book Medical Publishers.

Des Jardins, T.R. (1998). *Cardiopulmonary anatomy & physiology: Essentials for respiratory care* (3rd ed.). Albany, NY: Delmar Publishers.

Hunt, G.E. (1999). Gas therapy. In J.B. Fink & G.E. Hunt (eds.), *Clinical practice in respiratory care* (pp. 249–286). Philadelphia: J.B. Lippincott.

Martin, L. (1987). *Pulmonary physiology in clinical practice: The essentials in clinical practice* (p. 39). St. Louis: C.V. Mosby.

Shapiro B., Peruzzi, W.T., & Kozelowski-Templin, R. (1994). *Clinical application of blood gases* (5th ed.). St. Louis: C.V. Mosby.

Ulrich, S.P., Canale, S.W., & Wendell, S.A. (1998). *Medical–*

surgical nursing care planning guides (4th ed.). Philadelphia: W.B. Saunders.

Vollman, K.M., & Aulbach, R.K. (1998). Acute respiratory distress syndrome. In M.R. Kinney, S.B. Dunbar, J.A. Brooks-Brunn, N. Molter, & J.M. Vitello-Cicciu (eds.), *AACN clinical reference for critical care nursing* (4th ed.) (pp. 529–564). St. Louis: C.V. Mosby.

Von Rueden, P.A. (1998). Adult respiratory distress syndrome. In C.M. Hudak, B.M. Gallo, & P.G. Morton (eds.), *Critical care nursing: A holistic approach* (7th ed.) (pp. 513–524). Philadelphia: J.B. Lippincott.

Module 6

Arterial Blood Gas Analysis

Kathleen Dorman Wagner

This self-study module focuses on arterial blood gas analysis rather than on management of the patient with pulmonary dysfunction. The module is composed of eight distinct sections. Section One reviews factors affecting gas exchange. In Sections Two through Six, the focus shifts to acid–base physiology and compensation, normal arterial blood gas values, acid–base disturbances, and interpretation of arterial blood gases. Section Seven presents mixed acid–base disorders for those who wish to learn the basics of this more advanced concept. Section Eight briefly describes several noninvasive methods used in monitoring gas exchange. Each section includes a set of review questions or exercises to help the learner evaluate his or her understanding of each section before moving on to the next section. All Section Reviews and the Pretest and Posttest in the module include answers. It is suggested that the learner review those concepts answered incorrectly in the review questions before proceeding to the next section.

Objectives

Following completion of this module, the learner will be able to

1. Briefly discuss factors involved in gas exchange.
2. Identify mechanisms that the body uses to compensate for acid–base imbalances.
3. Identify normal values for arterial blood gases.
4. Differentiate between respiratory acidosis and alkalosis.
5. Differentiate between metabolic acidosis and alkalosis.
6. Interpret arterial blood gases for abnormalities of oxygenation, acid–base, and degree of compensation.
7. Recognize mixed acid–base disorders.
8. List noninvasive methods of monitoring gas exchange and applications.

Pretest

1. Common factors affecting gas exchange include all of the following EXCEPT
   - A. partial pressure
   - B. oxyhemoglobin dissociation
   - C. mixed venous saturation
   - D. diffusion
2. Which of the following reflects the natural movement of gas diffusion?
   - A. from low to high pressure
   - B. from high to low pressure
   - C. from equal to unequal pressure
   - D. from negative to positive pressure
3. The body compensates for acid–base imbalance by all of the following mechanisms EXCEPT
   - A. buffering
   - B. hepatic compensation
   - C. respiratory compensation
   - D. excretion of bicarbonate

4. Respiratory compensation involves excretion or retention of
   A. CO_2
   B. HCO_3
   C. H_2O
   D. K^+
5. Normal values for arterial blood gases (ABGs) include
   A. pH = 7.5
   B. $Paco_2$ = 20 mm Hg
   C. HCO_3 = 26 mm Hg
   D. Sao_2 = 75 mm Hg
6. According to the oxyhemoglobin dissociation curve, at a Pao_2 of less than 60 mm Hg, a large decrease in Pao_2 should produce what in the Sao_2?
   A. a small increase
   B. a large increase
   C. a small decrease
   D. a large decrease
7. Respiratory acidosis is caused by
   A. alveolar hyperventilation
   B. alveolar hypoventilation
   C. mechanical ventilation
   D. inadequate perfusion
8. Patient situations associated with respiratory alkalosis include
   A. anxiety
   B. sedation
   C. pulmonary edema
   D. neuromuscular blockade
9. Metabolic disturbances are reflected by changes in
   A. HCO_3, Sao_2
   B. Pao_2, base excess
   C. Base excess, HCO_3
   D. HCO_3, Pao_2
10. Metabolic acidosis results in
    A. increased $Paco_2$
    B. decreased pH
    C. increased base excess
    D. increased HCO_3
11. A patient has the following arterial blood gas results:

    pH = 7.58, $Paco_2$ = 38 mm Hg, HCO_3 = 30 mEq/L

    The correct acid–base interpretation of this ABG is
    A. uncompensated respiratory alkalosis
    B. partially compensated respiratory acidosis
    C. uncompensated metabolic alkalosis
    D. partially compensated metabolic acidosis
12. A patient has the following ABG results:

    pH = 7.48, $Paco_2$ = 33 mm Hg, HCO_3 = 25 mEq/L, Pao_2 = 68 mm Hg, Sao_2 = 98%

    The correct oxygenation status interpretation of this ABG is
    A. uncompensated respiratory alkalosis
    B. hypoxemia with normal saturation
    C. normal oxygenation status
    D. partially compensated metabolic acidosis
13. Which of the following statements most accurately describes a mixed acid–base disorder?
    A. it can have a nullifying effect on the pH
    B. it has no predictable effect on the pH
    C. it is primarily associated with respiratory disorders
    D. it has a respiratory as well as a metabolic acid–base component
14. The key to recognizing mixed acid–base disorders on an arterial blood gas is
    A. looking for pH extremes
    B. recognizing abnormal base excess levels
    C. knowing the predicted compensation relationships
    D. the presence of abnormal HCO_3 with a normal pH
15. Pulse oximetry measures
    A. mixed venous saturation
    B. transcutaneous oxygen saturation
    C. venous oxygen capillary hemoglobin saturation
    D. arterial oxygen capillary hemoglobin saturation
16. The end tidal CO_2 is an indicator of alveolar
    A. acid–base state
    B. ventilation
    C. oxygenation
    D. compensation

Pretest Answers: 1. C, 2. B, 3. B, 4. A, 5. C, 6. D, 7. B, 8. A, 9. C, 10. B, 11. C, 12. B, 13. A, 14. C, 15. D, 16. B

GLOSSARY

Acids. Substances that dissociate or lose ions

Bases. Substances capable of accepting ions

Buffer. A substance reacting with acids and bases to maintain a neutral environment of stable pH

Capnogram. Graphic representation of carbon dioxide levels during respiration

Capnometry. Measurement of carbon dioxide in expired gas

Compensated. A state in which the pH is within normal limits with the acid-base imbalance being neutralized but not corrected

Corrected. A state in which all acid-base parameters have returned to normal ranges after a state of acid-base imbalance

Diffusion. Movement of gas molecules from an area of high to an area of low partial pressure

2,3-DPG (diphosphoglycerate). A molecule produced by red blood cells that facilitates oxygen release to tissues

End tidal carbon dioxide (P_{ETCO_2} or $ETCO_2$). Concentration of carbon dioxide at the end of exhalation

Nonvolatile acids. Metabolic acids that cannot be converted to a gas, requiring excretion through the kidneys

Oxyhemoglobin dissociation curve. A graphic representation of the relationship between oxygen saturation of hemoglobin (Sa_{O_2}) and the partial pressure of oxygen (Pa_{O_2}) in the plasma

Partial pressure. Pressure each gas exerts in a total volume of gases

Partially compensated. A state in which the pH is abnormal but the body buffers and regulatory mechanisms have started to respond to the imbalance

pH. Represents free hydrogen ion concentration

Pressure gradient. Difference between the partial pressures of a gas; influences rate of diffusion

Pulse oximetry. Noninvasive technique for monitoring arterial capillary oxygen saturation

Volatile acids. Acids that can convert to a gas form for excretion

Uncompensated. An acid–base state in which the pH is abnormal because other buffer and regulatory mechanisms have not begun to correct the imbalance

ABBREVIATIONS

ABG. Arterial blood gas

BE. Base excess

CO_2. Carbon dioxide

H^+. Hydrogen ion

H_2CO_3. Carbonic acid

Hgb (Hb). Hemoglobin

HCO_3. Bicarbonate

mEq/L. Milliequivalents per liter

mm Hg. Millimeters of mercury

O_2. Oxygen

Pa_{CO_2}. Partial pressure of arterial carbon dioxide

Pa_{O_2}. Partial pressure of arterial oxygen

P_{ETCO_2}. Partial pressure of end tidal carbon dioxide

pH. Free hydrogen ion concentration

Pv_{CO_2}. Partial pressure of venous carbon dioxide

Pv_{O_2}. Partial pressure of venous oxygen

Sa_{O_2}. Saturation of arterial oxygen

Sp_{O_2}. Saturation of arterial capillary hemoglobin determined by pulse oximetry

SECTION ONE: Factors Affecting Gas Exchange

At the completion of this section, the learner will be able to briefly discuss factors involved in gas exchange.

Many factors affect gas exchange. This process occurs between the alveoli and pulmonary capillaries and between the capillaries and tissues. Concepts to be considered are partial pressure, diffusion, ventilation–perfusion matching, and oxyhemoglobin dissociation. Most of these concepts have been covered in the Respiratory Process module (Module 3) and are reviewed briefly in this module.

Partial Pressure

Partial pressure, or tension, is the pressure each individual gas exerts in a total volume of gases. For example, atmospheric pressure (the total pressure of gases) is 760 mm Hg at sea level, and oxygen (O_2) comprises 21 percent of room air. To determine the partial pressure of oxygen,

0.21 (percent of oxygen) × 760 mm Hg (atmospheric pressure) = 158 mm Hg (Pa_{O_2})

As the percentage of oxygen is increased, the pressure it exerts also increases.

Henry's law states that when a gas is exposed to liquid, some of it will dissolve in the liquid. The partial pressure of the gas and its solubility determine the amount of gas that dissolves. Oxygen is not very soluble in plasma. Only 3 percent of the total oxygen content dissolves in blood. It is the partial pressure of gases (oxygen and carbon dioxide) moving out of the plasma that is measured in a blood gas sample.

Diffusion

Diffusion of gas refers to the transfer of gas molecules from an area of high partial pressure to an area of lower partial pressure. The difference between the partial pressures is called the **pressure gradient.** Diffusion occurs at the alveolar and tissue levels to exchange oxygen and carbon dioxide. At the alveolar level, oxygen moves into blood, and carbon dioxide moves out. At the tissue level, oxygen leaves the blood to nourish the tissues, and carbon dioxide (waste) shifts into the capillaries for removal from the body by the lungs.

The alveolar–capillary membrane is very thin (0.5 μm), offering little resistance to diffusion in normal circumstances. The membrane can thicken when pulmonary pathologic processes exist, reducing diffusion (e.g., pulmonary edema, acute respiratory distress syndrome). Since carbon dioxide diffuses 20 times faster than oxygen, the carbon dioxide tension may remain at normal levels initially, but the oxygen tension decreases.

Ventilation–Perfusion Relationship

The relationship between ventilation and perfusion ($\dot{V}/\dot{Q}$ ratio) also affects gas exchange. Normally, ventilation is the greatest where perfusion is the greatest, thus optimizing gas exchange. Many pulmonary disorders interfere with this relationship, decreasing ventilation to the alveoli (pneumonia, atelectasis), decreasing perfusion of capillary blood flow by the alveoli (pulmonary embolus), or both (emphysema). The relationship of ventilation to perfusion is discussed in detail in Module 3.

Oxyhemoglobin Dissociation Curve

Hemoglobin is the primary carrier of oxygen in the blood. It has an affinity or attraction for oxygen molecules. In the pulmonary capillaries, oxygen binds loosely and reversibly to hemoglobin, forming oxyhemoglobin for transport to the tissues, where it can be released. The amount of oxygen that loads onto hemoglobin is expressed as a percentage of hemoglobin saturation by oxygen (% SaO_2). The affinity of hemoglobin for oxygen varies, depending on certain physiologic factors. A graph has been developed to represent the relationship of the partial pressure of arterial oxygen (PaO_2) and hemoglobin saturation (SaO_2). This graph is called the **oxyhemoglobin dissociation curve** (Fig. 6–1), which is depicted as an S-curve rather than a straight line, showing that the percentage saturation of hemoglobin does not maintain a direct relationship with the PaO_2.

The top portion of the curve ($PaO_2 \geq 60$ mm Hg) is flattened into a horizontal position. In this portion of the curve, a large alteration in PaO_2 produces only small alterations in percentage of hemoglobin saturation (% SaO_2). For example, note that a 10 mm Hg decrease of a patient's PaO_2 from 80 mm Hg to 70 mm Hg would produce very little change in SaO_2 (see Fig. 6–1). Clinically, this means that although administering supplemental oxygen may significantly increase the patient's PaO_2, the resulting SaO_2 increase will be small in proportion. The patient's oxygenation status is better protected at the top of the curve.

The bottom portion of the curve ($PaO_2 \leq 60$ mm Hg) is steep. In this portion, any alteration in PaO_2 yields a

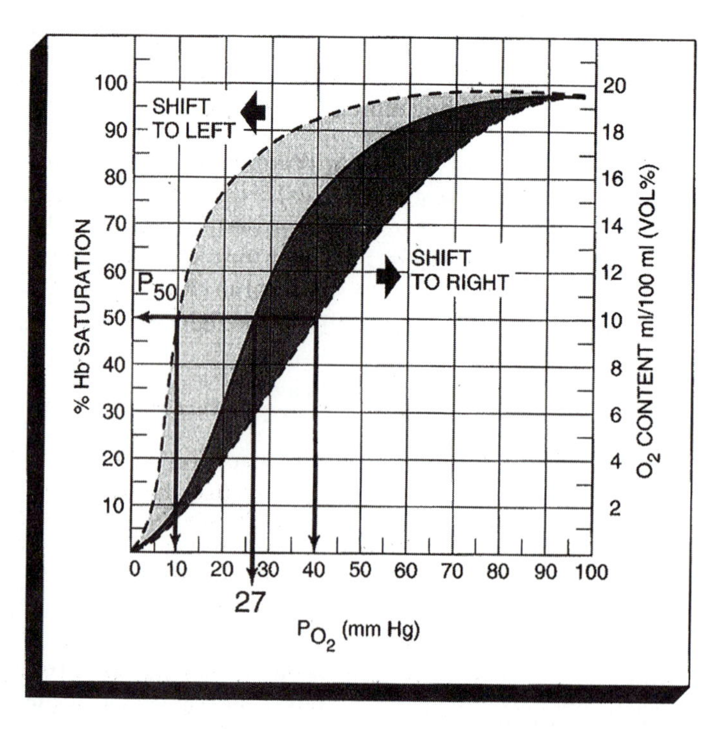

Figure 6–1. The P_{50} represents the partial pressure at which hemoglobin is 50 percent saturated with oxygen. When the oxygen dissociation curve shifts to the right, the P_{50} increases. When the oxygen dissociation curve shifts to the left, the P_{50} decreases. *(From* Cardiopulmonary Anatomy and Physiology, *2nd ed., by J. R. Des Jardins © 1993. Reprinted with permission of Delmar, a division of Thompson Learning. Fax (800) 730-2215.)*

large change in percentage of hemoglobin saturation (SaO_2). For example, a 10 mm Hg decrease in PaO_2 from 60 mm Hg to 50 mm Hg drops the SaO_2 from about 85 percent to about 75 percent (a decrease of approximately 10 percent SaO_2). Clinically, this means that administration of supplemental oxygen sufficient to increase the PaO_2 should yield large increases in SaO_2. However, abnormalities in the ventilation–perfusion relationship may exist, interfering with reoxygenation.

Low PaO_2 at the tissue level stimulates oxygen release from hemoglobin to the tissue. High PaO_2 at the pulmonary capillary level stimulates hemoglobin to bind with more oxygen. Other factors can change the curve, shifting it to the right or the left. A right shift prevents hemoglobin from binding as readily with oxygen, although oxygen is able to be released at the tissue level more readily. A left shift causes hemoglobin to bond more readily with oxygen in the lungs, but inhibits release at the tissue level. Factors that shift the curve to the right and left are listed in Table 6–1. Slight shifts are adaptive. For example, an increased body temperature increases oxygen demand, causing a slight right shift, which increases release of oxygen to the tissues to meet increasing tissue oxygen demand. Severe or rapid shifts, however, can produce life-threatening tissue hypoxia.

TABLE 6–1. FACTORS AFFECTING THE OXYHEMOGLOBIN DISSOCIATION CURVE

RIGHT SHIFT	LEFT SHIFT
Acidosis	Alkalosis
Hyperthermia	Hypothermia
Hypercarbia	Hypocarbia
Increased 2,3-DPG[a]	Decreased 2,3-DPG

[a]2,3-DPG = 52,3-diphosphoglycerate.

In summary, many factors affect gas exchange, including the partial pressure of a gas, ability to diffuse across the alveolar–capillary membrane, $\dot{V}/\dot{Q}$ ratio, and oxyhemoglobin dissociation. An understanding of these concepts assists in determining alternatives for clinical interventions.

SECTION ONE REVIEW

1. Common factors affecting gas exchange include all of the following EXCEPT
   A. partial pressure
   B. oxyhemoglobin dissociation
   C. mixed venous saturation
   D. diffusion
2. Partial pressure is defined as
   A. the difference between concentrations of gases
   B. the amount of pressure exerted by each gas
   C. the atmospheric pressure at sea level
   D. the amount of diffusion across alevolar membranes
3. Which of the following reflects the natural movement of gas diffusion?
   A. from low to high pressure
   B. from high to low pressure
   C. from equal to unequal pressure
   D. from negative to positive pressure
4. The oxyhemoglobin dissociation curve represents hemoglobin ability to
   A. transport heme
   B. react with carbon dioxide
   C. split off iron molecule
   D. chemically bind and release oxygen

Answers: 1. C, 2. B, 3. B, 4. D

SECTION TWO: Acid–Base Physiology and Compensation

At the completion of this section, the learner will be able to identify mechanisms that the body uses to compensate for acid–base imbalances.

Acid–base balance is crucial to the effective functioning of the body systems. Severe imbalances can be lethal to the patient. The body contains many acid and base substances. **Acids** are substances that dissociate or lose ions. **Bases** are substances capable of accepting ions. The **pH** represents the free hydrogen ion (H^+) concentration. An increase in H^+ concentration lowers pH and increases acidity. A decrease in H^+ concentration increases pH and increases alkalinity.

The body's acids include volatile acids and nonvolatile acids. **Volatile acids** can convert to a gas form for excretion (carbonic acid). Carbonic acid rapidly converts to carbon dioxide for excretion from the lungs. The lungs excrete a very large amount of acid each day in this manner. **Nonvolatile (metabolic) acids** cannot be converted to gas, so they must be excreted through the kidneys. Examples of nonvolatile acids include lactic acid and ketones. Unlike the lungs, the kidneys are capable of excreting only a small amount of acid each day and respond slowly to changes. Hydrogen ions are excreted in the proximal and distal tubules of the kidneys in exchange for sodium.

Buffer Systems

The body is not tolerant of wide changes in pH and is working constantly to maintain the pH range between 7.35 and 7.45. A normal pH is maintained if the ratio of bicarbonate (HCO_3) to carbon dioxide (CO_2) remains at approximately a 20:1 (HCO_3/CO_2) ratio (Fig. 6–2). The body has three mechanisms to maintain acid–base balance: the buffering mechanism, the respiratory compensation mechanism, and the metabolic or renal compensation mechanism.

The buffering mechanism represents chemical reactions between acids and bases to maintain a neutral environment. Bases react with excess hydrogen ions (H^+) to prevent shifts in pH, and acids react with excess HCO_3. This process starts immediately. The bicarbonate **buffer** system is the major buffering system in the body. Its components are regulated by the lungs (CO_2) and kidneys (HCO_3). The following reversible reaction represents the shifts that occur as carbonic acid (H_2CO_3) is shifted depending on body needs:

$$H^+ + HCO_3 \rightleftharpoons H_2CO_3 \rightleftharpoons CO_2 + H_2O$$

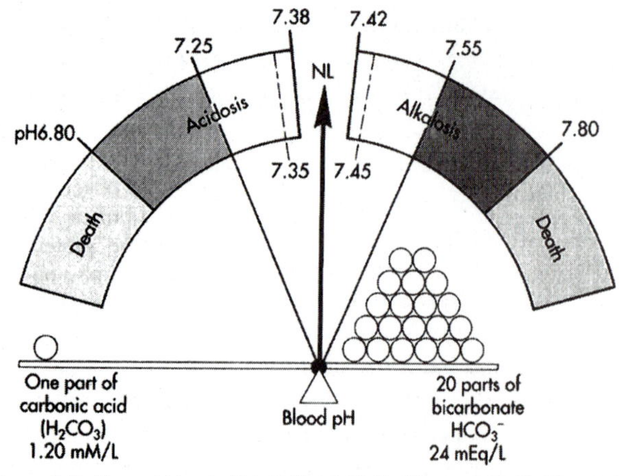

Figure 6–2. Normal blood pH is 7.40 ± 0.02 (1 SD) or ± 0.05 (2 SD). Acid–base balance occurs when the ratio of bicarbonate to carbonic acid is 20:1. Any change in this ratio tips the balance and swings the pointer to the acidosis or alkalosis side. A pH < 7.25 or > 7.55 is life-threatening, and the extremes of 6.8 or 7.8 cause death. *(From Price, S.A., & Wilson, L.M. [1992].* Pathophysiology: Clinical concepts of disease processes, *4th ed., p. 260. St. Louis: C.V. Mosby.)*

Additional nonbicarbonate buffers include hemoglobin, serum proteins, and the phosphate system, the latter of which is mainly a function of the kidneys.

The respiratory compensation mechanism increases or decreases alveolar ventilation. Hyperventilation excretes carbon dioxide, ridding the system of excessive acid (often called blowing off CO_2). Hypoventilation results in the retention of carbon dioxide, which increases the amount of acid available to combine with excess bicarbonate to form carbonic acid. Compensation begins rapidly in minutes but may take several hours for maximum effect.

The metabolic compensation mechanism controls the rate of elimination or reabsorption of hydrogen and bicarbonate ions in the kidney. In situations of increased acid loads (acidosis), H^+ elimination and bicarbonate reabsorption are increased. In alkalosis, H^+ is reabsorbed and HCO_3^- is excreted. Metabolic compensation is slow. It begins in hours but takes days to reach maximum compensation.

Levels of Compensation

- **Uncompensated:** The pH is abnormal because buffer and regulatory mechanisms have not begun to correct the imbalance. In these situations, the acid or base component is abnormal.
- **Partially compensated:** The pH is abnormal, but the body buffers and regulatory mechanisms have started to respond to the imbalance. In these situations, the acid and base components are abnormal.
- **Compensated:** The pH is within normal limits, ranging between 7.35 and 7.45. The acid–base imbalance has been neutralized but not corrected. In this situation, the acid and base components are abnormal but balanced.
- **Corrected:** The pH is within normal limits. All acid–base parameters have returned to normal ranges after a state of acid–base imbalance.

The body corrects imbalances with continual slight adjustments. However, it does not overcompensate for acid–base abnormalities. Thus, pH reflects the primary problem of acidosis or alkalosis. Clinically, when drugs are administered to correct an acid–base imbalance, the larger dose or adjustment may overshoot the neutral target point. For example, the administration of large amounts of sodium bicarbonate in a cardiac arrest (metabolic acidosis) situation can overshoot the neutral target pH (7.40) and place the patient in metabolic alkalosis.

In summary, the body attempts to maintain pH within a narrow range. Compensatory mechanisms include buffering, excretion or retention of carbon dioxide (respiratory), and excretion or retention of H^+/HCO_3^- (metabolic).

SECTION TWO REVIEW

1. The body compensates for acid–base imbalance by all of the following mechanisms EXCEPT
   A. buffering
   B. hepatic compensation
   C. respiratory compensation
   D. excretion of HCO_3
2. Respiratory compensation involves excretion or retention of
   A. CO_2
   B. HCO_3
   C. H_2O
   D. K^+
3. Metabolic compensation involves changes in excretion or reabsorption of
   A. H^+, CO_2
   B. HCO_3, H^+
   C. glucose, HCO_3
   D. CO_2, HCO_3
4. The body's buffering system continually works toward maintenance of a bicarbonate/carbon dioxide ratio of
   A. 1:5
   B. 1:20
   C. 5:1
   D. 20:1

Answers: 1. B, 2. A, 3. B, 4. D

SECTION THREE: Normal Values for Arterial Blood Gases

At the completion of this section, the learner will be able to identify normal values for arterial blood gases.

Indicators for Determination of Acid–Base State

pH

The pH represents the amount of free H^+ available in the blood (normal value 7.35 to 7.45). The body's normal state is slightly alkaline, and the body strives to maintain this range. Extreme deviation for long periods of time is incompatible with survival. pH reflects the body's total acid–base balance. It is shifted by changes in hydrogen (H^+) or bicarbonate (HCO_3) ion concentration. Gain of acid or loss of base shifts the acid–base balance to the acid side. Loss of acid or gain of base or both shift the balance to the alkaline side.

$Paco_2$

The $Paco_2$ is the partial pressure of carbon dioxide in arterial blood (normal value 35 to 45 mm Hg). $Paco_2$ represents the respiratory component of the arterial blood gases (ABGs). The lungs control the excretion or retention of carbon dioxide through alveolar ventilation. Elevated $Paco_2$ indicates hypoventilation of the alveoli. Decreased $Paco_2$ represents alveolar hyperventilation.

HCO_3

HCO_3 represents the concentration of bicarbonate in the blood (normal value 22 to 26 mEq/L). HCO_3 represents the renal or metabolic component of the arterial blood gases. It is influenced by metabolic processes.

Base Excess

The level of base excess (BE) can be measured as an indirect reflection of bicarbonate concentration in the body (normal value ±2 mEq/L). Base excess is considered a purely nonrespiratory measurement because it is not affected by carbonic acid concentrations. A base deficit is present if BE is greater than −2 mEq/L, reflecting an excess of fixed acids or a deficit in base. A base excess is present if the BE is greater than +2 mEq/L, reflecting either an excess of base or a deficit of fixed acids. Base excess measurement is not considered an essential step in basic ABG interpretation.

Indicators of Oxygenation Status

Pao_2

Pao_2 represents the partial pressure of the oxygen dissolved in arterial blood (3 percent of total oxygen) (normal value 80 to 100 mm Hg), not the total amount of oxygen available. Though it accounts for only a small percentage of total oxygen in the blood, it is an important indicator of oxygenation, since Pao_2 and oxygen saturation (Sao_2) maintain a relationship. This relationship is reflected in the oxyhemoglobin dissociation curve, making it an important indicator of oxygenation status.

Sao_2

Oxygen saturation (Sao_2) is the measure of percentage of oxygen combined with hemoglobin compared with the total amount it could carry (normal value > 95 percent). The degree of saturation is important in determining the amount of oxygen available for delivery to the tissues.

Hemoglobin

Hemoglobin (Hgb or Hb) is the major component of red blood cells (normal values 12 to 15 g/dL in women, 13.5

to 17 g/dL in men). It is composed of protein and heme, which contains iron. Oxygen binds to the iron atoms located on the four heme groups of each hemoglobin molecule. Hemoglobin is the major carrier of oxygen in the blood and is, therefore, an important factor in tissue oxygenation.

Arterial Blood Gas

Arterial blood gas (ABG) normal values typically are reported as normal at sea level (760 mm Hg) partial pressures, room air (21 percent oxygen), and a blood temperature of 37°C (98.6°F). Changes in these factors need to be considered during interpretation. Age also affects the normal values. Newborns have a lower PaO_2 (40 to 70 mm Hg), as do elderly people, whose PaO_2 decreases approximately 10 mm Hg per decade (in the 60- to 90-year age range). Normal ABG values are ranges for normal, healthy adults. It is important to establish a baseline for the individual, since abnormal values are normal for some individuals. A patient with chronic lung disease may have a PaO_2 of 60 mm Hg with a $PaCO_2$ of 50 mm Hg as a normal baseline. Attempts to return ABG values to those of a normal, healthy individual would have serious consequences.

A person receiving supplemental oxygen also can be evaluated without determining room air gas. The PaO_2 should rise approximately 50 mm Hg for each 10 percent rise in oxygen concentration. A simple way to estimate what the PaO_2 should be is to multiply 5 times the percent of oxygen. If the PaO_2 is less than this value, the patient would probably be inadequately oxygenated on room air. For example, 5 × 50% O_2 = 250 mm Hg PaO_2.

In summary, indicators of acid–base and oxygenation states have been presented. Included in the discussion were normal values and a brief description of each indicator. The concept of arterial blood gases was presented in regard to the basis of normal values, gas considerations, and alterations in normal blood gas values associated with the pathophysiologic changes of chronic obstructive pulmonary disease. Table 6–2 summarizes normal arterial blood gas values.

TABLE 6–2. NORMAL ARTERIAL BLOOD GAS VALUES

	RANGE
Acid–base	
pH	7.35–7.45
$PaCO_2$	35–45 mm Hg
HCO_3	22–26 mEq/L
BE	± 2 mEq/L
Oxygenation Status	
PaO_2	80–100 mm Hg
SaO_2	95–100%
Hgb*	13.5–17 g/dL (males) 12–15 g/dL (females)

*From Kee, J.L. (1999). Laboratory and diagnostic tests with nursing implications, 5th ed. Norwalk, CT: Appleton & Lange.

SECTION THREE REVIEW

1. Normal values for arterial blood gases include
   A. pH 7.5
   B. $PaCO_2$ 20 mm Hg
   C. HCO_3 26 mm Hg
   D. SaO_2 75 mm Hg
2. An increase in bicarbonate would cause the pH to become more
   A. acidic
   B. alkaline
   C. neutral
   D. no change
3. $PaCO_2$ is the _______ component, and HCO_3 is the _______ component.
   A. oxygenation, metabolic
   B. respiratory, metabolic
   C. metabolic, respiratory
   D. hepatic, oxygenation
4. According to the oxyhemoglobin dissociation curve, at a PaO_2 of less than 60 mm Hg, a large decrease in PaO_2 should produce what kind of change in the SaO_2?
   A. small increase
   B. large increase
   C. small decrease
   D. large decrease
5. What factor must you always evaluate to place ABGs in the proper context?
   A. laboratory values
   B. oxygen supplemental therapy
   C. mode of ventilation
   D. patient

Answers: 1. C, 2. B, 3. B, 4. D, 5. D

TABLE 6–3. COMMON CAUSES OF ACUTE RESPIRATORY ACIDOSIS

Alveolar hypoventilation, caused by
- Respiratory depression
  - Oversedation
  - Overdose
  - Head injury
- Decreased ventilation
  - Respiratory muscle fatigue
  - Neuromuscular diseases
  - Mechanical ventilation (underventilation)
- Altered diffusion/ventilation–perfusion mismatch
  - Pulmonary edema
  - Severe atelectasis
  - Pneumonia
  - Severe bronchospasm

SECTION FOUR: Respiratory Acid–Base Disturbances

At the completion of this section, the learner will be able to differentiate between respiratory acidosis and alkalosis.

Primary respiratory disturbances are reflected by changes in the $Paco_2$, being either above normal as in respiratory acidosis, or below normal as in respiratory alkalosis.

Respiratory Acidosis

Respiratory acidosis occurs when the $Paco_2$ moves above 45 mm Hg and the pH drops below 7.35. The elevated carbon dioxide (CO_2) indicates alveolar hypoventilation. The lungs are not blowing off enough carbon dioxide, causing a carbonic acid excess. Carbon dioxide is considered an acid because it combines with water to form carbonic acid. It is essential to determine the cause of hypoventilation and then to correct it when possible. Table 6–3 lists some of the major causes of acute respiratory acidosis.

A chronic acid–base state means that a state of compensation exists. Chronic respiratory acidosis usually is associated with a chronic obstructive pulmonary disease, such as chronic bronchitis or emphysema. The elevation of carbon dioxide occurs gradually over many years. Thus, the body is able to compensate to maintain a normal pH by elevating the bicarbonate. Since these individuals have little respiratory reserve, additional stressors can cause decompensation, which produces respiratory failure. Table 6–4 compares the effects of acute and chronic acidosis on ABG levels. (Respiratory failure is discussed in depth in Module 3.)

TABLE 6–4. COMPARISON OF ACUTE AND CHRONIC RESPIRATORY ACIDOSIS

	UNCOMPENSATED	COMPENSATED	
PARAMETER	Acute	Partial	Chronic
pH	↓	↓	Normal
$Paco_2$	↑	↑	↑
HCO_3	Normal	↑	↑

TABLE 6–5. COMMON CAUSES OF ACUTE RESPIRATORY ALKALOSIS

Alveolar hyperventilation, caused by
- Anxiety, fear
- Pain
- Hypoxia
- Head injury
- Fever
- Mechanical ventilation (overventilation)

Respiratory Alkalosis

Respiratory alkalosis occurs when the $Paco_2$ falls below 35 mm Hg with a corresponding rise in pH to > 7.45. The decreased carbon dioxide indicates alveolar hyperventilation. The lungs are eliminating too much carbon dioxide, causing a carbonic acid deficit. There are inadequate amounts of carbon dioxide available to combine with water to form carbonic acid (H_2CO_3). The key to effective treatment of respiratory alkalosis is to determine the cause of the hyperventilation and provide the intervention necessary to correct the problem. Common causes of acute respiratory alkalosis are listed in Table 6–5.

Chronic respiratory alkalosis is uncommon. The same factors causing acute respiratory alkalosis could cause a chronic state if the problem remained uncorrected. Table 6–6 compares the effects of acute and chronic respiratory alkalosis on ABG levels.

In summary, to differentiate between primary respiratory acidosis and alkalosis, the $Paco_2$ and pH must be

TABLE 6–6. COMPARISON OF ACUTE AND CHRONIC RESPIRATORY ALKALOSIS

	UNCOMPENSATED	COMPENSATED	
PARAMETER	Acute	Partial	Chronic
pH	↑	↑	Normal
$Paco_2$	↓	↓	↓
HCO_3	Normal	↓	↓

evaluated. The cause of respiratory acidosis is alveolar hypoventilation, and the cause of respiratory alkalosis is alveolar hyperventilation. Compensation of respiratory acid–base disturbances requires evaluation of changes in bicarbonate. Treatment includes correction of the underlying problem, when possible.

SECTION FOUR REVIEW

1. Respiratory acidosis is caused by which of the following?
   A. alveolar hyperventilation
   B. alveolar hypoventilation
   C. mechanical ventilation
   D. inadequate perfusion
2. Which of the following occurs as a result of acute respiratory acidosis?
   A. pH increases
   B. pH decreases
   C. CO_2 decreases
   D. HCO_3 decreases
3. Respiratory alkalosis is caused by which of the following?
   A. alveolar hyperventilation
   B. alveolar hypoventilation
   C. mechanical ventilation
   D. inadequate perfusion
4. Patient situations associated with respiratory alkalosis include
   A. sedation
   B. neuromuscular blockade
   C. pulmonary edema
   D. anxiety

Answers: 1. B, 2. B, 3. A, 4. D

SECTION FIVE: Metabolic Acid–Base Disturbances

At the completion of this section, the learner will be able to differentiate between metabolic acidosis and alkalosis.

Primary metabolic disturbances are reflected by changes in bicarbonate (HCO_3) levels and base excess (BE). Metabolic acidosis can be defined clinically as $HCO_3 = < 22$ mEq/L, pH < 7.35, with a base deficit (< -2). Metabolic acidosis can be caused by an increase in metabolic acids or excessive loss of base.

Examples of conditions precipitating an increase in hydrogen ion (H^+) concentrations include:

- Diabetic acidosis due to elevated ketones
- Uremia associated with increased levels of phosphates and sulfates
- Ingestion of acidic drugs, such as aspirin (salicylate) overdose
- Lactic acidosis caused by increased lactic acid production

Examples of conditions that precipitate a decrease in bicarbonate (HCO_3) levels include:

- Diarrhea, which causes loss of alkaline substances
- Gastrointestinal fistulas leading to loss of alkaline substances
- Loss of body fluids from drains below the umbilicus (except urinary catheter) causing loss of alkaline fluids
- Drugs causing loss of alkali, such as laxative overuse
- Hyperaldosteronism, which causes increased renal loss

Lactic Acidosis

Currently there is increased clinical interest in evaluating metabolic acidosis that is precipitated by elevated lactate levels. Acid metabolites, such as lactic acid (lactate), result from cellular breakdown and anaerobic metabolism. The normal range for serum lactate is 0.5 to 2.0 mEq/L. High-acuity patients are at particular risk for developing elevated levels of lactate since lactic acidosis is closely associated with shock and other severe physiologic insults. During a shock episode, cellular hypoxia drives serum lactate levels up rapidly, usually to > 5 mEq/L. This rise often precedes decompensatory signs such as decreased urine output and decreased blood pressure, and thus may be an indicator of impending shock. Other conditions that can cause lactic acidosis include severe dehydration, severe infection, severe trauma, diabetic ketoacidosis, and hepatic failure (Kee, 1999).

Table 6–7 compares the effects of acute and chronic metabolic acidosis on arterial blood gases.

TABLE 6–7. COMPARISON OF ACUTE AND CHRONIC METABOLIC ACIDOSIS

	UNCOMPENSATED	COMPENSATED	
PARAMETER	Acute	Partial	Chronic
pH	↓	↓	Normal
$Paco_2$	Normal	↓	↓
HCO_3	↓	↓	↓

Metabolic Alkalosis

Metabolic alkalosis can be defined clinically as a bicarbonate (HCO_3) > 26 mEq/L, pH > 7.45, and a base excess > +2). Metabolic alkalosis occurs when the amount of alkali (base) increases or excessive loss of acid occurs.

A common cause of increased alkali is in the ingestion of alkaline drugs associated with the overuse of antacids or overadministration of sodium bicarbonate during a cardiac arrest emergency.

Examples of conditions that result in a decrease in acid include:

- Loss of gastric fluids from vomiting or nasogastric suction
- Treatment with steroids, especially those with mineralocorticoid effects
- Diuretic therapy with certain drugs, such as furosemide (Lasix), causing loss of potassium
- Binge–purge syndrome

TABLE 6–8. COMPARISON OF ACUTE AND CHRONIC METABOLIC ALKALOSIS

	UNCOMPENSATED	COMPENSATED	
PARAMETER	Acute	Partial	Chronic
pH	↑	↑	Normal
$Paco_2$	Normal	↑	↑
HCO_3	↑	↑	↑

Table 6–8 compares the effects of acute and chronic metabolic alkalosis on arterial blood gases.

In summary, to differentiate between primary metabolic acidosis or alkalosis, the bicarbonate and pH must be evaluated. Base excess provides additional data. Conditions that cause each acid–base disturbance have been presented. Compensation of metabolic acid–base disturbance requires evaluation of the $Paco_2$.

SECTION FIVE REVIEW

1. Metabolic disturbances are reflected by changes in which of the following?
   A. HCO_3, FIO_2
   B. PaO_2, SaO_2
   C. HCO_3, BE
   D. BE, PaO_2
2. Metabolic acidosis results in
   A. increased $PaCO_2$
   B. decreased BE
   C. increased pH
   D. increased HCO_3
3. A condition that may cause metabolic acidosis due to a decrease in bicarbonate levels is
   A. diarrhea
   B. uremia
   C. aspirin ingestion
   D. diabetic ketoacidosis
4. Metabolic alkalosis is caused by a (an) ______ in acid or a (an)______ in base.
   A. increase, increase
   B. decrease, decrease
   C. decrease, increase
   D. increase, decrease

Answers: 1. C, 2. B, 3. A, 4. C

SECTION SIX: Arterial Blood Gas Interpretation

At the completion of this section, the learner will be able to interpret arterial blood gases for acid–base state, degree of compensation, and abnormalities of oxygenation.

A single ABG measurement represents only a single point in time. Arterial blood gases are most valuable when trends are evaluated over time, correlated with other values, and incorporated into the overall clinical picture. Interpretation of ABGs includes determination of acid–base state, level of compensation, and oxygenation status. The oxygenation status reflects alveolar ventilation, the amount of oxygen available in arterial blood for possible tissue use, oxygen-carrying capacity, and oxygen transport.

A step-by-step process for ABG interpretation evaluates each component to determine acid–base balance and oxygenation status. For the purpose of organizing this section, acid–base balance determination is discussed first. However, oxygenation status often is analyzed first, based on the needs of the patient and the preference of the person performing the analysis.

Acid–Base Balance Determination

Evaluate pH

The normal pH is 7.35 to 7.45, with the midpoint being 7.40. For the purpose of interpretation, consider all values higher than 7.4 to be alkaline and all values less than 7.4 to be acidic.

Ask: Is the pH within normal range? Does the pH deviate to the acid or alkaline side?

Evaluate $Paco_2$

Normal $Paco_2$ is 35 to 45 mm Hg. If the $Paco_2$ is < 35 mm Hg, consider it alkaline. If it is > 45 mm Hg, consider it acidic. Remember that CO_2 is the respiratory component.

Ask: Is $Paco_2$ within the normal range? If not, does it deviate to the acid or the alkaline side?

Evaluate HCO_3

The normal HCO_3 value is 22 to 26 mEq/L. If the HCO_3 is < 26 mEq/L, consider it acid. If it is > 26 mEq/L, consider it alkaline. Remember that HCO_3 is the metabolic component.

Ask: Is HCO_3 within the normal range? If not, does it deviate to the alkaline or acid side?

Determine the Acid–Base Status

The acid–base status has now been determined for the individual components of $Paco_2$ and HCO_3.

Ask: Which individual component matches the pH acid–base state? The match determines the primary acid–base disturbance.

Example: pH 7.21 (acid), $Paco_2$ 60 mm Hg (acid), HCO_3 22 mEq/L (normal). Interpretation: pH and $Paco_2$ match (acidosis). $Paco_2$ is the respiratory component. Thus, the primary disturbance is respiratory acidosis.

Figure 6–3 provides a summary algorithm of acid–base balance determination.

Determination of Compensation

Once the acid–balance has been analyzed, it is necessary to determine whether compensation for an acid–base disturbance is occurring and at what level. In discussing compensation, only three components need to be considered: pH, $Paco_2$, and HCO_3.

The pH indicates the degree of compensation. A normal pH indicates that either the ABG is normal or full compensation exists. In full compensation, the body has balanced the acid–base state. An abnormal pH indicates an uncompensated or partially compensated acid–base state.

Determine the Level of Compensation

UNCOMPENSATED (ACUTE). Abnormal pH plus one abnormal value plus a normal value.

Example: pH 7.20, $Paco_2$ 60 mm Hg, HCO_3 24 mEq/L. Interpretation: The pH and $Paco_2$ match (acid). HCO_3 is normal. No compensation is occurring. A state of uncompensated (acute) respiratory acidosis exists.

PARTIALLY COMPENSATED. Abnormal pH plus two abnormal values ($Paco_2$ and HCO_3 are moving in opposite directions). The body has initiated neutralizing the imbalance but has not yet fully compensated for it.

Example: pH 7.30, $Paco_2$ 60 mm Hg, HCO_3 30 mEq/L. Interpretation: The pH and $Paco_2$ match (acid). HCO_3 is alkaline or moving in the opposite direction from the $Paco_2$. The pH is still abnormal. A state of partially compensated respiratory acidosis exists.

COMPENSATED. Normal pH plus two abnormal values ($Paco_2$ and HCO_3 are moving in opposite directions).

Example: pH 7.38, $Paco_2$ 50 mm Hg, HCO_3 30 mEq/L. Interpretation: The pH and $Paco_2$ match (acid). HCO_3 is alkaline (opposite of $Paco_2$). pH is normal. A state of compensated respiratory acidosis exists.

CORRECTED. Normal pH and two normal values. No acid–base disturbance currently exists.

Example: pH 7.36, $Paco_2$ 43 mm Hg, HCO_3, 26 mEq/L. Interpretation: If this is the current acid–base state in a patient who, until recently, had an acid–base disturbance, this ABG would be called a corrected acid–base state.

Figure 6–4 provides a summary algorithm of determination of level of compensation.

In summary, analysis of the acid–base state has been described using a step-by-step approach. This approach allows problem solving without requiring memorization of all disturbance possibilities. Compensation states are classified as uncompensated (acute), partially compensated, compensated (chronic), or corrected.

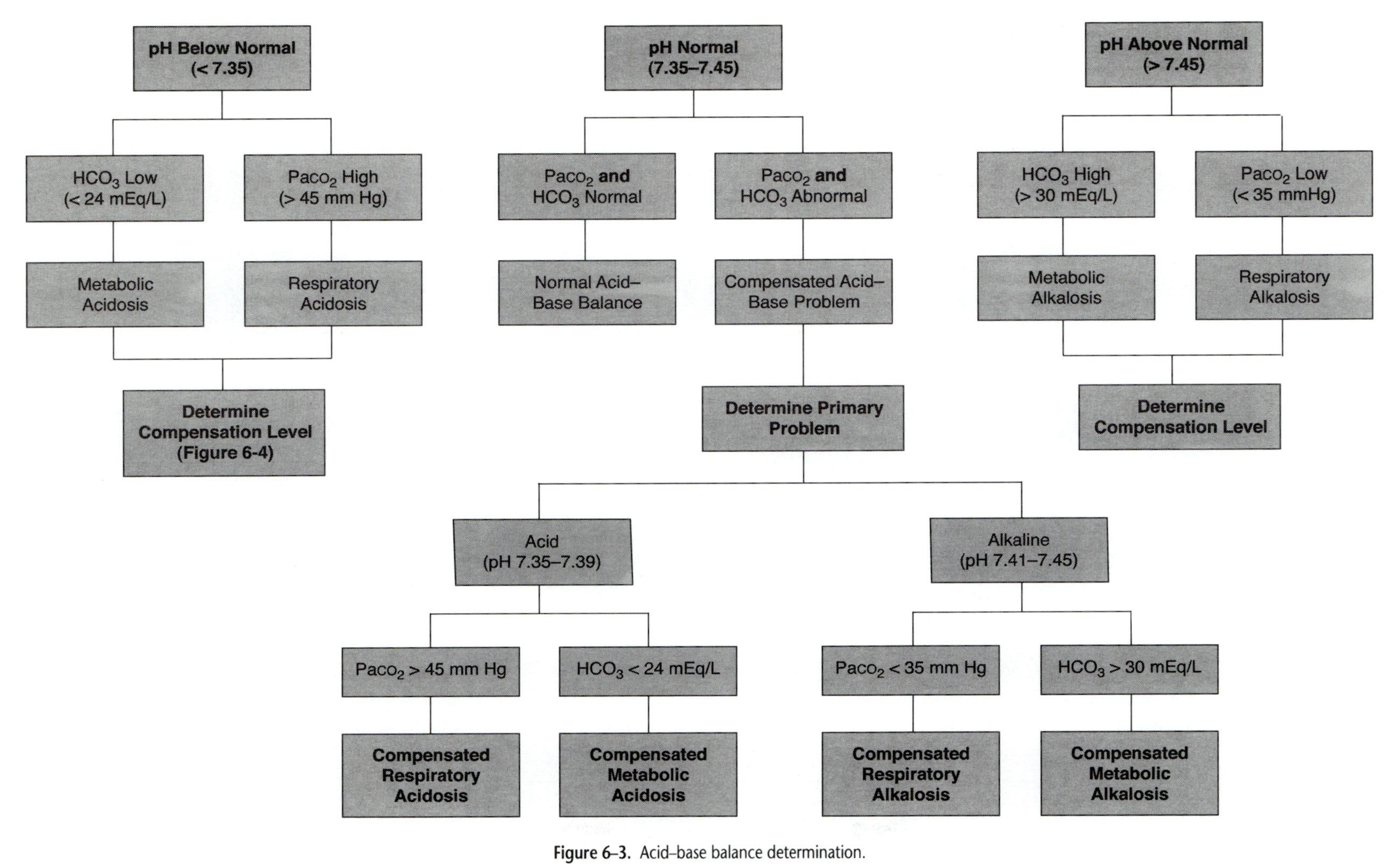

Figure 6–3. Acid–base balance determination.

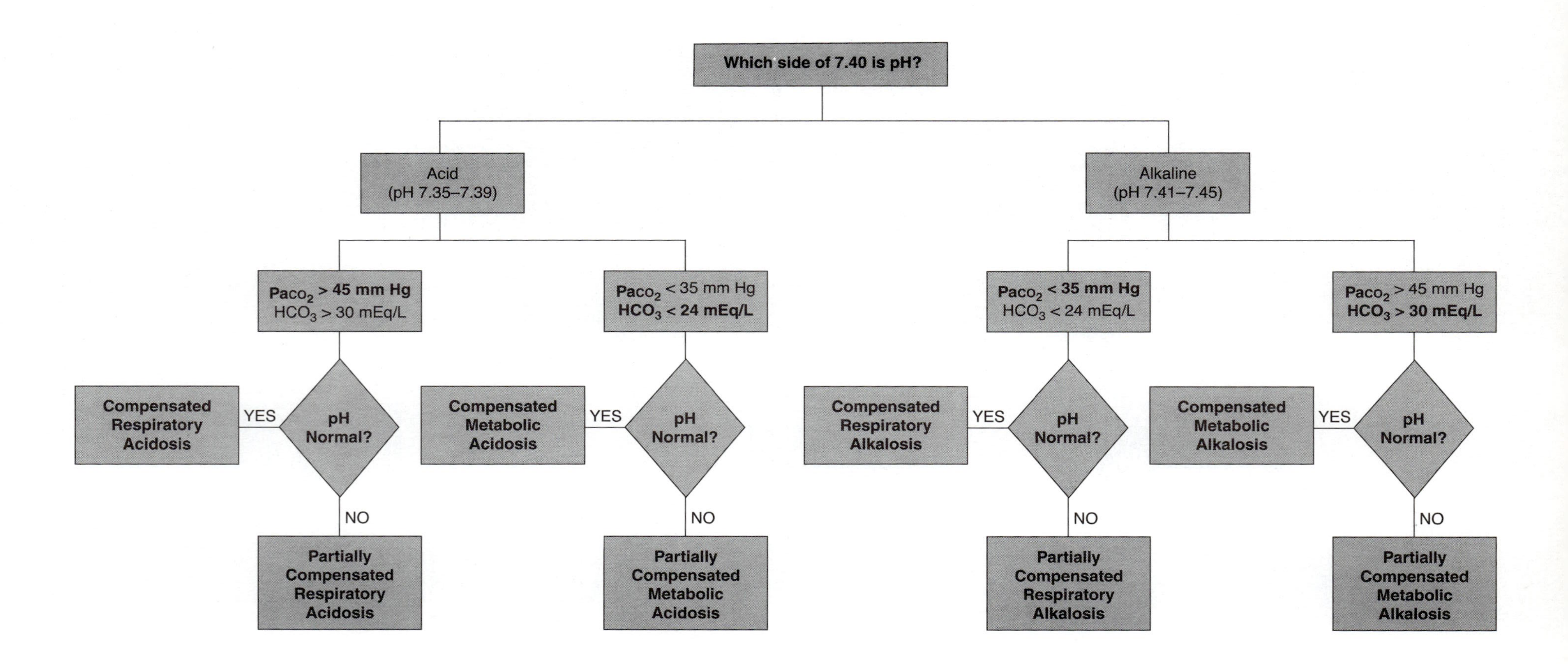

Figure 6–4. Determination of level of compensation.

ACID–BASE EXERCISE

Take time to practice determining acid–base and compensation using the steps outlined above. Interpret the acid–base status as normal, metabolic or respiratory, alkalosis or acidosis. Indicate the state of compensation as being uncompensated (acute state), partially compensated, or compensated (chronic state).

1. pH = 7.58, $Paco_2$ = 38 mm Hg, HCO_3 = 30 mEq/L
   Interpretation:

   Compensation:

2. pH = 7.20, $Paco_2$ = 60 mm Hg, HCO_3 = 26 mEq/L
   Interpretation:

   Compensation:

3. pH = 7.39, $Paco_2$ = 43 mm Hg, HCO_3 = 24 mEq/L
   Interpretation:

   Compensation:

4. pH = 7.32, $Paco_2$ = 60 mm Hg, HCO_3 = 30 mEq/L
   Interpretation:

   Compensation:

5. pH = 7.5, $Paco_2$ = 50 mm Hg, HCO_3 = 38 mEq/L
   Interpretation:

   Compensation:

6. pH = 7.45, $Paco_2$ = 30 mm Hg, HCO_3 = 20 mEq/L
   Interpretation:

   Compensation:

7. pH = 7.40, $Paco_2$ = 40 mm Hg, HCO_3 = 24 mEq/L
   Interpretation:

   Compensation:

ACID–BASE EXERCISE ANSWERS

1. pH 7.58 (alkaline) and HCO_3 30 mEq/L (alkaline) match. $Paco_2$ 38 mm Hg (normal). Interpretation: metabolic alkalosis. Compensation: uncompensated.
2. pH 7.20 (acid) and $Paco_2$ 60 mm Hg (acid) match. HCO_3 26 mEq/L (normal). Interpretation: respiratory acidosis. Compensation: uncompensated.
3. pH 7.39 (normal, slightly to acid side of 7.4) and $Paco_2$ 43 mm Hg (normal). HCO_3 24 (normal). Interpretation: normal. Compensation: none required.
4. pH 7.32 (acid) and $Paco_2$ 60 mm Hg (acid) match. HCO_3 30 mEq/L (alkaline) Interpretation: respiratory acidosis. Compensation: partial compensation.
5. pH 7.5 (alkaline) and HCO_3 38 mEq/L (alkaline) match. $Paco_2$ 50 mm Hg (acid). Interpretation: metabolic alkalosis. Compensation: partial compensation.
6. pH 7.45 (normal, alkaline side) and $Paco_2$ 30 mm Hg (alkaline) match. HCO_3 20 mEq/L (acid). Interpretation: respiratory alkalosis. Compensation: full compensation.
7. pH, $Paco_2$, and HCO_3 are all normal. Interpretation: normal. Compensation: none required.

Evaluation of Oxygenation Status

Evaluation of oxygenation has three components: partial pressure of arterial oxygen (Pao_2), percentage of hemoglobin saturation (Sao_2), and hemoglobin (Hgb or Hb). The following is a systematic approach to evaluating oxygenation status.

Evaluate the Pao_2
Ask: Is it normal (normal Pao_2 is 80 to 100 mm Hg)? What is baseline for this person? Is it within the acceptable range? If not, is it too low or too high?

Evaluate the Sao_2
Ask: Is it within the acceptable range? (Normal Sao_2 is > 95 percent.)

Evaluate the Hgb
Ask: Are there enough oxygen carriers? (Normal Hgb is 12 to 15 g/dL in women and 13.5 to 17 g/dL in men.)

Patient Assessment

Although ABG interpretation is an important adjunct to assessing a patient's status, it cannot take the place of direct evaluation of the patient. Does the patient's clinical picture match the acid–base and oxygenation interpretation? Many things can interfere with the validity of blood gas analysis and oximetric measurements, for example, a pulse oximetry sensor malfunction, a venous rather than an arterial blood sample, or incorrect ABG procedures. Does the patient have a chronic disorder that is associated with long-term alterations in ABGs? Are there any acute processes occurring that need to be taken into consideration? Does the patient have a fever?

In summary, ABG analysis is a step-by-step process. Each component is evaluated individually and then in relationship to other components. Although acid–base state, compensation, and oxygenation status are important factors, the most important step is applying the results to the individual patient and the particular clinical situation. Take time to practice determining acid–base state and oxygenation status using the steps outlined above. Interpret the acid–base status as normal, metabolic or respiratory, alkalosis or acidosis. Indicate the state of compensation as being uncompensated (acute state), partially compensated, or compensated (chronic state). Indicate the oxygenation status as adequate or inadequate.

OXYGENATION AND ACID–BASE ANALYSIS EXERCISE

1. pH = 7.37, $Paco_2$ = 48 mm Hg, HCO_3 = 29 mEq/L, Pao_2 = 80 mm Hg, Sao_2 = 95 percent
   Acid–base state:

   Oxygenation status:

2. pH = 7.48, $Paco_2$ = 30 mm Hg, HCO_3 = 24 mEq/L, Pao_2 = 90 mm Hg, Sao_2 = 98 percent
   Acid–base state:

   Oxygenation status:

3. pH = 7.48, $Paco_2$ = 33 mm Hg, HCO_3 = 25 mEq/L, Pao_2 = 68 mm Hg, Sao_2 = 98 percent
   Acid–base state:

   Oxygenation status:

4. pH = 7.38, $Paco_2$ = 38 mm Hg, HCO_3 = 24 mEq/L, Pao_2 = 269 mm Hg, Sao_2 = 100 percent
   Acid–base state:

   Oxygenation status:

5. pH = 7.17, $Paco_2$ = 18 mm Hg, HCO_3 = 7 mEq/L, Pao_2 = 100 mm Hg, Sao_2 = 99 percent
   Acid–base state:

   Oxygenation status:

OXYGENATION AND ACID–BASE EXERCISE ANSWERS

1. pH 7.37 (normal range, acid) and $Paco_2$ 48 mm Hg (acid) match. HCO_3 29 mEq/L (alkaline) is opposite. Pao_2 80 mm Hg and Sao_2 95 percent both are low normal. Acid–base state: compensated respiratory acidosis (pH normal). Oxygenation status: adequate. The Hgb is not known, but the relationship between Pao_2 and Sao_2 appears normal. Assessing trends is important. Is the $Paco_2$ continuing to increase and Pao_2 continuing to decrease? Continue to monitor.

2. pH 7.48 (alkaline) and $Paco_2$ 30 mm Hg (alkaline) match, HCO_3 24 mEq/L, Pao_2 90 mm Hg, and Sao_2 95 percent are all normal. Acid–base state: acute respiratory alkalosis (uncompensated). Oxygenation status: within normal limits and seems adequate. Look at your patient.

3. pH 7.48 (alkaline) and $Paco_2$ 33 mm Hg (alkaline) match. HCO_3 25 mEq/L is normal. Pao_2 68 mm Hg (low) and Sao_2 98 percent (normal). Acid–base state: acute respiratory alkalosis. Oxygenation status: low oxygen with high saturation. Hemoglobin is carrying a full load but needs more carriers. What is this patient's hemoglobin? Nursing interventions may focus on decreasing oxygen demand. Is this patient tachypneic? Is supplemental oxygen available? Is a transfusion ordered?

4. pH 7.38, $Paco_2$ 38 mm Hg, HCO_3 24 mEq/L are all normal. Pao_2 269 mm Hg is high, and Sao_2 100 percent is high normal. Acid–base state: normal. Oxygenation status: too high! What oxygen percentage is this patient on? Oxygenation supplement needs to be decreased.

5. pH 7.17 (acid) and HCO_3 7 mEq/L (acid) match. $Paco_2$ 18 mm Hg (alkaline) is opposite. Pao_2 100 mm Hg is high, and Sao_2 99 percent is high normal. Acid–base state: severe metabolic acidosis with partial compensation. Oxygenation status: adequate oxygen provided, but it is doubtful that the patient can use what is available efficiently due to the state of severe acidosis. Cellular metabolism is compromised and cannot function efficiently in the acid environment. Cardiovascular status is very likely compromised. The reactivity and effectiveness of many drugs are altered severely in an acidic environment such as this.

SECTION SEVEN: Interpretation of Mixed Acid–Base Disorders

At the completion of this section, the learner will be able to recognize mixed acid–base disorders.

It is not always clear whether the patient is experiencing a simple acid–base disorder with compensation or a mixed acid–base disorder. Recognition and analysis of mixed acid–base disorders is a more complex skill than basic blood gas analysis. This section focuses on the basic concepts involved in recognition of mixed acid–base disorders and provides four rules that help differentiate mixed acid–base disorders from simple (single) disorders with compensation.

The majority of acid–base disturbances have one primary origin with a single secondary acid–base compensatory response. The high-acuity patient, however, is at increased risk for more complex acid–base disorders and may have several different primary acid–base disturbances at the same time. For example, a patient with diabetic ketoacidosis (DKA), a primary metabolic acidosis, might also develop respiratory failure, a primary respiratory acidosis. This situation represents a mixed acid–base disorder. Mixed disorders can have an additive effect, such as seen with the above example (two forms of acidosis), which results in a major derangement in pH. Mixed disorders can also have a nullifying effect (e.g., a primary metabolic alkalosis in the presence of a primary respiratory acidosis), which may rebalance the pH. Table 6–9 lists some complex health problems that are frequently involved in mixed acid–base disorders.

Identifying a Mixed Acid–Base Disorder

Initial Recognition

Before the nurse can attempt to analyze an ABG for the presence of a mixed acid–base disorder, she or he must first recognize the characteristics of a mixed disorder. When either the $PaCO_2$ or the HCO_3 value appears to be out of the ordinary boundaries, a mixed disorder should be suspected. The following rule summarizes the initial recognition:

TABLE 6–9. EXAMPLES OF CLINICAL PROBLEMS ASSOCIATED WITH MIXED ACID–BASE DISORDERS

CLINICAL PROBLEM	ASSOCIATED MIXED DISORDERS
Cardiac arrest	Metabolic acidosis and respiratory acidosis
Salicylate toxicity	Metabolic acidosis and respiratory alkalosis
Renal failure with vomiting	Metabolic acidosis and metabolic alkalosis
Vomiting with chronic obstructive pulmonary disease	Metabolic alkalosis and respiratory acidosis

From Czekaj, L.A. (1998). Promoting acid–base balance. In M. R. Kinney, S.B. Dunbar, J.A. Brooks-Brunn, N. Molter, & J. M. Vitello-Cicciu (eds.), *AACN clinical reference for critical care nursing,* 4th ed. (pp. 135–144). St. Louis: C.V. Mosby.

RULE: A mixed acid–base disorder is present when either the $PaCO_2$ or the HCO_3 value is

1. In a direction opposite its predicted direction, or
2. Not close to the predicted value, during normal compensatory activity (see Table 6–10).

For example, a patient with DKA has an ABG drawn, which shows a pH of 7.05 and an HCO_3 of 16. In this instance, both the pH and the HCO_3 are acidotic. Depending on the level of compensation, one would predict that the $PaCO_2$ level should be either normal or predictably alkaline, as a secondary acid–base response to this situation. If, however, the same DKA patient develops ventilatory failure (hypercapnia), the $PaCO_2$ will also be acidotic (indicating respiratory acidosis), which is not a predicted alteration. The presence of both an acid HCO_3 and $PaCO_2$ is an example of an additive type of mixed acid–base problem, which would drop the pH significantly.

A second example is one that presents a situation in which a nullifying mixed acid–base problem might develop. If the same DKA patient develops severe vomiting or diarrhea (complications that can cause metabolic alkalosis), the patient will have metabolic acidosis (caused by ketoacidosis) and metabolic alkalosis (caused by vomiting or diarrhea). The opposing metabolic disturbances represent a nullifying mixed acid–base problem. In this situation, the pH will lean toward the predominant problem, but it will not be as severely deranged as one would predict based on the patient's DKA status. As a result of these opposing metabolic derangements, the patient's $PaCO_2$ compensatory changes will reflect the predominant acid–base disorder. The degree of $PaCO_2$ compensation, however, will not be as would be predicted for either metabolic disturbance existing alone. In this complex clinical situation, evaluation of the patient's condition must be an integral part of the acid–base assessment. In addition, the base excess and anion gap can be obtained to assist in the analysis of the situation. This type of complex interpretation is generally beyond the nurse's responsibility. It is more important that the nurse (1) recognizes that the patient's clinical picture does not coincide with the ABG results, and (2) contacts the physician to report the concern.

The key is learning how to predict the "normal" compensation relationships between $PaCO_2$, HCO_3, and pH so that you can recognize when the relationships are abnormal.

Systematic Evaluation

Once a mixed acid–base problem is suspected, a systematic approach should be used to interpret the disorder. The first two steps are common to all blood gas analyses. It is at Step Three that mixed acid–base analysis begins.

TABLE 6–10. A COMPARISON OF MIXED ACID–BASE DISORDERS[a]

PARAMETER	MIXED DISORDERS				
	Matching Derangements		Opposite Derangements		
	Metabolic acidosis + Respiratory acidosis	Metabolic alkalosis + Respiratory alkalosis	Metabolic acidosis + Respiratory alkalosis	Metabolic alkalosis + Respiratory acidosis	Metabolic acidosis + Metabolic alkalosis
pH	↓↓	↑↑	NL, ↓, or ↑	NL, ↓, or ↑	NL, ↓, or ↑
$Paco_2$	↑	↓	↓	↑	↓, or ↑
HCO_3	↓	↑	↓	↑	NL, ↓, or ↑

[a]The column on the left, Matching Derangements, illustrates the direction of the value trends when both primary disorders are the same (acidotic or alkalotic). This situation results in a severely deranged pH (as shown by two arrows). The three columns on the right, Opposite Derangements, illustrate the direction of value trends when the primary disorders are the opposite of each other (one is acidotic and the other is alkalotic). When opposite primary derangements coexist, they may fully or partially nullify the impact of the pH. If one disorder is predominant, the pH will lean toward the pH associated with that disorder, but to a lesser degree (as shown by single arrows). NL = normal.

Step 1: **Identification of the Primary Disorder**

Ask: Does the pH indicate acidosis or alkalosis? To which side of 7.40 does the pH lean?

Step 2: **Identification of the Primary Disorder as Metabolic or Respiratory**

Ask: Which value ($Paco_2$ or HCO_3) matches the acid–base state of the pH?

Discussion: If both values match the pH, a mixed acid–base disturbance is present. Several primary disorders are at work.

Example: pH = 7.30, $Paco_2$ = 50 mm Hg, HCO_3 = 20 mEq/L. All three indicators are acidotic, thus, the problem is a mixed acid–base disorder.

Step 3: **Estimate Expected Compensatory Responses Using Appropriate Rule**

Three pairs of relationships require analysis when seeking to differentiate the nature of a mixed acid–base disorder: pH to HCO_3, pH to $Paco_2$, and $Paco_2$ to HCO_3. Each pair is accompanied by a rule that defines the relationship.

If the calculated (predicted) values are similar to the actual values, a simple acid–base disturbance with compensation is present. If, however, the calculated (predicted) values are not similar to the actual values, a mixed disorder is present.

When a mixed acid–base disorder is suspected, the following questions should be asked:

- Is the relationship between pH and $Paco_2$ (respiratory component) as predicted?
- Is the relationship between pH and HCO_3 (metabolic component) as predicted?
- Is the relationship between $Paco_2$ and HCO_3 as predicted?
- If the relationships are not as predicted, has there been sufficient time for compensation to have taken place?

THE pH TO HCO_3 RELATIONSHIP. If a metabolic disturbance is present, the pH and HCO_3 should maintain a stable relationship.

RULE: If the acid–base problem is purely metabolic, a pH change of 0.15 will result in a corresponding change in HCO_3 of approximately 10 mEq/L (Pilbeam, 1998).

Example #1: Max Wilson had an ABG drawn revealing a pH of 7.55 and an HCO_3 of 34 mEq/L. The pH difference between the initial standard of 7.40 and Max's ABG pH of 7.55 is 0.15. The HCO_3 difference between the initial standard of 24 mEq/L and Max's HCO_3 is 10 mEq/L. Therefore, since Max's pH and HCO_3 altered within the parameters of the rule, the relationship has been maintained, indicating that a pure metabolic acidosis is present.

THE pH AND $Paco_2$ RELATIONSHIP. If the acid–base problem may have a primary respiratory origin, the relationship of pH to $Paco_2$ can be estimated.

RULE: For every 20 mm Hg increase in $Paco_2$ above 40, the pH will decrease by 0.10 unit.
For every 10 mm Hg decrease in $Paco_2$ below 40, the pH will increase by 0.10 unit.
pH decreases as $Paco_2$ increases; pH increases as $Paco_2$ decreases (Pilbeam, 1998).

Example #2: Jill Brown's $Paco_2$ is 60 mm Hg, which is 20 mm Hg above the standard of 40 mm Hg. In response, her pH should predictably decrease by 0.10 unit, dropping from 7.40 to 7.30.

Example #3: Lee Chong's $Paco_2$ is 30 mm Hg, which is 10 mm Hg below the standard of 40 mm Hg. In response, his pH should increase to 7.50 (an increase of 0.10 unit).

Example #4: Eva Thompson has a $Paco_2$ of 60 mm Hg, which is 20 mm Hg above the standard of 40 mm Hg, and a pH of 7.20. Her pH is NOT close to the predicted pH value of 7.30. Assuming that there has been sufficient time for compensatory mechanisms to take effect, a mixed disorder is present.

THE $PaCO_2$ TO HCO_3 RELATIONSHIP. Under normal conditions the $PaCO_2$ and HCO_3 maintain a stable relationship.

RULE: For every increase of 10 mm Hg in $PaCO_2$, there is a corresponding increase of 1 mEq/L of HCO_3.
For every decrease of 10 mm Hg in $PaCO_2$, there is corresponding decrease of 1.5 mEq/L of HCO_3 (Pilbeam, 1998).

Example #5. Richard Collins has an ABG drawn. The $PaCO_2$ was 60 mm Hg and the HCO_3 was 31.2 mEq/L. The difference between his $PaCO_2$ (60 mm Hg) and the standard of 40 mm Hg is 20 mm Hg. The predicted HCO_3 is 26 mEq/L. Richard's actual HCO_3 compensatory response level is 31.2 mEq/L, which is significantly different from the predicted answer.

Assuming that his compensatory mechanisms have had sufficient time to take effect, a mixed disorder is present.

Example #6: Joseph Brown has an ABG drawn. The $PaCO_2$ was 35 mm Hg and the HCO_3 was 26 mEq/L. The difference between Joseph's $PaCO_2$ (35 mm Hg) and the standard is 5 mm Hg. This means that for a $PaCO_2$ of 35 mm Hg, the predicted HCO_3 compensatory response level would be approximately 25 mEq/L. Joseph's HCO_3 is close to the predicted level. The appropriate level of compensation suggests a simple acid–base disorder.

Step 4: Compare the ABG with the Patient's Clinical Status

Knowledge of the patient's clinical status and possible metabolic and respiratory disorders is crucial when attempting to interpret mixed acid–base problems. Such knowledge allows for determination of the primary acid–base disturbance that is present in a single blood gas disorder, and helps to sort out the multiple primary disorders in a mixed acid–base disorder.

Ask: Is the patient at risk for:
Alveolar hyper- or hypoventilation?
Lactic acidosis?
Ketoacidosis?
Loss of bicarbonate?

In summary, high-acuity patients may develop mixed acid–base disorders. These complex derangements can be recognized and broadly differentiated by answering a series of questions and estimating expected predicted responses. Three rules of normal compensatory relationships have been presented, including pH to HCO_3, pH to $PaCO_2$, and $PaCO_2$ to HCO_3. A four-step mixed-gas interpretation approach provides a systematic method for identifying a mixed acid–base disorder. Once estimations have been made and relationships have been analyzed, data must be compared with the patient's clinical situation. For many nurses, the major responsibility in regard to mixed acid–base disorders is recognizing ABG values that are not congruent with predicted results, while taking the patient's clinical status into consideration. This recognition should then be followed up in a timely manner by contacting the physician.

SECTION EIGHT: Noninvasive Monitoring of Gas Exchange

At the completion of this section, the learner will be able to list noninvasive methods of monitoring gas exchange and applications.

Pulse Oximetry

Pulse oximetry is a noninvasive technique for monitoring arterial capillary hemoglobin saturation (SpO_2) and pulse rate. It uses light wavelengths to determine oxyhemoglobin saturation. It also detects pulsatile flow to differentiate between venous and arterial blood. A sensor is placed on a finger, nose, or ear, and an oximeter provides a constant assessment of arterial oxygen saturation. Pulse oximetry is best used as an adjunct to a variety of assessment modalities in providing continuous information for evaluation of oxygenation status. Ideally, the continuous arterial oxygen saturation readings reflect the patient's oxygenation status and alert the clinician to subtle or sudden changes. In some patients, use of oximetry may decrease the frequency of invasive ABG measurements if acid–base and ventilation are not problems.

Many factors can alter the accuracy of pulse oximetry in high-acuity patients. In general, these factors can be divided into problems of technical (mechanical) origin and those of physiologic origin. Technical problems include external light sources and improper sensor placement. Bright light sources within the patient's immediate environment can compete with the pulse oximetry sensor light source. When this is a problem, the sensor must be covered up to protect it from the external lighting. An improperly placed sensor may not be able to register arterial pulsations owing to lack of sufficient arterial flow. An additional technical problem is excessive patient movement, which can cause the sensor to misinterpret body movement as arterial pulsations. Mechanical problems are generally easy to correct once they are recognized (Messina, 1994; Thelan et al., 1998).

Physiologic factors that alter the accuracy of SpO_2 to predict blood oxygen content (and ultimately delivery of oxygen to the tissues) include hemoglobin level, acid–base imbalance, and vasoconstrictive situations (e.g., peripheral vascular disease, hypothermia, shock, hypovolemia, and vasopressors in high doses). The level of hemoglobin greatly affects the oxygen content of the blood. When a patient is severely anemic, the SpO_2 may remain high, indicating sufficient oxygen saturation of available hemoglobin. The actual oxygen content of the blood, however, may be inadequate to meet tissue oxygenation needs, thus increasing the risk of tissue hypoxia. Hemoglobin levels should be monitored and taken into consideration when analyzing SpO_2 measurements.

When an acid–base imbalance exists, acidosis may cause a lower saturation reading and alkalosis may cause a higher reading owing to shifts in the oxyhemoglobin dissociation curve. Severe peripheral vasoconstriction creates a low-flow arterial state in which the pulsatile force is too weak to be accurately read by pulse oximetry. When severe vasoconstriction is present, the sensor may read more accurately if it is removed from distal sites (fingers, toes) and attached to a more central location, such as the bridge of the nose or the ear lobes. The hypothermic patient generally requires warming to normothermic levels before pulse oximetry can be used. In addition, patients who have abnormal levels of carboxyhemoglobin (carbon dioxide and carbon monoxide) may have a high SpO_2 even though the oxyhemoglobin level is very low. This false reading occurs because pulse oximetry cannot differentiate carboxyhemoglobin from oxyhemoglobin. Other means of assessing oxygenation need to be used in cases of carbon dioxide and carbon monoxide toxicity (Messina, 1994).

End-Tidal Carbon Dioxide Monitoring

Capnometry is the noninvasive measurement of carbon dioxide (CO_2) concentration in expired gas. It results in a single value measurement called the $PETCO_2$ (partial pressure of end tidal CO_2). At this time, most continuous bedside monitoring of CO_2 is accomplished using infrared analyzers; however, continuous readings can also be obtained through mass spectrometry and spectrography. Infrared analyzers measure carbon dioxide based on its strong absorption band at a distinctive wavelength. A **capnogram** displays the capnometry measurements as a continuous waveform that can be read throughout the breathing cycle.

There are two types of $PETCO_2$ infrared analyzers, sidestream and mainstream. When a sidestream analyzer is used, a small volume of exhaled gas is diverted from the airway circuit through a small plastic tube and is analyzed in a special chamber apart from the airway circuit. This causes a time delay between the carbon dioxide sampling and the display of data. The small tubing may become obstructed with secretions or water. Mainstream infrared analyzers use a technology that is similar to sidestream analyzers. Mainstream analyzers, however, are placed in-line as part of the airway circuit, and $PETCO_2$ analysis occurs in-line. Mainstream devices are easier to damage and many are heavy and cumbersome additions to the artificial airway circuit (Shapiro, Peruzzi, & Templin, 1994; Pilbeam, 1998).

The normal capnogram shows a $PetCO_2$ within several mm Hg of arterial $PaCO_2$ at the end of the plateau phase (the end tidal CO_2). In a normal capnogram, the carbon dioxide concentration is zero at the beginning of expiration, gradually rising until it reaches a plateau. The end tidal carbon dioxide is the highest concentration at the end of exhalation. **End-tidal carbon dioxide ($PETCO_2$)** monitoring is used in the clinical setting as a noninvasive indirect method of measuring $PaCO_2$. In a normal person, $PETCO_2$ is typically 4 to 6 mm Hg below $PaCO_2$ (Pilbeam, 1998).

End-tidal carbon dioxide monitoring may be used to assess ventilatory status to provide an early warning of changes in ventilation. An abnormally low $PETCO_2$ (< 36 mm Hg) most commonly is associated with hyperventilation. Increased $PETCO_2$ (> 44 mm Hg) is associated with increased production of carbon dioxide or problems causing hypoventilation (e.g., respiratory center depression, neuromuscular diseases, COPD). Use of the capnogram may help detect improper intubation, ventilation patterns, mechanical problems, or failure in ventilators. Certain capnographic patterns are associated with hyperventilation, incomplete exhalation, and a variety of disease states. Anesthesiologists have used this technique in the operating room, and new applications are being explored in critical care, emergency care, and prehospital care.

In patients with ventilation–perfusion abnormalities, the $PETCO_2$ may not accurately reflect $PaCO_2$. However, it still may be helpful if a correlation between $PaCO_2$ and $PETCO_2$ can be established and used for trending. Unfortunately, high-acuity patients commonly have ventilation–perfusion abnormalities, which may limit the usefulness of $PETCO_2$ monitoring.

In summary, pulse oximetry and $PETCO_2$ monitoring are noninvasive tools to assist in monitoring oxygenation and ventilation parameters. They can be used singly, but dual use provides information on capillary arterial oxygen saturation (oxygenation) and $PaCO_2$ (ventilation). Advantages of use include continuous readings to trend conditions and less invasive procedures.

SECTION EIGHT REVIEW

1. Pulse oximetry measures
   - **A.** mixed venous saturation
   - **B.** transcutaneous oxygen saturation
   - **C.** venous oxygen capillary hemoglobin saturation
   - **D.** arterial oxygen capillary hemoglobin saturation
2. Conditions that impair the accuracy of pulse oximetry include all of the following EXCEPT
   - **A.** excessive movement
   - **B.** improper sensor placement
   - **C.** hypothermia
   - **D.** vasodilation

3. P_{ETCO_2} is used as a reflection of
   A. arterial carbon dioxide
   B. $\dot{V}/\dot{Q}$ ratio
   C. oxygenation status
   D. venous carbon dioxide

4. P_{ETCO_2} is an indicator of alveolar
   A. acid–base state
   B. compensation
   C. oxygenation
   D. ventilation

Answers: 1. D, 2. D, 3. A, 4. D

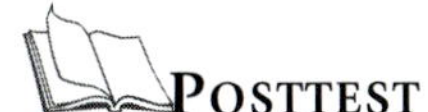

POSTTEST

The following Posttest is constructed in a case study format. Several patients are presented. Questions are asked based on available data. New data are presented as the case study progresses.

Juanita M, 32 years old, was admitted to the hospital last night with a diagnosis of pneumonia. She is receiving oxygen and mist through an aerosol face tent.

1. Juanita's febrile state would cause the oxyhemoglobin dissociation curve to shift away from the normal curve. Based on the direction of the shift associated with fever, which of the following statements is correct?
   A. oxygen binds rapidly to hemoglobin
   B. carbon dioxide binds rapidly to hemoglobin
   C. hemoglobin readily releases its oxygen to tissues
   D. hemoglobin is prevented from releasing its oxygen to tissues
2. Juanita has another arterial blood gas drawn. The nurse makes the following comment regarding the results: "The pH is abnormal, but the body buffers and regulatory mechanisms have begun to respond to the imbalance." This statement describes which of the following levels of acid–base compensation?
   A. uncompensated
   B. partially compensated
   C. compensated
   D. corrected
3. Juanita's normal bicarbonate–carbon dioxide ratio should remain at approximately
   A. 5:1
   B. 10:1
   C. 15:1
   D. 20:1
4. On the original arterial blood gas, Juanita's BE was +1.5. Which of the following statements is correct regarding base excess?
   A. it reflects only her metabolic status
   B. any value that is outside a BE of ±1 is abnormal
   C. it reflects only her respiratory status
   D. any value that is outside a BE of ±2.5 is abnormal

Juanita has a complete blood count (CBC) and ABG drawn. Her Hgb is currently 10 g/dL. Her latest temperature was 102.4°F. The ABG has the following results: pH = 7.47, Pa_{CO_2} = 32 mm Hg, HCO_3 = 25 mEq/L, BE = +1.5, Pa_{O_2} = 74 mm Hg, Sa_{O_2} = 89%. She is started on 40 percent oxygen.

5. If Juanita has normal gas exchange, her predicted response to initiation of 40 percent oxygen therapy would be an increased Pa_{O_2} to about
   A. 100 mm Hg
   B. 150 mm Hg
   C. 200 mm Hg
   D. 250 mm Hg
6. The underlying problem associated with Juanita's acid–base status is
   A. pulmonary edema
   B. alveolar hyperventilation
   C. atelectasis
   D. alveolar hypoventilation
7. Juanita's body is beginning to compensate for her Pa_{CO_2} of 32 mm Hg. The predicted compensation for her respiratory situation is
   A. increased Pa_{CO_2}
   B. increased HCO_3
   C. decreased Pa_{CO_2}
   D. decreased HCO_3

Thomas J, a 46-year-old type I diabetic, is admitted to the hospital with a serum glucose of 650 mg/dL and positive serum ketones. He is diagnosed with DKA. He has blood gases drawn with the following results: pH = 7.25, Pa_{CO_2} = 36 mm Hg, HCO_3 = 14 mEq/L.

8. Thomas's current pH is most likely due to which of the following?
   A. accumulating ketones
   B. lactic acidosis
   C. severe diarrhea
   D. severe hyperglycemia
9. If Thomas's acid–base status becomes fully compensated, the nurse would anticipate seeing which acid–base trends?

A. normal range of pH, normal HCO_3
B. elevated pH, low HCO_3
C. low pH, high $Paco_2$
D. normal range of pH, low $Paco_2$

10. The nurse would correctly interpret Thomas's arterial blood gas as
A. acute metabolic acidosis
B. partially compensated metabolic acidosis
C. compensated metabolic acidosis
D. corrected metabolic acidosis

11. Joshua K has the following arterial blood gas results: pH = 7.50, $Paco_2$ = 30 mm Hg, HCO_3 = 20 mEq/L, Pao_2 = 88 mm Hg, Sao_2 = 98%. The nurse would correctly interpret this ABG as
A. compensated metabolic alkalosis
B. partially compensated metabolic acidosis
C. partially compensated respiratory alkalosis
D. compensated respiratory acidosis

12. Carrie D has the following ABG results: pH = 6.83, $Paco_2$ = 50 mm Hg, HCO_3 = 20 mEq/L. The nurse would correctly conclude that these results are
A. suspicious of a mixed disorder
B. typical of acute metabolic acidosis
C. an impossible combination
D. within ordinary compensatory boundaries

13. The nurse believes that Wendell Q has a mixed acid–base disorder. When this type of acid–base disorder is suspected, it is crucial that the clinician obtain a
A. computer analysis
B. second sample of arterial blood
C. mixed venous blood sample
D. summary of the patient's medical status

Adam D is in hypovolemic shock secondary to a massive gastrointestinal bleed. The nurse is preparing to place him on pulse oximetry.

14. Based on the provided data, the best location for the pulse oximetry sensor would be a (an)
A. toe
B. earlobe
C. fingertip
D. forearm

15. Beverly P has been in a critical care unit for a week. She has $PETCO_2$ monitoring attached to her mechanical ventilator circuit. This type of monitoring is primarily used to assess
A. early tissue metabolic changes
B. oxygenation failure
C. early changes in ventilation
D. ventilator dependency

POSTTEST ANSWERS

Question	Answer	Section
1	C	One
2	B	Two
3	D	Two
4	A	Three
5	C	Three
6	B	Four
7	D	Four
8	A	Five
9	D	Five
10	A	Six
11	C	Six
12	C	Seven
13	D	Seven
14	B	Eight
15	C	Eight

REFERENCES

Czekaj, L.A. (1998). Promoting acid–base balance. In M.R. Kinney, S.B. Dunbar, J.A. Brooks-Brunn, N. Molter, & J.M. Vitello-Cicciu (eds.), *AACN clinical reference for critical care nursing*, 4th ed. (pp. 135–144). St. Louis: C.V. Mosby.

Des Jardins, T.R. (1993). *Cardiopulmonary anatomy and physiology: Essentials for respiratory care*, 2nd ed. Albany, NY: Delmar Publishers.

Kee, J.L. (1999). *Laboratory and diagnostic tests with nursing implications*, 5th ed. Stamford, CT: Appleton & Lange.

Messina, B.A. (1994). Pulse oximetry: Assuring accuracy. *J Post Anesth Nursing* 9(4):228–231.

Pilbeam, S.P. (1998). *Mechanical ventilation: Physiological and clinical applications*, 3rd ed. St. Louis: C.V. Mosby.

Price, S.A., & Wilson, L.M. (1992). *Pathophysiology: Clinical concepts of disease processes*, 4th ed. (p. 260). St. Louis: C.V. Mosby.

Shapiro, B.A., Peruzzi, W.T., & Templin, R. (1994). *Clinical application of blood gases*, 5th ed. St. Louis: C.V. Mosby.

Thelan, L., Urden, L.D., Lough, M.E., & Stacy K.M. (1998). *Critical care nursing: Diagnosis management*, 3rd ed. St. Louis: C.V. Mosby.

Module 7

Mechanical Ventilation

Kathleen Dorman Wagner

This self-study module focuses on a variety of concepts related to initiation of mechanical ventilation and management of the patient on a mechanical ventilator. This module uses information covered in two other modules: "*Respiratory Process*" and "*Arterial Blood Gas Analysis*." It is suggested that the reader become familiar with the material in those two modules before reading this one.

This module is divided into 10 sections. Sections One through Six include such topics as criteria used for determination of the need for mechanical ventilation, required equipment to initiate mechanical ventilation, various types of mechanical ventilators, a brief discussion of the more commonly monitored ventilator settings, and noninvasive ventilatory support. In Sections Seven and Eight, the focus shifts to a discussion of how mechanical ventilation and artificial airways affect various parts of the body, including information about potential complications and methods to avoid them. Section Nine describes the nursing management of the mechanically ventilated patient. This section focuses on respiratory-related nursing diagnoses. The final section briefly describes the weaning process. Each section includes a set of review questions to help the learner evaluate his or her understanding of the section's content before moving on to the next section. All Section Reviews and the module Pretest and Posttest include answers. It is suggested that the learner review those concepts answered incorrectly in the review questions before proceeding to the next section.

Objectives

Following completion of this module, the learner will be able to

1. Correctly state why a mechanical ventilator is not a mechanical respirator.
2. Identify criteria used to determine the need for mechanical ventilator support.
3. Discuss the equipment necessary to initiate mechanical ventilation.
4. Describe the types of mechanical ventilators, based on mechanism of force and cycling mechanism.
5. Explain the commonly monitored ventilator settings.
6. Briefly explain two methods of providing noninvasive ventilatory support.
7. Discuss the major complications of mechanical ventilation.
8. Explain the cause and prevention of artificial airways complications.
9. Describe care of the patient requiring mechanical ventilation.
10. Describe the weaning process.

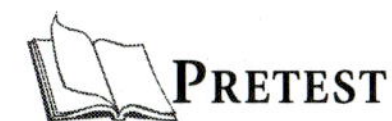 Pretest

1. Mechanical ventilators are responsible for
   A. diffusion
   B. ventilation
   C. perfusion
   D. respiration

2. The most common indication for use of a mechanical ventilator is
   A. pneumonia
   B. chronic obstructive pulmonary disease (COPD)
   C. acute asthmatic attack
   D. acute ventilatory failure
3. Acute ventilatory failure is associated with
   A. alveolar hypoventilation
   B. severe hypoxemia
   C. alveolar hyperventilation
   D. severe hypocarbia
4. Acute respiratory acidosis can be defined clinically as
   A. pH > 7.50, PaO_2 < 60 mm Hg
   B. pH < 7.30, $PaCO_2$ > 50 mm Hg
   C. pH > 7.50, PaO_2 < 60 mm Hg
   D. pH < 7.30, $PaCO_2$ < 30 mm Hg
5. The primary purpose of the endotracheal tube cuff is to seal off the
   A. lower airway from the upper airway
   B. lower airway from the esophagus
   C. oropharynx from the nasopharynx
   D. oropharynx from the esophagus
6. The most common type of airway access used during an emergency is
   A. tracheostomy
   B. nasal intubation
   C. pharyngeal airway
   D. oral intubation
7. A major advantage of volume-cycled ventilation is that it
   A. applies negative pressure to the thorax
   B. overcomes changes in lung compliance
   C. does not require an artificial airway
   D. automatically adjusts volume of gas delivered
8. A low tidal volume is associated most closely with which of the following?
   A. hypoventilation
   B. hypocapnia
   C. hypoxia
   D. hypotension
9. The fraction of inspired oxygen (FIO_2) is correctly measured in
   A. decimals
   B. percentages
   C. centimeters of water pressure (cm H_2O)
   D. millimeters of mercury (mm Hg)
10. Synchronized intermittent mandatory ventilation (SIMV) is sensitive to
    A. rate of airflow
    B. respiratory rate
    C. concentration of oxygen
    D. the patient's ventilatory cycle
11. A common side effect of positive end-expiratory pressure (PEEP) is
    A. increased blood pressure
    B. decreased cardiac output
    C. decreased lung compliance
    D. increased venous return to the heart
12. During positive pressure ventilation, airflow will be greatest
    A. in areas that are diseased
    B. in areas that are nondependent
    C. in the peripheral lung areas
    D. in the lung apices
13. In what way does positive pressure ventilation affect intracranial pressure (ICP)?
    A. it has no effect
    B. it decreases ICP
    C. it increases ICP
    D. its effects are unknown
14. What effect does positive pressure ventilation have on renal function?
    A. urine output is unaffected
    B. urine output is decreased
    C. urine output is increased
    D. its effects are unknown
15. The term *barotrauma* refers to injury caused by
    A. oxygen
    B. friction
    C. temperature
    D. pressure
16. Oxygen toxicity has what effect on lung tissue?
    A. it increases surfactant production
    B. it decreases mucous production
    C. it increases macrophage activity
    D. it increases lung compliance
17. Endotracheal cuff trauma can be avoided by maintaining cuff pressures at which of the following ranges?
    A. 5 to 10 mm Hg
    B. 10 to 20 mm Hg
    C. 20 to 25 mm Hg
    D. 25 to 30 mm Hg
18. Noninvasive intermittent positive pressure ventilation (NIPPV) is most useful for the patient who
    A. requires only support of tidal volume
    B. cannot fully support his or her own expiratory effort
    C. requires only support for nocturnal hypercapnia and hypoxemia
    D. cannot fully support his or her own ventilatory effort over long periods of time
19. Common complications of noninvasive methods of ventilatory support include all of the following EXCEPT
    A. conjunctivitis
    B. nasal congestion
    C. hypoventilation
    D. otitis media
20. The majority of difficult to wean patients have which of the following problems?
    A. pneumonia
    B. congestive heart failure

C. acute respiratory distress syndrome
D. chronic pulmonary disease

21. The term __________ weaning is used to refer to weaning by intermittently removing the patient from the ventilator for increasing periods of time.
A. manual
B. ventilator
C. IMV/SIMV
D. pressure support ventilation

Pretest Answers: 1. B, 2. D, 3. A, 4. B, 5. A, 6. D, 7. B, 8. A, 9. A, 10. D, 11. B, 12. B, 13. C, 14. B, 15. D, 16. B, 17. C, 18. D, 19. D, 20. D, 21. A

GLOSSARY

Acute ventilatory failure (AVF). A state of respiratory decompensation in which the lungs are unable to maintain adequate alveolar ventilation, losing the ability to eliminate carbon dioxide

Airway resistance (R_{aw}). The amount of opposition to airway flow through the conducting system

Alveolar ventilation (VA). The air that fills the alveoli and is available for gas exchange

Assist/control mode (A/C). A mechanical ventilation mode that combines two single modes: assist, a patient-sensitive mode; and control, a time-triggered mode

Auto-PEEP. The unintentional buildup of positive end-expiratory pressure caused by air-trapping

Barotrauma. Injury to pulmonary tissues due to excessive volumes or pressures

Compliance. The amount of force required to expand the lungs; measured in mL/cm H_2O; normal is 50 to 100 mL/cm H_2O

Continuous positive airway pressure (CPAP). The application of positive pressure to the airway of a spontaneously breathing person (see PEEP)

Cycle. The mechanisms by which the inspiratory phase is stopped and the expiratory phase is started

Deadspace ventilation (VD). Air that fills the conducting airways and does not take part in gas exchange

Extubation. Removal of an endotracheal or tracheostomy tube from the patient's airway

Fraction of inspired oxygen (FIO_2). That portion of the total gas being inspired that is composed of oxygen; expressed in decimals from 0.21 to 1.0

Intermittent mandatory ventilation (IMV). A mechanical ventilator mode that allows the patient to breathe spontaneously through ventilator circuitry while interspersing mandatory mechanical breaths at even intervals via a preset rate

Negative inspiratory force (NIF), also called **maximum inspiratory force (MIF).** The amount of negative pressure a person can exert during inspiration; normal is −50 to −100 cm H_2O

Noninvasive intermittent positive pressure ventilation (NIPPV). The application of positive pressure ventilation using a mechanical ventilator and a mask in place of an artificial airway

$PaCO_2$. The partial pressure of carbon dioxide as it exists in the arterial blood; normal range is 35 to 45 mm Hg

PaO_2. The partial pressure of oxygen as it exists in the arterial blood; normal range is 75 to 100 mm Hg

Peak airway pressure (PAP). Amount of pressure required to deliver a volume of gas

Positive end-expiratory pressure (PEEP). The application of positive pressure to the airway at the end of expiration such that the airway pressure never returns to ambient

Pressure support ventilation (PSV). A type of mechanical ventilatory support in which a preset level of positive pressure augments the inspiratory effort required to attain a tidal volume, thereby decreasing the work of breathing

Respiration. The exchange of oxygen and carbon dioxide across a semipermeable membrane

Shunting. The state in which pulmonary capillary perfusion is normal but alveolar ventilation is lacking

Sigh. Intermittent hyperinflation of the lungs

Spontaneous breaths. Breaths that use the patient's own respiratory effort and mechanics

Synchronous intermittent mandatory ventilation (SIMV). A form of intermittent mandatory ventilation (IMV) mode in which the mandatory breaths are synchronized to the patient's own breathing cycle

Tidal volume (VT). The volume of air moved in and out of the lungs during normal breathing

Ventilation. The gross movement of air in and out of the lungs

Ventilation–perfusion ratio ($\dot{V}/\dot{Q}$). The relationship of pulmonary ventilation to pulmonary perfusion expressed as a ratio in liters/minute; normal is 4:5 (0.8)

Ventilator (mechanical) breath. A breath, either patient or machine triggered, that delivers gas at prescribed ventilator settings

Vital capacity (VC). The volume of air that can be exhaled after maximum inhalation; an indication of respiratory muscle strength; normal is 65 to 75 mL/kg

Weaning. Gradual withdrawal of mechanical ventilation

ABBREVIATIONS

ABG. Arterial blood gases

A/C. Assist/control mode

ARDS. Acute respiratory distress syndrome

AVF. Acute ventilatory failure

BiPAP. Bi-level positive airway pressure

cm H_2O. Centimeters of water pressure

CNS. Central nervous system

CO_2. Carbon dioxide

COPD. Chronic obstructive pulmonary disease

CPAP. Continuous positive airway pressure

CPP. Cerebral perfusion pressure

CVP. Central venous pressure

EPAP. Expiratory positive airway pressure

ET tube. Endotracheal tube

f. Respiratory rate

FIO_2. Fraction of inspired oxygen

HFJV. High-frequency jet ventilation

ICP. Intracranial pressure

ILV. Independent lung ventilation

IMV. Intermittent mandatory ventilation

IPAP. Inspiratory positive airway pressure

MABP. Mean arterial blood pressure

MAP. Mean airway pressure

mm Hg. Millimeters of mercury

MPV. Microprocessor ventilator

NIF. Negative inspiratory force

NIPPV. Noninvasive intermittent positive pressure ventilation

O_2. Oxygen

$\overline{PA}$. Mean airway pressure

PaO_2. Partial pressure of arterial oxygen

PAP. Peak airway pressure; proximal airway pressure

PEEP. Positive end-expiratory pressure

pH. Hydrogen ion concentration

PIP. Peak inspiratory pressure

PPV. Positive pressure ventilation

PSV. Pressure support ventilation

SaO_2. Saturation of arterial oxygen

SILV. Synchronous independent lung ventilation

SIMV. Synchronous intermittent mandatory ventilation

SV. Spontaneous ventilation

SVR. Systemic vascular resistance

T-E. Tracheoesophageal

V_A. Alveolar ventilation

VC. Vital capacity

V_D. Deadspace ventilation

$\dot{V}_E$. Minute ventilation

$\dot{V}/\dot{Q}$. Ventilation–perfusion ratio

V_T. Tidal volume

SECTION ONE: Ventilator versus Respirator

At the completion of this section, the learner will be able to briefly explain why a mechanical ventilator is not a mechanical respirator.

To understand the concept of mechanical ventilation, one must first have a basic understanding of the difference between respiration and ventilation. **Ventilation** refers to the gross movement of air in and out of the lungs. It is composed of **deadspace ventilation (V_D)**, the air that fills the conducting airways and does not take part in gas exchange, and **alveolar ventilation (V_A)**, the air that fills the alveoli and is available for gas exchange (Fig. 7–1). Adequate alveolar ventilation is necessary to maintain normal arterial blood gas levels.

V_D is easily measured, since it is equivalent to the ideal body weight of the person. For example, if the patient's ideal body weight is 150 pounds, the V_D would be 150 mL. V_A is easily calculated as the person's tidal volume (V_T) minus V_D.

$$V_A = V_T - V_D$$

Respiration is the exchange of oxygen and carbon dioxide across a semipermeable membrane. Respiration occurs both in the lungs (external respiration) and in the tissues (internal respiration).

Mechanical ventilators are sometimes referred to as *respirators*. This is a misnomer. Though the technology has become very sophisticated, the machines only cause gases to be moved in and out of the lungs, using negative or positive pressure. Although certain ventilator settings help maintain alveoli in an open state to facilitate respiration, the machines do not have the capability to diffuse gases. Respiration, then, remains dependent on adequate functioning of the lung tissues and pulmonary capillaries.

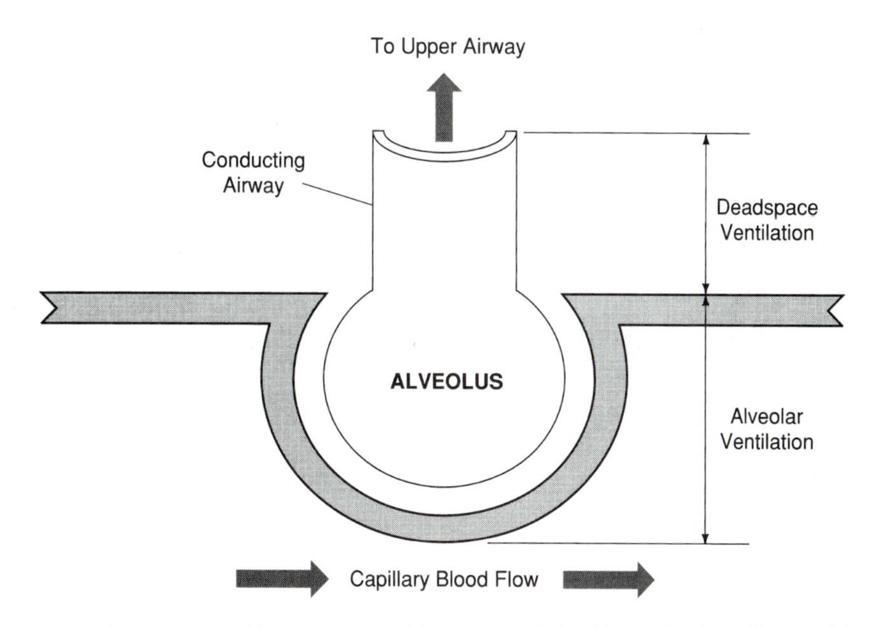

Figure 7–1. Components of ventilation. Ventilation is composed of deadspace ventilation (VD) and alveolar ventilation (VA). VD is the air located in the conducting airways. (The conducting airways begin at the mouth and nose and end at the terminal airways.) VA is the air that is present in the alveoli.

In summary, mechanical ventilation is a means by which the patient receives mechanical ventilatory support in maintaining adequate alveolar ventilation. Mechanical ventilators cannot cause diffusion of gases in the lungs. Rather, they facilitate the ventilatory process. Improved ventilatory status will enhance the ability of the gases to diffuse across the alveolar–capillary membrane.

SECTION ONE REVIEW

1. The primary purpose of mechanical ventilation is to
   A. support external respiration
   B. support alveolar ventilation
   C. prevent fatigue of the diaphragm
   D. prevent development of pneumonia
2. Deadspace ventilation refers to
   A. the amount of air left in the lungs after expiration
   B. the amount of carbon dioxide in venous blood
   C. the air in the lungs that does not take part in gas exchange
   D. the air in the lungs that leaks into the pulmonary interstitial space
3. Internal respiration refers to
   A. gas exchange between the blood and tissues
   B. gas exchange between the alveoli and blood
   C. the movement of air into the alveoli
   D. the movement of gases between alveoli
4. The term alveolar ventilation refers to
   A. gas exchange between the alveoli and the blood
   B. the intra-alveolar movement of air
   C. air in the alveoli that does not take part in gas exchange
   D. air that fills the alveoli and is available for gas exchange

Answers: 1. B, 2. C, 3. A, 4. D

SECTION TWO: Determining the Need for Ventilatory Support

At the completion of this section, the learner will be able to identify criteria used for determination of the need for mechanical ventilatory support.

The decision to place a patient on a mechanical ventilator is a very serious one. The invasiveness of the artificial airway as well as the physiologic alterations associated with mechanical ventilation place the patient at substantial risk for development of serious complications. Therefore, the relative benefits and costs must be weighed.

Mechanical ventilation is a supportive intervention only. It is meant to support the patient's oxygenation and ventilation status while curative interventions are initiated to correct the underlying problem. Ventilatory support is probably best initiated as a "semielective" procedure before the patient's condition is severely compromised (i.e., cardiopulmonary arrest). Early support is thought to improve the patient's outcome.

How then is the decision made to place a patient on a mechanical ventilator? A variety of criteria have been established by pulmonary experts to aid the health care team in establishing rapidly which patients may require ventilatory support. These criteria generally are not based on specific medical diagnoses but rather on respiratory function status.

Acute Ventilatory Failure

Acute ventilatory failure (AVF) is probably the most common indication for ventilator support. Acute ventilatory failure is the inability of the lungs to maintain adequate alveolar ventilation. It is diagnosed on the basis of the acid–base imbalance it creates—acute respiratory acidosis, which is expressed as **$Paco_2$** > 50 mm Hg and pH < 7.30. A variety of problems can cause AVF, such as head trauma, apnea of any etiology, neuromuscular dysfunction, and drug-induced central nervous system (CNS) depression. Essentially, any problem that decreases movement of air to and from the alveoli can precipitate AVF.

Generally speaking, AVF is a direct indication for rapid intubation and mechanical ventilatory support. A possible exception is the patient with chronic obstructive pulmonary disease (COPD, chronic airflow limitation). Patients with COPD live in a state of chronic (long-term) ventilatory insufficiency. They are at particularly high risk for development of complications if placed on a ventilator. For this reason, physicians often are reluctant to intubate and mechanically ventilate these patients unless it is absolutely necessary. Other criteria may be used, such as level of consciousness or a particular degree of respiratory acidosis, in making the decision to initiate mechanical support for this patient population.

Hypoxemia

The second major indication for mechanical ventilatory support is hypoxemia, which is frequently quantified as a **Pao_2** of < 50 mm Hg. A low **ventilation–perfusion ratio ($\dot{V}/\dot{Q}$)** is the most common cause of hypoxemia. A low $\dot{V}/\dot{Q}$ refers to a state in which there is an excess of perfusion in relation to ventilation. The cause of a low $\dot{V}/\dot{Q}$ often is an obstructing mucous plug in the distal airway, causing a reduction in alveolar ventilation. Examples of conditions that are associated with a low $\dot{V}/\dot{Q}$ include asthma, pneumonia, COPD, and atelectasis.

Low $\dot{V}/\dot{Q}$ is associated with a phenomenon called shunting. **Shunting** refers to the state in which pulmonary capillary perfusion is normal but alveolar ventilation is lacking. Pulmonary capillary blood that runs by a nonfunctioning alveolar unit cannot pick up oxygen from that alveolus. Although some shunting is normal, if many alveolar units become nonfunctioning, a significant decrease in oxygen saturation (Sao_2) will occur, causing hypoxemia. Severe shunting is associated with such conditions as respiratory distress syndromes of both the infant and adult and severe pneumonia.

Pulmonary Mechanics

Pulmonary function (pulmonary mechanics) testing may be used to decide if mechanical ventilatory support is needed. Such testing provides the clinician with crucial information about respiratory muscle strength and airflow. When evaluating the need for mechanical ventilation, pulmonary function tests can provide data regarding evidence of hypoventilation. Several of the more common tests used as criteria are **vital capacity (VC), negative inspiratory force (NIF),** and respiratory rate (f).

In summary, the decision as to whether or not to place a patient on a mechanical ventilator is a complex one, based on analysis of a variety of data. Actual criteria used to make this decision vary but generally include the patient's level of consciousness, arterial blood gas status, and pulmonary mechanics. A patient need not be in AVF or in severe hypoxemia to be placed on mechanical ventilation. If the clinician believes that the patient is in impending ventilatory failure, mechanical ventilation may be initiated as a semielective procedure. Table 7–1 summarizes some criteria that may be used to determine the need for mechanical ventilatory support.

TABLE 7–1. CRITERIA FOR VENTILATORY SUPPORT

CRITERIA	CRITICAL VALUES
Acute ventilatory failure (AVF)	$Paco_2$ > 50 mm Hg, pH < 7.30
Acute hypoxemia	Pao_2 < 50 mm Hg
Pulmonary mechanics	
Respiratory rate (f)	f > 35 breaths/min
Vital capacity (VC)	VC < 15 mL/kg (normal: 65–75 mL/kg)
Negative inspiratory force (NIF)	NIF < −20 cm H_2O (normal: −50 to −100 cm H_2O)
Minute ventilation ($\dot{V}_E$)	$\dot{V}_E$ > 10 L/min (normal: 5–10 L/min)

SECTION TWO REVIEW

1. The term *ventilatory failure* refers to the inability of the lungs to
   A. expand
   B. diffuse gases
   C. use oxygen and carbon dioxide
   D. maintain adequate alveolar ventilation
2. Acute respiratory acidosis is defined clinically as
   A. $PaCO_2 > 50$ mm Hg and pH < 7.30
   B. $PaO_2 < 60$ mm Hg
   C. $PaCO_2 > 45$ mm Hg and pH < 7.35
   D. $PaO_2 < 80$ mm Hg
3. Common causes of acute ventilatory failure include all of the following EXCEPT
   A. apnea
   B. head trauma
   C. mechanical ventilation
   D. neuromuscular dysfunction
4. A low V/Q exists when
   A. ventilation is in excess of perfusion
   B. perfusion is in excess of ventilation
   C. blood is shunted away from the alveoli
   D. there is an obstruction in the pulmonary capillaries
5. The term *pulmonary shunt* refers to
   A. movement of air directly from one alveolus to another
   B. normal pulmonary capillary perfusion, lacking alveolar ventilation
   C. an opening between the pulmonary artery and the heart
   D. normal alveolar ventilation, lacking pulmonary capillary perfusion

Answers: 1. D, 2. A, 3. C, 4. B, 5. B

SECTION THREE: Required Equipment for Mechanical Ventilation

At the completion of this section, the learner will be able to describe the equipment necessary for proper mechanical ventilation.

Mechanical ventilation is a complex intervention that requires a protocol of procedures and equipment. Adequate preparation before placement of the patient on the mechanical ventilator will facilitate smooth implemention.

Initial Equipment Necessary for Establishment of a Patent Airway

Mechanical ventilation requires the use of special artificial airways. Artificial airways can be divided into two groups: endotracheal tubes and tracheostomy tubes.

Endotracheal Tubes

The endotracheal (ET) tube is a specially designed semirigid radiopaque tube. Its slightly curved shaft is designed for ease of passage through the curved upper airway. In adults, the tubes require a cuff if positive pressure ventilation is to be initiated. The cuff is a balloon that is attached to the outside wall on the distal end of the ET tube. When inflated, the cuff seals off the lower airway from the upper airway and holds the tube in a stable position (Fig. 7–2). Neonatal and small pediatrics ET tubes do not have cuffs, since in children younger than 5 years, the cricoid cartilage offers a sufficient seal once the tube is inserted.

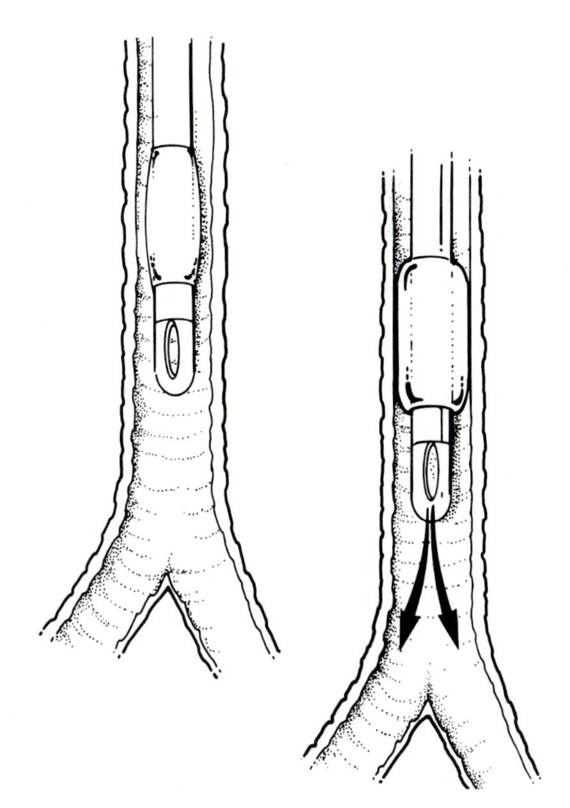

Figure 7–2. Endotracheal tube in the trachea. **A.** Balloon deflated. **B.** Balloon inflated. Air that is pushed through the tube enters the lungs, since it cannot escape around the tube when the balloon is inflated. *(From Martin, L. [1987].* Pulmonary physiology in clinical practice: The essentials for patient care and evaluation *[p. 198]. St. Louis: C.V. Mosby.)*

Choice of Endotracheal Tube Size. The size of the ET tube to be inserted will depend primarily on the age of the person to be intubated. ET tube sizes range from 2 mm to 11 mm, which reflects the diameter of the inside lumen. Table 7–2 lists recommended adult ET tube sizes by gender.

In the adult, the route of entry also determines ET tube size. A smaller sized tube is required if it is to be inserted nasally, since the nasal airway passage is significantly smaller than the oral airway passage. Many brands of ET tubes designate, on the tube, which route is appropriate for each size tube (i.e., nasal, nasal/oral, or oral).

Nasal intubation generally is performed blindly, that is, without viewing the vocal cords through a laryngoscope. It is most frequently performed when the procedure is a semielective (nonemergency) intubation. The nasal route is more comfortable for the patient once it is in place, and the tube is very stable. Oral intubation is most frequently used during an emergency, since direct visualization of the vocal cords assures rapid proper placement in the lower airway. Figure 7–3 provides an illustration of a properly positioned ET tube.

Intubation Equipment. The endotracheal tube is inserted by a specially trained member of the health care team. The following items must be gathered before intubation:

- Soft-cuffed ET tubes
- Stylet
- Topical anesthetic
- Laryngoscope handle with blade attached

TABLE 7–2. RECOMMENDED SIZES FOR ENDOTRACHEAL TUBES IN ADULTS

GENDER	INTERNAL DIAMETER (mm)	LENGTH (cm)
Female	8.0–9.0	19–24
Male	8.5–10.0	20–28

- Magill forceps
- Suction catheters, Yankauers suction tip
- Syringe for cuff inflation
- Water-soluble lubricant
- Adhesive tape

Tracheostomy Tubes

Generally, when mechanical ventilation is initiated, a tracheostomy is not the entry of choice because it is more invasive and takes longer to perform. However, tracheostomy might be performed initially if the patient has received head or neck surgery or has an upper airway obstruction resulting from severe edema (such as burns) or a tumor obstruction. Tracheostomy is more commonly performed on the patient who requires prolonged intubation (over 2 to 3 weeks) because of failure to wean from the ventilator. Many hospitals have established guidelines for limiting the length of time a person is allowed to have an ET tube in place before receiving a tracheostomy.

Prolonged use of an ET tube is associated with many complications. Some of these complications can be avoided if a tracheostomy is performed in a timely manner. It should be noted that tracheostomy also is associated with a variety of complications. Currently, there is

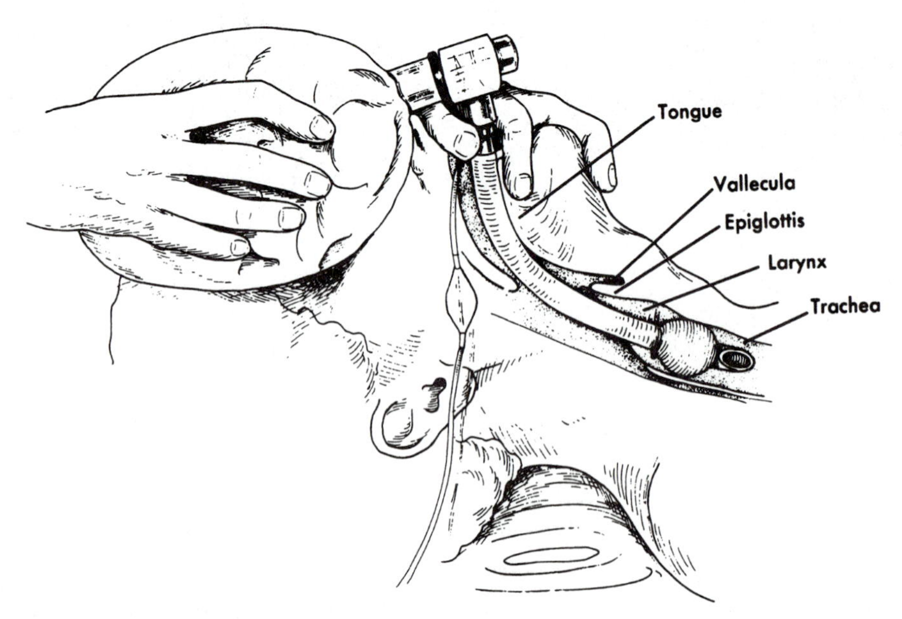

Figure 7–3. Orotracheal tube in place being used with a bag-valve resuscitator. *(From Marshak, A.B., & Scanlon, C.L. [1990]. Emergency life support. In C.L. Scanlon, R.L. Wilkins, & J.K. Stoller (eds.):* Egans fundamentals of respiratory care, *5th ed. [p. 533]. St. Louis: Mosby Year Book. Used by permission.)*

increasing controversy over when tracheostomy should be performed. (Artificial airway complications are discussed in Section Seven.)

Securing the Artificial Airway

Any type of artificial airway must be secured in place properly to prevent tube displacement and to minimize trauma to mucous membrane. Initially, in an emergency situation, the tube is secured with adhesive tape. Figure 7–4 illustrates one method of securing an ET tube. This technique can be used with either nasal or oral ET tubes. Twill tape and a variety of commercially available stabilizers may be used in place of adhesive tape, particularly for prolonged use. Whatever method is used, stabilization of the tube is imperative. Tracheostomy tubes commonly are secured with twill tape or a commercially available tracheostomy band. The tracheostomy tube also may be sutured in place to prevent accidental dislodgment. Once the airway is secured, a chest x-ray should be performed to confirm correct placement.

Supportive Equipment

In addition to the artificial airway and mechanical ventilator, other supplies and equipment must be readily available.

- Two oxygen sources
  - One for the ventilator
  - One for the resuscitation bag, to provide 100 percent oxygen
- Suction equipment and at least one suction source
- Disposable sterile suction kits or sterile suction catheters, gloves, containers, sterile water
- Oral pharyngeal airway or a bite block if the oral route is used (to prevent closure of the airway if the patient should bite down on the tube)—also facilitates access to the oropharynx for suctioning
- Cuff manometer to check the cuff pressure on a regular basis
- A manual resuscitation bag to provide adequate backup in case of ventilator failure and for suctioning

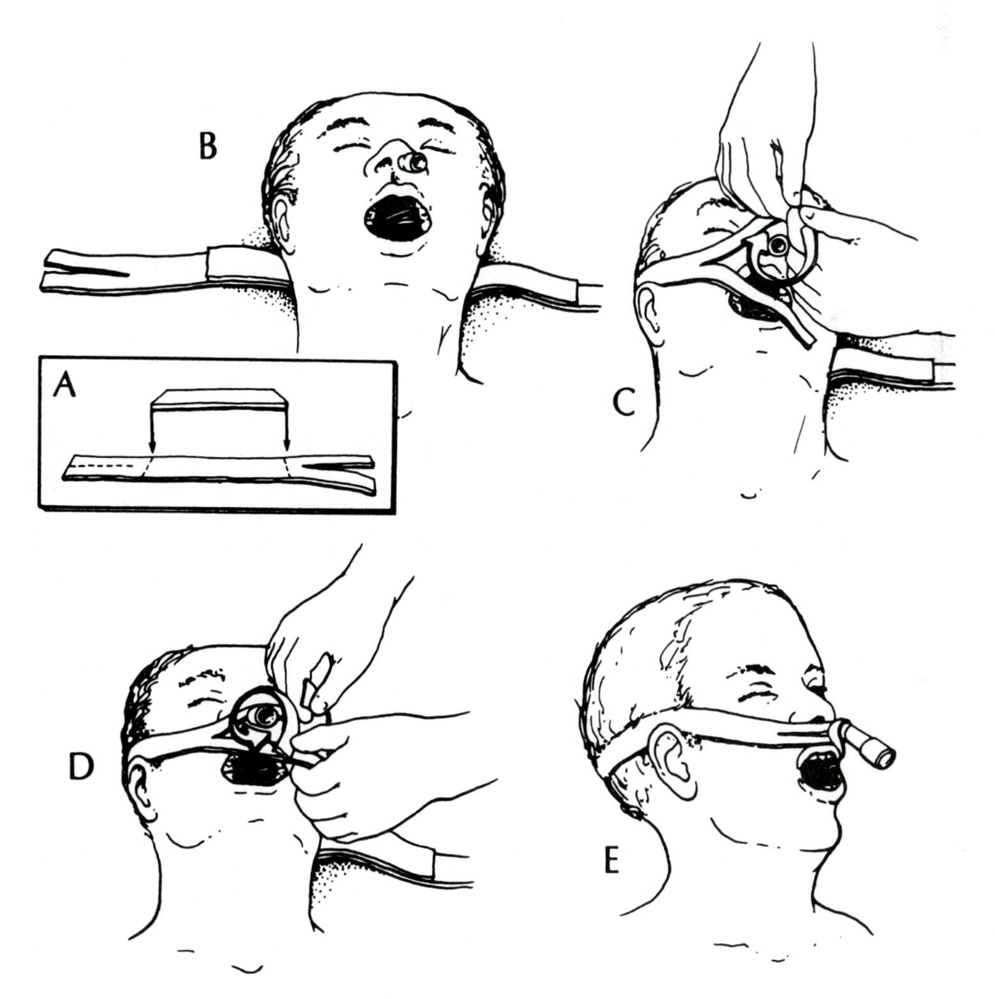

Figure 7–4. The "head halter" technique for securing a nasotracheal tube. **A** demonstrates how the tape is cut on both ends with the middle section apposed by a tape section so that hair will not stick to the halter. **B** shows the tape under the patient's head. **C** demonstrates how one side is brought over the ear and the top leaf is wrapped around the tube in a clockwise fashion. **D** demonstrates the bottom leaf wrapped around the tube in a counterclockwise fashion. The procedure is repeated for the other side of the tape. *(From Shapiro, B.A., et al. [1991].* Clinical application of respiratory care, *4th ed. [p. 164]. St. Louis: C.V. Mosby.)*

- If positive end-expiratory pressure (PEEP) is to be used on the ventilator, a manual resuscitation bag with a PEEP attachment is recommended
- Sedation and/or muscle relaxants

In summary, positive pressure mechanical ventilation requires the insertion of an artificial airway, either in the form of an ET tube, which can be inserted by the oral or nasal route, or by performing a tracheostomy. In an emergency, oral intubation using a laryngoscope most commonly is performed because of the speed and accuracy with which it can be placed. Adult artificial airways must have a cuff that is inflated for mechanical ventilation. Tracheostomy frequently is performed in those patients requiring prolonged mechanical ventilatory support or long-term assistance with airway clearance.

SECTION THREE REVIEW

1. In the adult, an inflated ET tube cuff is necessary for mechanical ventilation primarily because it
   A. prevents stomach contents from getting into the lungs
   B. seals off the nasopharynx from the oropharynx
   C. prevents air from getting into the stomach
   D. seals off the lower airway from the upper airway
2. The endotracheal tube size indicated on the tube reflects what measurement?
   A. the length of the tube
   B. the internal diameter of the tube
   C. the circumference size of the tube
   D. the length of the person's airway
3. In an emergency situation, the most common entry route for airway access is
   A. oral intubation
   B. nasal intubation
   C. tracheostomy
   D. oropharyngeal airway
4. Which of the following statements is true about securing the artificial airway?
   A. the inflated cuff provides sufficient securing
   B. the airway is generally sutured in place
   C. a nasotracheal tube does not require securing
   D. artificial airways must be secured directly to the patient.
5. When setting up a room for mechanical ventilator use, there must be
   A. one oxygen source
   B. two oxygen sources
   C. clean gloves for suctioning
   D. back-up ventilator in room

Answers: 1. D, 2. B, 3. A, 4. D, 5. B

SECTION FOUR: Types of Mechanical Ventilators

At the completion of this section, the learner will be able to describe the types of mechanical ventilators, based on mechanism of force and cycling mechanism.

A common classification of ventilators uses mechanism of force, which is either negative or positive pressure. Figure 7–5 compares the mechanics of spontaneous ventilation, negative pressure ventilation, and positive pressure ventilation.

Negative Pressure Ventilators

According to Pilbeam (1998), negative pressure ventilators were the first ventilators to be experimented with, as early as the middle 1800s. The first model that achieved widespread success was developed in the United States in 1928 by Dr. Drinker and his associates. This model completely encased the body in an airtight tank, with only the patient's head being exposed to the outside. As an alternative design, first French physicians and then the inventor Alexander Graham Bell designed the cuirass (a French word meaning "breastplate"). The cuirass negative pressure ventilator covers only the thoracic area (or the thorax and abdomen), somewhat like a turtle shell.

Negative pressure ventilation uses negatively applied pressure to the thorax by external means. To use a negative pressure ventilator, the patient's entire body (e.g., in an iron lung) or thoracic region (e.g., in a cuirass) is encased in an airtight unit. At regular intervals, the air pressure in the sealed unit is reduced to below atmospheric pressure. The resulting negative pressure is transmitted through the thorax, which results in a pressure gradient that causes air to move into the lungs. The amount of negative pressure used is based on the desired tidal volume (VT)—the higher the desired VT, the higher the negative pressure required.

Negative pressure ventilation has several major advantages: (1) it does not require an artificial airway; (2) the patient can eat and talk normally; and (3) breathing mechanics are more normal, thereby decreasing the risk of physiologic complications. This type of ventilation also has a number of disadvantages, including (1) decreases venous return to the heart; (2) it may cause abdominal pooling of blood; and (3) the patient is relatively inaccessible for performance of activities of daily living (ADLs).

With the advent of positive pressure ventilators, negative pressure ventilators rapidly lost favor. Today, negative pressure ventilators are primarily used in the home, for long-term use in patients with relatively normal lung function. Examples of patients who might benefit from negative pressure ventilation include those with chronic hypoventilation and/or respiratory failure associated with neuromuscular diseases; those who require intermittent ventilatory support, such as during sleep; and, in certain cases, those with COPD.

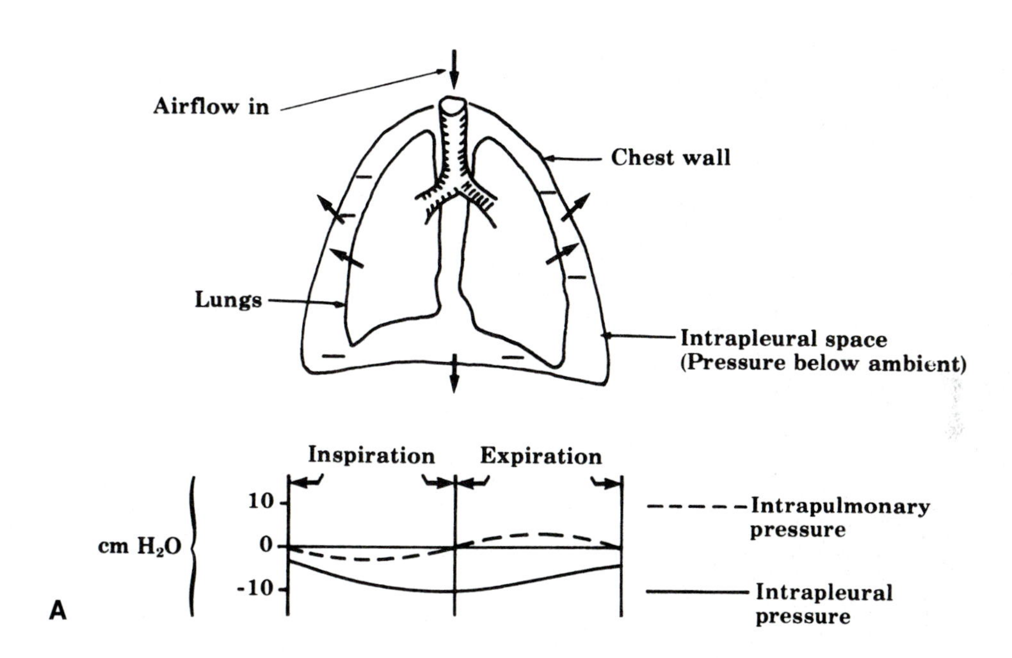

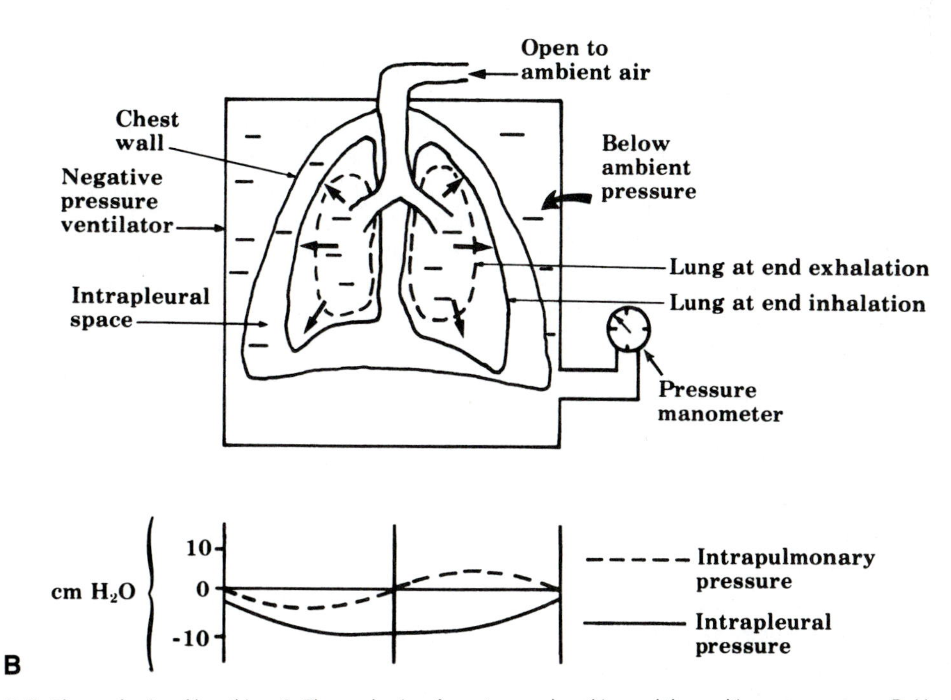

Figure 7-5. The mechanics of breathing. **A.** The mechanics of spontaneous breathing and the resulting pressure waves. **B.** Negative pressure ventilation and the resulting lung mechanics and pressures. *(From Pilbeam, S.P. [1998].* Mechanical ventilation: Physiological and clinical applications, *3rd ed. [pp. 31–35]. St. Louis: C.V. Mosby.) (continues)*

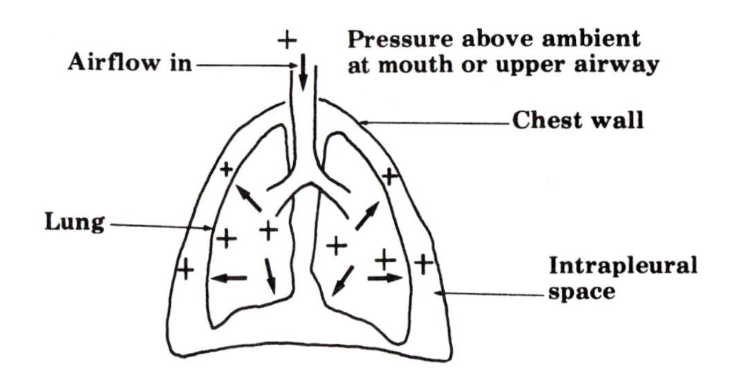

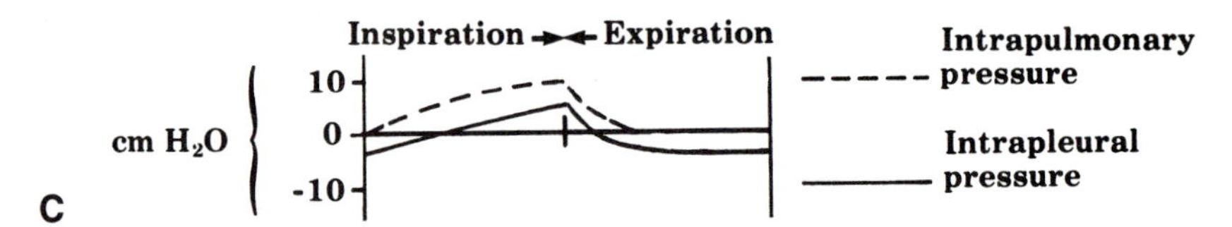

Figure 7–5 (cont'd). C. The mechanics and pressures associated with positive pressure ventilation. Intrapleural pressures are above ambient pressure during end-inspiration.

Positive Pressure Ventilators

Positive pressure ventilators require an artificial airway to deliver ventilatory support. Gases are driven into the lungs through the ventilator's circuitry, which is attached to an artificial airway (ET or tracheostomy tube). Figure 7–6 shows an example of a positive pressure ventilator.

Positive-pressure ventilators are commonly described on the basis of their cycling mechanism. The term **cycle** refers to the mechanism by which the inspiratory phase is stopped and the expiratory phase is started. There are four major cycling mechanisms: pressure-cycled, volume-cycled, time-cycled, and flow-cycled. Since the cycling mechanisms actually limit the length of inspiration, the term *cycle* is often replaced by the term *limit* (i.e., pressure-limited). The newer ventilators provide more than one cycling device; however, only one cycling mechanism can be used at a time. With this increased flexibility, the health care team can alter the type of cycling based on the changing needs of the patient without switching ventilators. The remainder of this section briefly describes ventilators based on the cycling mechanism being used.

Pressure-Cycled Ventilation

Pressure-cycled ventilation delivers a preset pressure of gas to the lungs. The pressure delivered (expressed in centimeters of H_2O) is constant. The volume of air it delivers varies with the lung's compliance and airway resistance. This presents potentially serious support problems, since stiffening lungs, a leak in the system, or a partially obstructed airway can significantly alter the volume of gas delivered. Maintaining an adequate VT is crucial for normal lung functioning. For this reason, use of pressure-cycled ventilation generally is reserved for short-term use, such as in postanesthesia recovery. An example of a pressure-cycled ventilator is the Bird-Mark-7.

Volume-Cycled Ventilation

Volume-cycled ventilation delivers a preset volume of gas (measured in milliliters or liters) to the lungs, making volume the constant and pressure the variable. Within a certain preset safety range (pressure limits), the ventilator will deliver the established volume of gas regardless of the amount of pressure it requires. This has the advantage of being able to overcome changes in lung **compliance** and airway resistance. For example, as lung compliance decreases or airway resistance increases, the pressure at which the gas is delivered to the lungs will increase sufficiently to deliver the desired volume of gas to the lungs.

Time-Cycled Ventilation

When time-cycled ventilation is used, the length of time allowed for inspiration is controlled. There are mechanical ventilators that solely use time-cycled ventilation, including the Servo 900c, Sechrist IV-100, and others. These ventilators hold time constant but volume and pressure may vary. Time-cycled ventilators frequently are referred to as time-cycled–pressure-limited ventilators, since they also limit the amount of pressure that can be delivered. The microprocessor ventilators can use time-cycling and also have the advantage of be-

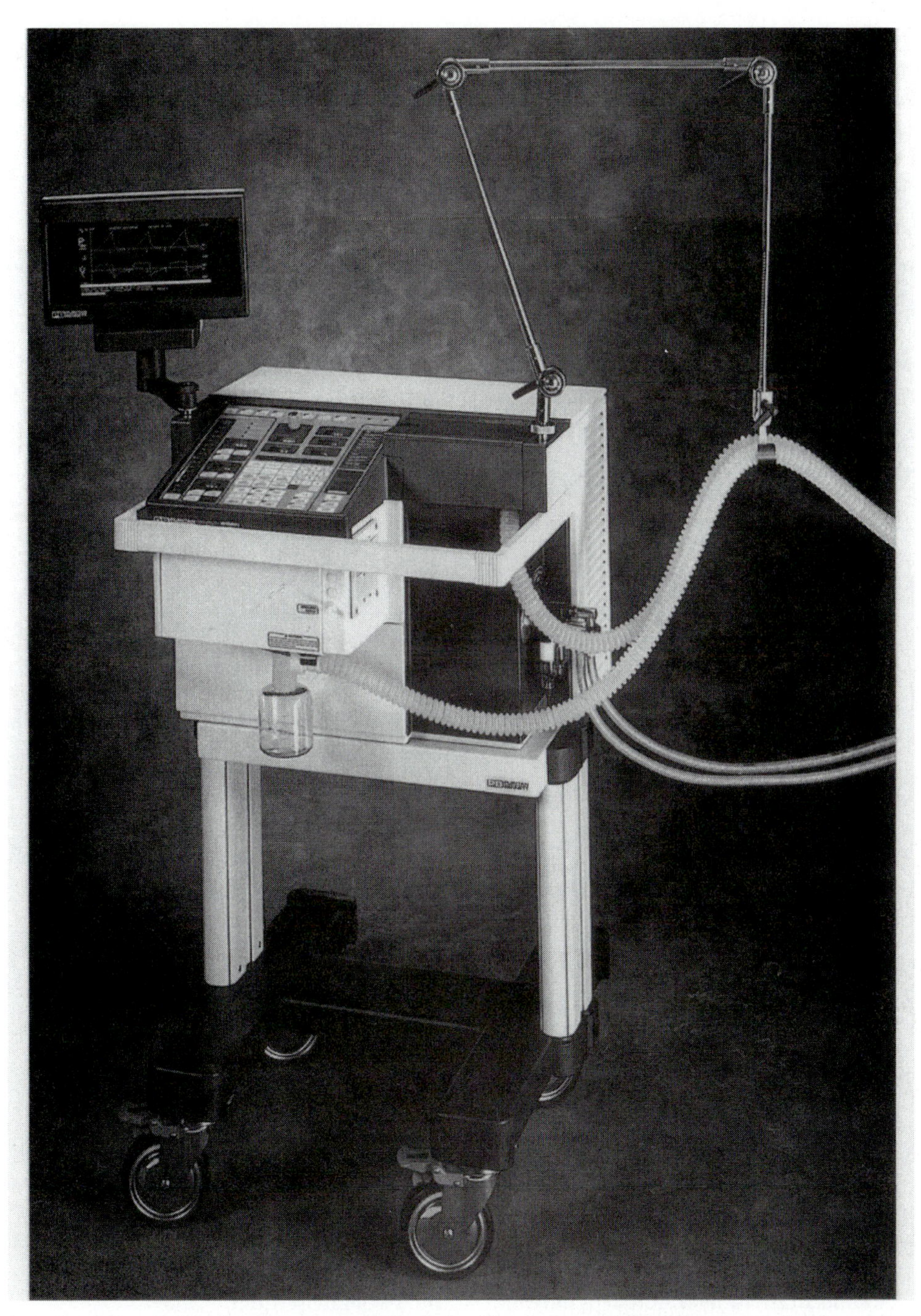

Figure 7–6. Puritan-Bennett 7200 series microprocessor-controlled positive pressure ventilator. *(Courtesy of Puritan-Bennett Corp., Carlsbad, CA.)*

ing able to limit volume and pressure. Time-cycling is often used during weaning.

Flow-Cycled Ventilation

Pilbeam (1998) explains that flow-cycled ventilation holds flow constant while time, pressure, and volume vary, depending on the patient's breathing effort and changing lung characteristics. Inspiration ends when the rate of gas flow decreases to a preset level (often 25 percent of peak inspiratory flow). Flow-cycled ventilation is most commonly used when the pressure support mode of ventilation is used.

In summary, negative pressure ventilators require sealing at least the chest of the patient in an airtight tank or shell. They do not require an artificial airway. Negative pressure ventilators are no longer seen commonly in acute care settings. Positive pressure ventilators directly force gases into the lungs using positive pressure. Various types of positive pressure cycling mechanisms are available. Pressure-cycled ventilation delivers a set amount of pressure to the lungs. Volume-cycled ventilation delivers a set amount of volume to the lungs. Volume cycling is commonly used, since it is possible to adjust pressure to meet changes in airway resistance and compliance. Time-cycled ventilation uses inspiratory time as its major cycling parameter. Flow-cycled ventilation uses a decrease in inspiratory flow rate to determine when expiration will begin.

SECTION FOUR REVIEW

1. Negative pressure ventilators adjust the tidal volume by
   A. adjusting the amount of negative airflow
   B. adjusting the amount of positive airflow
   C. altering the amount of negative pressure applied
   D. altering the amount of positive pressure applied
2. The term *cycle* as it applies to mechanical ventilation refers to the mechanism by which
   A. the ventilator turns on and off
   B. inspiration ceases and expiration starts
   C. the concentration of oxygen is controlled
   D. the rate of airflow is maintained
3. Volume-cycled ventilation has an advantage over pressure-cycled ventilation because it
   A. adjusts volume as pulmonary pressure changes
   B. increases airflow as compliance increases
   C. decreases airflow as airway resistance decreases
   D. can adjust pressure to changes in lung compliance
4. Pressure-cycled ventilation uses which of the following as a constant?
   A. pressure
   B. time
   C. volume
   D. flow rate
5. In adults, time-cycled ventilation is used primarily for which purpose?
   A. initial support
   B. pneumothorax
   C. IMV weaning
   D. acute respiratory distress syndrome
6. Flow-cycled ventilation is most commonly used for/with
   A. postanesthesia recovery
   B. pressure support mode
   C. atelectasis
   D. acute respiratory distress syndrome

Answers: 1. C, 2. B, 3. D, 4. A, 5. C, 6. B

SECTION FIVE: Commonly Monitored Ventilator Settings

At the completion of this section, the learner will be able to explain the commonly monitored ventilator settings.

Positive pressure ventilators offer many variables that can be manipulated to meet precisely the individual pulmonary needs of the patient. Certain settings and values related to each variable must be monitored by anyone taking care of a mechanically ventilated patient whether in a critical care unit, on a general floor, or in the home. The most commonly monitored settings include tidal volume (VT), fraction of inspired oxygen (FIO_2), ventilation mode, respiratory rate (f), positive end-expiratory pressure (PEEP), continuous positive airway pressure (CPAP), pressure support (PS), peak inspiratory pressure (PIP), and alarms. Figure 7–7 shows the ventilator settings on a Puritan-Bennett 7200 Control Panel.

Tidal Volume

Tidal volume (TV or VT) is the **amount** of air that moves in and out of the lungs in one normal breath. Normal VT ranges from 7 to 9 mL/kg (or 500 to 800 mL in an adult). If VT is too low, hypoventilation will occur. If VT is too high, the patient is at risk for pneumothorax and possible depression of the cardiovascular system.

If volume-cycled ventilation is to be used, the desired VT must be set when mechanical ventilation is initiated. Opinions vary regarding how high to set the VT. The major argument focuses on high-volume settings versus normal-volume settings.

High-Volume Settings

According to Pilbeam (1998), a tidal volume over 15 mL/kg is no longer recommended because it overdistends the alveoli, causing lung damage. Large tidal volumes can injure the basement membranes, epithelium, and endothelium of the lungs. Injured lung tissue increases the permeability of the lungs' microvasculature, which ultimately may result in lung rupture. The risk of lung injury increases as peak alveolar pressure increases. Though alveolar pressure is not measured directly, it can be approximated through measurement of the plateau pressure. Plateau pressure is easily measured at the end of inspiration by momentarily occluding the ventilatory circuit.

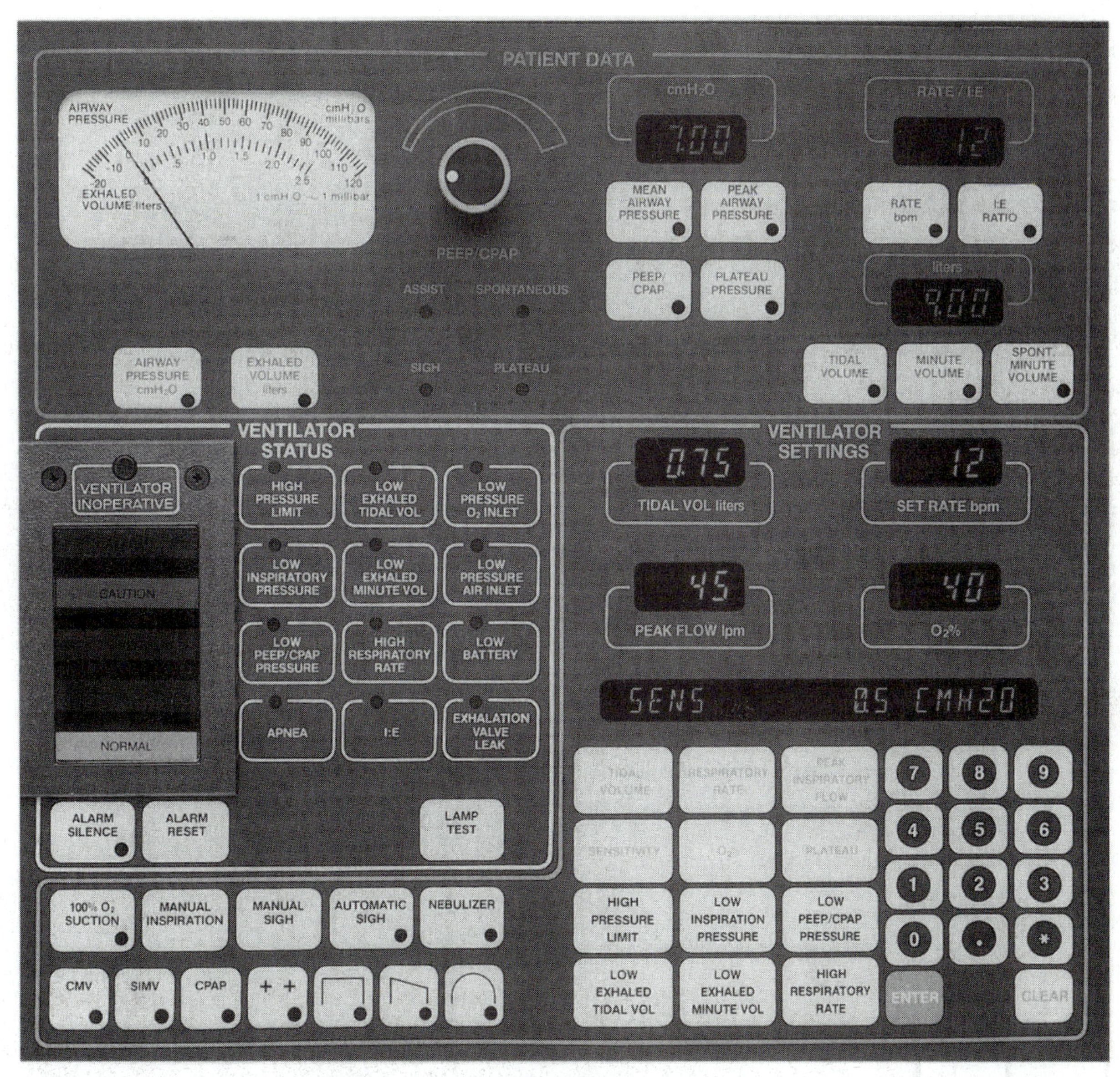

Figure 7–7. Mechanical ventilator Control Board. The control board of the Puritan-Bennett 7200 Microprocessor ventilator is divided into three sections. **A.** Patient data provides visual information regarding the patient's current ventilatory status. **B.** Ventilator status alerts the clinician to alarms and machine problems. **C.** Ventilator settings provide an active keyboard for manipulation of all the ventilator settings, such as mode, rate, volumes, and pressure limits. *(Courtesy of Puritan-Bennett Corp., Carlsbad, CA.)*

Normal-Volume Settings

Pilbeam (1998) suggests using 5 to 12 mL/kg of ideal body weight (adult) to establish an initial tidal volume setting. The goal is to adequately ventilate the lungs while maintaining a plateau pressure of less than 35 cm H_2O. Some patients with pulmonary diseases are at high risk for lung injury due to increased alveolar pressure and over distention. A technique called *permissive hypercapnia* may be considered for use in this patient population. The technique deliberately allows hypoventilation by using low tidal volumes. Vollman and Aulbach (1998) explain that the patient's $PaCO_2$ is allowed to slowly rise over a 24 to 48 hour period by slowly reducing minute ventilation. The healthcare team must determine how high the $PaCO_2$ and how low the pH will be permitted to drift.

Sigh

The term **sigh** refers to intermittent hyperinflation of the lungs. During normal spontaneous breathing, a person naturally takes an occasional deep breath (about one sigh every six minutes), which improves ventilation of the lungs. Use of manual and automatic sighs during mechanical ventilation was used widely in the 1960s to prevent development of atelectasis and to decrease shunt. When the practice of high tidal volume ventilation became common, use of the sigh controls was no longer considered necessary or desirable. Use of sighing remains controversial. When used, it is commonly set at a volume of 1.5 to 2 times the patient's VT and at a rate of 6 to 10 per hour.

Fraction of Inspired Oxygen

FIO_2 means the **fraction of inspired oxygen.** It is expressed as a decimal, although clinicians often discuss it in percentages, in terms of oxygen concentrations. At sea level, the room air that is inhaled into the alveoli is composed of oxygen that is 0.21 of the total concentration of gases in the alveoli. A mechanical ventilator is able to deliver a wide range of FIO_2, from 0.21 to 1.0 (an oxygen concentration of 21 percent to 100 percent).

Initially, in an emergency situation, FIO_2 is commonly set at 0.5 to 1.0 to deliver 50 percent to 100 percent oxygen to the patient. The setting is then increased or decreased based on the patient's PaO_2 and clinical picture. The goal is to maintain the PaO_2 within an acceptable range for the individual, using the lowest level of FIO_2. Prolonged use of $FIO_2 > 0.60$ may cause complications associated with oxygen toxicity (discussed in Section Seven).

In a semielective situation, the initial FIO_2 may be set at lower levels, based on more individualized oxygenation needs. The patient who has a carbon dioxide–retaining COPD requires special consideration. When maintenance of some degree of patient-initiated breathing is desirable, care must be taken to set the FIO_2 at the lowest level that will deliver an acceptable PaO_2. The use of high concentrations of oxygen on such an individual may obliterate the hypoxic drive to breathe.

Ventilation Mode

The ventilation mode refers to that which initiates the cycling of the ventilator to terminate expiration. The most common modes are **assist/control (A/C) mode** and **intermittent mandatory ventilation (IMV).**

Assist/Control Mode

Most ventilators have an assist mode, a control mode, and an assist/control mode. In assist mode, the ventilator is sensitive to the inspiratory effort of the patient. When the patient begins to inhale, the assist mode triggers the ventilator to deliver a breath at the prescribed settings (called a **ventilator** or **mechanical breath**). In the control mode, the ventilator delivers the breaths at a preset rate based on time. It is not sensitive to the patient's own ventilatory effort. Control mode generally is not used alone unless the patient is continuously apneic. A combination of assist and control modes generally is used. A/C mode protects the patient in the following manner. The assist part of the mode is sensitive to spontaneous inspiratory effort of the patient, allowing the patient to maintain some control over breathing. At the same time, the control part of the mode acts as a backup should the patient decrease the breathing effort below the preset rate. When A/C mode is used, every breath is a ventilator breath (VT, and so on, as set by the clinician), which differentiates it from IMV. A/C mode commonly is used initially, particularly in patients with acute respiratory failure or respiratory muscle fatigue, because A/C mode takes over the work of breathing.

Intermittent Mandatory Ventilation Mode

Using the IMV mode, the patient spontaneously breathes through the ventilator circuit, maintaining much of the work of breathing. Interspersed at regular intervals, the ventilator provides a preset ventilator breath. The intervals are based on the IMV rate set by the operator. For example, if the IMV is set at 12, the ventilator will deliver a breath approximately every 5 seconds. Between mandatory breaths, the patient's breathing will vary in VT and rate, since it is composed of **spontaneous breaths,** not ventilator breaths.

Synchronous intermittent mandatory ventilation (SIMV) is a type of IMV. The original IMV mode is not sensitive to the patient's own ventilatory cycle. Thus, an IMV breath can be stacked on top of the patient's own inhalation. SIMV synchronizes a mandatory breath to follow the patient's exhalation. The advantages of SIMV over IMV mode have not been proven, since stacking of breaths has not been shown to be a physiologic hazard. SIMV, however, is more comfortable for the patient because it does not interfere with the normal breathing cycle. IMV/SIMV have certain advantages over the other modes. They decrease the risk of hyperventilation and also provide a better ventilation–perfusion distribution. IMV/SIMV also facilitate the process of ventilator weaning.

Pressure Support Ventilation Mode

Pressure support ventilation (PSV) was introduced into the United States during the mid-1980s. Pressure support ventilation is defined as an adjunct weaning mode that enhances spontaneous inspiratory effort by application of positive pressure. Although clinical research has not yet clearly established the indications for effective use of PSV, it has gained rapid popularity and widespread use throughout the United States.

In principle, PSV is similar to intermittent positive pressure breathing (IPPB). Both are triggered by the patient's spontaneous breathing effort and both decrease the effort (work) required to achieve a VT. IPPB and PSV differ in what occurs upon achieving the preset level of pressure. IPPB ceases applying positive pressure as soon as the preset pressure is achieved. PSV, however, applies and maintains the preset pressure throughout the entire inspiration phase.

The purpose of PSV is to decrease the work of breathing by overcoming increased **airway resistance (R_{aw})** imposed by the presence of an artificial airway and ventilator circuitry. Pressure support ventilation is most often used as an aid to ventilator weaning. Patients on IMV/SIMV weaning mode are at increased risk for respiratory muscle fatigue and ventilatory failure because they must breathe harder than normal to maintain adequate tidal volumes due to increased airway resistance. In these patients, PSV decreases the work of breathing by supporting the tidal volume during spontaneous breaths. Pressure support ventilation can also be used to assist patients who are breathing spontaneously as long as an artificial airway is in place, including patients receiving continuous positive airway pressure. Pressure support ventilation is sometimes applied to the assist mode during ventilatory support. This application requires a stable lung condition as well as a reliable respiratory center. Should the patient have an apneic spell while on PSV using the assist mode, there is no timed back-up present to take over ventilation.

The level of PSV support can be based on the desired VT or on calculated airway resistance. Three factors predominantly determine the patient's VT: the preset pressure support level, the degree of patient effort, and the level of airway resistance and compliance (Pilbeam, 1998). When using desired VT as the basis for manipulating the level of PSV, the level is increased until the desired VT is reached. When the level of PSV is based on calculated airway resistance, the PSV level is adjusted to provide just enough support to overcome the calculated resistance. This, in effect, cancels out the impact of increased airway resistance. Pressure support ventilation frequently is adjusted in increments of 5 cm H_2O, with levels commonly ranging from 5 to 15 cm H_2O.

Rate

Properly setting the ventilator rate (f) is important in establishing adequate minute ventilation ($\dot{V}E$). Minute ventilation is the amount of air that moves in and out of the lungs in 1 minute. Normal $\dot{V}E$ is 5 to 7 L/min. VT and f are the two variables that make up $\dot{V}E$. It can be calculated using the following equation:

$$\dot{V}E = VT \times f$$

These variables are significant because if either one is manipulated, it will affect $\dot{V}E$. If $\dot{V}E$ becomes too low, hypoventilation will occur, possibly precipitating acute respiratory acidosis. In the carbon dioxide–retaining COPD patient, hyperventilation that results in decreased carbon dioxide levels can complicate weaning from the mechanical ventilator.

Pilbeam (1998) suggests that the rate depends on the characteristics of the patient's lungs. For example:

- Normal lungs
  VT: 12 mL/kg
  f: 8 to 12/min
- Lung disease with increased CL and R_{aw}
  VT: 8 to 12 mL/kg
  f: 6 to 10/min
- Restrictive lung disease
  VT: ≤ 8 to 10 mL/kg
  f: 12 to 20/min

The IMV rate also is based on providing adequate ventilation for the patient. If the rate is set too slow, hypoventilation may occur, precipitating acute ventilatory failure (respiratory acidosis). If the rate is set too high, it may precipitate respiratory alkalosis by blowing off too much carbon dioxide.

PEEP and CPAP

For many years there has been an interest in perfecting a method to keep the alveoli open throughout the breathing cycle. Although this method (called positive end-expiratory pressure) was first developed in the 1940s by the military, it was not used in medicine until 20 years later, in the late 1960s. In the early 1970s, it was introduced as a treatment for respiratory distress syndrome in newborns. Since that time, it has become the foundation for oxygenating the lungs in newborns and adults with respiratory distress syndrome (Pilbeam, 1998).

There are two methods by which positive end-expiratory pressure is applied to the lungs: **positive end-expiratory pressure (PEEP)** and **continuous positive airway pressure (CPAP)**. PEEP and CPAP are important ventilatory modes that are initiated for treatment of specific disease processes. When either is ordered, the nurse must monitor the level of PEEP as well as the therapeutic and nontherapeutic effects that PEEP has on the patient. PEEP and CPAP provide the alveoli with a constant (preset) amount of positive pressure at the end of each expiration. PEEP/CPAP prevents airway pressure from returning to zero; thus, it remains positive throughout the breathing cycle.

PEEP is used with patients who have part or all of their work of breathing supplied by a mechanical ventilator. It can be used in a variety of ventilator modes, including assist/control and IMV. CPAP is used on patients who are spontaneously breathing. It does not require an artificial airway or a mechanical ventilator, although many ventilators have a CPAP mode.

Normally, at the end of expiration, alveoli have a natural tendency to collapse. When positive pressure is provided during the expiration phase of the breathing cycle, it forces the alveoli to remain open, which (1) recruits previously collapsed alveoli, (2) prevents atelectasis, and (3) improves oxygenation (Fig. 7–8). The primary indication for use of PEEP/CPAP is the presence of refractory

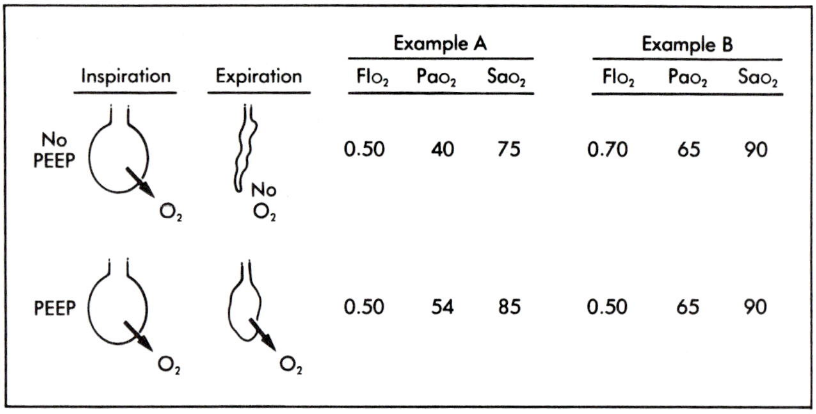

	Inspiration	Expiration	Example A			Example B		
			FIO_2	PaO_2	SaO_2	FIO_2	PaO_2	SaO_2
No PEEP	O_2	No O_2	0.50	40	75	0.70	65	90
PEEP	O_2	O_2	0.50	54	85	0.50	65	90

Figure 7–8 Effect of PEEP on oxygenation. During expiration with PEEP, airways that would otherwise collapse are kept open, allowing continued oxygen transfer. In **Example A,** the PaO_2 and SaO_2 improve, and FIO_2 is unchanged. In **Example B,** the PaO_2 is maintained at an acceptable level, whereas the FIO_2 is decreased from 0.70 to 0.50. *(From Martin, L. [1987]. Pulmonary physiology in clinical practice: The essentials for patient care and evaluation [p. 212]. St. Louis: C.V. Mosby.)*

hypoxemia (i.e., hypoxemia that is unresponsive to increasing concentrations of oxygen). PEEP is also useful in treating acute diffuse lung disease processes (e.g., severe diffuse pneumonia and cardiogenic pulmonary edema), and in treating postoperative atelectasis (Pilbeam, 1998).

The level of PEEP can be monitored on most ventilators by observing the airway pressure manometer. When no PEEP is being applied, the manometer needle should fall back to 0 at the end of each breath. When PEEP is present, the needle should fall back only to the level of PEEP. For example, if PEEP is set at 10 cm H_2O, the needle should fall to 10 $\pm$ 2 cm H_2O rather than to 0. The level of PEEP/CPAP is adjusted to meet the patient's oxygenation needs. The criteria used to determine when the desired level of positive pressure has been reached vary between clinicians. There is, however, some consensus regarding the approaches used (Pilbeam, 1998), including:

1. PEEP should be increased in increments of 3 to 5 cm H_2O per step in adults.
2. An optimal oxygenation point should be achieved which allows adequate tissue oxygenation (optimal oxygen transport) at a safe FIO_2.
3. Cardiovascular status must be closely monitored and maintained at an acceptable level.

PEEP can also be used to offset auto-PEEP. **Auto-PEEP** refers to an unintentional buildup of positive end-expiratory pressure caused by air-trapping. It is particularly associated with COPD. Air-trapping prevents the COPD patient from exhaling fully, which leaves a volume of air in the alveoli at the end of expiration. When a COPD patient's lungs become hyperinflated, he or she may not be able to inhale sufficiently to trigger the mechanical ventilator in an assist mode. Applying a small amount of PEEP externally, to match the level of auto-PEEP, can offset the effects of the auto-PEEP such that the patient can trigger the ventilator to cycle properly.

The level of positive pressure required depends primarily on the severity of lung injury. Mild forms of injury usually require between 5 and 15 cm H_2O. In cases of more severe injury, the patient may require 10 to 30 cm H_2O. In rare instances of extreme lung injury, the patient can require over 30 cm H_2O. There is a trend away from using PEEP levels over 30 cm H_2O in favor of newer ventilator modes such as inverse ratio ventilation (IRV) (Pilbeam, 1998).

Although PEEP and CPAP are important in the treatment of severe hypoxemia, their use is associated with significant complications that can be as detrimental to patient outcomes as severe hypoxemia. The risk of complications increases as the amount of PEEP or CPAP is increased. The complications associated with PEEP can be categorized into two groups: barotrauma to the lungs and decreased cardiac output. Complications are discussed in Section Seven.

Peak Airway Pressure or Peak Inspiratory Pressure

When using volume-cycled ventilation, the tidal volume is preset to deliver a certain number of milliliters or liters. The pressure it takes to deliver that amount of volume varies depending primarily on airway resistance and lung compliance. The amount of pressure required to deliver the volume is called the **peak airway pressure (PAP)** or peak inspiratory pressure (PIP). PIP is measured in centimeters of water pressure and may be visualized on an airway pressure manometer or on a data screen. In the adult, PIPs of < 40 cm H_2O are considered desirable. It is known that high PIPs greatly increase the risk of barotrauma and negative effects on other body systems (see Section Seven). PIP should be recorded at regular intervals for trending—taking multiple measurements over an extended period of time to evaluate the parameter for a pattern of change.

Increasing Peak Inspiratory Pressure Trend

This signifies that increasing amounts of pressure are necessary to deliver the preset tidal volume. It is most commonly indicative of increased airway resistance or decreased lung compliance.

Decreasing Peak Inspiratory Pressure Trend

This signifies that less pressure is needed to deliver the tidal volume. It may indicate an improvement in airway resistance or lung compliance.

Alarms

The patient's life depends on correct functioning of the ventilator and maintenance of a patent airway. To protect the patient, ventilators are equipped with a system of alarms to alert the caregiver to problems. Many variables may be equipped with alarms. Two frequently triggered alarms are the low exhaled volume and high pressure alarms.

The low exhaled volume alarm indicates that there is a loss of tidal volume or a leak in the system. When this alarm goes off, the nurse should focus rapidly on checking to see whether the ventilator tubing has become disconnected or whether the artificial airway cuff is inadequately filled with air or has a leak. The cuff can be checked by feeling for air leaking out of the nose and mouth. It may be noted that the patient can suddenly vocalize, which also indicates a leak or insufficiently inflated cuff. A leaking cuff may be checked by deflating and then reinflating the cuff to observe for its ability to attain and then maintain a tracheal seal. If the cuff is ruptured, the nurse must notify the medical team immediately and prepare for reintubation.

The high pressure alarm is the most commonly heard alarm. Anything that increases airway resistance can trigger it. Examples of clinical conditions that cause a high pressure alarm include coughing, biting on the tube, secretions in the airway, or water in the tubing. Clearing the airway or tubing most frequently will correct the problem.

TABLE 7–3. THE GOLDEN RULE OF VENTILATOR ALARMS

If the cause of an alarm is not immediately found or cannot be corrected immediately, the patient should be removed from the ventilator and manually ventilated using a resuscitation bag until the problem is corrected.

Alarms should never be ignored or turned off. Some alarms can be muted temporarily, for example, during suctioning. Table 7–3 presents the rule regarding the proper response to an alarm.

Initial Ventilator Settings

When a patient is first placed on the mechanical ventilator, certain standard settings may be used as a guideline. The settings are as follows:

Tidal volume	5–12 mL/kg ideal body weight
Rate	8–12/minute
Mode	A/C
FIO_2	0.5–1.0 (less in COPD, if possible)
Peak flow	40–60 L/min
Inspiratory sensitivity	−1 to −2 cm H_2O

In summary, positive pressure ventilators have many parameters that must be monitored by those persons who work directly with them. This section presents the most commonly monitored mechanical ventilator settings, including VT, FIO_2, modes, rate, PEEP/CPAP, pressure support, PIP, and alarms. Special consideration is given to ventilator setting alterations for management of the patient with carbon dioxide–retaining COPD.

SECTION FIVE REVIEW

1. The normal VT in a spontaneously breathing adult is_____ mL/kg.
   A. 2–5
   B. 5–7
   C. 7–9
   D. 10–15
2. The common volume VT setting range on a mechanical ventilator is _____ mL/kg.
   A. 2 to 5
   B. 5 to 12
   C. 7 to 9
   D. 10 to 15
3. If VT is set too low on the ventilator, it will cause
   A. hypoventilation
   B. pneumothorax
   C. hypoxemia
   D. hypocapnia
4. A high FIO_2 level (> 0.5) is avoided in patients with COPD when possible because it could
   A. cause hyperventilation
   B. lead to hypocapnia
   C. obliterate the hypoxic drive
   D. precipitate metabolic acidosis
5. A major advantage of initial use of A/C mode is that it allows
   A. the diaphragm to exercise
   B. the patient to rest
   C. increased work of breathing
   D. maintenance of some spontaneous breathing

6. SIMV is used primarily for
   A. weaning
   B. full support
   C. acute head injury
   D. acute pulmonary diseases
7. A low minute ventilation ($\dot{V}_E$) can cause which of the following?
   A. acute metabolic alkalosis
   B. acute respiratory alkalosis
   C. acute metabolic acidosis
   D. acute respiratory acidosis
8. PEEP affects the alveoli by
   A. increasing alveolar fluid
   B. decreasing their relative size
   C. sealing off nonfunctioning units
   D. maintaining them open at end expiration
9. PSV is used primarily for what purpose?
   A. to increase PIP
   B. to decrease oxygen need
   C. to decrease work of breathing
   D. to prevent atelectasis
10. An increasing PIP most commonly indicates which of the following?
   A. increasing airway resistance and/or decreasing lung compliance
   B. decreasing airway resistance and/or decreasing lung compliance
   C. increasing airway resistance and increasing lung compliance
   D. decreasing airway resistance and decreasing lung compliance
11. The ventilator low exhaled volume alarm will trigger when
   A. the patient is coughing
   B. there is water in the tubing
   C. the patient is biting the ET tube
   D. there is a leak in the system

Answers: 1. C, 2. B, 3. A, 4. C, 5. B, 6. A, 7. D, 8. D, 9. C, 10. A, 11. D

SECTION SIX: Noninvasive Alternatives to Mechanical Ventilation

At the completion of this section, the learner will be able to explain briefly three methods of providing noninvasive ventilatory support.

The physiologic effects of positive pressure ventilation (PPV), with its accompanying artificial airway, places the patient at increased risk for multiple complications. The combination of PPV and artificial airways significantly increases patient morbidity and mortality. In an effort to reduce some of the risks, several alternative noninvasive methods have been developed for delivery of positive airway pressure without requiring artificial airways. Noninvasive ventilatory methods have been shown to be an effective alternative to traditional invasive techniques in certain patient populations (Bonekat, 1998). This section presents an overview of three major noninvasive alternatives to conventional mechanical ventilatory support: **noninvasive intermittent positive pressure ventilation (NIPPV),** nasal continuous positive airway pressure (CPAP), and bilevel positive airway pressure (BiPAP).

Noninvasive Intermittent Positive Pressure Ventilation (NIPPV)

NIPPV is a relatively new means of providing ventilatory support without requiring intubation. It is more comfortable, is easier to apply and remove, and has a lower incidence of nosocomial pneumonia than conventional mechanical ventilation (Thelan et al., 1998). It requires use of a positive pressure mechanical ventilator and a mask.

Mechanical Ventilator

NIPPV can be provided by any positive pressure ventilator; however, small portable ventilators are most commonly used since NIPPV is predominantly used in the home setting. The ventilator may be either pressure-supported or volume-supported. The current trend is toward home ventilator systems that provide pressure-support with timed backup. Pressure support ventilation (PSV) works like an intermittent positive pressure breathing (IPPB) machine. Every time the patient inhales, the ventilator is triggered to deliver a preset level of positive pressure. The tidal volume changes from one breath to another since only pressure is controlled. PSV enhances the patient's tidal volume and decreases the work of breathing. The rate of breathing is not machine-controlled; however, timed backup provides a safety mechanism that triggers the machine if the patient fails to initiate a spontaneous breath within a specific time frame. If a portable volume-supported ventilator is used, the ventilator is preset with a tidal volume and a rate (A/C mode) or inspiratory time (assist mode). A/C mode is advisable if a minimum rate must be guaranteed (e.g., sleep apnea). Assist mode may be used when the NIPPV is required solely for enhancing tidal volumes (Pilbeam, 1998).

Masks

NIPPV, nasal CPAP, and BiPAP use either an oronasal mask or a nasal mask in place of the invasive endotracheal or tracheostomy tube. The oronasal mask covers up both the mouth and the nose, and the nasal mask covers only the nose. Currently, the nasal mask is the most common route of delivery. Since there is no artificial airway with an inflated cuff to guarantee positive pressure airflow from the ventilator into the lower airway, the mask must be strapped securely in place to minimize or eliminate air leakage.

Indications and Contraindications for Use

NIPPV is used primarily for therapy in patients who cannot fully support their own ventilatory effort for prolonged periods. Hicks and Scanlan (1999) suggest that NIPPV is an effective therapy for conscious patients who develop acute respiratory failure secondary to COPD, obstructive sleep apnea, or congestive heart failure (CHF). NIPPV may also be used as an alternative to intubation in patients who do not wish to be intubated (Pilbeam, 1998). Vanderwarf (1999) suggests that NIPPV may be useful in supporting patients whose respiratory status has deteriorated after having been withdrawn from conventional mechanical ventilation.

There are a variety of contraindications for using NIPPV, including an unstable hemodynamic status, cardiac dysrhythmias, apnea, the inability to clear one's own secretions or maintain airway patency, and the inability to attain a proper mask fit (Thelan et al., 1998). NIPPV is also contraindicated in patients whose respiratory status is worsening, as indicated by a decreased lung compliance or increased airway resistance (Hicks & Scanlan, 1999).

Nasal Continuous Positive Airway Pressure (CPAP)

CPAP provides a continuous level of positive airway pressure for a spontaneously breathing person. The level of pressure remains the same throughout the breathing cycle. Nasal CPAP does not require a mechanical ventilator; instead, it is delivered by a special flow generator (i.e., a blower). Other necessary equipment includes a nasal mask, a one-way valve or reservoir bag, and a PEEP/CPAP valve (threshold resistor). The CPAP level is adjustable from 2.5 to 20 cm H_2O.

Scanlan, Heuer, & Wyka (1999) suggest that several methods are used to determine the desired level of CPAP. When employed as a treatment of sleep apnea, the desirable level of CPAP is determined through a series of sleep studies in a laboratory setting. The goal is to establish the level of CPAP at which the patient stops having the apnea episodes or the frequency and duration of episodes is at an acceptable level. The CPAP level can also be determined by monitoring the patient's arterial desaturation level through pulse oximetry. Using this method, the CPAP level is adjusted to the lowest point at which the SpO_2 is ≥ 90 percent. Some of the newer CPAP units adjust airway pressure automatically, responding to snoring, apnea/hypopnea, or airflow limitation.

Nasal CPAP is used primarily to treat obstructive sleep apnea; however, it has also been shown to be effective for people who can support their own breathing during the day but become hypoxic and hypercapnic when they go to sleep. Nasal CPAP is restricted to people who do not require timed backup ventilation to protect them against prolonged apneic spells.

Bilevel Positive Airway Pressure (BiPAP)

BiPAP is a type of noninvasive positive pressure ventilation that is available using the Respironics BiPAP S/T. Positive pressure is applied through special nasal prongs, nasal mask, or full face mask (Burns, 1998). BiPAP has two pressure control settings that enable the user to set different pressures for the inspiratory positive airway pressure (IPAP) and the expiratory airway pressure (EPAP), whereas CPAP has only a single control setting. IPAP assists the inspiration phase in a manner similar to that provided by pressure support ventilation, which results in enhanced tidal volume and minute ventilation. The EPAP provides end-expiratory pressure to maintain open airways, thus enhancing oxygenation.

According to Burns (1998), BiPAP is best suited for patients with hypoventilatory problems resulting from a long-term chest deformity or disease when more invasive interventions are considered undesirable. It is useful in avoiding intubation in patients with hypercapnia and for respiratory failure; and may prevent the need for reintubation in patients whose condition might otherwise require it.

Complications

Many of the potential complications associated with positive pressure ventilation, as described in Section Seven, also apply to noninvasive ventilation, although the severity and frequency of the complications is significantly reduced. Additional patient problems are associated with delivery of positive pressure through a mask, including conjunctivitis, gastric distention, nasal problems, and skin irritation. In addition, hypoventilation is a common complication associated with mechanical problems.

Conjunctivitis is caused by air leaking out from the mask around the bridge of the nose and blowing on the eyes. This problem may be easily corrected by readjusting the mask to eliminate the leak or it may require the fitting of a new mask. Gastric distention is caused by air swallowing. Pilbeam (1998) suggests that distention may be relieved by altering the sleeping position and/or using an abdominal strap. Fortunately, with long-term use, gastric distention often becomes less of a problem. Nasal-related complaints include dryness, bleeding, and congestion. These problems may be relieved by use of humidification, either in-line, via nasal sprays, or room humidification. Skin irritation may develop under the straps and mask. To minimize or prevent this problem, the mask and straps require daily cleaning, and a good seal must be maintained. Hypoventilation is the major mechanical problem associated with noninvasive positive pressure ventilation therapy. Hypoventilation can occur through two mechanisms: (1) when there is an inadequate seal to attain the preset pressure, or (2) when there is inadequate airflow. Improving the seal or adjusting the flow (when possible) may relieve this problem. On some of the newer machines, such as the Respironics BiPAP S/T, the pressure adjusts automatically to overcome the problem of leakage, which reduces the risk of hypoventilation.

Home ventilatory support therapy requires careful, thorough instructions to the patient and/or the primary caregiver. Teaching needs include:

- Signs and symptoms of complications
- Under what circumstances to call the physician
- Proper use and maintenance of equipment
- Troubleshooting problems

Table 7–4 lists instructions for maintenance of nasal CPAP therapy equipment. Instructions regarding mask application and care also apply to NIPPV and BiPAP. Follow-up visits by a home health nurse and/or a respiratory therapist are usually ordered, as a means of monitoring both the equipment and the patient.

TABLE 7–4. TYPICAL PATIENT INSTRUCTIONS FOR HOME NASAL CPAP THERAPY

Equipment preparation

1. Place blower unit on a level surface (table or nightstand) close to where you sleep.
2. Make sure that the air exhaust and inlet vents are not obstructed.
3. Plug machine into a standard grounded (three-prong) electrical outlet.
4. Check air inlet filter to be sure it is in place and free of dust.
5. Connect one end of the tubing to the airflow outlet on the blower.
6. Connect the other end of the tubing to the mask. Then place the mask over the nose.
7. Adjust strap tightness to seat mask firmly over nose.
8. Turn on the blower and verify a flow of air.
9. Assure proper fit and adjustment of mask and headgear. Air should not be leaking out around the bridge of the nose into the eyes.
10. You are now ready to sleep with mask on.

In the morning

1. Remove mask by slipping strap off of back of head. (You may leave the headstrap connected between cleaning.)
2. Turn off blower.
3. Wash the mask every morning with a mild detergent, then rinse with water. This keeps the mask soft and airtight.
4. Store the mask in plastic bag to keep free of dust and dirt.

Weekly

1. Wipe off the blower unit with a clean, damp cloth.
2. Wash the headstrap and circuit tubing.
3. Service the filters according to the instructions in your patient manual.

From Scanlan, C.L., Heuer, A., & Wyka, K.A. (1999). Respiratory care in alternative settings. In C.L. Scanlan, R.L. Wilkins, & J.K. Stoller (eds.). Egan's fundamentals of respiratory care, *7th ed. [p. 1132]. St. Louis: C.V. Mosby.*

In summary, several noninvasive positive pressure ventilation systems have been described, including NIPPV, nasal CPAP, and BiPAP. These alternative methods are primarily used in the home setting, although BiPAP is being studied as a treatment for acute respiratory failure in certain patient populations. NIPPV requires use of a mechanical ventilator and has the potential for providing a higher level of support than CPAP or BiPAP. CPAP does not require the use of a mechanical ventilator and can only be used on patients who are spontaneously breathing and do not require timed backup ventilation. BiPAP provides control settings for inspiratory positive airway pressure (IPAP) and expiratory positive airway pressure (EPAP). The potential complications associated with NIPPV, CPAP, and BiPAP are similar to those associated with conventional mechanical ventilators although they are typically less severe. In addition, delivery of positive pressure through a mask is associated with multiple problems that, while not critical, decrease patient compliance unless they can be resolved. Patient and care provider teaching is crucial if home noninvasive ventilatory support is to be successful. Follow-up home visits by a home health nurse and/or respiratory therapist are also recommended, if not required.

SECTION SIX REVIEW

1. Which of the following statements describes NIPPV?
   A. it requires a flow-generator (blower)
   B. it combines negative and positive pressure principles
   C. it uses a positive pressure mechanical ventilator
   D. it independently manipulates inspiratory and expiratory pressures

2. NIPPV is most useful for the patient who
   A. requires only support of tidal volume
   B. cannot fully support his or her own expiratory effort
   C. requires only support for nocturnal hypercapnia and hypoxemia
   D. cannot fully support his or her own ventilatory effort over long periods of time
3. Which of the following statements best reflects nasal CPAP?
   A. it is used as a treatment of obstructive sleep apnea
   B. it requires a positive pressure mechanical ventilator
   C. the pressure level cannot be readjusted once it has been set
   D. it allows manipulation of inspiratory and expiratory pressures
4. BiPAP differs from CPAP because it
   A. requires an artificial airway
   B. can provide inspiratory positive pressure
   C. uses a standard positive pressure ventilator
   D. provides only nocturnal support
5. Common complications of noninvasive methods of ventilatory support include all of the following EXCEPT
   A. conjunctivitis
   B. nasal congestion
   C. hypoventilation
   D. otitis media

Answers: 1. C, 2. D, 3. A, 4. B, 5. D

SECTION SEVEN: Major Complications of Mechanical Ventilation

At the completion of this section, the learner will be able to discuss the major complications of mechanical ventilation.

Positive pressure ventilation (PPV) affects virtually all body systems. These effects can lead to multiple system complications. This section is a summary of the major effects of PPV, by system, as described by Pilbeam (1998), and the resulting potential major complications. Table 7–5 summarizes the multisystem effects of positive pressure ventilation.

Cardiovascular Complications

During normal spontaneous inhalation, air is drawn into the lungs due to a drop in intrathoracic pressure. At the same time, the decreased intrathoracic pressure increases venous return to the heart by drawing blood into the heart and the major thoracic vessels. As blood is moved into the right heart, the right heart chamber enlarges and stretches, enhancing right ventricular preload and stroke volume. During normal exhalation, there is an increase in the flow of blood from the pulmonary circulation to the left heart, increasing left ventricular preload and stroke volume. At the end of spontaneous exhalation, the output of blood decreases in both the right and left heart.

When PPV is used, the positive pressure being exerted on the lungs causes a relative increase in intratho-

TABLE 7–5. MULTISYSTEM EFFECTS OF POSITIVE PRESSURE VENTILATION

SYSTEM	EFFECTS OF PPV
Cardiovascular	Decreased cardiac output: Decreased right ventricular preload Decreased stroke volume Decreased left ventricular output *Clinical manifestations:* Decreased blood pressure (particularly in presence of hypovolemia) If compensation is present: normal blood pressure, increased heart rate, increased systemic vascular resistance
Pulmonary	Increased gas flow to nondependent lung and to central lung tissue Increased blood flow to peripheral lung tissues *Clinical manifestations:* Decreased Pa_{O_2}
Neurovascular	Decreased venous return from the head Decreased blood flow to head if cardiac output is decreased *Clinical manifestations:* Possible increased intracranial pressure Possible altered level of consciousness
Renal	Redistribution of blood flow through kidneys Decreased blood flow to the kidneys associated with decreased cardiac output *Clinical manifestations:* Decreased urine output Increased serum sodium and creatinine levels
Gastrointestinal	Decreased blood flow into the intestinal viscera Increased risk of Gastric ulcer formation Gastrointestinal bleed Hepatic dysfunction (increased bilirubin)

racic pressure, which is then transmitted to all structures in the thorax, including the heart, lungs, and major thoracic vessels. The major vessels become compressed, which creates an increase in central venous pressure (CVP). Blood return to the right heart is reduced owing to a decreased pressure gradient. The resulting reduction in venous return to the heart causes right preload and stroke volume to decrease. Left ventricular output falls as a direct result of decreased right ventricular output.

PPV reduces cardiac output by decreasing venous return to the heart in three major ways. First, as described earlier, the presence of positive intrathoracic pressure prevents blood from being pulled into the major thoracic vessels and into the heart. Second, cardiac output is reduced through a squeezing of the heart by the lungs during the inspiratory phase of PPV. Third, the amount of pressure being exerted on the alveoli is the single most important factor influencing cardiac output when considering pulmonary influences. As the level of pressure is increased, venous return to the heart decreases. The more the heart and pulmonary capillaries are squeezed by the presence of positive pressure, the lower the cardiac output. This helps explain why high levels of PEEP can dramatically reduce cardiac output. Other factors that influence the effects of PPV on the cardiovascular system include lung and thoracic compliance, airway resistance, and the patient's volemic state.

Decreased cardiac output may be manifested as a reduction in arterial blood pressure, particularly if the patient is hypovolemic. However, a normal blood pressure frequently is maintained in PPV patients through the compensatory mechanisms of increased heart rate and increased systemic vascular resistance (SVR). Hemodynamic monitoring usually shows a decreased cardiac output, increased pulmonary artery wedge pressure, and increased right atrial pressure.

Pulmonary Complications

Normally, during spontaneous breathing, the relationship between ventilation and perfusion ($\dot{V}/\dot{Q}$) is relatively balanced, with most inhaled gases flowing toward the diaphragm. The distribution of gases to the alveoli normally favors the peripheral and dependent lung areas. Likewise, pulmonary perfusion normally is the greatest in dependent areas, thus matching the lung zones with the most ventilation with the lung zones with the most perfusion.

Altered Ventilation and Perfusion

PPV alters the relationship of ventilation to perfusion in the lungs. Gases flow through the path of least resistance, which during PPV, increases ventilation to the nondependent lung areas and large airways. This is largely due to the decreased functioning and stiffening of the diaphragm associated with passive PPV. PPV gas flow increases ventilation to the healthy lung areas while flow decreases to the diseased areas, since it meets increased resistance in diseased lung tissue.

When PPV is being used, the positive pressure is transmitted to the pulmonary vessels, pushing the blood to the peripheral lung and to dependent areas. Since perfusion is now the greatest in the periphery and in the dependent lung areas and ventilation is greatest in the nondependent and larger airways, the relationship of ventilation to perfusion is altered to some degree. In areas with the most perfusion, there is decreased ventilation, and in areas with adequate ventilation, perfusion is reduced. This can create problems with oxygenation due to increased shunting which can be reflected in deteriorating $Pa{O_2}$ levels. Under certain circumstances, shunt and $\dot{V}/\dot{Q}$ matching can significantly improve during PPV. This is typically seen when PEEP is applied to treat refractory hypoxemia associated with increased shunt and decreased functional residual capacity (e.g., ARDS). In such a situation, shunt is often reduced, $\dot{V}/\dot{Q}$ matching is improved, and $Pa{O_2}$ levels may significantly improve.

Barotrauma/Volutrauma

There is increasing evidence that the pulmonary injury associated with PPV results from alveolar distention created by a combination of excessive alveolar pressure **(barotrauma)** and volume **(volutrauma).** The higher the positive pressure and/or volume applied, the greater the risk of trauma. Patients who are at the highest risk for development of barotrauma/volutrauma are those requiring high levels of PEEP and high peak airway pressures (PAP, PIP) or high tidal volumes. Barotrauma/volutrauma can manifest itself as pneumothorax, subcutaneous emphysema, or pneumomediastinum. Clinically, it should be suspected if (1) the patient has a sudden onset of agitation and cough associated with a frequent high pressure alarm, (2) the blood pressure and ABG rapidly deteriorate, (3) breath sounds suddenly are diminished or absent, or (4) subcutaneous emphysema can be palpated on the anterior neck or chest. If a pneumothorax or pneumomediastinum is diagnosed, insertion of a chest tube should be anticipated and prepared for.

Oxygen Toxicity

Oxygen toxicity is associated with the use of an oxygen concentration of ≥ 60 percent ($F{IO_2}$ of ≥ 0.6) for more than 48 hours. The use of 100 percent oxygen concentration ($F{IO_2}$ of 1.0) can cause pulmonary changes within 6 hours. Oxygen toxicity damages the endothelial lining of the lungs and decreases alveolar macrophage activity. It also decreases mucous and surfactant production. If it is allowed to continue for more than 72 hours, the patient may develop a pattern of symptoms similar to ARDS. The early signs and symptoms of oxygen toxicity are nonspecific (malaise, fatigue, and substernal discomfort). Because early symptoms are difficult to assess, the nurse should be aware of who is at risk for developing oxygen toxicity on the basis of the length of time that the patient has received an O_2 concentration of 60 percent (or even 50 percent) (Pilbeam, 1998). Changes in pulmonary mechanics are the best indicator of oxygen toxicity. A pattern of decreased lung compliance, decreased vital capacity, and increased PIP is noted.

Nosocomial Pulmonary Infection

Nosocomial pulmonary infection is a common major complication of mechanical ventilation. The passing of an ET tube from the upper airway into the lower airway introduces upper airway contaminants into the lower airway. The presence of an artificial airway bypasses the normal upper airway defense mechanisms. Contamination also occurs as a result of failure to maintain strict aseptic technique during pulmonary suctioning or use of contaminated equipment. These factors, coupled with the physiologically compromised state of most mechanically ventilated patients and tearing of the mucous membranes with tracheal suctioning, places them at high risk for development of a pulmonary infection. Signs and symptoms of a pulmonary infection include development of adventitious breath sounds and changes in sputum color or quantity. Systemically, infection may be evidenced by fever and increased white blood cell (WBC) count. Positive chest x-ray and sputum culture findings are important diagnostic tools.

Neurovascular Complications

PPV can cause a change in neurovascular status through two major mechanisms. First, intracranial pressure (ICP) can increase, and, second, cerebral perfusion pressure (CPP) can decrease. Patients who have existing intracranial or neurovascular problems are at particular risk when moderate to high ventilation pressures are required. The increased intrathoracic pressure associated with PPV decreases venous return from the head. The higher the pressure required to ventilate the patient, the greater the effects on the ICP.

Blood flow to the head (cerebral perfusion pressure) may be reduced. If cardiac output drops sufficiently to reduce systolic blood pressure, cerebral perfusion may become compromised. CPP is influenced by two factors: ICP and mean arterial blood pressure (MABP). This relationship is expressed in the statement

$$CPP = MABP - ICP$$

MABP is determined by the systolic and diastolic blood pressures. Therefore, if systolic blood pressure is reduced, so will MABP be, thus reducing CPP. If CPP drops too low, cerebral hypoxia can result.

Renal Complications

PPV is associated with decreased urinary output. The mechanisms for this decrease are multiple, and some are unclear. Two major mechanisms are decreased cardiac output and redistribution of renal blood flow.

Decreased cardiac output is associated with reduced renal perfusion and reduced glomerular filtration rate, which can cause decreased urine output. In patients who are receiving PPV, arterial blood pressure generally is maintained through compensatory mechanisms.

It is suggested that when cardiac output has not been reduced significantly, the cause of low urine output may be associated with the redistribution of intrarenal blood flow that occurs with PPV. The redistribution of blood causes changes in kidney function. PPV seems to alter renal perfusion by decreasing blood flow to the outer renal cortex and increasing flow to the inner cortex and outer medullary tissue, where the juxtamedullary nephrons are located. This results in a 40 percent net decrease in urinary output, and less sodium and creatinine are excreted. When sodium is reabsorbed, water also is reabsorbed to maintain homeostasis, thus reducing urine output.

Gastrointestinal Complications

PPV can decrease blood flow into the intestinal viscera by increasing visceral vascular resistance. The increased resistance to flow can result in tissue ischemia, which causes increased permeability of the protective mucosal lining. This predisposes the ventilator patient to gastric ulcer formation and gastrointestinal bleeding. In addition, some patients develop hepatic dysfunction even if there is no history of liver disease.

Gastrointestinal bleeding occurs in approximately 25 percent of patients on mechanical ventilators through development of stress ulcers. Stress ulcers develop as a result of either gastric hyperacidity or, more commonly, from a transient visceral hypoxic episode. In the mechanically ventilated patient, the tissue hypoxia may have occurred related to acute respiratory failure or may be the result of increased resistance to blood flow in the viscera. Stress ulcers, which usually are shallow erosions in the mucosal lining, often cause slow bleeds and may, therefore, not be diagnosed early in their development. For this reason, it is important to check all stools for guaiac.

Clinically, the patient exhibits a decreasing hematocrit and guaiac-positive stools. Stools may be black or dark red. If the ulcer formation is gastric, nasogastric aspirate will be guaiac-positive, and the aspirate appears bright red to dark red. Preventive interventions include the use of antacids, histamine (H_2) antagonists, or both to maintain a gastric pH of > 3.5.

In summary, there are many potential complications associated with mechanical ventilation. Cardiovascular complications are those associated with a significantly reduced cardiac output. PEEP is especially associated with cardiovascular compromise. Pulmonary complications include altered ventilation and perfusion and increased shunt, which can decrease oxygenation; barotrauma/volutrauma, associated mostly with higher levels of PEEP and high tidal volumes; oxygen toxicity, which occurs with higher levels of oxygen for a prolonged period of time (oxygen toxicity has been attributed to the development of ARDS); and nosocomial pulmonary infection. Neurovascular complications include increased intracranial pressure and decreased cerebral perfusion pressure. The primary renal complication is decreased urine output, which can be severely reduced. Gastrointestinal complications include development of stress ulcers, gastrointestinal bleeding, and hepatic dysfunction.

SECTION SEVEN REVIEW

1. PPV affects the cardiovascular system by
   A. increasing cardiac output
   B. decreasing venous return to the heart
   C. increasing arterial blood pressure
   D. increasing venous return to the heart
2. Changes in cardiac output resulting from positive pressure ventilation are associated with which of the following manifestations?
   A. increased arterial blood pressure
   B. increased urinary output
   C. arrhythmia development
   D. decreased pulse rate
3. PPV alters the relationship of ventilation to perfusion in what way?
   A. ventilation increases in nondependent lung areas
   B. ventilation increases in the small airways
   C. perfusion increases in the nondependent lung areas
   D. perfusion increases near the large airways
4. Which of the following are manifestations of pulmonary barotrauma/volutrauma secondary to mechanical ventilation?
   A. onset of increased lethargy
   B. increase in arterial blood pressure
   C. increase in breath sounds over a lung field
   D. increased cough with high pressure alarm triggering
5. Oxygen toxicity affects the pulmonary tissue in which of the following ways?
   A. decreasing macrophage activity
   B. increasing mucous production
   C. increasing surfactant production
   D. decreasing PIP
6. Patients receiving mechanical ventilation are at increased risk of developing a nosocomial pulmonary infection because
   A. the lower airway is defenseless
   B. macrophage activity has been bypassed
   C. normal upper airway defenses are bypassed
   D. normal pulmonary mechanics have been interfered with
7. PPV influences ICP by
   A. decreasing intrathoracic pressure
   B. increasing cerebral perfusion pressure
   C. decreasing venous drainage from the head
   D. increasing MABP
8. The kidneys are affected by PPV in what way?
   A. decreased sodium retention
   B. redistribution of renal blood flow
   C. renal effects of increased cardiac output
   D. redistribution of urine flow through the kidneys
9. The gastrointestinal system may be adversely affected by PPV due to
   A. increased visceral vascular resistance
   B. increased blood supply to the viscera
   C. increased venous pooling in the viscera
   D. decreased visceral vascular resistance
10. Gastrointestinal bleeding secondary to mechanical ventilation most frequently manifests itself as
    A. grossly bloody stools
    B. guaiac-positive stools
    C. grossly bloody nasogastric drainage
    D. guaiac-negative nasogastric drainage

Answers: 1. B, 2. C, 3. A, 4. D, 5. A, 6. C, 7. C, 8. B, 9. A, 10. B

SECTION EIGHT: Artificial Airway Complications

At the completion of this section, the learner will be able to explain the cause and prevention of artificial airway complications.

Artificial airways have their own set of complications that are primarily related to pressure damage.

Nasal Damage

Placing an artificial airway through the nasal passage is associated with trauma to nasal mucous membranes during the passing of the tube. In addition, ischemia and even necrosis of the nares may develop caused by the pressure the tube exerts against the internal nasal wall. Anchoring the tube to the cheeks rather than to the top of the nose helps prevent pressure damage. Choice of the proper size tube also is important in minimizing the risk of damage. Nasotracheal tubes can cause inner ear problems related to their location. The nasotracheal tube can occlude the eustachian tubes, which increases the risk of development of ear pressure problems or inner ear infection.

Cuff Trauma

Although the use of tracheal cuffs is necessary to mechanically ventilate the patient properly, they are associated with potentially severe tracheal and laryngeal injuries. The use of excessive cuff pressures is the major contributing factor in these injuries. Arterial capillary blood flow pressure through the trachea is low (< 30 mm Hg). A high-pressure force, such as is delivered by an overinflated cuff, exerts a pressure that is higher than capillary pressure, causing circulation in the cuffed area to be compromised. Decreased or obliterated blood flow to an area of tissue causes ischemia, which, if allowed to continue for an extended period, can produce necrosis. Necrosis of the trachea, larynx, or both is associated with the development of fistulas, fibrosis, and ulceration.

Proper monitoring and control of cuff pressures decreases the risk of complications significantly. Cuff pressures must be monitored at least once every shift. Safe cuff pressure ranges between 20 and 25 mm Hg (27 to 34 cm H_2O). If a cuff manometer is not available, it is simple to make one using a three-way or four-way stopcock, a 10-mL syringe, and a sphygmomanometer (Fig. 7–9).

A minimum occluding pressure technique may also be used to reduce the risk of pressure-related cuff damage. Using this technique, the cuff is inflated only to the point at which it seals the airway during the mechanical ventilation. Cuff pressure should be regularly checked using this technique and should not exceed 20 to 25 mm Hg.

Artificial airways can damage one or both vocal cords as a result of traumatic introduction of the tube or damage related to pressure of the tube against the cords. Fistula formation is also a major concern. Should tracheal injury from a cuff cause a fistula to form between the trachea and esophagus, gastric secretions can be aspirated into the lungs. Tracheoesophageal (TE) fistulas should be suspected if tube feeding or food is aspirated during tracheal suctioning. The patient can be tested for a TE fistula by placing food dye in food products, such as liquid drinks or tube feedings. During ET suctioning, the secretions are monitored for the presence of the food dye, which, if present, is indicative of esophageal contents in the lower airway. Proper cuff technique and use of correct tube size can minimize cuff-related complications.

In summary, the patient who requires an artificial airway is at risk for developing a complication related to its use. Artificial airway complications are primarily due to the effects of pressure on delicate mucous membranes. Nasal damage may occur during passage of the tube or

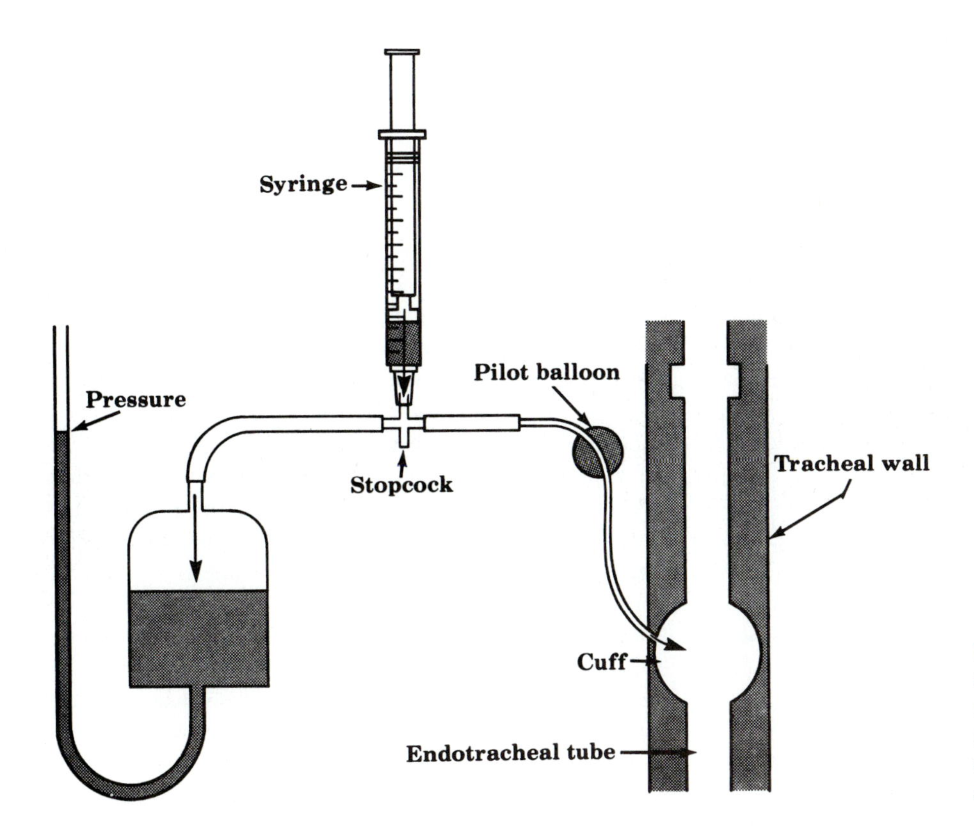

Figure 7–9. The use of syringe, mercury manometer, and three-way stopcock for measuring cuff pressure. *(From Pilbeam, S.P. [1992].* Mechanical ventilation: Physiological and clinical applications, *3rd ed. [p. 294]. St. Louis: C.V. Mosby.)*

may be caused by the pressure of the tube against the nares or nasal passage. Cuff trauma is caused by excessive pressure being exerted against the trachea, compromising blood flow to the surrounding mucosa. Cuff pressures should be measured on a regular basis and should be maintained at 20 to 25 mm Hg (27 to 34 cm H_2O). The use of a minimum occluding pressure technique also can be used to reduce the chances of damage to the trachea. The presence of an artificial airway can damage one or both vocal cords. The formation of a TE fistula is a potentially serious complication that can cause aspiration of esophageal or stomach contents into the lower airways. Placing food dye in oral or tube feedings can test for the presence of a TE fistula.

SECTION EIGHT REVIEW

1. The presence of a nasotracheal tube can affect the ears because it can
   A. occlude the eustachian tubes
   B. exert direct pressure on the inner ears
   C. cause inner ear ischemia
   D. directly damage the eustachian tubes
2. High endotracheal tube cuff pressures can damage the trachea when cuff pressure is
   A. increased during coughing
   B. reduced due to a leak
   C. lower than surrounding capillary pressure
   D. higher than surrounding capillary pressure
3. Normal tracheal capillary pressure is about _____ mm Hg.
   A. < 10
   B. < 20
   C. < 30
   D. < 40
4. Safe tracheal cuff pressure ranges are _____ mm Hg.
   A. 10 to 15
   B. 15 to 20
   C. 20 to 25
   D. 25 to 30
5. TE fistula formation secondary to tracheal cuff complications can cause
   A. sepsis
   B. aspiration pneumonia
   C. gastric ulcerations
   D. esophageal varices

Answers: 1. A, 2. D, 3. C, 4. C, 5. B

SECTION NINE: Care of the Patient Requiring Mechanical Ventilation

At the completion of this section, the learner will be able to describe care of the patient requiring mechanical ventilation.

Patient Care Goals

The general goals and outcome criteria appropriate to the management of a patient receiving mechanical ventilation may be divided into two major groupings: support of physiologic needs and support of psychosocial needs.

Support of Physiologic Needs
Support of the patient's physiologic needs is accomplished through interventions that promote optimal oxygenation, provide adequate ventilation, protect the airway, support tissue perfusion, and provide adequate nutrition.

Support of Psychosocial Needs
Support of the patient's psychosocial needs centers around interventions to reduce anxiety, provide a balance of sleep and activity, promote communication, and support the family.

Nursing Management of Physiologic Needs

The patient's nursing management is planned around interventions to attain the patient care goals. The first three goals—promote optimal oxygenation, provide adequate ventilation, and protect the patient's airway—are all addressed through implementation of the three pulmonary-related nursing diagnoses, as follows.

Ineffective Airway Clearance
The patient who requires conventional positive pressure ventilation will have an endotracheal or tracheostomy tube inserted to access and seal off the lower airway. The length and relatively small internal diameter of artificial airways (particularly ET tubes) make it difficult, if not impossible, for the patient to clear his or her own airway. The problem of airway clearance is often compounded by general weakness and fatigue or diminished level of responsiveness, any of which also hinders airway clearance.

Airway clearance is a top-priority nursing goal in management of the patient with an artificial airway. If airway patency is not maintained, the patient's breathing and cardiovascular status eventually will fail due to hypoxia or hypercarbia.

> Remember to apply the ABCs—Airway, Breathing, Circulation—in that order.

The primary reason that airway patency becomes compromised is airway obstruction caused by excessive, thick, or pooled secretions. Each of these situations must be managed properly by the nurse.

EXCESSIVE SECRETIONS. Excessive secretions are removed by suctioning the artificial airway on an as-necessary basis, which may be every few minutes during initial intubation to several times a shift in chronic intubation. The patient's breath sounds should be assessed every 1 to 2 hours for the presence of secretions. If adventitious breath sounds are auscultated in the large airways, suctioning should be performed. Coughing, whether or not it sets off the ventilator's high pressure alarm, may indicate a need for suctioning. The nurse often can hear the secretions without the use of a stethoscope, particularly during coughing. Coughing, however, can occur due to tracheal irritation or bronchospasm or because the tip of the airway is touching the carina. The last two situations can precipitate severe coughing spasms. Because coughing may occur without the presence of secretions in the large airways, the nurse should assess the situation first. Unnecessary suctioning causes needless trauma to the delicate mucous membranes in the trachea and also depletes oxygen levels.

Good rules to apply are:

- Always assess before suctioning.
- Do not suction unnecessarily.
- Follow approved protocols for suctioning.
- Monitor the patient closely for adverse effects of suctioning, such as arrhythmias and hypoxia.

In most circumstances, the nurse will maintain PaO_2 levels during suctioning if the following common protocol is maintained.

Step 1. Hyperoxygenate/hyperventilate. Deliver 100 percent oxygen accompanied by manually ventilating the patient with a resuscitation (Ambu) bag for four to five breaths (two-handed ventilating will give significantly larger breaths than one-handed ventilating).

Step 2. Suction. Use moderate, not high, suction pressure. If secretions are too thick to be aspirated, instill approximately 3 mL of sterile saline down the airway during hyperventilation. Apply suction only on withdrawal, rotating the catheter while using intermittent suction and withdrawing the catheter within 10 seconds. Repeat Steps 1 and 2 until the airway is cleared.

Step 3. Return the patient to the ventilator.

There are many variations to suctioning protocols. Some hospitals only hyperoxygenate by temporarily increasing the ventilator's oxygen concentration (FIO_2) to 100 percent (for 1 to 5 minutes). Hyperventilation may be part of such a policy. Hyperventilation can be accomplished through a sigh or other intermittent large inhaled volume mechanism on the ventilator that, when manually triggered, will deliver a breath that is 1.5 to ≥ 2 times the patient's set tidal volume. In patients with acute neurologic injury, protocol may call for initial hyperoxygenation/hyperventilation for 1 or more minutes before initiation of the suctioning protocol. The practice of instilling saline as part of the routine suctioning protocol remains controversial and may or may not be part of an institution's suctioning policy.

Suction catheters can be divided into two major groups: open and closed systems. Both systems are used for suctioning artificial airways, but only open systems are used without an artificial airway in place. Each type of system has its own suctioning protocol. Closed system catheters are self-contained within a sheath attached directly to the artificial airway. A closed catheter system remains in the artificial airway system between suctioning, allowing it to be used multiple times. Open systems generally are single-use catheters and require introduction of the catheter into the artificial airway from outside the artificial airway system. Further discussion of suctioning systems is beyond the scope of this module.

If the patient is receiving PEEP, a different suctioning protocol may be required. Patients on PEEP often do not tolerate being detached from the ventilator for any reason. Loss of PEEP can precipitate oxygen desaturation and may make the patient hemodynamically unstable. Several approaches may be used: (1) the usual suctioning protocol, (2) the usual suctioning protocol using a manual resuscitation bag that has a special PEEP attachment, set at the prescribed PEEP level, or (3) suctioning without removing the patient from the ventilator by either an in-line closed suction system or introducing a suction catheter into the closed system through a special port on top of the ventilator adaptor nozzle. Research is continuing on which type of suctioning system and protocol is best in specific situations. All types of suctioning have associated problems, including infection, hypoxia, trauma, arrhythmias, trauma to mucous membranes, and others.

THICK SECRETIONS. Thick secretions are a common challenge to maintaining effective airway clearance. Properly hydrating the patient is the most important means of thinning secretions, since secretions are composed primarily of water. A fluid intake of 2 to 2.5 L/day is recommended unless it is contraindicated. Mechanically ventilated patients receive warmed, humidified gases that facilitate liquefication of secretions. Intermittent nebulizer treatments of normal saline or mucolytics may be ordered to liquefy secretions.

POOLED SECRETIONS. Pooled secretions can cause obstruction of major airways or can plug the tip of the artificial airway. Proper suctioning, liquefying secretions, and turning the patient every 1 to 2 hours all help prevent obstruction by pooling.

Impaired Gas Exchange

Treatment of impaired gas exchange is the major reason for placing patients on a mechanical ventilator (i.e., impending ventilatory failure or acute respiratory failure). Ventilators can manipulate carbon dioxide levels directly by causing alveolar hyperventilation or hypoventilation.

Alveolar hyperventilation is associated with decreasing carbon dioxide levels and respiratory alkalosis. It can be patient induced if the patient is on the A/C mode and is hyperventilating for any reason (e.g., anxiety, pain, head injury), since he or she can blow off too much carbon dioxide. It also can be induced mechanically by setting the rate and/or tidal volume too high on the ventilator. Sometimes, as in patients with increased intracranial pressure, mild respiratory alkalosis is induced intentionally to facilitate cerebral vasoconstriction through low carbon dioxide levels.

Alveolar hypoventilation is associated with increasing carbon dioxide levels and respiratory acidosis. Hypoventilation may be patient induced, for example, in the patient on SIMV mode (or other spontaneous breathing mode) whose breathing is very shallow. It also can be induced mechanically by setting the rate and/or tidal volume too low on the ventilator.

A changing ABG trend may indicate a change in the patient's respiratory or metabolic status, reflecting improvement or deterioration in his or her condition. The cause of the imbalance must be found and treated to correct the imbalance. It is the nurse's responsibility to monitor the ABG trends, observe the patient's condition, notify the physician of increasing abnormalities, follow up on orders received, and monitor the ventilator settings at established intervals. The nurse also can facilitate gas exchange by taking actions to maintain airway clearance and effective breathing patterns.

Ineffective Breathing Patterns

Patients may be placed on the mechanical ventilator because of ineffective breathing patterns, which consist of any significant changes in the breathing rate, rhythm, or depth from the patient's baseline normals (e.g., tachypnea, bradypnea, apnea, hypoventilation, hyperventilation). Changes in breathing patterns can affect oxygenation and acid–base status, as previously described.

Breathing patterns that remain too rapid must be controlled once the patient is placed on the ventilator, to prevent hyperventilation problems. A variety of analgesics (e.g., IV morphine) or sedatives (e.g., benzodiazepines, such as Valium and Ativan) may be ordered. In some patients, a neuromuscular blocking agent (e.g., curare or pancuronium) may be ordered if the breathing pattern is adversely affecting the patient's progress and cannot be controlled using analgesics or sedatives. The nurse should assess for possible causes of the rapid pattern and take steps to relieve the problem when possible. Rapid breathing patterns may stem from fear, anxiety, pain, or such physiologic problems as acid–base imbalance or head injury.

Protection of the Airway

Protecting the airway is a major goal in caring for the mechanically ventilated patient. Any artificial airway can be fairly easily dislodged, either partially or completely. Because of this, the nurse must always take steps to minimize the possibility of dislodgment, which could precipitate respiratory compromise. During bedside care, dislodgment is at the highest risk while moving the patient from side to side in bed or when transferring the patient into or out of bed. Certain nursing actions minimize this risk, such as (1) maintaining sufficient slack on the ventilator tubing to minimize tension on the airway during moving, (2) disconnecting the patient from the ventilator and manually ventilating during transfer into and out of bed, and (3) adequately securing the airway through correct taping or other stabilizing device. Tracheostomy tubes often are sutured in place as well as being tied around the neck. Securing an ET tube using twill tape may not stabilize the tube sufficiently to prevent accidental dislodgment.

If the patient is not fully oriented or is uncooperative, he or she may pull the airway out. To prevent accidental or intentional dislodgment by the patient, many hospitals have a standard policy of applying soft wrist restraints at all times to patients on a mechanical ventilator. When restraints are in use, neurovascular checks should be performed routinely distal to the restraints. The purpose of the restraints must be explained and intermittently reinforced to both the patient and family, emphasizing that the restraints are in place for protection of the airway. Patients and families frequently view restraints as a punishment or unnecessary restriction of freedom.

Alteration in Cardiac Output

The general goal, support tissue perfusion, can be addressed using the nursing diagnosis *Alteration in cardiac output: decreased*. Positive pressure ventilation profoundly affects the normal hemodynamics of the body by increasing intrathoracic pressures and decreasing venous return to the heart, which decreases cardiac output. The use of PEEP further compromises cardiac output by further decreasing venous return. These effects are described in detail in Section Seven.

HEMODYNAMIC EFFECTS OF MECHANICAL VENTILATION. While on the mechanical ventilator, the patient may have a pulmonary artery flow-directed catheter inserted to closely monitor hemodynamic status, particularly if

TABLE 7–6. HEMODYNAMIC EFFECTS OF MECHANICAL VENTILATION

MEASURED PULMONARY ARTERY CATHETER PARAMETER	TREND
Right atrial pressure	Increased
Pulmonary artery pressure	Increased
Pulmonary artery wedge pressure	Usually increased
Left atrial pressure	Usually increased
Peripheral arterial pressure	Unchanged or decreased
Cardiac output	Decreased

there is a history of cardiovascular problems. Table 7–6 shows the hemodynamic trends associated with mechanical ventilation.

If the patient does not have a pulmonary artery catheter inserted, the nurse can assess for the clinical manifestations of decreased cardiac output, such as confusion, restlessness, decreased urine output, flattened neck veins, and clammy, cool skin. Management of the patient with decreased cardiac output is described in detail in the perfusion modules of the textbook.

Alteration in Nutrition

Many patients who require mechanical ventilation have preexisting malnutrition associated with chronic illness, with inadequate nutritional support, during hospitalization or a combination of both. This patient population is at high risk for *Alteration in nutrition: less than body requirements*. During the acute phase of illness, the patient will maintain an NPO status. The presence of an ET tube, even with a properly inflated cuff, places the patient at risk for aspiration of microparticles that can leak around the endotracheal cuff and contaminate the lower airway. This leakage can precipitate complications associated with aspiration. Avoiding food and fluids by the oral route and maintaining excellent oral hygiene, including frequent oral suctioning, reduce the risk of microaspiration.

Maintaining a malnourished state with its negative nitrogen balance will significantly decrease the patient's chances of successful weaning from the mechanical ventilator because of respiratory muscle atrophy and weakness. Regaining nutritional integrity is a crucial aspect of care management because it has a direct impact on the patient's ability to improve his or her condition.

While on mechanical ventilation, the patient has a small-bore feeding tube inserted, either nasogastric or nasoenteric. Feedings ideally are initiated within 3 days of artificial airway placement to prevent gastrointestinal complications and to initiate early nutritional support. Pulmonary patients may require special consideration of carbohydrate loading because of the high carbon dioxide by-product produced, which can further complicate acid–base balance. Management of the patient with alterations in nutrition is detailed in Module 22.

Nursing Management of Psychosocial Needs

The psychosocial needs of the high-acuity patient are presented in depth in Module 1. The following is a brief discussion of psychosocial needs specific to mechanical ventilation.

Anxiety

The patient who is being mechanically ventilated is usually experiencing a high level of anxiety associated with the insertion of the ET tube, the mechanical ventilator, and the critical care environment. Anxiety is a common complaint of patients who have chronic respiratory problems. Many chronic pulmonary diseases are progressive in nature, thus a pattern of increasing disability is experienced.

As many chronic pulmonary diseases progress, patients experience an increasing pattern of hospital admissions for complications of their disease. Ultimately, at end-stage disease, these patients most commonly die of complications of their disease, such as severe respiratory failure or cor pulmonale.

When patients are experiencing acute respiratory distress, they often are anxious. Severe dyspnea frequently is associated with fear of suffocation or dying. All energy is focused toward breathing when acute distress exists. Being placed on a mechanical ventilator may be received by the patient either with relief or with an increased state of anxiety. The nursing diagnosis to deal with this problem is *Anxiety*, which is associated with the unfamiliar environment, unfamiliar invasive breathing assist device, loss of control, painful procedures, lack of understanding or procedures, and fear of dying.

Management of the patient's anxiety while on the mechanical ventilator combines collaborative and independent nursing interventions. Sedation commonly is ordered to decrease anxiety levels, which, in turn, helps the patient breathe with the ventilator. The sedation may be in the form of narcotics or sedatives. A high-anxiety state must be brought under control if the patient is to decrease the work of breathing and oxygen consumption. Narcotics are particularly useful if the breathing pattern must be subdued, because they have a respiratory depressant side effect. This is sometimes the case in patients who have uncontrolled tachypnea. When oxygen consumption is very high, it may be decided to use a neuromuscular blocking agent to paralyze the respiratory muscles, producing rapid apnea and total skeletal muscle paralysis. Neuromuscular blocking agents do not alter the responsiveness level of the patient. Therefore, while in the paralyzed state, this group of patients should receive intermittent IV sedation at regular intervals to reduce anxiety and to enhance mental rest.

Nursing interventions regarding anxiety include

- Monitoring for anxiety status
- Implementing measures to reduce anxiety
- Maintaining a restful environment

- Explaining all procedures and diagnostic tests
- Assessing for therapeutic and nontherapeutic effects of sedation

Sleep Pattern Disturbance

While on the ventilator, the patient experiences interruptions throughout the 24-hour day. Airway clearance and other maintenance nursing interventions frequently require disturbing a resting or sleeping high-acuity patient. The nursing diagnosis addressing this problem is *Sleep pattern disturbance*.

Management of this problem often is a matter of careful planning on the part of the nurse. Clustering activities to allow for prolonged periods of undisturbed rest, particularly during the night hours, is a nursing goal. Minimizing interruptions at night for suctioning and turning and other high-priority interventions requires coordination and good communication among the entire nursing team.

Communication and Sensation

The presence of an artificial airway prevents the patient from communicating verbally. This alteration is addressed in the nursing diagnosis *Impaired verbal communication*. The patient may require frequent reminders that he or she will be able to talk once the tube is removed, with a brief explanation of why speech is not possible at this time. The patient who is fully responsive may become very frustrated when he or she cannot be understood. Alternative communication methods are available. To evaluate appropriate types of communication alternatives, the nurse must evaluate the patient's visual status. If eyesight is poor or glasses are not available, communication alternatives are reduced significantly.

The nurse has a variety of communication alternatives from which to experiment for effectiveness; for example, an alphabet or picture board for the patient to point to. Alphabet boards are not very satisfactory for many patients because they cannot concentrate sufficiently or do not have the strength to point to multiple letters for writing a message. Some facilities have a talking board, on which the patient touches the appropriate picture and the board verbally states the particular need. Use of any type of picture board depends on the patient's ability to see the pictures. Some patients are able to write on a board with paper and pencil or other type of writing board, such as a magic slate or small chalkboard.

Patience on the part of the nurse is a major component of successful communication with a mechanically ventilated patient. Simple needs often can be expressed through lip reading or hand signals. It is easier to lip read with a patient who has a nasotracheal tube rather than an orally placed tube.

Family Support

The psychosocial needs of the patient's family cannot be forgotten while he or she is being managed on the ventilator. Families vary on how they perceive the ventilator. The family may express relief that the patient's breathing status is now protected. This is particularly true of families of patients who have had several past intubations. The patient's family initially may find the presence of the artificial airway and mechanical ventilator a frightening experience. The frequent alarms and the patient's inability to communicate verbally are the basis of many of the questions asked of the nurse. Family members must be oriented to the equipment in direct simple terms. Frequent updates should be given on the patient's status in terms they can understand. It also is appropriate to remind the family, as necessary, that the patient will be able to talk once the tube is removed if a temporary tracheostomy or ET tube is in place. The nurse may have to translate communications from the patient to his or her family members.

In summary, care of the patient requiring mechanical ventilation involves interdisciplinary support of physiologic and psychosocial needs. Pulmonary physiologic needs focus on promoting optimal oxygenation, providing adequate ventilation, and protecting the patient's airway. In addition, the physiologic needs of tissue perfusion and nutritional support require aggressive attention. Psychosocial problems include anxiety, sleep pattern disturbance, and impaired verbal communication. The mechanically ventilated patient may require numerous additional nursing diagnoses based on specific functional needs associated with specific disease processes and multisystem dysfunction.

SECTION NINE REVIEW

1. The primary reason that airway patency becomes compromised in the mechanically ventilated patient is
   A. ineffective cough
   B. oversedation
   C. airway obstruction
   D. dehydration
2. Unless contraindicated, the patient should receive a fluid intake of _____ to _____ liters per day to combat thick secretions.

A. 1, 1.5
B. 2, 2.5
C. 3, 3.5
D. 4, 4.5

3. The mechanically ventilated patient can develop respiratory alkalosis if the _____ and _____ settings on the mechanical ventilator are set too high.
   A. rate, tidal volume
   B. peak airway pressure, rate
   C. O_2 concentration, peak airway pressure
   D. tidal volume, O_2 concentration
4. A mechanically ventilated patient who is malnourished is at high risk for failure to wean due to
   A. impaired gas exchange
   B. decreased cardiac output
   C. increased airway resistance
   D. respiratory muscle weakness
5. To treat the nursing diagnosis, *Sleep pattern disturbance*, while managing the care of a mechanically ventilated patient, the *best* nursing action would be to
   A. cluster activities
   B. administer sedatives
   C. administer neuromuscular blocking agents
   D. space activities evenly throughout the 24-hour day

Answers: 1. C, 2. B, 3. A, 4. D, 5. A

SECTION TEN: Weaning the Patient from the Mechanical Ventilator

At the completion of this section, the learner will be able to describe the **weaning** process.

The term *mechanical ventilator weaning* refers to the activities involved in withdrawing a patient from mechanical ventilator support and attaining total independence from the ventilator. Withdrawing mechanical ventilator support is a multidisciplinary effort that requires coordination between the physician, respiratory therapist, nurse, and patient. Ventilator weaning may be a relatively simple and rapid withdrawal process or it may be complex and extremely slow. The majority of patients requiring mechanical ventilator support are weaned rapidly with little difficulty. The remaining few are those who require prolonged weaning or are unable to wean. This small but significant group primarily consists of patients who have a history of chronic pulmonary disease or who have required prolonged mechanical ventilation. This section presents a brief overview of the weaning process that will familiarize the learner with major assessments and interventions that are an integral part of the process.

Shelledy (1999) divides patients who are being evaluated for ventilator weaning into three categories:

1. Patients whose removal is rapid and require only the routine weaning activities.
2. Patients whose removal is slow and gradual and require more deliberate planning than the usual routine weaning activities.
3. Patients who are considered unweanable (ventilator-dependent) and require special approaches to the weaning process.

The Weaning Process

Just as criteria are used in making the decision to place a patient on a mechanical ventilator, criteria are used when determining readiness for withdrawal from ventilator support. Successful weaning involves using a systematic approach, including determination of readiness to wean, weaning, and postextubation follow-up.

Determination of Readiness to Wean

Successful weaning is largely dependent on the physiologic and psychologic readiness of the patient. A variety of criteria are used to determine readiness; these criteria can be divided into simple and comprehensive patient screenings.

SIMPLE PATIENT SCREENING. According to Shelledy (1999), several simple questions can be asked that can rapidly identify patients who are *not* yet ready for weaning. These questions are

- Has the problem that precipitated the need for mechanical ventilation resolved?
- Is the patient's clinical condition stable?
- Is the patient's clinical condition improving?

If the answer to any of these questions is "no," the patient is at increased risk for failure to wean.

COMPREHENSIVE PATIENT SCREENING. The decision of when it is appropriate to start the weaning process is not necessarily a clear one. Generally, prior to making a final decision, a multisystem assessment review is conducted, focusing on those physiologic systems that are particularly associated with ventilator dependence (respiratory, cardiovascular, CNS, renal, and metabolic). Inadequate functioning of any of these systems increases the risk of failure to wean (Shelledy, 1999). Table 7–7 presents an

TABLE 7–7. MECHANICAL VENTILATOR WEANING CRITERIA

CRITERIA	RESPONSES
I. Initial Criteria:	
A. Is the patient clinically stable?	Yes/No
B. Is the patient's clinical condition improving?	Yes/No
C. Is precipitating problem resolved?	Yes/No
D. Is $\dot{V}_E$ < 10 L/min on A/C or SIMV of ≤ 14?	Yes/No
E. Is Spo_2 ≥ 90% at ≤ 0.40 Fio_2?	Yes/No
F. Is A-a gradient < 100 mm Hg?	Yes/No
If any "No" answers, quit here. Patient does not qualify for initiation of weaning. Reevaluate in 48 hours.	
II. Comprehensive Criteria: Is the patient:	
A. Hemodynamically stable?	
1. SBP 100–150, DBP 60–90 mm Hg at rest?	Yes/No
2. Heart rate 60–100 beats/min at rest?	Yes/No
3. Usual ECG pattern?	Yes/No
B. Systemically hydrated?	
1. I = O	Yes/No
2. Urinary output > 620 mL/24 hr	Yes/No
3. BUN and creatinine: WNL	Yes/No
C. Without fever or new/unresolved pulmonary infection? (Chest x-ray within past 48 hr; temp. < 100°F orally)	Yes/No
D. Receiving support for nutritional status?	Yes/No
E. Have drugs been discontinued that	
1. decrease respiratory drive?	Yes/No
2. increase muscle weakness?	Yes/No
3. increase anxiety?	Yes/No
III. Laboratory Values Are the following parameters in at least minimal acceptable ranges and current within the last 24 hours? Specify "Yes" if replacement therapy is occurring if value is below normal range.	
A. K^+ (normal, 3.5–5.0 mEq/L)	Yes/No
B. Na^+ (normal, 135–145 mEq/L)	Yes/No
C. PO_4 (normal, 3.0–4.5 mg/dL, acceptable > 2.0)	Yes/No
D. Ca^{++} (normal, 8.5–10.5 mg/dL)	Yes/No
E. Mg^{++} (normal, 1.5–4.5 mg/dL)	Yes/No
F. Prealbumin (normal, 24–30 mg/dL, acceptable ≥ 10)	Yes/No
G. CBC with differential, specifically:	
WBC (normal, 5,000–10,000/μL)	Yes/No
Hgb (normal, > 10 g/dL)	Yes/No
Hct (normal, > 30 g/dL)	Yes/No
Calculated total lymphocyte count (normal, ≥ 1500 or 2,000/μL)	Yes/No
H. Theophylline level (normal, < 20 μg/dL)	Yes/No
I. ABG while on ventilator within the past 12 hours:	
pH = 7.35–7.45	Yes/No
Po_2 = ≥ 60 mm Hg on Fio_2 of ≥ 0.4	Yes/No
Pco_2 = < 50 mm Hg or within 10 mm Hg of baseline	Yes/No
Sao_2 = ≥ 90% at ≤ 0.40 Fio_2	Yes/No

If there are any "No" answers to the criteria in Sections II and III, the decision to initiate weaning will be closely evaluated. If the problem is easily correctable, appropriate interventions will be taken to correct the problem and the patient will be reevaluated after 24 hours.

example of a combined simple and comprehensive assessment form that might be used in helping to determine readiness for weaning. Note the number of criteria that focus on nutrition and metabolic function.

Assessment data provided by the simple and comprehensive patient screenings identify potential barriers to successful weaning and actions that must be taken to resolve each problem. It is at this point in the weaning process that actions vary widely. Barriers to successful weaning are not necessarily considered equal and experts disagree regarding which criteria are absolute and which are relative contraindications. For this reason, weaning may be initiated on patients who do not meet all the simple or comprehensive criteria (e.g., presence of active but improving pneumonia; improving but not corrected malnutrition).

Alternative Indications of Readiness to Wean

The traditional criteria for readiness to wean are similar to the criteria used in deciding to place the patient on the mechanical ventilator. These criteria are useful primarily for assessing the readiness of short-term, relatively healthy individuals. They have not, however, been found to effectively predict weaning success in the elderly or those with chronic pulmonary disease (patients who make up a high proportion of the difficult-to-wean group). Interest in finding better indicators of weaning readiness is strong. It is hoped that these new indicators will be more predictive of successful weaning in the difficult-to-wean population.

Weaning

RAPID WEANING (SHORT-TERM). Frequently, a patient with no significant lung disease requires short-term mechanical ventilation (e.g., surgery, drug overdose). Once the underlying problem is corrected (e.g., reversal of anesthesia effects), the patient is evaluated for weaning. Shelledy (1999) suggests the following rapid weaning routine: If weaning criteria are met, the patient is removed from the ventilator and placed on a T-piece for 30 minutes. During the trial period, the patient is monitored for comfort, ECG status, and ABG status. If these criteria remain within acceptable limits (PaO_2 remaining stable, pH stable and above 7.30), the patient is extubated. Rapid weaning may also be accomplished using PSV or CPAP. The patient is given a brief trial period and then extubated.

SLOW WEANING (LONG-TERM). Patients who have underlying chronic lung disease (e.g., emphysema or pulmonary fibrosis) that is complicated by some acute problem (e.g., pneumonia) frequently cannot be weaned as rapidly as patients with normal lungs. Slow weaning is performed on patients who are resistant to weaning for a variety of reasons. Problems associated with difficult weaning include excessive respiratory muscle work of breathing, respiratory muscle fatigue, anemia, malnutrition, excessive secretions, infection, unstable hemodynamic state, fear, and anxiety. Difficult-to-wean patients often are in a poorer state of general health than the fast weaning group. Their ability to make the transition back to spontaneous negative pressure breathing from long-term positive pressure breathing is slow and requires retraining and restrengthening of the respiratory muscles.

Slow weaning is a complex and difficult process for all involved. Over time, multiple weaning alternatives (IMV/SIMV, MMV, PSV, manual weaning) may need to be employed in response to changes in the patient's clinical status. Long-term weaning requires close monitoring of the patient's multisystem functions, as well as his or her psychosocial status. Rapid, aggressive management of problems as they arise significantly improves the chances for successful weaning.

Methods of Weaning

Manual Weaning. Manual weaning was the original method of withdrawing a patient from a ventilator, and it is still used. Manual weaning is accomplished through following a schedule of removal from the mechanical ventilator for increasing periods of time. When this method is used the patient is taken off the ventilator and the artificial airway is attached to a humidified oxygen source using a T-piece. The nurse is responsible for closely monitoring the patient for signs of weaning intolerance, such as respiratory rate > 30/min, a significant increase in blood pressure and pulse, a minute ventilation of over 10 L/min, development of cyanosis, or a decrease in oxygen saturation on pulse oximetry to below the patient's acceptable level.

Manual weaning requires close patient contact throughout the weaning period, since the nurse plays a crucial part in patient monitoring and coaching correct breathing rate and depth for the trial period. The nurse's calm reassurance is instrumental in assisting the patient past the period of anxiety often associated with removal from the mechanical ventilator. Manual weaning is performed on an increasing schedule either throughout the 24-hour period or throughout the day and evening. The amount of time the patient is kept off the ventilator may start at 5 minutes and increase to the entire day, except at night, before full independence. Manual weaning must be individually designed, based on the patient's changing status from day to day.

Manual weaning is a strengthening exercise for the respiratory muscles. Complete removal from the ventilator forces the respiratory muscles to take over complete work of breathing, without any assistance from the ventilator for increasing blocks of time. Muscle strength is increased through use of the weaning procedure and good nutrition and hydration. There are several disadvantages to manual weaning. First, it may be a frightening experience to the patient, who is more accustomed to positive pressure breathing. Abrupt removal from the ventilator may precipitate high anxiety, which can hinder the weaning process. Second, manual weaning is time consuming for the nurse. During the period that the patient is off the ventilator, particularly in the early stages of weaning, the nurse is needed directly at the bedside to coach and monitor, and to give encouragement.

Ventilator Weaning. Today, ventilator weaning (weaning the patient using a ventilator mode) is more common than manual weaning. It is generally thought to be less traumatic to the patient because it does not involve intermittent removal from the ventilator. A variety of alternative modes are used for ventilator weaning. Four of the most common ones include intermittent (or synchronous intermittent) mandatory ventilation (IMV/SIMV), pressure support ventilation (PSV), and mandatory minute ventilation (MMV). The choice of weaning mode is based on the clinician's preferences, the type of mode available due to equipment constraints, and the patient's needs and clinical status. Table 7–8 provides a summary of the common ventilator weaning modes.

IMV/SIMV Weaning. The most common type of ventilator weaning at this time is the IMV/SIMV mode. The following is a brief description of one ventilator weaning protocol using IMV/SIMV. Using this ventilator mode, the patient is given mandatory mechanical (ventilator) breaths at preset intervals every minute. Between the mechanical breaths, the patient is able to exercise his or her respiratory muscles spontaneously. The IMV/SIMV rate initially may be set fairly high, near the patient's own respiratory rate. The rate of mandatory breaths is then decreased by two-breath increments one to two times per day (as tolerated) until the IMV/SIMV rate is down to four breaths per minute. Once the mandatory rate is at four breaths per minute, a spontaneous mode (such as PSV) or a T-piece trial is attempted for a minimum of 30 minutes. If the patient tolerates the weaning procedure and all parameters remain within acceptable boundaries, he or she can be extubated.

IMV/SIMV weaning is an endurance exercise for the respiratory muscles. The muscles work continuously over the entire day except when the IMV/SIMV breath triggers a positive pressure breath, which allows a single breath rest. Some patients do not tolerate decreasing IMV/SIMV rates. This tolerance may change on a day-to-day basis. Weaning often is not a smooth undertaking. In patients with underlying disease, changing status can require temporary cessation of weaning. This is particularly true if the patient should develop pneumonia. Such a status change may first manifest itself in a sudden intolerance to weaning.

Postextubation Follow-up

Extubation (removal of the artificial airway) is carried out as soon as it is determined that the patient can sustain his or her own spontaneous breathing. Rapid tube re-

TABLE 7–8. COMMON VENTILATOR WEANING MODES

WEANING MODE	DESCRIPTION	ADVANTAGES	DISADVANTAGES
IMV/SIMV	Frequency of mandatory ventilator breaths is slowly decreased, which requires the patient to gradually take over own work of breathing	Maintains respiratory muscle strength and reduces atrophy Maintains more normal gas distribution Reduces cardiovascular side effects Maintains some of the work of breathing	May increase the work of breathing due to demand valve system Rate must be manually manipulated
PSV	Provides positive pressure during the inspiration phase to support tidal volumes and decrease work of breathing	Decreased work of breathing Increased patient comfort Minimal cardiovascular side effects	All breaths are spontaneous Flow pattern may not be adequate Inspiratory flow rate may be too high or too low
MMV	Guarantees an ongoing stable level of minute ventilation ($\dot{V}_E$): as the patient increases or decreases his or her own ventilatory effort, the ventilator adjusts itself automatically to continue to provide the same level of $\dot{V}_E$	Good control of $Paco_2$ Protection from hypoventilation during weaning Facilitates transition from ventilator to spontaneous breathing	May not respond quickly enough to an apneic episode Potential for development of hypercapnea in presence of a rapid shallow breathing pattern

Data from Pilbeam, S.P. (1990). Mechanical ventilation: Physiological and clinical applications, *3rd ed. St. Louis: C.V. Mosby.*

moval is recommended because of the increased work of breathing imposed on the patient due to the presence of increased airway resistance associated with artificial airways, particularly ET tubes.

Following extubation, particular attention must be given to excellent pulmonary hygiene, including a routine of coughing, deep breathing, and incentive spirometry. Various aerosol therapies, percussion, and postural drainage may be ordered to prevent or treat complications, if necessary.

Shelledy (1999) suggests that postextubation stridor must be closely watched for following extubation. It results from glottic edema and can be mild or severe. When severe, it can cause total obstruction of the airway.

In summary, withdrawal from mechanical ventilation (weaning) is a three-step process, including (1) determination of readiness, an assessment phase; (2) weaning, an intervention phase; and (3) postextubation follow-up, an evaluation phase. Determination of readiness includes both simple and comprehensive weaning criteria that assess multiple body systems. There are two general types of weaning; rapid (short-term) and slow (long-term). Rapid weaning is performed on the majority of patients, usually those without significant lung disease. Slow weaning is required primarily in patients with significant lung disease and those with more serious health problems. Slow weaning may involve use of multiple weaning methodologies. The two general methods of weaning are manual and ventilator weaning. Manual weaning consists of intermittent removal of the patient from the ventilator for increasing periods of time. Ventilator weaning uses manipulation of certain ventilator modes to wean the patient without disconnecting him or her from the ventilator. Common ventilator weaning modes include IMV/SIMV, PSV, and MMV. Postextubation follow-up includes close monitoring of the patient for development of postextubation respiratory distress, as well as interventions to facilitate adequate ventilation and oxygenation.

SECTION TEN REVIEW

1. The vast majority of patients requiring mechanical ventilation are weaned
   A. rapidly, with difficulty
   B. rapidly, without difficulty
   C. slowly, with difficulty
   D. slowly, without difficulty
2. The majority of difficult-to-wean patients have which of the following conditions?
   A. pneumonia
   B. congestive heart failure
   C. acute respiratory distress syndrome
   D. chronic pulmonary disease
3. An example of a simple patient screening question is
   A. is the urinary output > 620 mL/24 hr?
   B. is the prealbumin ≥ 10 mg/dL?
   C. is the patient's clinical condition improving?
   D. have drugs been discontinued that decrease the respiratory drive?
4. Traditional weaning criteria most effectively predict readiness in patients who

A. are elderly
B. are relatively healthy
C. have chronic pulmonary disease
D. require prolonged mechanical ventilation

5. The term _________ weaning is used to refer to weaning by intermittently removing the patient from the ventilator for increasing periods of time.
A. manual
B. ventilator
C. IMV/SIMV
D. pressure support ventilation

6. IMV/SIMV weaning primarily is a(n) _____ exercise for the respiratory muscles.
A. supportive
B. resistance
C. strengthening
D. endurance

Answers: 1. B, 2. D, 3. C, 4. B, 5. A, 6. D

POSTTEST

The following posttest is constructed in a case study format. A patient is presented. Questions are asked based on available data. New data are presented as the case study progresses.

Mary R, 55 years of age, has a 20-year history of smoking. She has been treated medically for emphysema for several years. Mary weighs 115 pounds. She is admitted to the hospital with a diagnosis of acute respiratory failure.

1. If Mary's tidal volume was 300 mL, her alveolar ventilation would be _____ mL.
A. 8.4
B. 50
C. 185
D. 300

2. To be clinically called acute ventilatory failure, which of the following arterial blood gas results must be present?
A. pH < 7.35
B. $PaCO_2$ > 50 mm Hg
C. PaO_2 < 60 mm Hg
D. HCO_3 < 18 mm Hg

3. Mary has a low ventilation–perfusion ratio due to pulmonary shunting. Shunting refers to
A. blood that does not go through the heart
B. normal alveolar ventilation with poor perfusion
C. diminished pulmonary ventilation and perfusion
D. normal perfusion past unventilated alveoli

Mary is showing evidence of ventilatory fatigue. It is decided that she will require intubation and mechanical ventilation.

4. Mary's intubation is a semielective one. For increased comfort, she may have which type of artificial airway inserted?
A. oral endotracheal tube
B. nasotracheal tube
C. tracheostomy tube
D. oral pharyngeal airway

Mary is placed on volume-cycled ventilation.

5. The primary advantage of using volume-cycled ventilation is that it
A. overcomes changes in airway resistance
B. does not require a cuffed artificial airway
C. automatically alters volume as pressure changes
D. delivers higher levels of oxygen than other ventilators

6. Mary's tidal volume is set at 450 mL. A sufficiently large tidal volume is set on a mechanical ventilator to decrease
A. peak airway pressure
B. pneumothorax occurrence
C. ventilator breaths
D. atelectasis occurrence

Mary's minute ventilation is 5.6 L/min. Her ventilator settings are currently as follows: V_T 700 mL, f 8/min. Her $PaCO_2$ has increased from 45 mm Hg in the last hour to the latest level of 55 mm Hg.

7. Assuming that the tidal volume cannot be manipulated further, how can the rate be manipulated to increase the minute ventilation to 7 L/min?
A. decrease the rate to 6/min
B. increase the rate to 10/min
C. increase the rate to 12/min
D. increase the rate to 14/min

8. If Mary was placed on 10 cm H_2O of PEEP, the level of PEEP could be monitored by the nurse in which manner?
   A. the PIP should increase by 10 cm H_2O during inspiration
   B. the PIP should decrease by 10 cm H_2O during inspiration
   C. the airway pressure manometer needle should fall only to 10 cm H_2O during expiration
   D. the airway pressure manometer should fall to negative 10 cm H_2O during expiration

Mary has improved and weaning from the ventilator has begun. The decision is made to place Mary on synchronous intermittent mandatory ventilation (SIMV) of 12/min with pressure support of 10 cm H_2O.

9. Pressure support ventilation is used for which of the following reasons?
   A. it makes inspiration easier
   B. it makes expiration easier
   C. it keeps alveoli open through the breathing cycle
   D. it increases PIP during inspiration
10. Mary's PIP has increased steadily for the past 3 hours. This trend may indicate
    A. increased lung compliance
    B. decreased airway resistance
    C. decreased lung compliance
    D. increased lung ventilatory capacity
11. Mary's low exhaled volume alarm keeps triggering. The problem is not found immediately. The nurse should
    A. call the physician
    B. manually ventilate
    C. check connections again
    D. put more air in the tracheal cuff
12. When Mary was on PEEP, the nurse would expect which of the following trends secondary to changes in cardiac output?
    A. decreased blood pressure, increased pulse
    B. increased blood pressure, increased pulse
    C. decreased blood pressure, decreased pulse
    D. increased blood pressure, decreased pulse
13. If Mary developed a right lower lobe (RLL) pneumonia while receiving mechanical ventilation, how would airflow be affected?
    A. ventilation would not be affected
    B. ventilation to RLL would increase
    C. ventilation to all right lung fields would decrease
    D. ventilation to RLL would decrease
14. Mary's urine output before mechanical ventilation was approximately 100 mL/hour over a 24-hour period. Once mechanical ventilation was initiated, the nurse should expect which trend for urine output?
    A. decrease
    B. increase slightly
    C. increase significantly
    D. remain approximately the same
15. While Mary is on the mechanical ventilator, the nurse will need to monitor her closely for development of a stress ulcer related to
    A. visceral tissue ischemia
    B. increased visceral blood flow
    C. increased visceral venous return
    D. decreased visceral vascular resistance
16. The nurse will need to monitor Mary for development of a nosocomial pulmonary infection. An assessment that would best support this problem is
    A. sputum is green
    B. lung sounds are clear
    C. a large quantity of sputum
    D. an increased serum white blood cell count
17. To prevent complications associated with endotracheal trauma, the nurse should maintain the cuff pressure within what range?
    A. 10 to 15 mm Hg
    B. 15 to 20 mm Hg
    C. 20 to 25 mm Hg
    D. 25 to 30 mm Hg
18. The nurse is having difficulty clearing Mary's airway of thick secretions. The most effective means of enhancing Mary's airway clearance is to
    A. increase frequency of suctioning
    B. increase fluid intake
    C. reposition her every 2 hours
    D. administer nebulizer treatments

Mary's ventilator settings were changed earlier today. The changes were as follows:

V_T: increased from 500 mL to 700 mL
f: increased from 14 to 16 breaths/min

19. Mary has ABGs drawn. Based on the ventilator setting changes, which trend would be anticipated?
    A. increasing pH
    B. increasing $PaCO_2$
    C. decreasing pH
    D. decreasing SaO_2
20. The nurse is preparing to transfer Mary from her bed to a chair positioned next to the bed. Assuming Mary's respiratory status is stable, the safest method of transferring her is to
    A. closely observe the ventilator tubing during transfer
    B. have someone hold her head during transfer
    C. assure that the ET tube taping is secure prior to transfer
    D. disconnect her from the ventilator during transfer

The pulmonary team is considering initiating the weaning process. Mary's current status is as follows:

HR: 100/min, regular
RR: 28/min
Respiratory pattern: irregular
No palpable abdominal tensing on expiration

21. Which of Mary's assessments does not meet the simple criteria for weaning readiness?
    A. heart rate
    B. respiratory rate
    C. respiratory pattern
    D. abdominal tensing

22. Mary is weaned successfully using IMV/SIMV mode. This mode supports the weaning process by
    A. requiring Mary to gradually take over her own work of breathing
    B. supporting Mary's tidal volume during inspiration
    C. assuring that Mary maintains a stable minute ventilation
    D. supporting Mary by maintaining open alveoli at end expiration

POSTTEST ANSWERS

Question	Answer	Section	Question	Answer	Section
1	C	One	12	A	Five
2	B	Two	13	D	Seven
3	D	Two	14	A	Seven
4	B	Three	15	A	Seven
5	A	Four	16	A	Seven
6	D	Five	17	C	Eight
7	B	Five	18	B	Nine
8	C	Five	19	A	Nine
9	A	Five	20	D	Nine
10	C	Five	21	C	Ten
11	B	Five	22	A	Ten

REFERENCES

Bonekat, H.W. (1998). Noninvasive ventilation in neuromuscular disease. *Critical Care Clinics, 14*(4):775–795.

Burns, S.M. (1998). Mechanical ventilation and weaning. In M.R. Kinney, S.B. Dunbar, J.A. Brooks-Brunn, N. Molter, & J.M. Vitello-Cicciu (eds.), *AACN clinical reference for critical care nursing* (4th ed.) (pp. 607–633). St. Louis: C.V. Mosby.

Hicks, G.H., & Scanlan, C.L. (1999). Initiating and adjusting ventilatory support. In C.L. Scanlan, R.L. Wilkins, & J.K. Stoller (eds.), *Egan's fundamentals of respiratory care* (7th ed.) (pp. 893–920). St. Louis: C.V. Mosby.

Marshak, A.B., & Scanlan, C.L. (1999). Emergency life support. In C.L. Scanlan, R.L. Wilkins, & J.K. Stoller (eds.), *Egan's fundamentals of respiratory care* (7th ed.) (pp. 893–920). St. Louis: C.V. Mosby.

Martin, L. (1987). *Pulmonary physiology in clinical practice: The essentials for patient care and evaluation*. St. Louis: C.V. Mosby.

Pilbeam, S.P. (1992). *Mechanical ventilation: Physiological and clinical applications* (2nd ed.). St. Louis: C.V. Mosby/Multi-Media Publishing.

Pilbeam, S.P. (1998). *Mechanical ventilation: Physiological and clinical applications* (3rd ed.). St. Louis: C.V. Mosby.

Scanlan, C.L., Heuer, A., & Wyka, K.A. (1999). Respiratory care in alternative settings. In C.L. Scanlan, R.L. Wilkins, & J.K. Stoller (eds.). *Egan's fundamentals of respiratory care* (7th ed.) (pp. 1103–1140). St. Louis: C.V. Mosby.

Shapiro, B.A., Kacmarek, R.M., Cane, R.D., Peruzzi, W.T., & Hauptman, D. (1991). *Clinical application of respiratory care* (4th ed.). St. Louis: C.V. Mosby.

Shelledy, D.C. (1999). Discontinuing ventilatory support. In C.L. Scanlan, R.L. Wilkins, & J.K. Stoller (eds.). *Egan's fundamentals of respiratory care* (7th ed.) (pp. 967–992). St. Louis: C.V. Mosby.

Thelan, L.A., Urden, L.D., Lough, M.E., & Stacy, K.M. (1998). *Critical care nursing: Diagnosis and management* (3rd ed.). St. Louis: C.V. Mosby.

Vanderwarf, C.J. (1999). Mechanical ventilation. In J.B. Fink & G.E. Hunt (eds.), *Clinical practice in respiratory care* (pp. 405–435). Philadelphia: J.B. Lippincott.

Vollman, K.M., & Aulbach, R.K. (1998). Acute respiratory distress syndrome. In M.R. Kinney, S.B. Dunbar, J.A. Brooks-Brunn, N. Molter, & J.M. Vitello-Cicciu (eds.). *ACCN clinical reference for critical care nursing* (4th ed.) (pp. 529–564). St. Louis: C.V. Mosby.

Module 8

Nursing Care of the Patient with Altered Respiratory Function

Kathleen Dorman Wagner

This module is designed to integrate the major points discussed in the modules, "*Respiratory Process*," "*Arterial Blood Gas Analysis*," and "*Mechanical Ventilation*." This module summarizes relationships between key concepts and assists the learner in clustering information to facilitate clinical application. The module is divided into three sections. It applies content from Part II: Respiration and Ventilation in an interactive learning style. Using a case study format, the learner is encouraged to identify nursing actions based on the assessment of a patient with a restrictive pulmonary disease in Case Study One, a patient with an obstructive pulmonary disease in Case Study Two, and a patient requiring mechanical ventilation in Case Study Three. Case Studies One and Two include collaborative and independent nursing interventions typically used in planning the care of patients with restrictive and obstructive pulmonary disorders.

Objectives

Following completion of this module, given a specific clinical situation, the learner will be able to

1. Interpret the significance of laboratory data.
2. Interpret the significance of assessment data.
3. Develop appropriate expected patient outcomes.
4. Apply knowledge of the patient with altered respiratory function to develop a plan of nursing interventions.
5. Describe the nursing management of the patient with restrictive and obstructive pulmonary diseases.

Case Study 1

MARY R, A PATIENT WITH RESTRICTIVE DISEASE

You are the nurse assigned to admit Mary R, 38 years old, who is a direct admission from a family practice clinic. No other information is available. You have just been informed that Mary has been brought to the floor and has been assisted into bed.

Initial Appraisal

On walking into her room for the first time, you quickly note the following.

General Appearance. Mary is an African-American female of small stature. She appears well nourished and is tidy in appearance. She is still fully clothed except for her shoes. She is wearing glasses.

SIGNS OF DISTRESS. Mary's respirations are rapid and appear shallow. She is moving restlessly in the bed. A frequent, harsh cough is heard, and secretions are audible during coughing. Perspiration is noted on Mary's face.

OTHER. You do not note any intravenous lines or oxygen in use. A man of approximately the same age is in the room with Mary, talking quietly to her. He identifies himself as James, her husband.

Focused Respiratory Assessment

Mary's clothing is exchanged quickly for a hospital gown to make assessment easier and make her more comfortable. Because Mary appears to be in acute respiratory distress, you immediately perform a rapid assessment focusing first on her pulmonary status. The results are as follows:

Mary is restless and oriented to person, place, and time. Her respiratory rate is 32/min, shallow, and regular. Her mucous membranes are dusky. Her respirations are labored. She is using accessory muscles in her neck during inspiration. Crackles and wheezes are auscultated in the right middle and right lower lobes of her lungs. A pleural friction rub is auscultated at the right anterior axillary line, fifth intercostal space. Her current blood pressure is 140/88 (baseline, according to her husband, is 130/76), pulse is 120/min, and temperature is 102°F (orally). She is complaining of increased shortness of breath that does not improve when the head of the bed is raised. Though her cough is weak, she is expectorating a small amount of thick, green sputum.

After this initial assessment, you call her admitting physician. The physician gives the following stat phone orders:

- Arterial blood gas (ABG)
- Complete blood cell count (CBC)
- Electrolytes
- Portable chest x-ray
- Sputum for culture and Gram stain

QUESTION

Considering Mary's symptoms and assuming that the tests cannot all be performed at the same time, which test should you order to be done first?

A. electrolytes
B. portable chest x-ray
C. ABG
D. CBC

ANSWER

The correct answer is C. Since Mary appears to be in acute respiratory distress, priority tests would be, first, the ABG, which is a rapid, accurate method of measuring oxygenation and acid–base status. *Discussion of incorrect options:* The second priority is the chest x-ray, a rapidly performed diagnostic test that helps locate and differentiate the pulmonary problem. The CBC and electrolytes, although important, do not have a direct impact on Mary's respiratory status. The sputum specimen should be obtained as soon as possible. Results of the culture will not be available for several days.

Stat Test Results

Arterial blood gases (on room air)

pH = 7.45, Pa_{CO_2} = 33 mm Hg, Pa_{O_2} = 68 mm Hg, HCO_3 = 20 mEq/L, Sa_{O_2} = 90%

WBC = 15,000	(Normal range 4,500–10,000/μL)
RBC = 4.8	(Normal range 4.0–5.0 × 10^{12}/μL in females)
Hgb = 14	(Normal range 12–15 g/dL in females)
Hct = 42%	(Normal range 36%–46% in females)

Electrolytes (Normal ranges are from Kee, 1999)

Sodium (Na) = 142	(Normal range 135–145 mEq/L)
Potassium (K) = 4.5	(Normal range 3.5–5.3 mEq/L)
Chloride (Cl) = 104	(Normal range 95–105 mEq/L)
Calcium (Ca) = 9.2	(Normal range 9–11 mg/dL)

Portable chest x-ray results

Right middle lobe (RML) and right lower lobe (RLL) infiltrates are consistent with pneumonia

Sputum for culture and Gram stain

Results pending on culture

Gram stain: gram-positive clustered cocci

QUESTION

Which of the following statements is true regarding the laboratory or x-ray data?

A. The ABG shows evidence of acid–base balance with mild hypoxemia
B. The electrolytes show evidence of possible overhydration
C. The CBC does not show evidence of an infectious process
D. The Gram stain is consistent with a viral infection

ANSWER

The correct answer is A. The ABG shows acid–base balance with mild hypoxemia. *Discussion of incorrect options:*

The electrolytes show evidence of possible dehydration in high-normal sodium and chloride levels. The increased white blood cell count on the CBC is consistent with the presence of an infectious process. The high-normal hematocrit may suggest dehydration when considered with the high-normal sodium and chloride levels. The presence of gram-positive clustered cocci in the sputum Gram stain is consistent with staphylococci. The Gram stain helps differentiate the causative agent before confirmation by the sputum culture results, which take several days.

The results of the ABG are called to the physician immediately, and oxygen is initiated at 4 L/min per nasal cannula. The physician states that she will be at the hospital to see Mary shortly.

QUESTION

On closer examination of Mary's ABG results, the nurse would conclude that the acid–base values could best be explained by her

- **A.** crackles and wheezes
- **B.** pleural friction rub
- **C.** respiratory rate
- **D.** shallow breathing

ANSWER

The correct answer is C. Her rapid respiratory rate is blowing off CO_2, which has precipitated respiratory alkalosis (compensated). Though her breathing *appears* shallow, it is currently not causing her to hypoventilate. Respiratory alkalosis is a common early acid–base disturbance associated with conditions that cause a rapid respiratory rate (e.g., pneumonia, acute asthmatic episode). Crackles, wheezes, and pleural friction rub are adventitious breath sounds that do not directly affect acid–base balance.

QUESTION

You note that Mary is very restless in the bed. This assessment is most likely associated with her

- **A.** decreased $PaCO_2$
- **B.** decreased PaO_2
- **C.** increased pH
- **D.** decreased HCO_3

ANSWER

The correct answer is B. Restlessness is a sign commonly associated with hypoxemia and general discomfort. You should assess Mary for possible etiologies of her restlessness before sedation or analgesia is considered since use of these drugs may or may not be the best treatment. For example, if Mary's shallow breathing is secondary to her pleural pain, analgesia therapy may well facilitate deeper breaths and improve oxygenation. If, however, sedation or analgesic therapy should depress her respiratory pattern further, it could worsen her hypoxemia.

Focused Nursing History

Since Mary is in too much distress to be interviewed directly, you decide to talk with her husband to obtain the most important critical historical data that may have an impact on Mary's present situation. The complete nursing database will be completed within the first 24 hours postadmission. Her husband gives the following history:

> Mary began exhibiting common cold symptoms approximately 10 days ago. About 4 days ago, Mary's fever began to increase, accompanied by severe chilling. Her cough became productive, with green sputum. The cough has prevented Mary from sleeping very much for the past several nights. She has been complaining of a pattern of increasingly severe shortness of breath. Mary is not currently taking any prescription drugs. She has been taking several over-the-counter medications to relieve her symptoms: a nonnarcotic cough preparation and acetaminophen. For the past several days, she has been complaining of a transient sharp pain in her lower right chest that increases with breathing. Mary is allergic to penicillin. She has a 20-year history of smoking 1/2 to 1 pack of cigarettes per day but has not been able to smoke for several days because of shortness of breath. She rarely drinks any alcoholic beverages.

QUESTION

Additional priority nursing history data that the nurse should obtain from Mary's husband is

- **A.** dietary preferences
- **B.** usual weight
- **C.** preexisting medical conditions
- **D.** date of last menstrual period

ANSWER

The correct answer is C. It is crucial to be aware of any preexisting medical conditions. Many high-acuity patients have preexisting conditions such as diabetes mellitus, chronic pulmonary diseases, or congestive heart failure that must be monitored and taken into consideration when developing the plan of care. The existence of preexisting chronic conditions may place the patient at increased risk for development of complications during the current acute illness. The other pieces of data, while adding to the overall database, can be obtained at a later time, as appropriate.

Systematic Bedside Assessment

Before the physician's arrival, you initiate a head-to-toe assessment.

HEAD AND NECK. Mary's overall skin coloring is difficult to assess because it is dark. Therefore, her mucous membranes are assessed, and they are dusky in color. Mary continues to be completely oriented but remains restless. Slight nasal flaring is noted. She has nasal cannula oxygen delivering 4 L/min. She does not have jugular vein distention. No other abnormalities of the head or neck are noted.

CHEST. Pulmonary status is as previously noted in the Focused Respiratory Assessment.

Cardiac status is as follows. Pulmonary adventitious sounds make it somewhat difficult to clearly discriminate sounds. S_1 and S_2 and no murmur are auscultated. Sounds are regular, with a rate of 122/min.

ABDOMEN. The abdomen is flat. Positive bowel sounds are auscultated in all quadrants. Mary denies any abdominal tenderness. It is soft to palpation.

PELVIS. Mary voided 125 mL of clear, dark amber urine, with a specific gravity of 1.030.

EXTREMITIES. There is poor skin turgor. The skin is hot and diaphoretic. No peripheral edema is noted. The nailbeds are difficult to assess due to dark pigmentation. Peripheral pulses are palpable in all four distal extremities.

POSTERIOR. No skin breakdown is noted, and there is no sacral edema. Posterior breath sounds; crackles and wheezes present on the right side to midlung field.

QUESTION

Which of the following best states the cause of Mary's right-sided crackles? Her crackles

A. probably indicate exudate in the small airways
B. are suggestive of bronchoconstriction
C. are typical of secretions in the large airways
D. result from inflammation of the parietal pleura

ANSWER

The correct answer is A. Crackles are heard in the small airways and indicate the presence of fluid, exudate, or atelectasis. *Discussion of incorrect options:* Wheezing is a musical sound commonly heard on expiration, indicating airway narrowing usually from bronchoconstriction and/or bronchospasm. Rhonchi are auscultated in the larger airways and indicate the presence of secretions or fluid. Inflammation of the parietal pleura is associated with pleural pain. A pleural friction rub is sometimes present over the inflamed area.

Development of Nursing Diagnoses

Clustering Data

You have just completed your head-to-toe assessment and are now ready to develop a problem list based on the subjective and objective data that you have collected thus far. To cluster your data, you look for abnormalities found during the assessment. During the initial appraisal you immediately noted Mary's labored, rapid, shallow respirations. These symptoms are sufficient to begin clustering similar data that can support or refute the presence of a pulmonary problem.

CLUSTER 1. (from previous history and physical assessment data):

Subjective data: Patient complaining of dyspnea unaffected by position changes. Cold symptoms for 10 days. Increasing pattern of shortness of breath that does not seem to be affected by changing height of head of the bed. Cough with green sputum is noted. Chills and fever that have worsened over several days. Is complaining of a transient sharp pain in her lower right chest that increases with breathing. Has had difficulty sleeping due to frequent coughing.

Objective data: Labored, shallow respirations. Respiratory rate is 28/min. Accessory muscles are in use. Crackles and wheezes heard in RML and RLL in anterior fields and to midchest in posterior right field. Pleural friction rub is auscultated at right anterior axillary line, fifth intercostal space. ABG shows that mild hypoxemia is present. Chest x-ray indicates an RML/RLL infiltrate. Gram stain shows gram-positive clustered cocci. Her cough is weak. Secretions, which are very thick and green, are difficult for her to expectorate. Fever and chills are present.

QUESTION

Based on these data, which of the following nursing diagnoses would you select as being appropriate in planning Mary's care?

A. impaired gas exchange
B. ineffective airway clearance
C. ineffective breathing pattern
D. all of the above

ANSWER

The correct answer is D. Mary's pulmonary problem is a complex one that requires a wide variety of medical and nursing interventions. NANDA has approved all of the three presented pulmonary-related nursing diagnoses as individual diagnoses. However, because all three apply to Mary, it is suggested that you choose *Impaired respiratory function*.

- *Impaired gas exchange* related to alveolar consolidation, pooling of secretions
- *Ineffective airway clearance* related to thick secretions associated with pulmonary infection and dehydration, pleural pain, ineffective cough
- *Ineffective breathing pattern:* hypoventilation related to weakness, pleural pain, fatigue

QUESTION

List at least six expected outcomes (EPOs) that would be appropriate for Mary's nursing diagnosis, *Impaired respiratory function:*

Impaired gas exchange
Ineffective airway clearance
Ineffective breathing pattern

1.
2.
3.
4.
5.
6.

ANSWER

1. Normal respiratory rate, depth, and rhythm
2. Improved or clear breath sounds
3. Improving or no dyspnea
4. Usual mental status
5. Mucous membranes are pink
6. ABGs within acceptable limits for patient

For the purposes of Mary's case study, only the pulmonary-related nursing diagnoses are developed further. However, in a true clinical situation, as the nurse creating Mary's plan of care, you would continue to develop other clusters based on primary critical cues and supporting cues from the data already collected. If data are insufficient, you should follow through on collecting the necessary data to confirm or refute your hypotheses.

Based on the preliminary data collected on Mary, there is sufficient support to state the following nursing diagnoses (Ulrich et al., 1998).

- Pain: pleural
- Risk for fluid volume deficit
- Self-care deficit
- Sleep pattern disturbance
- Altered nutrition: less than body requirements
- Potential complications:
  1. Exudative pleural effusion
  2. Atelectasis

Developing the Plan of Care

Mary's pneumonia is a restrictive pulmonary disease process. She has many signs and symptoms consistent with restrictive diseases.

Treatment goals based on the restrictive nature of her disease include (1) optimizing her oxygenation status, (2) promoting airway clearance, and (3) maintaining functional alveoli. These general goals are reflected in the nursing diagnoses and desired patient outcomes (DPOs) on the nursing care plan. For example, optimizing oxygenation status is addressed in the nursing diagnoses *Impaired gas exchange* and *Ineffective airway clearance*. Accomplishment of the goal is measured in such criteria as ABGs within normal limits for patient, usual skin color, usual mental status, and improved lung sounds.

Nursing interventions are based on activities to help Mary meet her DPOs. They consist of collaborative interventions, which are activities ordered by the physician but require some actions by the nurse, and independent interventions, activities that are within the nursing scope of practice to write and carry out as nursing orders.

Collaborative Interventions Related to Pulmonary Status

The physician's orders may include the following:

1. *Pulmonary drug therapy*. Mary will be receiving several drugs while hospitalized. Oxygen therapy has been ordered to treat Mary's mild hypoxemia. In general, the minimal goal of oxygen therapy is to increase the PaO_2 to at least 60 mm Hg. Other types of drug therapy that probably will be ordered for Mary include antibiotics for treatment of pneumonia and analgesics for treatment of pleuritic pain. She may not receive a cough suppressant in this stage of her pneumonia because a productive cough is a protective reflex to help rid the lungs of unwanted secretions. If necessary, she also may receive drug therapy through handheld nebulizer or metered-dose inhaler.
2. *Laboratory and x-ray testing*. These may be ordered intermittently. Of particular interest will be the ABGs, CBC, and chest x-ray to follow progress of the therapeutic plan.
3. *Percussion and postural drainage*. P and PD may be ordered to facilitate airway clearance. In many hospitals, this is performed by a respiratory therapist. P and PD also can be done by the nurse if she or he is properly trained, as ordered by the physician, or it may be an independent nursing action, depending on hospital policy.
4. *Intravenous fluids*. These may be ordered to promote hydration, which is crucial in loosening secretions for improved airway clearance. An IV access site also is necessary for IV antibiotic therapy, if ordered.

Independent Nursing Interventions

A. Assess for decreased respiratory function (report abnormal)
   - Respirations < 8/min or > 30/min
   - Increasingly shallow, labored breathing
   - Increasing dyspnea or central cyanosis
   - Change in mental status
     - Increased restlessness
     - Increased lethargy
   - Increasingly abnormal ABGs
   - Increasingly abnormal breath sounds, adventitious sounds
   - Change in sputum
   - Accessory muscle use

QUESTION

Some of the remaining independent nursing interventions are incomplete. Fill in the spaces with the correct information as they apply to her impaired respiratory function.

B. Turn every _______ hours.
C. Cough and deep breathe every ____ to ____ hours.
D. Incentive spirometry every ____ to ____ hours.
E. Encourage fluids: to ____ to ____ L /24 hr, or 600 to 800 mL/8-hr shift, unless contraindicated.
F. Tracheal suction as needed.
G. Position of comfort with head of bed __________________________.
H. Monitor for effects of drug therapy (therapeutic and nontherapeutic).
I. Monitor test results (report abnormals).
J. Instruct patient and/or family regarding _______, _______, _______, and _______.
K. Encourage self-care as tolerated.
L. Assess for pleural pain every 4 hours and PRN. Administer analgesics as needed.

ANSWERS

B. 2
C. 1, 2
D. 1, 2
E. 2, 2.5
G. elevated > 30 degrees
J. condition, procedures, medications, and treatment

Plan Evaluation and Revision

Mary's pulmonary plan of care is now developed and ready to execute. Her progress is monitored at regular intervals to evaluate the effects of the various therapeutic actions. If progress is not being noted toward attainment of Mary's various desired patient outcomes, her plan may need revisions, examining alternative interventions that may be more effective.

Mary's plan of care is effective, and she responds rapidly to her antibiotic therapy and her pulmonary hygiene program. Because she does not have underlying pulmonary disease, her recovery is uncomplicated. Before discharge, she will need to receive teaching concerning continuing her antibiotic therapy as prescribed, increasing her activities slowly at home, smoking cessation, and pulmonary hygiene.

CASE STUDY 2

PETER M, A PATIENT WITH OBSTRUCTIVE PULMONARY DISEASE

You are a registered nurse working on a general surgical floor in a 300-bed community hospital. You have, as part of your assignment, Mr. Peter M, a 68-year-old patient who had a transurethral resection (TUR) 3 days ago. You have just heard the shift report, in which you received the following information about Peter.

At 2:00 P.M., vital signs are BP 150/90 (baseline is 130/84), pulse 100/min and slightly irregular, rate 38/min, temperature 98.6°F (oral). He has 2 L of oxygen ordered per nasal cannula. Peter's lungs sound a little more congested, and breathing seems more labored. He has been on bed rest since surgery. Peter has a history of emphysema and his post-TUR status is stable and his urinary status has been uneventful since surgery. Urine is clear, and a three-way Foley catheter is in place. It will probably be discontinued today. His appetite has been poor. He has an IV of 5% dextrose in 0.45% normal saline in a right peripheral line. The nurse reporting off suggests that you watch Peter closely this evening, stating that he seems weaker today. He has been fully alert and awake throughout the day. The nurse also reports that Peter has gained 4 pounds over the past several days.

Significant History

Peter is a retired teacher. He was diagnosed with pulmonary emphysema approximately 10 years ago and congestive heart failure approximately 2 years ago. He states that he drinks an occasional glass of beer or wine but not on a regular basis. Over the past year, Peter has had increasing difficulty passing urine. Tests showed benign prostatic hypertrophy. His TUR was an elective procedure. He has no known allergies. His appetite has been poor for the past several days due to complaints of nausea, though he has not been vomiting. Peter usually sleeps using two large pillows to help him breathe better.

QUESTION

In addition to what has already been obtained in the nursing history, the nurse should also obtain Peter's __________ history as a priority, at the time of admission.

A. smoking
B. complete medication
C. diet
D. usual activity level

ANSWER

The correct answer is B. Peter has a positive history of cardiopulmonary disease and is probably receiving long-term drug therapy to treat these medical conditions. It is important to know what medications he normally takes at home so that decisions can be made regarding continuation of his meds while hospitalized. In addition, certain drugs (e.g., digoxin, theophylline) may build up in the serum and precipitate adverse reactions. For this reason, the physician may order serum drug levels to be drawn to determine whether therapeutic levels are present. *Discussion of incorrect options:* While information regarding his smoking, activity level, and diet history will be a useful part of the database, they are not as high a priority in helping to meet his immediate needs.

New Data Obtained during the Nursing History

Peter informs the nurse that he has been taking theophylline (Theo-Dur), digoxin, furosemide (Lasix), terbutaline inhalant, and prednisone. He has also been receiving home oxygen therapy for about 1 year. Peter has a history of smoking 2 to $2^1/_2$ PPD for 40 years. This last year, he cut his intake to $^1/_2$ PPD. He has been on a low-sodium diet for at least 5 years. Peter states that he is "pretty good" at sticking with the diet. He indicates that he can usually perform his own ADLs. He complains that, over the past several months, he has become increasingly short of breath with climbing 15 steps to get to his bedroom, and he voices concern that he will not be able to do this much longer.

Initial Appraisal

It is now the beginning of your shift, and you are making your patient rounds with initial appraisals. On approaching Peter's bed, you note the following.

GENERAL APPEARANCE. Peter M is a Caucasian male. He is barrel-chested and poorly nourished in appearance, with little body fat noted. He is in bed sitting upright, leaning forward with his arms stretched out to his knees.

SIGNS OF DISTRESS. Respirations are rapid, with a prolonged expiratory phase. His breathing is noisy, with an expiratory wheeze heard while you are standing at the foot of the bed. His breathing appears labored and you note use of accessory muscles during inspiration. His coloring appears dusky.

OTHER. There is approximately 50 mL of urine in his Foley bag. You note a three-way Foley catheter in place. Urine is clear and yellow. A bladder irrigant bag is hanging but is not running. The IV fluid is infusing at the correct rate. He has oxygen running at 2 L/minute per nasal cannula. He is oriented to his name and the year but cannot tell you where he is. No one else is in the room with him.

QUESTION

Based only on Peter's history and initial appraisal, you would most appropriately perform a focused assessment of the _______ system as a priority.

A. genitourinary
B. integumentary
C. gastrointestinal
D. cardiopulmonary

ANSWER

D is correct. Because your initial appraisal of Peter included abnormal assessments that are overtly respiratory, you rapidly focus in on a more complete respiratory assessment followed by a cardiovascular assessment. You do this with the understanding that pulmonary signs and symptoms can be of pulmonary or cardiac origin.

Focused Assessment

His vital signs currently are respiratory rate 32/min and labored. Pulse 115/min; S_1 and S_2 are present though the sounds are hard to distinguish because of his loud adventitious breath sounds. BP is 156/92. You auscultate loud coarse rhonchi on both inspiration and expiration, and expiratory wheeze is heard bilaterally. Breath sounds can be heard distinctly in the apices but are progressively diminished from mid to low lung fields bilaterally. He has a full rolling cough, but he is unable to clear the secretions from his lungs. His bedside chart shows an imbalance of 1,500 mL of intake over output during the past 24 hours.

Following respiratory data collection and based on Peter's history, you decide that his signs and symptoms may not be completely of pulmonary origin. You, therefore, quickly assess his cardiovascular status further.

CARDIOVASCULAR STATUS. You note positive jugular vein distention. Peter has 3+ pitting edema of his lower legs. You cannot distinguish heart sounds sufficiently to assess for S_3 and S_4 reliably. His current urine output is 50 mL in a 2-hour period. Breath sounds are too diminished to clearly assess for presence of crackles in the bases.

Following your focused assessment, you call your report to the physician, who orders the following stat orders.

- Portable chest x-ray
- ABG
- Furosemide 40 mg IV now
- Aminophylline drip at 35 mg/hr
- Serum electrolytes
- Digoxin and theophylline levels
- Electrocardiogram (ECG)

QUESTION

Considering Peter's present condition and assuming that the orders cannot all be carried out at the same time, which stat physician order should you do first?

A. IV furosemide
B. ABG
C. digoxin and theophylline levels
D. chest x-ray

ANSWER

The correct answer is B. Obtaining the ABG first is a rapid and accurate method of measuring his oxygenation and acid–base status. *Discussion of incorrect options:* The IV furosemide would be next in priority to help relieve fluid volume excess problems. You should be aware, however, that Peter has been on long-standing digoxin therapy. It will be very important to check his electrolyte level at the earliest opportunity for possible hypokalemia, particularly since he is receiving furosemide, a potent loop diuretic that is very potassium depleting. Low serum potassium associated with digoxin therapy can precipitate digoxin toxicity. The portable chest x-ray and ECG also can be ordered rapidly, but there often is a delay before these procedures are actually performed.

Stat Test Results

Portable chest x-ray
Right heart enlargement consistent with cor pulmonale. Hyperlucency is present, with flattening of the diaphragm. Increased anteroposterior (A/P) diameter is present. Bullous lesions are noted.

Arterial blood gases

$$\text{pH} = 7.32,\ Pa_{CO_2} = 75\ \text{mm Hg},\ Pa_{O_2} = 70\ \text{mm Hg},\ HCO_3 = 36\ \text{mEq/L}$$

Electrolytes

$$Na = 138\ \text{mEq/L},\ K = 4.0\ \text{mEq/L},\ Cl = 102\ \text{mEq/L},\ Ca = 9.2\ \text{mg/dL}$$

Digoxin level

2.2 ng/mL (therapeutic range 0.5–2 ng/mL)

Theophylline level

15 μg/mL (therapeutic range 5–20 μg/mL)

ECG Right ventricular leads show changes consistent with cor pulmonale. Changes also are noted consistent with digitalis effects. Unifocal premature ventricular contractions are present.

(Therapeutic ranges are from Kee, 1999)

QUESTION

Which of the following statements is correct regarding the significance of laboratory and other test data?

A. The ABG shows metabolic acidosis with mild hypoxemia
B. The electrolytes are all within acceptable limits
C. The chest x-ray finding of cor pulmonale is an uncommon finding in COPD
D. The premature ventricular contractions are not of concern at this time

ANSWER

The correct answer is B. Peter's electrolyte levels are not significant at this time. However, they will need to be monitored carefully while he is receiving diuretics because of the potential for electrolyte depletion complications. *Discussion of incorrect options:* His portable chest x-ray showed evidence of cor pulmonale, right heart enlargement, and hypertrophy of pulmonary etiology. Cor pulmonale is frequently associated with some degree of right heart failure. The lung fields are consistent with emphysematous changes. His ABG showed acute respiratory acidosis with mild hypoxemia. Patients with chronic obstructive diseases frequently undergo progressive ABG alterations. Normal ABG values are relative numbers in patients with COPD.

If Peter has very severe emphysema, he may breathe normally on a hypoxic drive. He, like many COPD patients, may be tolerant of relatively low PaO_2 levels and high $PaCO_2$ levels. His current pH is below the normal range, however, which tells you that at this time, he for some reason has moved from a state of chronic insufficiency to acute respiratory failure. (For review, see Modules 5 and 6).

Peter's digoxin level is toxic. This is not uncommon in older patients receiving chronic digoxin therapy. Digoxin toxicity is potentially dangerous. As the nurse, you would hold the drug and inform the physician of the test results. Digoxin generally is held until levels return to therapeutic levels. His theophylline level is within the therapeutic range at this time. Patients on chronic theophylline therapy often become toxic, developing symptoms of nausea and vomiting, increased heart rate, dysrhythmias, insomnia, headache, and increased irritability.

Peter's ECG shows evidence of his chronic drug therapy and his cor pulmonale. The presence of premature ventricular contractions is significant because of his digoxin toxic state, which can precipitate many arrhythmias and conduction problems.

Systematic Bedside Assessment

Once you have completed the various stat activities on Peter, you begin your head-to-toe assessment.

HEAD AND NECK. Circumoral and earlobe duskiness is noted. Oxygen is in place at 2 L/min. *Responsiveness level:* He is oriented to name and month but not to place, although he has been reminded recently. His speech is breathless, and he is able to talk in one- to two-word phrases only. Purse-lipped breathing is noted. Positive jugular vein distention is noted at 45 degrees.

CHEST. The chest is as previously assessed in the focused pulmonary and cardiac assessment.

ABDOMEN. His abdomen is distended and tight. He complains of tenderness in his right upper quadrant. Bowel sounds are auscultated in all four quadrants but are hypoactive.

PELVIS. A three-way Foley catheter is present. He denies pain at this time. Urine output in the bag is 50 mL for a 1-hour period. The urine color is clear and amber. No drainage is noted around the catheter at the meatus.

EXTREMITIES. Mild digital clubbing is noted. His nailbeds are dusky, and capillary refill is < 3 seconds. His skin is warm and flaky dry. He has a peripheral IV in his right forearm. The site is negative for edema, redness, or heat; 1+ edema is noted in both hands, and 3+ edema is noted in the lower legs. He has positive peripheral pulses. When he is on his feet, you are able to palpate his dorsalis pedis pulses but not his posterior tibial pulses.

POSTERIOR. No skin breakdown is noted at this time, but redness is noted in several areas along the spinous processes of the vertebrae and on the coccyx. Scattered rhonchi are auscultated throughout the posterior fields, and sounds are diminished.

Development of Nursing Diagnoses

Clustering Data

Following the systematic bedside assessment, there are sufficient data to develop nursing diagnoses. The first step is to cluster data based on major abnormal cues.

EXERCISE

You have hypothesized that Peter has an acute pulmonary problem. In the space provided, list the major abnormal data that have been obtained thus far, supporting this hypothesis.

CLUSTER 1.

ANSWER

Subjective data: Peter has a long history of pulmonary emphysema. He continues to smoke, although he has decreased his intake to ½ pack per day. His at-home pulmonary medications include Theo-Dur, oxygen, prednisone, and terbutaline.

Objective data: Peter's respiratory rate is 32/min and labored. Pursed-lip breathing is noted. He is sitting upright in bed, leaning forward. His expiratory phase is noticeably longer than his inspiratory phase. He is using his accessory muscles to breathe. Loud rhonchi and wheezes are present. A full rolling cough is noted, but he is unable to cough up and expectorate the secretions. His pulse is 115/min, and blood pressure is 156/92. His theophylline level is within normal limits. His latest ABG showed acute respiratory acidosis with mild hypoxia. He has oxygen per nasal cannula running at 2 L/min. Circumoral and earlobe duskiness are noted.

QUESTION

Based on these data, which of the following nursing diagnoses would you select as being appropriate in planning Peter's care?

A. impaired gas exchange
B. ineffective airway clearance
C. ineffective breathing pattern
D. all of the above

ANSWER

The correct answer is D. Peter's critical cues show evidence of all three respiratory-related nursing diagnoses.

- *Impaired gas exchange* related to ineffective airway clearance, ineffective breathing pattern, and decrease in functional lung surface area
- *Ineffective airway clearance* related to excessive secretions, ineffective cough, and pooling of secretions
- *Ineffective breathing pattern* related to anxiety and dysfunction of the muscles of respirations

---

Desired patient outcomes (evaluative criteria) for Peter would include:

1. Normal respiratory rate, depth, and rhythm
2. Decreased dyspnea
3. Usual or improved breath sounds
4. Usual mental status
5. ABGs within normal limits for patient

If Peter's emphysema is severe, his blood gases may never attain the usual normals. ABG normal values often are altered in patients with chronic obstructive diseases. His acceptable ranges might be

- pH 7.35–7.45 (remains unchanged with disease)
- $Pa{CO_2}$ < 50 mm Hg (increases with obstructive disease)
- $Pa{O_2}$ > 50 mm Hg (decreases with obstructive disease)
- $Sa{O_2} \geq 85\%$ (decreases with obstructive disease)

QUESTION

In the space provided, state what additional effect Peter's age of 68 has on his $Pa{O_2}$.

ANSWER

Peter's age of 68 influences his acceptable $Pa{O_2}$ range. It is known that normal aging decreases the number of functioning alveoli. For this reason, $Pa{O_2}$ has a normal tendency to decrease with age.

Peter's assessment had sufficient evidence to develop a picture consistent with a pulmonary problem and a possible cardiovascular problem. Because the pulmonary and cardiovascular systems actually exist as a single cardiopulmonary circuit, the possible cardiovascular problem is briefly explored.

EXERCISE

You have also hypothesized that Peter may have an acute cardiac problem. In the space provided, list the major abnormal data obtained thus far that would support this hypothesis, and state the major nursing diagnosis based on the cluster.

CLUSTER 2.

NURSING DIAGNOSIS:

ANSWER

Subjective data: Peter has a 2-year history of congestive heart failure. At-home cardiac-related medications include digoxin and furosemide. He usually sleeps on two pillows.

Objective data: Jugular vein distention is present, and 3+ edema is noted in his lower legs. His current urine output is 50 mL in a 2-hour period. Chest x-ray shows evidence of cor pulmonale. Digoxin level is > 2.0 (toxic). ECG results were consistent with cor pulmonale and showed premature ventricular contractions. He has experienced a 4-pound weight gain over the past several days.

Based on these data, a nursing diagnosis of *Altered cardiac output: decreased,* related to ineffective right heart pumping associated with right heart hypertrophy, is noted. Appropriate patient outcomes would need to be decided on and interventions performed to address this problem. This second cluster of data was included to exemplify the common cardiac complications associated with chronic respiratory disease. Nursing management of the patient with cardiovascular problems is addressed in another module.

Other nursing diagnoses supported by the existing data include:

- Activity intolerance
- Altered comfort: nausea
- Altered nutrition: less than body requirements
- Anxiety
- Knowledge deficit
- Self-care deficit
- High risk for altered protection: impaired skin integrity

Developing the Plan of Care

Peter's emphysema is an obstructive pulmonary disease. He has many of the signs and symptoms that are typical of obstructive diseases.

Patients with chronic obstructive pulmonary disease (COPD) often are admitted to hospitals for reasons unrelated to their pulmonary disorder, such as was the case of Peter with his genitourinary problem. When a patient with COPD is admitted to the hospital for any reason, the health care team must incorporate management of the chronic problem with management of the acute problem if complications are to be avoided.

Many patients with COPD exist in a day-to-day state of chronic respiratory insufficiency; that is, they are able to maintain a relatively normal (balanced supply and demand) acid–base and oxygenation states only at the expense of the other body systems. Normalcy is maintained through compensatory mechanisms.

QUESTION

What are the major clinical manifestations that indicate the presence of compensation activities by the systems listed below?

A. cardiovascular system
B. renal system
C. pulmonary system
D. hematopoietic system

ANSWER

A. elevated BP and pulse
B. increased retention of bicarbonate
C. increased respiratory rate and depth
D. increased RBC production

Compensatory mechanisms, however, are finite in their abilities to compensate and vary in the length of time they take to respond to new demands. When a person, like Peter, is placed under an acute physiologic or psychologic stress (e.g., surgery, hospitalization, trauma, acute illness), the sudden increase in physiologic demand may go beyond the ability of the body to supply the necessary oxygen and eliminate the increased carbon dioxide. From the time of hospital admission, Peter has been under increased stress and thus is at increased risk for development of multiple complications.

Overall goals in planning Peter's pulmonary care are consistent with his obstructive pulmonary disease needs and include (1) optimizing ventilation and (2) maintaining adequate oxygenation. A plan using both collaborative and independent interventions will be developed to accomplish these goals.

Collaborative Interventions Related to Peter's Pulmonary Status

The physician's orders may include the following:

1. *Pulmonary drug therapy*. Peter, like many patients with COPD, is on long-term bronchodilator and steroid therapy. Bronchodilators dilate the smooth muscle of the bronchi, decreasing airway obstruction. There are two major groups of bronchodilators, the methylxanthines (e.g., aminophylline, theophylline) and the sympathomimetic bronchodilators (e.g., isoetharine, albuterol, terbutaline, metaproterenol). His bronchodilators may be administered orally, IV, by hand-held nebulizer, or by metered-dose inhaler. Corticosteroids sometimes are ordered for treatment of restrictive diseases but are used more commonly as treatment of obstructive diseases. This group of drugs reduces inflammation, promotes bronchodilation, and inhibits bronchoconstriction. In the presence of acute infection, corticosteroid therapy may be contraindicated because of its immunosuppressant activity. Prolonged use of corticosteroids is associated with many adverse effects, and thus their use is closely weighed in terms of benefits and risks before initiation of long-term therapy. Corticosteroids may be administered orally or by aerosol. Examples of commonly used drugs include prednisone, methylprednisone, and prednisolone.

   Oxygen therapy will be ordered carefully. If Peter is a carbon dioxide retainer, his respiratory center is driven by a hypoxic drive. Moderate to high oxygen concentrations may turn off his drive to breathe. Peter's oxygen concentration most likely will be maintained at 2 to 3 L/nasal cannula, or 28 percent VentiMask. Analgesic therapy may be ordered to control Peter's postsurgical pain. His respiratory status must be monitored closely for signs and symptoms of respiratory depression, such as slowing respiratory rate or increasingly shallow respirations. Many analgesics are associated with respiratory depression, increasing the risk of acute ventilatory failure. This is of particular concern in patients with severe pulmonary problems.
2. *Laboratory and x-ray tests*. Peter may have laboratory tests and x-rays ordered intermittently if significant clinical changes are noted in his status. They will, most likely, not be ordered on a regular basis. Of particular interest would be ABGs, electrolytes, and a CBC. A serum albumin may be ordered if the physician is concerned about possible malnutrition.
3. *Pulmonary function tests*. Pulmonary function tests may be ordered if the physician wants to either (1) obtain baseline data concerning Peter's cur-

rent pulmonary function status or (2) compare his current status with previously documented pulmonary function data.

4. *Diet.* A special diet may be ordered that is low in carbohydrate, high in protein, and high in fat. Patients with chronic respiratory diseases frequently experience a loss of appetite from coughing, shortness of breath, general fatigue, excessive mucous production, and the side effects of drug therapy. Hypoxia, associated with advanced pulmonary disease, decreases the endurance of the respiratory muscles and increases energy consumption due to increased work of breathing. The combination of anorexia and hypoxia causes the chronic respiratory patient to lose weight. Ultimately, there is a decreased supply associated with an ever-increasing demand.

   Chronic respiratory patients may need to control carbohydrate intake. Normally, carbohydrates comprise the majority of dietary intake. Carbohydrate metabolism causes CO_2 production that is higher than what is produced by fat or protein. A high carbohydrate diet may precipitate acute respiratory failure in the following way. The acutely ill respiratory patient is often in a malnourished state, which weakens the respiratory muscles, resulting in a decreased tidal volume. A decrease in tidal volume can result in alveolar hypoventilation. The combination of increased carbon dioxide in the alveoli and decreased alveolar ventilation causes increasing Pa_{CO_2} levels, which ultimately can cause acute respiratory acidosis.

   The malnourished respiratory patient has a lower than normal protein level. Protein is vital to proper body function. Serum albumin (normal 3.5 to 5 g/dL) determination is a frequently used laboratory test to measure nonmuscle protein. Albumin is one of the best malnutrition predictors. Approximately 55 percent of plasma proteins in the blood is albumin. A serum albumin level of < 2.5 g/dL is considered critically low, decreasing the patient's chance of survival through an acute illness.

Independent Nursing Interventions

Nursing management of Peter, a patient with obstructive pulmonary disease, is essentially the same as management of the patient with restrictive pulmonary disease (refer to Case Study One, Independent Nursing Interventions). Emphasis however, is placed on airway clearance and pulmonary hygiene. His nutritional status must be improved and monitored closely. His oxygenation status and therapy will require close assessment for therapeutic and nontherapeutic effects to prevent loss of his hypoxic drive to breathe if he is a CO_2 retainer. Encouraging him to maintain activities, such as getting up into a chair, walking in the room or hall, will help maintain or strengthen activity tolerance and reduce the risk of immobility complications.

Plan Evaluation and Revision

Peter's plan of care should be evaluated at regular intervals. Evaluation will be based on the status of specific expected patient outcomes. If evaluation shows lack of forward progress toward attaining or maintaining goals, the plan must be revised, seeking alternatives to care that will be more successful.

CASE STUDY 3

The Continuing Case of Peter M, the Patient Requiring Mechanical Ventilation

In the first two case studies, Mary R and Peter M were successful in meeting their outcome criteria and were subsequently discharged home without further complications. In this case study, we are going to assume that Peter developed a complication of bed rest—pneumonia—and his condition has deteriorated.

Status Update

Today, Peter has demonstrated increasing respiratory distress and has been transferred to the critical care unit for close observation. Stat arterial blood gases are drawn (obtained while breathing room air) and the following results are called back to the nurse:

$$pH = 7.28,\ Pa_{CO_2} = 82\ mm\ Hg,\ Pa_{O_2} = 48\ mm\ Hg,\ HCO_3 = 34\ mEq/L,\ Sa_{O_2} = 74\%$$

EXERCISE

In the space provided, interpret the preceding ABG:
Acid–base status:

Oxygenation status:

ANSWER

Peter is in respiratory acidosis, either acute or partially compensated with moderate hypoxemia. If his elevated HCO_3 represents his baseline value, he is in an acute acidotic state.

Focused Respiratory Assessment

Upon transfer to the medical ICU, the nurse quickly performs a focused assessment of Peter's pulmonary and cardiovascular status, with the following results: Respiratory rate is 28/min, labored, and regular. Little air movement is heard on auscultation with distant breath sounds heard only in the central airway. Tongue and oral mucous membranes are dark and dusky, as are his lips and nail beds. He is sitting up on the side of the bed leaning on his bed stand. He is making heavy use of his accessory muscles. The respiratory therapist performs pulmonary mechanics, which result in a vital capacity (VC) of 952 mL (Peter weighs 68 kg); a minute ventilation ($\dot{V}E$) of 12 L/min (normal is 5 to 10 L/min); and a negative inspiratory force (NIF) of −10 cm H_2O.

QUESTION

Based on the preceding assessment, which of Peter's data meet the criteria for ventilatory support? Circle "yes" or "no" beside each criteria.

1. Respiratory rate	Yes	No
2. pH and $PaCO_2$	Yes	No
3. PaO_2	Yes	No
4. VC	Yes	No
5. NIF	Yes	No
6. $\dot{V}E$	Yes	No

ANSWER

Some of the common critical values used for criteria for ventilatory support include $PaCO_2$ of > 50 mm Hg with a pH of < 7.30; PaO_2 of < 50 mm Hg; respiratory rate of > 35 breaths/min; vital capacity of < 15 mL/kg; NIF of < −20 cm H_2O; and a $\dot{V}E$ of > 10 L/min.

Based on these critical values, with the exception of respiratory rate, Peter currently meets all criteria. A person does not need to meet all of the criteria to be placed on a mechanical ventilator. Criteria are used to assist the clinician in decision making.

The decision is made to intubate Peter and place him on the mechanical ventilator to treat his acute respiratory failure. The nurse begins to assemble the necessary intubation equipment.

EXERCISE

List at least six pieces of equipment that must be assembled for an intubation:

1.
2.
3.
4.
5.
6.

ANSWER

Equipment needed for placement of an ET tube include soft-cuffed ET tubes, stylet, topical anesthetic, laryngoscope handle with blade attached, Magill forceps, suction catheters, Yankauer suction tip, syringe for cuff inflation, water-soluble lubricant, and adhesive tape.

While Peter's ET tube is being placed, a mechanical ventilator is set up with initial settings. Depending on available support staff in a facility, a variety of people may be trained to set initial settings, including the respiratory therapist, the physician, or the nurse.

QUESTION

In the spaces provided, fill in the typical standard setting as described in Section Five of the Mechanical Ventilation Module.

1. Tidal volume ____ to ____ mL/kg
2. Rate ____ to ____ breaths/min
3. FIO_2 ____ to ____
4. Mode A/C or SIMV (circle one)

ANSWER

1. Tidal volume: 5 to 7 mL/kg
2. Rate: 8 to 12 breaths/min
3. FIO_2 0.5 to 1.0 (50 to 100 percent oxygenation concentration)
4. Mode A/C (Assist/Control)

Though mechanical ventilation was a necessary intervention to protect Peter's life, it has placed him at high risk for development of complications. The nurse will particularly need to monitor his cardiovascular status closely now that he is receiving positive pressure ventilation (PPV).

QUESTION

Based on what you know about Peter's history and assessments, why is the nurse particularly concerned about monitoring his cardiovascular status?

ANSWER

PPV reduces cardiac output by decreasing venous return to the heart. Peter already has a history of congestive heart failure and he was recently treated for an acute episode. He is extremely vulnerable for development of a recurrent CHF episode and he could potentially develop multiple system problems associated with reduced cardiac output.

A major general patient care goal used in guiding Peter's nursing interventions while he is receiving mechanical ventilation is support of physiologic needs. More specifically, Peter's pulmonary support will focus on protecting his airway and promoting ventilation and oxygenation. Endotracheal suctioning is a major intervention that helps meet his pulmonary needs.

QUESTION

Which of the following open-system suctioning routines would best meet Peter's need for optimizing oxygenation? (*Note:* H/H = hyperoxygenate/hyperventilate)

A. Suction, H/H, return to ventilator
B. H/H, suction, suction, H/H, return to ventilator
C. Suction, H/H, suction, H/H, return to ventilator
D. H/H, suction, H/H, suction, H/H, return to ventilator

ANSWER

The correct answer is D. It is important to optimize oxygenation prior to initiating suctioning since the suction removes oxygenation as well as secretions. The hyperventilation/hyperoxygenation procedure should be repeated prior to each suctioning pass and prior to returning the patient to the ventilator to replace lost oxygen. Each suctioning pass should be limited to no longer than 10 seconds. As a reminder of the length of time for a single pass, some nurses hold their breath while suctioning. Breath holding becomes uncomfortable within 10 seconds for many people. If this easy procedure is used, the nurse can initially time her or his own breath holding to experience how it feels at 10 seconds. If the patient is attached to pulse oximetry, many nurses will also hyperoxygenate/ hyperventilate the patient until the SpO_2 has returned to > 95 percent.

Scenario Update

Peter's pneumonia is now resolved and it is believed that he is ready for removal from the mechanical ventilator. It has been 7 days since he was first placed on mechanical ventilation. To initiate the weaning process, the clinicians will first need to determine his readiness to wean.

EXERCISE

List three simple questions that can be asked that can rapidly identify if Peter is NOT ready for weaning.

1.
2.
3.

ANSWER

Initially, it is simpler to decide if he is **not** ready for weaning, since determination of actual readiness requires more thorough testing in patients with complex problems.

1. Has the problem that precipitated the need for mechanical ventilation resolved?
2. Is the patient's clinical condition stable?
3. Is the patient's clinical condition improving?

Peter's status does, in fact, meet the initial criteria. The clinicians decide to proceed with a more comprehensive patient screening. Since dysfunction of particular body systems increases the risk of Peter becoming ventilator dependent, the comprehensive screening focuses on function of those systems.

EXERCISE

List the five physiologic systems that are associated with failure-to-wean problems and list at least one test that might be performed to measure the function of each system:

Physiologic System	Test
1.	
2.	
3.	
4.	
5.	

ANSWER

Physiologic System	Test
1. Respiratory	ABG, $\dot{V}_E$, A-a gradient, SpO_2, chest x-ray
2. Cardiovascular	BP, heart rate, ECG pattern
3. CNS	Alert, cooperative, willing to be weaned
4. Renal	I = O, adequate urine output, BUN, and creatinine
5. Nutritional/Metabolic	Electrolytes, CBC with differential, albumin/ prealbumin

---

It is determined that Peter meets the comprehensive patient-screening criteria sufficiently to warrant initiating weaning. Due to his history of chronic lung disease, it is anticipated that he will require a slow ventilator weaning process, using SIMV mode with pressure support ventilation (PSV).

QUESTION

Which of the following statements best describes SIMV weaning mode?

A. Guarantees an ongoing stable level of minute ventilation.
B. Frequency of mandatory ventilator breaths is slowly decreased.
C. Patient is removed from ventilator for increasing lengths of time.
D. Provides positive pressure during the inspiration phase to support tidal volume.

ANSWER

The correct answer is B. SIMV allows Peter to take over his own work of breathing gradually, as he gains back his muscle strength. *Discussion of incorrect options:* A. Describes mandatory minute ventilation (MMV); C. Describes manual weaning; D. Describes pressure support ventilation (PSV).

Scenario Update

Peter has been successfully weaned from mechanical ventilation over a 5-day period. It is now time to extubate him.

QUESTION

Briefly explain the reason for rapid removal of the endotracheal tube once Peter no longer requires mechanical ventilation.

ANSWER

The presence of the endotracheal tube increases Peter's airway resistance and thus increases his work of breathing. It will be easier for him to breathe once the artificial therapy has been removed.

Following extubation, the nurse will monitor Peter closely for signs of acute respiratory distress. Such signs may occur immediately, due to swelling of the airway associated with the trauma of tube removal; or it may occur later, usually due to respiratory muscle fatigue. He will immediately be placed on low-flow humidified (usually per mask) oxygen to maintain his oxygenation status.

REFERENCES

Kee, J. (1999). *Laboratory and diagnostic tests with nursing implications*, (5th ed.). Stamford, CT: Appleton & Lange.

Ulrich, S.P., Canale, S.W., & Wendell, S.A. (1998). *Medical–surgical nursing care planning guides*. (4th ed.). Philadelphia: W.B. Saunders.

PART III

CELLULAR OXYGENATION

MODULE 9

Oxygenation

Karen L. Johnson

This self-study module focuses on the physiologic as well as the pathophysiologic processes involved in oxygenation. The module is composed of six sections. Section One considers the underlying general principles involved in the oxygenation process. Sections Two through Four review the processes of pulmonary gas exchange, oxygen delivery, and oxygen consumption. In Section Five, definitions of clinical conditions that occur as a result of impaired oxygenation are given. Section Six reviews oxygenation assessment techniques. Each section includes a set of review questions to help the learner evaluate his or her understanding of the section's content before moving on to the next section. All Section Reviews and the module Pretest and Posttest include answers. It is suggested that the learner review those concepts answered incorrectly in the review questions before proceeding to the next section.

OBJECTIVES

Following completion of this module, the learner will be able to

1. Explain the concept of oxygenation.
2. Discuss pulmonary gas exchange.
3. Describe the physiologic components of oxygen delivery.
4. Describe oxygen consumption in terms of aerobic and anaerobic metabolism.
5. Define pathophysiologic conditions that are a result of impaired oxygenation.
6. Identify techniques to assess oxygenation status in relation to pulmonary gas exchange, oxygen delivery, and oxygen consumption.

PRETEST

1. Oxygenation is
   - **A.** a concept that involves multisystem coordination of the intake, delivery, and use of oxygen for energy
   - **B.** a process that occurs in the lungs
   - **C.** a process that involves the transportation of oxygen to cells
   - **D.** a process dependent on ventilation, diffusion, and perfusion
2. Gas exchange is dependent on
   - **A.** ventilation and diffusion
   - **B.** ventilation, diffusion, and perfusion
   - **C.** PAO_2
   - **D.** oxygen diffusion across alveolar–capillary membranes
3. Oxygen delivery is affected by
   - **A.** hemoglobin and the oxygen content of arterial blood
   - **B.** cardiac output, autoregulation, and the oxygen content of arterial blood
   - **C.** cardiac output, autoregulation, and autonomic nervous system input
   - **D.** cardiac output, autoregulation, autonomic nervous system input, and oxygen content of arterial blood

4. Ninety-seven percent of oxygen carried to tissues is
   A. dissolved in the plasma
   B. carried as oxyhemoglobin
   C. unavailable for cellular use
   D. delivered to cells by the heart
5. The most effective mechanism of oxygen consumption occurs by
   A. aerobic metabolism
   B. anaerobic metabolism
   C. producing two ATP molecules, lactate and pyruvate
   D. oxygen extraction
6. Completion of a nursing assessment would have what impact on oxygen consumption?
   A. none
   B. increase consumption by 10 percent
   C. increase consumption by 20 percent
   D. increase consumption by 30 percent
7. Impaired oxygenation can result in
   A. hypoxemia and hypoxia
   B. hypoxemia, hypoxia, and dysoxia
   C. hypoxemia, hypoxia, dysoxia, and shock states
   D. hypoxemia, hypoxia, dysoxia, shock states, and multiple organ dysfunction
8. Hypoxemia is defined as
   A. a $PaO_2 > 50$ mm Hg
   B. a $PaCO_2 > 50$ mm Hg
   C. inadequate amount of oxygen in arterial blood
   D. hemoglobin < 10 mg/dL
9. Clinical assessment of oxygenation includes assessment of
   A. arterial blood gases
   B. assessment of the cardiovascular and pulmonary systems
   C. assessment of pulmonary gas exchange and oxygen delivery
   D. assessment of pulmonary gas exchange, oxygen delivery, and oxygen consumption
10. Assessment of oxygen consumption is made using
   A. serum lactate levels
   B. arterial blood gases
   C. serum hemoglobin levels
   D. serum adenosine triphosphate levels

Pretest answers: 1. A, 2. B, 3. D, 4. B, 5. A, 6. B, 7. D, 8. C, 9. D, 10. A

GLOSSARY

Aerobic metabolism. The mechanism used by the body for energy generation through the use of oxygen

Affinity. To what degree hemoglobin releases oxygen

Anaerobic metabolism. The mechanism used by the body for energy generation without the use of oxygen

Autoregulation. Mechanism used by tissues to regulate their own blood supply by dilating or constricting local blood vessels

Cardiac output. The amount of blood pumped by the ventricles each minute

Cyanosis. A bluish skin discoloration that results from decreased oxygen delivery

Diffusion. Movement of gases down a pressure gradient from an area of high concentration to low concentration

Dysoxia. Condition characterized by an inability of the cells to use oxygen properly despite adequate levels of oxygen delivery

Hypoxemia. A condition characterized by an inadequate amount of oxygen in the blood as a result of impaired gas exchange, frequently quantified as a PaO_2 of < 50 mm Hg

Hypoxia. An inadequate amount of oxygen available at the cellular level

Oxygen consumption (VO_2). The amount of oxygen used by cells

Oxygen delivery. The process of transportation of oxygen to cells, dependent on cardiac output, hemoglobin saturation with oxygen, and the partial pressure of oxygen in arterial blood (PaO_2)

Oxygen extraction. The process by which cells take oxygen from the blood

Pulmonary gas exchange. The process that involves the intake of oxygen from the external environment into the internal environment and is carried out by the processes of ventilation, diffusion, and perfusion

Ventilation. The mechanical movement of airflow to and from the atmosphere and the alveoli

ABBREVIATIONS

ABG. Arterial blood gas

AV. Alveolar ventilation

ARDS. Acute respiratory distress syndrome

ATP. Adenosine triphosphate

CO. Cardiac output

CO_2. Carbon dioxide

CaO_2. Oxygen content of arterial blood

DO_2. Oxygen delivery

FIO_2. Fraction of inspired oxygen

H_2O. Water

Hgb. Hemoglobin

Hgbo$_2$. Oxyhemoglobin

MODS. Multiple organ dysfunction syndrome

MV. Minute ventilation

O$_2$. Oxygen

Pao$_2$. The amount of oxygen physically dissolved in arterial blood, unattached to hemoglobin

PAO$_2$. The partial pressure of alveolar oxygen

PvO$_2$. The amount of oxygen physically dissolved in venous blood

Qsp/Qt. Intrapulmonary shunt

RR. Respiratory rate

Sao$_2$. Oxygen saturation of arterial blood

TV. Tidal volume

VC. Vital capacity

VO$_2$. Oxygen consumption

SECTION ONE: Oxygenation

At the completion of this section, the learner will be able to explain the concept of oxygenation.

Oxygenation is a concept of multisystem integration and coordination in the intake, delivery, and use of oxygen for energy metabolism. Oxygenation cannot be understood solely by understanding the pulmonary system or the cardiovascular system. Oxygenation involves the integration and coordination of pulmonary, cardiovascular, neurologic, hematologic, and metabolic processes.

Unlike the heart, which has intrinsic rhythmic properties to work independently, the respiratory system requires continuous input from the nervous system. Depending on various internal and external stimuli, the nervous system regulates the respiratory system to meet identified body needs for oxygen. Oxygen is brought into the internal environment via the respiratory system during the process of ventilation. Oxygen crosses alveolar–capillary membranes by diffusion, combines with hemoglobin, and is transported via the pulmonary vein to the left side of the heart. The cardiovascular system transports oxygenated blood to the tissues. Oxygenated blood then leaves the capillaries by diffusion and enters cells. Depending on cellular energy requirements, each cell extracts the amount of oxygen it needs to fulfill its metabolic requirements. The cells use oxygen to convert food substrates into energy. Carbon dioxide and "unused" oxygen are carried to the right side of the heart and back to the lungs for elimination and reuse.

The concept of oxygenation involves three physiologic components for the intake, delivery, and use of oxygen for energy: pulmonary gas exchange, oxygen delivery, and oxygen consumption, as summarized in Figure 9–1. Adequacy of oxygenation depends on the integration of these physiologic components. Pulmonary gas exchange involves the intake of oxygen from the external environment into the internal environment and is carried out by

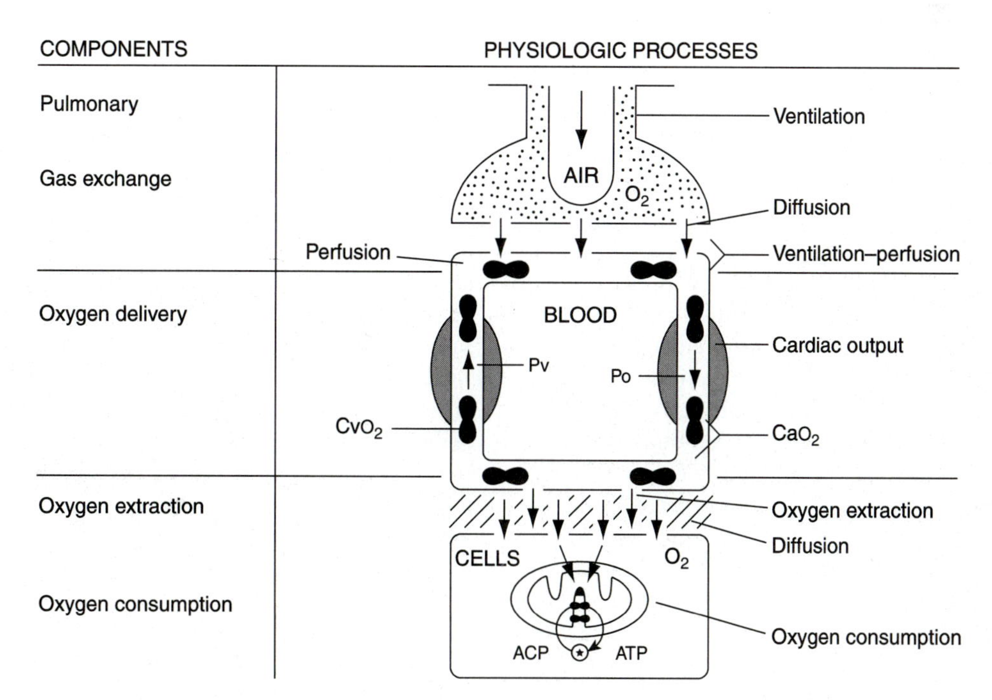

Figure 9–1. Johnson's conceptual model of oxygenation depicts oxygenation as a process involving the intake, delivery, and use of oxygen for energy metabolism. *(Adapted, with permission, from Taylor, C.R., & Weibel, E.R. [1981], Design of the mammalian respiratory system,* Respiration Physiology, *41 [p. 2]. Copyright © 1981 by Elsevier Science.)*

the processes of ventilation, diffusion, and perfusion. Oxygen delivery is the process of transportation of oxygen to cells and is dependent on cardiac output, hemoglobin saturation with oxygen, and the partial pressure of oxygen in arterial blood (PaO_2). Oxygen consumption involves the use of oxygen at the cellular level to generate energy for cells to use to perform their specific functions. Impaired oxygenation can result from impaired pulmonary gas exchange, decreased oxygen delivery, or impaired oxygen consumption.

In summary, the concept of oxygenation requires an understanding that the intake, delivery, and use of oxygen for energy involves multisystem integration and coordination involving three physiologic components: pulmonary gas exchange, oxygen delivery, and oxygen consumption. Adequacy of oxygenation is dependent on these three components. Any disease or condition that affects these processes will affect oxygenation.

SECTION ONE REVIEW

1. Oxygenation is
   A. a process that occurs in the pulmonary system
   B. a process that involves ventilation, diffusion, and perfusion
   C. a process that involves the transportation of oxygen to cells
   D. a concept that the intake, delivery, and use of oxygen requires multisystem integration and coordination
2. Which of the following are the physiologic processes involved with oxygenation?
   A. pulmonary gas exchange, oxygen delivery, and oxygen consumption
   B. diffusion, ventilation, and perfusion
   C. cardiac output and hemoglobin saturation with oxygen
   D. the pulmonary and cardiovascular systems
3. Pulmonary gas exchange is carried out by which of the following?
   A. inspiration of oxygen by the process of ventilation
   B. expiration of carbon dioxide by the process of diffusion
   C. ventilation, diffusion, and perfusion
   D. ventilation, oxygen consumption, and perfusion
4. Oxygen consumption
   A. is dependent on cardiac output and hemoglobin saturation with oxygen
   B. involves the use of oxygen to generate energy
   C. involves the intake of oxygen from the external environment
   D. is the process of transporting oxygen to cells

Answers: 1. D, 2. A, 3. C, 4. B

SECTION TWO: Pulmonary Gas Exchange

At the completion of this section, the learner will be able to discuss pulmonary gas exchange. For more detailed information, please refer to the Respiratory Process module (Module 5). An understanding of FIO_2, PAO_2, PaO_2, and PvO_2 is necessary to understand this section.

The initial component of oxygenation involves pulmonary gas exchange. **Pulmonary gas exchange** involves the inspiration and delivery of oxygen from the external environment to the alveoli and diffusion across the alveolar–capillary membrane, where oxygen combines with hemoglobin in the pulmonary capillaries. Adequate blood flow must exist to "carry away" the oxygenated blood to the left side of the heart and the systemic circulation. These functions are carried out by physiologic processes involving ventilation, diffusion, and perfusion (Fig. 9–2).

Ventilation is the movement of air to and from the atmosphere to the alveoli. It involves the actual work of breathing and requires adequate functioning of the ventilatory muscles, thorax, lungs, conducting airways, and nervous system. Decreased functioning of any one of these systems can affect ventilation and impair oxygenation.

Diffusion is the mechanism by which oxygen moves across the alveoli and into the pulmonary capillary. There are three factors that affect diffusion across the alveolar–capillary membrane: pressure gradient, surface area, and thickness. The greater the difference between alveolar oxygen and pulmonary capillary oxygen pressures, the greater the diffusion of oxygen from the alveoli to the pulmonary capillaries. The greater the available alveolar–capillary membrane surface area, the greater the amount of oxygen that can diffuse across it. Many conditions can cause a significant reduction in functional surface area. The thickness of the alveolar–capillary membrane affects diffusion of oxygen from the alveoli to the pulmonary capillary. Conditions that increase the thickness of the alveolar–capillary membrane can decrease diffusion.

The third component of gas exchange involves perfusion. Three factors affect perfusion: hemoglobin (Hgb) concentration, affinity of oxygen to Hgb, and blood flow. When oxygen diffuses across the alveolar–capillary mem-

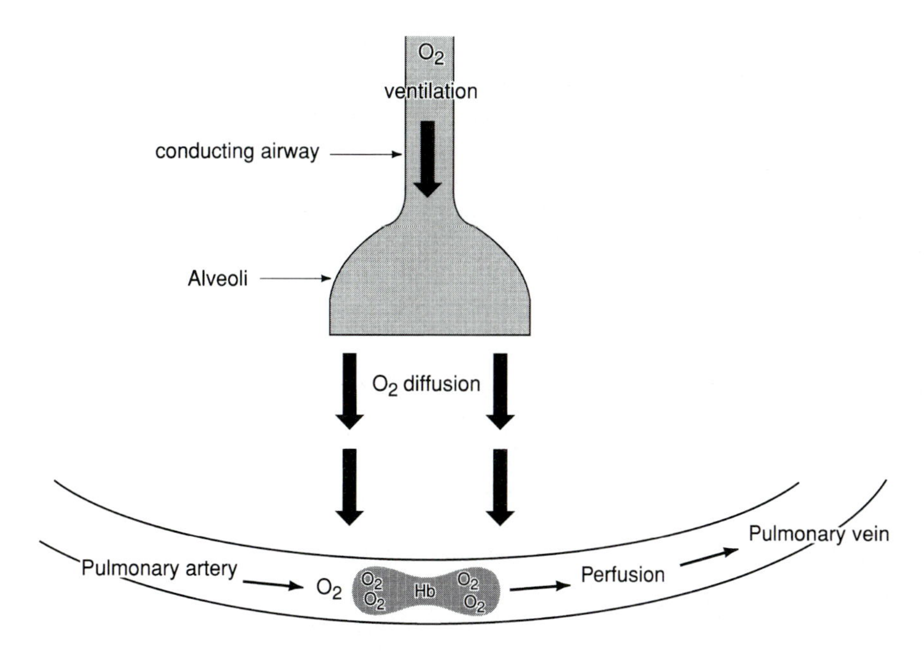

Figure 9–2. Initial process of oxygenation: pulmonary gas exchange.

brane it combines with hemoglobin in the pulmonary capillary and is carried to the left side of the heart. Factors that affect hemoglobin concentration or the affinity of oxygen to hemoglobin affect the amount of oxygen in the blood. Refer to Module 6 for factors that influence the oxyhemoglobin dissociation curve. Perfusion of alveoli has an effect on oxygenation. A decrease in blood flow through the pulmonary vasculature results in a ventilation–perfusion imbalance. Any disease or condition that impairs pulmonary perfusion impairs pulmonary gas exchange. Some conditions and diseases that affect oxygenation as a result of impaired gas exchange are summarized in Table 9–1.

In summary, the initial component of oxygenation is pulmonary gas exchange. Gas exchange is dependent on three processes: ventilation, diffusion, and perfusion. Any disease or condition that affects gas exchange can impair oxygenation.

TABLE 9–1. CONDITIONS THAT IMPAIR GAS EXCHANGE

Ventilation Impairment
Decreased pressure gradient for oxygen
Inspiratory muscle weakness or trauma (↑ Pa_{CO_2}, ↑ PA_{CO_2}, ↓ PA_{O_2})
Loss of consciousness
Obstruction or trauma to airways, lung, thorax
Restrictive pulmonary disorders

Diffusion Impairment
Decrease in alveolar–capillary membrane surface area (emphysema, lung tumors, pneumonia)
Increase in alveolar–capillary membrane thickness (acute respiratory distress syndrome, pulmonary edema, pneumonia)

Perfusion impairment
Decreased Hgb (anemia, carbon monoxide poisoning)
Decreased perfusion (hemorrhage, pulmonary embolism, pulmonary vasoconstriction)
Physiologic shunt (anatomic, capillary, shuntlike effect)
Vasoconstriction

SECTION TWO REVIEW

1. Which of the following conditions has an effect on ventilation?
   A. low hemoglobin levels
   B. upper airway obstruction
   C. pulmonary embolism
   D. hypovolemic shock
2. A PA_{O_2} of 100 mm Hg and a pulmonary Pa_{O_2} of 40 mm Hg would
   A. facilitate diffusion
   B. decrease diffusion
   C. decrease ventilation
   D. facilitate perfusion
3. Pneumonia results in a decrease in functional alveolar–capillary membrane surface area. This results in a(n)
   A. increased alveolar–capillary pressure gradient
   B. decreased alveolar–capillary pressure gradient
   C. decrease in oxygen diffusion across alveolar–capillary membranes
   D. increase in oxygen diffusion across alveolar–capillary membranes

4. Anemia affects which component of the gas exchange process?
   A. ventilation
   B. diffusion
   C. PAO_2
   D. perfusion

5. Impaired gas exchange results in
   A. oxygenation impairment
   B. ventilation impairment
   C. diffusion impairment
   D. perfusion impairment

Answers: 1. B, 2. A, 3. C, 4. D, 5. A

SECTION THREE: Oxygen Delivery

At the completion of this section, the learner will be able to describe the physiologic components of oxygen delivery.

The second component of oxygenation is oxygen delivery. **Oxygen delivery** involves the process of transporting oxygen to cells. The amount of oxygen delivered to tissues is approximately 1,000 mL/min. (When indexed to consider body surface area, oxygen delivery is approximately 600 mL/min/m^2.) Factors that affect oxygen delivery include cardiac output (CO), autoregulation, oxygen content of arterial blood (CaO_2), and autonomic nervous system innervation.

Cardiac output is the amount of blood pumped by the heart each minute (see Module 13). The greater the cardiac output, the greater the amount of oxygen delivered to the tissues per minute. Conversely, conditions that cause a decrease in cardiac output result in a decrease in the amount of oxygen delivered to tissues per minute.

Under normal circumstances, the volume of oxygenated blood pumped by the heart is proportional to the body's demands. When tissues require more oxygen, heart rate will increase in an attempt to augment cardiac output in the delivery of more oxygenated blood. Tissues have the ability to regulate their own blood supply by dilating or constricting local blood vessels through the mechanism of autoregulation. Tissues have varying energy requirements and use autoregulation to meet their metabolic demands. When the body is at rest, not all tissue capillaries are open at the same time. Increased metabolic rate (e.g., during exercise) and arterial hypoxemia (decreased PaO_2) open more tissue capillaries, thereby allowing more oxygen to be extracted by tissue beds. **Autoregulation** serves to protect tissues by controlling blood flow and oxygen delivery in response to individual tissue needs.

Oxygen is carried in arterial blood in two forms: It can be combined with hemoglobin or it can be dissolved in the plasma. Normally, 20 mL of oxygen is transported per 100 mL of blood. Almost 97 percent of all oxygen delivered to cells is in the form of oxyhemoglobin ($HgbO_2$), and the remaining 3 percent is delivered partially dissolved in plasma.

Each molecule of hemoglobin has the ability to carry four oxygen molecules. When hemoglobin is fully saturated with oxygen, oxyhemoglobin is formed. Each hemoglobin molecule can be thought of as a bus that carries four oxygen passengers to tissues. The measurement of SaO_2 by arterial blood gas (ABG) analysis is a measurement of the ratio of oxygenated hemoglobin to total hemoglobin (see Module 6). For example, if the SaO_2 is 95 percent, it can be interpreted that 95 percent of all the available seats on the "hemoglobin bus" are occupied by oxygen. Because the majority of oxygen is carried to tissues by hemoglobin, any condition or disease that decreases hemoglobin concentrations will severely decrease the amount of oxygen carried to tissues. (This will be discussed in further detail in Module 10.)

Many conditions impair oxygen delivery. An uncompensated decrease in cardiac output, hemoglobin, or SaO_2 can significantly reduce oxygen delivery. Patients who have what may appear to be clinically insignificant decreases in all three factors can have a significant decrease in oxygen delivery when they are considered together.

The autonomic nervous system exerts partial control of oxygen delivery through excitatory or inhibitory effects on the heart, lungs, and blood vessels. Specific cell mediators present in the cardiovascular and respiratory systems, when stimulated, result in a target cell response. The types of cell receptors and their physiologic responses are summarized in Table 9–2.

TABLE 9–2. ALPHA, BETA, AND DOPAMINERGIC RECEPTOR STIMULATION AND PHYSIOLOGIC RESPONSE

RECEPTOR	STIMULATION	PHYSIOLOGIC RESPONSE
$Alpha_1$	Vasoconstriction Intestinal relaxation	Increased vascular resistance Increased pressure and afterload
$Alpha_2$	Suppression of norepinephrine	Controls excess catecholamine release
$Beta_1$	Increased myocardial rate and contractility	Increased cardiac ouptut Increased myocardial oxygen consumption
$Beta_2$	Bronchodilation Vasodilation	Decreased airway resistance Decreased vascular resistance
Dopaminergic	Renal vasodilation Mesenteric vasodilation	Increased renal blood flow Increased mesenteric blood flow

In summary, oxygen delivery is the process of transporting oxygen to cells. Four factors affect oxygen delivery: cardiac output, autoregulation, oxygen content of arterial blood, and autonomic nervous system innervation. An uncompensated decrease in cardiac output, hemoglobin, or SaO_2 can cause a significant reduction in the amount of oxygen delivered to cells.

SECTION THREE REVIEW

1. Oxygen delivery is the
   - **A.** amount of oxygen in arterial blood
   - **B.** process of transporting oxygen to cells
   - **C.** process of utilizing oxygen for energy
   - **D.** amount of blood pumped by the heart per minute
2. Factors that affect oxygen delivery include
   - **A.** ventilation, diffusion, and perfusion
   - **B.** cardiac output, hemoglobin concentration, and ventilation
   - **C.** cardiac output, autoregulation, and oxygen content of arterial blood
   - **D.** cardiac output, autoregulation, oxygen content of arterial blood, and autonomic nervous system innervation
3. A patient who has suffered a myocardial infarction is at risk for impaired oxygenation primarily related to
   - **A.** overactive autoregulation
   - **B.** impaired autonomic nervous system innervation
   - **C.** decreased cardiac output
   - **D.** decreased oxygen content of arterial blood
4. Ninety-seven percent of all oxygen delivered to cells
   - **A.** is in the form of oxyhemoglobin
   - **B.** is dissolved in plasma
   - **C.** is carried as PaO_2
   - **D.** is carried as HCO_3
5. Administration of a drug that stimulates dopaminergic receptors would
   - **A.** decrease blood pressure
   - **B.** increase cardiac output
   - **C.** increase renal blood flow
   - **D.** decrease afterload

Answers: 1. B, 2. D, 3. C, 4. A, 5. C

SECTION FOUR: Oxygen Consumption

At the completion of this section, the learner will be able to describe oxygen consumption in terms of aerobic and anaerobic metabolism.

The third component of oxygenation is oxygen consumption. **Oxygen consumption (VO_2)** (Fig. 9–3) is the process by which cells use oxygen to generate energy. Oxygen enables the energy contained in food to be converted into a usable form of energy. Ingested carbohydrates, fats, and proteins are broken down into substrates that are converted in the Krebs' cycle into energy in the form of adenosine triphosphate (ATP). This process is called **aerobic metabolism** (Fig. 9–4). The purpose of forming ATP is to create intracellular energy stores. Fatty acids are primary energy substrates in aerobic metabolism. When energy is needed, ATP is broken down and energy is released. Aerobic metabolism results in the creation of 36 molecules of ATP. Cells use ATP molecules as their energy source to perform all their necessary functions. Without the ATP energy stores, cellular processes break down and cells cannot function. The primary value of oxygen is its ability to develop ATP.

As a "backup" mechanism, cells have the ability to

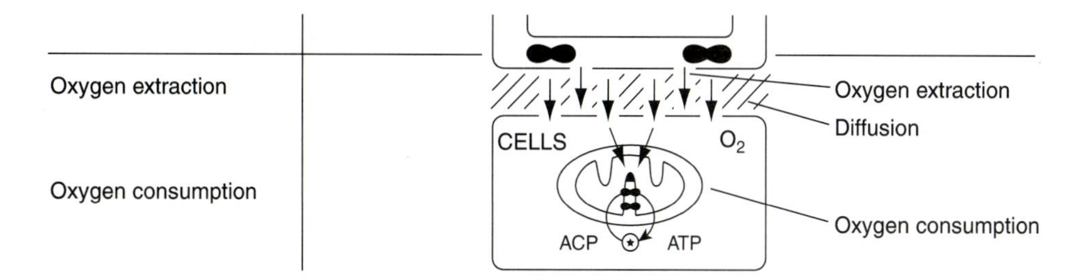

Figure 9–3. Johnson's conceptual model of oxygenation depicts oxygenation as a process involving the intake, delivery, and use of oxygen for energy metabolism. *(Adapted, with permission, from Taylor, C.R., & Weibel, E.R. [1981], Design of the mammalian respiratory system,* Respiration Physiology, *41 [p. 2]. Copyright © 1981 by Elsevier Science.)*

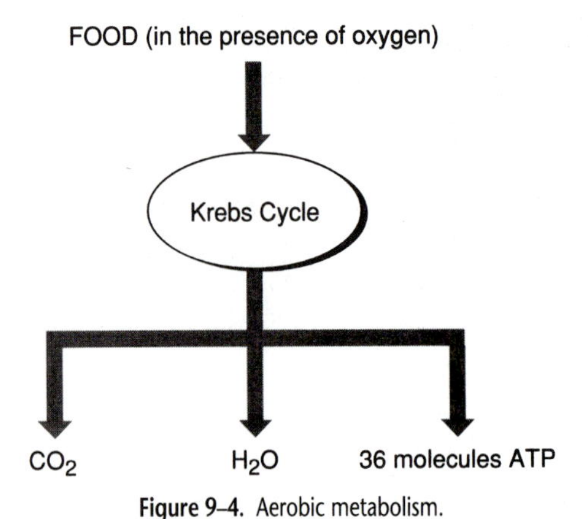

Figure 9–4. Aerobic metabolism.

generate energy in the absence of oxygen by the process of anaerobic metabolism (Fig. 9–5). When **anaerobic metabolism** is used, carbohydrates are broken down to generate ATP. Carbohydrates are the only food substrates that can be broken down to generate ATP without the use of oxygen. Anaerobic metabolism produces only two ATP molecules, and produces the by-products pyruvate and lactate. When cells use anaerobic metabolism, lactate (an acid) accumulates in the body and results in lactic acidosis. The acidic environment alters cellular structure and greatly impairs cellular function. Anaerobic metabolism is less efficient than aerobic metabolism and results in some potentially harmful byproducts. Table 9–3 compares aerobic and anaerobic metabolism.

The process by which cells take oxygen from the blood is called **oxygen extraction**. Under normal circumstances, oxygen is loosely attached to hemoglobin so that oxygen is readily removed from the hemoglobin. To what degree the hemoglobin releases oxygen is called **affinity**. The affinity of oxygen to hemoglobin is determined by the oxyhemoglobin dissociation curve (see Module 6). Oxygen dissociates from hemoglobin in response to local tissue oxygen demands. When cells have increased energy demands, they extract more oxygen from the blood. For

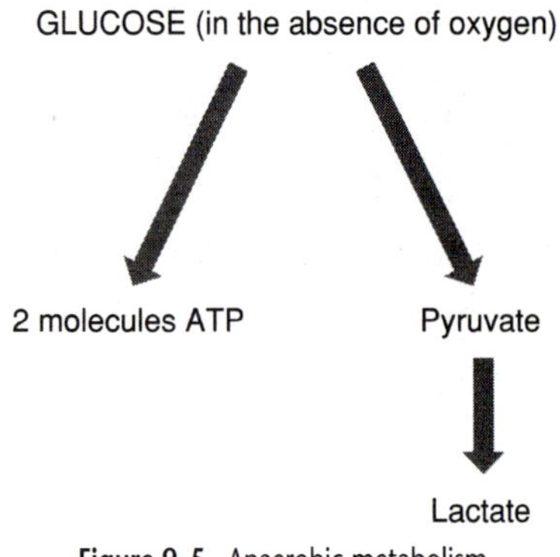

Figure 9–5. Anaerobic metabolism.

TABLE 9–3. AEROBIC VERSUS ANAEROBIC METABOLISM

AEROBIC METABOLISM	ANAEROBIC METABOLISM
Generation of energy through the use of oxygen	Generation of energy in the absence of oxygen
Carbohydrates, fats, proteins broken down into substrates	Carboyhydrates broken down into substrates
Produces 36 ATP molecules	Produces 2 ATP molecules, lactate and pyruvate
Generates large amount of energy	Generates small amount of energy

example, during exercise, muscle cells extract more oxygen than they do when at rest.

The amount of oxygen actually used (or "consumed") by cells is normally 250 mL/min. (When indexed to body surface area, oxygen consumption is 110 to 130 mL/min/m^2.)

Numerous conditions alter the oxygen consumption of critically ill patients (Table 9–4). Coexisting conditions can have an additive effect on oxygen consumption. For example, a patient with a fever, infection, and increased work of breathing can have an oxygen consumption two times the resting oxygen consumption.

Research has demonstrated that numerous activities frequently performed by nurses can increase oxygen consumption in critically ill patients (Swinamer et al., 1987). Table 9–5 lists some routine activities that increase oxygen consumption.

In summary, oxygen consumption is the process by which cells use oxygen to generate energy in the form of ATP. Under normal circumstances, this is done by aerobic

TABLE 9–4. CONDITIONS THAT ALTER OXYGEN CONSUMPTION

Increase O_2 consumption	Hyperventilation, hyperthermia, trauma, sepsis, anxiety, stress, hyperthyroidism, increased muscle activity
Decrease O_2 consumption	Hypoventilation, hypothermia, sedation, neuromuscular blocking agents, anesthesia, hypothyroidism, inactivity

TABLE 9–5. ACTIVITIES THAT INCREASE OXYGEN CONSUMPTION

ACTIVITY	APPROXIMATE INCREASE ABOVE RESTING OXYGEN CONSUMPTION (%)
Nursing assessment	10
Repositioning patient	30
Dressing change	10
Bed bath	20
Weighing patient on sling bed scale	40
Visitors	18
Restlessness/agitation	18

metabolism. When insufficient oxygen is available, cells use anaerobic metabolism. Anaerobic metabolism is inefficient and results in lactic acidosis. When cellular energy demands increase, oxygen extraction and oxygen consumption increase. Research has demonstrated that various clinical conditions and activities increase oxygen consumption.

SECTION FOUR REVIEW

1. A continuous supply of oxygen is
   A. not necessary, since oxygen is stored in cells
   B. required for adequate ATP synthesis
   C. dependent on the amount of blood ejected from the left ventricle
   D. dependent on adequate supplies of hemoglobin
2. A blood sample for a newly admitted trauma patient reveals a high level of lactate. This is indicative of
   A. adequate oxygen delivery
   B. anaerobic metabolism
   C. adequate oxygen consumption
   D. aerobic metabolism
3. Which of the following conditions increases oxygen consumption?
   A. pancuronium 10 mg IV
   B. morphine sulfate 5 mg IV
   C. bedrest
   D. temperature of 102°F
4. Which of the following have been shown to cause the most dramatic increase in oxygen consumption?
   A. dressing change
   B. agitation
   C. visitors
   D. weighing a patient on a sling bed scale

Answers: 1. B, 2. B, 3. D, 4. D

SECTION FIVE: Impaired Oxygenation

At the completion of this section, the learner will be able to define pathophysiologic conditions that are a result of impaired oxygenation.

Sections Two through Four of this module reviewed the three physiologic components of oxygenation: pulmonary gas exchange, oxygen delivery, and oxygen consumption. Any condition or disease that affects one or more of these components will result in impaired oxygenation (e.g., acute respiratory distress syndrome, anemia, hyperventilation). These conditions represent a "continuum" of oxygen disturbances. Life-threatening oxygenation impairments usually involve deficiencies of all three components of oxygenation.

Ventilation–perfusion matching is essential for gas exchange. Most abnormalities of gas exchange are due to ventilation–perfusion mismatching. Conditions such as pulmonary embolus or pneumothorax can produce ventilation–perfusion mismatching. The mismatching of ventilation to perfusion is a common cause of hypoxemia. **Hypoxemia** is a condition characterized by an inadequate amount of oxygen in the blood as a result of impaired gas exchange. Hypoxemia is frequently quantified as a PaO_2 of < 50 mm Hg (see Module 7). If allowed to progress, hypoxemia can result in hypoxia. **Hypoxia** is defined as an inadequate amount of oxygen available at the cellular level such that cells experience anaerobic metabolism (Third European Consensus Conference in Intensive Care Medicine, 1997). **Dysoxia** is a condition characterized by an inability of the cells to use oxygen properly despite adequate levels of oxygen delivery.

If left untreated, hypoxemia, hypoxia, or dysoxia can lead to more life-threatening oxygenation impairments, including shock states and multiple organ dysfunction syndrome (MODS). Shock states are characterized by an imbalance of oxygen supply and demand (see Module 10). MODS is characterized by a continuing impairment of oxygenation, mediated by the inflammatory process (refer to Module 11 for more information).

In summary, any disease or condition that affects one or more of the three components will result in impaired oxygenation. Impaired oxygenation can result in ventilation–perfusion disturbances, including hypoxemia, hypoxia, dysoxia, and shock states.

SECTION FIVE REVIEW

1. Hypoxemia is defined as
   A. an inadequate amount of oxygen in the blood
   B. an inadequate amount of oxygen available at the cellular level
   C. a $PaCO_2$ of < 50 mm Hg
   D. an imbalance of oxygen supply and demand

2. Hypoxia is defined as
   A. an inadequate amount of oxygen in the blood
   B. an inadequate amount of oxygen available at the cellular level
   C. a $PaCO_2$ of < 50 mm Hg
   D. the inability of cells to use oxygen properly
3. Dysoxia is defined as
   A. an inadequate amount of oxygen in the blood
   B. an inadequate amount of oxygen available at the cellular level
   C. a $PaCO_2$ of < 50 mm Hg
   D. the inability of cells to use oxygen properly
4. Shock states are characterized by
   A. an inadequate amount of oxygen in the blood
   B. an inadequate amount of oxygen available at the cellular level
   C. a $PaCO_2$ of < 50 mm Hg
   D. an imbalance of oxygen supply and demand
5. MODS is characterized by
   A. continuing hypoxemia
   B. continuing hypoxia
   C. continuing impairment of oxygenation mediated by the inflammatory response
   D. continuing dysoxia mediated by the inflammatory response

Answers: 1. A, 2. B, 3. D, 4. D, 5. C

SECTION SIX: Assessment of Oxygenation

At the completion of this section, the learner will be able to identify techniques to assess oxygenation status in relation to pulmonary gas exchange, oxygen delivery, and oxygen consumption.

Monitoring oxygenation is one of the most important components of a nursing assessment (Ahrens, 1993a). Accurate assessment and treatment of oxygenation disturbances may determine whether patients survive their intensive care unit stay (Ahrens, 1993b). The outcome of critical illness depends more on the adequacy of oxygenation than on any other factor (Pierson, 1993).

Identification of impaired oxygenation requires an understanding of the three aspects of oxygenation: pulmonary gas exchange, oxygen delivery, and oxygen consumption. Each of these three aspects of oxygenation may vary independently in response to pathophysiologic conditions and therapeutic interventions. Therefore, it is necessary to accurately assess all three levels of oxygenation.

There are two goals in the assessment of oxygenation: (1) to determine overall adequacy of oxygenation and (2) to determine which element of oxygenation dysfunction should be manipulated to improve patient outcome (Nelson, 1993). Oxygenation can be assessed in the critically ill patient using direct and indirect assessment techniques. It is imperative that impaired oxygenation be promptly recognized to ensure proper treatment. Assessment and treatment of impaired oxygenation must be directed toward improvement of all three components of oxygenation.

Pulmonary Gas Exchange

Assessment of gas exchange must include techniques to assess ventilation, diffusion, and perfusion. Techniques to assess for pulmonary gas exchange are summarized in Box 9–1.

Assessment of respiratory muscle efficiency is accomplished by pulmonary function tests (see Module 5) and includes measurements of tidal volume (TV), minute ventilation (MV), alveolar ventilation (AV), respiratory rate (RR), and vital capacity (VC).

Auscultation of the lungs is a common and easy assessment technique to use to assess gas exchange. The key physiologic disturbance that auscultation of the lungs is designed to detect is a change in airflow. Changes in airflow indicate a reduction in the ventilation–perfusion ratio; thus, auscultation may detect pulmonary shunting (Ahrens, 1993a). It is important for the nurse to convey the assessment accurately, using correct terminology. *Crackles* should be used to describe a discontinuous sound and *wheeze* should be used to describe a continuous sound.

Calculation of intrapulmonary shunt can be made in critical care areas for patients who have a peripheral arterial and pulmonary artery catheters. Intrapulmonary shunt (Qsp/Qt) is the proportion of blood that flows past alveoli without participating in gas exchange. An elevated intrapulmonary shunt indicates a large proportion of blood is flowing past alveoli without participating in gas exchange. Elevated intrapulmonary shunt can be attributed to a diffusion impairment or ventilation to perfusion abnormalities. Data needed to calculate Qsp/Qt are obtained by drawing simultaneous mixed venous and ar-

BOX 9–1 Assessment of Pulmonary Gas Exchange

ABG
Assessment of respiratory muscle efficiency (TV, MV, AV, RR, and VC)
Auscultation
Calculation of intrapulmonary shunt

terial blood gases. The formula for Qsp/Qt is complex to calculate, although most bedside monitoring systems in the ICU have the capability to calculate Qsp/Qt once the mixed venous and arterial blood gas data are available and the following data are entered into the system: Hb, SaO_2, PaO_2, PvO_2, and SvO_2. Normal intrapulmonary shunt is < 5% (Misasi & Keyes, 1996).

Oxygen Delivery

Assessment of **oxygen delivery** must include the components of oxygen delivery, including cardiac output, hemoglobin, SaO_2, and PaO_2.

Direct physical assessment of oxygen delivery is difficult because oxygen is a colorless, odorless gas. Indirect physical assessments of oxygen delivery can be made using skin color assessments and capillary refill. **Cyanosis**, a term used to describe bluish skin discoloration, is difficult to use because of subjectivity.

Direct measurement of PaO_2, SaO_2, and hemoglobin can be made through a blood sample analysis. Although PaO_2 minimally contributes to oxygen delivery (less than 3 percent of all oxygen delivered to tissues), it is still used in the evaluation of oxygen delivery. Arterial oxygen saturation is the ratio of oxygenated hemoglobin to total hemoglobin. It can be measured by arterial blood gas analysis (SaO_2) or by pulse oximetry ($SpaO_2$). Pulse oximetry is used for continous noninvasive measurement of arterial oxygenation saturation (Grap, 1998).

Cardiac output can be assessed directly or indirectly. An indirect assessment of cardiac output would include an evaluation of heart rate and stroke volume, including the components of preload and afterload (see Module 13). Direct measurement of cardiac output can be made in critical care areas by the use of a pulmonary artery catheter. Cardiac output measurements can be made using thermodilution techniques or by the use of a special pulmonary artery catheter that measures cardiac output continuously (see Module 13). Oxygen delivery (DO_2) can also be calculated for these patients. Calculation of oxygen delivery requires a cardiac output measurement, serum hemoglobin analysis, and ABG analysis for SaO_2 and PaO_2. Oxygen delivery can be calculated as the product of cardiac output and oxygen content of arterial blood as shown below.

$$DO_2 = (CO \times [Hgb \times 1.34 \times SaO_2] + [PaO_2 \times 0.003]) \times 10^*$$

*10 is a conversion factor

Oxygen Consumption

Assessment of oxygen consumption must include techniques that assess the availability and use of oxygen at the cellular level. Direct assessment of oxygen consumption in the clinical setting is currently not possible. Traditional means of assessing oxygenation (ABGs, cardiac output, etc.) do not reflect oxygen availability at the cellular level. Future technologies will focus on measures to assess oxygenation at the cellular level.

Current methods of assessing oxygen consumption are limited to indirect measurement techniques including measurement of serum lactate levels, base deficit, and mixed venous oxygen saturation monitoring.

Under conditions of inadequate oxygen delivery, cells convert from aerobic metabolism to anaerobic metabolism. The by-product of anaerobic metabolism is lactate. Normal serum lactate levels are < 2 mMol/L. The underlying cause of high serum lactate levels may be inadequate oxygen delivery to meet cellular oxygen needs (Porter & Ivatury, 1998). Serum lactate levels should be evaluated using serial measurements (every 4 to 8 hours) (Mikhail, 1999). These levels can be used as an indicator of improving or worsening oxygen delivery in relation to oxygen consumption (Cornwell et al., 1996).

Base deficit is defined as the amount of base (mMol) required to titrate 1 liter of whole arterial blood to a normal pH (Mikhail, 1999). It is calculated from an arterial blood gas analysis in the laboratory. Normal base deficit is +3 mMol to −3 mMol. It is used as an approximation of acidosis. A base deficit results from an imbalance between oxygen delivery and oxygen consumption, which results in a lactic acidosis secondary to anaerobic metabolism (Porter & Ivatury, 1998). Base deficit can be classified as: mild (2 to −5 mMol); moderate (−6 to −14 mMol); and severe (> −15 mMol). Base deficit has been shown to increase with ongoing oxygenation impairment and to decrease with improving oxygenation.

Mixed venous oxygen saturation (SvO_2) reflects the balance between oxygen supply and oxygen demand. SvO_2 is a clinical parameter that reflects a balance between the variables of oxygen delivery (CO, SaO_2, and Hgb) and oxygen consumption. SvO_2 can be measured intermittently by blood gas analysis of a mixed venous blood sample drawn from the distal port of a pulmonary artery catheter. SvO_2 can be measured continously through the use of a special fiber-optic pulmonary artery catheter. The oxygen saturation of mixed venous blood ranges from 60 percent to 80 percent, with "normal" being approximately 75 percent. Recall that the oxygen saturation of arterial blood (SaO_2) is normally 98 percent to 99 percent. Normally, 25 percent of the oxygen delivered to cells is extracted for cellular use.

To illustrate how SvO_2 monitoring can be used to assess oxygen consumption, consider the following patient examples using the data contained in Box 9–2.

BOX 9–2

Parameter	**Patient X**	**Patient Z**
SaO_2	100%	98%
SvO_2	75%	40%

Patient X's SaO_2 indicates that the oxygen content of arterial blood is fully saturated and that the oxygen saturation of the blood returning to the right side of the heart is 75 percent. If 100 percent was delivered and 75 percent was returned, it appears that the cells extracted 25 percent of the oxygen they received. This is a normal oxygen extraction. Patient X appears to have a normal oxygen supply-and-demand balance.

Now consider patient Z's values. The SvO_2 value is below normal. This can be interpreted as a decrease in oxygen delivery compared with oxygen demand. Thus, more oxygen is being extracted at the cellular level. The alteration in this SvO_2 value does not indicate which of the determinants of oxygen delivery has changed but implies an oxygenation impairment. The nurse should then assess for changes in cardiac output, SaO_2, and hemoglobin, or for conditions that cause an increase in oxygen consumption (e.g., fever). (Conditions that increase oxygen consumption were discussed in Section Four of this module.)

Monitoring SvO_2 trends in the critically ill patient can be used to adjust medical and nursing interventions in an effort to maximize oxygenation and prevent activities that produce an oxygenation impairment. Research has demonstrated that SvO_2 values can be used by nurses to assess when routine nursing care causes significant oxygen supply/demand imbalances, and that SvO_2 values can be used to determine whether modifications in care are needed and whether the activity should be aborted (Palmer & Grove, 1996). A decline in SvO_2 values during a nursing intervention implies that the oxygen demands of the nursing care have exceeded the patient's oxygen supply.

In summary, monitoring oxygenation is one of the most important components of a nursing assessment. Clinical assessment of oxygenation should include techniques that assess oxygenation at each of the three levels: pulmonary gas exchange, oxygen delivery, and oxygen consumption. Assessment of gas exchange must include techniques to assess ventilation, diffusion, and perfusion. Assessment of oxygen delivery includes cardiac output, hemoglobin, SaO_2, and PaO_2. Current methods of assessing oxygen consumption are limited to indirect measurement techniques, including serial measurements of lactate, base deficit, and SvO_2.

SECTION SIX REVIEW

1. Auscultation is an assessment tool to detect
   A. pulmonary shunt
   B. disturbances in oxygen delivery
   C. disturbances in oxygen consumption
   D. respiratory muscle efficiency
2. The "gold standard" for the assessment of oxygen delivery is
   A. PAO_2
   B. cardiac output
   C. SvO_2
   D. auscultation
3. Direct measurement of oxygen consumption
   A. is made using SvO_2 monitoring
   B. is made using transcutaneous oxygen measurements
   C. is not clinically possible
   D. can be calculated as the product of cardiac output and oxygen content of arterial blood
4. A patient has the following values: SaO_2 100 percent and SvO_2 55 percent. Which one of the following assessments would be helpful in determining the source of his oxygenation imbalance?
   A. auscultate lung fields
   B. take his temperature
   C. draw an arterial blood gas
   D. measure preload
5. Calculation of oxygen delivery requires all of the following EXCEPT
   A. cardiac output measurement
   B. serum hemoglobin analysis
   C. ABG analysis
   D. measurement of blood pressure

Answers: 1. A, 2. B, 3. C, 4. B, 5. D

POSTTEST

1. The concept of oxygenation involves
   A. pulmonary gas exchange, oxygen delivery, and oxygen consumption
   B. integration of the pulmonary and cardiovascular systems
   C. ventilation, diffusion, and perfusion
   D. oxygen extraction and oxygen consumption
2. Your patient's postoperative hemoglobin is 10 mg/dL. What impact would this have on the initial component of oxygenation?

A. none
B. ventilation impairment
C. diffusion impairment
D. perfusion impairment

3. A pulmonary embolism would result in impaired gas exchange as a result of
A. ventilation impairment
B. diffusion impairment
C. perfusion impairment
D. decreased oxygen content of arterial blood

4. Which of the following contributes minimally to oxygen delivery?
A. PaO_2-50 mm Hg
B. SaO_2-70 percent
C. CO-3 L/min
D. Hgb-10 mg/dL

Mr. B is admitted with a diagnosis of pneumonia. His data on admission are as follows:

ABG	PaO_2 45 PaO_2 50 SaO_2 70 percent pH 7.30 HCO_3 28
Lactate	8 mMol/L
Hgb	10 mg/dL
CO	3 L/min
SvO_2	60 percent

Questions 5, 6, and 7 pertain to Mr. B.

5. Based on the preceding data, Mr. B has impaired oxygen consumption as evidenced by
A. PaO_2 of 45, PaO_2 of 50
B. PaO_2 of 50, SaO_2 of 70 percent
C. lactate 8 mMol/L and SvO_2 of 60 percent
D. Hgb 10 mg/dL and CO of 3 L/min

6. Based on the data preceding question 5, you determine that Mr. B has
A. multiple organ dysfunction syndrome
B. shock
C. hypoxemia and hypoxia
D. dysoxia

7. Based on the data preceding question 5, calculate the oxygen delivery.
A. 283 mL/min
B. 28,142 mL/min
C. 125 mL/min
D. 243 mL/min

8. Which of the following would decrease oxygen consumption?
A. administration of an antibiotic
B. preoperative anxiety
C. nursing assessment
D. administration of a sedative

9. The clinical condition characterized by inadequate oxygen in arterial blood is
A. hypoxia
B. hypoxemia
C. dysoxia
D. shock

10. Which of the following represents the most complete oxygenation assessment?
A. arterial blood gas, auscultation, and calculation of intrapulmonary shunt
B. auscultation of lung fields, measurement of cardiac output, and SvO_2
C. cardiac output, serum measurement of hemoglobin, SaO_2, and PaO_2
D. serum lactate level, SvO_2, and arterial blood gas

POSTTEST ANSWERS

Question	Answer	Section	Question	Answer	Section
1	A	One	6	C	Five
2	D	Two	7	A	Six
3	C	Two	8	D	Four
4	A	Three	9	B	Five
5	C	Four	10	B	Six

REFERENCES

Ahrens, T. (1993a). Respiratory monitoring in critical care. *AACN Clin Issues Crit Care* 4:56–65.

Ahrens, T. (1993b). Changing perspectives in the assessment of oxygenation. *Crit Care Nursing* 13:78–83.

Cornwell, E.E., Kennedy, F., & Rodriguez, J. (1996). The critical care of the severely injured patient. *Surg Clin North Am* 76: 959–969.

Grap, M.J. (1998). Protocols for practice: Applying research at the bedside. *Crit Care Nurse* 18 (1):94–99.

Mikhail, J. (1999). Resuscitation endpoints in trauma. *AACN Clin Issues Crit Care* 10 (1):10–21.

Misasi, R.S., & Keyes, J.L. (1996). Matching and mismatching ventilation and perfusion in the lungs. *Crit Care Nurse*, 16 (3):23–38.

Nelson, L.D. (1993). Assessment of oxygenation: Oxygenation indices. *Resp Care* 38:631–645.

Palmer, C.L.K., & Grove, S.K. (1996). Developing the nursing diagnosis of impaired oxygenation: abnormally low SvO_2 value. *Crit Care Nurse 16* (1):69–76.

Porter, J.M., & Ivatury, R.R. (1998). In search of optimal endpoints of resuscitation in trauma patients: A review. *J Trauma 44*:908–914.

Pierson, D.J. (1993). Normal and abnormal oxygenation: Physiology and clinical syndromes. *Resp Care 38*:587–602.

Swinamer, D.L., Phang, P.T., Jones, R.L., Grace, M., & King, E.G. (1987). Twenty-four hour energy expenditure in critically ill patients. *Crit Care Med 15*:637–643.

Third European Consensus Conference in Intensive Care Medicine. (1997). Tissue hypoxia: How to detect, how to correct, how to prevent. *J Crit Care 12* (1):39–47.

Module 10

Shock States

Karen L. Johnson

The major function of the cardiovascular system is to deliver blood, oxygen, and nutrients to the cells, tissues, and organs of the body and to remove metabolic wastes. When this fails to occur, a state of shock occurs.

Defining *shock* is more difficult than defining other disease entities. No one seems to agree on one concise definition because shock is a syndrome, a complex of signs and symptoms that describe a sequence of changes that occur when the circulation fails to meet its major objective. One of the best definitions of shock, primarily because it is nonspecific, was offered by Samuel Gross over 100 years ago. He characterized shock as a "rude unhinging of the machinery of life." Continuing research has improved the understanding of the basic concepts of shock. Clinically, shock can be defined as a "complex syndrome of decreased blood flow to body tissues resulting in cellular dysfunction and eventual organ failure" (Rice, 1991a). Shock states represent an imbalance of oxygen supply and demand. The relationship between oxygen supply (delivery) and oxygen demand (consumption) serves as the conceptual framework for shock in this module.

This self-study module is composed of four sections. Section One describes the mechanisms of impaired oxygenation for each of four functional classifications of shock. Section Two reviews the compensatory mechanisms that occur in response to shock states. In Section Three, clinical manifestations for each of the four functional shock states are given. The final section describes medical and nursing interventions that optimize oxygen delivery and decrease oxygen consumption. Each section includes a set of review questions to help the learner evaluate his or her understanding of the section's content before moving on to the next section. All Section Reviews and the module Pretest and Posttest include answers. It is suggested that the learner review those concepts answered incorrectly in the review questions before proceeding to the next section.

Objectives

Following completion of this module, the learner will be able to

1. Describe the pathologic mechanisms of impaired oxygen delivery and oxygen consumption for each of the four functional classifications of shock states.
2. Describe the physiologic compensatory mechanisms that occur to correct the imbalance of oxygen delivery and consumption in shock.
3. List the clinical manifestations of each of the four functional shock states.
4. State the medical and nursing interventions used in the treatment of shock states that optimize oxygen delivery and decrease oxygen consumption.

PRETEST

1. Common to all shock states is
   - A. blood pressure of 90 mm Hg, heart rate greater than 100 bpm
   - B. loss of blood volume
   - C. decreased oxygen delivery with decreased oxygen consumption
   - D. inadequate oxygen delivery to meet cellular oxygen demands
2. Which of the following shock states have similar pathologic mechanisms?
   - A. neurogenic and septic shocks
   - B. anaphylactic and cardiogenic shocks
   - C. left ventricular myocardial infarction and cardiac tamponade
   - D. carbon monoxide poisoning and cardiac tamponade
3. Which of the following is NOT one of the sympathetic nervous system's fight-or-flight responses?
   - A. increased heart rate
   - B. dilation of pupils
   - C. increased respiratory rate
   - D. increased intestinal peristalsis
4. Which of the following is a potent vasoconstrictor?
   - A. renin
   - B. aldosterone
   - C. angiotensin II
   - D. antidiuretic hormone (ADH)
5. In neurogenic shock, signs and symptoms are related to
   - A. loss of spinal fluid
   - B. damaged parasympathetic cells
   - C. loss of hypothalamic control
   - D. loss of sympathetic innervation
6. Shock states result from
   - A. an imbalance of oxygen delivery and oxygen consumption
   - B. an increase in oxygen delivery and oxygen consumption
   - C. a decrease in oxygen delivery and oxygen consumption
   - D. inadequate blood pressure, heart rate, and urine output
7. Transport shock states are the result of
   - A. an increase in vessel diameter
   - B. dysfunctional or inadequate amount of hemoglobin
   - C. a barrier to flow of oxygenated blood
   - D. failure of the heart to adequately pump blood
8. All of the following are stages of shock EXCEPT
   - A. initial
   - B. compensatory
   - C. noncompensatory
   - D. progressive
9. A systemic response to infection that includes a temperature > 30°C and a heart rate > 90 bpm characterizes
   - A. sepsis
   - B. severe sepsis
   - C. septic shock
   - D. septic syndrome
10. All of the following may be used in the treatment of cardiogenic shock EXCEPT
    - A. ventricular assist device
    - B. intra-aortic balloon pump
    - C. cardiac transplantation
    - D. isoproterenol

Pretest answers: 1. D, 2. A, 3. D, 4. C, 5. D, 6. A, 7. B, 8. C, 9. A, 10. D

GLOSSARY

Oxygen consumption. The amount of oxygen used by the body; described as a product of cardiac output and the difference between arterial oxygen content and venous oxygen content

Oxygen delivery. The product of cardiac output and arterial oxygen content

ABBREVIATIONS

ACTH. Adrenocorticotropic hormone

ADH. Antidiuretic hormone

CO. Cardiac output

CVP. Central venous pressure

GI. Gastrointestinal

Hct. Hematocrit

Hgb. Hemoglobin

HR. Heart rate

IABP. Intra-aortic balloon counterpulsation

MAP. Mean arterial pressure

MDF. Myocardial depressant factor

MSO_4. Morphine sulfate

O_2. Oxygen

$Paco_2$. Partial pressure of dissolved carbon dioxide in the plasma of arterial blood

PAP. Pulmonary artery pressure

PAWP. Pulmonary artery wedge pressure

RAP. Right atrial pressure

SVR. Systemic vascular resistance

VAD. Ventricular assist device

WBC. White blood cell

SECTION ONE: Functional Classifications of Shock States

At the completion of this section, the learner will be able to describe the mechanism of impaired oxygenation for each of the four functional classifications of shock.

Common to all shock states is inadequate oxygen delivery to meet cellular oxygen demand. Traditionally, shock states have been classified according to their etiology (e.g., septic shock, hemorrhagic shock, neurogenic shock). More recently, shock states have been categorized into functional shock states. Several functional classifications have been used. For this module, shock is classified into four categories: hypovolemic, transport, obstructive, and cardiogenic (Clochesy, 1988). This classification system groups shock states not according to the cause of the shock state but according to similar mechanisms responsible for impaired oxygenation.

Hypovolemic shock states have impaired oxygenation because of inadequate cardiac output (CO) as a result of decreased intravascular volume. Transport shock states have impaired oxygenation due to a diminished supply of hemoglobin in which to carry oxygen to tissues. Obstructive shock states have impaired oxygenation because of a mechanical barrier to blood flow. Cardiogenic shock states have impaired oxygenation because the heart fails to function as a pump to deliver oxygenated blood. The functional states, causes, and mechanisms of impaired oxygen delivery are summarized in Table 10–1.

Hypovolemic Shock States

Hypovolemia can result from two conditions: the fluid volume in the circulation has decreased or the size of the intravascular compartment has increased in proportion to the fluid volume. When either or both of these conditions occur, there is decreased venous return to the right heart. This reduces ventricular filling pressure, stroke volume, cardiac output, and blood pressure.

Loss of intravascular volume can be caused by loss of blood volume (hemorrhage), loss of intravascular fluid from the skin (as with dehydration or burns), loss of fluid from persistent vomiting or diarrhea, or loss of fluid from the intravascular compartment to interstitial spaces (third spacing). A diminished fluid volume leads to a decreased cardiac output, resulting in impaired oxygen delivery.

When the size of the intravascular compartment has increased in proportion to the amount of fluid in the intravascular compartment, the body interprets this as a state of hypovolemia. The blood volume may be "normal," but the intravascular space has increased without a

TABLE 10–1. FUNCTIONAL STATES OF SHOCK, CAUSES, AND PATHOLOGIC MECHANISMS

FUNCTIONAL STATE	ETIOLOGY	MECHANISM OF IMPAIRED O_2 DELIVERY
Hypovolemic	Fluid volume loss (dehydration, burn injuries, third spacing) Vasodilation (neurogenic shock, anaphylactic shock, septic shock)	Loss of intravascular volume Increase in vessel diameter due to: Loss of sympathetic tone Histamine release Endotoxin release
Transport	Diminished supply of Hgb to carry O_2 (anemia, hemorrhage, carbon monoxide poisoning)	Dysfunction or inadequate amount of Hgb to bind with O_2
Obstructive	Mechanical barriers to blood flow (pulmonary embolism, tension pneumothorax, cardiac tamponade)	Barrier to flow of oxygenated blood due to: Pulmonary artery blocked Great vessels kinked Ventricles unable to fill or eject blood volume
Cardiogenic	Heart fails to function as a pump (myocardial infarction, dysrhythmias)	Ischemic muscles fail to contract Irregular rate/rhythm causes heart to fail its function as a pump

Adapted from Clochesy, J.M. (ed). 1988. Essentials of critical care nursing (p. 127). Rockville, MD: Aspen Publishing.

proportional increase in blood volume. Vasodilation causes the intravascular compartment to increase without a corresponding increase in volume. Vasodilation can occur with neurogenic shock, anaphylactic shock, and septic shock.

Neurogenic shock may occur with a spinal cord injury. When there is injury to the spinal cord above the midthoracic region, impulses from the sympathetic nervous system cannot reach the arterioles. The loss of sympathetic innervation prohibits vasoconstriction of blood vessels, but blood vessels continue to receive parasympathetic innervation, allowing vasodilation. Blood then pools in the dilated peripheral venous system. The right heart receives an inadequate venous return, and cardiac output decreases. As cardiac output decreases, delivery of oxygen-carrying blood decreases.

Anaphylactic shock occurs in response to a severe allergic reaction to such things as foods (peanuts, fish, eggs, milk), drugs (nonsteroidal anti-inflammatory drugs, aspirin, antibiotics, blood products), insect venoms, and latex (Wyatt, 1996). Massive amounts of vasoactive substances (e.g., histamine and kinins) are released, which cause vasodilation and an increase in capillary permeability. Vasodilation increases the size of the intravascular compartment. Increased capillary permeability allows fluid to move from intravascular spaces to interstitial spaces. As fluid is lost from the vascular compartment, a relative hypovolemia develops. The net consequences of combined massive vasodilation and increased capillary permeability are a decrease in venous return, decreased cardiac output, and a decrease in oxygen delivery.

Septic shock is a systemic response to invading microorganisms of all types: gram-positive and gram-negative bacteria, fungi, or viruses. The systemic response to infection triggers a complex series of cellular and humoral events (Fig. 10–1). These organisms release endotoxins that invade the bloodstream and stimulate the release of cytokines (tumor necrosis factor and interleukins). These substances produce vasodilation and increased capillary permeability. This reduces venous return and lowers diastolic filling pressures in the heart. A second fluid alteration seen in septic shock is a maldistribution of circulating blood volume. Some organs receive more blood than needed as a result of vasodilation, whereas others (skin, lungs, kidneys) do not receive the blood flow they need. Altered fluid volume related to vasodilation, increased capillary permeability, and maldistribution of circulating volume characterize septic shock.

Transport Shock States

The common pathologic mechanism in transport shock states is a diminished supply of hemoglobin available to carry oxygen to tissues. Recall that hemoglobin is the bus that carries oxygen molecules to tissues (Module 7). Anemia and hemorrhage are characterized by a decrease in red blood cells and hemoglobin for oxygen to bind to.

Carbon monoxide toxicity represents another form of transport shock state. Carbon monoxide is a colorless, odorless gas that when inhaled rapidly binds to hemoglobin to form carboxyhemoglobin. The hemoglobin bus

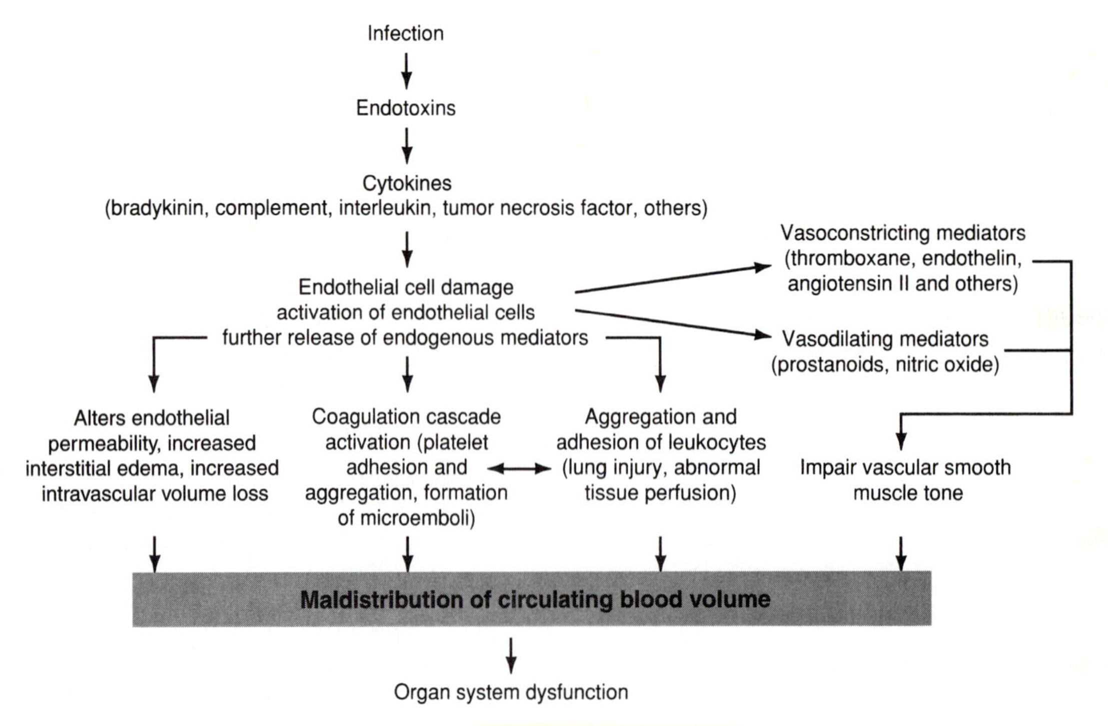

Figure 10–1. Pathophysiology of septic shock.

seats are occupied by carbon monoxide, leaving little room for oxygen. Oxygen cannot be transported to tissues. The presence of carbon monoxide interferes with the release of oxygen from hemoglobin and also interferes with the cell's ability to use oxygen properly (Weaver, 1999). A state of shock occurs as the transport of oxygen to tissues is severely limited.

Obstructive Shock States

Obstructive shock states occur as a result of a mechanical barrier to blood flow that blocks oxygen delivery to tissues. Causes may be attributed to pulmonary embolism, tension pneumothorax, or cardiac tamponade.

Pulmonary embolism can range from clinically unimportant thromboembolism to massive embolism with sudden death. Hypercoagulability leads to formation of thrombi in the deep veins of the legs, pelvis, or arms. The thrombi dislodge and embolize to the pulmonary arteries. Pulmonary arteries become partially obstructed, which results in an increase in alveolar dead space and a ventilation–perfusion mismatch, which impairs gas exchange. Platelets release vasoactive substances (serotonin) that increase pulmonary vascular resistance (Goldhaber, 1998). As right ventricular afterload increases, right ventricular dysfunction can occur. Shock states in response to a pulmonary embolism can result from inadequate systemic oxygen delivery due to impaired gas exchange and cardiac dysfunction.

A tension pneumothorax occurs when air enters the pleural space during inspiration but cannot leave during expiration. The progressive accumulation of air within the thoracic cavity leads to a shift of the mediastinal structures and compression of the opposite lung. The increased pleural pressure impedes venous return and serves as a barrier to oxygen delivery.

Cardiac tamponade is caused by bleeding into a nonflexible pericardial sac. The accumulating pressure around the heart increases intracardiac pressures, impairing ventricular filling and decreasing cardiac output.

Cardiogenic Shock States

Cardiogenic shock states occur as a result of impaired oxygen delivery due to cardiac dysfunction. Dysfunction of either the right or left ventricle can lead to cardiogenic shock. Failure can occur when the right ventricle fails to pump the volume of venous blood returned to it or when the left ventricle fails to pump oxygenated blood to the systemic circulation. Causes of cardiogenic shock include extensive acute myocardial infarction, mechanical complications (papillary muscle rupture), or other conditions (end-stage cardiomyopathy). Among patients with myocardial infarction, shock is more likely to develop in those who are elderly, diabetic, and have anterior infarction (Hollenberg, Kavinsky, & Parillo, 1999).

A left ventricular myocardial infarction produces a necrotic area that impairs contractility and cardiac output. The ventricle cannot propel oxygenated blood forward into the systemic circulation for delivery to tissues. As stroke volume decreases, so do cardiac output and blood pressure. Because the damaged left ventricle cannot propel all of its contents forward, blood begins to "back up" into the pulmonary system, causing pulmonary congestion. Increased pulmonary congestion leads to increased afterload for the right ventricle. These changes can occur rapidly or can progress over several days.

In cardiogenic shock caused by dysfunction of the right ventricle, the right ventricle ejects too little blood and therefore less oxygenated blood enters the left ventricle. As left ventricular stroke volume decreases, cardiac output and blood pressure fall. Because the right ventricle cannot effectively pump all the blood it receives, blood begins to "back up" into the systemic circulation.

In summary, shock states can be classified according to the common pathologic mechanisms that produce impaired oxygenation: hypovolemic, transport, obstructive, and cardiogenic shock states. Independent of etiology or pathologic mechanisms, altered tissue perfusion with impaired oxygen delivery in relation to oxygen consumption is common to all forms of shock.

SECTION ONE REVIEW

1. Which of the following conditions produces a hypovolemic shock state?
   - **A.** carbon monoxide poisoning
   - **B.** tension pneumothorax
   - **C.** pulmonary emboli
   - **D.** third spacing (movement of fluid from the vascular to the interstitial space)
2. Which of the following conditions can produce a transport shock state?
   - **A.** carbon monoxide poisoning
   - **B.** dehydration
   - **C.** cardiac tamponade
   - **D.** anaphylactic shock
3. Which of the following conditions can produce an obstructive shock state?
   - **A.** myocardial infarction
   - **B.** anemia
   - **C.** pulmonary emboli
   - **D.** sepsis

4. Which of the following statements characterizes septic shock?
   A. occurs as a result of fluid shifts and vasoconstriction
   B. inadequate oxygen delivery and impaired oxygen consumption
   C. loss of sympathetic nerve innervation prohibits vasoconstriction
   D. occurs in response to an allergic reaction
5. Which of the following statements characterizes cardiogenic shock?
   A. increasing stroke volume in face of decreasing cardiac output
   B. the heart fails to function as a pump
   C. increasing stroke volume in face of increasing cardiac output
   D. cardiogenic shock is the result of a massive myocardial infarction

Answers: 1. D, 2. A, 3. C, 4. B, 5. B

SECTION TWO: Physiologic Response to Shock

At the completion of this section, the learner will be able to describe the compensatory mechanisms that occur in response to shock states.

Shock occurs when oxygen delivery does not support tissue metabolic demands. In an attempt to stabilize this life-threatening situation, a pattern of responses, or compensatory mechanisms, occurs.

Compensation in Shock

Complex neuroendocrine responses are triggered to overcome ineffective circulating blood volume. Low-pressure stretch receptors in the right atrium sense a decrease in circulating blood volume when there is a decrease in venous return to the right atrium. Baroreceptors in the aorta and carotid arteries sense a decrease in blood volume and cardiac output. Carotid body chemoreceptors sense alterations in pH and $PaCO_2$. These receptors alert the hypothalamus to what could be a life-threatening situation. The baroreceptors and chemoreceptors alert the hypothalamus to activate the sympathetic nervous system's fight-or-flight response. This system releases a massive amount of norepinephrine, which produces several compensatory mechanisms (Table 10–2). The beneficial effects of these mechanisms are an increase in venous return, increase in cardiac output, and increase in oxygen delivery.

In response to shock states, the endocrine system attempts to increase **oxygen delivery** by increasing blood volume (Fig. 10–2). The hypothalamus releases adrenocorticotropic hormone (ACTH), which activates the adrenals to secrete aldosterone. Aldosterone causes sodium and water retention in efforts to increase the blood volume and blood pressure. Sodium and water retention stimulates the release of antidiuretic hormone (ADH), which increases reabsorption of water in the kidney tubules and thus increases the blood volume. The goal of the release of these hormones is to preserve blood volume by conserving the amount of fluid excreted by the kidneys.

Cardiac output must be augmented in shock to ensure adequate tissue perfusion. Cardiac output is proportional to venous return. To increase venous return, sodium and water are retained by aldosterone and ADH. In addition to these hormones, another mechanism, the renin–angiotensin–aldosterone cycle, is activated to increase blood volume and venous return. As a result of decreased blood flow to the kidneys, the juxtaglomerular cells in the kidneys excrete renin. Renin catalyzes angiotensinogen in the liver, which then converts to angiotensin I in the circulation. Once in the lungs, angiotensin I converts to angiotensin II, which is a potent

TABLE 10–2. SYMPATHETIC NERVOUS SYSTEM'S FIGHT-OR-FLIGHT RESPONSE

PHYSIOLOGIC RESPONSE	PHYSIOLOGIC RATIONALE
Increased heart rate	For rapid delivery of needed oxygen
Increased respiratory rate	To receive more oxygen and correct acidosis
Increased glycolysis	To increase availability of glucose for energy
Decreased urine output	To conserve fluid volume, return more blood volume to cardiovascular system to increase volume and blood pressure
Decreased blood flow to internal organs (e.g., kidneys, gastrointestinal tract, liver)	To allow more blood flow to more vital organs (e.g., heart and lungs)
Decreased intestinal peristalsis	Shunting of blood to vital organs, no need for digestion as body energy is redirected to lifesaving measures
Cool skin	Alpha receptors produce peripheral vasoconstriction to shunt blood to more vital organs
Diaphoresis	To release heat as a by-product of energy use

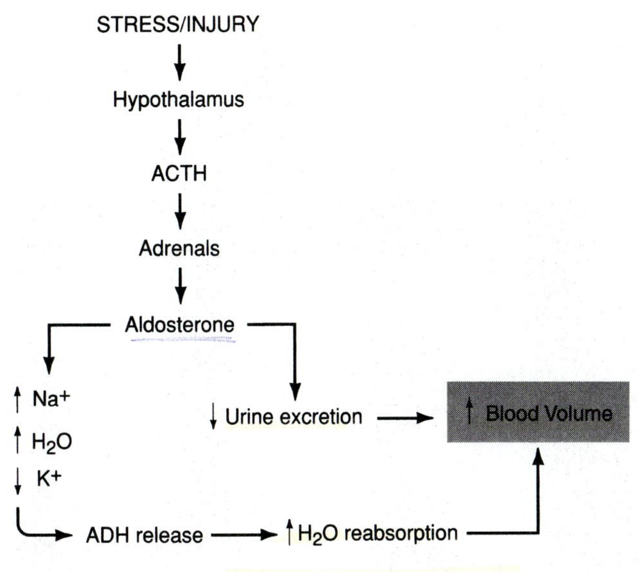

Figure 10–2. ACTH, aldosterone, and ADH release.

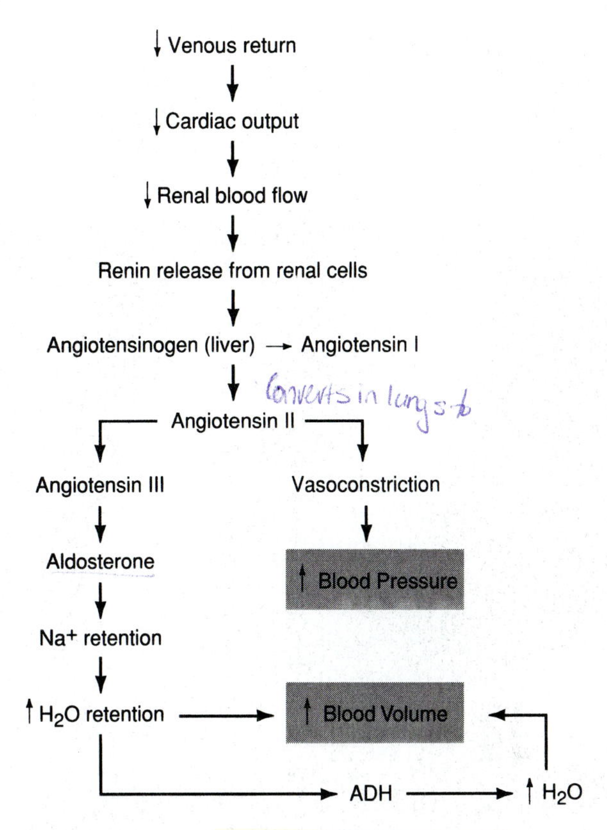

Figure 10–3. Renin–angiotensin–aldosterone cycle.

vasoconstrictor. The vasoconstriction produced by angiotensin II increases blood pressure by increasing afterload. Angiotensin II is converted to angiotensin III, which stimulates the release of aldosterone. The renin–angiotensin–aldosterone cycle is depicted in Figure 10–3. The net effects of these hormonal mechanisms are increased blood pressure through vasoconstriction and increase in venous return through retention of sodium and water, and decreased urine output.

Compensatory mechanisms that occur in response to shock are designed to restore oxygen delivery by augmenting cardiac output, redistributing blood flow, and restoring blood volume.

Progression of Shock

There are four stages of shock: initial, compensatory, progressive, and refractory. In the initial stage, decreased cardiac output and decreased tissue perfusion are evident. Decreased oxygen delivery to cells results in anaerobic metabolism and lactic acidosis. In the compensatory stage, neuroendocrine responses are activated to restore cardiac output and oxygen delivery. Clinical signs and symptoms of these mechanisms are evident.

When compensatory mechanisms cannot restore homeostasis and if prompt and proper treatment has not been instituted, the third stage of shock can occur. Progressive shock results in major dysfunction of many organs. The continued low blood flow, poor tissue perfusion, inadequate oxygen delivery, and buildup of metabolic wastes over time lead to multiple organ dysfunction syndrome (MODS, Module 11).

The final stage of shock is the refractory stage. In this stage, the shock state is so profound and cell destruction is so severe that death is inevitable (Rice, 1991b). The patient, although alive, has become refractory to conventional therapy. Profound hypotension occurs despite administration of potent vasoactive drugs. The patient remains hypoxemic despite oxygen therapy. A state of intractable circulatory failure leads to total body failure and death.

Not every patient progresses through all four stages. Often, the progression from one stage to the next is not obvious. If the shock state is assessed early and appropriate treatment is instituted the progression of shock is halted, the oxygen supply-and-demand balance is restored, and the patient recovers.

In summary, compensatory mechanisms occur in response to shock in an attempt to prevent further deterioration and restore homeostasis. Complex neuroendocrine responses are triggered to overcome ineffective circulating blood volume. The hormones ACTH, aldosterone, and ADH are released to increase cardiac output. The sympathetic nervous system releases a massive amount of norepinephrine, which produces multiorgan responses in an effort to sustain a life-threatening situation. The cardiovascular system tries to restore arterial blood pressure by augmenting CO through increased venous return. The renin–angiotensin–aldosterone cycle is initiated to enhance preload through increased venous return and increased afterload through vasoconstriction. When compensatory mechanisms cannot restore the system to normal, shock can progress to a phase of continued inadequate tissue oxygenation in relation to demand. Cells become ineffective and die, metabolic wastes accumulate, and MODS occurs. Eventually, shock can progress to a refractory phase where death is inevitable.

SECTION TWO REVIEW

1. Aldosterone increases blood volume by all of the following EXCEPT
   A. increasing sodium retention
   B. increasing water retention
   C. decreasing potassium retention
   D. increasing calcium retention
2. Angiotensin II
   A. is a vasoconstrictor
   B. is a vasodilator
   C. is released by ADH
   D. causes the release of ACTH
3. ACTH, aldosterone, and ADH
   A. sense alterations in pH and $Paco_2$
   B. alert the hypothalamus to what could be a life-threatening situation
   C. conserve the amount of fluid excreted by the kidneys
   D. increase the heart rate for rapid delivery of oxygen
4. Norepinephrine produces which of the following compensatory mechanisms?
   A. decreased blood pressure
   B. increased intestinal peristalsis
   C. increased glycolysis
   D. decreased heart rate
5. Continued low blood flow, poor tissue perfusion, and inadequate oxygen delivery cause
   A. multisystem organ dysfunction
   B. the hypothalamus to release ACTH
   C. the release of renin from renal cells
   D. decreased urine output

Answers: 1. D, 2. A, 3. C, 4. C, 5. A

SECTION THREE: Clinical Findings Associated with Shock States

At the completion of this section, the learner will be able to list the clinical manifestations for each of the functional shock states.

Clinical manifestations of all shock states are the result of inadequate oxygen delivery and the compensatory mechanisms of the neuroendocrine and cardiovascular systems.

Traditional signs used to assess for shock include blood pressure, heart rate, mentation, and urine output. However, these signs often underestimate the degree of physiologic abnormalities. Blood pressure is hard to assess because it is so individualized. A blood pressure of 90/60 may be normal in one patient but hypotensive in another patient. There are many factors that cause tachycardia, including anxiety, pain, arrhythmia, and fever. Mentation may be hard to assess due to the presence of head injury, alcohol, drugs, or chronic diseases (Alzheimer's). Several factors may produce a false sense of security when adequate urine output is present (Cornwell, Kennedy, & Rodriguez, 1996). These can include the neuroendocrine response to shock, hyperglycemia, and diabetes insipidus. Research is ongoing, but evidence is mounting that shock states persist despite normalization of blood pressure, heart rate, and urine output (Porter & Ivatury, 1998).

Serum lactate levels can be used as an indirect measure of impaired oxygenation and shock. Normal serum lactate levels are < 2 mMol/L. However, during shock states when there is impaired oxygen delivery to meet cellular oxygen demand, anaerobic metabolism occurs (see Module 9, Section Four). The by-product of this is lactate. Hyperlactatemia can produce metabolic acidosis. Hyperlactatemia can serve as an approximation of the magnitude of hypoperfusion and the severity of shock (Mikhail, 1999). Serial measurements of serum lactate levels, as an indicator of improving or worsening of shock states, has been advocated (Porter & Ivatury, 1988).

Base deficit is the amount of base (mMol) required to titrate one liter of arterial blood to a normal pH. It is calculated from an arterial blood gas. Normal base deficit is +3 mMol to −3 mMol. A base deficit results from an imbalance between oxygen delivery and oxygen consumption producing a lactic acidosis secondary to anaerobic metabolism. Base deficit has been classified as mild (2 to −5), moderate (−6 to −14) and severe (< −15). Ongoing or worsening base deficit may indicate further evaluation for an ongoing shock state.

A major focus in shock research has been in the evaluation of new technologies to assess the severity of shock state. These include gastric tonometry, infrared spectroscopy, and a modified pulmonary artery catheter, which measures right ventricular end-diastolic volume index (Mikhail, 1999).

Hypovolemic Shock States

In hypovolemic shock states due to fluid loss, the signs and symptoms are related to the degree of volume depletion. The skin will be cool, and capillary refill will be poor. Depending on the amount of fluid volume lost, the blood pressure may be low, and orthostatic changes in blood pressure may be noted. Tachycardia will be evident, and urine output will be low. Hemodynamically, as less volume is returned to the right atrium, the right atrial pressure (RAP) will be low. As less fluid is delivered to the pulmonary vasculature and the left ventricle, pressures will be low, as evidenced by a low pulmonary artery wedge pressure (PAWP), low pulmonary artery pressure (PAP), and low cardiac output (CO). The systemic vascular resistance (SVR) will be elevated as vasoconstriction occurs in efforts to increase venous return and CO.

In neurogenic shock, signs and symptoms are related to the loss of sympathetic innervation. Persistent vasodilation produces a decreased SVR. Pooling of blood in dilated vessels results in diminished venous return, producing a lower RAP, PAP, PAWP, and CO. Heart rate (HR) will be decreased as a result of parasympathetic innervation. Peripheral vasodilation produces warm skin. Hypothermia and absence of sweating below the level of the spinal cord injury may be present.

Severe anaphylactic shock frequently involves multiple organ systems of the body, but the most life threatening are those involving the cardiovascular and pulmonary systems. Anaphylactic shock can develop rapidly (5 to 30 minutes) or slowly (6 to 12 hours) but follows a typical pattern of generalized itching followed by cutaneous flushing, urticaria, a fullness in the throat, "anxiety," tightness in the chest, faintness, and loss of consciousness (Friday & Fireman, 1996). Severe upper airway obstruction by edema can lead to asphyxia, while lower airway obstruction with wheezing and chest tightness is caused by bronchospasm (Wyatt, 1996).

A multitude of metabolic, hematologic, and hemodynamic abnormalities occur as a systemic response to the invasion of microorganisms in the bloodstream. These abnormalities are part of a complex syndrome that may ultimately culminate in septic shock. Early recognition and treatment of septic shock are crucial. Broad definitions of sepsis and septic shock have been developed to assist in the early recognition and treatment of these disorders (Bone et al., 1992). These definitions are summarized in Table 10–3.

Septic shock is initially characterized by a low PAWP, low CO, and normal or elevated SVR before fluid resuscitation, and a high CO, low SVR after fluid resuscitation (Wheeler & Bernard, 1999). Hypotension that persists despite fluid resuscitation is frequently the result of low SVR and reduced CO, which stems from myocardial depressant factors. Lactic acidosis may be present.

TABLE 10–3. DEFINITIONS OF SEPSIS, SEVERE SEPSIS, AND SEPTIC SHOCK

Sepsis	The systemic response to infection manifested by two or more of the following conditions: 1. Temperature > 30°C or < 36°C 2. HR > 90 bpm 3. Respiratory rate > 20 breaths/min or $Paco_2$ < 32 mm Hg 4. WBC count > 12,000/µL or < 4,000/µL or > 10% immature (band) forms
Severe sepsis	Sepsis associated with organ dysfunction, hypoperfusion, or hypotension. Hypoperfusion and perfusion abnormalities may include, but are not limited to, lactic acidosis, oliguria, or an acute alteration in mental status.
Septic shock	Sepsis associated with hypotension despite adequate fluid resuscitation along with the presence of perfusion abnormalities that may include but are not limited to lactic acidosis,oliguria, or an acute alteration in mental status.

Transport Shock States

Diminished oxygen-carrying capacity of the blood produces the clinical manifestations seen in transport shock states. In shock caused by anemia or hemorrhage, a low hematocrit and hemoglobin will be present. RAP and PAWP may be normal, depending on the patient's volume status.

Symptoms caused by carbon monoxide poisoning can be a result of exposure to low levels of carbon monoxide for prolonged periods or can arise from exposure to higher levels for a shorter duration (Weaver, 1999). The severity of poisoning is dependent on several factors including underlying health. The most common symptoms of carbon monoxide poisoning are headache, malaise, nausea, difficulties with memory, and personality changes, as well as gross neurologic dysfunction (Weaver, 1999). An elevated carboxyhemoglobin level confirms carbon monoxide poisoning. Carboxyhemoglobin levels are usually in excess of 70 percent; however, even with low levels of carboxyhemoglobin (6 percent), cardiac dysfunction and ischemia are increased in older patients who have underlying coronary artery disease (Weaver, 1999).

Obstructive Shock States

The clinical manifestations of obstructive shock states are the result of a mechanical barrier to blood flow resulting in inadequate oxygen delivery.

Pulsus paradoxus is one of the classic signs of cardiac tamponade. Pulsus paradoxus is an exaggerated decrease (> 10 mm Hg) of the systolic blood pressure during inspiration. Other clinical manifestations of cardiac tamponade are distant heart sounds (muffled by the increased pericardial fluid) and a pericardial friction rub. In tamponade, RAP usually is elevated and is equaled by the PAWP. Beck's triad, consisting of elevated RAP, decreased BP, and muffled heart sounds, may be present.

Increased pleural pressure as a result of a tension pneumothorax puts direct pressure on the heart, vena cava, and contralateral lung. As a result, there will be decreased breath sounds, tracheal deviation, and bradycardia. This results in poor ventilation, decreased venous return, and decreased CO.

Dyspnea is the most frequent symptom of pulmonary embolism, and tachypnea is the most frequent sign. The presence of pleuritic pain, cough, or hemoptysis suggests a small embolism near the pleura, and the presence of dyspnea, syncope, or cyanosis usually indicate a massive pulmonary embolism (Goldhaber, 1998). The most frequent electrocardiographic abnormality is T wave inversion in the anterior leads (V1 to V4) (Ferrari et al., 1997). ABGs may be normal or indicate hypoxemia or hypercapnia. Perfusion lung scans, pulmonary angiography, spiral CT of the chest with contrast, or transthoracic echocardiography may be used in the diagnostic workup.

Cardiogenic Shock States

Clinical manifestations produced in cardiogenic shock states depend on whether heart failure is left-sided or right-sided.

Left ventricular failure produces clinical manifestations associated with hypoperfusion and pulmonary congestion, including dyspnea, bilateral rales (crackles), distant heart sounds, and third or fourth heart sounds are usually present. The hemodynamic profile of cardiogenic shock includes an elevated PAWP (> 15 mm Hg) and a low cardiac index (< 2.2 L/min/m^2) (Hollenberg, Kavinsky, & Parillo, 1999).

Clinical manifestations of right ventricular failure are associated with systemic venous congestion. Peripheral edema may be evident. Lung sounds will be clear unless there is also left ventricular dysfunction. A split second heart sound may be heard. This sound, produced by delayed closure of the tricuspid valve, is indicative of a distended right ventricle. The hemodynamic profile of right ventricular failure includes elevated RAPs in the presence of normal or low PAWP (Hollenberg, Kavinsky, & Parillo, 1999).

In summary, clinical manifestations associated with shock states are the result of impaired oxygenation and the compensatory mechanisms of the neuroendocrine and cardiovascular systems. In hypovolemic shock states due to fluid loss, the signs and symptoms are related to the degree of volume depletion. In neurogenic shock, anaphylactic shock, and septic shock, signs and symptoms are related to vasodilation. A diminished supply of hemoglobin produces the clinical manifestations seen in transport shock states. The clinical manifestations of obstructive shock states are the result of a mechanical barrier to blood flow. Clinical manifestations of cardiogenic shock states depend on whether there is left or right ventricular failure. Right ventricular failure produces signs associated with systemic venous congestion. Left ventricular failure produces clinical manifestations associated with hypoperfusion and pulmonary congestion.

SECTION THREE REVIEW

1. The signs and symptoms of anaphylactic shock are
   A. related to the loss of sympathetic tone
   B. related to the release of chemical mediators
   C. decreased SVR, PAWP, and increased temperature
   D. decreased RAP, increased CO, and increased temperature
2. A low Hct and Hgb will be present in shock caused by
   A. a pulmonary embolism
   B. cardiac tamponade
   C. anemia
   D. right ventricular failure
3. Mr. G was involved in a motor vehicle crash. He sustained a spinal cord injury. Which of the following are clinical manifestations of a spinal cord injury?
   A. increased heart rate, SVR, and RAP
   B. decreased heart rate, decreased SVR, and increased RAP
   C. increased heart rate, increased SVR, and decreased RAP
   D. decreased heart rate, SVR, and RAP
4. Mr. T has candida sepsis. Which of the following clinical manifestations would he likely demonstrate in the warm phase?
   A. decreased SVR, decreased CO
   B. increased SVR, decreased CO
   C. decreased SVR, increased CO
   D. increased SVR, increased CO
5. Which of the following would characterize right-sided heart failure?
   A. RAP will be high and much higher than PAWP
   B. RAP will be low
   C. PAWP will be high and much higher than RAP
   D. RAP and PAWP will be greatly elevated

Answers: 1. B, 2. C, 3. D, 4. C, 5. A

SECTION FOUR: Treatment of Shock

At the completion of this section, the learner will be able to list the medical and nursing interventions used in the treatment of shock states that optimize oxygen delivery and decrease oxygen consumption.

The primary goals of treatment are to identify and treat the underlying cause of shock, optimize oxygen delivery, and decrease oxygen consumption.

Interventions to Optimize Oxygen Delivery

Supplemental oxygen may be administered in an attempt to improve oxygen delivery to hypoxic tissues. For patients who are conscious, are spontaneously breathing, and have adequate arterial blood gases, oxygen delivered by nasal cannula or mask may be all that is necessary. However, in the unconscious patient or in the patient demonstrating respiratory distress, intubation and mechanical ventilation may be required.

Administration of IV fluids assists in restoring optimal tissue perfusion by restoring preload and increasing the cardiac output component of oxygen delivery. The fluid best suited for shock states remains controversial. Usually, a combination of crystalloids and colloids is administered. Crystalloid solutions (i.e., lactated Ringer's solution) restore interstitial and intravascular fluid volumes and increase preload and cardiac output. Administration of colloids enhances the blood's oxygen-carrying capacity. Colloids have oncotic capabilities not inherent in crystalloids. Whole blood is administered in a volume of 500 mL and can increase the hematocrit by 2 to 3 percent. Packed red blood cells are administered in a volume of 250 mL and can elevate the hematocrit by 3 to 4 percent (Greenburg, 1988). Packed red blood cells usually are given to provide adequate hemoglobin concentration and are supplemented with crystalloids to maintain an adequate circulatory volume. Inotropic medications may be necessary if volume administration is not sufficient to improve oxygenation.

Positive inotropic drugs increase contractility by stimulating the $beta_1$-receptors in the heart. Increased contraction results in increased stroke volume as the ventricles eject more completely. Inotropic drugs that increase cardiac output and enhance tissue perfusion include dopamine, dobutamine, norepinephrine, and isoproterenol. Dopamine has both alpha- and beta-receptor effects. In low doses (1 to 2 mg/kg/min), it causes renal vasodilation, improves renal blood flow, and increases urine output. In moderate doses (2 to 5 mg/kg/min), $beta_1$-receptors are activated, and cardiac output increases. Larger doses stimulate alpha-receptors and increase blood pressure. Dobutamine selectively acts on $beta_1$-receptors to increase contractility and cardiac output. Dobutamine also decreases SVR. Isoproterenol acts on $beta_1$- and $beta_2$-receptors to increase cardiac output, increase heart rate, and decrease SVR. All inotropic drugs must be used with caution, since they increase myocardial oxygen consumption.

Vasoactive drugs are drugs that act on the smooth muscle layer of blood vessels, which affects preload and afterload. These drugs are either vasoconstrictors or vasodilators. Vasoconstrictors, or vasopressors, mimic the sympathetic nervous system to increase blood flow to vital organs by increasing blood pressure and cardiac output. Vasopressors include epinephrine, norepinephrine, and dopamine. These drugs increase SVR and blood pressure. Vasopressors should not be given unless the SVR is abnormally low, as in septic shock or anaphylactic shock. These drugs should be given only when the patient's volume status is adequate (as reflected by RAP or PAWP or both).

Afterload reducing (vasodilating) drugs improve cardiac output and oxygen delivery. Peripheral arterial vasodilators (nitroprusside, nitroglycerine) decrease SVR. When afterload is decreased, stroke volume is improved. The ventricles have less resistance to overcome and eject blood with less force. These drugs decrease preload as well as afterload. Therefore, these drugs should be used with caution in shock. Afterload reducing drugs should be given only to patients who have adequate fluid volume. The patient must be monitored carefully so that the blood pressure does not become so low that reflex tachycardia occurs and coronary perfusion suffers.

In most circumstances, a combination of drugs may be advantageous. Combining an inotropic drug with a vasodilating drug can maximize oxygen delivery by increasing contractility and decreasing afterload. Sympathomimetic drugs are temporary agents, since they do not treat the underlying cause of shock. They have a relatively short duration of action and can be easily titrated to the patient's rapidly changing condition.

Placing the patient in Trendelenburg's position is a controversial intervention used for the treatment of hypotension. Some authors advocate that this position displaces blood from the systemic venules and small veins into the right heart and thus serves to increase stroke volume and cardiac output. Others believe that the Trendelenburg's position increases afterload to the left ventricle and thus decreases cardiac output. Further research is needed to evaluate the effects of Trendelenburg's position on cardiac output and blood pressure.

The patient's response to treatment must be assessed frequently for signs of improved oxygen delivery. Signs of improved oxygen delivery include improvements in cardiac index, urine output, and mean arterial pressure.

Interventions to Decrease Oxygen Consumption

In addition to optimizing oxygen delivery, interventions also should include measures to decrease **oxygen consumption.** Interventions to decrease oxygen consumption should be directed toward decreasing total body work, decreasing pain and anxiety, and decreasing temperature.

Decreasing total body work is an attempt to decrease oxygen demands of all tissues. Hyperventilation occurs in an effort to increase oxygen delivery to meet demands, but this requires a great deal of effort, and the patient can rapidly develop respiratory alkalosis and respiratory distress. Effective ventilation is ensured with intubation and mechanical ventilation. Mechanical ventilation also decreases the respiratory muscle oxygen demands. A tidal volume of 9 to 13 mL/kg (twice the norm) often is needed to respond to increased metabolic and oxygen demands. Decreasing oxygen consumption of voluntary muscles can be achieved with neuromuscular blocking agents such as pancuronium (Pavulon) or vecuronium (Norcuron). These drugs eliminate unnecessary muscle activity and allow oxygen to be redirected for use in involuntary muscles, such as the heart.

Pain and anxiety initiate the sympathetic nervous system's fight-or-flight response, which causes the release of catecholamines. Catecholamines increase metabolic rates and oxygen consumption. Measures should be taken to minimize pain and anxiety. Appropriate analgesics should be administered. It is important to recognize that pain and anxiety are present in the patient receiving neuromuscular blocking agents.

Hyperthermia increases metabolic demands and oxygen requirements. This should be controlled with antipyretic drugs, such as acetaminophen, and/or physical cooling measures (such as a fan or cooling blanket).

Interventions to optimize oxygen delivery and minimize oxygen consumption should be applied to all patients in shock. Individualized interventions should be initiated to treat the underlying cause of shock. These interventions are described briefly in the following paragraphs.

Hypovolemic Shock States

The treatment goal for hypovolemic shock states is restoration of fluid volume. In hypovolemic shock, the source of the fluid loss should be identified and controlled. Additional intravenous fluid (crystalloid and/or colloid) is administered. The nurse should assess for an improvement in heart rate, blood pressure, and urine output. If no response is noted, additional fluids may be required.

The goal of treatment in neurogenic shock (see Module 20) is to maintain stability of the spine and provide cardiovascular stability. Because of unopposed parasympathetic innervation, patients with complete, high spinal cord injuries have decreased blood pressure and pulse. These patients often require fluid administration to establish preload or a vasopressor if adequate volume has been given. A slight bradycardia requires close monitoring. If a marked bradycardia occurs, appropriate medications to increase heart rate and avoid hypoxia will be necessary.

The immediate goal in the treatment of anaphylactic shock is to maintain an adequate airway and to support the blood pressure. Oxygen may be administered. Epinephrine (subcutaneous or intravenous routes) may be given to restore vascular tone and blood pressure. Hypotension is treated with IV fluids to restore intravascular volume. Antihistamines (diphenhydramine), H_2 histamine antagonists (cimetidine), and bronchodilators (inhaled or IV) may be used (Wyatt, 1996).

Conventional treatment of sepsis centers on early recognition, removal of the source of infection, appropriate antibiotic therapy, and hemodynamic support with the administration of volume and vasoactive medications (Colletti, Dew, & Goulart, 1993). Appropriate antibiotic therapy requires monitoring serum drug levels, especially of aminoglycosides, to maintain adequate bacterial killing while minimizing toxicity. Volume replacement attempts to correct the maldistribution of circulating volume and augment cardiac output and blood pressure. Vasoactive medications may be administered to enhance afterload (norepinephrine, dopamine, phenylephrine). Inotropic agents (dobutamine) may be given to augment myocardial contractility. Treatment of hyperthermia with antipyretics (aspirin, acetaminophen) will decrease oxygen consumption.

Recent advances in the understanding of some of the pathophysiologic processes involved in sepsis and septic shock (see Fig. 10–1) have resulted in the development of a variety of pharmacologic agents that are given to manipulate the sequelae of the systemic response to infection. Many of these drugs (Table 10–4) are still being investigated in human clinical trials. The reader is referred to more in-depth reviews of trends in agents used for the management of sepsis (Wheeler & Bernard, 1999; Zeni, Freeman, & Natanson, 1997). Antibiotics are necessary but not sufficient for the treatment of sepsis. Antibiotics may also precipitate septic changes by liberating microbial products (Wheeler & Bernard, 1999). Prevention of organ failure is imperative to survival (see MODS, Module 11).

TABLE 10–4. AGENTS USED IN THE MANAGEMENT OF SEPSIS AND SEPTIC SHOCK

Antiendotoxin agents	Antiendotoxin monoclonal antibodies
Anticytokine agents	Antitumor necrosis factor monoclonal antibodies Interleukin-1 receptor monoclonal antibodies Interleukin-1 receptor agonists Interleukin-1 inhibitors Anti-interleukin-6 monoclonal antibodies Interleukin-6 inhibitor
Antieicosanoid agents	Cyclooxygenase inhibitors Platelet-activating factor receptor antagonists Thromboxane A_2 synthase inhibitor
Others	Nitric oxide synthetase inhibitors

Transport Shock States

The treatment goal in transport shock states is to restore the oxygen-carrying capacity of red blood cells. For the treatment of anemia or hemorrhage, packed red blood cells may be administered in an effort to provide an adequate hemoglobin concentration.

The treatment for carbon monoxide poisoning consists of the administration of high fractional concentrations of supplemental oxygen. There is considerable controversy over whether the use of hyperbaric oxygen therapy is advantageous in carbon monoxide poisoning (Weaver, 1999). Serial carboxyhemoglobin levels should be monitored to evaluate patient response to treatment.

Obstructive Shock States

The treatment goal in obstructive shock states is to remove the mechanical barrier to blood flow. For a tension pneumothorax, trapped air is decompressed by a physician with the insertion of a 14-gauge needle or a chest tube. Needle pericardiocentesis may decompress the pericardium for cardiac tamponade. This decompression should improve the heart's pumping ability. If not, a thoracotomy may be required to surgically control and decompress the tamponade.

The cornerstone of management for pulmonary embolism is heparin as it prevents additional thrombus from forming and permits endogenous fibrinolysis to dissolve some of the clot (Goldhaber, 1998). Inferior vena cava filters may be used in the presence of active hemorrhage or recurrent pulmonary embolism despite intensive prolonged anticoagulation (Goldhaber, 1998). Thrombolysis can be lifesaving in patients with massive pulmonary embolism, cardiogenic shock or overt hemodynamic instability (Jerjes-Sanchez, Ramirez, & Garcia, 1995).

Cardiogenic Shock States

The specific treatment for cardiogenic shock is based on the cardiac abnormality and whether the shock is caused by left-sided or right-sided heart failure. Nursing and medical interventions for patients in cardiogenic shock are directed toward decreasing myocardial oxygen demand and improving myocardial oxygen supply.

The initial management of the patient in cardiogenic shock may include fluid resuscitation (unless pulmonary edema is present), central venous and arterial access, urinary catheterization, pulse oximetry, oxygenation, and airway protection, correction of electrolyte abnormalities and relief of pain and anxiety (Hollenberg, Kavinsky, & Parillo, 1999).

Inotropic agents may be used in patients with inadequate tissue perfusion and adequate intravascular volume. Dobutamine can be used to improve myocardial contractility and increase cardiac output without markedly changing heart rate (Hollenberg, Kavinsky, & Parillo, 1999). Sympathomimetic infusions must be carefully titrated in an effort to maximize coronary perfusion pressure and minimize myocardial oxygen demand. Hemodynamic monitoring using a pulmonary artery catheter permits serial measurements of cardiac output which allows titration of inotropic and vasopressor drugs to the minimum dose required to achieve therapeutic goals. Diuretics may be used to treat pulmonary congestion. Vasodilators may be used (after blood pressure has been stabilized) to decrease both preload and afterload. Further treatment may include thrombolytic therapy, intra-aortic balloon pumping and revascularization (angioplasty or coronary artery bypass surgery).

Although it has been demonstrated that thrombolytic therapy reduces mortality rates in patients with acute MI, the benefits of this therapy in patients with cardiogenic shock are less certain. Thrombolytic therapy can reduce the likelihood of developing cardiogenic shock after initial presentation (Hollenberg, Kavinsky, & Parillo, 1999). Intra-aortic balloon pumping (IABP) reduces afterload and augments coronary perfusion, which increase cardiac output and improve coronary blood flow. The IABP is inserted into the femoral artery and advanced until it is in the descending thoracic aorta. The IABP is synchronized with the patient's heart rate. During ventricular diastole, the balloon inflates. With the balloon inflated, the blood distal to the balloon is forced back toward the aortic valve. This supplies the coronary arteries with additional oxygenated blood to meet myocardial oxygen needs. Before ventricular systole, the balloon deflates, which decreases pressure in the aorta. This makes it easier for the left ventricle to contract and expel its oxygenated blood. In hospitals without direct angioplasty capabilities, stabilization with IABP and thrombolysis followed by transfer to a tertiary care facility may be the best treatment option (Hollenberg, Kavinsky, & Parillo, 1999).

Mechanical revascularization for patients with cardiogenic shock caused by MI can be done. Direct percutaneous transluminal coronary angioplasty (PTCA) may be used to improve wall motion in the infarct area and increase perfusion of the infarct zone. In patients with cardiogenic shock who have left main and three vessel coronary disease, coronary artery bypass surgery may be performed (Hollenberg, Kavinsky, & Parillo, 1999).

In summary, the primary goals for treatment of shock are to optimize oxygen delivery and decrease oxygen consumption. Interventions that optimize oxygen delivery include supplemental oxygen administration, restoration of intravascular fluid volume, administration of inotropic and vasoactive drugs, and Trendelenburg's position. Improved oxygen delivery should be assessed in terms of improved cardiac output, increased urine output, a decrease in heart rate, and an increase in blood pressure. Interventions that decrease oxygen consumption include decreasing total body work through adequate ventilation and neuromuscular blocking agents, minimizing pain and stress, and correcting hyperthermia. Further and more individualized interventions are directed at treating the underlying cause of shock for each of the four functional shock states.

SECTION FOUR REVIEW

You have been assigned to provide nursing care to Mr. J, a 74-year-old male with a diagnosis of septic shock of unknown etiology. During the change of shift report, you are given the following information:

- Vital signs: BP 70/42, pulse 140 sinus tachycardia, respirations 38, temperature 103°F
- Recent laboratory results: ABGs: pH 7.25, $PaCO_2$ 30, PaO_2 60, HCO_3^- 18, base deficit 8, Hct 27, Hgb 8, Na^+ 140, K^+ 4.5
- Hemodynamic readings: MAP 51, RAP 3, PAP 18/8, PAWP 8, CO 4, SVR 356
- IV fluids: D_5 and ½ NS +20 mEq KCl at 100 mL/hr
- Urine output past 8 hours: 160 mL/hr

As you walk to Mr. J's bedside, you note that he is pale and restless. He is lying in the semi-Fowler's position. Answer the following questions based on the information provided about Mr. J.

1. Which of the following could best increase Mr. J's cardiac output and restore preload?
   A. D_5 and ½ NS + 20 mEq KCl at 75 mL/hr
   B. D_5 and ½ NS + 20 mEq KCl at 100 mL/hr
   C. Lactated Ringer's (LR) at 50 mL/hr
   D. LR at 200 mL/hr
2. Which of the following would indicate that Mr. J's oxygen delivery was improving?
   A. urine output of 50 mL/hr
   B. RAP 1 mm Hg
   C. Hct 27
   D. respiratory rate of 38/min
3. Mr. J currently is receiving a total volume (TV) of 350 mL/hr. Based on what you know about oxygen consumption during shock, which of the following orders might you expect the physician to write?
   A. decrease the TV
   B. increase the TV
   C. eliminate the TV
   D. leave the TV at 350
4. Which of the following drugs would NOT decrease Mr. J's oxygen consumption?
   A. norepinephrine
   B. pancuronium
   C. acetaminophen
   D. MSO_4
5. What effect would be produced if dopamine 1 mg/kg/min was added to Mr. J's treatment?
   A. increased myocardial oxygen demands
   B. increased blood pressure
   C. decreased urine output
   D. increased urine output

Answers: 1. D, 2. A, 3. B, 4. A, 5. D

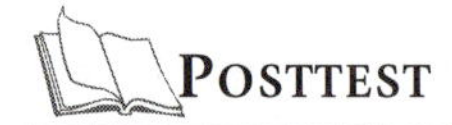

POSTTEST

1. Conditions common to all shock states are
   A. decreased blood pressure, heart rate, and urine output
   B. increased oxygen delivery with increased oxygen consumption
   C. impaired oxygen delivery with altered oxygen consumption
   D. decreased blood pressure, increased heart rate, and decreased urine output
2. Transport shock states have impaired oxygen delivery because
   A. a barrier impedes blood flow to tissues
   B. there is a loss of intravascular volume
   C. hemoglobin is unavailable to carry oxygen
   D. decreased sympathetic tone produces vasoconstriction
3. Vasodilation and maldistribution of circulating volume characterize
   A. anaphylactic shock
   B. septic shock
   C. neurogenic shock
   D. obstructive shock
4. ACTH and ADH
   A. cause sodium and water depletion
   B. are chemoreceptors that sense alterations in pH and $PaCO_2$

C. release norepinephrine
D. preserve blood volume by conserving fluid

5. Clinical signs of hypovolemic shock include
   A. cool skin, increased pulse, and low RAP
   B. warm skin, decreased pulse, and decreased CO
   C. cool skin, increased pulse, and increased CO
   D. warm skin, increased pulse, and low RAP
6. Systemic venous congestion is a manifestation of
   A. left ventricular failure
   B. right ventricular failure
   C. anaphylactic shock
   D. cardiac tamponade
7. Crystalloid solutions
   A. can increase the Hct by 2 to 3 percent
   B. are given to supplement Hgb concentrations
   C. restore fluid volumes and increase preload
   D. possess oncotic capabilities
8. Afterload reducing drugs
   A. increase blood pressure and CO
   B. restrict blood flow to internal organs
   C. produce vasodilation and improve cardiac performance
   D. produce vasoconstriction and increase myocardial oxygen consumption

POSTTEST ANSWERS

Question	Answer	Section	Question	Answer	Section
1	C	One	5	A	Three
2	C	One	6	B	Three
3	B	One	7	C	Four
4	D	Two	8	C	Four

REFERENCES

Bone, R.C., et al. Definitions for sepsis and organ failure and guidelines for the use of innovative therapies in sepsis. *Chest 101*:1644–1655.

Clochesy, J.M. (1988). Understanding shock states. In J.M. Clochesy (ed.), *Essentials of critical care nursing* (pp. 16–21). Rockville, MD: Aspen Publishing.

Colletti, R.C., Dew, R.B., & Goulart, A.E. (1993). Antiendotoxin therapy in sepsis. *Crit Care Nurs Clin North Am* 5:345–353.

Cornwell, E.E., Kennedy, F., & Rodriguez, J. (1996). The critical care of the severely injured patient. *Surg Clin North Am* 76:956–969.

Ferrari, E., Imbert, A., Chevalier, T., Mihoubi, A., Morand, P., & Baudouy, M. (1997). The ECG in pulmonary embolism. *Chest 111*:537–543.

Friday, G.A., & Fireman, P. (1996). Anaphylaxis. *Ear, Nose, Throat 75*(1):21–24.

Goldhaber, S.Z. (1998). Pulmonary embolism. *N Engl J Med* 339(2):93–104.

Greenburg, A.G. (1988). Pathophysiology of shock. In T.A. Miller (ed.), *Physiologic basis of modern surgical care* (pp. 154–172). St. Louis: C.V. Mosby.

Hollenberg, S.M., Kavinsky, C.J., & Parillo, J.E. (1999). Cardiogenic shock. *Ann Intern Med 131*:47–59.

Jerjes-Sanchez, C., Ramirez, A., & Garcia, M.L. (1995). Streptokinase and heparin versus heparin alone in massive pulmonary embolism. *Thrombolytics Thrombolysis 2*:227–229.

Mikhail, J. (1999). Resuscitation endpoints in trauma. *AACN Clin Issues 10*(1):10–21.

Porter, J.M., & Ivatury, R.R. (1998). In search of the optimal endpoints of resuscitation in trauma patients: A review. *J Trauma 44*:908–914.

Rice, V. (1991a). Shock: A clinical syndrome. An update. Part 1. *Crit Care Nurse 11*(4):20–27.

Rice, V. (1991b). Shock: A clinical syndrome. An update. Part 2. *Crit Care Nurse 11*(5):74–82.

Weaver, L.K. (1999). Carbon monoxide poisoning. *Crit Care Clin 15*:297–317.

Wheeler, A.P., & Bernard, G.R. (1999). Treating patients with severe sepsis. *N Eng J Med 340*:207–214.

Wyatt, R. (1996). Anaphylaxis. *Postgrad Med 100*(2):87–99.

Zeni, F., Freeman, B., & Natanson, C. (1997). Anti-inflammatory therapies to treat sepsis and septic shock: A reassessment. *Crit Care Med 25*:1095–1100.

Module 11

Multiple Organ Dysfunction Syndrome

Karen L. Johnson

Multiple organ dysfunction syndrome (MODS) is a syndrome characterized by the progressive dysfunction of two or more organ systems. The clinical course of MODS typically results in prolonged intensive care unit (ICU) stays, during which potentially enormous resources are utilized. Despite the expenditure of significant time, resources, and technology, the mortality rate from MODS remains high. Through identification of risk factors and timely interventions, critical care nurses can have an important role in detecting and preventing this highly lethal cascade of events.

This self-study module describes the local inflammatory response to injury (Section One), how the local response can progress to pathophysiologic changes associated with a systemic inflammatory response (Section Two), and the progression to multiple organ system dysfunction syndrome (Section Three). As pathophysiologic changes continue, organ involvement and failure can occur remote from the initial site of injury (Section Four). Nursing management of the patient with MODS and organ failure is presented in Section Five.

Each section includes a set of review questions to help the learner evaluate his or her understanding of the section's content before moving on to the next section. All Section Reviews and the module Pretest and Posttest include answers. It is suggested that the learner review those concepts answered incorrectly in the review questions before proceeding to the next section.

Objectives

Following completion of this module, the learner will be able to

1. State the physiologic changes that occur during the local inflammatory process.
2. Contrast the physiologic changes that occur with the local inflammatory response with those that occur with the systemic inflammatory response syndrome.
3. State three pathophysiologic changes that occur with multiple organ dysfunction syndrome.
4. Identify the six most common organ systems that fail as a result of the SIRS process.
5. Describe management of the patient with multiple organ dysfunction syndrome.

Pretest

1. All of the following can initiate inflammation EXCEPT
   A. fever
   B. injury
   C. bacteria
   D. ischemia
2. Which of the following squeeze through vessels walls to perform phagocytosis?
   A. immune mediators
   B. inflammatory mediators
   C. red blood cells (RBCs)
   D. white blood cells (WBCs)

3. Systemic inflammatory response syndrome (SIRS) can be characterized by all of the following EXCEPT
   A. temperature > 38°C (100°F)
   B. heart rate < 80 bpm
   C. WBC > 12,000 cells/mm^3
   D. immature bands (> 10%)
4. Vasodilation, microvascular permeability, cellular activation, and coagulation characterize
   A. sepsis
   B. septic shock
   C. the local immune response
   D. the local and systemic inflammatory response
5. MODS is a progressive dysfunction of at least
   A. one organ
   B. two organ systems
   C. three organ systems
   D. four organ systems
6. Two forms of MODS are
   A. initial and progressive
   B. progressive and refractory
   C. local and systemic
   D. primary and secondary
7. A principal contributor to the progression of SIRS and MODS is
   A. mediator-induced organ interaction
   B. mediator-induced thrombocytopenia
   C. progressive organ dysfunction
   D. bacterial translocation
8. Jaundice and coagulopathy characterize
   A. renal failure
   B. hematologic failure
   C. liver failure
   D. MODS

Pretest answers: 1. A, 2. D, 3. B, 4. D, 5. B, 6. D, 7. A, 8. C

GLOSSARY

Mediators. A broad category of bioactive substances that stimulate physiologic change in cells

Multiple organ dysfunction syndrome (MODS). The presence of altered organ function in an acutely ill patient such that homeostasis cannot be maintained without intervention

Primary MODS. Organ dysfunction directly related to an organ insult

Secondary MODS. An abnormal and excessive inflammatory response as a consequence of the patient's response to a secondary insult

Sepsis. A subcategory of systemic inflammatory response syndrome

Systemic inflammatory response syndrome (SIRS). The systemic inflammatory response to an initiating event

ABBREVIATIONS

ARDS. Acute respiratory distress syndrome

Bpm. Beats per minute

CO. Cardiac output

CNS. Central nervous system

GI. Gastrointestinal

ICU. Intensive care unit

MODS. Multisystem organ dysfunction syndrome

MOF. Multiple organ failure

SIRS. Systemic inflammatory response syndrome

WBC. White blood cell

SECTION ONE: Local Inflammatory Response

At the completion of this section, the learner will be able to state the physiologic changes that occur during the local inflammatory process.

An initiating event such as an injury, invading organism, or ischemia can trigger inflammation. The goal of inflammation is to limit the extent of injury and promote healing. This is accomplished by the production and elimination of biologically active mediators. **Mediators** are endogenous bioactive substances that stimulate physiologic and pathophysiologic changes in cells. There are numerous inflammatory response mediators.

Four physiologic changes occur during the local inflammatory process: vasodilation, increased microcirculatory permeability, cellular activation/adhesion, and coagulation (Secor, 1996) (Fig. 11–1). Vasodilation increases delivery of oxygen, white blood cells, and nutrients to the injured site. Increased microvascular permeability allows nutrients and other factors to leave the vascular space

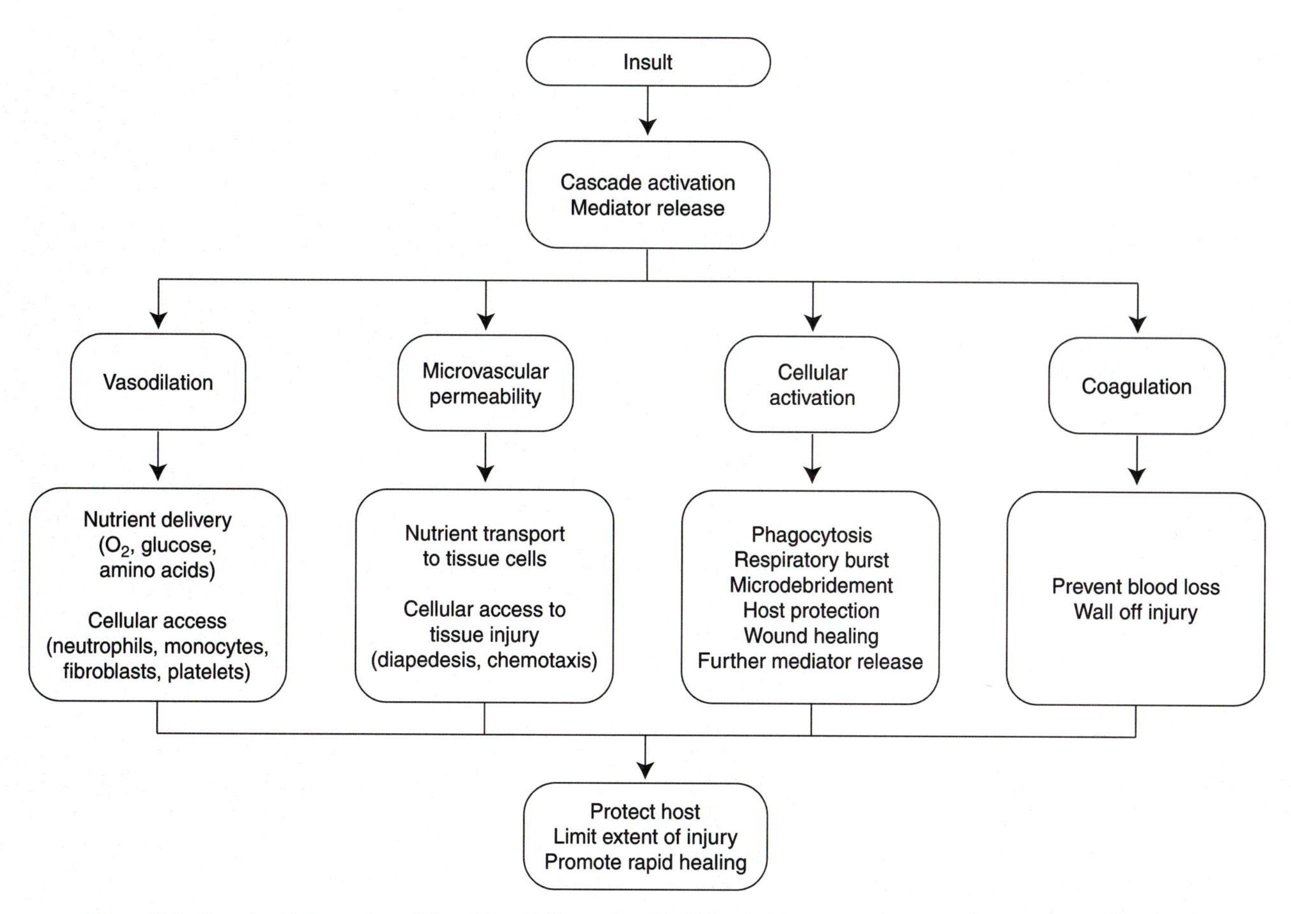

Figure 11–1. Cascade of inflammation. *(Adapted from Huddleston, V.B. [1992].* Multisystem organ failure: Pathophysiology and clinical implications *[p. 21]. St. Louis: C.V. Mosby.)*

and enter the injured tissue area. For example, WBCs squeeze through openings in vessel walls, move into the injured areas, and phagocytose necrotic tissue and invading pathogens. Coagulation occurs in an effort to minimize blood loss and repair injured vessels.

The inflammatory response triggers an immune response. The immune response is mediated by T lymphocytes and B lymphocytes, whose action primarily takes place in lymph tissue. T and B cells react only with specific antigens they recognize. After exposure to antigens, most T and B cells carry out specific functions. Others return to lymph tissue and reside as memory cells. The memory cells enable the host to mount a more rapid and vigorous response with repeated exposures to the same antigen (Secor, 1996).

In summary, an initiating event triggers an inflammatory response at the area of injury in an effort to limit the extent of injury and promote healing. This is accomplished by various mediators that are released after injury to tissues and cells. Mediators produce physiologic changes in cells at the injury site to limit further injury and repair damaged tissue. The immune response is also activated to help fight invading pathogens. When localized to the site of injury, the inflammatory and immune responses are very effective.

Section One Review

1. A local inflammatory response can be initiated by all of the following except
   A. injury
   B. ischemia
   C. bacteria
   D. biologically active mediators

2. The inflammatory process does all of the following EXCEPT
   A. remove debris
   B. limit mediator release
   C. control bleeding
   D. limit infection

3. Which of the following allow the host to mount a rapid and vigorous response with repeated antigen exposures?
   A. T cells and B cells
   B. bradykinin
   C. thromboxane
   D. prostaglandins

Answers: 1, D. 2, B. 3, A

SECTION TWO: Systemic Inflammatory Response Syndrome

At the completion of this section, the learner will be able to contrast the physiologic changes that occur with the local inflammatory response with those that occur with the systemic inflammatory response syndrome.

As discussed in Section One, localized inflammation is a physiologic defense mechanism that occurs in response to an injury, ischemia, or an invading pathogen. Four physiologic mechanisms occur to protect the host, limit the extent of injury, and promote rapid healing. These include: vasodilation, increased microvascular permeability, cellular activation, and coagulation. However, this response must be tightly controlled by the body at the local injury site or the response becomes overly activated, leading to an exaggerated, systemic response in each of these four physiologic mechanisms (Secor, 1996).

The **systemic inflammatory response syndrome (SIRS)** is defined as a systemic inflammatory response to an initiating event (trauma, shock, sepsis, ischemia). This systemic response is manifested by two or more of the following conditions: alteration in body temperature (> 38°C [100°F] or < 36°C [96.8°F]), tachycardia (> 90 bpm), tachypnea (> 20 breaths/min or $PaCO_2$ < 32 torr), and altered WBC count (> 12,000 cells/mm^3, or < 4,000 cells/mm^3 or > 10% immature bands) (American College of Chest Physicians & Society of Critical Care Medicine, 1992). Patients with SIRS may or may not have positive cultures, and typically present in a hyperdynamic, hypermetabolic state (Wheeler & Bernard, 1999). They may exhibit an elevated cardiac output (CO), decreased systemic vascular resistance (SVR), leukocytosis, tachycardia, and fever.

SIRS is characterized by an exaggerated inflammatory response of that which occurs at the local injury site (Table 11–1). Major alterations in tissue perfusion, metabolism, and oxygen utilization occur. It is difficult to stop these physiologic mechanisms because the pathophysiology is self-perpetuating and can spiral out of control. SIRS is now recognized as a major etiologic factor in the development of organ dysfunction and failure, especially if a second insult (shock, infection, ischemia) follows the initial injury (Secor, 1996) (Fig. 11–2).

It is currently believed that multiple organ dysfunction syndrome (MODS) represents only the most severe or end stage of uncontrolled SIRS (Zimmerman et al.,

TABLE 11–1. EXAGGERATED MECHANISMS OF INFLAMMATION IN SIRS

MECHANISM	RESPONSE
Excessive vasodilation	↓ SVR, ↓ BP, often refractory to fluids
Increased microvascular permeability	Generalized peripheral edema, third spacing, edema in organ beds
Exaggerated cellular activation	↑ Cellular aggregation, vascular obstruction, tissue infiltration, excessive mediator production. WBCs release toxic by-products
Accelerated coagulation	Excessive formation of microthrombi

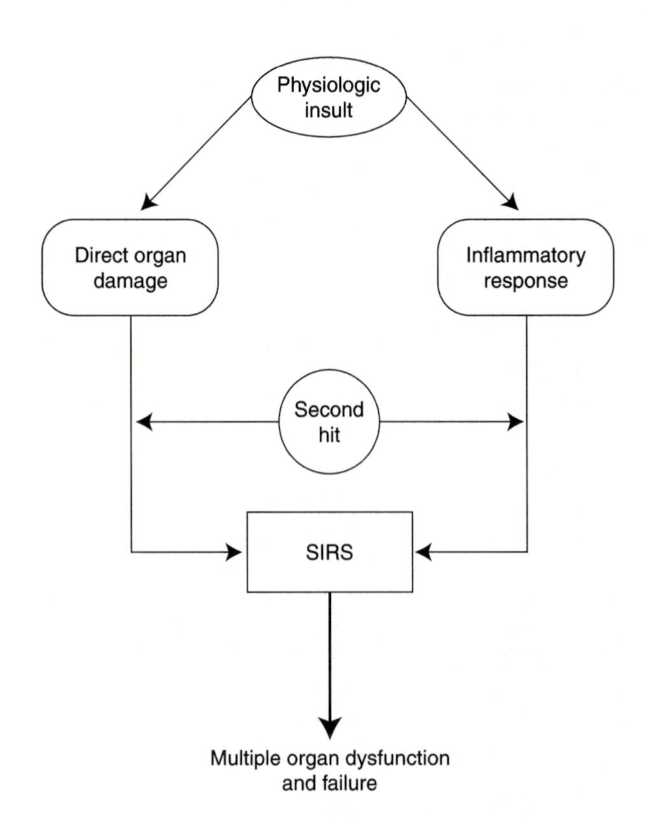

Figure 11–2. Relationship between Initial Insult, Second Hit, and SIRS. *(From Secor, V.H. [1994]. The inflammatory/immune response in critical illness: Role of the systemic inflammatory response syndrome.* Crit Care Nurs Clin North Am *6:259.)*

1996). This makes prevention, early detection and prompt management of SIRS so crucial in the prevention of MODS.

In summary, localized inflammation occurs in response to an injury. Physiologic mechanisms initiated to protect the host include vasodilation, microvascular permeability, cellular activation, and coagulation. In SIRS, an exaggerated systemic response in each of these four mechanisms occur. SIRS may be manifested by alterations in body temperature, fever, heart rate, and WBC count. The pathophysiology of SIRS is self-perpetuating. It is now recognized SIRS is a major etiologic factor in the development of MODS.

SECTION TWO REVIEW

1. Excessive vasodilation that occurs with SIRS produces
   - **A.** decreased systemic vascular resistance, decreased blood pressure
   - **B.** generalized edema
   - **C.** fever
   - **D.** erythema
2. Your patient is assessed to have the following: temperature 39.5°C, heart rate 110 BPM, respiratory rate 12/min, WBC 15,000 cells/mm^3 with > 10% bands. This patient may have which of the following?
   - **A.** MODS
   - **B.** bacteremia
   - **C.** SIRS
   - **D.** a local inflammatory response
3. Prevention, early detection, and prompt management of SIRS is crucial because
   - **A.** it has a high mortality
   - **B.** it can progress to MODS
   - **C.** long-term treatment is costly
   - **D.** rehabilitation is extensive

Answers: 1. A, 2. C, 3. B

SECTION THREE: Multiple Organ Dysfunction Syndrome

At the completion of this section, the learner will be able to state three pathophysiologic changes that occur with MODS.

Multiple organ dysfunction syndrome (MODS) is defined as the presence of altered organ function in an acutely ill patient such that homeostasis cannot be maintained without interventions (American College of Chest Physicians & Society of Critical Care Medicine, 1992). MODS is a nonspecific expression of critical illness involving progressive dysfunction of two or more organ systems, which is driven by the presence of numerous mediators and conditions, most notably SIRS (Secor, 1996). As organs become further dysfunctional and they irreversibly fail, multiply organ failure (MOF) can occur.

Theories about the etiology and clinical presentation of MODS have changed over the past several decades. It is now apparent that a clinical infection is not needed to initiate MOF. Less than half of all patients have positive blood cultures (Wheeler & Bernard, 1999).

A "hit" model has been developed to describe different stages or forms of MODS (Fig. 11–3). Single-hit, or **primary MODS,** is thought to occur in response to the initial insult and subsequent resuscitation measures. Death occurs within several days after ICU admission. Direct pulmonary trauma (such as hemothorax/pneumothorax, pulmonary contusions), severe head injury, and delayed or inadequate resuscitative measures greatly contribute to primary MODS (Secor, 1996). In double-hit or **secondary MODS**, secondary complications occur (sepsis, shock, myocardial infarction), which perpetuate SIRS. The initial shock is thought to prime the inflammatory response and a secondary insult reactivates it at an exaggerated level (Secor, 1996) (Fig. 11–3).

MODS is characterized by three pathophysiologic changes: maldistribution of circulating volume, imbalance of oxygen supply and demand, and alterations in metabolism (Fig. 11–4). These three pathophysiologic changes incite ischemia, tissue damage, and organ dysfunction and failure. If these pathophysiologic changes cannot be reversed or slowed, MODS and MOF ensue (Secor, 1996).

Inflammatory mediators release a variety of vasoactive substances that cause a maldistribution of blood flow to the tissues. In **sepsis** and inflammation, mediators produce vasodilation and increased vascular permeability at the microcirculatory level (Robins, 1996). Vasodilation produces peripheral blood pooling, decreased venous return, and decreased preload. Other mediators and catecholamines from the sympathetic nervous system produce vasoconstriction.

One of the common factors in the pathophysiologic

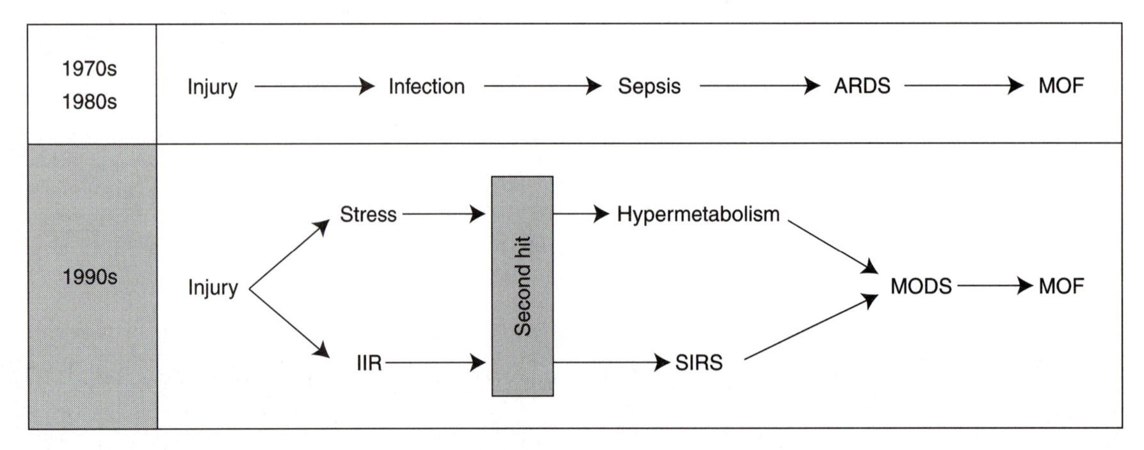

Figure 11–3. Current and Past Theories of the Etiology and Clinical Progression of MODS. ARDS, Acute respiratory distress syndrome; MOF, multiple organ failure; IIR, inflammatory/immune response; SIRS, systemic inflammatory response syndrome; MODS, multiple organ dysfunction syndrome. *(From: Secor, V.H. [1996].* Multiple organ dysfunction & failure. *2nd ed. [p. 6]. St. Louis: C.V. Mosby.)*

progression of MODS appears to be an unrecognized mismatch between oxygen delivery and oxygen consumption (Kearney, 1996). Regional blood flow maldistribution contributes to impaired oxygen delivery. Sluggish microvascular blood flow produces mechanical blockades in the microvasculature. Toxic damage to mitochondrial cell membranes impair oxygen utilization and consumption. Currently, there is no clear understanding of the etiology and effects of impaired oxygenation on MODS. However, it is likely that numerous factors affect the intake, delivery, and use of oxygen during the genesis and progression of MODS.

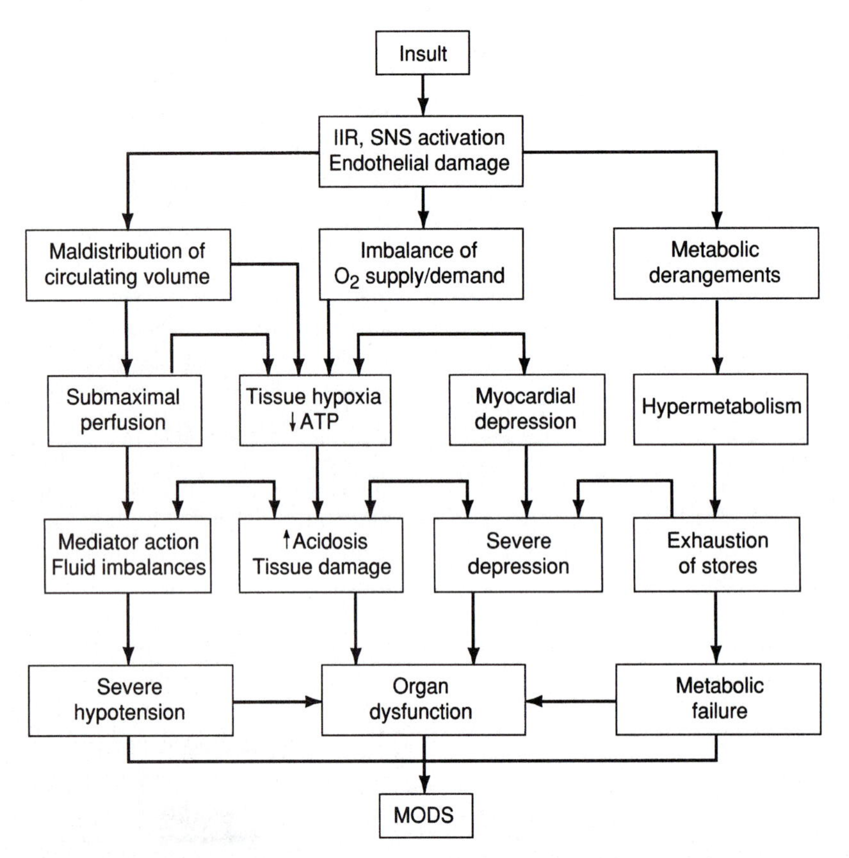

Figure 11–4. Pathophysiologic cascade mechanism organ failure. (*Modified from Huddleston, V.B. [1991].* Multisystem organ failure: A pathophysiologic approach. *Paper presented at the National Teaching Institute, American Association of Critical Care Nurses. Boston, MA.*)

A hypermetabolic state occurs in response to injury. This physiologic mechanism is designed to meet short-term energy needs. Prolongation of the hypermetabolic state occurs in MODS. This results in excessive catabolism of protein and fat stores and a negative nitrogen balance. Malnutrition resulting from the metabolic response is associated with delayed recovery, increased susceptibility to infection, and increased mortality and morbidity (Kimbrell, 1996).

In summary, MODS is a syndrome characterized by the progressive dysfunction of two or more organ systems. Theories about the clinical progression of MODS have changed over the decades. Two forms of MODS are thought to exist: primary and secondary. MODS is characterized by three physiologic changes: maldistribution of circulating volume, impaired oxygenation, and hypermetabolism.

Section Three Review

1. MODS is characterized by the dysfunction of how many organ systems?
   A. 1
   B. ≥ 2
   C. ≥ 3
   D. ≥ 4
2. What percentage of patients have a positive blood culture?
   A. < 10%
   B. < 50%
   C. > 50%
   D. > 90%
3. Primary MODS can occur in response to
   A the insult itself
   B. secondary complications
   C. an exaggerated SIRS
   D. septic shock
4. All of the following are pathophysiologic changes that occur with MODS EXCEPT
   A. impaired oxygenation
   B. hypermetabolism
   C. maldistribution of circulating blood volume
   D. hypotension, tachycardia, fever

Answers: 1, B. 2, B. 3, A. 4, D

SECTION FOUR: Organ Involvement and Failure

At the completion of this section, the learner will be able to identify the six most common organ systems that fail as a result of the SIRS process.

As the pathophysiologic changes discussed in Section Three continue, organ dysfunction continues. Organ dysfunction can occur far from the initial injury site as a result of SIRS. Mediators enable organ-to-organ interaction. This interaction is thought to be a principal contributor to the progression of SIRS and MODS (Secor, 1996). Organ ischemia and cellular damage perpetuate SIRS, which perpetuates MODS. A vicious cycle develops. As each additional organ fails, mortality escalates. The average risk of death increases 15 percent to 20 percent with failure of each additional organ (Wheeler & Bernard, 1999). It is not clear whether a hierarchical relationship exists among the various organ systems in terms of mortality (Kollef & Sherman, 1999). Definitions of organ system failure in the six most common systems are presented in Table 11–2.

The lungs are usually the first to show signs of dysfunction and respiratory failure rapidly progresses to acute respiratory distress syndrome (ARDS). Certain risk factors have a higher associated frequency of ARDS, and there is an additive effect of two or more risk factors. These include sepsis, pancreatitis, hypertransfusion, aspiration of gastric contents, abdominal trauma and multiple fractures (Brandstetter et al., 1997). The clinical pattern of ARDS occurs within a few days of the initiating event. Fluid resuscitation given to maintain circulating volume, coupled with increased capillary permeability, contributes to the development of ARDS. ARDS may also develop due to microemboli that form as a result of sluggish blood flow through pulmonary capillaries. Increased oxygen demand places additional stress on the pulmonary system. This inevitably results in respiratory failure and the need for mechanical ventilation.

In cardiovascular failure, the transition from a hyperdynamic to hypodynamic state is a very late occurrence in MODS. It is characterized by increased SVR and decreased cardiac output (CO). Reductions in myocardial contractility stem from myocardial depressant factors (Wheeler & Bernard, 1999).

Central nervous system (CNS) dysfunction can manifest as restlessness, agitation, confusion, or coma. The exact etiology of CNS dysfunction associated with SIRS is not known, although two hypotheses have been postulated: (1) formation of brain microabscesses and (2) occurrence of cerebral edema (Briones, 1996).

Renal failure may be secondary to (1) administration

TABLE 11–2. DEFINITIONS OF ORGAN SYSTEM FAILURE

Cardiovascular failure (presence of one or more)	Heart rate ≤ 54 bpm Mean arterial pressure ≤ 59 mm Hg Occurrence of ventricular tachycardia and/or ventricular fibrillation Arterial pH of ≤ 7.24 with a $Paco_2$ ≤ 49 torr
Respiratory failure (presence of one or more)	Respiratory rate of ≤ 5 breaths/min or ≥ 49 breaths/min $Paco_2$ of ≥ 50 torr P(A–a) O_2 of 350 torr Dependent of ventilator on day 4 of organ system failure
Renal failure (presence of one or more)	Urine output of ≤ 479 mL/24 hr or ≥ 159 mL/8 hr Serum BUN of ≥ 100 mg/dL Serum creatinine ≥ 3.5 mg/dL
Hematologic failure (presence of one or more)	WBC count of ≤ 1000 cells/mm^3 Platelets of ≤ 20,000 cells/mm^3 Hematocrit ≤ 20%
Neurologic failure (presence of one or more)	Glasgow Coma Scale score ≤ 6 (in absence of sedation at one point in day)

From Zimmerman, J.E., Kraus, W.A., Wagner, D.P., et al. (1996). A comparison of risks and outcomes for patients with organ failure: 1982–1990. *Crit Care Med 24*:1634.

of nephrotoxic antibiotics, (2) presence of mediators and cellular alterations, or (3) decreased renal perfusion. Progressive renal failure is manifested by oliguria and elevated blood urea nitrogen (BUN) and creatinine. When the kidney is the only organ to fail, mortality is < 10 percent (Toto, 1996). However, in the face of pulmonary or liver failure, the mortality rate increases. The majority of patients who survive renal failure, and MODS fully recover renal function (Toto, 1996).

Hepatic failure involves progressive failure in liver function. Hepatic failure develops in 10 percent to 40 percent of patients with SIRS (Lohrman, 1996). Because the liver performs so many functions, liver dysfunction affects almost all other organ systems. The liver, as a mechanical and immunologic filter, may be the source of mediators that cause lung injury (Wheeler & Bernard, 1999). Hepatic failure is manifested by jaundice and coagulopathy. Once liver failure occurs in the setting of MODS, mortality approaches 90 percent to 100 percent (Lohrman, 1996).

An increasing body of evidence suggests that the gastrointestinal (GI) system may play a pivotal role in "fueling" MODS. Gut organs are vulnerable to decreased perfusion during stress and SIRS. In the presence of ischemia, the protective gut barrier is damaged, allowing bacteria, mediators, and endotoxins to enter the peritoneal cavity and portal circulation. As a result, the gut extends the damage to the whole body and exacerbates MODS (O'Neill, 1996).

In summary, organ dysfunction can occur remote from the initial injury site because mediators enable organ-to-organ interaction. Organ ischemia and cellular damage perpetuate SIRS, which perpetuates MODS. Any organ system can manifest dysfunction, and six of the most common organ systems were presented. As additional organs fail, mortality escalates.

SECTION FOUR REVIEW

1. A principal contributor to the progression of SIRS and MODS is
   A. xanthine oxidase
   B. organ-to-organ communication
   C. septic shock
   D. ARDS
2. One of the last organ systems to fail in MODS is the
   A. CNS system
   B. pulmonary system
   C. renal system
   D. cardiovascular system
3. Which of the following systems plays a pivotal role in "fueling" MODS?
   A. GI system
   B. pulmonary system
   C. CNS system
   D. renal system

Answers: 1, B. 2, D. 3, A

SECTION FIVE: Nursing Management of MODS

At the completion of this section, the learner will be able to describe the management of the patient with MODS.

In Section Four, the progression of SIRS to MODS was reviewed. An awareness of this natural progression may help the nurse to identify patients at risk and prevent the progression of SIRS, MODS, and MOF. There is no cure for MODS. Supportive care has been emphasized in three general areas: source control, restoration and maintenance of oxygenation, and metabolic support (Reilly & Yucha, 1994).

Source control is directed at eliminating the initiating events that trigger SIRS. Recall from Section Two that these events include trauma, shock, sepsis, and ischemia. Strategies can include fracture stabilization, control of hemorrhage, drainage of infection, and debridement of necrotic tissue. A major goal is to prevent sepsis. Whenever possible, an infective source must be identified, corrected, and treated (see Module 10, Section Four). Critically ill patients are at high risk for infection because of indwelling tubes, catheters, and open wounds. Meticulous aseptic techniques must be used in the care of indwelling tubes and catheters.

The second goal of treatment is to restore and promote adequate oxygenation. The nurse must assess oxygenation status in relation to pulmonary gas exchange, oxygen delivery, and oxygen consumption (as discussed in Module 9, Section Six). Interventions to optimize oxygen delivery and decrease oxygen consumption must be promptly instituted (see Module 10, Section Four).

The last goal of treatment is to provide metabolic support. Total energy expenditure in MODS can be 1.5 to 2 times the normal metabolic rate (Reilly & Yucha, 1994). Nurses must encourage the initiation of supplemental nutrition within 48 hours to 96 hours after the onset of critical illness (McMahon, 1995). The consequences of inadequate nutrition can include electrolyte imbalances, muscle atrophy, poor wound healing, skin breakdown, clotting abnormalities, and gut atrophy. Recall from Section Four that the GI system may "fuel" MODS. Early enteral feedings with the feeding tube placed distal to the pylorus must be initiated (Reilly & Yucha, 1994).

Other supportive care measures may be taken to maintain the functions of individual organ systems. For example, supportive care for respiratory failure may include mechanical ventilation. Supportive care for renal failure may include dialysis.

In summary, it is important for the nurse to identify patients at risk and prevent the progression of SIRS, MODS, and MOF. Because there is no cure, supportive care is required in three areas: source control, restoration and maintenance of oxygenation, and metabolic support. Other supportive care measures are directed at maintaining the functions of individual organ systems.

SECTION FIVE REVIEW

1. The cure for renal failure is
   - **A.** dialysis
   - **B.** prevention
   - **C.** an improvement in renal perfusion
   - **D.** not available
2. Supportive care for MODS includes all of the following EXCEPT
   - **A.** organ transplantation
   - **B.** source control
   - **C.** restoring and maintaining oxygenation
   - **D.** metabolic support
3. Enteral feeding
   - **A.** is not possible when patients are on a ventilator
   - **B.** may prevent gut atrophy
   - **C.** contributes to fueling of MODS
   - **D.** causes gastric distention

Answers: 1, D. 2, A. 3, B

POSTTEST

1. The goal of inflammation is to
   - **A.** produce heat
   - **B.** produce swelling
   - **C.** kill bacteria
   - **D.** limit the extent of injury and promote healing
2. Endogenous substances that stimulate physiologic and pathophysiologic changes are called
   - **A.** endotoxins
   - **B.** mediators
   - **C.** white blood cells
   - **D.** neurotransmitters

3. SIRS is an exaggerated systemic response to
   A. bacteria
   B. sepsis
   C. local inflammation
   D. endotoxins
4. Which of the following is a major etiologic factor in the development of MODS?
   A. SIRS
   B. ARDS
   C. disseminated intravascular coagulation (DIC)
   D. MOF
5. MODS is characterized by progressive dysfunction of
   A. the immune system
   B. the inflammatory response
   C. the lungs and one other organ
   D. two or more organ systems
6. MODS is characterized by all of the following pathophysiologic changes EXCEPT
   A. maldistribution of circulating blood volume
   B. hypotension, increased CO
   C. imbalance of oxygen supply and demand
   D. hypermetabolism
7. A major contributor of the progression of SIRS to MODS is
   A. organ-to-organ communication
   B. renal failure
   C. improper treatment of septic shock
   D. inadequate perfusion
8. The "fuel" of MODS may be
   A. antibiotics
   B. liver failure
   C. failure of gut barrier
   D. renal failure
9. Goals for supportive care for MODS includes all of the following EXCEPT
   A. source control
   B. dialysis
   C. restoration of oxygenation
   D. metabolic support
10. Supplemental nutrition should be
   A. withheld until bowel sounds are present
   B. given by nasogastric route
   C. given by parenteral route
   D. initiated early after onset of critical illness

POSTTEST ANSWERS

Question	Answer	Section	Question	Answer	Section
1	D	One	6	B	Three
2	B	One	7	A	Four
3	C	Two	8	C	Four
4	A	Two	9	B	Five
5	D	Three	10	D	Five

REFERENCES

American College of Chest Physicians & Society of Critical Care Medicine. (1992). The AACP/SCCM consensus conference on sepsis and organ failure. *Chest, 101*:1481–1483.

Brandstetter, R.D., Sharma, K.C., DellaBadia, M., Cabreors, L.J., & Kabinoff, G.S. (1997). Acute respiratory distress syndrome: A disorder in need of improved outcome. *Heart Lung, 26*:3–14.

Briones, T.L. (1996). Central nervous system dysfunction in multiple organ dysfunction syndrome. In V.H. Secor (ed.), *Multiple organ dysfunction & failure* (2nd ed.) (pp. 304–322). St. Louis: C.V. Mosby.

Kearney, M.L. (1996). Imbalance of oxygen supply and oxygen demand. In V.H. Secor (ed.), *Multiple organ dysfunction & failure* (2nd ed.) (pp. 135–146). St. Louis: C.V. Mosby.

Kimbrell, J.D. (1996). Alterations in metabolism. In V.H. Secor (ed.), *Multiple organ dysfunction & failure* (2nd ed.) (pp. 148–161). St. Louis: C.V. Mosby.

Kollef, M.H., & Sherman, G. (1999). Acquired organ system derangements and hospital mortality: Are all organ systems created equally? *Am J Crit Care 8*:180–188.

Lohrman, J. (1996). Hepatic dysfunction, hypermetabolism, and multiple organ dysfunction syndrome. In V.H. Secor (ed.), *Multiple organ dysfunction & failure* (2nd ed.) (pp. 196–211). St. Louis: C.V. Mosby.

McMahon, K. (1995, December). Multiple organ failure: The final complication of critical illness. *Crit Care Nurse*, pp. 20–29.

O'Neill, P.L. (1996). Gastrointestinal system: Target organ and source of multiple organ dysfunction syndrome. In V.H. Secor (ed.), *Multiple organ dysfunction & failure* (2nd ed.) (pp. 215–234). St. Louis: C.V. Mosby.

Reilly E., & Yucha, C.B. (1994, April). Multiple organ failure syndrome. *Crit Care Nurse*, pp. 25–33.

Robins, E.V. (1996). Maldistribution of Circulating Volume. In V.H. Secor (ed.), *Multiple organ dysfunction & failure* (2nd ed.) (pp. 107–134). St. Louis: C.V. Mosby.

Secor, V.H. (1996). Multiple organ dysfunction syndrome: Background, etiology, and sequence of events. In V.H. Secor (ed.), *Multiple organ dysfunction & failure* (2nd ed.) (pp. 3–18). St. Louis: C.V. Mosby.

Toto, K.H. (1996). The kidney in multiple organ dysfunction syndrome. In V.H. Secor (ed.), *Multiple organ dysfunction & failure* (2nd ed.) (pp. 276–301). St. Louis: C.V. Mosby.

Wheeler, A.P., & Bernard, G.R. (1999). Treating patients with severe sepsis. *N Engl J Med 340*:201–214.

Zimmerman, J.E., Knaus, W.A., Wagner, D.P., et al. (1996). A comparison of risks and outcomes for patients with organ failure: 1982–1990. *Crit Care Med 24*:1633–1641.

Module 12

Nursing Care of the Patient with Impaired Oxygenation

Karen Johnson, Pamela Stinson Kidd

This self-study module is designed to integrate the major points discussed in Modules 9, 10, and 11, as well as assist the learner in clustering information to facilitate clinical application. Content is applied in an interactive learning style. Using a case study format, the learner is encouraged to identify nursing actions based on the assessment of a patient with impaired oxygenation. Consequences of selecting a particular action are discussed. Rationale for all answers is presented. The module ends with a brief summary of major points.

Objectives

Following completion of this module, the learner will be able to

1. Describe an appropriate database for a patient experiencing impaired oxygenation related to inflammation.
2. Discuss development of nursing diagnoses appropriate to patients with multiple organ dysfunction syndrome (MODS).
3. Explain the development of a plan of care for the patient with MODS.
4. Analyze outcomes of care in a patient with MODS.

Glossary

Continuous arteriovenous hemofiltration (CAVH). The use of a transmembrane pressure gradient to remove water, electrolytes, and small-to-medium-molecular-weight molecules from the vascular space. Blood enters the extracorporeal circuit by arterial access and returns by venous access. The patient's hydrostatic blood pressure drives the blood flow; no external pump is used

Extracorporeal membrane oxygenation (ECMO). A process that uses a mechanical device to replace cardiac and lung function

Abbreviations

CAVH. Continuous arteriovenous hemofiltration

CI. Cardiac index

CO. Cardiac output

CVP. Central venous pressure

ECMO. Extracorporeal membrane oxygenation

FIO_2. Fraction of inspired oxygen

PAD. Pulmonary artery diastolic pressure

PAS. Pulmonary artery systolic pressure

PAWP. Pulmonary artery wedge pressure

PEEP. Positive end-expiratory pressure

TNF. Tumor necrosis factor

CASE STUDY

Dale F is admitted to your unit with a diagnosis of pneumonia. He presented to the emergency department (ED) after having 2 weeks of low-grade fever and chills. He complained of a cough. Mr. F had completed 3 days of oral cephalosporin treatment given to him by a physician at an urgent care center. His chest x-ray in the ED showed bilateral pneumonia with greater involvement of the left lung than the right.

Initial Appraisal

On walking into the room, you note the following:

GENERAL APPEARANCE. Mr. F is around 40 years of age. He appears as a "healthy," well-nourished man. He has well-developed arm muscles and dark skin from spending a lot of time outdoors. He is wearing glasses.

SIGNS OF DISTRESS. Mr. F is diaphoretic and breathing rapidly. He is sitting upright and coughs frequently. Secretions are audible during coughing.

OTHER. You note an intravenous line in his right dorsal hand. Oxygen is running at 2 L through a nasal cannula. A woman who identifies herself as his wife is in the room.

Focused Assessment

You quickly introduce yourself and immediately perform a rapid assessment, focusing on Mr. F's pulmonary status and oxygenation. The results are as follows:

Dale is restless but is oriented to person, place, and time. His respiratory rate is 30/min. Respirations are regular and shallow. He asks to be allowed to sit upright to ease his breathing. He is using accessory muscles in his neck while breathing, but no retractions are noted. Diffuse medium crackles are auscultated in the middle and lower lung fields bilaterally. S_1 and S_2 are auscultated without rub or murmur. His current blood pressure is 140/90 mm Hg, pulse is 110, and his temperature is 101.5°F (38.6°C) orally. He coughs up some white mucus.

QUESTION

What additional information could you obtain that would help you assess oxygen delivery?

A. urine output
B. arterial oxygen saturation
C. mean arterial pressure
D. sputum culture

ANSWER

The correct answer is B. To assess oxygenation, you must have information about Mr. F's oxygen delivery. This can easily be accomplished by application of a pulse oximeter. Knowing his urine output will help you assess whether he is receiving adequate blood flow and oxygen to his kidneys, but adequate flow does not guarantee adequate oxygenation. Mean arterial pressure will tell you about afterload (the resistance that his heart must pump and fill against). A sputum culture will provide information regarding the cause of his pneumonia. Arterial oxygen saturation is the ratio of oxygenated hemoglobin to total hemoglobin. Over 97 percent of all oxygen delivered to cells is delivered as oxyhemoglobin.

After the initial assessment you connect Mr. F to the pulse oximeter. You look through his chart to see if any lab work was completed in the ED. You find the following:

CBC

WBC = 18,000/mL	(Normal, 4,500 to 10,000/mL)
RBC = 5.33 × 10^{12}L	(Normal, 4.6 to 6.0 × 10^{12}L)
Hgb = 15.3 g/dL	(Normal, 13.5 to 17 g/dL
Hct = 43.8%	(Normal, 40 to 54%)
Platelets = 397,000/mL	(Normal, 150,000 to 400,000/mL)

Electrolytes

Glucose = 95 mg/dL	(Normal, 70 to 110 mg/dL)
BUN = 30 mg/dL	(Normal, 5 to 25 mg/dL)
Creatinine = 0.9 mg/dL	(Normal, 0.5 to 1.5 mg/dL)
Sodium = 139 mEq/L	(Normal, 135 to 145 mEq/L)
Potassium = 4.6 mEq/L	(Normal, 3.5 to 5.3 mEq/L)
Chloride = 110 mEq/L	(Normal, 95 to 105 mEq/L)

Urine
Specific gravity = 1.030 (Normal, 1.005 to 1.030)

Arterial Blood Gases

pH = 7.37	(Normal, 7.35 to 7.45)
$PaCO_2$ = 42 mm Hg	(Normal, 35 to 45 mm Hg)
PaO_2 = 82 mm Hg	(Normal, 75 to 100 mm Hg)
HCO_3 = 26 mEq/L	(Normal, 24 to 28 mEq/L)
SaO_2 = 92%	(Normal, 95% or greater)

QUESTION

Which of the following statements are true about Dale's condition?

A. he shows evidence of an infection
B. he is in respiratory acidosis
C. he may be dehydrated
D. he is anemic

ANSWER

In this case, both A and C are correct. Dale shows signs of infection as evidenced by elevation in WBC count and fever. He may also be dehydrated as evidenced by hyperchloremia, elevated specific gravity, and elevated BUN in face of a normal creatinine. Although Dale's oxygen saturation level is low, he is compensating well and is not in respiratory acidosis since his pH is normal. His RBC and Hgb counts are normal, so he is not anemic.

You check the orders that have accompanied Dale and find that he needs several things:

- IV D_5LR @ 200 mL/hr
- IV erythromycin 500 mg q6h
- Sputum culture
- Pulmonary function tests
- Acetaminophen 325 mg q4h PRN fever

QUESTION

Which of these orders should you implement first?

ANSWER

You should initiate the IV fluids and simultaneously hang the first dose of the IV erythromycin. These actions address both the dehydration and infection suggested by Dale's laboratory data, x-ray reading, and your assessment findings. Your actions will help promote oxygenation by increasing oxygen delivery through increased blood flow, improving pulmonary gas exchange by eliminating lung infiltrates and increasing lung surface area for diffusion. If Dale is dehydrated, it will be more difficult to obtain a sputum culture, plus it will take several days to obtain information from this test. The pulmonary function tests will require Dale's cooperation. In addition to being in minor distress, he is breathing too fast to perform these tests presently. Dale is febrile. Fever increases oxygen consumption. Since Dale alredy has impaired gas exchange from pneumonia, and decreased oxygen delivery from dehydration, his fever should be treated with antipyretics as soon as the IV and antibiotic interventions have been initiated.

Focused Nursing History

Dale started feeling bad about 2 weeks ago. His shortness of breath has been increasing and 3 days ago he went to an urgent care center. After starting on cephalosporin, he initially felt better. Yesterday his fever went up and his chills began. His cough prevents him from sleeping at night and eating as well as normal. Over-the-counter cough medicine has not relieved it. He occasionally brings up white, thick sputum.

He is allergic to penicillin, and nonsteroidal anti-inflammatory agents hurt his stomach. He denies smoking or using drugs. He has a history of gout and lumbar disc problems from a motor vehicle crash in 1989.

Systematic Bedside Assessment

You perform a head-to-toe assessment.

HEAD AND NECK. Dale is tanned and it is difficult to assess for cyanosis. His mucous membranes are pink but dry. His lips are cracked. He has slight nasal flaring. His neck veins are full, not distended or flat.

CHEST. His pulmonary and cardiac exam is as previously stated.

ABDOMEN. His abdomen is slightly obese. Positive bowel sounds are auscultated in all quadrants. His abdomen is not tender on palpation. It is supple without rigidity.

PELVIS. Dale voided 100 mL of clear, dark urine that smells strong. He denies any penile discharge or voiding discomfort.

EXTREMITIES. His skin turgor is adequate. He is warm and diaphoretic. No peripheral edema is noted. Sensation and motor function are present in all extremities. Peripheral pulses are palpated in all extremities.

POSTERIOR. He complains of slight tenderness on palpation of his lumbar–sacral area but says "it is normal." Posterior breath sounds are diminished greater in the left lower lung fields than in the right, with bilateral crackles.

Development of Nursing Diagnoses

Clustering Data

You have just completed your head-to-toe assessment and are ready to develop a problem list based on the subjective and objective data you have collected thus far. To cluster your data, you look for abnormalities found during your assessment. Dale's major symptom at this time is his labored breathing. This symptom can initiate your first cluster of critical clues.

CLUSTER 1

Subjective data. Patient complaining of shortness of breath (SOB) with greater breathing comfort sitting at 90 degrees. Malaise for 2 weeks. Increasing cough and fever for 3 days. Occasional white sputum produced. Has difficulty sleeping and eating due to cough. Symptoms not relieved with cough medicine or antibiotic.

Objective data. Labored, shallow respirations at 30/min. Some accessory muscle use. Diminished breath sounds in lower lung fields with left greater than right. Crackles auscultated bilaterally. Chest x-ray indicates bilateral pneumonia. Low oxygen saturation on 2 L of oxygen. Fever present.

QUESTION

Based on these data, which of the following nursing diagnoses would you select as being appropriate in planning Dale's plan of care?

A. impaired gas exchange
B. ineffective breathing pattern
C. ineffective airway clearance
D. all of the above

ANSWER

This is a tough question. The data supports only C at present. Because of Dale's increased production of secretions due to the inflammatory process and his inability to cough up these secretions consistently, pneumonia has developed. He may be fatigued from lack of sleep, and this may contribute to ineffective clearing of secretions. He is also dehydrated, which makes the secretions thicker. Because his ABGs are normal, he is not experiencing impaired gas exchange yet. He is at risk for this problem due to a decrease in lung surface area available for oxygen diffusion. His breathing pattern is effective at present to meet cellular oxygen needs but his oxygen saturation is dropping, suggesting that he may decompensate shortly.

Desired patient outcomes for Dale (evaluative criteria) would include:

1. normal rate and depth of respirations
2. decreased SOB
3. improved breath sounds
4. improved oxygen saturation

CLUSTER 2

Subjective data. Patient complaining of increasing cough that prevents normal eating. The patient has had a fever for 3 days.

Objective data. Confirmed pneumonia on chest x-ray. Temperature 101.5°F. Respiratory rate 30/min. Urine dark and clear with strong smell. Specific gravity high normal. The patient is diaphoretic with full neck veins. Serum chloride 110 mEq/L. Mucous membranes are dry and lips are cracked. Pulse is 110.

You make the nursing diagnosis of *High risk for fluid volume deficit* related to decreased oral intake and excessive fluid loss due to hyperventilation and diaphoresis. Because of Dale's inflammation, you realize that he is in a hypermetabolic state in an attempt to mobilize the immune response to limit the infection and clean up debris. Because a greater number of metabolic reactions are occurring, more heat is generated and more water is used. At present, his hematocrit and specific gravity are normal, suggesting that his dehydration is minimal.

Developing the Plan of Care

The goals in Dale's plan of care are to (1) optimize his oxygenation, (2) promote his airway clearance, (3) provide adequate hydration, (4) maintain functioning alveoli, and (5) limit the infection. Nursing interventions consist of collaborative actions to fulfill orders written by the health care practitioner focused on treating the pathology and independent interventions aimed at treating Dale's responses to the pneumonia that are within the nursing scope of practice and can be initiated without a health care practitioner's order.

Collaborative Interventions

The health care practitioner's orders may include the following:

1. *Pulmonary drug therapy*: Beta-adrenergic agents that promote bronchodilation may be ordered. These may be administered through nebulization or by metered-dose inhaler. Anticholinergic agents may also be used, such as ipratropium bromide. Steroids and xanthine derivatives (such as aminophylline) may be ordered. Oxygen will be administered until Dale can maintain a normal oxygen saturation level. Antibiotics will be started and changed as necessary based on the findings of sputum and blood cultures. An expectorant and mucolytic agent may be ordered to help liquefy Dale's mucus and assist him in clearing his airway. A cough suppressant may be ordered for nighttime use to facilitate sleeping.
2. *Laboratory and x-ray testing*: Of particular interest will be the results of a sputum culture and blood cultures. Blood cultures have not yet been ordered for Dale. They may be initiated upon admission of the patient or in situations in which the patient does not respond to initial treatment.

Pulmonary function tests may help determine the degree of volume change associated with the decreased lung surface area due to the infiltrates. Chest x-rays and ABGs will be monitored intermittently.

3. *Intravenous fluids*: Because of IV access for antibiotics and Dale's risk for dehydration, IV have been ordered. The patency of this line should remain a nursing priority.

Independent Nursing Interventions

1. Assess for decreased respiratory function. Report:
   - Respirations < 8/min or > 30/min
   - Increasing dyspnea
   - A change in level of consciousness
   - A change in accessory muscle use
   - Decreasing oxygen saturation
2. Try to improve respiratory function:
   - Decrease patient oxygen needs by relieving fever, pain, and anxiety
   - Promote position of comfort and prevent slumping to improve diaphragmatic excursion
   - Promote incentive spirometer use q2h
   - Perform tracheal suctioning as needed
   - Maintain oxygen therapy
   - Perform percussion and postural drainage q8h
3. Prevent dehydration:
   - Encourage oral fluids
   - Monitor BUN, Hct, urine output, fever

Dale initially improves and plans are made to discharge him. The night before his discharge, Dale's fever increased to 102.4°F (39°C). His oxygen saturation dropped to 82 percent. He became severely dyspneic. A stat chest x-ray was obtained and showed diffuse bilateral infiltrates. His ABG on 2 L of oxygen was pH 7.45, PCO_2 35, and PO_2 44. SaO_2 was 82. The decision was made to transfer Dale to the intensive care unit.

Dale is exhibiting acute respiratory distress syndrome (ARDS). The inflammatory process was initiated with the development of the infiltrates in the lung (evidence of neutrophil migration), the slightly elevated WBC count, and his fever. Damage has occurred to the alevolar–capillary membrane from the release of mediators. First, the capillary endothelium is injured, allowing fluid to enter the interstitial spaces; then, as osmotic pressure builds in the interstitium, fluid enters the alveoli, damaging type II cells that produce surfactant. The alveoli collapse, decreasing the surface area available for oxygen diffusion.

QUESTION

If Dale is experiencing ARDS, why is he not in respiratory acidosis?

ANSWER

Dale is exhibiting hypoxemia (PaO_2 44). He is probably hyperventilating, which is why his PCO_2 is borderline low and his pH is borderline for respiratory alkalosis. Eventually the $PaCO_2$ will increase as Dale fatigues.

The sputum culture was negative, suggesting a viral form of pneumonia. Because Dale was improving, additional diagnostic tests were not performed. Now with his sudden deterioration, several orders are written:

1. 50 percent oxygen by simple face mask
2. Diagnostic bronchoscopy with lung biopsy
3. Blood cultures
4. Tuberculosis (TB) testing
5. Titers for *Mycoplasma*, *Pneumocystis*, Hantavirus, and *Legionella*
6. Ceftazidime 1 g IV q8h
7. Heparin 5,000 U SC q12h
8. Venous Doppler studies of legs

QUESTION

Of the following orders, which should be implemented first?

A. obtaining blood for the titers
B. administering the heparin
C. administering the ceftazidime
D. administering the oxygen

ANSWER

The correct answer is D. The oxygen should be given first. Inadequate oxygen to meet cellular demands will cause more inflammation and mediator release, thus greater alveoli damage.

Dale continues to deteriorate in spite of the 50 percent oxygen. He is now in respiratory acidosis (pH 7.3, PCO_2 49, PaO_2 50). Due to his fatigue, he could not continue hyperventilating to compensate for his respiratory failure. He is intubated, and a pulmonary artery catheter is inserted. He receives pancuronium (a neuromuscular blocking agent), lorazepam (for anterograde amnesia and sedation), and morphine sulfate (for pain and sedation). His initial ventilator settings are tidal volume 800 mL, FIO_2 60 percent, synchronous intermittent mandatory ventilation (SIMV) mode, with 10 cm H_2O of positive end-expiratory pressure (PEEP) and 5 cm H_2O pressure support. His pulmonary artery pressures are 48/28 mm Hg, central venous pressure (CVP) 10 mm Hg, pulmonary artery wedge pressure (PAWP) 14 mm Hg, cardiac output (CO) 15.3 L/min, and cardiac index (CI) 6.1 L/min.

Systematic Bedside Assessment

Once you have implemented the various stat activities for Dale, you begin a head-to-toe assessment.

HEAD AND NECK. Dale is in a chemically induced coma. An endotracheal tube is taped in his right nares and connected to ventilator tubing. His jugular veins are full.

CHEST. Breath sounds are auscultated bilaterally. Coarse crackles are present bilaterally. S_1 and S_2 are auscultated. No extra heart sounds are noted. A pulmonary arterial catheter is inserted in the right subclavian vein. Dressing is dry and intact.

ABDOMEN. No bowel sounds are auscultated. Abdomen is soft. No bruits auscultated.

PELVIS. A urinary catheter is present draining clear, dark amber urine. There is 50 mL for a 1-hour period.

EXTREMITIES. His skin is warm and dry. No peripheral edema is noted. Peripheral pulses are palpable.

POSTERIOR. No skin breakdown is noted. Scattered crackles are auscultated bilaterally throughout the posterior lung fields.

Development of Nursing Diagnoses

Clustering Data

The following data should be clustered based on abnormal findings.

CLUSTER 3

Subjective data. None due to Dale's comatose state.

Objective data. Bilateral diffuse infiltrates on chest x-ray. Respiratory acidosis. Low oxygen saturation level. Crackles auscultated bilaterally. Failure to respond to antibiotic therapy.

Based on these data, the diagnosis of *Impaired gas exchange* related to pulmonary alveoli membrane permeability and damage is appropriate. He is also at risk for *Ineffective airway clearance* due to intubation, chemical paralysis, and increased secretion production. Dale is also at risk for *Fluid volume excess* related to noncardiac pulmonary edema (if the inflammatory process continues) and PEEP, since PEEP may cause pulmonary hypertension, right heart failure, and decreased cardiac output.

Developing the Plan of Care

The goals in caring for a patient in ARDS are to (1) support tissue oxygenation, (2) prevent infection, and (3) treat the underlying cause. Interventions are both collaborative and independent.

Collaborative Interventions

1. *Pulmonary drug therapy*: The same bronchodilator therapy may be used as discussed earlier in the case. Surfactant replacement therapy may be started. Oxygen levels will be increased until the patient's PaO_2 level is 60 mm Hg. The goal is to keep the FIO_2 below 60 percent. Antibiotics will be given and changed pending the results of the lung biopsy and titers.
2. *Ventilatory management*: Pressure support was added to decrease Dale's work of breathing. Exploratory ventilator settings may be used, such as high-frequency jet ventilation or inverse ratio ventilation.
3. *Cardiovascular drug therapy*: The aim is to optimize cardiac output without causing pulmonary edema so that peripheral tissue remains adequately oxygenated. Diuretics will be given if the PAWP increases, or blood may be administered if the PAWP and CI decrease below normal.

Independent Interventions

Maintain Airway Patency

1. Suction ET tube as needed using sterile technique; note color, amount, and consistency of secretions
2. Check ET tube placement and anchoring every shift and PRN; check cuff pressure as per unit protocol
3. Change patient's position q2h
4. Assess breath sounds qh and PRN
5. Elevate head of bed for tube feedings (once initiated)

Maintain Hemodynamic Stability

1. Weigh patient daily
2. Assess hemodynamic parameters q1h and PRN
3. Monitor intake and output
4. Assess for signs of fluid overload (dependent edema, increased weight, increased crackles, increased CVP, decreased CI)
5. Assess for signs of decreased CI (decreased urine output)

Dale's venous Doppler studies are negative, while his lung biopsy shows interstitial pneumonia with marked diffuse alveolar damage. His titers are negative. His cultures fail to grow any specific organism. The reason for his ARDS is not known. His lactate level is 5.2 mMol/L. His glucose level increases to 320 mg/dL. Dale's BUN and creatinine elevate (70 and 2.8, respectively). His albumin level is 2.9 mg/dL. His WBC count is 25,100, while his hemoglobin is 7.5 and his hematocrit is 22.4 percent. Platelets are 86,000. His hemodynamic readings are PCWP 14 mm Hg, CO 14.2 L/min, CI 6 L/min. His systemic vascular resistance (SVR) is 907. Oxygen saturation is 92 percent on an FIO_2 of 100 and PEEP level of 15 cm H_2O. He is in metabolic acidosis but his latest ABGs have improved: pH 7.22, PCO_2 55, PaO_2 116, HCO_3 20. Oxygen saturation is 98%. His temperature is 99.1°F (37.2°C). The physician places Dale on **extracorporeal membrane oxygenation (ECMO)** to remove carbon dioxide. He is started on **continuous arteriovenous hemofiltration (CAVH)**. Dale begins to bleed from his mouth, ET tube, and IV lines. You place a stat call to the physician.

Relating Dale's Symptoms to the Inflammatory Process

Dale is probably in anaerobic metabolism as evidenced by high lactate and metabolic levels. As the amount of ATP produced decreases, active transport processes across the cell membrane cannot operate, the cell does not receive adequate nutrients, and cell death occurs. Sodium is allowed to enter the cell passively, water follows the sodium, and eventually the ribosomes of the cell detach, making it unable to make proteins. The cell membrane ruptures and intracellular enzymes are released (mediators). Simultaneously, Dale's sympathetic nervous system is responding to increased glucose production and improved peripheral circulation. This is why his cardiac index is elevated and he is hyperglycemic. Epinephrine (sympathetic nervous system neurotransmitter) stimulates platelet aggregation. The fever is less than what you would expect with the high WBC count and may indicate that Dale is unable to mount an adequate immune response. This is an ominous sign. Thus, Dale has gone from dysfunction of one organ, the lungs, into a cascade of events producing dysfunction in multiple systems. He is experiencing MODS.

QUESTION

Dale's BUN and creatinine are elevated. Which of the following statements provides the best rationale for this elevation?

- **A.** he is experiencing tubular cell necrosis from mediator destruction of the cell membrane and decreased renal blood flow
- **B.** he is exhibiting nephrotoxicity from drugs
- **C.** he is breaking down protein for glucose production
- **D.** BUN and creatine reflect the breakdown of RBCs due to his bleeding

ANSWER

The correct answer is A. As nephrons die, they release debris that form casts. These casts obstruct the renal tubules, decreasing the glomerular filtration rate. B may also be true in some patients with MODS. However, Dale has not received aminoglycosides, the group of antibiotics most notorious for nephrotoxicity. Protein breakdown is occurring but this would not elevate the creatinine level. Destruction of RBCs produces bilirubin.

Systematic Bedside Assessment

As you await the call from the physician you complete a head-to-toe assessment.

HEAD AND NECK. Dale is still in a chemically induced coma. There is blood in his ventilator tubing and some is oozing from his mouth.

CHEST. Coarse crackles are auscultated bilaterally with the ventilatory cycle. S_1 and S_2 are present. His apical rate is 116.

ABDOMEN. No bowel sounds are auscultated. His abdomen is distended.

PELVIS. He had 8,318 mL intake and 17,033 output via his continuous arteriovenous hemofiltration dialysis (CAVD) catheter in the last 24-hour period. No drainage is noted from the penis. His last bowel movement was loose and positive for blood.

EXTREMITIES. He has 3+ edema of both legs extending up to the shins. Pulses are palpable. Petechiae are noted on all extremities.

POSTERIOR. No skin breakdown is noted but there is redness in several areas along the vertebrae and the coccyx. Coarse crackles are auscultated bilaterally in the posterior lung fields.

Development of Nursing Diagnoses

Clustering Data

You cluster the major abnormal findings to derive the nursing diagnoses.

CLUSTER 1

Subjective data. None.

Objective data. Metabolic acidosis, elevated PCO_2 level. Coarse crackles bilaterally. Blood in the ET tube and ventilator tubing.

Based on these data you derive the nursing diagnoses of *Impaired gas exchange*, *Ineffective airway clearance*, and *High risk for aspiration.*

CLUSTER 2

Subjective data. None.

Objective data. Elevated CI. Sinus tachycardia. Decreased platelets. Bleeding from mouth, IV lines, ET tube, and in stool. Petechiae on all extremities.

QUESTION

Which of the following nursing diagnoses is most appropriate at this time?

A. *Fluid volume excess*
B. *Alteration in tissue perfusion: Cardiopulmonary*
C. *Fluid volume deficit*
D. *Decreased cardiac output*

ANSWER

The correct answer is C. Dale is experiencing active blood loss. He may consume all his clotting factors and progress into hypovolemic shock. Due to the inflammatory process, fluid has been shifting out of the vessels into the interstitial spaces and ultimately into the cells, contributing to decreased circulating volume. Currently, he does not have enough fluid in the alveoli to produce pulmonary hypertension and reduce coronary circulation and ultimate left heart filling. This may occur, at which time cardiac output will decrease. Massive blood loss and vasodilation from mediator release will also reduce venous return, decreasing cardiac output.

Clusters could be developed to support *Altered tissue perfusion: Renal; High risk for impaired skin integrity: Pressure ulcer;* and *Altered nutrition: Less than body protein–calorie requirements* (due to Dale's hypermetabolic state and need for glucose).

Developing the Plan of Care

Collaborative Interventions

1. *Cardiovascular drug therapy*: As cardiac output decreases secondary to pulmonary hypertension, dobutamine and nitroglycerin continuous infusions may be initiated. Dobutamine will augment contractility. Nitroglycerin will produce pulmonary venous vasodilation. This will decrease right heart afterload and augment right heart stroke volume.
2. *Maintaining oxygen supply*: Ventilatory settings will be adjusted to gradually decrease the FIO_2, PEEP, and pressure support as long as the PaO_2 remains above 60 mm Hg and the oxygen saturation is normal. ECMO may be used to remove carbon dioxide until Dale is able to respond to the ventilator settings. Because of Dale's active bleeding, packed RBCs, fresh frozen plasma, and platelets will be administered to replace volume loss, proteins, and platelets.

Independent Interventions

1. *Decreasing oxygen demands*: The nurse must ensure that neuromuscular blockade is adequate to prevent any voluntary movement. This can be accomplished through train-of-four monitoring. The peripheral nerves are stimulated to see degree of blockade. Complete blockade (no twitch) is recorded as 0/4. One twitch out of four stimulations is 1/4 or 90 percent. No blockade is recorded as 4/4 (Smith, 1998). Studies have shown patients can hear and remember events that occur during therapeutic paralysis (Johnson, Cheung, & Johnson, 1999). It is important that health care providers monitor their conversation at the bedside. Family should be encouraged to touch and talk with the patient. The nurse will continue to administer pancuronium and lorazepam until Dale's metabolic demands drop. The continuation of the morphine decreases Dale's pain since he is unable to convey his discomfort.
2. *Limiting the source of inflammation*: The nurse should maintain closed systems (such as in-line suction, capped IV ports). Proper suctioning can reduce Dale's chance for aspiration and promote his pulmonary hygiene. Turning and repositioning Dale may prevent pressure ulcer formation and another site for infection. Careful skin and oral care can prevent further bleeding and infection.
3. *Promoting nutrition*: Although not ordered yet due to his active GI bleeding (melena), enteric feedings will be started when the bleeding stops. Enteral feeding maintains the intestinal mucosa and prevents disruption of the normal gut flora. Elevating the head of the bed prior to tube feedings, assuring tube patency and proper placement prior to feeding, and keeping the tube feeding infusing at the proper rate will help increase Dale's albumin level and protein stores. Sucralfate or an H_2 histamine blocker (ranitidine) may be used to prevent stress ulcer formation.
4. *Maintaining oxygen supply:* Proper ET tube suctioning will also promote oxygenation. Ensuring that the ventilator system is operating correctly and that the patient remains connected are priorities.

Plan: Evaluation and Revision

Dale's treatment plan requires multiple revisions based on his changing status. His condition slowly improves and he is finally allowed to regain consciousness. Assuming that he continues to improve, the following indicators of progress will occur. Dale will return to a normal acid–base state and the ECMO will be stopped. His blood glucose will return to normal as his metabolic state slows down. His protein stores will improve and his WBC count will return to normal. Dale's bleeding will stop and his cardiac output will improve. As these events occur, renal function will improve and he will be weaned from the CAVD. The last sign of progress will be ventilator weaning. This will be the most difficult to accomplish owing to Dale's alveoli damage, respiratory muscle wasting (due to conversion of protein into glucose), and the possible psychologic dependence on the ventilator.

Dale did improve and was discharged to a rehabilitation facility after a 3-month hospital stay for the admitting diagnosis of pneumonia. Now 1 year after his illness, Dale has resumed full-time farming. Dale is one of the lucky ones who survived MODS.

REFERENCES

Johnson, K.L., Cheung, R.C., Johnson, S.B., et. al. (1999). Therapeutic paralysis of critically ill trauma patients: Perceptions of patients and their family members. *Am J Care*, 8:490–498.

Smith, R.N. (1998). Concepts of monitoring and surveillance. In M.R. Kinney, S.B. Dunbar, J.A. Brook-Brunn, N. Molter, & J.M. Vitello-Cicciu. *AACN clinical reference for critical care nursing* (4th ed.) (pp. 3–37). St. Louis: C.V. Mosby.

PART IV

Perfusion

MODULE 13

Determinants of Cardiac Output

James P. McGraw, Pamela Stinson Kidd

This self-study module is intended for the novice nurse caring for the acutely ill patient. The focus of this module is the physiologic concepts that influence the performance of the cardiovascular system, with particular focus on the heart. An understanding of these concepts will allow the nurse to apply them to a variety of clinical situations in order to understand and predict cardiovascular performance.

The module is composed of six sections that define terms and normal values, describe key relationships between variables, identify common clinical conditions that influence these variables, and present the clinical assessments that can be made of these variables. Each section includes a set of review questions to help the learner evaluate his or her understanding of the section's content before moving on to the next section. All Section Reviews and the module Pretest and Posttest include answers. It is suggested that the learner review those concepts answered incorrectly in the review questions before proceeding to the next section.

OBJECTIVES

Following completion of this module, the learner will be able to

1. Define and state adult normal values for cardiac output, heart rate, and stroke volume.
2. Define *preload*, *contractility*, and *afterload*.
3. Describe the effect of the Frank–Starling law on cardiac output.
4. Describe the relationship among pressure, flow, and resistance.
5. State some of the conditions that affect heart rate, preload, contractility, and afterload.
6. Identify the common clinical assessments made to evaluate heart rate, preload, contractility, and afterload.

PRETEST

1. The stroke volume multiplied by the heart rate equals the
   - A. cardiac output (CO)
   - B. cardiac index (CI)
   - C. pulse pressure product
   - D. left ventricular stroke work index
2. The normal cardiac output for an adult at rest is approximately
   - A. 1.2 L/min
   - B. 3.4 L/min
   - C. 5.0 L/min
   - D. 7.0 L/min
3. The resistance against which the heart must pump blood is known as the
   - A. preload
   - B. afterload
   - C. upload
   - D. download

4. The Frank–Starling law states that within physiologic limits, the heart will
   A. beat no faster than the body's demand for oxygen dictates
   B. pump all of the blood delivered to it
   C. completely empty of blood with each beat
   D. extract only the amount of oxygen needed from its blood supply
5. Pressure is the mathematical product of
   A. flow and volume
   B. flow and resistance
   C. viscosity and resistance
   D. viscosity and volume
6. Which of the following will depress myocardial contractility?
   A. epinephrine
   B. digitalis
   C. sympathetic nervous system activity
   D. hypoxia
7. Profound hemorrhage initially would result in
   A. decreased afterload
   B. decreased preload
   C. increased preload
   D. increased pulse pressure
8. The number of heartbeats too weak to be transmitted to the periphery can be measured by
   A. pulse pressure
   B. brachiopopliteal gradient
   C. electrocardiogram
   D. apical–radial pulse deficit
9. Heart rate may be slowed by
   A. straining to move bowels
   B. sympathetic nervous system stimulation
   C. physical exertion
   D. loss of 20 percent of circulating blood volume
10. Which of the following is consistent with diminished preload to the right ventricle?
    A. ascites
    B. jugular venous distention
    C. hepatic engorgement
    D. poor skin turgor

Pretest answers: 1. A (SV × HR = CO), 2. C, 3. B, 4. B, 5. B, 6. D, 7. B, 8. D, 9. A, 10. D

GLOSSARY

Afterload. The resistance against which the heart pumps blood

Aldosteronism. A disorder caused by increased secretion of an adrenal hormone, aldosterone, which results in retention of sodium and water and loss of potassium and hydrogen ions by the kidneys

Anaphylaxis. An abrupt, transient, allergic reaction with contraction of the smooth muscle and dilation of the capillaries

Aortic valve. The valve between the left ventricle and the aorta

Apical–radial pulse deficit. The difference between the apical and radial pulse rates, which reflects the number of heartbeats too weak to be transmitted to the periphery

Arterioles. Terminal arteries that have a muscular wall that feeds directly into the capillaries

Ascites. An accumulation of serous fluid in the peritoneal cavity

Body surface area (BSA). A measure of overall body size using both height and weight in its calculation

Cardiac index (CI). Cardiac output divided by body surface area

Cardiac output (CO). The amount of blood pumped by the heart each minute

Cardiomyopathy. Disease of the myocardium

Compliance. The change in volume resulting from an incremental increase in pressure within a structure

Contractility. The ability of a muscle to shorten when stimulated; in particular, the force of myocardial contraction

Dyspnea. A subjective sensation of shortness of breath

Ejection fraction. The portion of ventricular end-diastolic volume that is pumped from the ventricle in one beat

Flow. The volume of blood passing a point per unit of time, specifically, cardiac output

Frank–Starling law. The principle that states that within physiologic limits, the heart will pump as much blood as is delivered to it

Hypoxia. Subnormal levels of oxygen in tissue

Mitral valve. The valve between the left atrium and left ventricle

Myocarditis. Inflammation of the myocardium

Nomograms. Series of scales arranged so that calculations can be performed graphically

Orthostatic hypotension. Subnormal blood pressure caused by a change in body position, such as rising from supine to standing

Parasympathetic nervous system. The part of the autonomic nervous system that tends to increase secretions, increase tone in smooth muscle, and dilate blood vessels; in particular, it slows the heart rate

Preload. The degree of stretch in myocardial fibers at the end of diastole

Pulmonic valve. The valve between the right ventricle and the pulmonary artery

Septic shock. Shock resulting from an acute infection, associated with dilation of the peripheral vasculature

Stroke volume (SV). The volume of blood pumped with each heartbeat

Sympathetic nervous system. The part of the autonomic nervous system that tends to decrease secretions, decrease smooth muscle tone, and contract blood vessels; in particular, it increases the rate and strength of myocardial contraction.

Tricuspid valve. The valve between the right atrium and right ventricle

Abbreviations

bpm. Beats per minute

BSA. Body surface area

CI. Cardiac index

CO. Cardiac output

HR. Heart rate

S_3. Third heart sound, which is commonly found in normal youths and frequently is associated with congestive heart failure in later life

S_4. Fourth heart sound, which frequently is associated with congestive heart failure, myocardial infarction, and hypertension

SV. Stroke volume

SECTION ONE: Cardiac Output

At the completion of this section, the learner will be able to define and state adult normal values for cardiac output, heart rate, and stroke volume. These definitions and values will be applied to the content of later sections.

Cardiac output (CO) is the amount of blood pumped by the heart each minute. CO is a critical aspect of cardiovascular performance in both health and illness. Understanding how CO changes in response to changing conditions in the body will allow you to predict how the body will respond to different effects of injury or disease.

The normal CO is approximately 4.0 to 6.0 L/min (Funkhouser, 1994). The normal CO for individuals can vary significantly depending on body size. A tall, heavy person needs more CO to feed all of his or her cells than does a short, light person. Because of this, when CO is measured, it usually is corrected to account for body size. The correction is calculated by dividing the CO **by the body surface area (BSA)** and is called the **cardiac index (CI).** The normal CI is 2.5 to 4.5 L/min/m^2 (Funkhouser, 1994). The BSA is calculated via the use of **nomograms** or computer programs from the patient's height and weight. For example, if two patients each have a CO of 5.0 L/min but one has a BSA of 1.0 m^2 and the other has a BSA of 2.0 m^2, their CIs (5.0 L/m^2 and 2.5 L/m^2, respectively) illustrate that the perfusion of tissue is quite different despite their equal COs.

The heart pumps blood one burst at a time, with each heartbeat. The volume of blood pumped with each heartbeat is called the **stroke volume (SV).** The CO is the volume of each beat (SV) times the heart rate (HR):

$$SV \times HR = CO$$

Given a normal heart rate of approximately 72 bpm (range, 60 to 100) and CO of approximately 5 L/min, it is possible using this equation to determine that the usual stroke volume for an adult is approximately 70 mL.

$$\frac{5{,}000 \text{ mL/min}}{72 \text{ bpm}} = 69 \text{ mL/beat}$$

Changes in either the HR or SV will alter the CO. Fortunately, the body uses the interrelationship between these two factors to keep the CO at the level needed. For example, if the SV should fall, the body would immediately increase the HR to compensate and keep the CO unchanged. Conversely, if the HR should drop, the SV will increase and may allow the CO to remain unchanged. Of course, there is a limit to the capacity of the body to use these compensatory efforts to maintain CO.

In summary, the CO is the product of SV and HR. Both SV and HR can be modified to ensure that the CO is adequate to meet the body's needs.

Section One Review

1. The volume of blood pumped by the heart each minute is the

A. stroke volume
B. cardiac output
C. cardiac index
D. ejection fraction

2. A normal cardiac output for an adult at rest is approximately
   A. 1.2 L/min
   B. 3.4 L/min
   C. 5.0 L/min
   D. 7.0 L/min
3. The normal adult stroke volume is approximately
   A. 7 mL
   B. 17 mL
   C. 70 mL
   D. 700 mL
4. A patient has a stroke volume of 60 mL and a heart rate of 70 bpm. What is his cardiac output?
   A. 420 mL/min
   B. 1.1 L/min
   C. 4.2 L/min
   D. 150 mL/min

Answers: 1. B, 2. C, 3. C, 4. C, (SV × HR = CO).

$$\frac{60\text{ mL}}{\text{beat}} \times \frac{70\text{ beats}}{\text{minute}} = \frac{4{,}200\text{ mL}}{\text{minute}} \text{ or } 4.2\text{ L/min}$$

SECTION TWO: Preload, Afterload, and Contractility

At the completion of this section, the learner will be able to define preload, contractility, and afterload.

A great number of factors affect CO. If you understand how the four determinants of CO affect CO, you will understand easily how each of the multitude of factors in injury and disease affects CO.

The four determinants of CO are:

- Heart rate (HR)
- Preload
- Contractility
- Afterload

"Where," you may ask, "is stroke volume?" SV is determined by the interplay of preload, contractility, and afterload:

HR × SV = CO

Preload
Contractility
Afterload

Heart Rate

If the SV is held constant, any change in the HR will result in an immediate change in the CO. For example, if the SV is 70 mL and the HR drops from 70 bpm to 50 bpm, the CO will drop from 4.9 L/min to 3.5 L/min. If the pulse should rise from 70 bpm to 100 bpm and the SV should stay at 70 mL, the CO would rise from 4.9 L/min to 7.0 L/min.

Although the most effective way to manipulate CO is through HR, this manipulation has limits. If the pulse rises too high (approximately > 150 bpm), the SV will begin to drop because the heart has too little time during diastole to fill with blood properly.

Preload

Preload is the amount of stretch in the myocardial fibers at the end of diastole (just before the onset of systole). Usually, this is thought of as the volume of blood in the ventricle at end diastole (Ramsey & Tisdale, 1995). The greater the volume of blood in the ventricle, the greater the amount of stretch that the fibers experience. Preload is greatly affected by the volume of blood delivered to the heart by the venous system. If the venous system brings a large volume of blood to the ventricle, there will be much stretch and high preload. If the venous system brings a small volume of blood to the ventricle, there will be less stretch and less preload.

Injury or illness of the myocardium can make the myocardial cells less stretchable. If this should occur, increased volume within the ventricle may be required to stretch the myocardial cells to the same degree. This situation is known as diminished myocardial compliance. **Compliance** is a measure of stiffness. A certain amount of stiffness or tone is necessary for the ventricle to be able to eject. However, too much stiffness (compliance) as well as too little can affect preload.

In addition, if the heart should fail to eject the usual volume from the ventricle, any excess volume will remain in the ventricle at the end of systole. When the usual amount of venous blood rushes in during diastole, it will be added to the remainder from the previous beat. This will result in an unusually large volume of blood in the ventricle at the end of diastole, resulting in increased preload.

Contractility

Contractility is the force with which the heart pumps blood. If the heart contracts forcefully, it will push out much of the blood in the ventricle. If the heart is pumping poorly, the result will be a drop in the SV. Many variables affect the force with which the heart muscle contracts. Contractility is the result of the contractile activity of the myocardial cells. It is the ability of the heart muscle to work independently of preload and afterload (Ramsey & Tisdale, 1995, Headley, 1998). However, anything that enhances or diminishes the ability of these cells to contract vigorously will affect contractility. **Hypoxia** and acidosis diminish the contractile activity of myocardial cells.

Even when working perfectly, the ventricle does not eject all the blood it contains. Usually, the ventricle ejects only 60 percent of the blood that it contains at the end of diastole. This measure of the portion of blood ejected is known as the **ejection fraction** and is a commonly measured index of myocardial function.

Afterload

Afterload is the resistance against which the ventricle must pump blood. There is an optimal amount of resistance necessary for the system to work properly. The major influence on afterload is the mechanical resistance to flow offered by the arterial system. Other variables include the **pulmonic** and **aortic valves**, which may become stenotic and unable to fully open during systole.

HR affects CO directly if the SV does not change. SV has a direct effect on CO. SV is determined by preload, contractility, and afterload. An increase in the HR to compensate for diminished SV is common.

Section Two Review

1. The degree of stretch of myocardial cells at the end of diastole is known as
   A. preload
   B. contractility
   C. compliance
   D. distensibility
2. The vigor of myocardial cells' muscular activity is known as
   A. automaticity
   B. conduction
   C. contractility
   D. afterload
3. The resistance against which the ventricle pumps blood is known as
   A. preload
   B. blood pressure
   C. compliance
   D. afterload

Answers: 1. A, 2. C, 3. D

SECTION THREE: The Frank–Starling Law

At the completion of this section, the learner will be able to describe the effect of the Frank–Starling law on CO. All of the four factors mentioned earlier are related to CO. However, there is a particular relationship between preload and SV that is so important it deserves special attention.

Within limits, the heart will pump the amount of blood delivered to it with each beat. This is known as the **Frank–Starling law** of the heart. In other words, as preload increases, so does SV, and as preload decreases, SV falls (Fig. 13–1A). Unfortunately, this law only applies within a range of normal.

You will note that until a critical point is reached, as preload increases, so does SV. As you can see, there is an optimal preload for the heart to have maximal SV. If the patient's cardiovascular system is too far to the right past the optimal point, we can improve SV by lowering preload. Conversely, if the patient is on the far left part of the curve, we can improve SV by increasing preload.

It is important to realize that the Frank–Starling curve can change depending on the condition of the myocardium.

Note that with poor contractility shown in Figure 13–1B, the curve has moved down so that SV is less than normal at each point along the curve.

In summary, under normal conditions, SV increases and decreases as preload increases and decreases. Injury or disease can alter the response of the myocardium to changes in preload.

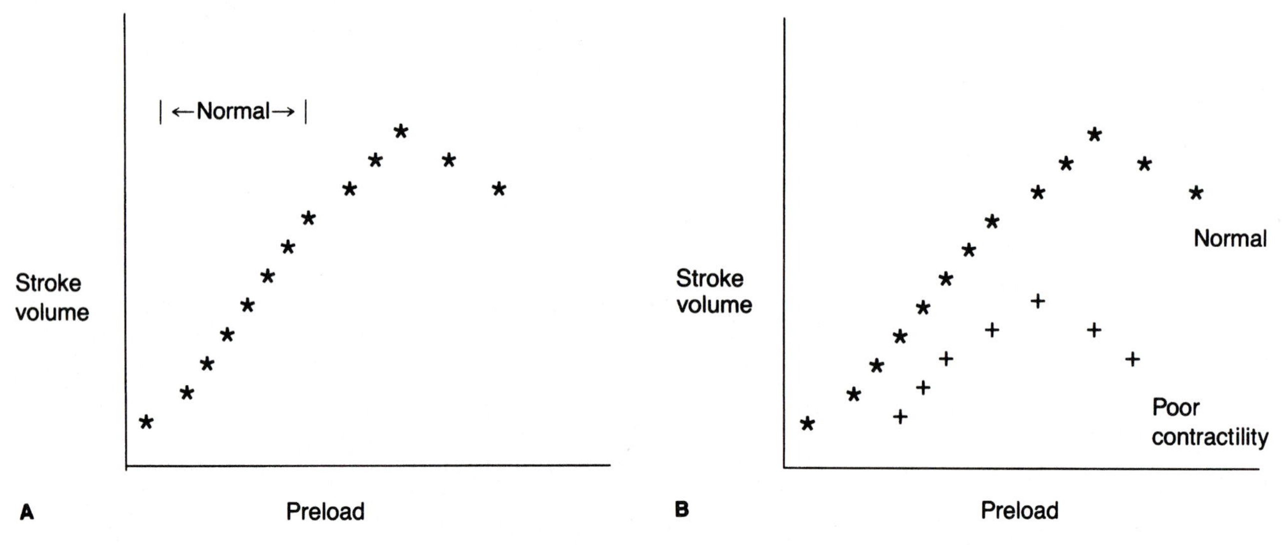

Figure 13–1. Graphs demonstrating the Frank–Starling law of the heart.

SECTION THREE REVIEW

1. The Frank–Starling law states that within physiologic limits the heart
   A. pumps as fast as it receives more blood
   B. pumps as much blood as it receives
   C. pumps less blood as it receives more blood
   D. pumps an unchanging amount of blood regardless of how much it receives

2. Disease may decrease the contractility of the myocardium. This means that if the preload decreases, the SV will
   A. increase
   B. decrease
   C. stay the same
   D. it cannot be determined from this information

Answers: 1. B, 2. B

SECTION FOUR: Pressure, Flow, and Resistance

At the completion of this section, the learner will be able to describe the relationship among pressure, **flow,** and resistance. This relationship will help you to understand how cardiac output and vascular resistance relate to blood pressure. These are relationships that often are manipulated in acutely ill patients.

Many aspects of cardiovascular physiology are similar to the plumbing that we use every day. One critical concept of hemodynamics that can be thought of in this way is the relationship among flow, pressure, and resistance.

Imagine a system with a pump, a rigid tube, and a valve some distance from the pump, as shown in Figure 13–2. If the valve is half closed, the pressure in the tube will increase as the rate of the liquid pumped is increased. If the pump were to run very fast with the valve partially closed, the pressure in the pipe would become great. If, on the other hand, the pump output remained constant and the valve were opened completely, there would be

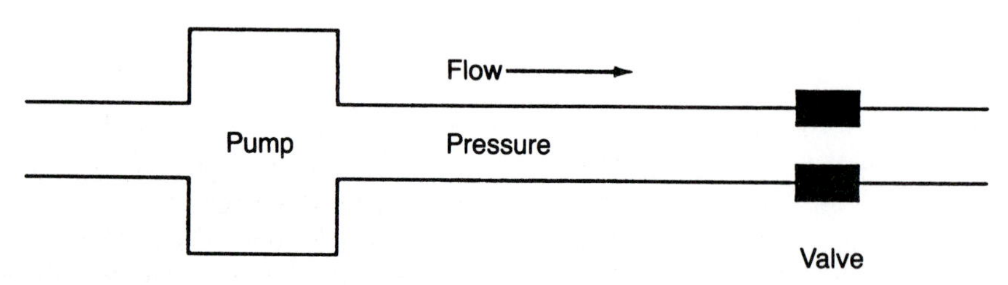

Figure 13–2. Diagram demonstrating the hemodynamic concept of the relationship among flow, pressure, and resistance.

little pressure in the tube. This relationship among flow, resistance, and pressure can be mathematically expressed as:

$$\text{Flow} \times \text{resistance} = \text{pressure}$$

In other words, just as SV and HR could compensate for each other to keep CO unchanged, flow and resistance can be adjusted to keep pressure steady. The flow in the cardiovascular system is the CO, the resistance is the afterload (the vascular resistance usually is the major component of this), and the pressure is the blood pressure.

In summary, blood pressure is the product of CO and vascular resistance. Blood pressure can be changed by adjustments in both CO and vascular resistance.

Section Four Review

1. The mathematical relationship among flow, resistance, and pressure is
   A. $\text{flow} = \dfrac{\text{resistance}}{\text{pressure}}$
   B. $\text{resistance} = \dfrac{\text{flow}}{\text{pressure}}$
   C. pressure × flow = resistance
   D. flow × resistance = pressure
2. What is the flow in the cardiovascular system?
   A. cardiac output
   B. heart rate
   C. stroke volume
   D. blood pressure
3. What is the resistance in the cardiovascular system?
   A. preload
   B. afterload
   C. contractility
   D. compliance
4. If pressure drops and flow remains unchanged, resistance would ______ to increase pressure.
   A. increase
   B. decrease
   C. be unchanged
   D. cannot be determined

Answers: 1. D, 2. A, 3. B, 4. A

SECTION FIVE: Conditions That Affect Cardiac Output

At the end of this section, the learner will be able to state some of the conditions that affect HR, preload, contractility, and afterload. This information will allow you to apply these concepts in clinical situations.

Heart Rate

HR is controlled predominantly by the heart's pacemaker sites, which are influenced by the interplay of the sympathetic and parasympathetic nervous systems. The **sympathetic nervous system** causes the fight-or-flight reaction, in which the body's resources are mobilized to counteract a real or perceived threat. The cardiovascular effects of sympathetic nervous system stimulation include increased HR, increased contractility, and vasoconstriction. The **parasympathetic nervous system** causes generally the opposite effects, with a slowing and retarding of cardiovascular performance.

Any stresses that cause the activation of the sympathetic nervous system will cause an increased HR. The stressors that can be responsible for this include anything that is perceived as a threat, ranging from speaking in front of large groups to fleeing a burning house. In the hospital environment, stimuli that activate the sympathetic nervous system include pain, anxiety, and sensory overstimulation, in addition to the physiologic causes. On a physiologic level, anything that causes a drop in SV is likely to cause an increase in HR in an effort to compensate and hold CO constant. In addition, there are numerous other causes of increased HR, including cardiac conduction system dysfunction, drug effects, and hormone imbalances.

HR is slowed most commonly by increased activity of the parasympathetic nervous system. There are numerous causes of this, ranging from drug effects and poisoning to straining hard to have a bowel movement. Other sources of a low HR include impaired impulse generation or conduction in the heart. HR may also be slowed by administration of drugs that either block sympathetic activity (beta blockers) or that inhibit calcium influx into myocardial cells (calcium channel blockers).

Preload

As you learned earlier, preload is the amount of stretch of myocardial fibers at the end of diastole, and preload can be thought of as being the amount of blood in the ventricle at end-diastole. Thus, preload can be altered by changing the amount of blood delivered to the heart by the venous system and the compliance or stiffness of the ventricles.

Loss of blood volume from hemorrhage, dehydration, diuretic use, or movement of fluid out of the vascular space into the extravascular compartment will result in a drop in preload. Diminished preload also can be caused by failure of the atrioventricular **valve** (either **tricuspid** or **mitral**) to allow free flow of blood into the ventricle. Loss of tone in the venous system can cause the venous vessels to dilate and hold more blood, which will result in less blood being delivered to the ventricle and a drop in preload. In addition, very fast HRs can so shorten diastole that there is insufficient time for the ventricle to fill adequately, resulting in diminished preload (Headley, 1998).

Increased blood volume will result in increased preload. Conditions that can cause increased blood volume are renal failure, fluid overload from IV therapy, **aldosteronism** (with retention of sodium and water), and excess sodium in the diet. Increased preload also occurs when the heart is unable to pump out the amount of blood received from the venous system. When this occurs, the remaining blood is still in the ventricle when the new flood of venous blood arrives to be pumped. As a result, the end-diastolic volume rises. One can imagine that if the heart continued to fail to pump the amount of blood delivered to it, there would be increasing congestion as the venous blood returned to the heart but was not promptly ejected into the arteries. This is precisely what happens in congestive heart failure: the heart pumps less blood than is delivered to it, and there is congestion in the venous system that drains into the affected ventricle. The tone of the ventricle is diminished. If the left ventricle fails, this congestion occurs in the pulmonary vascular bed. If the right ventricle fails, the congestion occurs in the systemic venous system.

Contractility

Contractility is the force with which the heart pumps blood. Contractility is much like HR in that it is heavily influenced by the autonomic nervous system. Sympathetic stimulation of the heart results in increased contractility, and conversely, parasympathetic stimulation causes decreased contractility. Other major determinants of contractility include oxygenation (hypoxia or ischemia decrease contractility), myocardial disease (**myocarditis, cardiomyopathy**), and drug effects (many narcotics and anesthetic agents are direct myocardial depressants) (Headley, 1998). Drugs that increase myocardial contractility include digitalis, epinephrine, and dopamine.

Afterload

Afterload is the resistance against which the heart must pump blood. The major determinant of afterload is the resistance to flow caused by the arterial system. Most of the arterial resistance is at the **arterioles** and is due to the tone in the muscles of their walls (Headley, 1998). Anything that causes changes in the arteriolar vascular tone can cause changes in afterload. For example, stimulation of the sympathetic nervous system will cause constriction of the arterioles and increase afterload. Drugs can relax or constrict the arterioles and cause a prompt drop or rise in afterload. The arterioles can be dilated by **septic shock,** spinal cord injury, or **anaphylaxis.**

Further resistance to flow can be caused by failure of the pulmonic or aortic valve to allow free flow of blood from the ventricle to the artery. In this case, the stenosed valve would cause an increase in afterload.

Each determinant of CO can be affected by numerous clinical conditions. Thus, clinical conditions can have an impact on CO by their influence on preload, afterload, contractility, and HR.

SECTION FIVE REVIEW

1. Decreased HR can be caused by
   A. decreased SV
   B. anxiety
   C. parasympathetic stimulation
   D. pain
2. Increased preload can be caused by
   A. mitral stenosis
   B. loss of venous vascular tone
   C. very fast HRs
   D. congestive heart failure
3. Increased contractility can be caused by
   A. ischemia
   B. hypoxia
   C. cardiomyopathy
   D. sympathetic stimulation
4. Increased afterload can be caused by
   A. sympathetic stimulation
   B. septic shock
   C. anaphylaxis
   D. spinal cord injury

Answers: 1. C, 2. D, 3. D, 4. A

SECTION SIX: Assessment of Cardiac Output

At the completion of this section, the learner will be able to identify the common clinical assessments made to evaluate the determinants of CO discussed in previous sections.

Heart Rate

Evaluating the HR is relatively easy. A simple count of the radial pulse is useful for determining the number of heartbeats that are strong enough to reach the periphery. A count of the apical HR is useful to determine the total HR. Usually, these two rates are equal, but there may be a deficit between the apical rate and the radial rate caused by irregular heart rhythms that result in SV varying from beat to beat, which results in some beats being too weak to be felt at the radial artery (this is called the **apical–radial pulse deficit**). For example, a radial pulse would give a better indication of the adequacy of peripheral perfusion in a person complaining of dizziness than an apical pulse. Electronic monitoring of the electrocardiogram (ECG) is a useful but incomplete assessment of HR, for one cannot determine the character of the pulse from the ECG.

To accurately obtain HR:

- Begin the counting interval with a beat and label that beat as zero.
- Use a 60-second counting interval when you are assessing a patient for the first time, the patient is unstable, the cardiac rhythm is irregular; or treatment decisions are based on HR (Sneed & Hollerbach, 1995).

Preload, like contractility and afterload, is infrequently measured directly at the bedside. Usually, we must rely on indirect measures that allow us to estimate or infer the preload, contractility, or afterload. The methods of directly measuring these factors that require invasive tests and devices (such as a pulmonary artery catheter) are not discussed here. You will note that the right ventricular contractility, right ventricular afterload, and left ventricular preload are difficult to assess at the bedside because the cardiovascular structures where these exist are embedded deeply in the chest and are unavailable for examination.

Preload

Preload for the right ventricle is assessed by looking at the systemic venous system. The assessment items include the following (Bates, 1994):

Increased Right Heart Preload

- Jugular venous distention (JVD)
- **Ascites**
- Hepatic engorgement
- Peripheral edema

(immediate sign requires several hours to days to appear)

Decreased Right Heart Preload

- Poor skin turgor
- Dry mucous membranes
- **Orthostatic hypotension**
- Flat jugular veins

Preload for the left heart is assessed by looking at the pulmonary venous system. These assessment items include the following.

Increased Left Heart Preload

- **Dyspnea**
- Cough
- Third heart sound (S_3)
- Fourth heart sound (S_4). S_4 is the sound heard as blood bounces off stiff, noncompliant ventricle walls. Thus, it may also indicate decreased contractility (Murphy & Bennett, 1992).

Decreased Left Heart Preload

Unfortunately, there are no noninvasive assessments that indicate specifically diminished left ventricular preload. Usually, if the left heart has insufficient preload, the right heart has the same situation, and we can rely on signs of diminished right ventricular preload. In some situations S_1 and S_2 may be muffled.

Contractility

Assessing the force of myocardial contraction is done by looking at the quality of the heartbeat when isolated from HR.

Pulse

The character of the pulse is noted at the radial artery. Increased contractility will demonstrate a bounding, vigorous pulse, whereas diminished contractility will demonstrate a weak, thready pulse. A splitting of S_2 indicates that one ventricle is emptying earlier or later than the other, usually due to a structural (e.g., valve defect), mechanical (e.g., heart failure), or electrical (e.g., alternate pacemaker) problem. Contractility may be diminished. It is important to note that contractility is difficult to measure indirectly by physical signs, since so many other factors may alter the character of the pulse. Decreased contractility usually is determined by exclusion of other causes of poor cardiac output.

Pulse Pressure

The pulse pressure is the difference between diastolic and systolic blood pressures. The pulse pressure reflects how much the heart is able to raise the pressure in the arterial system with each beat. Pulse pressure will increase when SV increases and/or in arteriole vasconstriction. Pulse pressure drops with decreased SV and/or arteriole vasodilation (e.g., some shock states). The normal pulse pressure is approximately 40 mm Hg (Thomas, 1993). Within the restrictions noted, the pulse pressure can be a useful, objective, and noninvasive indicator of myocardial contractility.

Afterload

As was mentioned previously, indirect assessment of right ventricle afterload is difficult because of the location of the pulmonary arterial system deep in the chest. However, it is possible for us to assess the systemic arterial system for signs of increased or decreased afterload. Even though we may find signs of altered afterload in some patients, they will not be present in all patients with altered afterload. It is necessary to remember once again that all of these determinants of CO are interrelated, and it can be difficult to isolate individual factors at the bedside without invasive tests.

Increased Systemic Afterload

Cool, clammy extremities may indicate that the arterioles to the skin have been constricted.

Systemic hypertension may indicate that the heart is pushing blood out against great resistance.

Nonhealing wounds on the extremities and thick brittle nails are indicators of chronic poor perfusion of the extremities, which may imply high vascular resistance.

Decreased Systemic Afterload

Warm, flushed extremities may indicate that the arterioles have relaxed and are offering little resistance to blood flow.

The status of preload, afterload, contractility, and HR can be assessed partially by clinical examination. Comprehensive assessment of these determinants can assist the clinician to identify the cause of altered CO.

SECTION SIX REVIEW

1. The total number of heartbeats is reflected in the pulse counted at the
   A. femoral artery
   B. cardiac apex
   C. carotid artery
   D. radial artery
2. Signs of increased preload for the right ventricle include
   A. jugular venous distention
   B. cool, clammy skin
   C. bounding pulse
   D. dry mucous membranes
3. Signs of decreased contractility include
   A. bounding pulse
   B. diminished pulse pressure
   C. ascites
   D. poor skin turgor
4. Signs of increased afterload for the left ventricle include
   A. cool, moist skin
   B. thin, flexible toenails
   C. liver engorgement
   D. peripheral edema

Answers: 1. B, 2. A, 3. B, 4. A

POSTTEST

Do not refer back to the text to answer these questions.

1. What is the relationship among stroke volume, cardiac output, and heart rate?
   A. SV × CO = HR
   B. SV × HR = CO
   C. CO × HR = SV
   D. $CO = \frac{HR}{SV}$
2. The degree of stretch in the myocardial fibers at the end of diastole is called
   A. preload
   B. contractility
   C. afterload
   D. compliance
3. In the healthy heart, the response to an increase in preload is for SV to
   A. increase
   B. decrease
   C. stay the same
   D. cannot be determined from the available data
4. If afterload increases and CO remains the same, what will happen to blood pressure?
   A. increase
   B. decrease
   C. stay the same
   D. cannot be determined from the available data

5. Myocardial ischemia will most directly influence
   A. preload
   B. afterload
   C. contractility
   D. vascular tone
6. Physical examination reveals jugular vein distention, ascites, and liver engorgement. These suggest
   A. increased left ventricular preload
   B. decreased left ventricular preload
   C. increased right ventricular preload
   D. decreased right ventricular preload
7. Sudden physiologic stress, such as escaping a burning building, will result in
   A. increased heart rate and increased afterload
   B. increased heart rate and decreased afterload
   C. decreased heart rate and increased afterload
   D. decreased heart rate and decreased afterload
8. Extremely rapid heart rate can decrease CO because there is inadequate time in each cycle for
   A. systolic ejection
   B. diastolic filling
   C. valve closure
   D. intraventricular conduction
9. If an adult patient has a blood pressure of 80/60 mm Hg, the pulse pressure is
   A. increased
   B. decreased
   C. normal
   D. unknown from these limited data
10. Following hemorrhage, cool, clammy skin most suggests
   A. increased contractility
   B. decreased contractility
   C. increased afterload
   D. decreased afterload

POSTTEST ANSWERS

Question	Answer	Section	Question	Answer	Section
1	B	One	6	C	Six
2	A	Two	7	A	Five
3	A	Three	8	B	Five
4	A	Four	9	B	Six
5	C	Five	10	C	Six

REFERENCES

Bates, B. (1994). *A guide to physical examination and history taking* (5th ed.). Philadelphia: J.B. Lippincott.

Funkhouser, S. (1994). Cardiovascular anatomy and physiology. In L. Thelan, J. Daire, L. Urden, & M. Lough (eds.) *Critical care nursing: Diagnosis and management* (2nd ed.), pp. 147–168. St. Louis: C.V. Mosby.

Headley, J.M. (1998). Invasive hemodynamic monitoring: Applying advanced technologies. *Crit Care Nurs Q 21*(3):73–84.

Ramsey, J., & Tisdale, L. (1995). Use of ventricular stroke work index and ventricular function curves in assessing myocardial contractility. *Crit Care Nurs 15*(1):61–67.

Sneed, N., & Hollerbach, A. (1995). Measurement error in counting heart rate: Potential sources and solutions. *Crit Care Nurs 15*(1):36–40.

Thomas, C.L. (ed). (1993). *Taber's cyclopedic medical dictionary* (17th ed.). Philadelphia: F.A. Davis Co.

Module 14

Hemodynamic Monitoring

Paula Hogsten, Megan Switzer

The high-acuity patient has complex nursing needs. This self-study module focuses on the integration of hemodynamic concepts and physical findings in the nursing assessment of the high-acuity patient. The nurse requires a working knowledge of the determinants of cardiac output: preload, afterload, and contractility. These determinants of cardiac output will be linked to the data available through hemodynamic monitoring with a pulmonary artery catheter. Mixed venous oxygen saturation will be discussed as one method to evaluate the adequacy of cardiac output and the patient's response to interventions. This knowledge, coupled with astute observation and sharp assessment skills, can guide critical thinking at the bedside and provide a higher level of nursing care for the high-acuity patient. The module is composed of nine sections. Each section includes a set of review questions to help the learner evaluate his or her understanding of the section's content before moving on to the next section. All Section Reviews and the module Pretest and Posttest include answers. It is suggested that the learner review those concepts answered incorrectly in the review questions before proceeding to the next section.

Objectives

Following completion of this module, the learner will be able to

1. Describe the purpose and functional components of a basic pulmonary artery catheter.
2. Understand the concept of thermodilution and continuous cardiac output determination.
3. Recognize the normal right atrial waveform pattern.
4. Relate right ventricular preload to the right atrial pressure.
5. Identify common physical findings and appropriate nursing interventions related to abnormal right atrial pressure.
6. Recognize the normal right ventricular waveform pattern.
7. Identify appropriate nursing interventions related to right ventricular waveforms.
8. Recognize the normal pulmonary artery waveform pattern.
9. Identify common physical findings and appropriate nursing interventions related to abnormal pulmonary artery pressures.
10. Recognize the normal pulmonary artery wedge pattern.
11. Relate left ventricular preload to pulmonary artery wedge pressure.
12. Identify common physical findings and appropriate nursing interventions related to abnormal wedge pressures.
13. Understand the physiology underlying the arterial waveform.
14. Identify the components of a normal arterial waveform.
15. Understand the implications of selected derived hemodynamic parameters.
16. Calculate mean arterial pressure, cardiac index, and systemic vascular resistance.
17. Relate the mixed venous oxygen saturation to the adequacy of the patient's cardiac output.
18. Recognize extraneous causes of abnormal mixed venous oxygen saturation values.

PRETEST

1. Filling pressure of the right ventricle (right ventricular preload) is measured through the pulmonary artery catheter port opening into the
   A. superior vena cava
   B. right atrium
   C. right ventricle
   D. pulmonary artery
2. The greatest potential for dysrhythmias occurs when the pulmonary artery catheter passes through the
   A. superior vena cava
   B. right atrium
   C. right ventricle
   D. pulmonary artery
3. The BEST definition of preload is
   A. the ejection fraction
   B. the volume of blood returning to the heart
   C. stretch exerted on the ventricular walls at end diastole
   D. the resistance the ventricle must overcome to eject its contents
4. Preload of the left ventricle is measured indirectly by
   A. cardiac output
   B. pulmonary artery systolic pressure
   C. pulmonary artery diastolic pressure
   D. pulmonary artery wedge pressure (PAWP)
5. Afterload is estimated by determining the
   A. PAWP
   B. right atrial pressure
   C. cardiac index
   D. systemic vascular resistance
6. Which of the following pulmonary artery pressures (PAPs) fall within the normal range?
   A. PAP = 40/22, PAWP = 18
   B. PAP = 26/12, PAWP = 10
   C. PAP = 18/7, PAWP = 3
   D. PAP = 34/26, PAWP = 23
7. Normal range for cardiac output is
   A. 2 to 6 L/min
   B. 4 to 8 L/min
   C. 6 to 10 L/min
   D. 8 to 12 L/min
8. The dicrotic notch on the pulmonary artery waveform represents
   A. atrial contraction
   B. closure of the pulmonic valve
   C. closure of the aortic valve
   D. the beginning of ventricular systole
9. The right atrial waveform and the __________ waveform are similar in appearance.
   A. pulmonary artery wedge
   B. right ventricular
   C. pulmonary artery
   D. systemic arterial
10. Mixed venous oxygen saturation represents oxygen saturation of the blood in the
    A. pulmonary artery
    B. superior vena cava
    C. right atrium
    D. coronary sinus
11. The left ventricle stroke work index is compared with which of the following, when assessing left ventricle function?
    A. right atrial pressure
    B. cardiac output
    C. cardiac index
    D. pulmonary artery wedge pressure
12. Which of the following parameters is most useful in evaluating the effects of nursing interventions?
    A. Sa_{O_2}
    B. CO
    C. Pa_{O_2}
    D. V_{O_2}

Pretest answers: 1. B, 2. C, 3. C, 4. D, 5. D, 6. B, 7. B, 8. B, 9. A, 10. A, 11. D, 12. D

GLOSSARY

Afterload. The resistance against which the heart pumps. Afterload is calculated as the systemic vascular resistance (SVR) for the left ventricle, and as pulmonary vascular resistance (PVR) for the right ventricle

Arterial oxygen content (Ca_{O_2}). The amount of oxygen present in the arterial blood; includes the oxygen dissolved in plasma (Pa_{O_2}) and the oxygen bound to hemoglobin (Sa_{O_2}) (normal Ca_{O_2} = 20.1 vol %)

Cardiac index (CI). Cardiac output (CO) divided by body surface area (2.4 to 4.0 L/min/m^2)

Cardiac output (CO). The amount of blood pumped by the heart each min (4 to 8 L/min)

Frank–Starling law. The principle that states that within physiologic limits, the heart will pump as much blood as is delivered to it

Mean arterial pressure (MAP). Directly measured by arterial line, or calculated from systolic and diastolic cuff readings (normal, 70 to 90 mm Hg)

Mixed venous oxygen saturation (Sv_{O_2}). The oxygen saturation of blood in the pulmonary artery (normal, 60 to 80%)

Oxygen consumption (VO_2). The amount of oxygen actually used by the tissues; it is the best indicator of tissue oxygen requirements (normal VO_2, 225 to 275 mL/min in a resting adult)

Oxygen delivery (DO_2). The oxygen supply; the DO_2 is the volume of oxygen delivered each minute to the tissues (normal DO_2, 640 to 1,400 mL/min in a resting adult)

Phlebostatic axis. An imaginary point determined by the intersection of two lines. One line is drawn directly across the chest from the fourth intercostal space at the sternum to near the posterior axillary line. The other line is drawn down the center of the lateral chest wall extending from the axilla to the last rib. The intersection of these two lines is the phlebostatic axis, and is the correct level for positioning transducers used for hemodynamic monitoring

Preload. The degree of stretch in myocardial fibers at the end of diastole. Left ventricular preload is measured indirectly by the pulmonary artery wedge pressure (PAWP); right ventricular preload is measured directly by the right atrial pressure (RAP)

Pulmonary artery diastolic (PAD) pressure. Reflects diastolic filling pressure in left ventricle (normal, 8 to 15 mm Hg)*

Pulmonary artery systolic (PAS) pressure. Pressure generated by the right ventricle during systole (normal, 20 to 30 mm Hg)

Pulmonary artery wedge pressure (PAWP). Pressure obtained when the inflated balloon wedges in a small branch of the pulmonary artery, reflecting pressures from left heart (normal, 4 to 12 mm Hg)†

Right atrial pressure (RAP or CVP). A measure of the pressure in the right ventricle at end diastole; this is right ventricular preload (normal, ~ 2 to 8 mm Hg)

Stroke volume (SV). The volume of blood pumped with each heartbeat (normal, 60 to 130 mL/beat); adjusting for body size provides the index (SVI = 33 to 47 mL/beat/m^2)

Systemic vascular resistance (SVR). Afterload of left ventricle; the resistance the left ventricle must overcome to open the aortic valve and eject the stroke volume into the aorta (800 to 1200 dynes • sec/cm^{-5}); adjusting for body size provides the index of this parameter (SVRI = 1,970 to 2,390 dynes • sec/cm^{-5}/m^2)

Venous oxygen content (CvO_2). The amount of oxygen present in the venous blood; it includes the oxygen dissolved in plasma (PvO_2) and oxygen bound to hemoglobin (SvO_2) (normal CvO_2, 15.5 vol %)

CARDIAC PRESSURES

Mean RAP	2 to 6 mm Hg	PAD	8 to 15 mm Hg
RV	20 to 30 mm Hg	PAWP	4 to 12 mm Hg
PAS	20 to 30 mm Hg		

COMMON FORMULAS

$$CaO_2 = (PaO_2 \times 0.003) + (1.34 \times Hgb \times SaO_2)$$

$$CO = SV \times HR$$

$$CI = \frac{CO}{BSA}$$

$$CvO_2 = (PvO_2 \times 0.003) + (1.34 \times Hgb \times SvO_2)$$

$$DO_2 = CO \times CaO_2 \times 10$$

$$MAP = \frac{SBP + 2\,(DBP)}{3}$$

$$SVR = \frac{[(MAP) - (RAP) \times 80]}{CO}$$

$$VO_2 = CO \times Hgb \times 13.4\,(SaO_2 - SvO_2)$$

*The pulmonary artery diastolic (PAD) pressure approximates the left ventricular end-diastolic pressure; normally, PAD is 2 to 5 mm Hg higher than pulmonary artery wedge pressure (PAWP).

†PAWP reflects the preload status of the left ventricle; a high PAWP suggests a relative or actual hypervolemia (a high filling pressure), and a low PAWP suggests hypovolemia (low filling pressure).

NORMAL VALUES

CaO_2	20.1 vol %	SVI	33 to 47 mL/beat/m^2
CO	4 to 8 L/min	SVR	800 to 1,200 dynes • sec/cm^{-5}
CI	2.4 to 4.0 L/min/m^2	SVRI	1,970 to 2,390 dynes • sec/cm^{-5}/m^2
CvO_2	15.5 vol %	PVR	37 to 250 dynes • sec/cm^{-5}
DO_2	640 to 1,400 mL/min	PVRI	255 to 285 dynes • sec/cm^{-5}/m^2
SV	60 to 100 mL/beat	VO_2	225 to 275 mL/min

ABBREVIATIONS

AOEDP. Aortic end-diastolic pressure

BSA. Body surface area

CI. Cardiac index

CO. Cardiac output

CVP. Central venous pressure

DBP. Diastolic blood pressure

Hgb. Hemoglobin

HR. Heart rate

LA. Left atrium

LV. Left ventricle

LVEDP. Left ventricular end-diastolic pressure

MAP. Mean arterial pressure

PA. Pulmonary artery

PAD. Pulmonary artery diastolic

PaO_2. Partial pressure of oxygen in arterial blood

PAP. Pulmonary artery pressure

PAS. Pulmonary artery systolic

PAWP. Pulmonary artery wedge pressure

PvO_2. Partial pressure of oxygen in venous blood

RA. Right atrium

RV. Right ventricle

RAP. Right atrial pressure (also known as central venous pressure, CVP)

RVEDP. Right ventricular end-diastolic pressure

SaO_2. Arterial oxygen saturation

SBP. Systolic blood pressure

SV. Stroke volume

SvO_2. Mixed venous oxygen saturation

SVR. Systemic vascular resistance

SVRI. Systemic vascular resistance index

VO_2. Oxygen consumption

SECTION ONE: The Pulmonary Artery Catheter

At the completion of this section, the learner will be able to describe the purpose and functional components of a basic pulmonary artery catheter. Various terms are used by health care professionals to refer to a pulmonary artery catheter, including right heart catheter, Swan or Swan–Ganz catheter, flow-directed thermodilution catheter, and pulmonary artery catheter. This module uses the term *pulmonary artery catheter*.

Purpose

The pulmonary artery catheter is an invasive diagnostic tool that can be used at the bedside for the following purposes:

1. Determination of the pressures within the right heart and pulmonary artery and indirect measurement of left heart pressures
2. Determination of cardiac output (CO)
3. Sampling of mixed venous blood from the pulmonary artery (SvO_2)
4. Infusion of fluids

Basic Construction

The pulmonary artery catheter is constructed of a radiopaque polyvinylchloride. Several sizes and various options are available to meet the needs of an adult or pediatric population. Most have a heparin coating to reduce the risk of thrombus formation. All pulmonary artery catheters have color-coded extrusions or "ports" on the proximal end that provide access to the various catheter lumens. The catheter is marked at 10-cm intervals to facilitate correct placement. A typical pulmonary artery catheter has five lumens, as shown in Figure 14–1.

Special Pulmonary Artery Catheters

Special pulmonary artery catheters are also available. These catheters are almost identical to the one pictured in Figure 14–1. However, additional options are present. One special catheter has integrated pacing wires that allow for synchronized atrial and ventricular pacing. Another catheter uses special technology to provide continuous monitoring of the cardiac output, as opposed to the individual "spot check" measurements traditionally obtained by the clinician. This technology is discussed in Section Two. Another special pulmonary artery catheter allows for continuous measurement of the **mixed venous oxygen saturation (SvO_2).** These catheters have special sending and receiving fiberoptics that permit continuous monitoring of the oxygen saturation in the pulmonary artery. As we will find in Section Nine, knowledge of the SvO_2 provides the clinician with information about the adequacy of the cardiac output. Other catheters will allow for recording an intracardiac electrocardiogram (ECG). Keep in mind that these special catheters provide all the functions of the basic catheter described in this section, but include special features that permit additional functions.

Components and Pertinent Points

Each section of the basic pulmonary artery catheter is listed and described below. When indicated, special nursing considerations are included with the descriptive information.

Proximal Injectate Lumen/Hub

- This lumen terminates in the most proximal chamber of the heart, the right atrium.
- Most catheter manufacturers imprint the word "proximal" on either the hub or the tubing close to the hub. Look for it.
- On most catheters, the tubing of this port is blue for rapid visual identification. One way to remember this is to link the blue tubing of this port to the "blue" desaturated blood found in the right atrium.
- This port allows for monitoring or sampling of the **right atrial pressure (RAP)** when it is connected to a transducer. Right atrial pressure is also referred to as the central venous pressure, or **CVP.**
- The injectate used for determination of cardiac output is pushed through this lumen.
- IV fluids can also be infused through this port, but keep in mind the precautions listed below.

Proximal Infusion Lumen/Hub (Optional)

- When present, this extra lumen terminates in the right atrium and is labeled "infusion" on the hub or the tubing near the hub.
- On most catheters, the tubing of this port is white or clear for rapid visual identification.
- This port is primarily used as the "central line" for IV fluid infusions. This is especially helpful in critically ill patients with poor venous access.
- This port can be used for obtaining cardiac output determinations if the proximal injectate lumen occludes. However, the individual values from this port may not be as reproducible as those obtained from the proximal injectate port.*

Distal Lumen/Hub

- This lumen terminates distally in the pulmonary artery.
- Most catheter manufacturers imprint the word *distal* on either the hub or the tubing close to the hub. Look for it.
- On most catheters, the tubing of this port is yellow for rapid visual identification.

* To avoid inadvertent bolus of potent medications, do not infuse vasoactive drips through the port selected for cardiac output determinations.

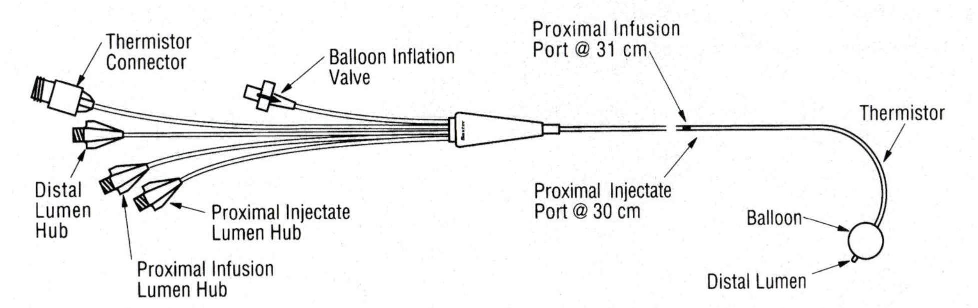

Figure 14–1. A five-lumen pulmonary artery catheter. *(Reprinted with permission. Copyright © 2000 Edwards Lifesciences, Swan-Ganz® is a trademark of Edwards Lifesciences Corporation, registered in the U.S. Patent and Trademark Office.)*

- This port is always connected to a transducer for continuous monitoring of the pulmonary artery pressure (PAP) and waveform.
- Pulmonary artery wedge pressure (PAWP) is obtained through this port by careful balloon inflation (discussed below).
- Mixed venous blood oxygen saturation (SvO_2) is obtained or "sampled" from this port. Remember that this port terminates in the pulmonary artery. The venous blood returning from all parts of the body has been "well mixed" in the right atrium and ventricle before it is pumped into the pulmonary artery.
- Patency of this important port is maintained by keeping 300 mm Hg pressure on the continuous flush solution attached to the hub.
- Medications are *not* infused through this port, except under certain conditions by a physician.

Thermistor Wire/Connector

- The thermistor wire terminates near the tip of the catheter and is exposed to the blood flowing through the pulmonary artery.
- This wire detects changes in the temperature of the blood, which is an essential part of cardiac output determination.
- It allows for continuous monitoring of core body temperature.
- The proximal end attaches to a cable linking it with the device used for measuring cardiac output. This will either be a cardiac output module compatible with the patient monitoring system or a freestanding cardiac output computer.[†]

Balloon Inflation Lumen/Valve

- This lumen is contiguous with the small balloon at the distal end of the catheter.
- A "gate valve" mechanism on the hub locks this port in an open or closed position.
- This balloon is slowly inflated using a syringe provided with the catheter, while the pulmonary artery waveform is continuously monitored. Inflation is stopped as soon as the waveform changes to a pulmonary artery wedge pattern.
- The maximum recommended inflation volume provided with catheter instructions should not be exceeded.
- Deflation is always passive. Manual deflation may damage balloon integrity.
- Never leave the balloon in the inflated position.

† The pulmonary artery catheter is a fluid-filled line with a thermistor wire terminating near the distal end. If the thermistor hub must be disconnected from the cardiac output computer, cover with the original cap or a finger cot to protect the patient from microshock.

General Considerations for the Pulmonary Artery Catheter

Insertion of a pulmonary artery catheter is a common procedure in critical care units, cardiac catheterization laboratories, and in surgery. The complication rate related to this procedure is low; however, the insertion of a pulmonary artery catheter is not without risks. Potential risks include pneumothorax, damage to the blood vessels or heart, arrhythmias, infection or bleeding, or bleeding at the insertion site and death. Except in emergency situations, informed consent should be obtained by the physician prior to catheter insertion.

Patient Teaching

Most patients are awake when the catheter is inserted, and it can be a frightening experience if the patient does not know what to expect. The patient should know that the purpose of the catheter is to assess heart function and fluid status, allowing more precise management of his or her condition. Explain to the patient that the site will be scrubbed with an antiseptic solution, and that a pinch, sting, or burning sensation may be felt when the local anesthetic is injected. A temporary sensation of pressure should be expected when a large IV catheter (the sheath) is inserted into the subclavian, jugular, or femoral vein. Once positioned, the sheath is typically sutured in place. The patient should know that the long, thin, balloon-tipped catheter will not be felt as it is threaded through the sheath, floated through the right heart, and positioned in the pulmonary artery. Most patients find it helpful during the procedure to receive general information on how things are going and an estimated time to completion. After the procedure the patient should expect to be attached to multiple IV lines that will restrict some freedom of movement. The family should be prepared to see additional equipment prior to the first visit postprocedure.

Nursing Responsibilities

In most hospitals, the critical care nurse is responsible for preparing the patient, the equipment, and all necessary supplies prior to the insertion of a pulmonary artery catheter. This includes careful flushing of all catheter ports, verifying the integrity of the catheter balloon, correctly attaching all necessary cables, zeroing the transducers at the level of the **phlebostatic axis,** and calibrating the equipment. Readings should be obtained with the transducer at catheter tip level. The phlebostatic axis approximates the level of the right atrium, and is considered to represent catheter tip level. Measurement of pressures in the heart and the pulmonary artery is accomplished by the use of transducers. Simply stated, a transducer senses changes in pressure and converts this information to an electrical signal. The electrical signal is then relayed to a monitor, where it is converted into a waveform and a numerical readout. The proximal and distal ports of the catheter are routinely attached to one or more transducers.

The insertion of a pulmonary artery catheter is always a sterile procedure. Along with the physician, the nurse is responsible for careful observation and monitoring of the patient during the insertion process. Once the physician has inserted the catheter, the nurse assumes responsibility for patient safety, comfort, and system maintenance. The nurse is responsible for catheter site maintenance, documentation of pressures in the heart and pulmonary artery, and obtaining valid cardiac output measurements. Postprocedure, a chest x-ray is obtained to confirm catheter position and assess for pneumothorax. It is the nurse's responsibility to recognize abnormal waveforms and trends, and intervene appropriately, including notification of the physician when indicated. The clinician must be aware of unit-specific policies and procedures related to hemodynamic monitoring.

Important Concept

Data collection is not the end point of hemodynamic monitoring. Abnormal pressures and changes in trends must be recognized, correlated with the patient's condition, and acted upon. Careful clinical assessment, integrated with the data collected from a pulmonary artery catheter, provides a good basis for nursing interventions and manipulation of potent vasoactive medications and/or fluids.

Several complications may occur from invasive hemodynamic monitoring. Infection may result. Air emboli or thromboembolism can occur from loose connections or improper flushing, respectively. Never flush a port if resistance is met. Fluid overload may result from fluid infusion through multiple lumens or lack of surveillance of IV pumps. Exsanguination may occur from any hemodynamic monitoring line if a stopcock remains open or tubing becomes disconnected.

The following guidelines can be used when interpreting readings.

1. Always look at patient trends and not an isolated reading.
2. Question abnormal readings. Recheck the reading after zeroing and calibrating the equipment. Assess the patient for additional data to support the reading.
3. Compare the patient with his or her normal values and not the textbook.
4. Do not be fooled by normal readings. The patient may have normal readings temporarily because of compensatory mechanisms. Continue to assess the patient.
5. Assess the interrelationships between the readings. You are trying to obtain a picture of the patient's hemodynamic status and not just a PAWP or a CVP reading.

In summary, the pulmonary artery catheter is a tool that has enhanced the care of critically ill patients. Changes in therapy can be guided by the information obtained from a pulmonary artery catheter with the goal of producing improved patient outcomes. An understanding of the functional components of a pulmonary artery catheter and the clinical interpretation of the data obtained from a pulmonary artery is important, and will be expanded upon in each section of this module.

SECTION ONE REVIEW

1. Which port of the pulmonary artery catheter is used to obtain a right atrial pressure (RAP)?
   A. proximal port
   B. distal port
   C. thermistor wire port
   D. balloon inflation port
2. Which lumen is used for obtaining CO determinations?
   A. proximal port lumen
   B. distal port lumen
   C. thermistor wire lumen
   D. balloon inflation port lumen
3. The purpose of protecting the thermistor hub whenever it must be disconnected from the CO computer cable is to
   A. prevent IV fluid leaks
   B. decrease the potential for an air embolism
   C. avoid inaccurate CO readings
   D. provide for the electrical safety of the patient
4. The pressure reading from which lumen is always continuously monitored?
   A. proximal
   B. distal
   C. thermistor wire
   D. balloon port
5. Why should vasoactive drugs never be infused through the port used for CO determinations?
   A. the size of the lumen is too small
   B. a bolus injection of a potent drug will occur every time CO is obtained
   C. CO readings will be less accurate
   D. some vasoactive drugs are not compatible with the catheter material

6. What is the best way to deflate the balloon on the PA catheter?
   - **A.** slowly pull back on the syringe plunger
   - **B.** quickly pull back on the plunger to limit inflation time
   - **C.** allow the balloon to deflate passively
   - **D.** remove the syringe from the hub directly after inflation

7. Which lumen is used to monitor PAP?
   - **A.** proximal port lumen
   - **B.** distal port lumen
   - **C.** thermistor wire lumen
   - **D.** balloon inflation port lumen

Answers: 1. A, 2. A, 3. D, 4. B, 5. B, 6. C, 7. B

SECTION TWO: Cardiac Output

At the completion of this section, the learner will understand the concept of thermodilution cardiac output determination.

Cardiac output (CO) is the amount of blood ejected from the heart into the systemic circulation each minute. It is expressed in liters per minute.

The formula used to derive the CO is simple. CO is the product of the heart rate (HR) multiplied by the stroke volume (SV) (i.e., the amount of blood ejected by each heart beat). The formula for CO then is $CO = HR \times SV$. Changes in the heart rate will affect the CO; in fact acceleration of the heart rate is one of the first compensatory mechanisms when the CO is depressed. The stroke volume is also variable and is altered by the effects of preload, afterload, and contractility. Understanding the concepts of preload, afterload, and contractility is key to the understanding of hemodynamics. These terms are introduced in the following sections and will be discussed throughout the module.

Preload

Preload is the pressure or stretch exerted on the walls of the ventricle by the volume of blood filling the ventricle at the end of diastole. Preload is typically used as an indication of the volume status of the patient. Too little preload (volume) will not adequately stretch the ventricular muscle to get the best contraction (i.e., the best stroke volume). Too much preload (volume) acts to overstretch the ventricular muscle, resulting in poor contractility, a reduced stroke volume, and a drop in CO. Preload, then, has to be "just right" to maximize Starling's law and get the best contraction and the most favorable CO. Although emphasis is often placed on left ventricular preload, keep in mind that both ventricles have the property of preload.

An estimate of preload can be quickly obtained from a PA catheter. For the left heart, the **pulmonary artery wedge pressure (PAWP)** is used as an indirect measurement of the pressure in the left ventricle at the end of diastole. This left ventricular end-diastolic pressure provides an estimate of the "volume status" of the patient. It is obtained from the distal port after the catheter balloon has been inflated and allowed to float into "wedge" position. The normal range of the PAWP is 4 to 12 mm Hg. However, every patient must be considered in the context of his or her health history. Patients with previous cardiac problems such as myocardial infarctions may need more volume to stretch an impaired ventricle to get the best contraction. Consequently, a higher PAWP of 15 mm Hg may be necessary to get the best possible squeeze from the ventricle. Right heart preload is obtained by using a transducer to measure the mean right atrial pressure from the proximal port of the PA catheter. The right atrial pressure (RAP) is also referred to as the central venous pressure (CVP). Normal is 2 to 6 mm Hg. RAP and PAWP are the topics of Sections Three and Six, respectively.

Afterload

Afterload is the resistance to ventricular contraction or systole. Simply stated, afterload is the pressure the ventricle has to overcome to open the aortic valve and push blood out of the ventricle into the systemic circulation. An estimate of afterload is obtained by using a formula to calculate the **systemic vascular resistance (SVR).** Afterload can be viewed as the pressure in the aorta pushing against the aortic valve to hold it in the closed position. However, fixed lesions such as aortic stenosis, and anomalies such as coarctation of the aorta, also represent afterload that must be overcome by the ventricle before it can eject the stroke volume. As afterload increases, the heart has to work harder, which requires more oxygen. When afterload is high, the ventricle does not empty well, which translates into a reduced stroke volume and low CO.

Afterload can also be too low. When the pressure or resistance in the aorta is low, the left ventricle needs to generate very little pressure to open the aortic valve and eject blood into the circulation. It will not contract vigorously. The net effect is a weak contraction, resulting in a reduced CO and a low systolic blood pressure. Like preload, afterload needs to be "just right" for the best CO.

Contractility

Contractility is the property of the heart that allows it to shorten muscle fibers and squeeze or contract. A vigorous contraction will improve CO by increasing the **stroke volume (SV).** Contractility is at its best when preload and afterload are optimal, as described above. If the CO remains low after both preload and afterload have been optimized, it is time to consider inotropic support. Increasing the contractile force of a weak ventricle will improve stroke volume, and the net result will be improved CO.

Contractility is assessed by calculating the ventricular stroke work index. The stroke work index is the work involved in moving blood in the left ventricle with each heartbeat against the resistance in the aorta (Ramsey & Tisdale, 1995). The left ventricular stroke work index (LVSWI) is the most sensitive indicator of left ventricle function. We will discuss how to calculate the LVSWI and how to plot it against the pulmonary artery wedge pressure in Section Eight.

It becomes clear that preload, afterload, and contractility interact to determine the CO by their effects on the stroke volume (see Fig. 14–2). Traditionally, primary emphasis has been placed on the left ventricle, because it is the capacity of the left ventricle to function as a pump that determines patient outcome. It is important to keep in mind that these properties are important to the function of both ventricles.

Cardiac Output

The normal range for CO is 4 to 8 L/min. This range allows the clinician to place a patient's CO inside or outside the normal range. However, this important parameter does not address the effect of body size on CO requirements. Consider the CO required by a large and muscular professional football player versus the CO needed by a petite female. If each one had a CO of 4 L/min, then technically both COs fall within the "normal range" of 4 to 8 L/min. A quick bedside physical assessment would tell us that more information is needed. While 4 L/min may well serve the needs of the petite female, it would likely be inadequate for the needs of a large, muscular professional football player.

The **cardiac index (CI)** references the CO to body size. This information is more useful to us because the CO is now individualized to a specific patient. The CI is obtained by dividing the CO by the patient's body surface area (BSA) to individualize the CO to the patient. A normal CI is 2.4 to 4.0 L/min. Most monitors calculate the CI if the patient's height and weight are entered. The CI is far more meaningful than the CO during bedside clinical decision making. As a derived parameter, the CI will be discussed further in Section Eight.

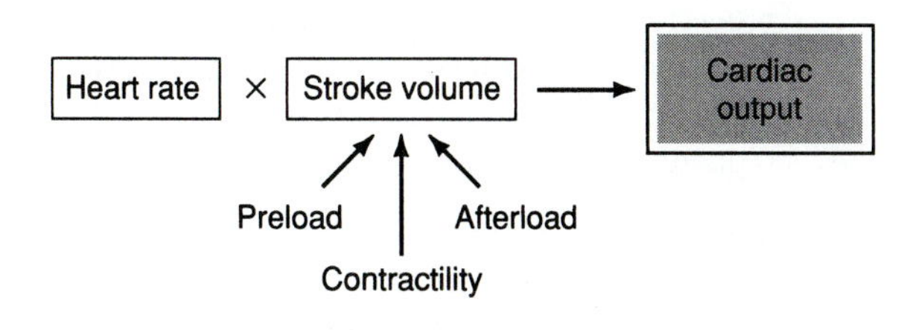

Figure 14–2. The determinants of cardiac output.

How Is Cardiac Output Obtained?

Various methods exist for determining CO. The focus of this section will be the traditional "bolus" thermodilution method of CO measurement. This is the most common technique in use today and is considered the "gold standard" for bedside assessment of CO. With this method, intermittent "spot" checks of CO are obtained at the discretion of the clinician or by a schedule dictated by policy or procedure. Other methods of obtaining CO will be briefly discussed at the end of this section.

The thermodilution method uses the theory of temperature change over time to calculate CO. The distal end of the thermistor wire terminates in an exposed bead 1.6 inches (4 cm) below the tip of the catheter (refer to Fig. 14–1). This thermistor bead is exposed to the blood flowing past it in the pulmonary artery. It senses the temperature of the blood and allows for constant monitoring of core body temperature. It also monitors changes in the temperature of the blood and the duration of the temperature change. This information is relayed to the computer through a special cable attached to the thermistor connector at the proximal end of the pulmonary artery catheter.

In the traditional method of "thermodilution" CO, a 10-mL bolus of fluid is injected through the proximal injectate port of the pulmonary artery catheter into the right atrium. The temperature of this fluid is cooler than the blood temperature. The injectate fluid temperature is sensed by an in-line temperature probe and then relayed to the CO computer. The CO computer now has two temperatures stored in it: the temperature of the blood and the temperature of the fluid bolus. The injection of the fluid bolus must be smooth, rapid, and completed within a 4-second interval. This fluid "bolus" mixes with blood as it is pumped through the right ventricle and into the pulmonary artery. The mixture of the cooler fluid bolus with the blood results in a transient drop in the temperature of the blood flowing through the pulmonary artery. As blood continues to be pumped into the pulmonary artery, the blood temperature will warm to prebolus level. The blood temperature change and the duration of the blood temperature change are sensed by the exposed thermistor bead positioned in the pulmonary artery. This information is relayed to the CO computer where it is analyzed and a time–temperature CO "curve" is formed (Fig. 14–3). The area under the curve represents the CO.

This area is calculated by the computer and displayed digitally in liters per min. There is an inverse relationship between the size of the curve and the CO. A small curve indicates a rapid return of the blood to its baseline tem-

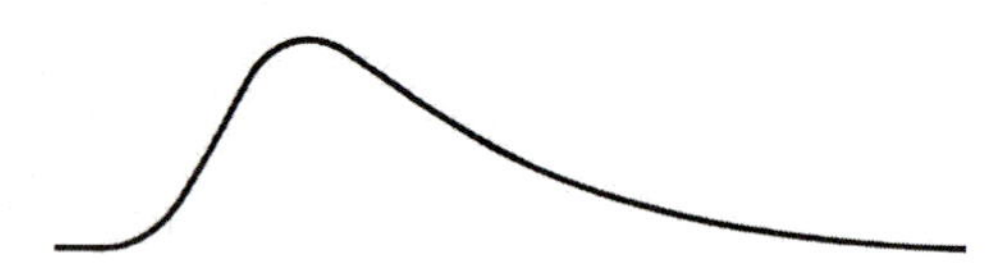

Figure 14–3. A normal cardiac output curve. *(Reprinted with permission. Copyright © 2000 Edwards Lifesciences, Swan-Ganz® is a trademark of Edwards Lifesciences Corporation, registered in the U.S. Patent and Trademark Office.)*

perature and therefore a high CO. A large curve indicates a "slow" return to baseline temperature and therefore a low CO. A notched or uneven curve indicates poor injection technique, and the value obtained should not be accepted.

General Considerations

Equipment Preparation

Obtaining valid CO determinations is an important nursing responsibility. To calculate CO accurately, the computer must know the catheter model, fluid bolus volume, and fluid temperature selected for use. A number or "constant" that represents this information must be entered into the computer before starting. This constant is obtained from a chart on a package insert provided with the catheter. It is important that the correct constant be entered prior to obtaining COs. If the volume or temperature of the injectate must be changed during the course of hemodynamic monitoring, a new constant must be entered or the CO determinations will be inaccurate.

Fluid Bolus

The volume of the "bolus" injectate used will vary according to hospital policy and patient condition. A common practice is for three sequential COs to be obtained, using 10 mL of saline or dextrose for each determination. If one of the results varies more than 10 percent it is rejected. The most common volume is 10 mL; however, if volume overload is a problem, 5 mL can be used. The literature reports that a 10-mL bolus provides the most reproducibility. An important nursing consideration is to be consistent and not vary the volume of the bolus. An average of at least two "similar" values is accepted for the CO.

Bolus Temperature

Selection of either room temperature or iced injectate is generally considered acceptable (according to unit policy), as long as the proper constant is used. Although there remains some controversy, research suggests that there is no significant difference between iced injectate and room temperature injectate, unless the patient is hypothermic or has a low (≤ 3.5 L/min) or high (≥ 8.0 L/min) CO (Wallace & Winslow, 1993). In hypothermia the temperature difference between the injectate and the patient's temperature may not be wide enough to ensure accuracy. Once the choice is made to use either iced or room temperature injectate, that decision should be followed through the course of that patient's hemodynamic monitoring. If the temperature must be changed, a new constant must be entered into the CO computer.

Patient Positioning

There has been debate on the importance of patient positioning on the accuracy of CO results. Traditionally, measurements were obtained with the patient in a supine and flat position. Unfortunately, this position is not well tolerated by many critically ill patients. The literature suggests that in patients with stable hemodynamics, there is no significant difference in measurements as long as the transducer is at the level of the phlebostatic axis and the elevation of the backrest is 45 degrees or less. In a patient with unstable hemodynamics, backrest elevation is recommended to be 20 degrees or less.

Timing of Bolus Injection

The timing of the bolus injection should coincide with the end-expiration phase of the patient's breathing cycle. This is thought to provide more consistency in the results.

Conditions Affecting Pulmonary Artery Temperature

Many conditions produce a change in venous return that can alter the pulmonary artery (PA) temperature. These include coughing, restlessness, shivering, and the administration of peripheral intravenous fluids of a different temperature through the venous infusion port of the pulmonary artery catheter.

Method of Bolus Injection

The bolus injection should be rapid and smooth. The entire bolus should be injected within a 4-second interval. Improper injection technique will affect accuracy.

Continuous Cardiac Output Measurement

The most widely accepted method for measuring CO is the traditional thermodilution method previously described. This is often considered the "gold standard" for measuring CO. Some concerns with traditional bolus thermodilution CO are listed below:

1. Interventions are based on the last hemodynamic profile, which may not reflect the patient's current hemodynamic status.
2. Frequent CO measurement subjects the patient to additional fluid, which may be contraindicated.
3. Accuracy is affected by user technique.
4. Frequent measurement of CO is time consuming.

Pulmonary artery catheters capable of continuous CO monitoring are available. This type of catheter utilizes a modified thermodilution method. Like a traditional catheter, there is a balloon tip, a proximal injectate port, an infusion port, a thermistor wire, and a distal port. The primary difference is a thermal filament on the exterior of the catheter between the infusion port and the balloon tip. When the catheter is properly positioned, this heating filament lies in the right ventricle. Random pulses of energy from the monitor raise the temperature of the filament to 44°C (111°F). The thermistor located downstream near the catheter tip detects the blood temperature change and relays it to the computer, which uses a formula to develop the familiar CO curve. The small amount of heat emitted has been found to be safe for the patient and has not been found to have an adverse effect on blood cells.

The CO and systemic vascular resistance (SVR) are displayed every 3 to 6 minutes. The displayed values represent an average of the CO and SVR of the previous 3 to 5 minutes. An updated average of the CO is provided 10 to 20 times every hour. By entering the patient's height and weight, a continuous CI can also be displayed (Headley, 1998). The accuracy of this modified technique, using heat "pulses" to replace the traditional fluid bolus, is not dependent on user technique. The patient is spared multiple fluid boluses, which may be detrimental for some patients. This catheter also permits traditional intermittent bolus COs and continuous monitoring of the SvO_2. SvO_2 will be introduced in Section Nine.

Several research studies compared this method to the traditional intermittent bolus thermodilution method. Data support an acceptable correlation (Boldt et al., 1994). Fever and prolonged insertion do not appear to affect accuracy. Further studies are needed, and this arena provides a good opportunity for nursing research involving a variety of patient populations.

In summary, cardiac output is the amount of blood ejected from the heart per min. Preload, afterload, and contractility determine cardiac output. Cardiac index references cardiac output to body size. Cardiac output can be measured through a thermistor wire in a pulmonary arterial catheter. In the traditional thermodilution method of measurement, a 10-mL fluid bolus is injected through the proximal injectate port of the pulmonary arterial catheter. In the continuous measurement method, heat pulses replace the fluid bolus. There is a good correlation between both methods.

SECTION TWO REVIEW

1. The normal CO is
   A. 1 to 4 L/min
   B. 2 to 6 L/min
   C. 4 to 8 L/min
   D. 6 to 10 L/min
2. The thermodilution method of CO determination is based on
   A. a blood temperature change over time
   B. the length of time it takes for dye to be circulated
   C. the temperature of the injectate
   D. the volume of the injectate
3. To increase the accuracy of CO determinations, which of the following techniques of injecting the fluid bolus is considered best?
   A. inject slowly and smoothly over 1 min
   B. inject smoothly within a 4-second interval
   C. inject rapidly over 8 seconds
   D. intermittently inject the volume over 30 seconds
4. Failure to provide the computer with a correct computation constant will
   A. not significantly alter the CO result
   B. result in inaccurate CO determinations
   C. be compensated for by throwing out grossly abnormal values
   D. not be a problem because the computer will not work without a constant
5. Continuous CO monitoring
   A. uses a modified thermodilution technique
   B. provides two updates on CO readings every hour
   C. is dependent on user technique for accuracy
   D. utilizes heating filament positioned in the right ventricle

Answers: 1. C, 2. A, 3. B, 4. B, 5. D

SECTION THREE: Right Atrial Pressure

At the completion of this section, the learner will be able to relate right ventricular preload to the mean right atrial pressure, recognize the normal pressure/morphology of a right atrial waveform, and identify common physical findings and nursing interventions related to abnormal right atrial pressures.

Right atrial pressure (RAP) is obtained from the proximal port of the pulmonary artery catheter, which opens into the right atrium. The RAP is always read as a mean pressure, and the normal range is 2 to 8 mm Hg (Fig. 14–4).

The importance of RAP is its use as an estimate of right ventricular preload (i.e., the volume status of the right heart). Recall from Section Two that preload is the

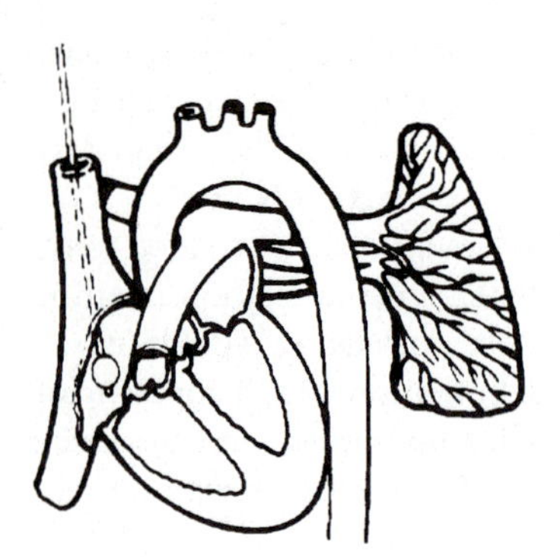

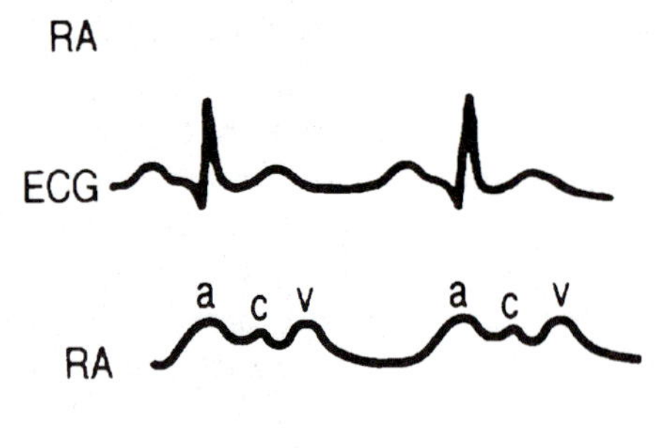

Figure 14–4. A right atrial waveform with the *a* and *v* wave components identified. *(Reprinted with permission. Copyright © 2000 Edwards Lifesciences, Swan-Ganz® is a trademark of Edwards Lifesciences Corporation, registered in the U.S. Patent and Trademark Office.)*

stretch exerted on the walls of the ventricle by the volume of blood filling the ventricle at the end of diastole. Although the blood volume in the right ventricle at the end of diastole cannot be measured, the pressure exerted by that volume can be measured. RAP then reflects the pressure in the right ventricle at the end of diastole. RAP is also known as right ventricular end-diastolic pressure (RVEDP). Measurement of the RVEDP is possible because the tricuspid valve remains open until the end of right ventricular diastole, allowing right ventricular pressure to be transmitted to the right atrium. This is why the RAP can be used to evaluate right heart preload. It is not a reliable indicator of left heart preload.

The right atrial waveform has a characteristic undulating pattern, consisting of three positive and two negative excursions. These undulations are a result of mechanical events in the cardiac cycle. The positive excursions consist of *a*, *c*, and *v* waves. The rise in atrial pressure during atrial systole forms an *a* wave. Closure of the tricuspid valve early in systole produces a *c* wave, which is not always well seen. The *v* wave is produced by the increase in pressure from passive atrial filling during ventricular systole. The negative excursions consist of an *x* and a *y* deflection. The *x* descent follows the *a* and *c* waves, and is a result of the drop in atrial pressure after atrial systole. The *y* descent is a result of passive right atrial emptying into the right ventricle when the tricuspid valve opens just prior to atrial systole. Refer to Figure 14–5 for a labeled atrial waveform.

The RAP and waveform can be monitored by attaching a transducer to the proximal (blue) port of the pulmonary artery catheter. The RAP will be used later in the hemodynamic calculations addressed in another section of this module.

Conditions Leading to an Elevated Right Atrial Pressure

Fluid overload increases intravascular volume (actual hypervolemia) and, therefore, the preload. In right heart failure, decreased contractility increases preload by causing a relative hypervolemia. The failing right ventricle just cannot empty itself well. The resultant resistance to further ventricular filling is evidenced by an elevated RAP, indicating an excess in preload.

Pulmonic Valve Stenosis

The right ventricle has to overcome the fixed resistance (fixed afterload) of a stenotic or "tight" pulmonary valve to eject the stroke volume into the pulmonary artery. As a result, there is reduced emptying of the right ventricle and an increase in the resistance to further ventricular filling. This is reflected by an elevated RAP.

Pulmonary Hypertension

Pulmonary hypertension can be primary or secondary. Examples of secondary pulmonary hypertension include pulmonary embolism and chronic lung disease. Pulmonary hypertension from any cause increases the pressure that must be overcome by the right heart to eject blood into the pulmonary artery and pulmonary circulation. As a result of the higher pressure or "afterload" in the pulmonary circuit, there is reduced emptying of the right ventricle, and this is reflected by an elevated RAP.

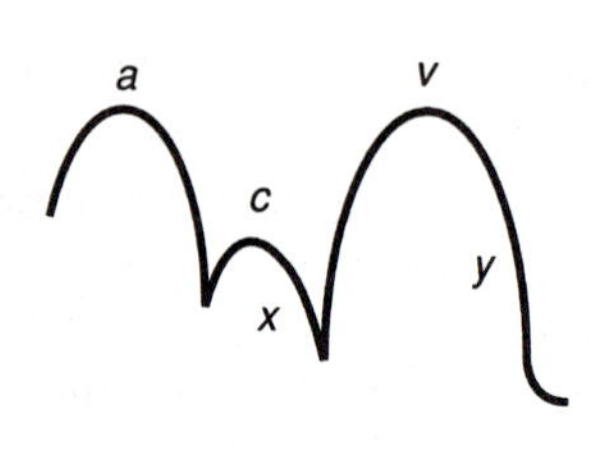

Figure 14–5. A labeled right atrial waveform.

Chronic or Severe Left Heart Failure
Inadequate cardiac output from the left ventricle will result in "backward failure." The increased volume in the pulmonary circulation will result in inadequate emptying of the right ventricle and increased resistance to ventricular filling. An elevated RAP will be seen.

Cardiac Tamponade
The right heart is a low pressure system. As a result of this, any rapid fluid buildup in the pericardial space will result in resistance to right ventricular filling. The RAP will be elevated.

Clinical Findings
Clinical findings associated with an increased RAP vary according to the cause and duration. Signs and symptoms may include all or some of the following: distended neck veins, tachycardia, a right ventricular gallop (S_3, S_4, or both), right upper quadrant tenderness from liver engorgement, dependent or generalized edema, and ascites.

When elevated RAP is a result of left heart failure, signs and symptoms of left ventricular failure also will be found. These are discussed later in this module.

Interventions
Interventions for an elevated RAP are determined by the cause. In general, care is directed toward optimizing preload by reducing volume. Overall goals are to decrease venous return to the right heart, increase contractility, and decrease the workload of the heart. Preload can be reduced by fluid and sodium restrictions, and administration of diuretics or vasodilating medications. Contractility is enhanced with medications such as digoxin and angiotensin-converting enzyme (ACE) inhibitors.

Nursing care includes careful and frequent assessment of the patient's response to interventions. The clinician should keep meticulous intake and output records, and obtain daily weights. A plan of care to decrease patient energy requirements should be implemented. Obtain a dietary consult for the patient and family on sodium and fluid restrictions. The provision of information about the purpose and importance of each medication may increase compliance.

Conditions Leading to a Low Right Atrial Pressure

A low right atrial pressure indicates low preload of the right heart. This is the result of either an actual or relative hypovolemia. Poor venous return to the heart for any reason will be demonstrated in a low RAP.

Fluid Deficit
There are two types of fluid deficit. First, an *actual* hypovolemia results from loss of volume from the vascular system. Causes include hemorrhage, overly vigorous diuresis, dehydration from vomiting or diarrhea, or loss of fluids from extensive burns.

Second, a *relative* hypovolemia can result from overly aggressive use of medications that dilate the venous beds. These medications include both intravenous and oral nitrates, some calcium channel blockers, ACE medications, and hydralazine. Although intravenous nitroprusside is primarily used for its action on the arterioles, it is included here because it also dilates the venous bed. Excessive use of these important medications causes a relative hypovolemia because the fluid volume is not lost but only temporarily displaced. This reduces venous return to the right heart and produces a low RAP, reflecting low preload.

Sepsis
The action of endotoxins at the cellular level can result in dilation of the venous beds. Volume is displaced, reducing venous return to the heart. Third spacing of fluid can also occur with sepsis, and through this mechanism volume is actually lost from the vascular system. The low preload seen with sepsis can be a result of both actual and relative volume loss. Both result in a low RAP.

Clinical Findings
Clinical findings accompanying low right heart filling pressures depend on the severity of the condition. Typical findings include tachycardia, hypotension, diminished pulse amplitude, flat neck veins in a supine position, reduced CO, thirst, poor skin turgor, dry mucous membranes, and decreased urine output.

If right heart preload (volume) is severely reduced, the signs and symptoms of shock also will be present.

Interventions
Interventions for a low RAP are determined by the cause. Activities are directed toward optimizing preload by restoring volume. Dehydration from overly vigorous diuresis, burns, vomiting, or diarrhea is corrected by oral replacement when possible or by careful intravenous hydration. Hemorrhage may need surgical correction. Clear fluids can replace volume lost by hemorrhage; however, when hemorrhage is significant, blood replacement is necessary to provide the oxygen-related capacity needed by the patient. The hypovolemia or low preload state related to sepsis is treated with replacement fluids, the administration of appropriate antibiotics to treat the sepsis, and careful adjustment of vasoconstricting medications such as dopamine and neosynephrine when these are indicated. Vasodilating medications are also a potential cause of low preload, as pooling of blood in a dilated vascular system reduces venous return to the heart. Intravenous nitrates and nitroprusside are typically titrated by the clinician, based on unit protocols. Oral medications

with vasodilating properties should be identified and discussed with the physician prior to administration.

The clinician should provide careful and frequent assessment of the patient's response to the interventions described above. Intake and output should be monitored and evaluated. Daily weights provide important information. Patients should be educated about the purpose of their outpatient medication, including signs or symptoms that require reporting.

In summary, the RAP is an indicator of right heart preload. It is obtained from the proximal port of the pulmonary artery catheter, and the normal range is 2 to 8 mm Hg. Treatment of either low or high RAP is guided by an ongoing evaluation of the hemodynamic response to interventions. Nursing care consists of both collaborative and independent nursing actions. The provision of information and emotional support to the patient and family is an important nursing function.

SECTION THREE REVIEW

1. RAP is measured through which port of the catheter?
   A. proximal port
   B. distal port
   C. thermistor wire port
   D. balloon inflation port
2. RAP is a reflection of
   A. PAWP
   B. preload of the right heart
   C. afterload of the right heart
   D. left heart function
3. Normal mean RAP is
   A. < 4 mm Hg
   B. 2 to 8 mm Hg
   C. 6 to 12 mm Hg
   D. 14 to 20 mm Hg
4. Right heart failure would result in a RAP that was
   A. lower than normal
   B. above normal
   C. within normal range
   D. unchanged
5. Hypovolemia would result in a RAP that was
   A. lower than normal
   B. above normal
   C. within normal range
   D. unchanged
6. With chronic lung disease, one would expect to find a RAP that was
   A. lower than normal
   B. above normal
   C. within normal range
   D. unchanged

Answers: 1. A, 2. B, 3. B, 4. B, 5. A, 6. B

SECTION FOUR: Right Ventricular Pressure

At the completion of this section, the learner will be able to recognize the normal right ventricular (RV) waveform pattern, state normal right ventricular pressure, and identify appropriate nursing interventions related to right ventricular waveforms.

Right ventricular pressure is not continuously monitored but should be observed and documented as the catheter is floated through the right ventricle into the pulmonary artery. It is the responsibility of the clinician to recognize a right ventricular waveform. If this waveform is seen during routine hemodynamic monitoring, it means that the catheter has become incorrectly positioned. The patient may be at risk for significant arrhythmias; and hemodynamic parameters, including COs, will be inaccurate.

The normal RV systolic pressure is 20 to 30 mm Hg. This represents the pressure necessary to exceed the pressure in the pulmonary artery (RV afterload), open the pulmonary valve, and eject blood into the pulmonary circulation. RV diastolic pressure range is low (2 to 8 mm Hg). This right end-diastolic pressure directly reflects the preload status of the right ventricle and should approximate the right atrial pressure (RAP).

The RV waveform has a characteristic pattern. It consists of a steep upstroke and a sharp downstroke (Fig. 14–6). Compare this waveform to the right atrial waveform in Figure 14–4. Although there is a marked increase in systolic pressure, the RV diastolic pressure remains essentially the same as the RAP. That is important information in identifying the waveform of a catheter that has slipped back into the right ventricle.

The RV waveform typically is seen by the nurse on only two occasions:

1. During insertion, as the catheter is floated through the right ventricle
2. If the catheter tip retreats from its proper position in the pulmonary artery into the right ventricle

Seeing this waveform at any time other than insertion indicates that the catheter tip has retreated from its proper position in the pulmonary artery. This has important implications from both a technical and a patient safety

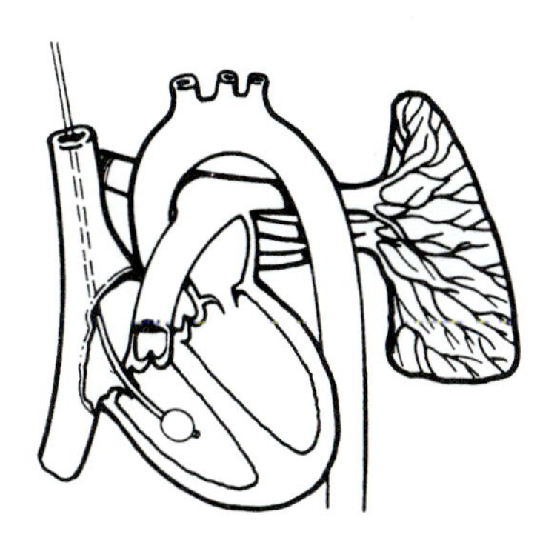

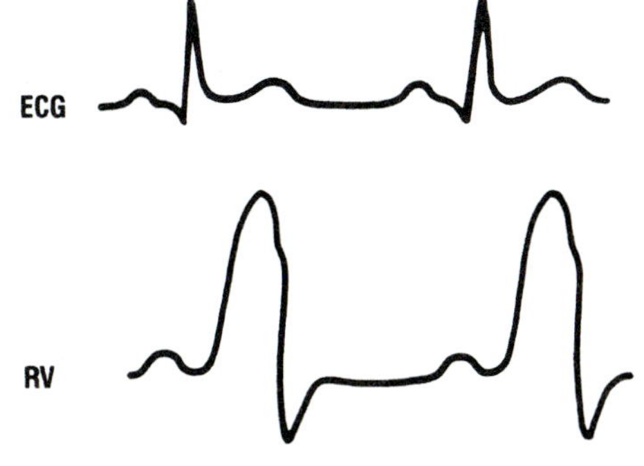

Figure 14–6. Right ventricular (RV) waveform. *(Reprinted with permission. Copyright © 2000 Edwards Lifesciences, Swan-Ganz® is a trademark of Edwards Lifesciences Corporation, registered in the U.S. Patent and Trademark Office.)*

standpoint. All parameters obtained from the catheter, including the CO, would now be incorrect. Most importantly, the patient would be at risk for arrhythmias. Irritation of the right ventricular endothelium by the catheter tip may cause premature ventricular contractions (PVCs) and could potentially elicit ventricular tachycardia. In addition, the right bundle branch portion of the cardiac conduction system lies close to the surface of the right ventricular septum. A patient with preexisting left bundle branch block on ECG could potentially develop complete heart block if the right ventricular septum and therefore the right bundle branch were irritated or stunned. For this reason, it is important to recognize the RV waveform and its corresponding pressures.

The cardiac rhythm and waveforms should be monitored by the nurse as the catheter is floated into the pulmonary artery. Once the catheter has been properly positioned in the pulmonary artery, a change to an RV waveform should be reported immediately to the physician to expedite repositioning of the catheter. Some hospitals or units have specific nursing protocols to follow when a pulmonary artery catheter retreats into the right ventricle. It is the responsibility of the nurse to be aware of unit policy and state licensure guidelines related to this event. In addition to observing for dysrhythmias and notifying the physician for repositioning, some facilities have specific protocols that may instruct the nurse to pull the catheter back into the right atrium or inflate the balloon to foster flotation of the catheter tip back into the pulmonary artery.

Close observation of the cardiac rhythm is indicated whenever the catheter tip is in the right ventricle. Once the catheter has been inserted, the exposed portion of the catheter is considered contaminated and should not be advanced unless a sterile sleeve was placed over the catheter before insertion. Use of these optional sleeves allows repositioning of the catheter without increasing the risk of infection.

In summary, RV waveforms should be seen only during insertion and removal of the catheter. The presence of the RV waveform at any other time indicates improper positioning, and puts the patient at an increased risk for the development of dysrhythmias. Careful observation of the patient and the cardiac rhythm is indicated when the catheter is in the right ventricle. Once the catheter has been inserted, the exposed portion of the catheter is considered contaminated and should not be advanced unless a sterile "sleeve" was placed over the catheter prior to insertion. Use of these optional sleeves allows repositioning of the catheter without increasing the risk of infection. The nurse is responsible for quick recognition of this problem and knowledge of unit protocol and state licensure guidelines related to this situation.

SECTION FOUR REVIEW

1. The normal range for RV systolic pressure is
   A. 10 to 20 mm Hg
   B. 20 to 30 mm Hg
   C. 30 to 40 mm Hg
   D. 40 to 50 mm Hg
2. The normal range for RV diastolic pressure is
   A. 2 to 8 mm Hg
   B. 4 to 10 mm Hg
   C. 6 to 12 mm Hg
   D. 8 to 14 mm Hg
3. The BEST description of an RV waveform is
   A. a soft undulating pattern
   B. a steep upstroke followed by a sharp downstroke
   C. sharply notched with a slow downstroke
   D. almost flat

4. The greatest potential for dysrhythmias occurs when the PA catheter is in the
   A. superior vena cava
   B. right atrium
   C. right ventricle
   D. pulmonary artery

Answers: 1. B, 2. A, 3. B, 4. C

SECTION FIVE: Pulmonary Artery Pressure

At the completion of this section, the learner will be able to state normal pulmonary artery pressure, recognize the typical morphology of a pulmonary artery waveform, and identify common physical findings and nursing interventions related to abnormal pulmonary artery pressures.

Pulmonary artery pressure (PAP) is read as a systolic and diastolic pressure. It is obtained from the distal port of the pulmonary artery catheter. Under normal conditions, the PAP is considered to reflect both right and left heart pressures.

The **pulmonary artery systolic (PAS) pressure** reflects the highest pressure generated by the right ventricle during systole. The normal range is 20 to 30 mm Hg. The **pulmonary artery diastolic (PAD) pressure** is normally 2 to 5 mm Hg higher than the PAWP. In the absence of chronic obstructive pulmonary disease, pulmonary embolism, mitral stenosis, and heart rates greater than 125, the PAD pressure can be used to estimate the left ventricular preload status. This is possible because there are no valves to impede the transmission of left atrial pressure to the pulmonary artery. The normal range for PAD pressure is 8 to 15 mm Hg. Once the PAD pressure has been demonstrated to correlate with the PAWP, it can be used to follow the left ventricular preload status.

The PA waveform is always monitored continuously by a transducer attached to the distal port of the catheter. The pulmonary artery waveform has a characteristic pattern (Fig. 14–7). It consists of a steep upstroke and a downstroke that is distinguished by a dicrotic notch formed by the closure of the pulmonic valve.

Review the RV waveform (Fig. 14–6) and compare it with the PA waveform in Figure 14–7. The systolic peaks of the RV and PA waveforms are approximately equal. That makes sense because the PAS pressure is generated by the right ventricle. However, the diastolic pressure in the pulmonary artery (8 to 15 mm Hg) normally reflects the left heart pressures, and will be higher than the diastolic pressure in the right ventricle (2 to 8 mm Hg).

On entering the pulmonary artery from the right ventricle, the top of the waveform will stay essentially the same height, but the bottom or diastolic portion of the waveform will elevate. Another identifying feature of the pulmonary artery waveform is the dicrotic notch on the downstroke. The dicrotic notch is formed by the closure of the pulmonic valve. If the catheter tip retreats into the right ventricle, the diastolic pressure will drop, and the dicrotic notch will be lost. Knowledge of these waveform properties allows the nurse to identify catheter position correctly. This is important because catheter retreat into the right ventricle could result in dysrhythmias (see Section Four).

Elevated Pulmonary Artery Systolic Pressure

The pulmonary artery pressure is generated by the right ventricle. Anything that increases the afterload of the right ventricle (i.e., increases the pulmonary vascular resistance) will result in an elevated pulmonary artery systolic pressure. Examples include pulmonary hypertension from any cause, including chronic lung disease, pulmonary embolism, and hypoxemia.

Clinical Findings

Symptoms vary according to the cause, severity, and duration of the elevated pressure. Assessment of the patient with pulmonary hypertension may reveal signs of right heart failure, including distended neck veins, peripheral edema, a tender liver, and ascites. Palpation may reveal a

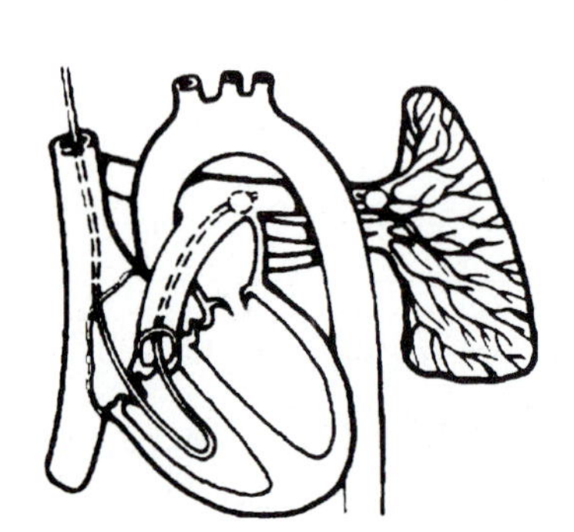

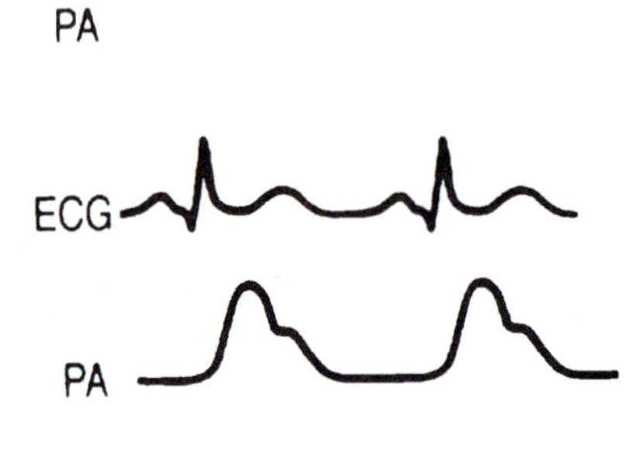

Figure 14–7. Pulmonary artery (PA) waveform. *(Reprinted with permission. Copyright © 2000 Edwards Lifesciences, Swan-Ganz® is a trademark of Edwards Lifesciences Corporation, registered in the U.S. Patent and Trademark Office.)*

right ventricular lift; and a right ventricular S_3 or S_4 gallop may be auscultated. Patients with chronic lung disease have a chronically elevated PAS pressure. Continuous oxygen therapy has been shown in some studies to reduce pulmonary vascular resistance and thus reduce the PAS pressure. A pulmonary embolus will increase the PAS pressure. The patient with a pulmonary embolus may present as a medical emergency with dyspnea, chest pain, hemoptysis, and hemodynamic instability. Oxygen therapy, hemodynamic support, and rapid intravenous anticoagulation are important.

Elevated Pulmonary Artery Diastolic Pressure

Conditions that affect the left heart, such as angina or myocardial infarction, fluid overload, mitral stenosis, and left-to-right intracardiac shunts, are associated with a high PAD pressure.

Clinical Findings

Clinical findings associated with left heart failure may result in some or all of the following signs and symptoms: dyspnea, tachycardia, LV gallop (S_3 or S_4), and bilateral crackles (rales) in the lungs. CO will be reduced and the PAWP will be elevated.

Interventions

Interventions for an elevated PAS or PAD pressure are determined by the cause. In general, care is directed toward reducing preload by administering diuretics and imposing fluid and sodium restrictions. Cardiac contractility may be improved by the use of inotropic medications, such as digoxin, dobutamine, dopamine, and amrinone. When indicated, the use of an intraaortic balloon pump can help reduce the afterload of a failing heart as well as increase the blood supply to the heart by augmenting the patient's diastolic pressure. Nursing care includes careful administration of potent medications, intake and output measurements, and daily weights. Care is directed also toward reducing the workload of the heart by planning activities to allow rest periods. The educational needs of the patient and family related to care, diet, medications, and activity should be incorporated into the plan of care.

Low Pulmonary Artery Diastolic Pressure

Low PAD pressure typically indicates an actual or relative hypovolemia, that is, a low preload state related to inadequate venous return to the left heart.

Clinical Findings

Clinical findings associated with low preload states include tachycardia, flat neck veins, clear lungs, dry oral mucosa, poor skin turgor, hypotension, and decreased urine output. If severe, the signs and symptoms of advanced shock, such as cool and clammy skin, also may be seen.

Interventions

Interventions are directed toward improving LV preload through volume replacement. Nursing care includes managing fluid replacement through an ongoing assessment of the patient's hydration status and hemodynamic parameters. Daily weights and accurate intake and output records are important.

In summary, under normal conditions, the PAS and PAD pressures provide a means for assessing both right and left heart function. Knowledge of the typical PA waveform helps the nurse to recognize incorrect catheter placement. Normal hemodynamics must be understood before abnormal ones can be explored. Integrating hemodynamic parameters with careful physical assessment findings allows the nurse to plan interventions to improve patient outcome.

SECTION FIVE REVIEW

1. The normal range for PAS pressure is
   - A. 10 to 20 mm Hg
   - B. 20 to 30 mm Hg
   - C. 30 to 40 mm Hg
   - D. 40 to 50 mm Hg
2. The normal range for PAD pressure is
   - A. 2 to 8 mm Hg
   - B. 4 to 10 mm Hg
   - C. 6 to 12 mm Hg
   - D. 8 to 15 mm Hg
3. The BEST description of a PA waveform is a
   - A. soft undulating pattern
   - B. steep upstroke followed by a sharp downstroke
   - C. sharply notched upstroke with a steep downstroke
   - D. steep upstroke and a downstroke distinguished by a dicrotic notch
4. Under normal conditions, a high PAD pressure suggests
   - A. hypovolemia (low preload)
   - B. hypervolemia (high preload)
   - C. good left heart function
   - D. right heart failure

5. The nurse should expect primary interventions for a PAD pressure of 2 mm Hg to be
   A. administering diuretics and implementing fluid restrictions
   B. managing and assessing the effects of volume replacement
   C. administering medications to increase contractility
   D. no intervention because 2 mm Hg is acceptable

Answers: 1. B, 2. D, 3. D, 4. B, 5. B

SECTION SIX: Pulmonary Artery Wedge Pressure

At the completion of this section, the learner will be able to recognize the normal pulmonary artery wedge pressure pattern, state normal PAWP, relate left ventricular preload to PAWP, and identify common physical findings and appropriate nursing interventions related to abnormal wedge pressures.

Preload is defined as the pressure or stretch exerted on the wall of the ventricle by the volume of blood filling it at end diastole. The **Frank–Starling law** of the heart states that the more myocardial fibers are stretched during diastole, the more they will shorten (contract) during systole, and the greater will be the force of contraction until a physiologic limit has been reached. The way myocardial fibers are stretched is through preload or volume.

This concept of preload applies to both the right and left ventricles, but emphasis is placed on the left ventricle because it is the capacity of the left ventricle to function as a pump that determines patient outcome. Left ventricular preload can be measured directly only during a cardiac catheterization or following open heart surgery when a left atrial line is placed. However, the PAWP provides an indirect estimate of left ventricular preload. It is obtained through the distal port of the pulmonary artery catheter. The normal range is 4 to 12 mm Hg. Like the RAP, the PAWP is always read as a mean pressure.

The pulmonary artery wedge waveform (Fig. 14–8) is similar in appearance to the right atrial waveform (Fig. 14–4).

To obtain a wedge pressure, the catheter balloon is inflated slowly, allowing the catheter to float and wedge in a small branch of the pulmonary artery. Inflation is stopped as soon as the characteristic PAWP pattern is observed (Fig. 14–9). The inflated balloon stops the forward flow of blood through that vessel. As there are no valves in the pulmonary circulation, the catheter can "see" the pressure in the left atrium. Since the mitral valve remains open until the end of ventricular diastole, the left atrium and ventricle essentially function as one open chamber until the mitral valve closes. This is why the PAWP reflects the pressure in the left ventricle at end diastole (LVEDP). In the absence of mitral valve disease, the PAWP is considered an accurate estimate of left ventricular preload. It provides information about the volume status of the left ventricle and aids in the evaluation of left ventricular compliance. An elevated PAWP suggests a stiff, noncompliant left ventricle that is poorly contractile. A low PAWP indicates that preload is low and volume is needed.

The normal pulmonary artery wedge waveform closely resembles the right atrial waveform. Compare Figure 14–8 with Figure 14–4. These waveforms are similar because they are propagated by the same mechanical cardiac events. Typically, two positive and two negative waves are seen on the PAWP waveform.

The first positive wave is the *a* wave, produced by the rise in atrial pressure caused by left atrial contraction. The second positive wave is the *v* wave, formed as the left atrium fills during ventricular systole. The *c* wave sometimes seen on the right atrial waveform is not typically seen on the PAWP trace. When the *c* wave is present, it is in the same location as the *c* wave on the right atrial waveform, and presents as a notch on the *x* descent of the *a* wave. The *c* wave of a PAWP waveform is produced by closure of the mitral valve at the initiation of ventricular systole.

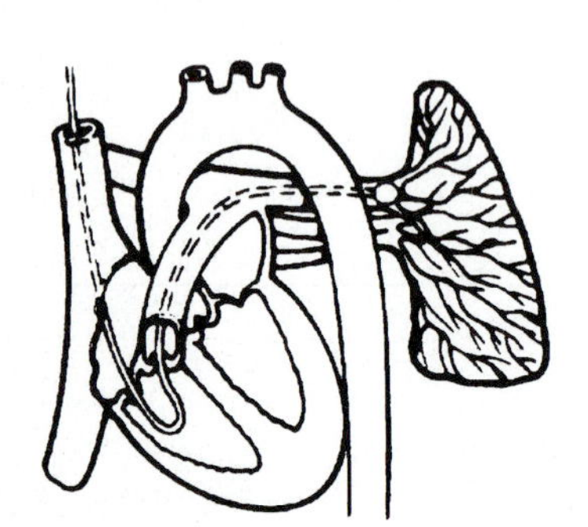

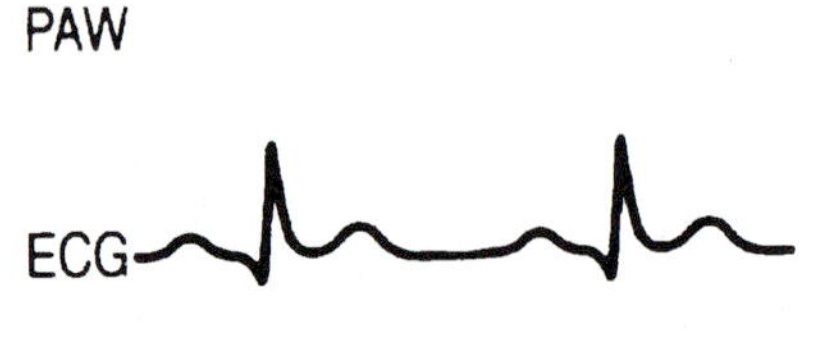

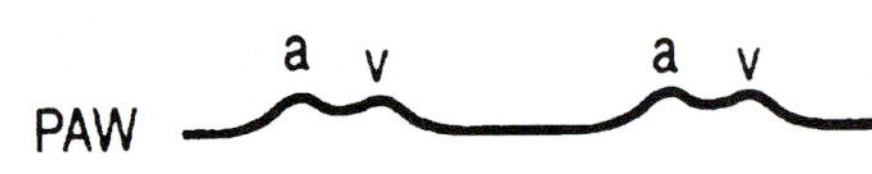

Figure 14–8. Pulmonary artery wedge (PAW) waveform. *(Reprinted with permission. Copyright © 2000 Edwards Lifesciences, Swan-Ganz® is a trademark of Edwards Lifesciences Corporation, registered in the U.S. Patent and Trademark Office.)*

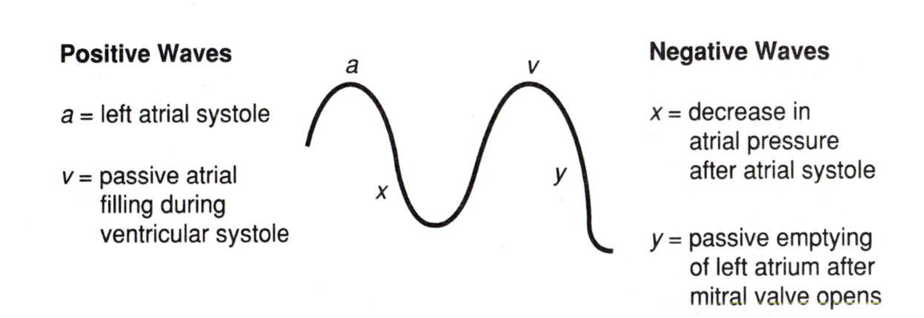

Figure 14–9. A labeled PAW waveform.

The two negative PAWP waveforms are the *x* and *y* descents. The first negative descent is the *x* wave, which reflects decreased volume in the left atrium after atrial systole. The *y* descent results from the pressure drop in the left atrium when the mitral valve opens just prior to atrial contraction, permitting passive emptying of the left atrium (see Fig. 14–9).

There are two primary differences in the right atrial and PAWP waveforms. First, the *c* wave sometimes present on the RA trace is rarely seen on a PAWP waveform. Secondly, the normal pressure of a PAWP trace is higher at 4 to 12 mm Hg than the normal RAP of 2 to 6 mm Hg.

Key Points to Follow When Obtaining Pulmonary Artery Wedge Pressure

- Observe the waveform constantly during inflation, and stop inflation as soon as the PAWP is identified.
- Use the smallest inflation volume possible, and do not exceed the maximum recommended volume (typically ≤ 1.5 mL), to reduce the risk of balloon rupture.
- Maintain inflation only long enough to obtain a stable reading.
- Obtain the PAWP at end expiration, when the pressure is most stable and less affected by respiratory variation.
- Allow the balloon to deflate passively to avoid damaging the balloon.

Pulmonary infarction can result from leaving the PA balloon inflated or when a deflated balloon becomes lodged in the pulmonary capillary bed. A wedging waveform will appear on the monitor. The patient should be turned or made to cough to relieve a lodged balloon. Open the stopcock on the port and remove the syringe to allow passive deflation of the balloon. The balloon may rupture from repeated overfilling of the balloon. If you are unable to obtain a wedge waveform after instilling the proper amount of air through the PA catheter balloon port, turn the lumen off to the patient, mark the line *Do not use*, and notify the physician.

Elevated Pulmonary Artery Wedge Pressure

Any condition that increases the left ventricular end-diastolic blood volume will result in an elevated PAWP. This can occur with:

- *Fluid overload.* An actual volume overload, elevated preload related to excess volume. This can be seen with overly aggressive fluid replacement, although normal kidneys usually compensate. Patients with acute and chronic renal failure often present with this type of overload.
- *Left ventricular failure.* This is a relative fluid overload; that is, an increased preload caused by inadequate emptying of the ventricle, caused by poor contractility.
- *Ischemia.* An ischemic myocardium becomes "stiff" and resistant to ventricular filling.
- *Mitral stenosis.* This creates a high left atrial pressure, which is transmitted back into the pulmonary vasculature.
- *Cardiac tamponade.* The pressure exerted by the fluid between the pericardium and the heart results in resistance to ventricular filling. The RAP, PAD, and PAWP will elevate, and all three values will be similar. This is known as *diastolic equalization*, and is a hallmark of cardiac tamponade.

Clinical Findings

Clinical findings related to an elevated PAWP will vary according to the degree of elevation, but typically include tachycardia, exertional dyspnea, orthopnea, paroxysmal nocturnal dyspnea (PND), crackles (rales) in the lung fields, and an S_3 or S_4 gallop at the apex. Neck veins will be distended. Untreated, a failing left ventricle can deteriorate until the symptoms of profound cardiogenic shock are seen.

Interventions

Interventions are directed toward optimizing preload by administration of diuretics and vasodilators along with sodium and fluid restrictions. Intravenous nitrates (Tridil) as well as oral nitrates will dilate the venous bed and displace fluid, which will lower preload by reducing the venous return to the heart. Control of dysrhythmias will help the heart to pump more effectively. Afterload, the resistance that the heart has to overcome to open the aortic valve and eject the stroke volume, is reduced by administration of arteriole vasodilators, such as nitroprusside (Nipride) and ACE inhibitors such as captopril (Capoten). By dilating the peripheral arterioles, these drugs reduce afterload, promote emptying of the ventricle, and effectively reduce cardiac work and oxygen need. Contractility is enhanced by careful titration of inotropic medications, such as digoxin, dobutamine (Dobutrex), and amrinone (Inocor).

Cardiac decompensation that does not respond readily to the above interventions may require the use of an intra-aortic balloon pump (IABP). This cardiac assist device can be inserted at the bedside percutaneously through the femoral artery. Deflation is timed to maximize afterload reduction to improve emptying of the ventricle. The heart receives its blood supply primarily during diastole, so balloon inflation is timed to augment diastolic pressure, improving blood supply to the heart.

The nurse is responsible for careful titration of potent vasoactive medications to improve hemodynamics. Manipulation of medications and treatments must be based on astute physical assessments correlated with current hemodynamic parameters obtained from the pulmonary artery catheter. Critical thinking at the bedside is crucial to improved patient outcomes. Frequent nursing assessments, meticulous intake and output records, and daily weights are crucial to follow the response to treatment. Activities should be limited and paced to the tolerance of the patient.

Low Pulmonary Artery Wedge Pressure (Low Preload)

A low PAWP typically is related to inadequate circulating blood volume.

Clinical Findings

Clinical findings include flat neck veins, clear lungs, low pulse pressure, decreased urine output, hypotension, tachycardia, and likely complaints of thirst.

Interventions

Interventions include careful replacement of fluid or blood products by correlating the PAWP with an ongoing assessment of the patient's response to treatment. Hourly urine output, careful intake and output records, and daily weights are indicated.

SECTION SIX REVIEW

1. What is the normal range of the PAWP?
   A. 2 to 10 mm Hg
   B. 4 to 12 mm Hg
   C. 8 to 16 mm Hg
   D. 10 to 18 mm Hg
2. The BEST description of a PAWP waveform is a
   A. soft undulating pattern
   B. steep upstroke followed by a sharp downstroke
   C. sharply notched with a slow downstroke
   D. sawtooth pattern
3. In a hypovolemic patient, the PAWP would be expected to fall in which range?
   A. well within the normal range
   B. low normal or below normal range
   C. high normal or above normal range
   D. high or low
4. In congestive heart failure, the expected PAWP would be
   A. well within the normal range
   B. low normal or below normal range
   C. high normal or above normal range
   D. high or low
5. Which waveform most closely resembles the PAWP waveform?
   A. right atrial waveform
   B. right ventricular waveform
   C. pulmonary artery waveform
   D. systemic arterial waveform

Answers: 1. B, 2. A, 3. B, 4. C, 5. A

SECTION SEVEN: Systemic Arterial Pressure

At the completion of this section, the learner will be able to understand the physiology underlying the arterial waveform and identify the components of a normal arterial waveform.

Blood pressure is a function of blood flow (CO) and the elasticity of the blood vessels. Systolic blood pressure normally ranges between 100 and 140 mm Hg. Systolic pressure reflects the highest pressure exerted by the left ventricle as it ejects the stroke volume into the aorta. Diastolic blood pressure normally ranges between 60 and 80 mm Hg. The **mean arterial pressure (MAP)** normally ranges between 70 and 90 mm Hg (Section Eight). The basic concept of blood pressure and the physiology related to an arterial waveform are the focus of this section.

Advantages of direct (invasive) blood pressure monitoring in the critically ill patient include:

- Knowledge of minute-to-minute changes in blood pressure
- Increased accuracy of measurement in the hypotensive patient
- More precise titration of medications and fluids

- The capacity to obtain arterial blood gases (ABGs) and blood samples without pain and discomfort to the patient

The arterial waveform has a characteristic morphology that is related to the cardiac cycle (Fig. 14–10). When the aortic valve opens, blood is ejected into the aorta. This forms a steep upstroke on the arterial waveform, called the anacrotic limb. The top of this limb represents the peak, or highest systolic pressure, which appears digitally on the monitor as the systolic pressure. After this peak pressure, the waveform descends. This descent forms the dicrotic limb and represents systolic ejection of blood that is continuing at a reduced force. The descending, or dicrotic, limb is disrupted by the dicrotic notch, which is an important point on the waveform. The dicrotic notch represents closure of the aortic valve and the beginning of ventricular diastole. The dicrotic notch is an important landmark in the timing of IABPs. Balloon inflation should occur when the dicrotic notch appears. The lowest portion of the waveform (baseline) represents the diastolic pressure, and is reflected digitally on the monitor.

Arterial monitoring occurs frequently in high-acuity settings. The nurse typically is responsible for setting up the equipment for an arterial insertion, calibrating the equipment to ensure accurate readings, and assisting the physician with the procedure. The two most common sites for arterial monitoring are the radial artery and the femoral artery.

Once the arterial catheter is placed, the nurse is responsible for patient safety and comfort, and the maintenance of the system. Securing the pressure tubing to prevent dislodgement and possible exsanguination is an important nursing responsibility. To overcome the arterial pressure and prevent the blood from backing up into the pressure tubing, a pressure bag is placed around the flush solution bag and inflated to about 300 mm Hg. Depending on hospital policy, the flush solution may or may not contain an anticoagulant (heparin or sodium citrate).

Monitoring circulation distal to the insertion site is another important nursing function. The skin color and temperature distal to the insertion site should be assessed and documented along with the pulse at regular intervals. Any alteration in circulation should be brought to the attention of the physician promptly. The site should be observed frequently for signs of infection: redness, warmth, edema, and drainage. Unit-specific protocols and responsibilities related to arterial monitoring are typically described in unit policy and procedure manuals.

Arterial monitoring provides the capacity to follow the patient's blood pressure on an almost continuous basis. Depending on specific monitor characteristics, digital blood pressure readings usually are updated at 4- to 6-second intervals. This allows the nurse to monitor the patient's response to interventions without having to disturb the patient to take a manual reading. Additionally, arterial blood gases and blood samples can be drawn without pain or discomfort to the patient. Manual baseline blood pressures should be taken at least once per shift to correlate with the arterial readings. It is helpful to be aware of significant variations between the manual cuff pressure and the arterial pressure before the arterial line is removed.

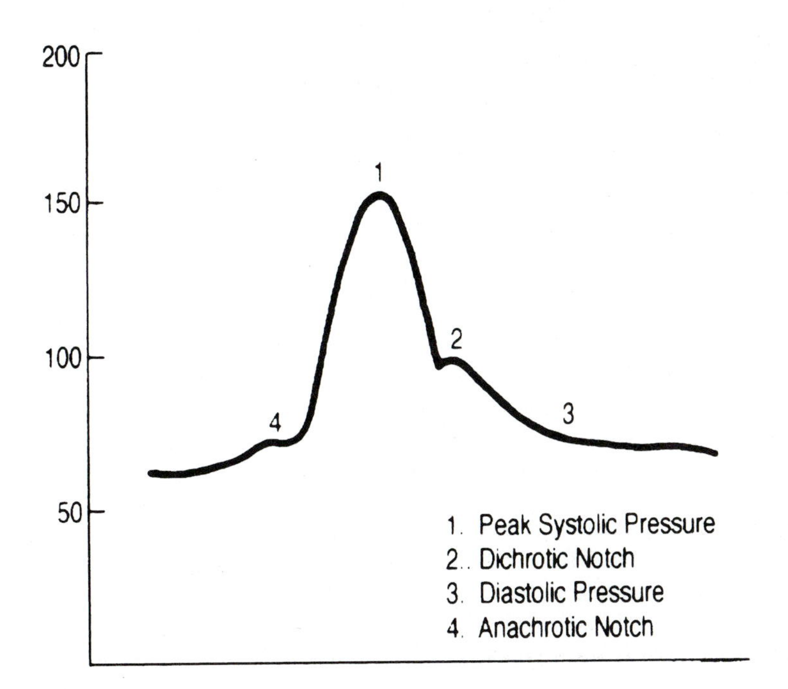

Figure 14–10. Components of the arterial waveform. *(Reprinted with permission. Copyright © 2000 Edwards Lifesciences, Swan-Ganz® is a trademark of Edwards Lifesciences Corporation, registered in the U.S. Patent and Trademark Office.)*

SECTION SEVEN REVIEW

1. The dicrotic notch on the descending limb of the arterial waveform represents
   A. opening of the aortic valve
   B. closure of the aortic valve
   C. the beginning of ventricular systole
   D. the diastolic pressure
2. The highest point on the arterial waveform denotes the
   A. anacrotic limb
   B. peak systolic pressure
   C. mean arterial pressure
   D. diastolic pressure
3. The lowest point on the arterial waveform represents the
   A. anacrotic limb
   B. peak systolic pressure
   C. mean arterial pressure
   D. diastolic pressure
4. The indentation on the descending limb of the arterial waveform is called the
   A. anacrotic limb
   B. dicrotic notch
   C. peak systolic pressure
   D. dicrotic limb

Answers: 1. B, 2. B, 3. D, 4. B

SECTION EIGHT: Derived Parameters

At the completion of this section, the learner will be able to understand the use and implications of selected derived hemodynamic parameters, and calculate mean cardiac index, arterial pressure, and systemic vascular resistance.

Cardiac Index

As discussed in Section Two, CO is the amount of blood ejected from the heart in 1 minute. The normal range is 4 to 8 L/min. As a generic or raw value, the CO does not take the size of the patient into account. The CI individualizes the CO to the patient by taking body size into consideration. Knowledge of the CO and body surface area (BSA) is all that is necessary to determine the CI. The formula is:

$$CI = \frac{CO}{BSA}$$

The normal CI is 2.4 to 4.0 L/min/m^2.

The BSA is simply a function of height and weight. Most monitors will calculate the BSA when the patient's height and weight have been entered. This method provides the most accurate estimate of BSA. An alternative method for obtaining the BSA is to use the Dubois body surface area chart (Fig. 14–11). This chart is comprised of three columns, one listing weight, one listing height, and one with the BSA estimate. A ruler placed across the three-column chart in a manner that connects the patient's height and weight will intersect the BSA of the patient.

The following example demonstrates the importance of calculating the CI.

	Patient A	Patient B
Height	6′0″	5′0″
Weight	216 lb	118 lb
BSA	2.22 m^2	1.50 m^2
CO	4.0 L/min	4.0 L/min
CI	1.89 L/min/m^2	2.4 L/min/m^2

Both patients have a CO of 4.0 L/min, which falls within the normal range, but the CI of Patient A is well below normal and suggests a shock state. Using the CO alone would not have indicated the gravity of the patient's hemodynamic status. The CI provides meaning to the CO, and is the more important parameter to consider when making clinical decisions at the bedside.

Mean Arterial Pressure

The MAP is an approximation of the average pressure in the systemic circulation throughout the cardiac cycle. Normal range is 70 to 90 mm Hg. MAP is a function of CO and the resistance of the blood vessels. The MAP is provided as a digital readout when an arterial line or automatic blood pressure equipment is in use. The MAP obtained from an arterial line is the most accurate, because the mean actually is measured rather than calculated.

When direct arterial monitoring is not available, the MAP must be calculated. Keep in mind that MAPs calculated from cuff pressures (automatic or manual) have a potential for error because of extraneous factors, such as the wrong size cuff, differences in hearing or sensitivity of the instrument, and patient movement.

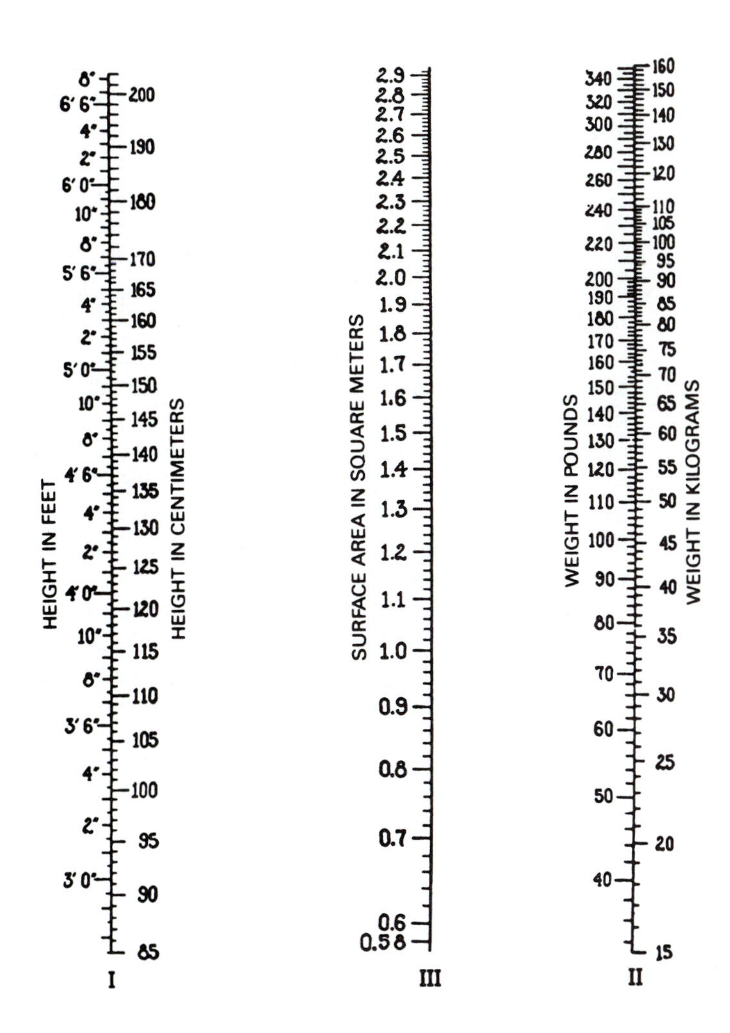

Figure 14–11. Dubois body surface chart. *(By Boothby and Sandiford of the Mayo Clinic; with permission of the Mayo Foundation.)*

The formula for MAP reflects the components of the cardiac cycle. In normal heart rates, systole accounts for one third of the cycle and diastole for two thirds of the cycle.

$$\text{MAP} = \frac{\text{SBP} + 2\ (\text{DBP})}{3}$$

Normal MAP is 70 to 90 mm Hg.

Systemic Vascular Resistance

SVR is an estimate of left ventricular afterload. It represents an average of the resistance of all the vascular beds. Recall from Section Two that afterload is the resistance the left ventricle must overcome to open the aortic valve and eject the stroke volume into the systemic circulation. Afterload, then, is one of the primary determinants of myocardial oxygen demand. The harder the heart must work to pump blood out of the ventricle, the higher the oxygen requirements become. A high SVR can reduce the stroke volume and cause a drop in CO. This is an important aspect to consider during regulation of potent vasoactive medications.

Although afterload generally is considered to be the resistance provided by the systemic vascular bed, anything that impedes ejection from the ventricle, including a stenotic aortic valve, constitutes afterload. Afterload is not measured directly. At the bedside, SVR is used to estimate afterload.

Most monitors will calculate the SVR. However, it is helpful to understand the components that make up the simple formula. The effect of the right heart (i.e., the RAP) is subtracted from the MAP. The result is multiplied by 80, which is a conversion constant. That product is then divided by the CO.

$$\text{SVR} = \frac{(\text{MAP} - \text{RAP}) \times 80}{\text{CO}}$$

The SVR is expressed in dynes · sec · cm^{-5}, and the normal range is 800 to 1,200 dynes · sec · cm^{-5}. Like the CO, the SVR is a generic, or raw, value. To individualize it to the patient, the CI is substituted for the CO in the formula. The patient's body surface is now taken into account. The formula for the SVR index (SVRI) is as follows:

$$\text{SVRI} = \frac{(\text{MAP} - \text{RAP}) \times 80}{\text{CI}}$$

The normal range for the SVRI is 1,970 to 2,390 dynes · sec/cm^{-5}/m^2. The indices of CI and SVRI are far better indicators of the patient's hemodynamic status than the CO and SVR alone because the indices are referenced to body size.

Elevated Systemic Vascular Resistance

A high SVR may be the result of multiple causes, and interventions must be directed at the cause. In hypothermia, peripheral vasoconstriction occurs as a compensatory mechanism intended to keep the central core warm. In this circumstance, warming the patient may be the only intervention necessary to dilate the constricted peripheral vasculature, normalize the SVR, and improve the CO.

Hypovolemia also results in an elevated SVR. Inadequate circulating blood volume induces several compensatory mechanisms, one of which is to induce the peripheral vascular beds to constrict. This mechanism results in the shunting of as much peripheral blood volume as possible back to the vital organs (heart, lung, and brain) to keep the patient alive. The increased SVR is needed to raise the blood pressure. Careful fluid or blood volume replacement should normalize the SVR.

In cardiac failure, hypotension initiates similar compensatory mechanisms. The peripheral vascular beds constrict in an attempt to increase the blood return to the heart and thereby increase the blood pressure. However, in this situation, returning more blood (more preload) to an already failing heart does not help. The vasoconstriction itself results in an increased afterload, which means the already struggling heart must now overcome more pressure to open the aortic valve and eject the stroke volume. This patient will need help on both preload and afterload reduction. Diuretics and nitrates will reduce preload. Afterload reduction must be undertaken cautiously in a patient with low blood pressure. Careful administration of a vasodilator such as nitroprusside (Nipride), or an ACE inhibitor such as captopril (Capoten) is warranted. Reducing an elevated afterload makes it easier for the heart to eject the stroke volume, lessens cardiac work and oxygen demand, and improves the CO. A very weak heart may need afterload adjusted to the lower limits of normal, and occasionally less than normal. This patient may also need help with contractility. Amrinone (Inocor) is an inotrope that improves myocardial contractility and causes vasodilation to reduce both afterload and preload.

Low Systemic Vascular Resistance

Low SVR is also a problem. During the isovolumetric phase of contraction, the ventricle begins to contract with both valves closed. The pressure increases in the ventricle until it exceeds the afterload on the other side of the aortic valve. The aortic valve opens and the stroke volume is ejected. The problem with low afterload is that the ventricle has to generate very little pressure to open the aortic valve, and that means the arterial pressure will be low. Physiologic responses to conditions such as sepsis, neurogenic shock, and anaphylactic shock initiate inappropriate vasodilation, resulting in a low SVR and a low blood pressure.

In sepsis, the treatment is appropriate antibiotic therapy and supportive measures to keep the patient alive until the antibiotics can work. SVR can be improved with careful titration of vasoconstricting medications such as dopamine, neosynephrine, or norepinephrine (Levophed). In anaphylactic shock, intravenous corticosteroids, antihistamines, epinephrine, and vasoconstricting medications are used. In neurogenic shock, corticosteroids and vasoconstricting medications are used. Vasodilator therapy is another cause of low preload. The patient's medications may need to be reviewed, and vasodilators may need to be reduced or eliminated. It becomes clear that afterload, just like preload, needs to be maintained in a range appropriate for the patient.

Left Ventricular Stroke Work Index

Left ventricular stroke work index (LVSWI) is the amount of work involved in moving blood in the left ventricle with each heartbeat. A lot of information goes into calculating the LVSWI, since it represents work performed that is influenced by both pressure the heart beats against and the volume the heart must pump. First, the stroke volume index (SVI) is calculated. Most monitors and software systems are capable of calculating the SVI. The formula is:

$$SVI = \frac{CI}{HR}$$

Once the SVI is calculated, the MAP must be calculated. Again, most monitor systems will do this for you. The PAWP is also needed, which you can obtain from the balloon port on the pulmonary artery catheter (see Section Six). Once you have all the information, it is placed in the following equation:

$$LVSWI = (MAP - PAWP) \times SVI \times 0.0136 \text{ (constant)}$$

MAP – PAWP = a measure of the pressure the left ventricle is ejecting against
SVI = the volume the left ventricle must eject
0.0136 = converts work to pressure

Normal values for LVSWI range from 35 to 80 g/m^2/beat. There are situations in which it helps to compare the LVSWI with the PAWP. In these situations, the PAWP does not accurately reflect left ventricle work (see Section Six). If the patient develops cardiac tamponade or pleural effusion, or is on high levels of positive end-expiratory pressure (PEEP) while being mechanically ventilated, the resistance that the left ventricle must work under is greater. Because the PAWP reflects the volume and not directly the pressure, it is not as sensitive as a parameter that accounts for both volume and pressure (LVSWI). When the left ventricle becomes stiffer (decreased compliance), the PAWP does not accurately reflect the workload of the left ventricle, because the relationship between volume and pressure is not direct. It is best to calculate contractility and not depend on the "volume" (PAWP), the left ventricle preload reading.

Once the LVSWI is obtained, it is plotted on the Y axis while the PAWP is plotted on the X axis (Fig. 14–12). This provides a picture of how well the left ventricle is performing work in light of the pressure and volume conditions it is under. As noted in the figure, an LVSWI between 40 and 60 g/m²/beat, and a PAWP between 8 and 20 mm Hg, is best for left ventricular ejection.

Low LVSWI indicates the patient is hypovolemic or has cardiac failure. If the PAWP is high, inotropic drugs are needed to increase contractility. However, in situations in which both the LVSWI and the PAWP are low, the patient needs more volume and may be able to improve contractility through this route based on Starling's law. IV fluids and blood products may be given. High LVSWI indicates hypervolemia and usually occurs as a compensatory phase prior to the beginning of heart failure. In cases in which both the LVSWI and the PAWP are high, diuretics and vasodilators may be needed. You will not have a situation in which the LVSWI is high and the PAWP is low unless the catheter is malfunctioning. This is because volume is incorporated into the LVSWI calculation; and if there is less volume, there is less work performed even if the left ventricle is facing great resistance in ejecting.

Now you can see why both the LVSWI and the PAWP are helpful in examining contractility. What if we look only at the PAWP? Let's suppose the PAWP is high (24 mm Hg). We would assume the patient needed diuretics. But if the patient's LVSWI is low while the PAWP is elevated, the patient needs inotropic medicine to enhance contractility. Once contractility is enhanced, the volume can be managed. The patient may need all of the volume for adequate oxygen delivery (see Section Nine) or to keep grafts open.

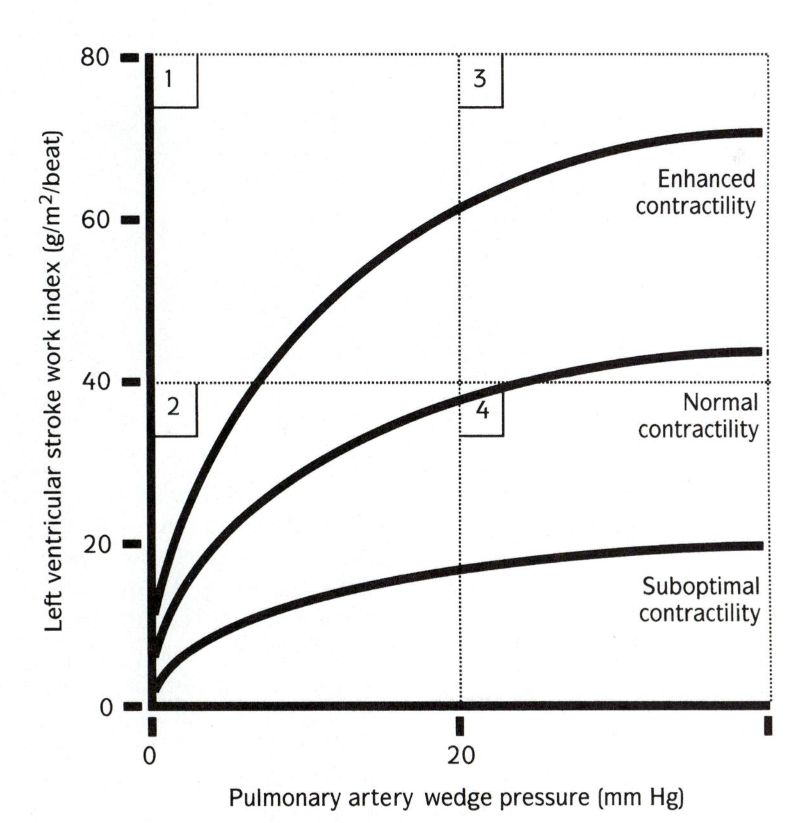

Quadrant 1: Optimal function; Quadrant 2: Hypovolemia;
Quadrant 3: Hypervolemia; Quadrant 4: Cardiac failure

Figure 14–12. Venticular function curve.

In summary, the derived parameters of mean arterial pressure, CI, systemic vascular resistance, and left ventricular stroke work index provide important information about cardiac status. Recall from Section Two that CO is determined by preload, afterload, and contractility. The PAWP is an estimate of left ventricular preload, and the systemic vascular resistance provides an estimate of afterload. In some situations, a more precise measure of contractility than volume estimate alone is needed. Correlating hemodynamic parameters with physical assessment can assist the nurse in clinical decision making at the bedside. Integration of this knowledge can enable the nurse to provide both independent and collaborative nursing interventions. These are the derived hemodynamic parameters most commonly seen in critical care units. The reader is referred to a cardiac hemodynamics text for more in-depth information on these and other derived parameters.

SECTION EIGHT REVIEW

1. Normal range for MAP is
   A. 60 to 80 mm Hg
   B. 70 to 90 mm Hg
   C. 80 to 100 mm Hg
   D. 90 to 110 mm Hg
2. Using the Dubois chart (Fig. 14–11), determine the BSA for a patient who is 5′0″ tall and weighs 140 pounds.
   A. 1.60
   B. 1.80
   C. 2.40
   D. 1.82
3. Using the following hemodynamic parameters: MAP = 90 mm Hg, RAP = 6 mm Hg, CO = 6.2 L/min, BSA = 1.8 m^2, calculate the CI.
   A. 2.00
   B. 3.44
   C. 4.50
   D. 2.96
4. Using the hemodynamic parameters in Question 3, calculate the SVR.
   A. 1,832 dynes · sec/cm^{-5}
   B. 622 dynes · sec/cm^{-5}
   C. 1,083 dynes · sec/cm^{-5}
   D. 1,274 dynes · sec/cm^{-5}
5. What would be the SVRI?
   A. 3,200 dynes · $sec/cm^{-5}/m^2$
   B. 1,020 dynes · $sec/cm^{-5}/m^2$
   C. 2,195 dynes · $sec/cm^{-5}/m^2$
   D. 1,953 dynes · $sec/cm^{-5}/m^2$
6. What is the normal range for the SVRI?
   A. 800 to 1,200 dynes · sec/cm^{-5}
   B. 250 to 680 dynes · sec/cm^{-5}
   C. 1,970 to 2,390 dynes · sec/cm^{-5}
   D. 1,200 to 1,500 dynes · sec/cm^{-5}
7. The LVSWI should be used instead of the PAWP in assessing left ventricular function in cases of
   A. hypovolemia
   B. congestive heart failure
   C. cardiac tamponade
   D. hypervolemia

Answers: 1. B, 2. A, 3. B, 4. C, 5. D, 6. C, 7. C

SECTION NINE: An Introduction to Continuous Svo_2 Monitoring: Pulling It All Together

Behavioral Objectives

At the end of this section, the learner will be able to

1. Relate the mixed venous oxygen saturation to the adequacy of the patient's CO.
2. State the normal range for the Svo_2.
3. Recognize extraneous causes of abnormal Svo_2 values.

For over a decade, hemodynamic profiles have been used to evaluate the status of critically ill patients. CI and arterial blood gases provide a feel for how well or how poorly the patient's heart and lungs are functioning. When these indicators fall within an accepted range, the patient is generally considered to be hemodynamically stable. However, that is not always the case. How often has a nurse stood at the bedside and looked at the patient's hemodynamic profile, then looked at the patient and said, "Something is not right here. How can this patient be so sick and yet look so good on paper?"

The physiology to keep in mind is that the primary function of the heart and lungs is to deliver oxygen—not to generate a good blood pressure or a good CO, but to deliver oxygen in whatever amount is necessary to meet the demands of the tissue. This is a key concept. A very important issue is whether or not the patient's CO meets the current oxygen demand of the tissues.

The purpose of this section is to introduce the concept of monitoring SvO_2. Understanding and evaluating SvO_2 can help to explain the patient who looks good on paper but not on physical assessment. Continuous SvO_2 monitoring has been found to provide quick feedback on the patient's response to interventions to increase the patient's oxygen supply and lower the oxygen demand. Monitoring SvO_2 can provide early warning of a change in the patient's condition, and prompt a timely reevaluation of the patient's hemodynamic status.

Included in this section is an overview of the fundamentals of oxygen transport. The reader is referred to Module 7, as well as the bibliography at the end of this chapter, for more in-depth information on this important topic.

What Is SvO_2?

Measuring continuous pulse oximetry, or the oxygen saturation of the arterial blood, is a common practice in critical care. The normal oxygen saturation of arterial blood is expected to be ≥ 95 percent. Much time is appropriately spent looking at the arterial side of the patient's hemodynamics (i.e., blood pressure, CI, ABGs, and SVR). SvO_2 monitoring now shifts the focus to the venous side to evaluate whether the effort of the heart and lungs to supply oxygen to the tissues is sufficient to meet the tissue demands.

When the supply of oxygen delivered to the tissues is sufficient, the tissues will extract the amount of oxygen needed for their metabolic processes. Each organ system requires a different amount of oxygen for functioning. The kidneys actually have a relatively low demand for oxygen because much of their function utilizes a passive transport. The oxygen saturation of the venous blood leaving the kidney averages 74 percent. Conversely, the heart requires a large amount of oxygen for its work. The oxygen saturation of blood leaving the coronary circulation averages only 30 percent. Each body part will extract a certain percent of the oxygen provided to it depending on the metabolic rate of that organ system. The venous blood returned from all organ systems is transported to the right heart, where it mixes as it is pumped through the right atrium and the right ventricle. The venous blood from all body systems is considered "mixed" when it has reached the pulmonary artery. The saturation of this mixed venous blood (SvO_2) represents an average of the venous saturation of blood from all parts of the body. Normal mixed venous oxygen saturation is 60 percent to 80 percent.

Why Measure SvO_2?

If the oxygen supplied to the tissues is adequate for tissue needs, the oxygen saturation of the blood in the PA will be in the normal range of 60 to 80 percent. Monitoring the SvO_2 will allow the clinician to know whether the demands of the tissues are being met. The SvO_2 provides information about the adequacy of the CO. The patient's blood gases and CI may "look good on paper," but if the SvO_2 is below 60 percent, the tissues are demanding more than the heart and lungs are providing. A low SvO_2 tells us the tissues need more oxygen delivered to them regardless of the blood gases or the CI. Conversely, a low CI of only 2.0 in a fresh post–open heart patient may actually not be of concern if the patient's SvO_2 is between 60 and 80 percent. These patients are hypothermic, sedated, intubated, and mechanically ventilated. Consequently, their tissue demands are very low. Their normal SvO_2 indicates that their tissues are currently satisfied with the oxygen supplied by the low CI of 2.0. Again, the SvO_2 provides information about the adequacy of the CO. This can provide immediate feedback on the results of interventions, or provide an early warning of changes in the patient's condition.

How Is the SvO_2 Measured?

The distal port of the basic PA catheter opens into the PA, permitting intermittent sampling of the blood in the PA. However, tissue needs often change quickly in a critically ill patient, and spot checks are not the best way to monitor this parameter. Just as continuous CO monitoring provides more information than intermittent bolus CO, continuous SvO_2 monitoring is the optimal method of evaluating the adequacy of the CO. As sedated patients wake up, get agitated, and begin the work of breathing, rapid changes occur in their need for oxygen. A drop in the SvO_2 prompts a recheck of the hemodynamic parameters that may have looked good 30 minutes ago. This early warning allows for early intervention.

Special oximetric PA catheters can provide continuous monitoring of the SvO_2. The clinician can obtain right atrial pressure, PA pressure, wedge pressure, CO, and core blood temperature in addition to continuous SvO_2 monitoring. A fiber-optic filament in the catheter emits a constant beam of light on the red blood cells flowing past it in the PA. The amount of emitted light reflected back to the computer through a receiving fiber-optic depends on the oxygen saturation of the red blood cells flowing past it. The computer uses this information to determine the oxygen saturation of mixed venous blood. A digital readout of the SvO_2 is updated several times each minute.

Fundamentals of Oxygenation

Oxygen delivery to the tissues and oxygen consumption by the tissues are important considerations for a critically ill patient. These are among the most important numbers calculated in critical care units. We are going to work through the formulas so we will have an understanding of what is involved, but keep in mind the concepts discussed rather than the formulas. Most monitors will provide these numbers for us in a timely fashion, but it is important to understand what this information represents.

Oxygen Supply

The first step is starting with oxygen supply. Two pieces of familiar information are needed to determine how much oxygen is being delivered to the tissues:

1. How much oxygen is in the arterial blood? This is the oxygen content (CaO_2). Oxygen content includes the oxygen combined with hemoglobin (the SaO_2 or oxygen saturation) and the oxygen dissolved in the plasma (PaO_2).
2. How fast is it flowing? CO is used to look at oxygen delivery (DO_2).

First, how much oxygen is in the blood? Oxygen in the blood is either carried on the hemoglobin or dissolved in the plasma. Oxygen carried on the hemoglobin is the oxygen saturation (SaO_2). The SaO_2 represents 98 percent of the oxygen content of the blood. This is clearly where most of the oxygen is located. The SaO_2 is routinely monitored with pulse or ear oximetry and can also be found on the arterial blood gas slip. Oxygen is also carried in the blood dissolved in the plasma. Oxygen dissolved in plasma comprises a very minuscule part of the arterial oxygen content (CaO_2). Oxygen dissolved in the plasma (PaO_2) is available on the arterial blood gas slip. The PaO_2 comprises only 2 percent of the oxygen content in the blood.

Arterial blood oxygen content (CaO_2) is measured in volume percent, which represents the amount of oxygen in 100 mL of blood. Normal is 20.1 vol %. Most critical care monitors calculate the CaO_2, requiring only the input of the patient's hemoglobin, SaO_2, and PaO_2. The formula is listed below:

Arterial oxygen content (normal = 20.1 vol %)

$$CaO_2 = 1.34 \times Hgb \times SaO_2 \quad + \quad 0.0031 \times PaO_2$$

(represents O_2 attached to hemoglobin) (represents O_2 dissolved in plasma)

The constant (1.34) represents the maximum amount of oxygen carried by 1 g of hemoglobin (Hgb). An example is provided to demonstrate the importance of considering the CaO_2 content.

Mark P is a 22-year-old trauma patient. His hemodynamic profile is good, with a CO of 6.8 and an index of 3.1. The SaO_2 is 98 percent and the PaO_2 is 94 mm Hg. Hemoglobin is 9.0/dL. Vital signs are stable and he clearly looks good on paper. However, Mark is tachypneic, tachycardic, and dusky, and his SvO_2 has been dropping. Taking the trouble to learn his oxygen content provides an answer and direction for intervention.

$$1.34 \times Hgb\ (9) \times SaO_2\ (0.98) = 11.8 \text{ vol } \%$$

Normal oxygen content, or CaO_2, is 20.1 vol %. Mark's CaO_2 is only 58 percent of normal.

Clearly, oxygen content is a problem. Notice that the content of the oxygen dissolved in the plasma (PaO_2) was omitted from the formula. In the example provided above, the amount of oxygen dissolved in Mark's plasma (PaO_2 = 94 mm Hg) calculates to be only 0.29 ($0.0031 \times 94 = 0.29$). Added to the CaO_2 of 11.8 vol %, Mark's oxygen content would increase to only 12.09 vol %. Although the PaO_2 is an important parameter, it is only a minuscule part of the oxygen content formula and is often omitted with minimal effect.

NURSING IMPLICATIONS. Mark's dropping SvO_2 prompted further evaluation in the face of good hemodynamics and vital signs. He is symptomatic and clearly needs more oxygen-carrying capacity. Interventions should be directed toward reducing the oxygen demand by actions that include relieving pain, reducing fever, reducing the work of breathing, and providing for rest. The oxygen supply side can be addressed by determining and correcting any source of blood loss and by transfusing blood as ordered.

(*Note:* **Venous oxygen content [CvO_2]** can also be calculated. The same formula is used, but the SvO_2 is substituted for the SaO_2 in the formula. The normal venous oxygen content is 15.5 vol % based on a normal venous oxygen saturation of 75 percent.)

Oxygen Delivery

Now that oxygen content is known, we need to know how fast the oxygen is delivered to the tissues. This is the second piece of information needed to determine the amount of oxygen supplied to the tissues. CO is the method through which oxygen is delivered to the tissues. **Oxygen delivery (DO_2)** is measured in milliliters of oxygen per minute. Normal DO_2 is 1,000 to 1,200 mL O_2/min. Most critical care monitors calculate the DO_2. The formula is listed below:

Oxygen delivery (DO_2) (normal = 1,000–1,200 mL O_2/min)

$$DO_2 = CO \times CaO_2 \times 10$$

In this formula, CO represents CO and CaO_2 represents the oxygen content. The number 10 is a factor necessary to provide a common denominator for CO, which is expressed in liters per minute, and oxygen content, which is expressed in milliliters of oxygen per 100 mL blood. An example is provided to demonstrate the importance of oxygen delivery.

Kathy P is a 22-year-old college student admitted to the ICU with hypothermia and a suspected cardiac contusion following a motorcycle crash. Core temperature is 96°F (35.5°C). CO is 4.0 L/min and hemoglobin is 13.5. Wedge pressure is elevated at 18, and the systemic vascular resistance index is up, at 3,500. SaO_2 is 98 percent. PaO_2

is 96 mm Hg. She is tachycardic and shivering. Her SvO_2 has been dropping. Taking the trouble to learn her oxygen delivery provides an answer and direction for intervention.

$$DO_2 = CO\ (4.0) \times CaO_2\ (17.7) \times 10 = 708\ mL/O_2/min$$

Normal DO_2 is 1,000 to 1,200 $mL/O_2/min$. Kathy's oxygen delivery is only 708 $mL/O_2/min$, which is less than 70 percent of normal. Her hemoglobin is 13.5, which is good for a young female of menstruation age. Tachycardia is her body's attempt to increase CO and thereby improve oxygen delivery. In spite of the tachycardia, CO is only 4.0, which is the lower limit of normal. Preload is too high at 18 (normal is 8 to 12), and elevated preload is likely a result of cardiac contusion, which is treated much like a myocardial infarction. Afterload also is way too high: the SVRI is 3,500 (normal is 1,979 to 2,390). Usually, afterload is not that important in a 22 year old, but Kathy has a cardiac contusion. Vasoconstriction is the normal physiologic response to hypothermia. Peripheral vasoconstriction shunts blood back to the core, and increases preload, which is already evidenced in a PAWP of 18 mm Hg. Vasoconstriction also increases the SVR, and Kathy's elevated afterload reduces CO. Shivering significantly increases the oxygen demand of the muscles. Clearly, there are multiple reasons for a dropping SvO_2.

NURSING IMPLICATIONS. Kathy needs a higher CO to improve oxygen delivery. Immediate interventions include supplemental oxygen to increase supply, along with measures that will reduce oxygen demand until the CO can be improved. Of primary importance is warming Kathy to normothermia. Correcting hypothermia will accomplish several things. Shivering will stop and this will reduce a high oxygen demand by the muscles. The vasoconstriction caused by hypothermia will resolve and directly reduce afterload. Reversal of vasoconstriction will also reduce preload. Blood previously shifted to the core by hypothermia created a relative hypervolemia, which may correct when blood flows back to the warmer periphery. With less afterload, the heart should be able to increase the stroke volume, which will further reduce preload and importantly increase the CO. Hemodynamics

A. Endotracheal Suctioning

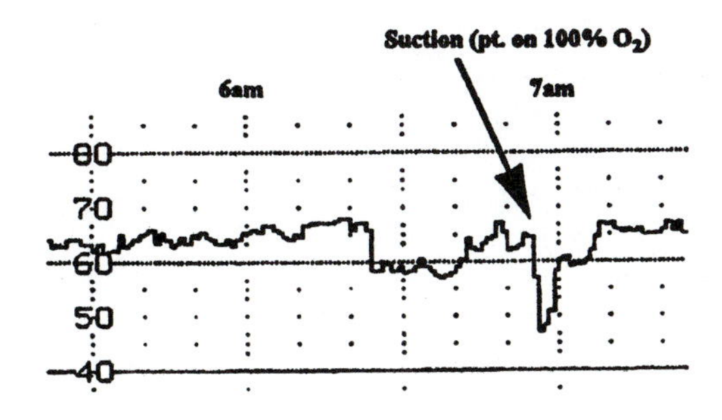

B. Cardiac Tamponade

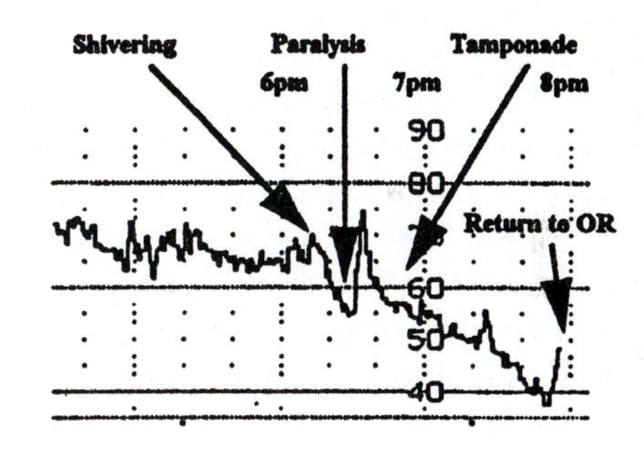

C. Fluid Volume Deficit

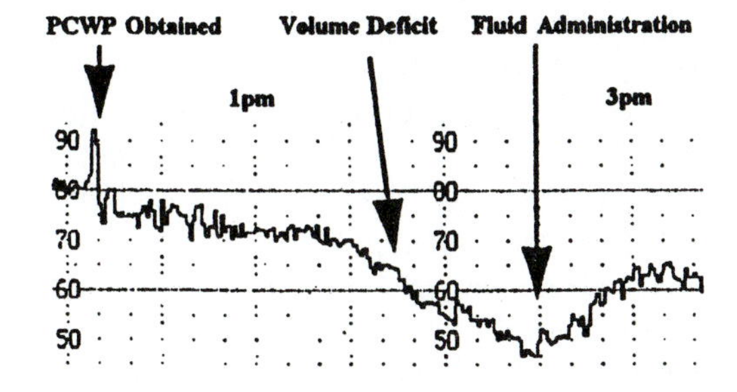

D. Increased O_2 Consumption

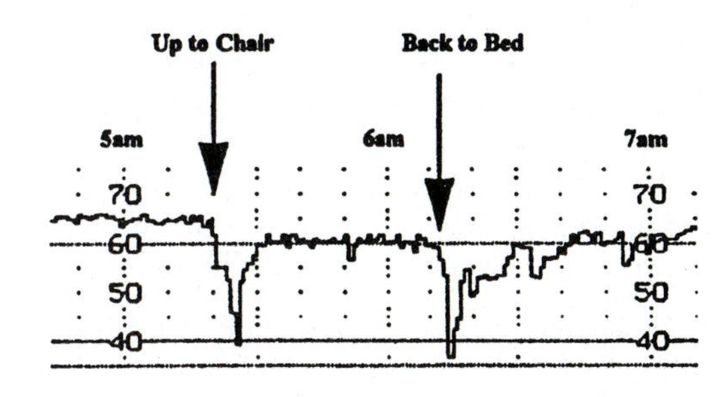

Figure 14–13. Comparison of SvO_2 patterns. *(Used with permission from Cathelyn, J.L., & Samples, D.A. (1998) SvO_2 monitoring: Tool for evaluating patient outcomes.* Dimensions Crit Care Nurs *17(2):58–66. Copyright © Springhouse Corporation/www.springnet.com.)*

and oxygenation should be reassessed after these measures for further direction. Following the SvO_2 will let the nurse know how Kathy is responding to interventions.

Oxygen Consumption

Oxygen consumption (VO_2) is the amount of oxygen that is actually utilized by the tissues. Oxygen consumption is measured in milliliters of oxygen per minute, and is the difference between the oxygen delivered to the tissues (DO_2) and the oxygen transported in the mixed venous blood (SvO_2). Normal oxygen consumption by the tissues is 250 to 300 mL/O_2/min.

Most critical care computers calculate the VO_2 as a part of the hemodynamics and oxygenation program. The formula is listed below:

Oxygen consumption (VO_2)

$$VO_2 = \underset{\text{cardiac output}}{CO} \times \underset{\text{hemoglobin}}{Hgb} \times \underset{\text{K factor (a constant)}}{13.4} \times (SaO_2 - SvO_2)$$

Tissues normally consume 250 to 300 mL of oxygen each minute. Oxygen consumption is an important nursing consideration, because it is not uncommon to see critically ill patients, regardless of diagnosis, double their metabolic rate. Stress alone can do that. Shivering can double the oxygen need. Fever increases the metabolic rate by 10 percent for each degree Celsius. Severe infections can increase oxygen demand by 60 percent.

Small increases in activity can result in a significant increase in the tissues' need for oxygen. Nurses must be aware of common activities that increase oxygen consumption, and space the timing of these activities. Getting a bed bath can increase oxygen consumption by 18 percent. Weighing on a sling scale can temporarily increase the oxygen demand by 36 percent. Repositioning and chest x-rays increase the demand another 25 to 30 percent.

A CO that falls well within the "normal" range may not be adequate to meet the tissues' demands for oxygen. As the demand for oxygen to fuel these needs goes up, the first result seen may be a dropping SvO_2. These patients are using their "reserve" oxygen supply. Knowledge of oxygenation and use of SvO_2 as an early warning signal can allow earlier intervention and an opportunity to improve outcomes. This is an important consideration in planning how care is delivered to patients who cannot effectively increase their oxygen supply (DO_2) to meet their oxygen demand (VO_2). The inability to regulate CO to meet tissue needs will be evidenced by a falling SvO_2.

NURSING CONSIDERATIONS. There are a few differences to note during insertion of this special PA catheter that is capable of reading SvO_2. The subclavian approach may not work as well as the jugular approach, because the bend under the clavicle sometimes interrupts the transmission of light. The optic catheter is fairly tough and holds up well to stretching, but tight bends or tight sutures can break the fiber-optic. Also, pulling on the catheter sharply where the optic attaches to the computer cable can break the connection and turn the catheter into a basic PA catheter. The SvO_2 catheter should be calibrated before insertion and at least once daily according to unit policy.

Figure 14–13 compares SvO_2 patterns of a patient experiencing changes in oxygenation due to nursing procedures (endotracheal suctioning and transfer) and clinical

TABLE 14–1. CAUSES OF DECREASED AND INCREASED SvO_2

Decreased SvO_2

1. Decreased oxygen supply
   - Decreased cardiac output
     - Heart failure
     - Hypovolemia
     - Dysrhythmias
     - Cardiac depressants (i.e., beta blockers)
   - Decreased oxygen saturation
     - Respiratory failure
     - Pulmonary infiltrates
     - Suctioning
     - Ventilator disconnection
   - Decreased hemoglobin
     - Anemia
     - Hemorrhage
2. Increased oxygen consumption
   - Hyperthermia
   - Seizures
   - Shivering
   - Pain
   - Increased work of breathing
   - Increased metabolic rate
   - Exercise
   - Agitation

Increased SvO_2[a]

1. Increased oxygen supply
   - Increased cardiac output
     - Inotropic drugs
     - Intra-aortic balloon pump
     - Afterload reduction
     - Early septic shock
   - Increased oxygen saturation
     - Increased FIO_2 (inspired oxygen)
     - Improvement in lung problem
   - Increased hemoglobin
     - Blood transfusion
2. Decreased oxygen demand
   - Hypothermia
   - Fever reduction
   - Sepsis (late stages)
   - Paralysis
   - Pain relief
   - Anesthesia

[a]A wedged pulmonary artery catheter may result in a falsely elevated SvO_2.

conditions (cardiac tamponade and fluid volume deficit). By assessing drops in SvO_2, the nurse can judge when the patient is able to tolerate interventions (Cathelyn & Samples, 1998).

In summary, SvO_2 provides information about the adequacy of the CO in meeting the oxygen needs of the tissues. It may provide an early warning of a deteriorating hemodynamic status, prompting the clinician to obtain current hemodynamic parameters. SvO_2 can provide current information on the patient's response to titration of vasoactive drips, volume loading, ventilator changes, suctioning, and the effects of patient activity. Table 14–1 lists some causes of decreased and increased SvO_2.

SECTION NINE REVIEW

1. If a person's CO is normal but the SvO_2 is abnormal, what does this indicate?
   A. the current oxygen supply is inadequate to match current oxygen demands
   B. decreased contractility
   C. fluid volume excess
   D. oxygen supply exceeds oxygen demands
2. SvO_2 is measured by
   A. peripheral venous blood gas
   B. peripheral arterial blood gas diluted with a peripheral venous blood gas
   C. pulmonary arterial catheter with an oximetry port
   D. central venous catheter
3. A patient with a 10 g/dL hemoglobin level and a SvO_2 level of 60 percent has a venous oxygen content of the blood of
   A. 8.0 vol %
   B. 2.2 vol %
   C. 80 vol %
   D. 22 vol %
4. A person who is tachycardic with a normal hemoglobin and a normal CO may be exhibiting signs of
   A. decreased oxygen delivery
   B. decreased contractility
   C. anemia
   D. increased oxygen supply

Answers: 1. A, 2. C, 3. A, 4. A

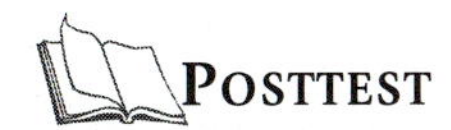

POSTTEST

Do not refer to the text to answer these questions.

1. In viewing a CO curve, a large curve indicates
   A. a normal CO
   B. a high CO
   C. a low CO
   D. an error in technique
2. CI is more specific than CO because
   A. CI is a direct measurement instead of an estimate
   B. CI takes the size of the patient into consideration
   C. CO can be affected by afterload
   D. CO is dependent on patient position
3. The hemodynamic measurement for right heart preload is
   A. PAWP
   B. PAS pressure
   C. right atrial pressure
   D. CO
4. Afterload is best defined as the
   A. volume filling the ventricle at end diastole
   B. blood ejected from the heart in 1 minute
   C. resistance to ventricular ejection
   D. ability of the cardiac muscle to contract
5. It is important to recognize a right ventricular waveform because
   A. a catheter in the right ventricle can induce dysrhythmias
   B. this pattern is the one that should be monitored constantly
   C. this is the best indicator of hemodynamic status
   D. the catheter tip should be in the right ventricle at all times
6. A normal PA pressure waveform will demonstrate which of the following characteristics?
   A. soft undulating pattern
   B. steep upstroke followed by a sharp downstroke
   C. sharply notched upstroke with a steep downstroke
   D. steep upstroke and a downstroke distinguished by a dicrotic notch
7. PAWP is the hemodynamic measurement for
   A. right ventricular preload
   B. right ventricular contractility
   C. left ventricular preload
   D. left ventricular afterload

8. The nurse would expect primary intervention for a symptomatic patient with a PAWP of 3 mm Hg to be
   A. fluid restriction
   B. decreasing preload
   C. volume replacement
   D. decreasing afterload
9. To assess the afterload status of the left ventricle, one should
   A. calculate the pulmonary vascular resistance
   B. calculate the systemic vascular resistance
   C. determine the mean arterial pressure
   D. determine the CI
10. Which is the most important parameter to follow when titrating inotropic drugs on a patient with poor left ventricular function?
    A. CO
    B. CI
    C. MAP
    D. RAP
11. Mixed venous oxygen saturation provides information about
    A. the arterial oxygen content
    B. oxygen delivery
    C. the adequacy of the CO
    D. contractility of the heart
12. Left ventricular stroke work index provides information about
    A. left ventricle preload
    B. contractility
    C. afterload
    D. right heart function
13. A person with a high V_{O_2} level may require all of the following EXCEPT
    A. frequent rest periods between nursing interventions
    B. less oxygen supply
    C. nonrebreather oxygen mask
    D. repositioning

POSTTEST ANSWERS

Question	Answer	Section	Question	Answer	Section
1	C	Two	8	C	Six
2	B	Two	9	B	Eight
3	C	Three	10	B	Eight
4	C	Three	11	C	Nine
5	A	Four	12	B	Nine
6	D	Five	13	B	Nine
7	C	Six			

REFERENCES

Boldt, J., Menges, T., Wollbruck, M., Hammermann, H., & Hempelmann, G. (1994). Is continuous CO measurement using thermodilution reliable in the critically ill patient? *Crit Care Med 22*(12):1913–1918.

Cathelyn, J.L., & Samples, D.A. (1998). $S\bar{v}O_2$ monitoring: Tool for evaluating patient outcomes. *Dimensions Crit Care Nurs 17*(2):58–66.

Headley, J.M. (1998). Invasive hemodynamic monitoring: Applying advanced technologies. *Crit Care Nurs Q 21*(3):73–84.

Ramsey, J.D., & Tisdale, L.A. (1995). Use of ventricular stroke work index and ventricular function curves: Assessing myocardial contractility. *Crit Care Nurse 15*(2):61–67.

Wallace, D., & Winslow, E. (1993). Effects of iced and room temperature injectate on cardiac output measurements in critically ill patients with low and high cardiac outputs. *Heart Lung* 22:55–63.

MODULE 15

Acute Cardiac Dysfunction and Electrocardiographic Monitoring

Pamela Stinson Kidd, Megan Switzer

This self-study module is written at the core knowledge level for individuals who provide nursing care for acutely ill patients. It consists of two parts. Part I (Sections One through Ten) provides a basic review of common dysrhythmias. The module translates the cardiac cycle in order to promote understanding of the implications of dysrhythmias. Guidelines for electrocardiogram (ECG) interpretations are included. The module does not attempt to discuss every potential dysrhythmia a nurse may encounter in the clinical setting. Instead, it provides a systematic approach to understanding automaticity and conduction that can then be applied to practical situations. The learner must go to outside sources for additional experience in ECG interpretation. Section One discusses automaticity. Sections Two and Three include guidelines for interpreting ECG patterns and normal sinus rhythm. Section Four addresses who is at risk for dysrhythmias. Sections Five through Ten cover basic dysrhythmias. Part II (Sections Eleven through Sixteen) discusses interventions that promote perfusion. Section Eleven describes the events associated with acute coronary syndromes, including myocardial infarction. Section Twelve provides a review of thrombolytic therapy. Basic pharmacology and electrical treatment of common dysrhythmias are addressed in Sections Thirteen and Fourteen, respectively. Section Fifteen describes new procedures used to maximize the pumping action and/or vascular supply of the heart. The module ends with a discussion of nursing assessment for the patient with a perfusion problem (Section Sixteen). Each section includes a set of review questions to help the learner evaluate his or her understanding of the section's content before moving on to the next section. All Section Reviews and the module Pretest and Posttest include answers. It is suggested that the learner review those concepts answered incorrectly in the review questions before proceeding to the next section.

OBJECTIVES

Following completion of this module, the learner will be able to

1. Describe the membrane permeability changes of cardiac cells.
2. Discuss the relationship between membrane permeability and serum electrolyte levels.
3. Describe the normal cardiac conduction system.
4. Identify common ECG patterns reflecting abnormal cardiac automaticity (sinus, atrial, junctional, and ventricular origin).
5. Identify common ECG patterns reflecting abnormal cardiac conduction.
6. Describe ECG patterns commonly associated with acute coronary syndromes including myocardial infarction.
7. Discuss indications for thrombolytic therapy.
8. Identify nursing responsibilities in thrombolytic therapy.
9. Discuss medications frequently used in treating cardiac pumping and rhythm problems.
10. Identify nursing responsibilities associated with cardiac pacing and caring for the patient with an implantable cardioverter defibrillator (ICD).
11. Identify nursing responsibilities when caring for a patient having cardiac monitoring.

12. Describe new procedures designed to improve coronary perfusion.
13. Discuss nursing assessment of a patient with a coronary perfusion problem.

PRETEST

1. The isoelectric line on the ECG pattern represents
   A. depolarization of cardiac cells
   B. an ectopic pacemaker
   C. the resting membrane potential
   D. cellular influx of potassium
2. Which of the following statements reflects events during the relative refractory period?
   A. there is a temporary decrease in excitability
   B. the cell can respond to a stimulus of greater intensity than normal
   C. depolarization occurs
   D. a flux of negatively charged ions out of the cell occurs
3. Failure to sense means that an artificial pacing device is
   A. not producing depolarization
   B. competing with the patient's own rhythm
   C. allowing ectopic beats to occur
   D. producing conduction delays
4. Digitalis glycosides may do all of the following EXCEPT
   A. increase the heart's sensitivity to electrical shock
   B. slow impulse conduction
   C. decrease automaticity of junction
   D. block the effect of catecholamines
5. P waves in sinus rhythms
   A. are always positively deflected
   B. should precede the QRS complex
   C. are 0.08 second in length
   D. are followed immediately by a T wave
6. Hyperkalemia produces
   A. tall, peaked T waves
   B. absent T waves
   C. flat T waves
   D. inverted T waves
7. Junctional rhythms commonly occur
   A. as a protective mechanism in sinoatrial (SA) node abnormalities
   B. in response to ventricular escape beats
   C. as an indication of reperfusion in thrombolytic therapy
   D. when a pacing device fails to capture
8. In a fast-paced rhythm (> 100 bpm), which of the following is the most plausible?
   A. the parasympathetic nervous system is stimulated
   B. the atrioventicular (AV) node is pacing the heart
   C. ventricular conduction is slowed
   D. decreased cardiac output may occur
9. Sinus dysrhythmia is usually
   A. a warning sign of impending heart failure
   B. life threatening
   C. harmless
   D. related to chronic coronary problems
10. The main difference between ventricular tachycardia and ventricular fibrillation is
    A. absence of P waves
    B. regularity of R–R interval
    C. widening of the QRS complex
    D. lengthening of the PR interval
11. Supraventricular tachycardia is
    A. produced by a ventricular pacemaker
    B. the result of delayed atrioventricular conduction
    C. produced by a cell functioning as a pacemaker above the ventricles
    D. associated with sympathetic response to pain
12. The ventricular rate in atrial flutter is
    A. greater than 250 bpm
    B. dependent on the number of impulses that pass through the AV node
    C. regular
    D. greater than the atrial rate
13. In ventricular tachycardia, the
    A. P waves are inverted
    B. QRS complexes are less than 0.12 second
    C. R–R interval is irregular
    D. P waves are usually buried in the QRS complexes
14. The difference between type I and type II second-degree heart block is
    A. dropping of a QRS complex
    B. rate of the rhythm
    C. progressive lengthening of the PR interval
    D. widening of the QRS complex
15. Premature ventricular contractions (PVCs) may be treated in all of the following circumstances EXCEPT when
    A. the patient is asymptomatic
    B. they occur in a couplet only
    C. they are multiformed
    D. they occur in a bigeminy pattern
16. Complete heart block is characterized by
    A. lengthening of the PR interval
    B. dropping of the QRS complex
    C. regular P–P and R–R intervals
    D. QRS complexes greater than 0.12 second
17. Which of the following individuals would be eligible for thrombolytic therapy?
    A. 50 year old with a history of a CVA 2 months ago
    B. 65 year old with chest pain relieved by three nitroglycerin tablets

C. 60 year old with chest pain of 2 hours' duration and ST elevation in two contiguous leads
D. 30 year old with ST elevation in two contiguous leads and blood pressure 220/120 mm Hg

18. An elevated ST segment suggests
A. ventricular irritability
B. impaired ventricular depolarization
C. impaired atrial depolarization
D. impaired ventricular repolarization

19. Which of the following ECG changes usually are present in myocardial infarction?
A. T wave and ST segment changes
B. P wave changes
C. lengthening of the PR and ST segments
D. PVCs

20. Tissue plasminogen activator (t-PA) may produce which of the following complications?
A. anaphylaxis
B. hives
C. hematuria
D. vomiting

21. Which of the following patients may need the skin prepared in order to obtain a good connection for the monitoring electrode?
A. dyspneic patient
B. diaphoretic patient
C. obese patient
D. elderly patient

22. If a patient presents in sinus tachycardia, which of the following would NOT be important to note in his history?
A. caffeine intake
B. takes Lasix PRN for "bloating"
C. history of mitral valve prolapse
D. presence and character of cough

23. Bypass-supported angioplasty is used for patients
A. undergoing coronary artery bypass graft (CABG)
B. with chronic hypertension
C. who are at high surgical risk
D. with chronic supraventicular tachycardia (SVT)

24. The circumflex artery
A. is a branch of the right coronary artery
B. perfuses the right ventricle
C. may perfuse the posterior of the heart
D. is a branch of the left anterior descending artery

25. If a patient has a blockage of the right coronary artery (RCA), the nurse should anticipate
A. bundle branch blocks
B. atrial arrhythmias
C. complete heart block
D. anterior wall myocardial infarction

Pretest answers: 1. C, 2. B, 3. B, 4. D, 5. B, 6. A, 7. A, 8. D, 9. C, 10. B, 11. C, 12. B, 13. D, 14. C, 15. A, 16. C, 17. C, 18. D, 19. A, 20. C, 21. B, 22. D, 23. C, 24. C, 25. B

GLOSSARY

Absolute refractory period. The period after an action potential when a stimulus cannot produce a second action potential no matter how strong the stimulus is

Action potential. Signal produced from rapid change in membrane permeability that is transmitted from one part of the nerve or muscle cell to another

Automaticity. Ability to initiate an impulse

Bigeminy. A cardiac rhythm of one SA node–generated beat followed by one premature ventricular contraction

Cardioversion. A synchronized direct current electrical countershock that depolarizes all the cells simultaneously, allowing the SA node to resume the pacemaker role

Contractility. The ability of a muscle to shorten when stimulated; in particular, the force of myocardial contraction

Defibrillation. An unsynchronized direct current electrical countershock that depolarizes all the cells simultaneously, allowing the SA node to resume the pacemaker role

Depolarization. A state where the membrane potential is less negative than the resting membrane potential

Edema. Accumulation of excessive fluid in the interstitial spaces

Excitability. Ability to respond to an impulse

Excitation–contraction coupling. Linking of the electrical and mechanical events in the heart; each individual myocardial cell is stimulated to contract sequentially so that contraction of the atria is followed by contraction of the ventricles

Fast response action potential. Action potential of a myocardial working cell. Created by a more negative resting membrane potential, which encourages the rapid entry of sodium into the cell

Isoelectric. Occurs when the muscle is completely polarized or depolarized; no potential is recorded on the ECG

Murmurs. Audible vibrations produced by turbulent blood flow in the heart

Palpitations. Cardiac rhythm abnormalities that produce a skipping sensation in the heart

Plateau phase. Part of the repolarization when the calcium channels open to allow movement of calcium into the cell to help maintain the cell in a depolarized state

Relative refractory period. The period after an action potential when a stimulus can produce a second action potential if the stimulus is greater than threshold level

Repolarization. Return of the cellular membrane to its resting membrane potential

Resting membrane potential. Point at the end of repolarization when the membrane is relatively permeable to potassium but is almost impermeable to sodium; thus, intracellular concentration of potassium is greater than extracellular concentration

S_1. Heart sound produced by closure of the mitral and tricuspid valves

S_2. Heart sound produced by closure of the aortic and pulmonic valves

S_3. Abnormal heart sound in persons over the age of 30 produced by ventricular filling against increased ventricular pressure; appears immediately after S_2 in the cardiac cycle

S_4. Abnormal heart sound produced by decreased ventricular compliance; appears immediately before S_1 in the cardiac cycle

Sarcolemma. Cell membrane of a muscle fiber

Slow response action potential. Action potential of a pacemaker cell characterized by the slow movement of sodium into the cell because the sarcolemma is permeable to sodium ions

Supranormal period. The period after an action potential during which a stimulus that is slightly less than normal can precipitate another action potential

Syncope. A temporary loss of consciousness usually related to decreased cardiac output

Trigeminy. A cardiac rhythm of two SA node–generated beats followed by one premature ventricular contraction

ABBREVIATIONS

ACS. Acute coronary syndromes

AMI. Acute myocardial infarction

AV node. Atrioventricular node

ASPAC. Anisoylated plasminogen streptokinase activator complex

CABG. Coronary artery bypass graft

CO. Cardiac output

CPK. Creatine phosphokinase

CVA. Cerebrovascular attack

ECG. Electrocardiogram

J. Joules

ICD. Implantable cardioverter defibrillator

mV. Millivolts

PAC. Premature atrial contraction

PAP. Pulmonary artery pressure

PAWP. Pulmonary artery wedge pressure

PTCA. Percutaneous transluminal coronary angioplasty

PVC. Premature ventricular contraction

SA node. Sinoatrial node

SVR. Systemic vascular resistance

SVT. Supraventricular tachycardia

t-PA. Tissue plasminogen activator

UA. Unstable angina

PART I: CARDIAC MONITORING

SECTION ONE: Membrane Permeability

At the completion of this section, the learner will be able to explain briefly membrane permeability changes in cardiac cells.

The resting membrane potential of cardiac cells is represented by an **isoelectric** line on the ECG pattern. There is no deflection, since there is no movement of ions across the **sarcolemma.** Normally, the intracellular concentration of potassium is greater than the extracellular concentration. The concentration of sodium ions is greater extracellularly. Calcium also has a much higher concentration outside of the cell. The intracellular potential becomes increasingly negative because potassium diffuses externally. In addition, proteins and phosphates remain internally, and they are negatively charged.

There are five phases of an **action potential:** depolarization (phase 0), early repolarization (phase 1), plateau phase (phase 2), repolarization (phase 3), and resting membrane potential (phase 4). During **depolarization,** the cell is almost impermeable to sodium unless a stimulus occurs. This stimulus may be electrical in origin, such as the firing of the sinoatrial (SA) node or defibrillation. Chemical changes also may precipitate depolarization. Hypoxia and its accompanying respiratory acidosis as well as pharmaceutical agents (i.e., sodium bicarbonate) may serve as chemical stimuli. In depolarization, more sodium moves into the cell through the fast sodium channels and creates a **fast response action potential.** The inside of the cell becomes positively charged.

The process of **repolarization** takes place over phases 1, 2, and 3. In early repolarization, sodium channels close. During the **plateau phase,** calcium channels open. These channels are slow in relation to the preceding sodium channels. The influx of calcium helps to maintain the positive charge (depolarization) a little longer. Chemical blockage of the channels may be used to treat cardiac abnormalities. In phase 3, repolarization, potassium moves back into the cell to create the original electrochemical gradient.

During the **resting membrane potential** phase (phase 4), repolarization is completed, and the original electrochemical gradient is in place. The cell is ready to be depolarized again. The **absolute refractory period** begins in phase 0 and lasts until the midpoint of phase 3. During this period, the cell cannot respond to another stimulus regardless of the strength of the stimulus. The **relative refractory period** begins at the midpoint of phase 3 and lasts until the beginning of phase 4. A stronger than normal stimulus may produce depolarization. During the **supranormal period** (phase 4), a weaker than normal stimulus can produce depolarization. A common example of a stimulus producing depolarization during the supranormal or relative refractory period is premature atrial and ventricular beats. These are discussed later in the module. Table 15–1 summarizes the phases of the action potential. The pacemaker cells in the sinoatrial node have a constant sodium influx; thus, they slowly depolarize at a steady rate until threshold is reached and an action potential created. These pacemaker cells do not have a "true" resting membrane phase (Funkhouser, 1994).

TABLE 15–1. PHASES OF AN ACTION POTENTIAL

Phase 0	Depolarization	Movement of sodium into cell (fast channels open)
Phase 1	Early repolarization	Closure of fast sodium channels
Phase 2	Plateau	Calcium moves into cell (slow channels open)
Phase 3	Repolarization	Potassium moves into cell
Phase 4	Resting membrane potential	Electrochemical gradient returned to normal Sarcolemma almost impermeable to sodium

In summary, it is helpful to remember that sodium, calcium, and potassium always are located both intracellularly and extracellularly. The total of these electrolytes remains the same. The action potential changes where the total is distributed, at the location of the ions. Figure 15–1 depicts the ion changes throughout the action potential.

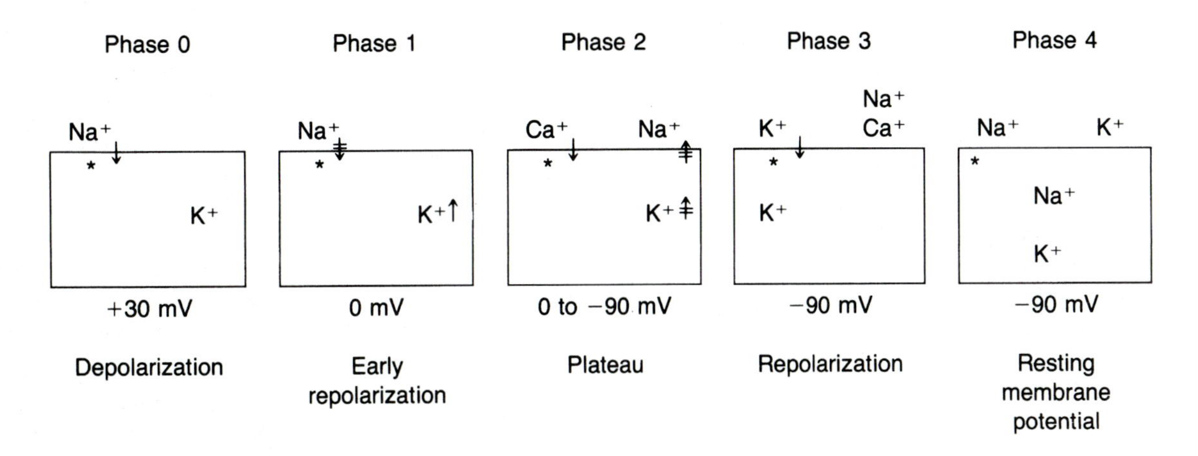

Figure 15–1. Membrane permeability changes in nonpacemaker myocardial cells. Cell membrane permeability changes throughout depolarization and repolarization. * = protein⁻, phosphate⁻; ↑↓ = rapid; ⇞⇟ = slow.

SECTION ONE REVIEW

1. Depolarization may occur in direct response to all of the following EXCEPT
   A. chemical stimuli
   B. acidosis
   C. defibrillation
   D. hyperglycemia
2. Potassium is located primarily
   A. intracellularly
   B. in skeletal muscle
   C. extracellularly
   D. in cardiac muscle
3. During the relative refractory period
   A. a larger than normal stimulus occurs
   B. the SA node fires
   C. depolarization may occur
   D. the cardiac cell is not able to be stimulated
4. The three major electrolytes associated with automaticity are
   A. sodium, potassium, and calcium
   B. potassium, glucose, and sodium
   C. calcium, phosphate, and proteins
   D. potassium, calcium, and phosphate
5. The movement of calcium into the cell promotes
   A. depolarization
   B. repolarization
   C. the refractory period
   D. closure of the slow channels

Answers: 1. D, 2. A, 3. C, 4. A, 5. A

SECTION TWO: Cardiac Conduction

At the completion of this section, the learner will be able to describe the cardiac conduction system and the normal ECG complex.

There are two types of myocardial cells: working cells and pacemaker cells. Pacemaker cells have a **slow response action potential.** The resting membrane potential of pacemaker cells is unstable, and the cell membrane is somewhat permeable to sodium. The slow diffusion of sodium into the cell precipitates depolarization without a preceding impulse. Only pacemaker cells possess **automaticity,** or the ability to initiate an impulse. Conversely, the working cells have a stable resting membrane potential. In order for depolarization to occur, a stimulus must be present. Working cells are responsible for **contractility.** Both working and pacemaker cells have the ability to respond to stimuli **(excitability)** and regularity (rhythmicity) and to conduct impulses.

The SA node is considered to be the pacemaker of the heart, since it controls the heart rate normally between 60 and 100 beats per minute (bpm). When abnormalities occur with the firing of the SA node, another cardiac cell will discharge. An ectopic pacemaker is a new site of impulse formation within the heart. The impulse is transmitted from the atria to the ventricles along a cardiac conduction pathway (Fig. 15–2). Myocardial contraction occurs when the ventricular muscle is stimulated. The combined events of depolarization and repolarization comprise the electrical phases of the cardiac cycle.

The normal ECG complex consists of several components. The P wave indicates atrial depolarization, stimulated by the firing of the SA node. The PR interval depicts atrial conduction of the impulse, through the AV node to the ventricles. The normal length of the PR interval is 0.12 to 0.20 second. A longer PR interval suggests a conduction delay, usually in the area of the AV node.

The QRS complex reflects ventricular depolarization and atrial repolarization. The atrial repolarization is overpowered by the ventricular depolarization because the ventricular muscle mass is larger than that of the atria. Therefore, atrial repolarization is not seen on the ECG. QRS complexes may be of various sizes and configurations. Figure 15–3 illustrates common QRS configurations. The QRS segment is 0.10 second or less in length. A prolonged QRS complex indicates abnormal impulse conduction through the ventricles.

The ST segment demonstrates ventricular conduction. It represents the completion of ventricular depolarization and the beginning of ventricular repolarization. The segment should be isoelectric, with no deflections present, because positive and negative charges are balanced. Deflections in the ST segment usually indicate ventricular muscle injury. The T wave depicts ventricular repolarization. T waves also are affected by ventricular muscle injury because of interference with repolarization. An example of a clinical condition with potential ventricular muscle injury is acute myocardial infarction.

The QT interval represents ventricular depolarization and repolarization. It is measured from the beginning of the QRS complex to the end of the T wave. The QT interval is usually less than 0.40 second in length, depending on heart rate. The QT interval is less than half the R–R interval. As heart rate increases, the QT interval will shorten. If the heart rate decreases, the QT interval will lengthen.

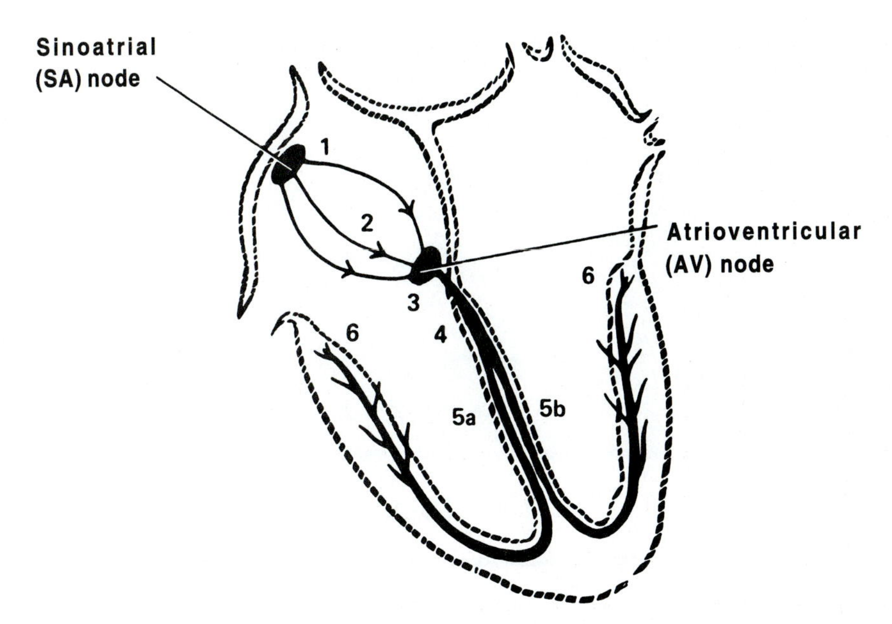

Figure 15–2. Conduction system of the heart. The impulse originates in the SA node (1). It spreads through the atrial muscles along three bands of tissue known as the internodal tracts (2), causing atrial contraction. It reaches the AV node (3), where it is momentarily slowed before passing on to the bundle of His (4). The impulse descends through the bundle of His and down the right and left bundle branches (5a, 5b). Reaching the terminal Purkinje fibers (6), the impulse stimulates the ventricular myocardial cells at the Purkinje–myocardial junction. Ventricular contraction then occurs. *(From Meltzer, L., Pinneo, R., & Kitchell, J. [1983].* Intensive coronary care: A manual for nurses *[p. 116]. (Reprinted by permission of Prentice-Hall, Inc., Upper Saddle River, NJ.)*

Electrical transmission can be connected with mechanical events of the heart. Diastole occurs during atrial depolarization and at the end of ventricular repolarization. This is depicted by the end of the T wave to the R wave on the ECG. During diastole the aortic and pulmonic valves close and the mitral and tricuspid valves open, allowing ventricle filling. Systole begins at the peak of the QRS complex (ventricular depolarization) and continues to the end of the T wave (ventricular repolarization). During systole, the ventricles contract. The increased intraventricular pressure causes the mitral and tricuspid valves to close. The intraventricular pressure exceeds the pressure within the aorta and pulmonary arteries, causing the pulmonic and aortic valves to open. The ventricles eject blood (known as the stroke volume) into the aorta and pulmonary arteries. Some blood remains in the ventricle (known as left ventricular end-diastolic volume, LVEDV). The ejection fraction is the ratio of blood ejected per beat to the LVEDV. Normal ejection fraction is greater than 50 percent (Funkhouser, 1994). Thus, abnormalities in ventricle depolarization decrease

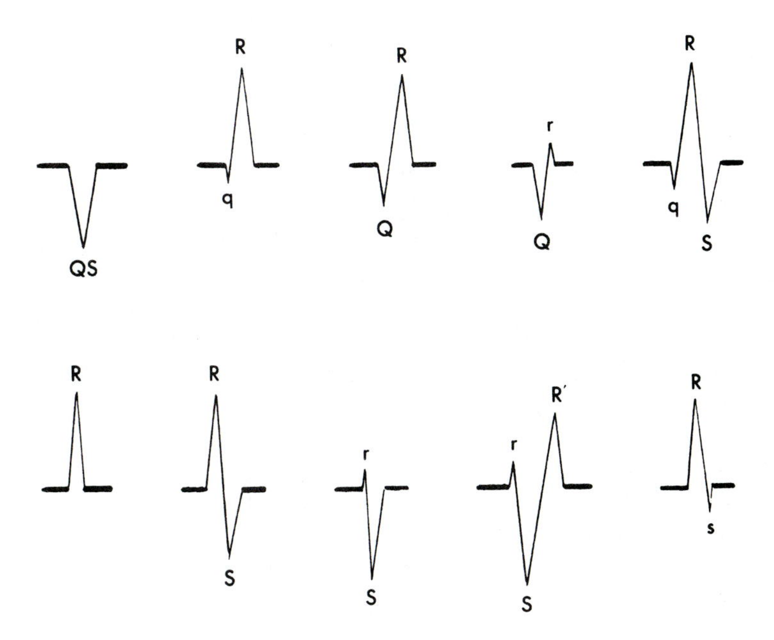

Figure 15–3. Common QRS complex configurations. Lower case letters indicate less-than-normal amplitude. *(From Goldberger, A.L., & Goldberg, E. [1986].* Clinical electrocardiography: A simplified approach, *3rd ed. St. Louis: C.V. Mosby.)*

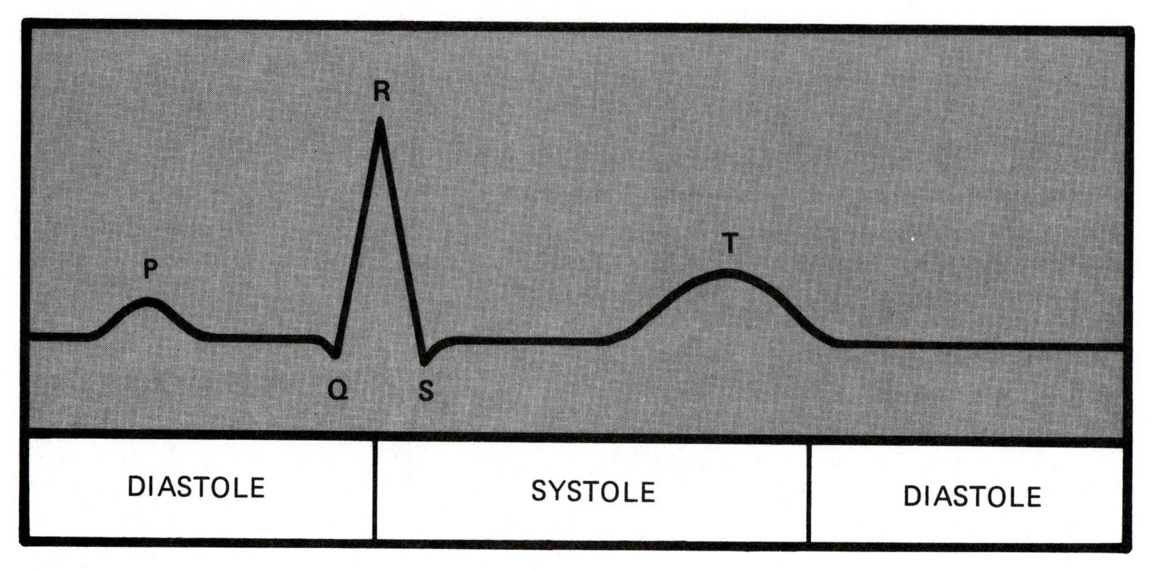

Figure 15–4. Relationship between ECG and cardiac cycle (diastole and systole). (*From Dracup, K. [1995].* Meltzer's intensive coronary care: A manual for nurses, *5th ed. [p. 127]. East Norwalk, CT: Appleton & Lange.)*

stroke volume and the ejection fraction. This relationship helps to explain why cardiac output is affected when a dysrhythmia occurs. Figure 15–4 illustrates the relationship between the ECG and the cardiac cycle.

Nursing Care of a Patient Being Cardiac Monitored

There are several nursing actions for a patient requiring cardiac monitoring. The chest wall should be shaved and treated with an adhesive (i.e., tincture of benzoin, skin preparation) before placement of the electrodes, especially for individuals who are sweating profusely. This will help ensure a good connection. Sites may be rotated every 24 hours to prevent skin breakdown. The sensitivity knob of the cardiac monitor may need to be adjusted to view complexes. Alarms on the monitor should be set and left on and be audible to the nurse. An ECG strip should be recorded and placed in the nursing record on a regular basis.

The patient should have explained to him or her why cardiac monitoring is required. Patients may need to be reassured that they are protected from electric shocks from the equipment. They may need to know that the alarms may sound as a result of patient movement and other factors, in addition to cardiac abnormalities.

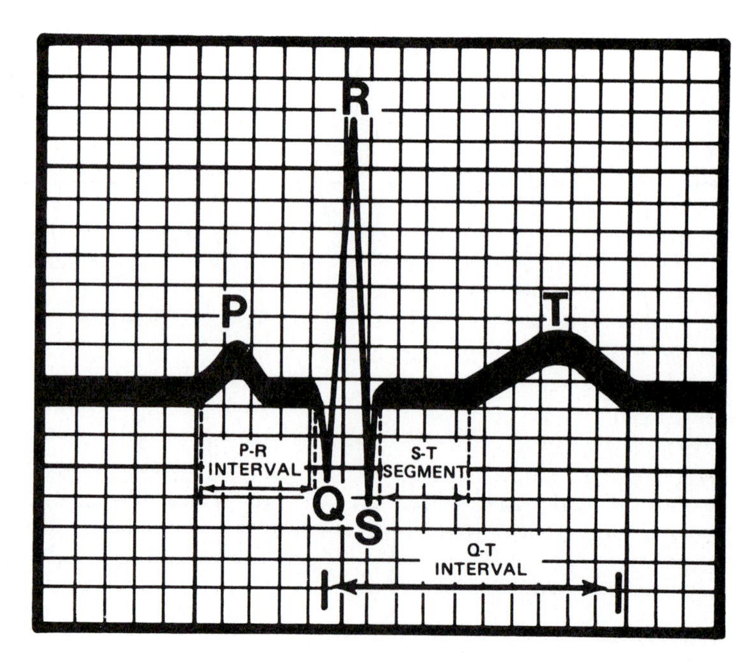

Figure 15–5. Normal cardiac cycle on the ECG. (*From Dracup, K. [1995].* Meltzer's intensive coronary care: A manual for nurses, *5th ed. [p. 127]. East Norwalk, CT: Appleton & Lange.)*

In summary, the ECG reflects the cardiac conduction pathway. Abnormalities in conduction will appear on the ECG. The cardiac cycle depends on proper electrical transmission and conduction in order to maintain an adequate cardiac output. The normal ECG (normal sinus rhythm) has a rate between 60 and 100 bpm. The SA node paces the rhythm (P wave), and the impulse is transmitted to the ventricles within 0.20 second (PR interval). The ventricles depolarize, representing contraction or systole, within 0.10 second. The complete sequence of ventricular events occur within 0.40 second (QT interval). Figure 15–5 is a diagram of a normal ECG.

The nursing care of a patient being cardiac monitored includes decreasing the patient's fear and increasing his or her knowledge regarding the procedure. Interventions can be conducted in a humanistic manner, thereby decreasing anxiety and myocardial oxygen demands through all available routes.

Section Two Review

1. Abnormalities in the firing of the SA node usually
   - A. result in cardiac arrest
   - B. result in the discharging of another pacemaker cell
   - C. produce tachydysrhythmias
   - D. result in heart blocks
2. A PR interval greater than 0.20 second
   - A. is normal
   - B. indicates a pacemaker other than the SA node is firing
   - C. indicates a delay in conduction
   - D. is too fast to maintain adequate cardiac output
3. Atrial repolarization is reflected in the
   - A. P wave
   - B. PR interval
   - C. T wave
   - D. QRS complex
4. The QT interval indicates all of the following EXCEPT
   - A. atrial recovery
   - B. ventricular depolarization
   - C. ventricular recovery
   - D. atrial depolarization
5. Systole is associated with
   - A. ventricular depolarization
   - B. atrial depolarization
   - C. AV nodal conduction
   - D. P wave on the ECG
6. A decreased ejection fraction occurs when
   - A. the atria depolarize abnormally
   - B. the PR interval is prolonged
   - C. the ventricles depolarize abnormally
   - D. the SA node fires abnormally

Answers: 1. B, 2. C, 3. D, 4. D, 5. A, 6. C

SECTION THREE: Interpretation Guidelines

At the completion of this section, the learner will be able to identify a system for interpreting ECG patterns.

The ECG is printed on graph paper. Each small block of the graph paper is equal to 1 mm, or 0.04 second on the horizontal axis. The horizontal axis of the graph paper represents time. The vertical axis of the graph paper represents voltage. Each small block is equivalent to 1 mm (0.1 mV) on the vertical axis. Each large box is 5 mm (0.5 mV). Adjusting the gain control on the ECG monitor alters the height. For the purposes of basic ECG interpretation, time is the most important factor to consider. Since each small block equals 0.04 second, a large block, composed of five small blocks, equals 0.20 second. Five large blocks represent 1 second (Figure 15–6).

There are six steps to follow in interpreting an ECG:

1. Measure the atrial and ventricular rate.
2. Examine the R–R interval.
3. Examine the P wave.
4. Measure the PR interval.
5. Check to see whether P waves are followed by a QRS complex.
6. Examine the QRS complex.

There are three ways the rate can be calculated. The first two methods discussed can be used only when the rate is regular. The number of 0.04-second boxes can be counted between two R waves and divided into 1,500. The number of 0.20-second boxes can be counted between two R waves and divided into 300. The last method is based on a 6-second cardiac strip. ECG paper is marked at the top margin in 3-second intervals. QRS complexes in a 6-second strip (30 large blocks, 150 small blocks) is multiplied by 10 to get the heart rate by minute ($6 \times 10 = 60$ seconds). Figure 15–7 demonstrates all three methods of rate calculation.

Next, the R waves should be examined. If the R waves appear in regular intervals (are constant), the rhythm is described as a regular rhythm. If the R waves do not occur in a regular pattern a dysrhythmia is present.

Normally, P waves precede each QRS complex. If the SA node is not serving as pacemaker and a cell other

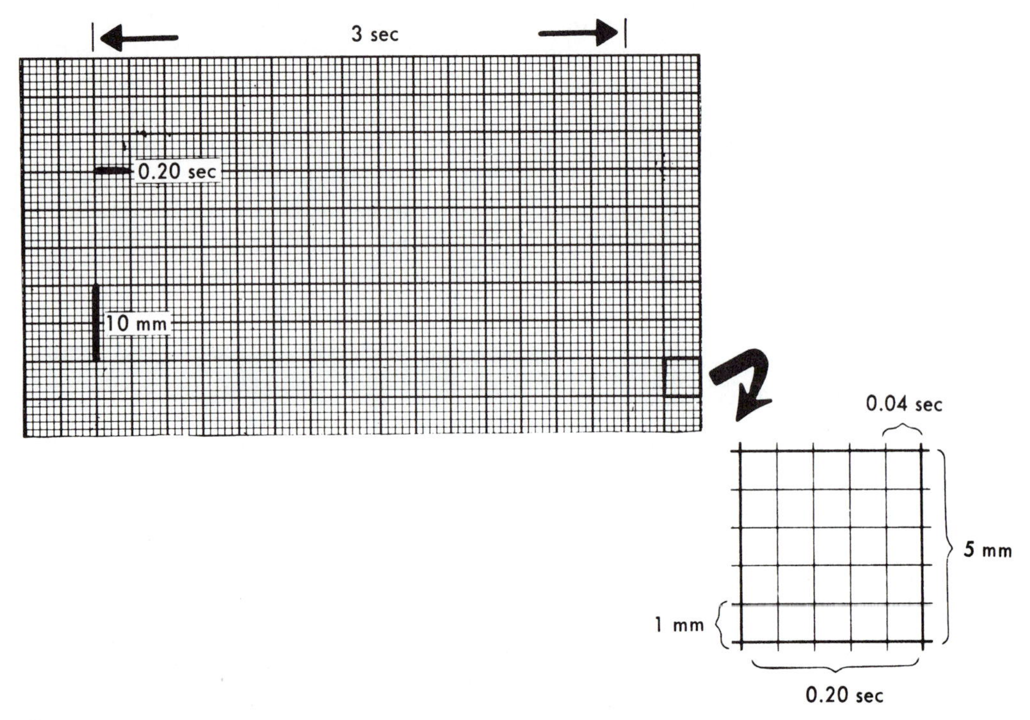

Figure 15–6. ECG paper is a graph divided into millimeter squares. Time is measured on the horizontal axis. With a paper speed of 25 mm/sec, each small (millimeter) box side equals 0.04 second and each larger (5-mm) box side equals 0.2 second. The amplitude of any wave is measured on the vertical axis in millimeters. *(From Goldberger, A.L., & Goldberger, E. [1994].* Clinical electrocardiography: A simplified approach, *5th ed. [p. 25]. St. Louis: C.V. Mosby.)*

than the SA node is serving as the pacemaker, P waves may be absent. Cardiac cells in the area of the AV node can pace the heart at a rate of 40 to 60 bpm. Pacemaker cells in the Purkinje fibers and ventricles pace at a rate less than 40 bpm. Generally, if the atria are discharging chaotically, the rate will be greater than 60 bpm. If the atria are not discharging and the pacer is outside the SA node, the rate is usually less than 60 bpm.

The next step in ECG interpretation is to measure the PR interval. If it is greater than 0.20 second in length, a delay in conduction is present. QRS complexes are always present.

Next, check to see whether P waves are followed by a QRS complex. If P waves are present but they are not followed consistently by a QRS complex, a second- or third-degree heart block (Section Ten) may be present.

The final step is examination of the QRS complexes. The complex should be 0.10 second or less in length unless there is a delay in the impulse reaching the ventricles. A widened QRS complex may mean delayed conduction through the bundle branches, abnormal conduction within the ventricles, or early activation of the ventricles through a bypass route (Lipman & Cascio, 1994).

Figure 15–8 illustrates the application of the principles discussed in this section. The system outlined in this section should provide a consistent and comprehensive approach to ECG interpretation.

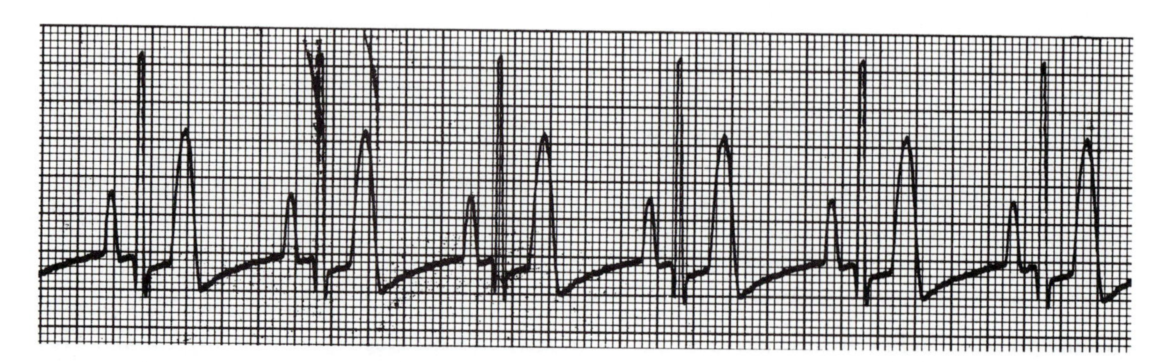

Figure 15–7. Calculation of heart rate. Method 1: Using 0.04-second boxes between R waves: 24 (0.04) boxes: 1,500 divided by 24 = 63 bpm. Method 2: Using 0.20-second boxes between R waves: 4.5 (0.20) boxes: 300 divided by 4.5 = 66 bpm. Method 3: Number of QRS complexes in a 6-second strip = 6:6 times 10 = 60 bpm.

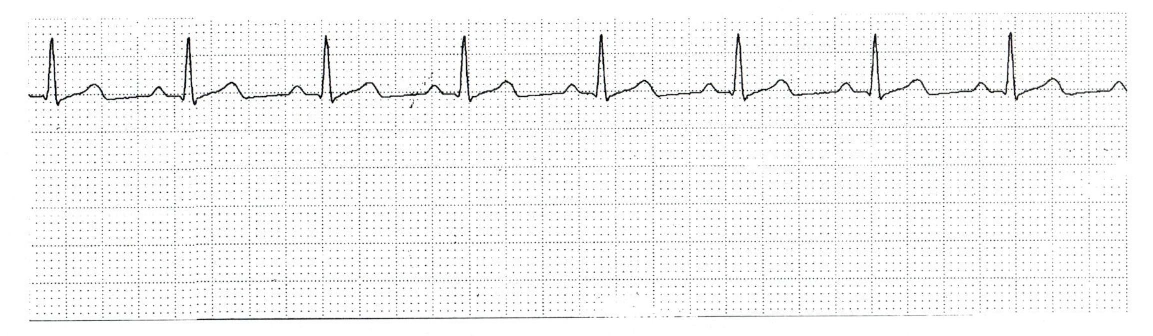

Figure 15–8. Interpretation of ECG using six-step process.

1. Measure the rate. There are 12 QRS complexes in the 6-second strip: $12 \times 10 = 120$. There are 12 small boxes (0.04) between two R waves: $\frac{1,500}{12} = 125$. There are approximately 2.5 large boxes (0.20) between two R waves: $\frac{300}{2.5} = 120$
2. Examine the R–R interval. The interval is regular; therefore, the rhythm is regular.
3. Examine the P wave. The P waves are the same configuration.
4. Measure the PR interval. The interval is constant and measures 4 small boxes (0.4) or 16 seconds.
5. Check to see whether the P waves are followed by a QRS complex. P waves are followed by QRS complex.
6. Examine the QRS complex. The complexes are the same configuration and measure 2 small boxes (0.04) or 8 seconds.

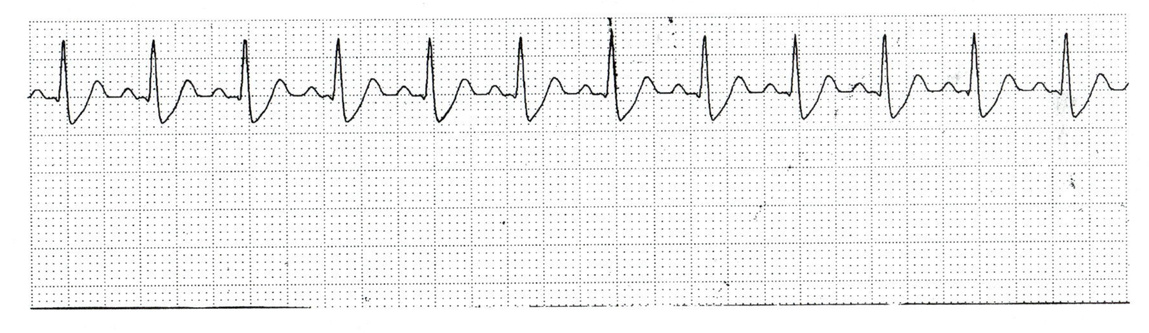

Figure 15–9. Normal sinus rhythm rate equals 1,500 divided by 19 × 0.04-second boxes = 83.

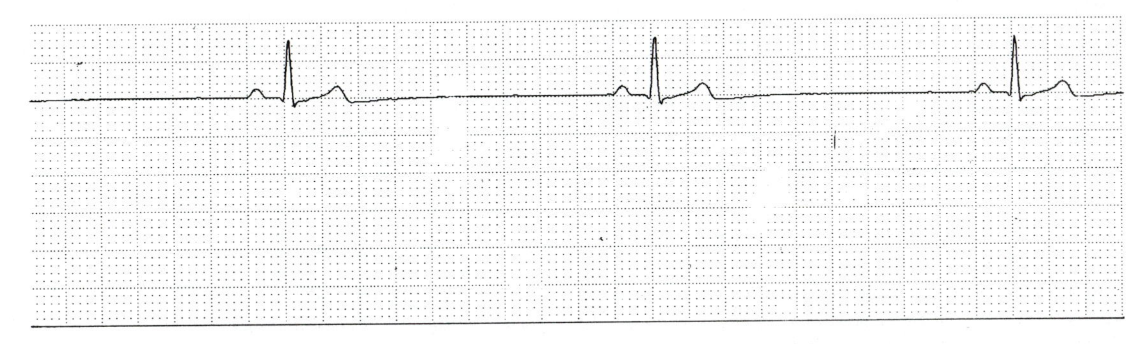

Figure 15–10. Sinus bradycardia rate equals 300 divided by 10 × 0.20-second boxes = 30.

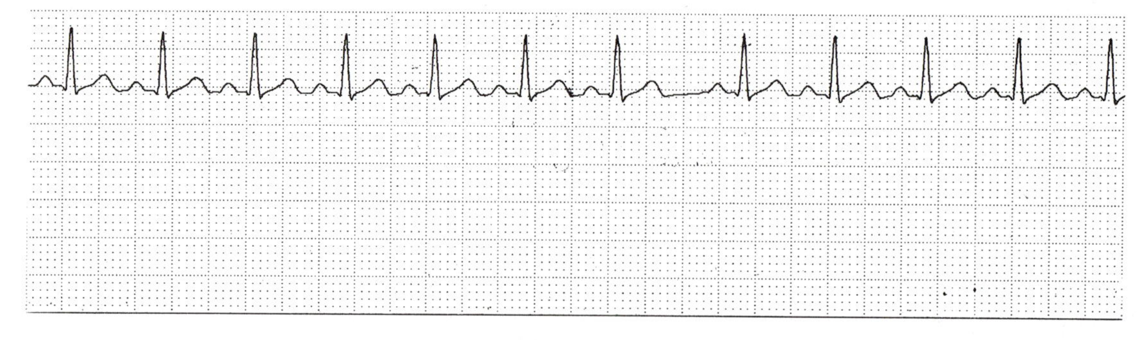

Figure 15–11. The sinus tachycardia rate equals 12 QRS complexes × 10 = 120.

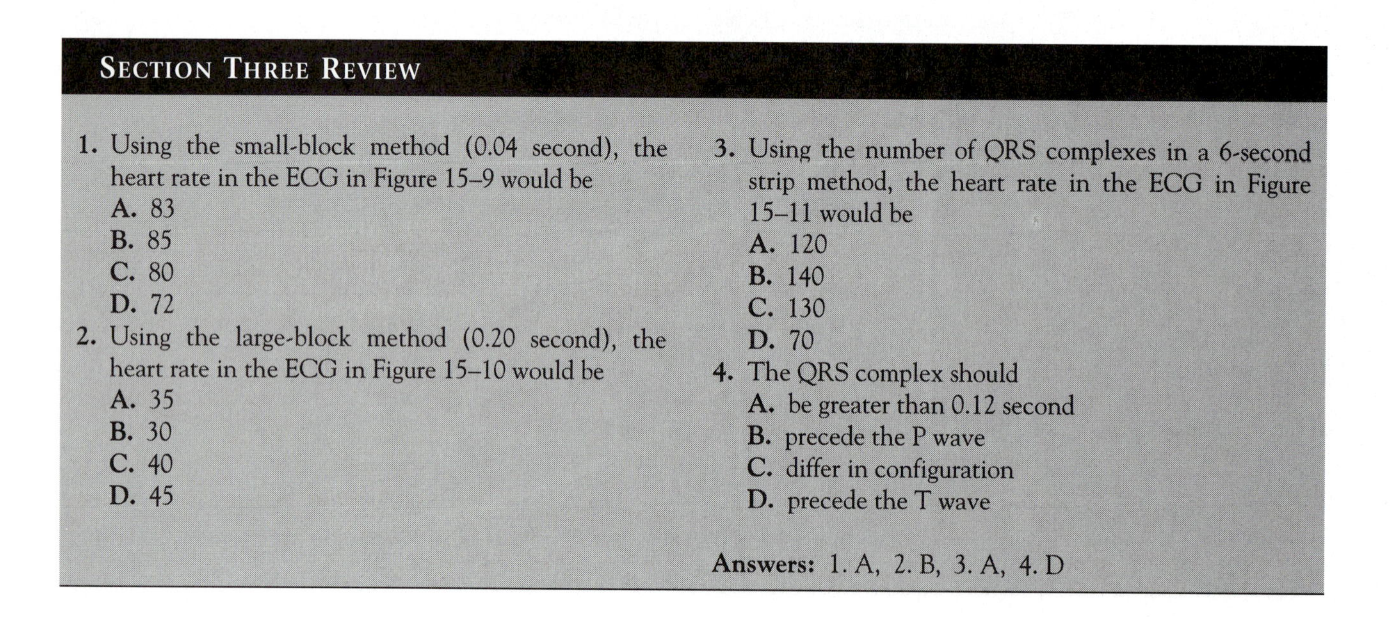

SECTION THREE REVIEW

1. Using the small-block method (0.04 second), the heart rate in the ECG in Figure 15–9 would be
   A. 83
   B. 85
   C. 80
   D. 72
2. Using the large-block method (0.20 second), the heart rate in the ECG in Figure 15–10 would be
   A. 35
   B. 30
   C. 40
   D. 45
3. Using the number of QRS complexes in a 6-second strip method, the heart rate in the ECG in Figure 15–11 would be
   A. 120
   B. 140
   C. 130
   D. 70
4. The QRS complex should
   A. be greater than 0.12 second
   B. precede the P wave
   C. differ in configuration
   D. precede the T wave

Answers: 1. A, 2. B, 3. A, 4. D

SECTION FOUR: At-Risk Factors

At the completion of this section, the learner will be able to identify factors that place a person at risk for developing dysrhythmias.

Anyone who has an alteration in tissue perfusion is at risk for a dysrhythmia. The alteration may be peripheral in nature, as in chronic hypertension. The increased afterload or resistance the heart must pump against in order to maintain an adequate cardiac output (CO) eventually produces ventricular enlargement and decreased contractility (Starling's law). The heart rate will try to increase as a way of maintaining CO, since the stroke volume (SV) is diminished. An alteration in cardiac perfusion due to coronary artery disease predisposes to dysrhythmias because of potential myocardial ischemia. The ventricles will not be able to depolarize as effectively (QRS complex), and repolarization may be inefficient (T wave). Thus, abnormal ventricular beats or blocks in conduction may occur.

A fluid volume deficit encourages the appearance of tachydysrhythmias. The heart rate increases, again in response to a diminished CO. Fluid volume overload eventually will result in ventricular enlargement and decreased contractility. Premature beats, cardiac conduction blocks, and abnormalities in heart rate may appear in response to the excess fluid volume.

Electrolyte abnormalities place a person at risk for dysrhythmias. Hypokalemia decreases the amount of positive ions available to produce depolarization. Depolarization becomes more difficult and repolarization is extended. Therefore, the PR interval may be longer, and the T wave may be flat. The QT interval may lengthen. An extra wave may follow the T wave (U wave). Bradydysrhythmias and conduction blocks are common. Premature ventricular contractions (PVCs) may occur if the heart rate is too slow. Hyperkalemia produces easier depolarization and short repolarization. Tall, peaked T waves are present. The QT interval shortens. Eventually the cell becomes too positive to respond and depolarize, and asystole occurs. Before asystole, the PR interval lengthens, and the QRS complex widens.

Increased levels of calcium strengthen contractility and shorten ventricular repolarization, shortening the QT interval. Hypocalcemia prolongs the QT interval (Love, 1994).

Magnesium is required for intracellular enzyme reactions. A deficit of magnesium will increase the irritability of the nervous system and can produce dysrhythmias. Prominent U waves and a flattening of the T wave may occur (Lipman & Cascio, 1994). Hypermagnesemia is associated with renal failure. Central nervous system depression results. The ECG may demonstrate a prolonged PR interval, wide QRS complexes, bradycardia, and tall, peaked T waves.

Hypothermia decreases the electrical activity of the heart. Thus, bradycardia, prolongation of the PR and QT intervals, and wide QRS complexes may occur.

In summary, a person may be at risk for developing cardiac dysrhythmias if an alteration in tissue perfusion, fluid volume, electrolyte values, or temperature is present.

SECTION FOUR REVIEW

1. Increased afterload increases the risk for dysrhythmias because
   - **A.** it increases automaticity
   - **B.** increasing pressure stimulates ectopic pacemakers
   - **C.** it delays cardiac conduction
   - **D.** it produces an influx of potassium ions
2. Excess fluid volume increases the risk for dysrhythmias because it
   - **A.** increases automaticity
   - **B.** decreases contractility
   - **C.** increases cardiac conduction
   - **D.** produces an influx of sodium ions
3. Hypokalemia results in
   - **A.** delayed conduction
   - **B.** increased automaticity
   - **C.** widened QRS complexes
   - **D.** inverted P waves
4. Hypocalcemia results in
   - **A.** decreased sodium influx into the cell
   - **B.** delayed repolarization
   - **C.** prolonged QT interval
   - **D.** spontaneous conduction
5. Hypermagnesemia may produce
   - **A.** tachydysrhythmias
   - **B.** bradycardia
   - **C.** shortened PR intervals
   - **D.** ST segment depression

Answers: 1. A, 2. B, 3. A, 4. C, 5. B

SECTION FIVE: Sinus Dysrhythmias

At the completion of this section, the learner will be able to describe common dysrhythmias arising from the SA node and their treatment.

Sinus node dysfunction (SND) is associated with heart disease. It usually results from blockages to the right coronary artery or the circumflex artery, since one of these provides the blood flow to the SA node. Usually the first indication of SND is sinus bradycardia (Moungey, 1994).

Sinus bradycardia is described as a heart rate less than 60 bpm and originating from the SA node, as evidenced by a regular P wave preceding each QRS complex. The only abnormality noted in this rhythm is the rate. This rhythm may be present in athletes because they have improved their cardiac muscle and thus their stroke volume (SV). The heart rate can decrease and still maintain an efficient CO. Sinus bradycardia may not be treated unless the person experiences symptoms of decreased CO, such as syncope, hypotension, and angina. If the rate drops too low, the chance of ectopic pacemakers firing increases. Lethal ventricular dysrhythmias may result. Sinus bradycardia is treated by administering atropine because it blocks the parasympathetic innervation to the SA node, allowing normal sympathetic innervation to gain control and increase SA node firing. Figure 15–12 illustrates sinus bradycardia.

Sinus tachycardia has a rapid rate, from 100 to 150 bpm. There are no other abnormal characteristics associated with this rhythm. The rapid rate results from sympathetic nervous stimulation. This stimulation may be in response to fear, increased activity, hypermetabolic states (such as fever), pain, and decreased CO due to hypovolemia or ventricular failure. Sinus tachycardia may produce angina if the CO decreases to the point of decreasing coronary circulation or if myocardial oxygen demand is increased without an increase in coronary circulation. Treatment is aimed at relieving the cause of increased sympathetic stimulation. Nursing measures, such as imagery, distraction, and promoting a calm environment, as well as drug therapy may be necessary. Sedatives, tranquilizers, antianxiety agents, analgesics, and antipyretics may be used. Figure 15–13 is an ECG tracing of sinus tachycardia.

In cases of SND, atrial conduction becomes less effective, and "rescue" rhythms originating elsewhere in the atria

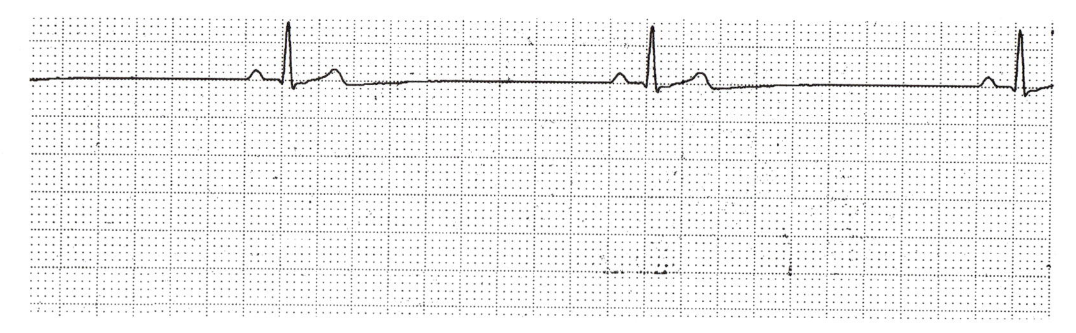

Figure 15–12. Interpretation of sinus bradycardia using the six-step process.
1. Rate = 30
2. R–R interval regular
3. P wave has same configuration
4. PR interval = 0.20
5. P wave precedes QRS: yes
6. QRS complex = 0.04

may occur to maintain cardiac output (e.g., atrial flutter and atrial fibrillation; see Section Six). Ultimately, SND is treated by pacemaker insertion (see Section Fifteen).

In summary, sinus dysrhythmias are characterized by regular rates. They usually are harmless unless CO becomes compromised. The nurse should assess the patient for signs of decreasing level of consciousness, hypotension, and angina. When these symptoms occur, the dysrhythmia is treated. Table 15–2 compares sinus dysrhythmias.

TABLE 15–2. SUMMARY OF DIFFERENCES IN SINUS DYSRHYTHMIAS

RHYTHM	CHARACTERISTICS	TREATMENT STRATEGIES
Sinus bradycardia	Rate < 60 bpm	Atropine
Sinus tachycardia	Rate > 100 bpm and < 150 bpm	Antianxiety measures Pain relief measures Antipyretics Oxygen Digitalis Beta-blocking agents

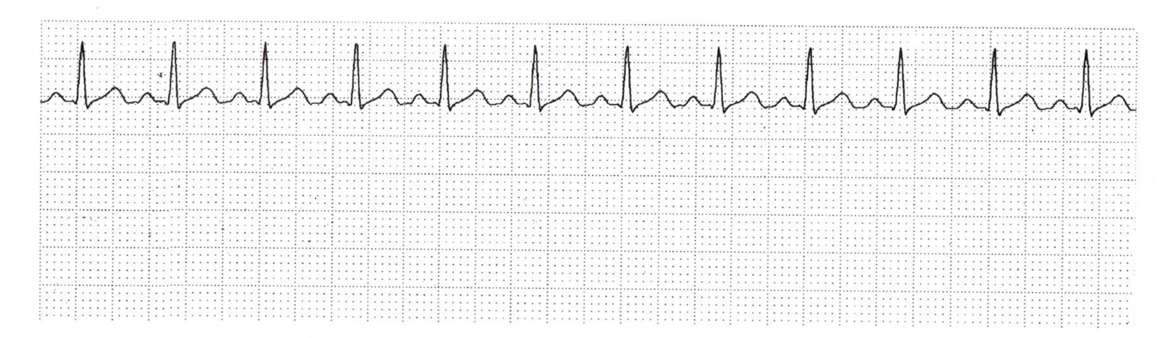

Figure 15–13. Interpretation of sinus tachycardia using the six-step process.
1. Rate = 120
2. R–R interval: regular
3. P wave has same configuration
4. PR interval = 0.12
5. P wave precedes QRS: yes
6. QRS complex = 0.04

SECTION FIVE REVIEW

1. Sinus bradycardia originates from
   A. delayed AV conduction
   B. AV nodal area
   C. Purkinje fibers
   D. SA node

2. Atropine is used to treat sinus bradycardia because it
   A. inhibits the AV node
   B. stimulates the sympathetic nervous system
   C. blocks the parasympathetic nervous system
   D. enhances ventricular conduction
3. Sinus tachycardia may result from all the following EXCEPT
   A. parasympathetic stimulation
   B. anxiety
   C. pain
   D. fever
4. Decreasing level of consciousness associated with sinus tachycardia indicates
   A. decreased ventricular contractility
   B. decreased cardiac output
   C. increased atrial filling
   D. decreased AV conduction

Answers: 1. D, 2. C, 3. A, 4. B

SECTION SIX: Atrial Dysrhythmias

At the completion of this section, the learner will be able to identify basic atrial dysrhythmias.

Common atrial dysrhythmias are supraventricular tachycardia (SVT), atrial flutter, and atrial fibrillation. Each of these dysrhythmias is characterized by a rapid rate. Most patients describe a fluttering sensation in the chest, dyspnea, lightheadedness, or angina when experiencing these dysrhythmias. The rapid heart rate decreases ventricular filling time and CO.

SVT has a rate between 150 and 250 bpm. The rhythm is regular, but P waves are not distinguishable, since they are buried in the preceding T wave. The QRS complex appears normal (≤ 0.14 second), because ventricular conduction is not affected. Normal QRS complexes indicate that the ectopic pacemaker is located above the ventricles. The exact location may not be distinguishable without having a 12-lead ECG available. At times SVT may be mistaken for ventricular tachycardia (VT) (see Section Eight). However, in VT, the QRS complex is > 0.14 second, and the rate is usually between 130 and 170 bpm. Treatment remains the same regardless of pacemaker origin. If the patient is not experiencing symptoms, drug therapy is initiated to slow the rate. SVT may be treated with Valsalva's maneuver and/or adenosine, an endogenous nucleoside. Because it is a naturally occurring body substance, it is rapidly removed from the circulation. Adenosine temporarily inhibits AV node conduction and prohibits reentry of impulses from the ventricles. Consequently, heart rate decreases and conduction of impulses through the AV node is slowed. Adenosine will help clarify whether the ECG pattern is SVT or VT. Only dysrhythmias involving the AV node will convert. Thus, VT will remain unchanged. Adenosine has a very short half-life (approximately 10 seconds). If the rhythm does not convert, advanced cardiac life support measures are initiated (see Section Eight). Adenosine is administered as a 6-mg intravenous push (IVP) dose given over 1 to 3 seconds, and followed by a rapid 20-mL normal saline IVP flush. It is administered through the IV port closest to the patient. A brief period of asystole (up to 15 seconds) is common after rapid administration. An additional 12-mg dose can be given peripherally if the rhythm does not convert within 2 minutes post initial administration (American Heart Association [AHA], 1997). Side effects include facial flushing, dyspnea, and chest pressure. Calcium channel blocking agents may be used to prevent the influx of calcium, and thus positive charges, into the cell, discouraging depolarization. Verapamil, digitalis preparations, propranolol, or quinidine also may be used. In cases in which the patient is experiencing distress or is unresponsive to drug therapy, cardioversion is used to rapidly correct the dysrhythmia. Figure 15–14 is an example of SVT.

Atrial flutter has a faster rate than SVT. The atrial rate will be greater than 250 bpm. The ventricular rate depends on the number of impulses that pass through the AV node. The ventricular rate may be irregular if some of the impulses are blocked. The atrial oscillations appear as sawtooth waves. A fast ventricular rate decreases CO in the absence of digitalis toxicity. Cardioversion is the preferred method of treating this dysrhythmia. Calcium channel blockers, beta-blocking agents, and digitalis preparations may be used (Section Thirteen). Atrial flutter is described by the number of atrial oscillations between each QRS complex (Fig. 15–15).

Atrial fibrillation is one of the most common heart disturbances in clinical practice, and the incidence is expected to increase as the population ages (Sargent, 1999). Atrial fibrillation is a condition in which the atria are contracting so fast that they are unable to refill before ejection. Therefore, the ventricles are filled inadequately and CO is diminished. The atria are not able to empty completely because of the fast rate of depolarization. Blood that remains in the atria is prone to forming clots, predisposing the person to stroke.

Atrial fibrillation has an irregular ventricular response. The QRS complexes are normal in appearance but occur at irregular intervals. This is manifested clinically as a difference between the apical heart rate and the peripheral pulse rate because the SV may be inadequate with some beats to produce a peripheral pulse. The atria may be discharging at a rate greater than 400 bpm. Absent P waves and irregular QRS intervals are characteris-

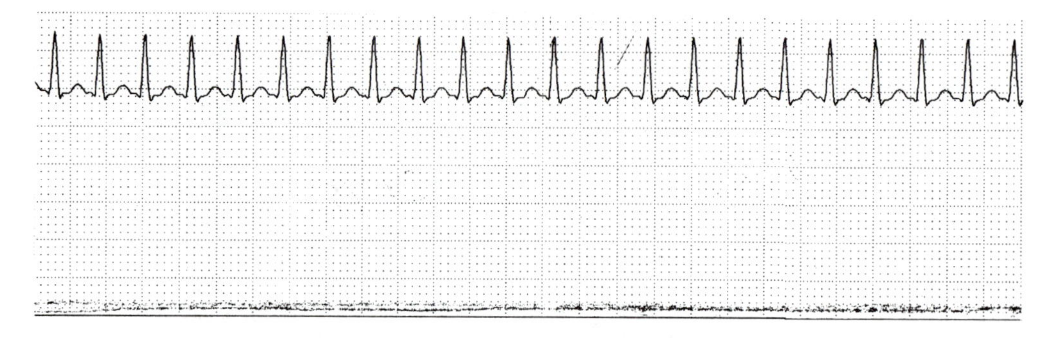

Figure 15–14. Interpretation of supraventricular tachycardia using the six-step process. (*Note:* This is not a 6-second strip.)

1. Rate = 250
2. R–R interval: regular
3. P wave: difficult to distinguish
4. PR interval: cannot calculate
5. P wave precedes each QRS: cannot identify
6. QRS complex = 0.04

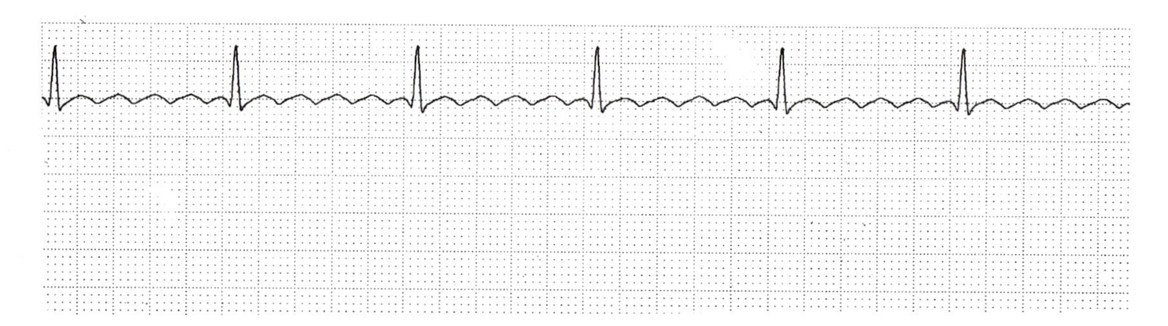

Figure 15–15. Interpretation of atrial flutter with 5.1 conduction using the six-step process.

1. Rate: atrial ~250
   ventricular = 60
2. R–R interval: regular
3. P wave: cannot distinguish, flutter wave present
4. PR interval: cannot calculate
5. P wave precedes each QRS: cannot identify
6. QRS complex = 0.06

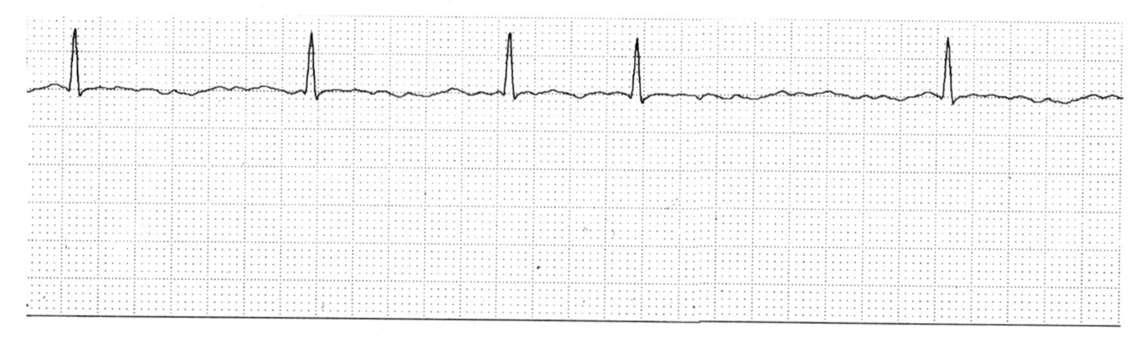

Figure 15–16. Interpretation of atrial fibrillation using the six-step process.

1. Rate: atrial: unable to calculate
   ventricular = 50
2. R–R interval: irregular
3. P wave: undistinguishable
4. PR interval: cannot calculate
5. P wave precedes each QRS: cannot identify
6. QRS complex = 0.06

TABLE 15–3. SUMMARY OF DIFFERENCES IN ATRIAL DYSRHYTHMIAS

RHYTHM	CHARACTERISTICS	TREATMENT STRATEGIES
Superventricular tachycardia	R–R interval regular Atrial rate 150–250 bpm	Adenosine Beta-blocking agents (propranolol) Calcium channel blocking agents Digitalis Cardioversion Overdrive pacing
Atrial flutter	R–R interval may be regular or irregular Atrial rate may be up to 350 bpm Sawtoothed waves	Cardioversion Digitalis
Atrial fibrillation	R–R interval irregular Atrial rate > 350 bpm	Digitalis Cardioversion Calcium channel blocking agents Class IA, IC, and III agents

tic of this dysrhythmia. Control of the ventricular rate is important in atrial fibrillation. Drugs that are particularly effective in controlling ventricular rate are digoxin, beta-adrenergic blocking agents, and calcium channel blocking agents. Conversion of the atrial fibrillation to a normal sinus rhythm will improve hemodynamics and help patients to feel better. Conversion can be achieved by direct current cardioversion and class IA, IC, and III antiarrhythmics. Class IA drugs are successful in converting atrial fibrillation in 40 to 80 percent of cases (Kayser, 1996). Class IA drugs include quinidine and procainamide (IV and PO). Class IC agents include flecanide. These drugs are successful in converting atrial fibrillation in 50 to 90 percent of cases. Class III drugs include amiodarone and ibutilide and are successful in 40 to 100 percent of cases. Atrial fibrillation may not be treated if it is of long-standing duration and does not produce symptoms. Figure 15–16 is an example of atrial fibrillation.

In summary, atrial dysrhythmias have a rapid atrial response and are characterized by absent P waves. A complication of these dysrhythmias may be decreased CO if the ventricular response also is rapid, resulting in inadequate ventricular filling. Table 15–3 compares atrial dysrhythmias.

Section Six Review

1. Atrial dysrhythmias produce symptoms of lightheadedness or angina because
   A. cardiac output is decreased
   B. ventricular conduction is delayed
   C. SA node is competing for pacemaker status
   D. coronary vasodilation occurs
2. Adenosine may be used to treat supraventricular tachycardia because it
   A. increases AV conduction
   B. prevents reentry of impulses from the ventricles
   C. prolongs repolarization
   D. blocks potassium movement extracellularly
3. Atrial fibrillation predisposes a person to a cerebrovascular attack because it produces
   A. cardiac fatigue
   B. inadequate emptying of the atria
   C. ventricular exhaustion
   D. decreased cerebral circulation

Answers: 1. A, 2. B, 3. B

SECTION SEVEN: Junctional Dysrhythmias

At the completion of this section, the learner will be able to identify common junctional dysrhythmias.

Junctional dysrhythmias occur because the SA node fails to fire. They have a protective function. The junctional area is located around the AV node. Pacemaker cells in this area have an intrinsic rate of 40 to 60 bpm. Once the pacemaker cell discharges, it spreads upward to depolarize the atria and downward to depolarize the ventricles. Since the ventricles usually are depolarized in a downward fashion, the QRS complex will appear normal. The atria are depolarized in an abnormal manner. Therefore, the P wave will be inverted (in lead II). The timing of the P wave is abnormal. It may precede the QRS complex, but the PR interval is shorter. The P wave may be buried in the QRS complex and be indistinguishable. It is possible that the P wave follows the QRS complex.

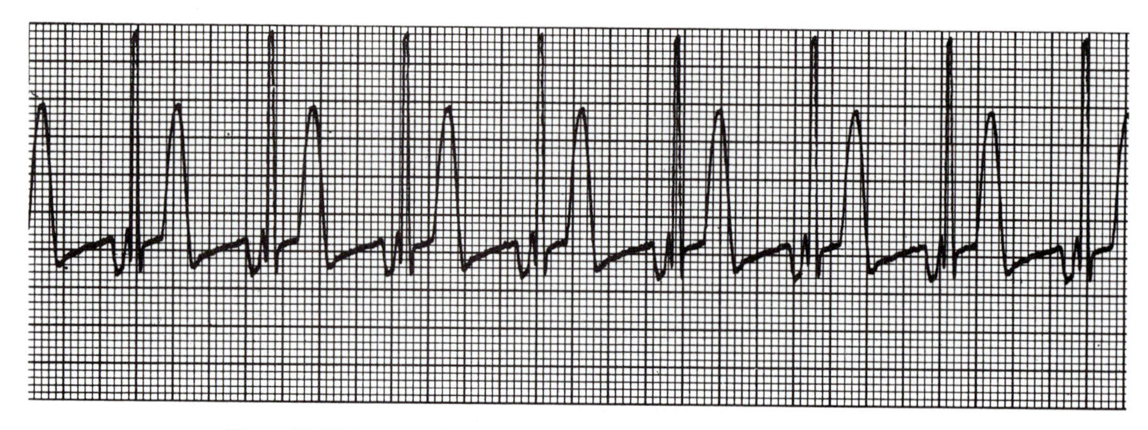

Figure 15–17. Interpretation of accelerated junctional rhythm using the six-step process.
1. Rate = 80
2. R–R interval: regular
3. P wave: same configuration, inverted
4. PR interval = 0.04
5. P wave precedes QRS: yes
6. QRS complex = 0.08

The term junctional tachycardia refers to a junctional rhythm with a rate greater than 100 bpm. If the rate of the rhythm is between 60 and 100 bpm, it is called an accelerated junctional rhythm. Figure 15–17 shows an accelerated junctional rhythm pattern.

Digitalis increases the automaticity of the AV node. Therefore, digitalis toxicity may precipitate junctional rhythms. The dysrhythmia is treated by withholding the medication. Usually the patient can tolerate junctional rhythms. However, if the patient experiences symptoms of decreased CO because the rate is too slow, atropine may be administered. A pacemaker may be inserted as a protective measure in case the junction fails or if the patient is symptomatic. Table 15–4 compares junctional rhythms.

In summary, junctional rhythms are a protective mechanism when the SA node fails to discharge appropriately. Depolarization of the atria is abnormal. Therefore, the P wave may fall before, during, or after the QRS complex.

TABLE 15–4. SUMMARY OF DIFFERENCES IN JUNCTIONAL DYSRHYTHMIAS

RHYTHM	CHARACTERISTICS	TREATMENT STRATEGIES
Junctional rhythm	Rate 40–60 bpm Inverted or absent P waves	May not be treated if patient is asymptomatic Atropine Pacemaker insertion
Junctional tachycardia	Rate > 100 bpm Inverted or absent P waves	May not be treated if patient is asymptomatic Pacemaker insertion Withhold digitalis if associated with digitalis toxicity

SECTION SEVEN REVIEW

1. Junctional rhythms are
   A. precursors to ventricular dysrhythmias
   B. a protective mechanism
   C. generated by the SA node
   D. considered an atrial dysrhythmia
2. Junctional tachycardia is classified as a junctional rhythm with a rate
   A. greater than 40 bpm
   B. greater than 60 bpm
   C. greater than 100 bpm
   D. between 60 and 100 bpm
3. The P wave in a junctional rhythm
   A. is bizarre in configuration
   B. is always abnormal in location
   C. can appear anywhere in relation to the QRS complex
   D. is flat

Answers: 1. B, 2. C, 3. C

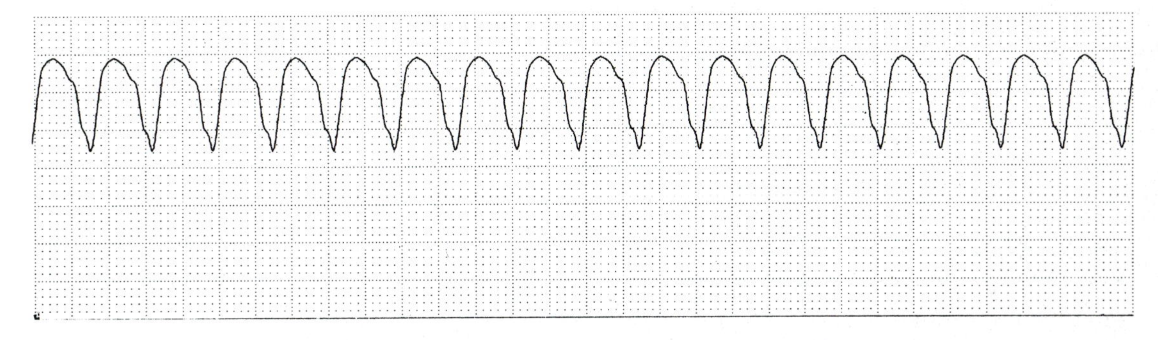

Figure 15–18. Interpretation of ventricular tachycardia using the six-step process.
1. Rate: atrial: unable to calculate
   ventricular = 180
2. R–R interval: regular
3. P wave: undistinguishable
4. PR interval: unable to calculate
5. P wave precedes each QRS: no
6. QRS complex = 0.28

SECTION EIGHT: Ventricular Dysrhythmias

At the completion of this section, the learner will be able to identify common ventricular dysrhythmias.

Ventricular dysrhythmias are considered the most lethal. Inadequate ventricular ejection produces inadequate CO. Coronary and peripheral ischemia results, producing necrosis and cell death. Two common ventricular dysrhythmias are ventricular tachycardia and ventricular fibrillation.

Ventricular tachycardia may follow PVCs (Section Nine). It is classified as three or more consecutive PVCs occurring at a rapid rate, usually > 140 bpm. Although the SA node continues to fire, ectopic pacemakers in the ventricles fire spontaneously and bear no relationship to the SA node–initiated impulse. P waves may not be identifiable because they are buried in the QRS complexes. The R–R interval may be regular. The QRS complex is greater than 0.12 second. Short runs of VT can be tolerated. A danger of VT is that it may develop into ventricular fibrillation. Patients may be alert while experiencing VT, and a carotid pulse may still be present. As CO diminishes, loss of consciousness ensues. Witnessed VT is treated with a precordial thump over the sternum. **Cardioversion** may be used. Lidocaine is the drug of choice in decreasing ventricular irritability. Bretylium may also be used. Figure 15–18 is an example of VT.

Ventricular fibrillation is the most common cause of sudden death. The patient will be unresponsive and without a pulse and requires emergency treatment. Cardiopulmonary resuscitation is initiated. **Defibrillation** is the treatment of choice and is used beginning with 200 J and

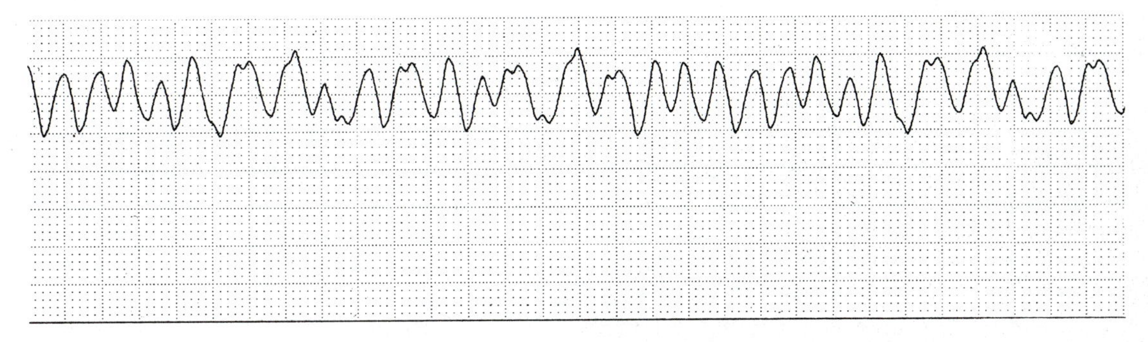

Figure 15–19. Interpretation of ventricular fibrillation using the six-step process.
1. Rate: atrial: unable to calculate
   ventricular: unable to calculate
2. R–R interval: irregular
3. P wave: undistinguishable
4. PR interval: unable to calculate
5. P wave precedes each QRS: no
6. QRS complex: no uniformity, unable to calculate

TABLE 15–5. SUMMARY OF DIFFERENCES IN VENTRICULAR DYSRHYTHMIAS

RHYTHM	CHARACTERISTICS	TREATMENT STRATEGIES
Ventricular tachycardia	R–R interval usually regular, but can be irregular Absent P waves or P waves not associated with QRS complex Wide QRS but somewhat uniform Rate > 150 bpm	Lidocaine Cardioversion
Ventricular fibrillation	R–R interval irregular Absent P wave Wide QRS, no uniformity Rate undeterminable	Cardiopulmonary resuscitation Defibrillation Epinephrine Lidocaine Bretylium

progressing up to 360 for a total of three times (AHA, 1997). A bolus of epinephrine is administered. If the patient remains pulseless, an IV lidocaine bolus is administered. For persistent or recurrent pulseless ventricular tachycardia or fibrillation, bretylium, magnesium, and procainamide should be used. Once the patient has converted from ventricular fibrillation and has a pulse, a continuous infusion of the last drug used to convert the rhythm is initiated. Myocardial infarction and premature ventricular beats may precede the development of ventricular fibrillation. The ECG pattern is chaotic. It is impossible to identify any PQRST waves, and the rhythm is grossly irregular. Figure 15–19 is an example of ventricular fibrillation.

In summary, ventricular dysrhythmias are more life threatening than other dysrhythmias and require immediate treatment. They are recognizable by absent P waves and regular, wide QRS complexes or, if P waves are present, they are not associated with the QRS complex. In the case of ventricular fibrillation, chaotic waveforms are seen. Table 15–5 compares ventricular dysrhythmias.

SECTION EIGHT REVIEW

1. Ventricular tachycardia
   A. may be harmless
   B. usually follows PVCs
   C. results from SA node fatigue
   D. produces ventricular rates < 100 bpm
2. In ventricular fibrillation, the ECG pattern
   A. is chaotic
   B. has recognizable QRS complexes
   C. has inverted T waves
   D. has a regular atrial rate
3. The treatment of choice in ventricular fibrillation is
   A. lidocaine
   B. epinephrine
   C. cardioversion
   D. defibrillation

Answers: 1. B, 2. A, 3. D

SECTION NINE: Premature Contractions

At the completion of this section, the learner will be able to distinguish premature beats and identify their origin.

Premature beats may originate in the atria, junctional area (AV node), or ventricles. Since premature junctional beats are treated in the same manner as premature atrial beats (PACs), discussion is limited to PACs and premature ventricular beats (PVCs).

In PACs, the P wave is abnormal in shape, since a focus other than the SA node is initiating the impulse. Therefore, there will be differences in the P wave configurations. The rhythm is irregular because there is a slight pause after the premature beat to allow for the SA node to get ready to initiate a beat after it responded to the premature stimulus. The remaining components of the ECG are normal. PACs do not pose a serious threat unless they occur at a rate greater than six per minute. This rate suggests the future development of atrial tachycardia or atrial fibrillation. Digitalis preparations usually are used to treat multiple PACs. Figure 15–20 is an example of a PAC.

PVCs originate in the ventricles and do not usually stimulate the atria retrospectively. Thus, P waves are absent in a PVC. The rhythm is irregular because of the compensatory pause before the next stimulus arrives to initiate a normal ventricular beat. The QRS complex is wide, greater than 0.12 second in length, and distorted. PVCs may originate from one irritable cell in the ventricles. Unifocal PVCs originate from the same location,

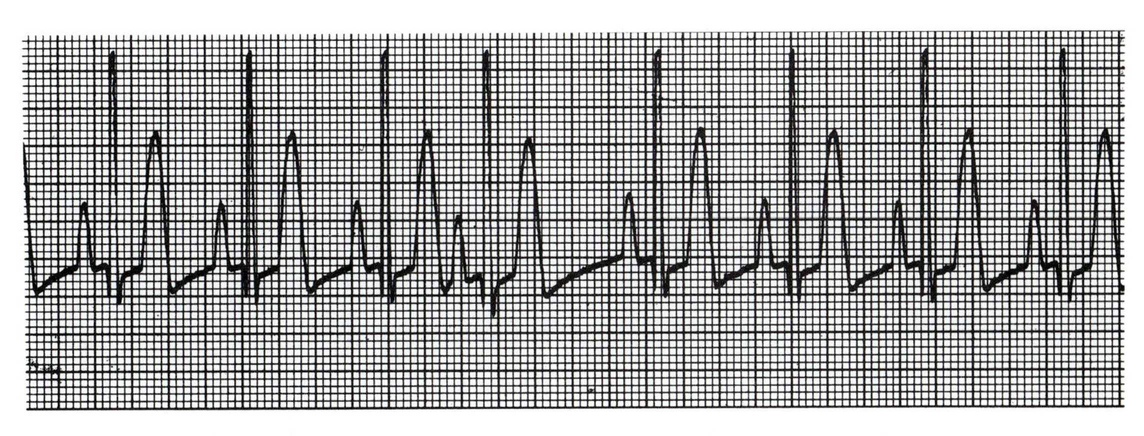

Figure 15–20. Interpretation of sinus rhythm with premature atrial contraction using the six-step process.
1. Rate = 80
2. R–R interval: irregular
3. P wave: same configuration
4. PR interval = 0.16
5. P wave precedes QRS: yes
6. QRS complex = 0.08

and thus they appear the same in configuration. Multifocal PVCs may originate from multiple irritable ventricular cells or they may originate from the same site but are conducted differently. Therefore, they have various shapes. Thus, all the premature beats have wide and chaotic QRS complexes, but they are not identical to one another unless they arise from the same site or are conducted in the same manner.

PVCs may appear in healthy individuals. Caffeine, alcohol intake, and stress may produce ventricular irritability. A major responsibility of the nurse is determining factors contributing to their occurrence. Ischemia is the most dangerous cause of PVCs. Hypoxia, acidosis, hypokalemia, and digitalis toxicity also are associated with PVCs. It is important to remember that not all PVCs are treated. This is especially true in cases in which PVCs originate because the underlying cardiac rhythm is too slow. Treating the PVCs may decrease CO further.

Certain circumstances warrant close observation of PVCs because they are associated with future development of VT and ventricular fibrillation. In the situations listed, lidocaine may be administered prophylactically if the patient has underlying cardiac disease. Treatment of PVCs remains controversial (AHA, 1997).

1. Greater than six PVCs/min
2. PVCs occurring together (couplet)
3. Multifocal PVCs
4. A run of ventricular tachycardia (more than three PVCs in a row)

Procainamide, followed by bretylium, may be administered if the PVCs are refractory to lidocaine. Amio-

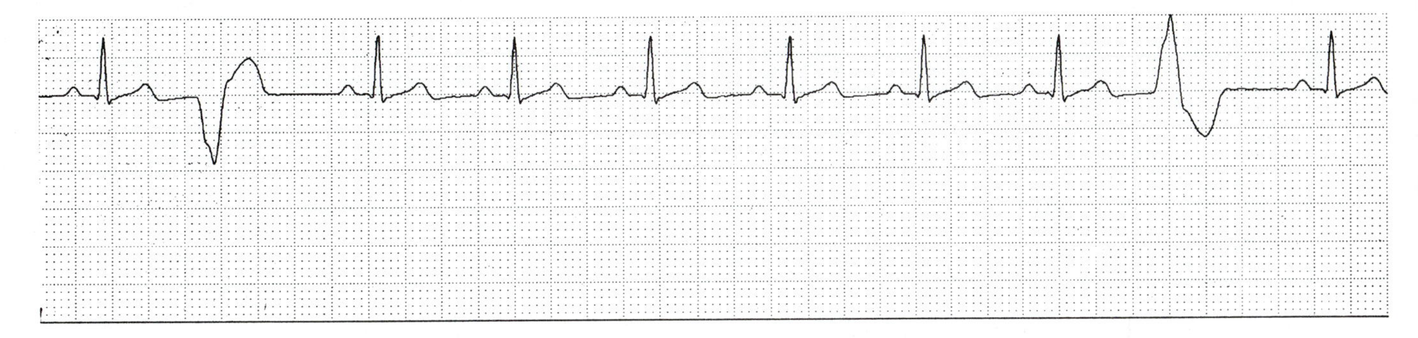

Figure 15–21. Interpretation of sinus rhythm with multifocal PVCs using the six-step process.
[*Note:* Strip is longer than 6 seconds = 37 (0.20) boxes.]
1. Rate = 70
2. R–R interval: irregular
3. P wave: same configuration
4. PR interval: 0.16
5. P wave precedes each QRS: no
6. QRS complex varies, 0.06 to 0.32

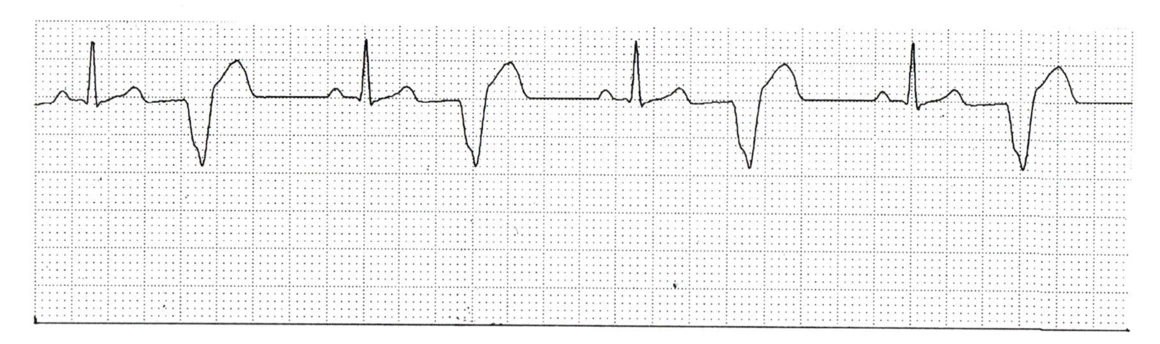

Figure 15–22. Interpretation of ventricular bigeminy using the six-step process.
1. Rate = 40
2. R–R interval: regular
3. P wave: same configuration
4. PR interval = 0.16
5. P wave precedes each QRS: no
6. QRS complex varies, 0.08 to 0.36

darone may be administered. Figure 15–21 is an example of sinus rhythm with multifocal PVCs.

The patient's underlying cardiac rhythm and the type of PVC (uniformed versus multiformed) should be described. The timing of the PVCs can be described if they occur in a repeatable pattern. For example, **bigeminy** is a pattern of one normal SA node–initiated beat followed by one PVC. **Trigeminy** is a pattern of two normal beats followed by one PVC. Figure 15–22 is an example of ventricular bigeminy.

In summary, PACs usually are harmless and are not treated unless they are present at a rate of six or greater a minute. PVCs may be life threatening, since they indicate ventricular irritability. Multiple PVCs, multifocal PVCs, a couplet of PVCs, and a run of VT may be treated with lidocaine if the patient has underlying cardiac disease, since they may predispose to life-threatening dysrhythmias. Table 15–6 compares premature contractions.

TABLE 15–6. SUMMARY OF DIFFERENCES IN PREMATURE CONTRACTIONS

CONTRACTION	CHARACTERISTICS	TREATMENT STRATEGIES
Premature atrial contraction	PR interval may be normal or prolonged QRS may be absent after P wave	May not be treated if patient is asymptomatic Reduce caffeine intake Beta-blocking agents (propranolol)
Premature ventricular contraction	PR interval absent in premature beat QRS > 0.12	May not be treated if patient is asymptomatic Reduce caffeine intake Decrease stress Lidocaine

SECTION NINE REVIEW

1. Which of the following statements best describes premature beats?
   A. they originate anywhere along the cardiac conduction pathway
   B. they originate in the atria
   C. they originate in the ventricles
   D. they originate in the junctional (AV nodal) area
2. PACs should be treated when they
   A. occur as a pair
   B. originate from different sites
   C. occur greater than six per minute
   D. occur in a repeatable pattern
3. Premature ventricular contractions (PVCs) may be associated with
   A. hyponatremia
   B. hypocalcemia
   C. hypoglycemia
   D. hypokalemia
4. In PVCs, the QRS complex is
   A. > 0.12 second
   B. negatively deflected
   C. isoelectric
   D. preceded by a T wave

Answers: 1. A, 2. C, 3. D, 4. A

SECTION TEN: Conduction Abnormalities

At the completion of this section, the learner will be able to distinguish the three most common and life-threatening conduction abnormalities.

Conduction can be inhibited anywhere along the cardiac conduction pathway. Normally, conduction of the impulse will be blocked in its transmission from the SA node to the ventricles. Delays may occur at the AV nodal area. Acute AV blocks are associated with myocardial infarction. Chronic AV blocks occur with coronary artery disease. Ischemia to the AV node, digitalis, antiarrhythmic agents, and increased parasympathetic activity can produce blocks in conduction.

A first-degree heart block is denoted by a prolonged PR interval (> 0.20 second.) There is a delay in conduction through the AV node. The rest of the ECG is normal. If the patient is asymptomatic, no treatment usually is necessary. If symptomatic, atropine may be administered, or a transcutaneous or a temporary pacing catheter may be placed. A permanent pacing device is placed later if necessary. Figure 15–23 is an example of first-degree heart block.

In second-degree heart block, an impulse is not transmitted to the ventricles because it is completely blocked in the AV nodal area. Therefore, a P wave will be present, but a QRS complex will not follow. The rhythm is irregular because of the missing QRS complexes. In some cases, the PR interval will lengthen progressively before the dropping of the QRS complex (Wenckebach or Mobitz type I second-degree heart block). In Mobitz type II second-degree heart block, the PR intervals are of constant duration before the dropping of the QRS complex. ORS complexes are wide because the block is usually lower in the conduction system (bundles). This type of heart block is less common but is considered more serious, because it is associated with third-degree heart block and asystole (AHA, 1997). The nurse should determine the ventricular rate (number of QRS complexes) of the rhythm and the frequency of dropped beats. Angina, lightheadedness, and dyspnea may occur because of decreased cardiac output. In the case of type I second-degree heart block, if the rate is below 60 bpm and the patient is asymptomatic, no treatment may be initiated. The patient is observed. A patient with type II second-degree heart block, whether symptomatic or asymptomatic, usually will receive a transvenous pacemaker. The point at which the pacemaker is inserted may vary, since symptoms are managed with medications initially. Regardless of the type of second-degree block, if the patient experiences symptoms, atropine is administered. If isoproterenol (considered possibly helpful) is used, it should be used with extreme caution (AHA, 1997). Dopamine or epinephrine may be used in severe symptomatic bradycardia. A transvenous pacemaker may need to be inserted for symptomatic patients with type I second-degree heart block. Transcutaneous pacing can be extremely effective. If bradycardia is severe and the patient is unstable, transcutaneous pacing should be performed immediately (AHA, 1997). Figure 15–24 is an example of type I second-degree heart block, and Figure 15–25 is an example of type II second-degree heart block. If two QRSs are dropped in a row, the heart block is called advanced heart block (Fig. 15–26).

Complete heart block requires emergency treatment because the atria and ventricles are contracting independently. Thus, CO is greatly diminished because of inadequate filling of the ventricles. Impulses are not conducted through the AV node. The atria and ventricles may fire at a regular rate, but they do not function as a single unit. The P–P wave interval will be regular, as will the R–R wave interval, but the PR interval will vary. There is no relationship between the P wave and the QRS complex, since the atria and the ventricles are being paced by a

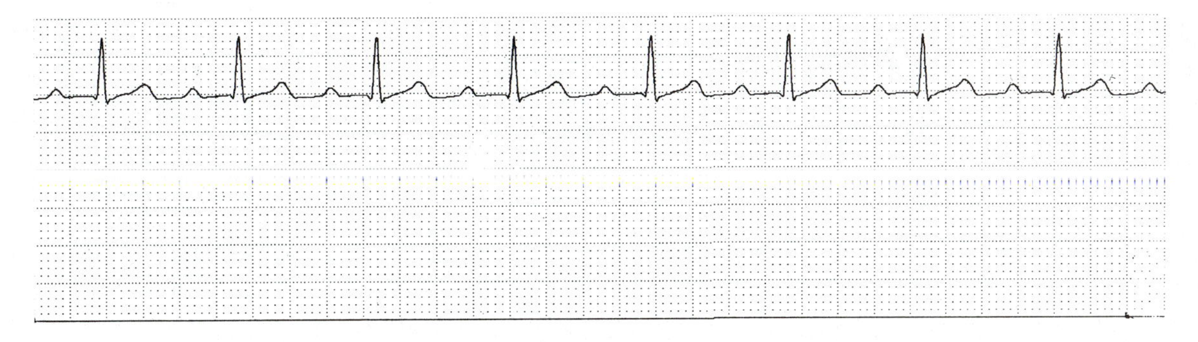

Figure 15–23. Interpretation of first-degree heart block using the six-step process.

1. Rate = 80
2. R–R interval: regular
3. P wave: same configuration
4. PR interval = 0.24
5. P wave precedes QRS: yes
6. QRS complex = 0.06

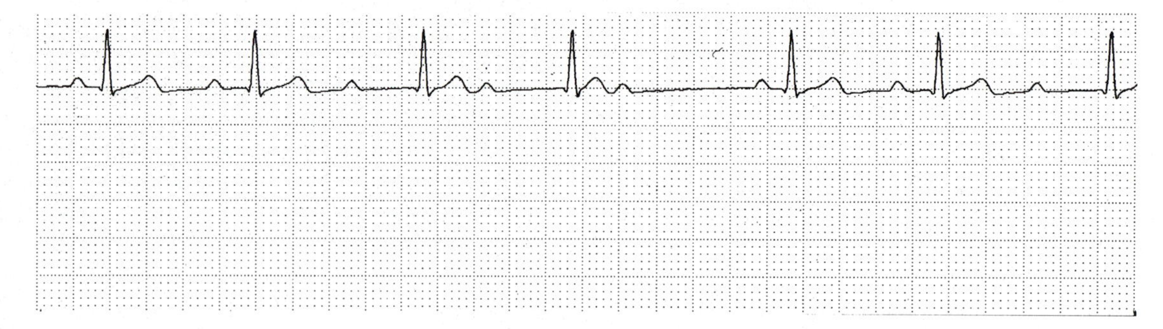

Figure 15–24. Interpretation of type I second-degree heart block using the six-step process.

1. Rate: ventricular = 70
   atrial = 80
2. R–R interval: irregular
3. P wave: same configuration
4. PR interval varies, 0.20 to 0.48
5. P wave precedes QRS: yes, but QRS does not always follow P wave
6. QRS complex = 0.06

separate pacemaker. The QRS complex is usually wide due to the ventricular origin of the stimulus. Complete heart block usually is associated with myocardial infarction. In rare cases, the ventricular rate is fast enough to maintain CO, and symptoms may be less severe. Usually, the patient experiences confusion and syncope. Complete heart block may progress to ventricular fibrillation. Treatment of complete heart block is the same as that for type II second-degree heart block. If symptomatic, the patient is administered atropine, dopamine, epinephrine, and if isoproterenol is used, it should be used with extreme caution. External pacing, and transvenous pacing may also be used. Figure 15–27 is an example of complete heart block.

Bundle branch blocks (BBBs) are caused by defects in intraventricular conduction. The bundle branches are divided into right and left. The impulse travels slowly through the blocked side; thus, one ventricle depolarizes faster than the other. The morphology of the QRS complex changes. Treatment is not necessary except in the case of a new onset left BBB in which the patient may be experiencing AMI. In the setting of BBB and diagnosis of myocardial infarction, the ST segment becomes distorted, therefore, significant ST segment elevation cannot be defined (AHA, 1997). BBBs may precede AV blocks.

In summary, abnormalities can occur along the cardiac conduction pathway that interfere with transmission of the

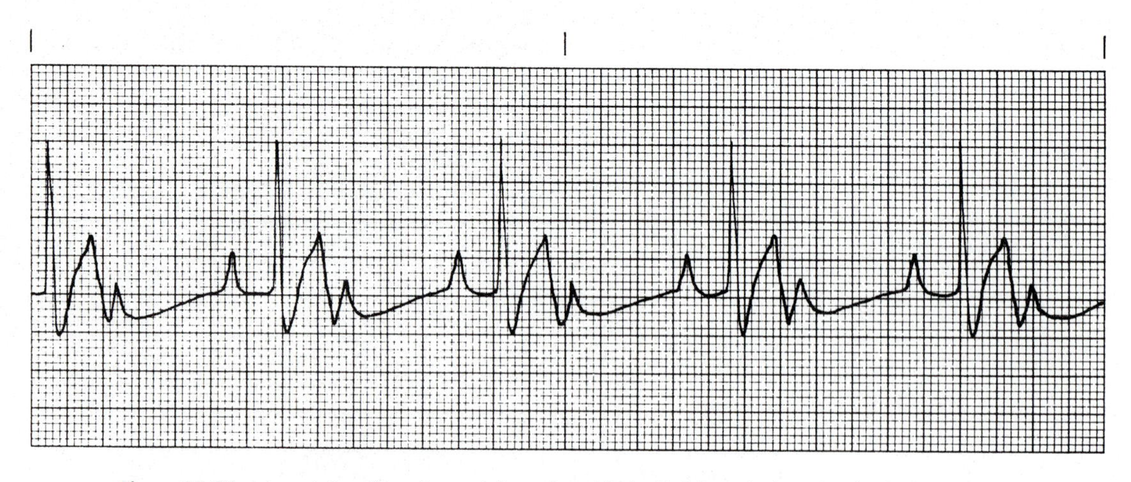

Figure 15–25. Interpretation of type II second-degree heart block with 2:1 conduction using the six-step process.

1. Rate: ventricular = 47
   atrial = 94
2. R–R interval: regular
3. P wave: same configuration
4. PR interval = 0.28
5. Every other P wave is not conducted
6. QRS complex = 0.12

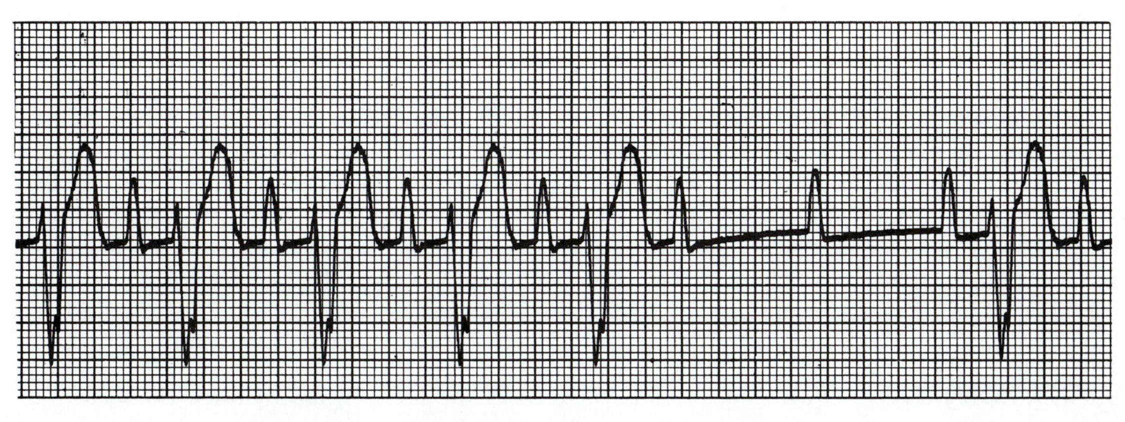

Figure 15–26. Interpretation of advanced AV heart block using the six-step process.
1. Rate: ventricular = 60
   atrial = 80
2. R–R interval: irregular
3. P wave: same configuration
4. PR interval = 0.28
5. P waves are not followed by QRS complex in two places
6. QRS complex = 0.12

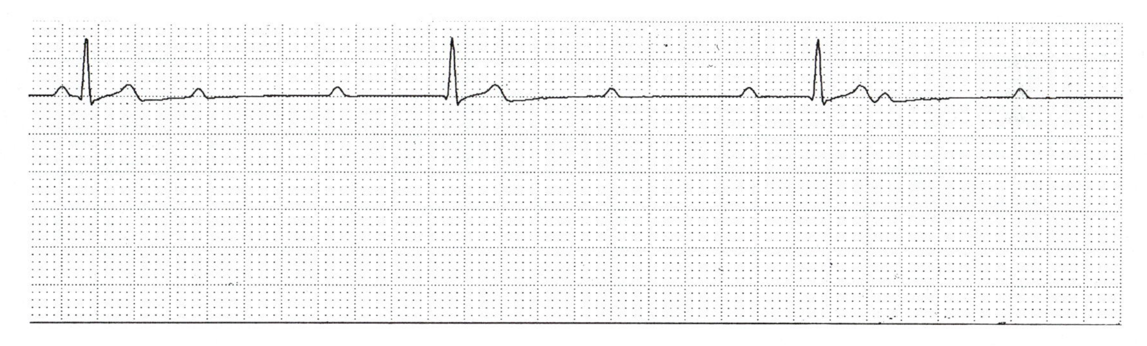

Figure 15–27. Interpretation of complete heart block using the six-step process.
1. Rate: ventricular = 30
   atrial = 70
2. R–R interval: regular
3. P wave: same configuration
4. PR interval varies
5. P wave precedes each QRS: no
6. QRS complex = 0.06

TABLE 15–7. SUMMARY OF DIFFERENCES IN ATRIOVENTRICULAR (AV) BLOCKS

BLOCK	CHARACTERISTICS	TREATMENT STRATEGIES
First degree	PR interval > 0.20 R–R interval is regular	May not be treated if patient is asymptomatic Atropine
Second degree, Mobitz type I	Atrial rate is greater than ventricular rate R–R interval is irregular PR interval gradually lengthens until a P wave is blocked (no QRS follows the P wave)	Withhold digitalis associated with digitalis toxicity Atropine Transcutaneous pacemaker Permanent pacemaker insertion
Second degree, Mobitz type II	Atrial rate is greater than ventricular rate No consistent pattern to the blocking of the P wave R–R interval usually irregular	Atropine Transcutaneous pacemaker Permanent pacemaker insertion
Advanced AV block	Atrial rate is greater than ventricular rate Two QRS complexes in a row are blocked R–R interval is irregular	Atropine Transcutaneous pacemaker Permanent pacemaker insertion
Third degree, complete	PR interval varies R–R interval regular QRS may be widened	Transcutaneous pacemaker Permanent pacemaker insertion

impulse from the atria to the ventricles. The least severe of these abnormalities is first-degree heart block. The impulse is transmitted to the ventricles, but there is a delay at the AV nodal area. Impulses from the atria to the ventricles are periodically blocked in second-degree heart block. In type I, the PR interval progressively lengthens before the blocked impulse. In type II, the PR interval remains constant. Complete heart block is a medical emergency. It is treated with the placement of a transcutaneous pacing catheter followed by a temporary cardiac pacemaker, since the atria and ventricles are contracting independently, decreasing CO. Table 15–7 compares atrioventricular blocks.

SECTION TEN REVIEW

1. Which of the following may produce blocks in impulse conduction?
   A. ischemia
   B. sympathetic stimulation
   C. fever
   D. antipyretic agents
2. The difference between type I and type II second-degree heart block is
   A. dropping of the QRS complex
   B. regularity of the rhythm
   C. length of the PR interval
   D. P wave configuration
3. Complete heart block is characterized by
   A. constant PR interval
   B. heart rate < 50 bpm
   C. QRS complexes < 0.12 second
   D. regular P–P and R–R intervals
4. First-degree heart block should be treated if the
   A. PR interval is irregular
   B. patient is symptomatic
   C. PR interval is isoelectric
   D. PR interval is negatively deflected
5. Advanced AV heart block is characterized by
   A. two blocked QRS complexes in a row
   B. a heart rate less than 60 bpm
   C. dropping of P waves
   D. shortening of the PR interval

Answers: 1. A, 2. C, 3. D, 4. B, 5. A

PART II: RELATED INTERVENTIONS

SECTION ELEVEN: Acute Coronary Syndromes

At the completion of this section, the learner will be able to describe ECG changes and diagnostic tests associated with acute coronary syndromes.

Acute coronary syndromes (ACS) represent a continuum of the disease process that is initiated by the rupture of an unstable, lipid-rich, atheromatous plaque in a coronary or epicardial artery. Plaque disruption and fissuring activates platelet adhesion, fibrin clot formation, and coronary thrombosis. The interplay between continuing clot formation and spontaneous fibrinolysis will determine whether the thrombus will resolve and the plaque will stabilize or the thrombus will progress and the artery will occlude. Occlusion will result in an acute coronary syndrome. Thrombotic occlusions can be either intermittent, resulting in unstable angina, or completely occlusive, resulting in acute myocardial infarction (AMI). The three major syndromes within the ACS are unstable angina, non–Q wave MI, and Q wave MI. It is important to restate that these syndromes represent a dynamic spectrum of disease and are part of a continuum. Unstable angina is a change in the pattern of predictability of stable angina. Unstable angina is defined as having three possible presentations: symptoms of angina at rest (usually prolonged, > 20 minutes), new onset (< 2 months) exertional angina of at least Canadian Cardiovascular Society Classification (CCSC) class III in severity, or recent (< 2 months) acceleration of angina as reflected by an increase in severity of at least one CCSC class to at least CCSC class III (Braunwald, 1997) (Table 15–8). Whether the AMI is Q wave or non–Q wave depends on the degree and duration of occlusion and the presence or absence of coronary collaterals. This classification can only be made after 24 hours. Q wave infarcts are diagnosed by the development of abnormal Q waves in serial tracings (or equivalent loss of R waves in anterior infarcts and development of abnormal R waves in lead V_1 in posterior infarcts). Q wave infarcts tend to be larger and occur in approximately 60 percent of all infarcts. Non–Q wave infarcts occur when an abnormal level of cardiac serum markers is released and only ST segment deviation or T wave abnormalities occur on the ECG. Non–Q wave MIs have a lower in-hospital mortality and complication rate but an increased incidence of subsequent cardiac events such as reinfarction, ischemia, and death (AHA, 1997).

TABLE 15–8. GRADING OF ANGINA PECTORIS BY THE CANADIAN CARDIOVASCULAR SOCIETY CLASSIFICATION SYSTEM

CLASS	DESCRIPTION OF STAGE
Class I	Ordinary physical activity does not cause angina, such as walking, climbing stairs. Angina [occurs] with strenuous, rapid, or prolonged exertion at work or recreation.
Class II	Slight limitation of ordinary activity. Angina occurs on walking or climbing stairs rapidly, walking uphill, walking or stair climbing after meals, or in cold, or in wind, or under emotional stress, or only during the few hours after awakening. Walking more than two blocks on the level and climbing more than one flight of ordinary stairs at a normal pace and in normal condition.
Class III	Marked limitations of ordinary physical activity. Angina occurs on walking one to two blocks on the level and climbing one flight of stairs in normal conditions and at a normal pace.
Class IV	Inability to carry on any physical activity without discomfort—anginal symptoms may be present at rest.

From Campeau, L. (1976). Grading of angina pectoris [letter]. Circulation *54:522–523. Copyright © 1976, American Heart Association, Inc. Used with permission.*

Diagnosis of Acute Coronary Syndrome

The heart is mainly supplied by three coronary arteries: anterior descending, circumflex, and right coronary artery. The anterior descending artery supplies the anterior left and right ventricle. The circumflex artery supplies the left atria and left lateral and posterior ventricle. The right coronary artery supplies the right atria and ventricle. There are four basic areas where an infarction can occur: the anterior, inferior, lateral, or posterior aspect of the heart. When results are available from echocardiography and/or cardiac catheterization, the nurse can anticipate dysrhythmias and the type of infarction to which the patient is most susceptible. Table 15–9 compares the relationship between location of perfusion problem, infarction, and ECG changes. This information can help the novice to focus on the most important ECG leads. Although this module does not discuss 12- or 15-lead ECG interpretation, certain leads have changes depending on the location of the infarct. For example, an anterior myocardial infarction will demonstrate changes in leads I, aVL, V_2, and V_3.

The ECG continues to be used as a primary diagnostic tool for detecting AMI. The hallmark of injury is ST segment deviation. ECG criteria indicative of AMI include: ST segment elevation ≥ 1 mm in two contiguous leads, the presence of new onset LBBB, a Q wave > 0.04 seconds of duration, and > 25 percent of R wave amplitude (AHA, 1997).

Ischemic changes may be visible in a single monitored lead, but it is not possible to confirm the presence and location of an infarction. Ischemia may impair repolarization. Thus, the T wave may be changed, since it corresponds with ventricular repolarization. The T wave may be inverted. As ischemia progresses into injury, repolarization is impaired even further. The ST segment may demonstrate changes. It may be either elevated or depressed depending on the lead that the cardiac monitor is displaying. Diagnosis of infarction requires a 12- or 15-lead ECG. Figure 15–28 is an example of ischemic changes in lead II.

As injury progresses into infarction, the area becomes necrotic and is without electrical activity. The Q wave may be deep and wide, since the area over the infarcted site is unable to exhibit electrical activity. The Q wave may be 25 percent of the height of the R wave and have a duration of 0.03 or 0.04 second (AHA, 1997). The ECG pattern depicted is produced by the area opposite the infarcted site. The infarcted site serves as a window through

TABLE 15–9. ASSOCIATIONS OF ECG LEAD CHANGES OF INJURY OR INFARCT WITH CORONARY ARTERY, ANATOMIC AREA OF DAMAGE, AND ASSOCIATED COMPLICATIONS

LEADS WITH ECG CHANGES	INJURY/INFARCT-RELATED ARTERY	AREA OF DAMAGE	ASSOCIATED COMPLICATIONS
V_1–V_2	LCA: LAD-septal branch	Septum; His bundle; bundle branches	Infranodal and BBBs
V_3–V_4	LCA: LAD-diagonal branch	Anterior wall LV	LV dysfunction; CHF, BBBs; complete heart block; PVCs
V_5–V_6 plus I and aVL	LCA-circumflex branch	High lateral wall LV	LV dysfunction; AV nodal block in some
II, III, aVF	RCA-posterior descending branch	Inferior wall LV; posterior wall LV	Hypotension; sensitivity to nitroglycerin and morphine sulfate
V_{4R} (II, III, aVF)	RCA-proximal branches	RV; inferior wall LV; posterior wall LV	Hypotension; supranodal and AV nodal blocks; atrial fibrillation/flutter; PACs; adverse medical reactions
V_1–V_4 (marked depression)	Either LCA-circumflex *or* RCA posterior descending branch	Posterior wall LV	LV dysfunction

LCA, left coronary artery; LAD, left anterior descending artery; RCA, right coronary artery; LV, left ventricle (left ventricular); RV, right ventricle; BBB, bundle branch block; CHF, congestive heart failure; PVC, premature ventricular complex; AV, atrioventricular; and PAC, premature atrial complex.

From American Heart Association. (1997). Textbook of Advanced Cardiac Life Support. *Dallas, TX: Author.*

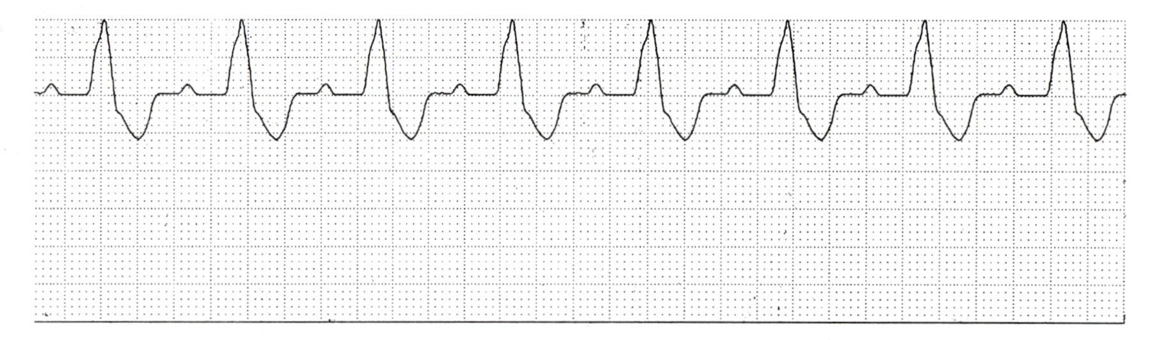

Figure 15–28. Characteristics of ischemia in lead II. Note the severe ST depression. Interpretation using the six-step process.
1. Rate = 80
2. R–R interval: regular
3. P wave: same configuration
4. PR interval = 0.20
5. P wave precedes QRS: yes
6. QRS complex = 0.12 to 0.16

which the electrical activity of the opposite side is transmitted. The electrical activity moves away from the necrotic zone, producing a deep, wide, negatively deflected Q wave. Serial ECG monitoring should be performed to monitor for progression of ischemia to infarction (Doering, 1999).

Echocardiography is used to assist in identifying infarcts based on evaluation of ventricular wall motion and global systolic function. They can be used as a tool in the emergency department to aid in diagnosis of patients with chest pain.

Serum cardiac markers are useful for confirming the diagnosis of AMI when patients present without ST segment changes, when the diagnosis is unclear, and when clinicians must distinquish patients with unstable angina from those with non–Q wave MI. Creatine phosphokinase (CPK) and its MB isoenzyme (CPK-MB) are being replaced by more cardiac specific markers such as troponin I and troponin T. Of these two markers, troponin T is more cardiac specific. CPK-MB isoforms (subcomponents of the isoenzyme) are also useful for evaluating patients with ACS. Myoglobin, as a serum cardiac marker, is not cardiac specific but is released more rapidly from infarcted myocardium than CPK-MB and it may be detected as early as 2 hours post-MI. The 1999 ACC/AHA Task Force reported that CPK-M isoforms and troponin reliably triages patients with chest pain. For patients presenting within the first 2 to 3 hours of symptom onset, myoglobin and CPK-MB isoforms are most appropriate (ACC/AHA Task Force, 1999).

Treatment of Acute Coronary Syndromes

Treatment of ACS varies depending on whether the patient has ischemia only as in unstable angina (UA) or necrosis as in non–Q wave or Q wave MI. Management of the patient with unstable angina and non–Q wave MI includes oxygen; analgesics; nitrates; beta blockers; antiplatelet agents such as aspirin, clopidogrel, and glycoprotein (GP) IIb/IIIa receptor antagonists; and antithrombins such as unfractionated heparin or low-molecular-weight heparins (LMWHs). Oxygen is administered to increase the supply of oxygen to ischemic tissues. Analgesics, such as morphine sulfate, are administered to reduce the pain of ischemia, reduce anxiety, increase venous capitance, and decrease systemic vascular resistance. These actions lead to reduced oxygen demands on the heart, which leads to less ischemia and infarct extension. Nitrates, such as nitroglycerin, decrease the pain of ischemia, increase venous dilation, dilate coronary arteries, and increase collateral blood flow. The clinical goal in nitroglycerin administration is not just to relieve pain but to produce improved hemodynamics. Aspirin blocks formation of thromboxane A_2, thereby preventing the platelet aggregation and constriction of arteries. It should be given as soon as possible. Beta blockers are administered to reduce myocardial oxygen consumption, block catecholamine stimulation, and decrease arrhythmias with the goal of reducing the area of ischemia. Beta blockers should be used cautiously, if at all, in patients with congestive heart failure/pulmonary edema, history of asthma, bradycardia, and hypotension. Commonly used beta blockers are metoprolol and atenolol. GP IIb/IIIa receptor antagonists are selective antagonists of ADP-induced platelet aggregation, blocking GP IIb/IIIa activation and are indicated for patients with UA or non–Q wave MI. They are given intravenously via a continuous infusion and are the most potent platelet inhibitors available. GP IIb/IIIa antagonists currently available include abciximab (ReoPro), tirofiban (Aggrastat), and eptifibatide (Integrelin). Adverse side effects include bleeding and the patient must be closely monitored for signs and/or symptoms of bleeding. Unfractionated heparin has been available for many years as an adjuvant therapy to UA and AMI.

LMWHs are a more recently available therapy and include enoxaparin (Lovenox) and dalteparin (Fragmin). LMWHs are replacing unfractionated heparin in the setting of UA and non–Q wave MI due to the ability to achieve full anticoagulation more quickly with subcutaneous dosing. Serial laboratory monitoring with activated partial thromboplastin times (aPTTs) is also not necessary. LMWH has had a greater impact on decreasing mortality and incidence of MI compared to unfractionated heparin (Robert, 1999; Schussheim & Fuster, 1997; Weitz, 1997). Use of LMWH in the setting of AMI is currently being researched.

Treatment of AMI includes oxygen, analgesics, aspirin, beta blockers, angiotensin-converting enzyme (ACE) inhibitors, antiplatelets, and antithrombins and magnesium (in certain instances). GP IIb/IIIa receptor antagonists are currently only approved in the setting of UA and non–Q wave MI. However, multiple research trials are underway to determine the effectiveness of a combination therapy of GP IIb/IIIa inhibitors and thrombolytic therapy in the MI patient. Thrombolytic therapy is indicated in the presence of ST elevation of at least 1 mm in two contiguous leads or new onset LBBB in patients without contraindications to thrombolytics (see Section Eleven). Thrombolytic therapy actually changes the course of infarctions originally destined to become Q wave infarctions, causing them instead to remain as non–Q waves or no infarction at all. As a result, the incidence of non–Q wave MIs has increased in the thrombolytic era. The presence of Q waves does not preclude thrombolytic therapy. The early development of Q waves appears to predict the size of infarction but does not negate the benefits of thrombolytic therapy. Beta blockers should be administered IV in the first four hours of an AMI and thereafter may be given orally. ACE inhibitors are recommended within the first 24 hours for patients with anterior infarcts or with clinical heart failure to reduce mortality via prevention of ventricular remodeling (Hoffman & Reeder, 1998). LMWH may be used for the non–Q wave MI but is currently not indicated for patients presenting with acute ST segment elevation and/or new onset LBBB. Unfractionated heparin should be used in this population and should be weight adjusted as follows: 60 U/kg as a bolus, then a maintenance of 12 U/kg to maintain the aPTT at 1.5 to 2.0 for 48 hours. Maximum dose should not exceed 4,000-U bolus or 1,000 U/hr in patients weighing greater than 70 kg (ACC/AHA Task Force, 1999). Lidocaine, an antiarrhythmic, is not recommended for prophylactic control of ventricular arrhythmias. It should be used only in the event of ventricular tachycardia, ventricular fibrillation and/or ventricular ectopy. Magnesium should only be used in patients with known or suspected magnesium deficiency. Magnesium deficiency should be expected in patients who use diuretics and in patients with poor nutrition and chronic diseases (AHA, 1997).

In summary, any of the ECG and echocardiography changes discussed in this section indicate myocardial circulatory compromise. Serum cardiac markers are essential in diagnosis of patients presenting with non–ST segment elevation. Prompt intervention may stop or reverse the sequence of events. The nurse should alert the physician to the occurrence of T wave and ST segment changes, since these may indicate impending or actual myocardial infarction.

Section Eleven Review

1. Ischemia produces changes in
   A. ventricular depolarization
   B. atrial depolarization
   C. ventricular repolarization
   D. AV conduction
2. Ischemia may be reflected by
   A. wide QRS complexes
   B. T wave changes
   C. isoelectric ST segment
   D. pathologic Q waves
3. A wide, deep Q wave may represent
   A. lack of electrical activity over a necrotic area
   B. slowed ventricular conduction
   C. impaired atrial repolarization
   D. ventricular irritability
4. A myocardial infarction usually will produce
   A. changes in the P and T wave configurations
   B. changes in the QRS complex
   C. T wave and ST segment changes
   D. lengthening of the PR and QT intervals
5. Serum cardiac markers are useful in distinquishing
   A. Q wave from non–Q wave infarction
   B. angina from non–Q wave infarction
   C. posterior from inferior infarction
   D. angina from chest wall pain
6. Treatment of ACS differs from AMI in which of the following medications being administered?
   A. aspirin
   B. beta blockers
   C. oxygen
   D. GP IIb/IIIa receptor antagonists

Answers: 1. C, 2. B, 3. A, 4. C, 5. B, 6. D

SECTION TWELVE: Thrombolytic Therapy

At the completion of this section, the learner will be able to identify selection criteria for thrombolytic therapy and nursing responsibilities associated with thrombolytic therapy.

Treatment of myocardial infarction has shifted from reducing myocardial oxygen demand to augmenting supply by improving perfusion to the infarcted area. Thrombolytic therapy has been used to lyse a clot in the coronary artery to prevent necrosis of the cardiac muscle. The goals of thrombolytic therapy are to maintain patency of the coronary artery, assess and prevent bleeding, avoid myocardial ischemia, prevent reocclusion, preserve left ventricular function, and reduce mortality. Thrombolytics work by converting plasminogen to plasma, which then breaks down the fibrin strands that hold the thrombosis together. Because of the ability of these agents to break down fibrin, they are also referred to as fibrinolytics. Several fibrinolytics are currently available: streptokinase (Kabikinase), anistreplase (Eminase), alteplase (t-PA, Activase), reteplase (r-PA, Retavase), recombinant plasminogen activator, and tenecteplase (TNK-t-PA, TNKase).

Table 15–10 summarizes the eligibility criteria used to determine which patients are suitable for thrombolytic therapy. Treating patients aged 75 years and older is a class IIB indication according to ACC/AHA 1999 guidelines. Despite higher morbidity and mortality as compared to younger patients who receive thrombolytics, the number of lives saved in those older than 75 years of age is greater than the number of lives saved in those younger than age 75. Contraindications generally are categorized as absolute or relative based on the degree of risk of bleeding. Table 15–11 summarizes contraindications to thrombolytic therapy. The learner should be aware that the literature is not conclusive for contraindications or the classification of contraindications as absolute or relative. For example, pregnancy may be considered as either a relative or an absolute contraindication. Risks and benefits must be carefully weighed. Where the risks outweigh the benefits, other reperfusion procedures (e.g., angioplasty or CABG) should be used. Table 15–12 serves as a summary of medications. Physician preference and patient stability also are factors to be considered.

Primary percutaneous coronary angioplasty (PCTA) is an alternative to thrombolytic therapy in patients with AMI and ST segment elevation or new or presumed new LBBB only when it can be performed within 12 hours of symptom onset. The procedure must be performed within 90 minutes of admission (AHA/ACC Task Force, 1999).

Nursing responsibilities include identifying which patients are suitable for thombolytic therapy. Prophylactic pressure dressings may need to be applied to wounds and arterial and venous puncture sites. The nurse must assess for signs of bleeding. The risk for intracranial bleeding is the greatest in the first 24 hours post thrombolytic administration. Neurologic checks should be performed routinely to detect signs of intracranial bleeding. All drainage should be tested for blood. Monitoring vital signs and laboratory tests is another responsibility. Menstrual flow may be heavier in women receiving thrombolytic therapy. Sanitary napkins should be used to monitor bleeding. A drop in the hematocrit may indicate the need for a transfusion. Partial thromboplastin time and prothrombin time should be monitored, and anticoagu-

TABLE 15–10. ELIGIBILITY CRITERIA FOR THROMBOLYTIC THERAPY

Chest pain of > 30 minutes' and < 12 hours' duration, unrelieved with nitroglycerin
ST segment elevation of at least 1 mm in two contiguous leads or new LBBB
Presentation time is < 12 hours from when pain became constant

TABLE 15–11. CONTRAINDICATIONS TO THROMBOLYTIC THERAPY

ABSOLUTE CONTRAINDICATIONS
Acute myocardial infarction
Active internal bleeding
History of cerebrovascular accident
Recent intracranial or intraspinal surgery or trauma (see WARNINGS)
Intracranial neoplasm, arteriovenous malformation, or aneurysm
Known bleeding diathesis
Severe uncontrolled hypertension
RELATIVE WARNINGS
Recent major surgery (e.g., coronary artery bypass graft, obstetrical delivery, organ biopsy, previous puncture of noncompressible vessels)
Cerebrovascular disease
Recent gastrointestinal or genitourinary bleeding
Recent trauma
Hypertension: systolic BP ≥ 180 mm Hg and/or diastolic BP ≥ 110 mm Hg
High likelihood of left heart thrombus (e.g., mitral stenosis with atrial fibrillation)
Acute pericarditis
Subacute bacterial endocarditis
Hemostatic defects including those secondary to severe hepatic or renal disease
Significant hepatic dysfunction
Pregnancy
Diabetic hemorrhagic retinopathy, or other hemorrhagic ophthalmic conditions
Septic thrombophlebitis or occluded AV cannula at seriously infected site
Advanced age (e.g., over 75 years old)
Patients currently receiving oral anticoagulants, e.g., warfarin sodium
Any other condition in which bleeding constitutes a significant hazard or would be particularly difficult to manage because of its location
Recent administration of GP IIb/IIIa inhibitors

From Genentech, Inc. (2000). Tenecteplase package insert. San Francisco: Author.

TABLE 15–12. COMPARISON OF THROMBOLYTIC AGENTS

AGENT	CHARACTERISTICS	DOSAGE
Streptokinase	Synthetic protein derived from group C beta-hemolytic streptococci Lyses clots by activating plasminogen at the clot site and in the circulation Nonspecific, thus may produce systemic symptoms if patient has experienced a prior streptococcal infection or has previously received streptokinase and has developed antibodies	1.5 million units IV infused over 60 minutes
Anisoylated plasminogen streptokinase activator complex (APSAC)	Binds with fibrin before activation so long-term infusions are contraindicated Antibody formation may occur with use of this agent	30 units IV infused over 5 minutes
Tissue plasminogen activator	Affinity for plasminogen that has been incorporated into the clot Because it is clot specific, hemorrhage is less likely No antibody formation, so may be administered more than once	A total of 100 mg is given, with 65 mg IV in the first hour of administration, of which 15 mg is given IVP over 2 minutes. Then a 50-mg/hr IV infusion is given over 1 hour. A 35-mg/hr infusion is given for the second hour. Weight adjusted dosing should be used for patients ≤ 147 lb.

lant therapy should be discontinued if these are elevated > 2.5 times normal values. Packed red blood cells, cryoprecipitate, or plasma may be administered. Protamine sulfate may be administered to counteract anticoagulant therapy. The patient may need computed tomography scanning to detect bleeding sources. Patients who develop an allergic reaction may need IV antihistamines and steroids.

Nursing responsibility also includes assessing for reperfusion. There are several signs of reperfusion. The patient experiences pain relief. Vital signs may change, with bradycardia and hypotension occurring. The ST segment on the ECG may return to baseline. The patient may have PVCs. Creatinine phosphokinase (CPK) levels may peak rapidly, since the artery is reopened, and the enzyme that is released from the necrotic tissue is able to flow into the general circulation. Reocclusion is indicated by chest pain and ST elevation and most commonly occurs within the first 24 hours.

Long-term treatment includes beta blockers, ACE inhibitors, nitrates, antiplatelet agents (aspirin), and anticoagulants. The patient may not understand why treatment is long term, because he or she may have been told that the damage was stopped or the infarction was prevented.

In summary, thrombolytic therapy when initiated within 12 hours of the onset of myocardial infarction helps to prevent necrosis of cardiac muscle. Four thrombolytic agents currently are being used: streptokinase, anisoylated plasminogen streptokinase activator complex (APSAC), tissue plasminogen activator (t-PA), and recombinant plasminogen activator (r-PA). Nursing responsibilities focus on identifying suitable patients, administering thrombolytic agents, monitoring for bleeding complications, and assessing the degree of reperfusion.

SECTION TWELVE REVIEW

1. Which of the following patients would be most eligible for thrombolytic therapy?
   A. 45-year-old patient with chest pain relieved by three nitroglycerin tablets
   B. 70-year-old patient with chest pain of 15 minutes' duration
   C. 50-year-old patient with ST elevation in two continuous leads
   D. 60-year-old patient with ST depression in lead II
2. Nursing interventions for a patient receiving thrombolytic therapy should include
   A. urinary catheter care
   B. neurologic checks
   C. vigorous mouth care
   D. preparing IV sites with a straight razor
3. A complication NOT associated with t-PA is
   A. bleeding from IV sites
   B. antibody reaction
   C. cerebrovascular attack
   D. hematuria
4. Which of the following patients is contraindicated for thrombolytic therapy with streptokinase?
   A. 20-year-old patient with history of gastrointestinal bleeding 15 days ago
   B. 55-year-old patient with history of bleeding gums
   C. 65-year-old who received streptokinase 3 months ago
   D. 30-year-old patient who was pulseless and received CPR for less than a minute

5. Reperfusion is indicated by which of the following symptoms?
   A. hypertension
   B. decrease in CPK level
   C. chest pain relief
   D. tachycardia

Answers: 1. C, 2. B, 3. B, 4. A, 5. C

SECTION THIRTEEN: Pharmacologic Interventions and Nursing Implications

At the completion of this section, the learner will be able to identify common drug classifications used in treating cardiac dysrhythmias and failure. The learner is referred to a pharmacology text to get specific information on dosage and administration. Nursing implications associated with administration of these agents are addressed briefly. Cardioversion and defibrillation are discussed because of the relationship between drug therapy and electric shock with some agents.

Treatment of Dysrhythmias

Antiarrhythmic agents are used in treating cardiac disturbances. The antiarrhythmics have several subcategories, class I through class IV. Additionally, class I has three subcategories, A, B, and C. Each of these drugs is capable of producing new dysrhythmias or worsening current dysrhythmias. Therefore, constant ECG monitoring is required as these medications are initiated (Table 15–13).

Class IA drugs reduce automaticity and prolong the refractory period of the heart. They are indicated in the treatment of atrial dysrhythmias and PVCs. Class IB drugs decrease refractory periods but do not affect automaticity to a great extent. These drugs are used chiefly in the treatment of ventricular dysrhythmias. Class IC agents decrease spontaneous depolarization. They are also used in treating ventricular dysrhythmias. These drugs have shown a proarrhythmic effect in some studies. Therefore, they are still under investigation (Hudak & Gallo, 1994).

Class II agents block the effects of the catecholamines (i.e., epinephrine). They decrease automatic-

TABLE 15–13. COMPARISON OF ANTIARRHYTHMIC AGENTS

CATEGORY	EXAMPLES	EFFECT	INDICATIONS
Class IA	Quinidine (Cardioquin)	Reduce automaticity	PVCs
	Procainamide (Pronestyl)	Prolong refractory period	Atrial fibrillation and flutter
	Disopyramide (Norpace)		
Class IB	Lidocaine (Xylocaine)	Decrease refractory period	PVCs
	Mexiletine (Mexitil)		Ventricular tachycardia or fibrillation
	Tocainide (Tonocard)		
Class IC	Encainide (Enkaid)	Decrease spontaneous depolarization	PVCs
	Flecainide (Tambocor)		Ventricular tachycardia
	Propafenone Moricizine (Ethmozine)		
Class II	Propanolol (Inderal) (beta blockers)	Decrease automaticity	Atrial/supraventricular dysrhythmias
	Esmolol (Brevibloc)	Decrease conduction	
	Acebutolol (Sectral)		
Class III	Amiodarone (Cordarone)	Prolong refractory period	Ventricular tachycardia or fibrillation
	Bretylium (Bretylol)		
	Sotalol (Butilide)		Atrial fibrillation/flutter
Class IV	Verapamil (Calan)	Decrease conduction	Supraventricular dysrhythmias and hypertension
	Diltiazem (Cardiazem)		
	Nifedipine (Procardia)		
Digitalis glycosides	Digoxin (Lanoxin)	Decrease conduction through AV node	Congestive heart failure
Endogenous nucleoside	Adenosine (Adenocard)	Blocks reentry of ventricular impulses through the AV node into the atria	Supraventricular dysrhythmias

ity and slow conduction. Their exact effects depend on which catecholamine receptor they block. Catecholamines may affect four different receptors: $alpha_1$ vasoconstriction, $alpha_2$ norepinephrine release, $beta_1$ cardiac stimulation, and $beta_2$ vasodilation and bronchodilation. For example, phentolamine (Regitine) is an alpha-blocking agent. Therefore, it produces vasodilation. However, most of the agents used to treat dysrhythmias in this category are beta-blocking agents. Thus, they decrease cardiac stimulation and may produce vasoconstriction and bronchoconstriction. Drugs in this category are used in treating tachydysrhythmias. These drugs may not be used in patients with congestive heart failure, severe bradycardia, and second degree or higher heart block because of decreased cardiac stimulation. They may be contraindicated in asthma due to bronchoconstriction. Since class II drugs decrease the heart rate, the heart rate may be unable to increase to maintain CO in some situations, such as exercise. In cases of cardiac arrest, the heart may be less sensitive to sympathomimetic drugs (i.e., epinephrine) because of the beta-blocking effect.

Class III agents prolong refractory periods, the direct opposite effect of class IB drugs. They increase the fibrillation threshold (making the cell more resistant) of the cells. Thus, they are indicated in the treatment of ventricular dysrhythmias. Sotalol is an agent in this category. Amiodarone is used when SVT and VT do not respond to conventional therapy, because of the seriousness of its side effects.

Class IV agents are calcium channel blockers. These drugs block the entry of calcium through the cell membranes, thereby decreasing depolarization. Verapamil is the most commonly used calcium channel blocker for dysrhythmias. Nifedipine is another drug in this category that is used to treat hypertension.

Cardioversion and Defibrillation

Cardioversion is used to treat supraventricular tachycardia that is resistant to medication and ventricular tachycardia in an unstable patient. The unstable patient may be hypotensive, dyspneic, experiencing chest pain, or have evidence of congestive heart failure, myocardial infarction, or ischemia. Analgesia may be provided before the electric shock. A synchronizer knob is pushed on the defibrillator machine, which allows the machine to discharge during firing of the ectopic impulse. Low voltages are tried initially (50 J to 100 J depending on the size of the patient). Cardioversion can be repeated using larger voltages if it is unsuccessful. Defibrillation is used to treat ventricular tachycardia in an unresponsive patient and ventricular fibrillation. Defibrillation is an unsynchronized electric shock that usually administers a larger number of joules than cardioversion (200 J up to 360 J). Defibrillation may be repeated.

Treatment of Heart Failure

Heart failure is classified according to the degree of dyspnea experienced (Table 15–14). ACE I inhibitors and angiotensin II receptor blockers are the main line treatment of congestive heart failure. ACE I drugs prevent the conversion of angiotensin I to II, thus preventing an increase in venous constriction. They also decrease the release of aldosterone, decreasing plasma volume. ACE inhibitors decrease preload and afterload simultaneously. In congestive heart failure, catecholamine secretion is increased as a compensatory mechanism for the decreased contractility. Atrial natriuretic factor is released in response to atrial distention. This factor enhances aldosterone to maximize blood volume. Organs react as if there is not enough blood, rather than a maldistribution of blood. Commonly used ACE inhibitors are captopril, enalapril, lisinopril, and fosinopril. The side effects of ACE inhibitors are cough and renal failure (Moser, 1996). Angiotensin II receptor blockers block the angiotensin receptor directly. The primary advantage over ACE I is that coughing does not occur as a side effect. Current ACE II blockers are losartan, irbisartan, valsartan, cardisartan, and telmasartan.

Digitalis glycosides may be used to treat decreased contractility seen in congestive heart failure. These drugs also slow impulse conduction through the AV node. They may also be used in the treatment of atrial or supraventricular dysrhythmias, although adenosine and verapamil are the preferred drugs for SVT and diltiazem, verapamil,

TABLE 15–14. NEW YORK HEART ASSOCIATION FUNCTIONAL CRITERIA FOR PATIENTS WITH HEART DISEASE

CLASS	FUNCTIONAL LIMITATION	DESCRIPTION
I	No limitation	Ordinary physical activity does not cause undue fatigue, dyspnea, or palpitation. Tolerance to intensive physical activity may be reduced.
II	Slight activity limitation	Comfortable at rest. Moderate physical activity (e.g., climbing stairs) results in fatigue, palpitation, dyspnea, or angina.
III	Marked activity limitation	Comfortable at rest. Very modest physical activity will lead to symptoms.
IV	Inability to carry out any physical activity without discomfort	Dyspnea due to congestive heart failure is present at rest. Any physical activity results in increased discomfort.

Adapted from Braunwald, E. (ed.). (1988). Heart disease, *3rd ed. (p. 12). Philadelphia: W.B. Saunders.*

or beta blockers are preferred for treating atrial fibrillation (AHA, 1997). Digitalis increases the heart's sensitivity to electric shock and may precipitate ventricular fibrillation. Thus, cardioversion should be attempted before administering digitalis, or the drug should be withheld 1 to 2 days before cardioversion. Vasodilators are recommended in patients who cannot tolerate ACE I drugs or in whom they are contraindicated.

Beta blockers such as carvedilol, a nonselective beta blocker with alpha F blocking has been found to reduce mortality rates and reduce worsening of heart failure (Konstam & Remme, 1998). As LV function declines in patients with heart failure, several compensating mechanisms are activated in an attempt to maintain adequate systemic blood pressure and perfusion of vital organs. Beta blockers are administered to control the compensating tachycardia that patients may develop. Not all heart failure patients are able to tolerate beta blockers and careful monitoring is important when initiating therapy (Michael & Parnell, 1998).

Surgical alternatives are available to help augment cardiac function. Although cardiac transplantation has become the therapy of choice for patients with advanced heart failure, scarcity of donors and age limitations prohibits its widespread use. Coronary artery bypass surgery, dynamic cardioplasty, and partial left ventriculectomy are currently surgical interventions (Dimengo, 1998). The nursing care of patients undergoing any of these procedures is beyond the scope of this book.

Nursing responsibilities in drug therapy focus on monitoring the ECG pattern to determine the response to drug therapy. Drug serum levels should be examined before administering the drug to prevent toxicity. The patient's pulse must be assessed for 1 minute before administering each dose, since many of these agents decrease the heart rate. If the heart rate is too slow (i.e., below 60 bpm), the physician should be notified, since the medication may need to be withheld. The nurse must teach patients how to obtain their heart rate and to determine regularity by assessing their pulse for 1 minute. The need to take the medications as prescribed and to report cardiac-related symptoms, such as palpitations, chest pain, wheezing, fatigue, and syncope, must be stressed.

In summary, antiarrhythmic agents are classified in four large categories. They usually act by decreasing automaticity or by affecting the refractory period. Impulse conduction may be delayed. They may help correct or worsen a dysrhythmia. Thus, nursing responsibilities include careful monitoring of the patient's ECG pattern and clinical response.

SECTION THIRTEEN REVIEW

1. Beta blockers (class II agents) may produce which of the following side effects?
   A. weight gain
   B. hypokalemia
   C. wheezing
   D. hives
2. Cardioversion should not be attempted in a digitalized patient because
   A. digitalis increases the heart's sensitivity to electric shock
   B. digitalis prevents electric stimulation of the heart
   C. extra voltage is required to produce the desired effect
   D. defibrillation is indicated
3. A patient on a beta-blocking agent may not respond to sympathomimetic agents in cardiac arrest because
   A. the beta blocker competes with the sympathomimetic agent for the beta receptor site
   B. beta-blocking agents inhibit the effect of catecholamines
   C. alpha receptors are also blocked
   D. the sympathomimetic agent is administered too late in the arrest
4. The difference between cardioversion and defibrillation is
   A. defibrillation uses a lower amount of joules
   B. cardioversion is synchronized
   C. defibrillation cannot be repeated
   D. cardioversion is used only to treat atrial dysrhythmias
5. Nursing responsibilities in administering antiarrhythmic agents include
   A. administering all agents by IV route
   B. obtaining a 12-lead ECG before each administration
   C. monitoring the patient's pulse for 30 seconds before administration
   D. checking drug serum levels

Answers: 1. C, 2. A, 3. B, 4. B, 5. D

SECTION FOURTEEN: Electrical Therapy

At the completion of this section, the learner will be able to identify indications for pacemaker and defibrillation therapy, types of devices, and nursing implications for the patient being electrically paced or rhythm reorganized.

Pacemakers

Pacemakers may be inserted in addition to drug therapy. An artificial pacemaker is indicated when one of three conditions exists: failure of the conduction system, failure to initiate an impulse spontaneously, and failure to maintain primary pacing control (spontaneous impulses may occur, but they are not synchronized). There are three commonly used pacing mechanisms: external, epicardial, and endocardial.

External pacing can be used in the same circumstances as an internal pacing device. The major difference is that it is always a temporary measure. The external pacer can be set for continuous or demand pacing. It delivers electric impulses to the myocardium transthoracically through two electrode pads placed anteriorly and posteriorly on the chest (Fig. 15–29). External pacers should be placed and used without hesitation. As hypoxia and acidosis increase, the myocardium is less responsive to external pacing (AHA, 1997). The date and time external pacing is initiated, as well as pacing rate, mode, current needed for capture, and a pacing strip should be documented. The presence of an adequate pulse and blood pressure demonstrates mechanical capture (the ability of the heart to respond to the electrical impulse).

An endocardial or epicardial pacer is placed later. Epicardial pacing is inserted during open heart surgery by placing electrodes directly on the surface of the heart. Endocardial pacers usually are inserted through the subclavian, jugular, or femoral veins into the right ventricle, where they are lodged.

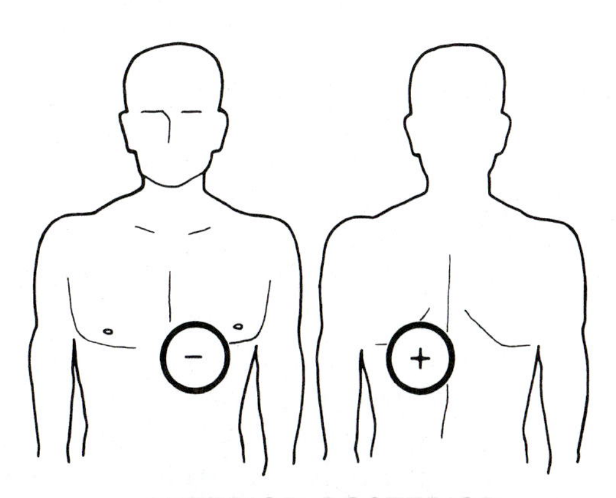

Figure 15–29. Anterior–posterior electrode placement. The most effective electrode placement is the anterior–posterior position. The negative electrode is placed anteriorly halfway between the xiphoid process and the left nipple. The positive electrode is placed beneath the scapula and to the left of the spine. *(Source: Journal of Emergency Nursing, Beeler, Vol 19, No. 3, p. 204. Mosby Yearbook.)*

Pacemakers can be programmed to pace different areas of the heart at specific time intervals and to respond to a level of stimulation. Most pacemakers are designed to pace the ventricles. In this case, a spike will occur before the QRS complex. This method of pacing may be used when transmission of impulses from the atria is being blocked (i.e., complete heart block, Section Ten). The atria also may be paced. A spike will appear before the P wave. This method of pacing may be used with sinus node disease. AV sequential pacing may be used to synchronize heart depolarization in order to maintain CO (Fig. 15–30). In this type of pacing, both the atria and the ventricles are paced (dual chamber). Spikes appear before the P wave and the QRS complex.

A pacemaker may be programmed to function in the inhibited mode, where a pacing impulse is initiated when an intrinsic beat is not sensed. If it is programmed in a triggered mode, it fires an impulse in response to sensing electrical activity (e.g., ventricular fibrillation). A double-function pacemaker reacts to both inhibition and triggering.

The number of times the pacemaker will fire is determined by the sensitivity setting of the pacemaker. If the sensitivity is low, the pacemaker basically ignores the patient's ventricles and will pace more frequently. If the sensitivity is high, the patient's ventricles will be allowed to discharge. Most patients are set on demand, with a high sensitivity setting. A paced beat occurs only when the patient's atria or ventricles fail to discharge. Fixed-rate pacing is used only with individuals whose inherent rhythm is exceedingly slow. If the pacemaker competes with the patient's own impulse generation, the term *failure to sense* is used. This is a potentially dangerous situation, because the pacemaker may discharge an impulse during the relative refractory or supranormal periods of ventricular repolarization, precipitating ventricular fibrillation. The term *failure to capture* is used to describe the situation in which the pacemaker initiates an impulse, but the stimulus is not strong enough to produce depolarization. A pacing spike may be present, but P waves or QRS complexes or both are absent. Figure 15–30 is an example of artificially paced ECG patterns. For sensing and capturing to occur, the pulse generator must have adequate battery function, the leads must be firmly attached to the pacemaker and the myocardium, and the lead wires must be intact (Witherall, 1994).

Pacemakers are classified according to a uniform system (Table 15–15). For example, a DDD pacemaker is a dual-chamber pacemaker that is able to pace and sense (Fig. 15–30). A DDDR pacemaker is rate responsive, which means that it can detect the metabolic need for rate adjustment (e.g., during exercise) and adjust accordingly if the native pacemaker fails to achieve this rate.

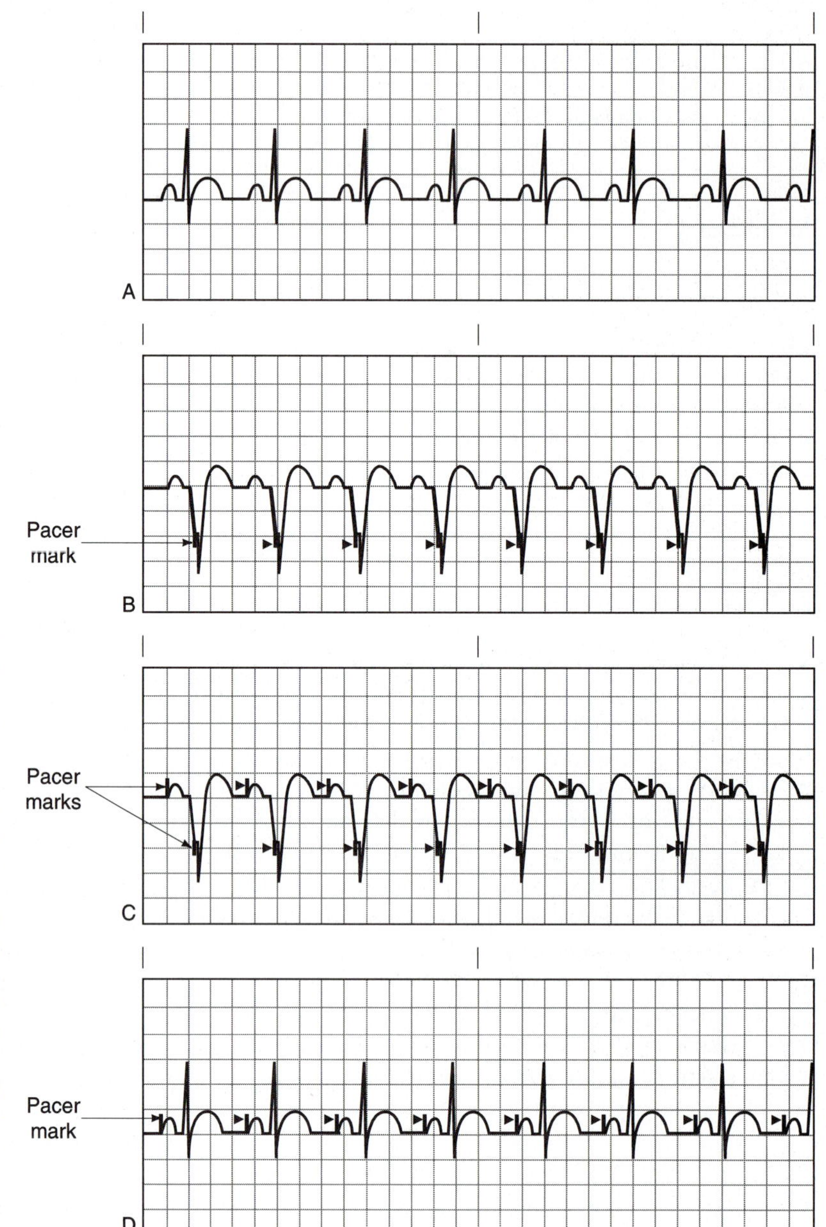

Figure 15–30. A pacemaker in DDD mode is capable of exhibiting any of four pacing patterns, all within a brief period of time. **A.** Atrial and ventricular sensing. In this situation, the patient's SA node is pacing at a higher rate than that programmed for the atrial pacemaker to kick in. The PR interval is less than the programmed delay, indicating that the ventricles are responding normally. The pacemaker is sensing the patient's own rhythm. Both atrial and ventricular pacing are inhibited. **B.** Atrial sensing and ventricular pacing. The patient's SA node is pacing, but the PR interval is greater than the programmed delay. The ventricles are being artificially paced. **C.** Atrial and ventricular pacing. The patient's SA node is firing less often than the pacemaker's programmed rate. The PR interval is greater than the programmed delay. Both atria and ventricles are being artificially paced. (Capture is evident by depolarization immediately after the pacing strikes.) **D.** Atrial pacing and ventricular sensing. The patient's SA node is firing less often than the pacemaker's programmed rate. The PR interval is less than the programmed delay. The atria are being artificially paced, while the ventricles are responding normally.

Defibrillators

An implantable cardioverter/defibrillator (ICD) may be implanted in patients who have had prior aborted sudden cardiac death or proven sustained ventricular tachycardia (Knight et al., 1997). It also may be placed prophylactally in high-risk groups. The device is a fully implantable, battery-operated system designed to recognize and terminate ventricular tachyarrhythmias that can cause sudden death (Fig. 15–31). The device will discharge to override the ectopic ventricular pacemaker. The most recent ICDs are capable of distinguishing ventricular tachycardia (VT) from ventricular fibrillation (VF) (thus delivering defibrillation shocks only when absolutely necessary); antitachycardia pacing (to treat VT without resorting to cardioversion shocks unless necessary); providing back-up bradycardia pacing (eliminating the need for a standard pacemaker); and storing cardiac events so that they can be retrieved for analyzing the patient's response to treatment. Battery life depends on the frequency of discharges but generally is 3 to 5 years (Knight et al., 1997).

Implantation of the ICD used to require an open chest procedure or subxiphoid approach. It now can be

TABLE 15–15. COMPARISON OF PAIN ASSESSMENT DATA

	CARDIAC ORIGIN	PULMONARY ORIGIN
Precipitating factors	Activity Changes in environmental temperature Eating Emotional stress Hypertension Traumatic injury to heart Infection	Immobility Fractures of ribs or long bones Upper or lower respiratory infection
Quality	Pressure-like tightness Burning nature Stabbing and sharp, may increase with anxiety	Changes with respiratory cycle May increase with cough May increase with activity
Region and radiation	Substernal Precordial Radiation to neck, arms, back, and abdomen	Lateral chest Radiation to shoulder and neck
Associated symptoms	Diaphoresis Nausea and vomiting Dyspnea Change in level of consciousness Abnormal heart sounds Apprehension	Dyspnea Cough Decreased or adventitious breath sounds Apprehension (but usually less than that seen with cardiac origin)
Timing and treatment strategies	May be sudden or gradual May be relieved with rest or vasodilators	May be sudden or gradual May be relieved with change in position Usually not relieved with rest or vasodilators

accomplished through a nonthoracic approach through the subclavian or cephalic vein. A unipolar system that uses the pectorally implanted pulse generator may be used which simplifies implantation. Once placed the device must be programmed and tested, using electrophysiologic studies. In essence, VF is intentionally induced in a controlled environment. The ICD is set to deliver shocks at the rate necessary to convert the VF to a sinus rhythm. The placement of the ICD is a frightening experience for some patients.

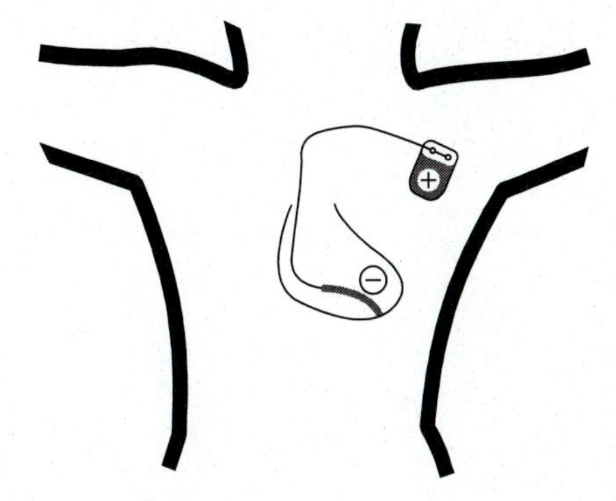

Figure 15-31. Nonthoracotomy lead system with the pectorally implanted pulse generator used as the anode of the defibrillating circuit.

If the ICD is malfunctioning, it may be necessary to deactivate the device by applying a doughnut-shaped magnet over the ICD. Reprogramming may be necessary. The magnet mode varies by manufacturers. The nurse must be familiar with the correct procedure for deactivating the device via the magnet. If the ICD is malfunctioning, or if the heart is not responding to delivered shocks, life-support measures should be initiated. During CPR, the rescuer may feel a mild shock (similar to a static electricity shock) if the device fires. External defibrillation is performed using anterior–posterior paddle placement. If temporary external pacing is required, the ICD should be deactivated with a magnet.

Patient teaching with ICD placement is extensive. Patients must understand the difference between heart attack and cardiac arrest. The ICD will not prevent an MI (heart attack), but it will help prevent cardiac arrest. The patient should be taught that the ICD can "reorganize" his or her heart rhythm as well as stimulate the heart (pacemaker action is available on most recent models). Patients should keep a diary of shocks received, activities before and after treatment, symptoms, and response after shock. They should contact their physician when they receive a shock.

Patients with ICDs may be restricted from driving in some states (Finch et al., 1997). They must avoid high magnetic fields because these may deactivate the device. These patients should not receive diathermy treatment, magnetic resonance imaging, or lithotripsy. Arc welders and large industrial motors should be avoided. Cellular phones can interfere with the operation of all defibrillators if held closer than six inches from the pulse generator.

An automatic external defibrillator may be used by some medical and nursing service personnel and laypersons to treat ventricular tachycardia and ventricular fibrillation. The ECG pattern is detected through paddles placed on the patient's chest. If a lethal dysrhythmia is detected, the paddles will discharge to defibrillate the patient.

Nursing care includes preparing the patient for insertion of an endocardial pacemaker, or applying an external pacing device correctly. The ECG pattern must be monitored to determine that the pacemaker is pacing at the correct rate (demand versus fixed), capturing with each impulse, and sensing the patient's own rhythm. Additionally, the nurse assesses the threshold (minimal amount of output required to initiate depolarization) of the pacemaker. The learner is referred to the literature associated with each pacing and defibrillation device to determine the correct method of checking the threshold for that device. It is helpful if patients with a history of dysrhythmias carry a copy of their most recent ECG. Patients should be encouraged to get a MedicAlert bracelet to identify that they have a pacemaker or ICD. They should have the type of device, manufacturer, and model number readily available. The nurse should identify who programs the device and how the device can be shut down if necessary.

In summary, there are three routes of electrical therapy: external, epicardial, and endocardial. The atria or the ventricles may be paced. The rate may be set on a demand or continuous setting. The pacing device may fail to sense and compete with the patient's own rhythm. The device may fail to capture by initiating an impulse that is not sufficient to depolarize myocardial cells. ICD devices are capable of pacing, cardioverting, and defibrillating (unless they are an older model). In cases in which the device malfunctions or the heart does not respond mechanically to treatment, CPR is initiated without hesitation. Nursing care focuses on assisting with insertion or application, and monitoring the threshold, capture, and sensitivity of the device.

Section Fourteen Review

1. An external pacing device
   - **A.** is used only to treat supraventricular dysrhythmias
   - **B.** is a temporary measure
   - **C.** requires the patient to be alert in order to function
   - **D.** can be set only in continuous mode
2. An epicardial pacing device is
   - **A.** placed through the subclavian vein
   - **B.** applied to the chest wall
   - **C.** inserted in open heart surgery
   - **D.** used exclusively for AV sequential pacing
3. Failure to sense means
   - **A.** the pacing device is turned off
   - **B.** depolarization is not occurring
   - **C.** the patient is tachycardic
   - **D.** the pacing device is competing with the patient's own rhythm
4. Failure to capture means
   - **A.** depolarization does not occur after a pacer-generated impulse
   - **B.** atria and ventricles are not contracting in a synchronous manner
   - **C.** the pacing device needs to be replaced
   - **D.** the patient will require cardioversion
5. When a pacemaker is functioning in an inhibited mode,
   - **A.** a pacing impulse is generated when an intrinsic beat is not sensed
   - **B.** it fires an impulse in response to sensing electrical activity
   - **C.** the SA node is overriding the pacing rate
   - **D.** the device is malfunctioning
6. A patient with an ICD complains of multiple repeated shocks. He is in sinus tachycardia on the heart monitor. The nurse should
   - **A.** hold a magnet over the ICD
   - **B.** cardiovert the patient
   - **C.** notify the physician to obtain a deactivation order
   - **D.** roll the patient to his left side

Answers: 1. B, 2. C, 3. D, 4. A, 5. A, 6. C

SECTION FIFTEEN: Improving Cardiac Perfusion and Pumping

At the completion of this section, the learner will be able to explain the relationship between dysrhythmia, infarction, and heart failure. New treatment modalities in caring for patients with perfusion problems will be addressed.

The cardiovascular system consists of three interrelated subsystems: (1) a pumping system to push fluid throughout the body; (2) a network of electrical wiring; and (3) a series of vascular conduits that supply the heart muscle and the electrical subsystem (Kollisch & Sloane, 1994). Dysrhythmias interfere with the normal rhythm of the pump. Pump problems develop when the pumping action is altered and/or when the pump is asked to perform more work than its vascular supply can support by way of the coronary arteries. Myocardial oxygen demand is a function of the work the pump performs (contractility) and heart rate. When contractility or heart rate increases, vascular supply must improve to meet these demands, or angina will occur. Infarction results from lack of blood being pumped through the coronary arteries to supply the heart. Thus, infarction may be caused by coronary artery occlusion (due to clot or spasm), or decreased contractility (as in heart failure), where heart rate alone is inadequate to maintain the cardiac output. Conversely, infarction may cause heart failure in cases where enough of the pump muscle is damaged and unable to contract. Dysrhythmias can precipitate infarction and subsequently heart failure, by increasing myocardial oxygen demands (tachycardia), or by decreasing vascular supply (fibrillation, complete heart block) due to inadequate pump action.

Procedures to Improve Coronary Artery Perfusion

Section Twelve discussed the use of thrombolytics in dissolving coronary artery clots. They are used in the acute situation. Blockages of the coronary arteries may be detected before cardiac ischemia and infarction occur through diagnostic testing (e.g., thallium scans, echocardiography, cardiac catheterization). Percutaneous transluminal coronary angioplasty (PTCA) has been used for over a decade in treating blockages and lesions in nonacute situations. The aim of PTCA is to dilate a stenotic segment of the artery to the same diameter as the surrounding areas by inflating a balloon catheter that is passed through a guide catheter. Although it was initially designed for single-vessel disease, it is now used for multiple-vessel disease. Contraindications for PTCA include left main stem coronary artery disease without collateral circulation (to protect the left ventricle when the balloon is inflated), and arteries with aneurysm formation (to prevent rupture). Dissection of the artery is a risk for any of the invasive procedures described in this section. Facilities performing PCTA must have the capability to perform open heart surgery in the event of a dissection or other complication. The patient may be premedicated with calcium channel blockers (to prevent coronary artery spasm) and aspirin, heparin, clopridogrel, and/or GP IIb/IIIa inhibitors (IV medication to prevent platelet aggregation).

A nursing care priority is to minimize bleeding from the insertion site and to monitor for other sources of bleeding. Mechanical compression devices (e.g., FemoStop) can be applied to maintain consistent pressure to the insertion site. Peripheral circulation must be checked prior to and during use of these devices. Patients should also be monitored for hematoma or pseudoaneurysm formation, embolism (shortness of breath [SOB], chest pain, tachycardia), thrombosis (diminished peripheral pulses, change in skin color and temperature), and hypersensitivity to the contrast dye (rash, SOB, decreased urine output). Stools, urine, and emesis should be tested for the presence of blood. Any changes in the patient's level of consciousness should be reported.

Percutaneous cardiopulmonary support (PCPS) may be used in acute situations for patients who are poor surgical risks for CABG. These patients are extremely ill, with ejection fractions less than 30 percent (Dukovcic, Daleiden-Burns, & Shaul, 1998). In essence, the patient is placed on extracorporeal circulation prior to the procedure to provide for more effective pumping and oxygenation of the blood. This increases the patient's ability to meet the extra myocardial demands from the procedure. After angioplasty is completed, the patient is weaned off the machine.

Laser coronary angioplasty is very similar to rotational ablation therapy. The laser catheter is flexible, allowing it to be used in tortuous arteries. Lesions are vaporized. Postprocedure care is the same as for ablation therapy.

Stents may be inserted to keep arteries open once they have been cleared. The most common stents in use are balloon expandable, made of a variety of materials such as stainless steel, and heparin coated. When the balloon is expanded, the stent is embedded into the vessel wall. Postprocedure care again focuses on minimizing blood loss and monitoring for internal bleeding. Prevention of restenosis is achieved with aspirin, antiplatelet agents such as ticlopidine or clopidogrel, anticoagulants such as heparin or LMWH, GP IIb/IIIa inhibitors such as abciximab and integrilin (Lefkovits & Topol, 1997).

Procedures to Improve Pumping Action

Radiofrequency catheter ablation therapy is used to interrupt electrical reentry paths in the heart that precipitate episodes of SVT and atrial fibrillation with a rapid ventricular response rate (Guaglianone & Tyndall, 1995). Before an area is electrically damaged by the catheter, the entire cardiac conduction system is examined and electrical pathways of the heart are mapped. This may take up to 6 hours, during which the patient must be immobile. The catheter is inserted, using a femoral or subclavian approach, and positioned near the site of abnormal conduction. Radiofrequency current is applied between the tip of the catheter and a skin electrode. Postprocedure nursing care focuses on dysrhythmia detection and treatment.

Cardiac transplants may be performed to improve pumping action. For information regarding this procedure, refer to Module 4.

Dynamic cardiomyoplasty is a procedure in which a section of the latissimus dorsi skeletal muscle is brought through the ribs and wrapped around the weakened heart muscle. The skeletal muscle is electrically paced to contract in synchrony with the left ventricle (Dimengo, 1998). Postprocedure nursing care centers on enhancing cardiac output, because the underlying problem precipitating the failure has not been treated. Inotropic drugs and vasopressors are given. Breath sounds are assessed frequently, and ABGs are monitored for symptoms of pulmonary edema and hypoxia.

In summary, several new procedures are available to treat the pumping ability, electrical wiring, and vascular conduits of the heart. Drug therapy as explained in Section Thirteen, and electrical therapy as explained in Section Fourteen, may be used in conjunction with these new procedures. Nursing's role in caring for these patients is to improve oxygen supply by preventing bleeding, treating dysrhythmias, and enhancing cardiac output, usually through drug and fluid therapy.

SECTION FIFTEEN REVIEW

1. The greatest risk of postprocedure bleeding is with the performance of
   A. radiofrequency ablation therapy
   B. PTCA
   C. coronary rotation ablation therapy
   D. stent placement
2. Which of the following best describes the relationship between infarction and heart failure?
   A. infarction occurs first, then heart failure follows
   B. either may occur first and lead to the other condition
   C. they are not related unless there is a dysrhythmia
   D. heart failure occurs first, then infarction follows
3. Which of the following may indicate postprocedure internal bleeding?
   A. increased urine output
   B. diminished peripheral pulse in cannulated extremity
   C. decreased bowel sounds
   D. change in level of consciousness

Answers: 1. C, 2. B, 3. D

SECTION SIXTEEN: The Focused Perfusion Assessment

At the completion of this section, the learner will be able to describe information to collect in a history and examination that is relevant to the perfusion status of the patient.

Nursing History

Precipitating Event

It is considered a priority to assess perfusion whether or not your patient has a history of a perfusion abnormality. Airway, breathing, and circulation should be assessed before eliciting a nursing history. A brief, limited assessment can be performed systematically in less than 60 seconds. A head-to-toe format or systems approach can be used to cluster assessment data. Regardless of the format used, the nurse is ensuring that the patient is able to provide subjective information without further compromising his or her physical integrity.

It is important to focus on the event that led to the present admission of the patient. Focusing on this area will provide information on the patient's ability to compensate to a cardiovascular stressor. Nursing interventions are targeted toward increasing myocardial oxygen supply while decreasing myocardial demands. Information about the precipitating event can be used to identify areas where the patient needs external support in order to compensate.

Past Medical History

The patient's past medical history is important. Certain conditions, such as hypertension, diabetes, congenital heart anomalies, mitral valve prolapse, and rheumatic fever, may produce vascular changes that impede the patient's ability to compensate. Medical management of previous perfusion abnormalities is important to note. A history of cardiac surgery, angioplasty, or administration of thrombolytics can alert the nurse to the patient's state of cardiovascular health and the patient's potential to compensate to an additional cardiovascular stressor.

It is essential to differentiate chronic symptoms from current symptoms. This is especially true in the elderly patient. For example, an elderly patient may have chronic pedal edema secondary to a decreased glomerular filtration rate or decreased venous compliance associated with normal aging. The edema may not be related to acute cardiovascular changes.

Diet History

A diet history should be elicited in a patient with a perfusion disorder. Cholesterol, fat, sodium, and potassium intake may be related to a hypertensive episode or a dysrhythmia. If the patient is on cardiovascular medications or thiazide diuretics, a diet history is crucial to assessing the patient's degree of compliance with the long-term management plan and perhaps understanding of the perfusion disorder and treatment modalities.

Medication History

A medication history will help the nurse evaluate the patient's response to interventions as well as identify potential sources for assessment findings. If the patient is taking beta blockers, such as propranolol (Inderal), depolarization is depressed. Beta-blocking agents inhibit sympathetic nervous stimulation and atrioventricular conduction and decrease cardiac contractility and arterial pressure. Thus, the cardiac rhythm is slower than what the patient may have experienced previously. If the patient's rhythm converts to complete heart block, a ventricular pattern, or asystole, it may be more difficult to convert the pattern to a sinus rhythm. The beta-blocking agent decreases the ability of the cardiac cells to respond to cardiac stimulating drugs. If the patient has been using over-the-counter stimulants, drinking or eating excessive caffeine-containing substances, or has a history of smoking tobacco, tachydysrhythmias and hypertension may result. These symptoms may occur in direct response to previous treatments or lifestyle patterns and not as a result of the presenting perfusion disorder.

In summary, a pertinent nursing history of a patient with a perfusion disorder includes a brief history of the present event, previously diagnosed conditions and medical management, comparison of current symptoms with previous symptoms, dietary intake, use of prescribed and over-the-counter medications, and a smoking/lifestyle profile.

Frequent Symptoms Associated with Perfusion Disorders

If a perfusion disorder is suspected, the nurse should focus on eliciting the most common circulatory complaints: pain, edema, palpitations, and a change in level of consciousness.

Pain

Although chest pain is discussed in Module 8, it warrants further discussion in order to discriminate pain of cardiac origin from that of pulmonary origin. The mnemonic PQRST is helpful in organizing assessment data related to pain. Eliciting information about precipitating factors (P), quality (Q), radiation and region (R), associated symptoms (S), and timing and treatment strategies (T) will clue the nurse to the origin of the pain. Table 15–15 compares pain assessment data. Pain should be measured consistently using the same scaling device each time (see Module 2).

The pain associated with perfusion disorders usually is related to an imbalance between myocardial oxygen supply and myocardial oxygen demands. This imbalance may be due to coronary artery vasoconstriction, coronary artery occlusion, a chronic narrowing of the coronary artery, or inadequate electrical activity of the heart. Myocardial oxygen supply also can be decreased because of decreased hemoglobin or decreased oxygen saturation of the hemoglobin. Fluid volume excess conditions can produce pain because the myocardium cannot permanently circulate the additional volume, and the oxygen demands of the myocardium increase. Although there may not be changes in the coronary arteries or hemoglobin, the normal supply may be inadequate to meet the increased demand. The pain associated with perfusion disorders must be relieved, since it is an indirect measurement of myocardial oxygen. Pain relief usually is achieved by using a combination of vasodilators and narcotics. Pain may not always be present in all patients with perfusion problems. Diabetic patients and the elderly may not feel pain. Women may have "atypical" pain such as abdominal pain and fatigue. These patients should be thoroughly evaluated with additional tests such as ECG and cardiac serum markers.

Edema

Edema may be manifested directly (as in shortness of breath) in a patient with a perfusion disorder. Increased ventricular and atrial pressures eventually result in heart failure (Starling's law) that leads to increased hydrostatic pressure due to fluid stasis. Venous obstruction, as in the case of thrombosis, can also increase hydrostatic pressure. Elevated hydrostatic pressure in the capillaries produces fluid movement out of the capillary and into the interstitial spaces. Edema is usually not detectable until the interstitial fluid volume is 30 percent above normal. This translates approximately to a 5- to 10-pound (2.3- to 4.5-kg) weight gain.

Shortness of breath results from fluid movement out of the pulmonary capillaries and into the lung interstitial space, thereby decreasing oxygen diffusion from the alevoli into the pulmonary capillaries. The presence of wet-sounding crackles (rales) on auscultation of the lungs indicates pulmonary edema. Severe pulmonary edema will be associated with frothy, pink sputum production.

Edema is measured on a 1 to 4 scale, with 4 being most severe. It is described as pitting or nonpitting in nature. Nonpitting edema is associated with protein coagulation in the tissue and is seen more frequently in conditions of decreased plasma proteins. Pitting edema, interstitial fluid with less protein content, is frequently associated with perfusion disorders. Assessment of edema includes direct observation and palpation of the skin, particularly in the sacrum and lower legs.

Edema has been discussed as a distribution problem. There are other signs of distribution abnormalities that should be evaluated in a patient with a perfusion problem. Jugular venous distention (JVD) may indicate a fluid distribution problem. The venous system is a low pressure system, and it is sensitive to right atrial pressure. Retention of blood in the right side of the heart (as in the case of heart failure or cor pulmonale) will increase right atrial pressure and subsequently produce jugular venous distention due to backflow through the vena cavae. In assessing for venous distention, elevate the head of the bed to approximately 45 degrees. The patient's head should be turned slightly away from the examiner. A penlight can be used to shine a light tangentially across the neck. Figure 15–32 illustrates measurement of JVD.

Invasive measurement of fluid distribution can be obtained through a pulmonary arterial catheter. An elevated pulmonary artery wedge pressure (PAWP) indicates left ventricle failure (increased left heart preload) and may be associated with crackles or rales because of backflow of blood into the lungs and subsequent fluid shifts. An elevated right atrial pressure (increased right heart preload) is seen commonly in right heart failure (cor pulmonale) and may be associated with jugular venous distention and peripheral edema. In cases of severe heart failure, the PAWP, right atrial pressure (RAP), and pulmonary artery pressure (PAP) will remain elevated while the CO decreases secondary to decreased contractility (Starling's law). This decreased contractility is assessed by calculating the left ventricular stroke work index (LVSWI) and plotting this value and the PAWP valve. In cases of elevated PAWP and decreased LVSWI, inotropic support is needed, not diuretics and vasodilators (Ramsey & Tisdale, 1995).

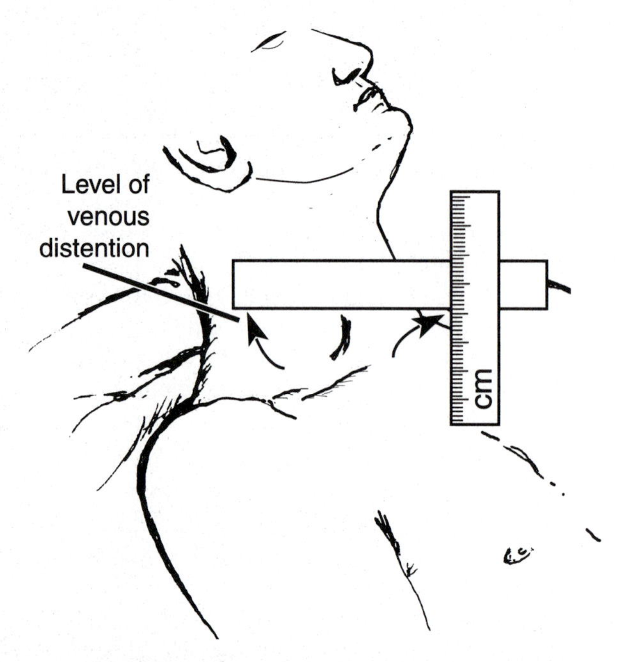

Figure 15–32. Measurement of jugular venous distention.

Palpitations

A patient with a perfusion disorder may complain of his or her heart "skipping" or "thumping" **(palpitations)**. This symptom is related to the occurrence of premature cardiac beats. The best way of detecting premature beats is by obtaining an ECG and monitoring the patient's cardiac rhythm. However, at times, the patient may be removed from the cardiac monitor in anticipation of transport out of an intensive or intermediate care setting. Palpation of the pulse will reveal premature beats. There will be irregular pulse amplitude due to the decreased blood volume associated with premature beats and larger-than-normal volume of the beat immediately after the premature beat related to prolonged diastolic filling.

Auscultation of heart sounds can confirm the presence of extra beats. $\mathbf{S_1}$ represents ventricular systole and occurs at the closure of the mitral and tricuspid valves. It is heard best at the apex of the heart because of the direction of blood flow during systole. The blood flow is out of the right ventricle into the pulmonary artery and out of the left ventricle into the aorta. $\mathbf{S_2}$ is the end of systole and represents the closure of the aortic and pulmonic valves. It is heard best at the aortic area. Diastole is longer than systole, so the pause between S_1 and S_2 is shorter than the pause between S_2 and S_1.

Extra heart sounds may appear during diastole because of rapid deceleration of blood against increased ventricular pressure, as encountered in heart failure. This increased pressure is due to remaining blood volume that is not ejected, related to overstretching of the myocardium. An $\mathbf{S_3}$ occurs immediately after the S_2 and is associated with heart failure and cardiomyopathy in individuals over 30 years of age. An $\mathbf{S_4}$ occurs immediately before an S_1. An S_4 may be present in the elderly patient due to decreased distensibility of the left ventricle associated with aging. An S_4 usually is associated with hypertension or myocardial infarction. In severe failure, both an S_3 and S_4 may be heard.

It is important to auscultate for the presence of **murmurs** in the patient with a perfusion disorder. A cardiology consultation and additional cardiovascular diagnostic tests may be necessary to determine the exact cause and classification of a murmur. The nurse should note the appearance of a new murmur, especially in patients who have experienced a myocardial infarction. A murmur in this situation may indicate abnormal atrioventricular venous communication due to ventricular septum rupture or acute mitral regurgitation due to papillary muscle rupture.

It is impossible to confirm the type or pattern of premature impulse by palpation alone. Only an ECG tracing will identify the number of premature beats occurring and their origin.

Change in Level of Responsiveness

A patient with a perfusion disorder may experience a change in level of responsiveness related to a decreased CO or blockage of cerebral circulation. Dysrhythmias, heart failure, myocardial infarction, or a cerebrovascular attack may be the initial event that precipitated the circulatory changes. The brain receives blood flow from the carotid and vertebral arteries. Fifteen percent of the total CO goes to the brain each minute. If the arterial pressure falls below 60 mm Hg, cerebral blood flow is compromised. A fluid volume deficit or a blood distribution problem ultimately can compromise cerebral blood flow. Changes in level of responsiveness can be subtle and may range from reduced wakefulness and decreased concentration to coma. The patient may experience **syncope** (a temporary loss of consciousness, followed by complete, spontaneous recovery).

The Perfusion Assessment

As stated earlier, the assessment begins with a primary overview that focuses on the assessment of airway, breathing, and circulation. Circulation is assessed initially by palpation of a pulse. If a pulse is absent, cardiopulmonary resuscitation and advanced life-support measures are initiated. These measures include insertion of an IV catheter and use of IV cardiac medications. The learner is referred to the American Heart Association's *Textbook of Advanced Cardiac Life Support* (1997) for a complete discussion of cardiopulmonary resuscitation.

When a pulse is verified as present, the nurse completes a rapid perfusion assessment. This assessment includes determining the degree of patient responsiveness, assessing for bleeding from invasive lines or tubes, examining the neck veins for distention, and inspecting the skin for adequate perfusion. Inspecting the skin involves assessment of capillary refill, the presence of peripheral pulses, and skin temperature.

Vital Signs

The nurse obtains a full set of vital signs. In the acutely ill patient, baseline vital signs are essential in order to determine the trend of subsequent data. The pulse can be evaluated using auscultation. The integrity of the heart sounds and the presence of extra heart sounds can be assessed at the same time. When a patient is on a mechanical ventilator and has a restrictive pulmonary disorder (presence of crackles and rhonchi), it may be impossible to hear heart sounds adequately. Palpation is used to calculate the heart rate and to assess the pulse integrity. Even in situations in which the pulse can be auscultated, the pulse should also be palpated. This provides data about the pulse amplitude and can provide clues to the presence of a fluid volume deficit condition (weak, thready pulse) or a fluid volume excess disorder (bounding pulse). A rhythm strip from the cardiac monitor should be obtained and interpreted. The strip usually is placed on the nursing assessment record. Additionally, peripheral pulses in all extremities should be assessed.

The patient's blood pressure can be obtained by using a variety of methods. An arterial line may be present to provide a direct measurement of arterial pressure. A mechanical external cuff blood pressure device may be used that records the blood pressure automatically. A traditional stethoscope and sphygmomanometer can be used. A Doppler device may be used to amplify sound in low flow states or noisy environments. Finally, the blood pressure can be obtained by using a sphygmomanometer and palpation, especially in noisy environments where it is difficult to hear, for example, during ground and air transport or in a busy emergency department. In patients with hypovolemia, increased systemic vascular resistance, or both, indirect measurements of blood pressure may be lower than invasive intra-arterial measurements because of diminution of sounds. Systolic pressure may be underestimated, and diastolic pressure may be overestimated.

A patient may have invasive measurement of heart pressure if a central venous line or a pulmonary arterial catheter is in place. Module 14 discusses these heart pressures in detail. If either of these lines is present, the nurse should obtain measurements of RAP, PAP, PAWP, CO, and derived parameters (cardiac index, mean arterial pressure, SVR, LVSWI) after the equipment is checked and calibrated. Strips of these hemodynamic patterns may be obtained and placed in the nursing assessment record for future comparison.

Temperature should be assessed. Fever increases myocardial oxygen demands and may precipitate an acute perfusion problem in a patient who has a history of cardiac disease. Fever should be treated with antipyretics, and the patient's temperature should be reevaluated to determine the degree of effectiveness of the medication.

Respirations are assessed for rate and character. Shortness of breath may accompany perfusion disorders, as in left ventricular failure. A detailed review of breath sounds is provided in Module 8.

Oxygen Saturation

Although oxygen saturation may be viewed as part of a ventilation assessment, this value also relates to perfusion. Continual pulse oximetry monitoring provides information about the degree to which hemoglobin is binding with oxygen. In situations in which oxygen is needed in the tissue, oxygen saturation will decrease since oxygen "jumps off" the hemoglobin to supply other cells and metabolic processes. In cases of myocardial demand (e.g., myocardial infarction) oxygen saturation will decrease in response to tissue needs.

Skin Integrity

The skin is assessed for temperature, edema, open wounds, and color. Pale, cool, clammy skin occurs from decreased peripheral perfusion, usually related to hypovolemia. These symptoms are in direct response to the sympathetic nervous system's attempt to maintain CO with a decrease in stroke volume. Pale, hairless skin that is taut from edema accompanies decreased peripheral perfusion related to the presence of fluid in the interstitial spaces. Edema is discussed in greater detail earlier in this module. The presence of nonhealing wounds may indicate decreased tissue perfusion from either a blockage of peripheral vessels or decreased CO. Capillary refill can be examined as a method of determining adequacy of peripheral perfusion. Normal refilling time of the nailbeds can fluctuate dramatically based on sex, history of peripheral vascular disease, and temperature of the extremities. The following parameters can be used for a standard of comparison: 2 seconds for adult male, 2.9 seconds for adult female, greater than 3 seconds for pediatric patients, and 4.5 seconds for the elderly patient (62 years of age or greater) (Schriger & Baraff, 1991).

Urine Output

Because 21 percent of a person's CO is distributed to the kidneys, renal perfusion is directly affected by decreased CO. Patients who are hemodynamically unstable should have their urine measured precisely. Urimeters may be placed on the urinary collection device to monitor output. A urine output of less than 30 mL/hr in the acutely ill adult patient indicates decreased blood renal perfusion.

In summary, an acute perfusion abnormality may occur rapidly. The nurse must know the patient's baseline data in order to appreciate changes in perfusion status. The following assessment data indicate an acute alteration in circulatory function:

- Presence of uncontrolled external bleeding
- Decreasing level of responsiveness, restlessness (decreased cerebral perfusion)
- Irregular, thready pulse
- Resting pulse rate of > 120 bpm
- Chest pain with shortness of breath
- Flat or distended neck veins (may indicate hypovolemia or pericardiac tamponade)
- Cool, clammy, pale skin
- Changing trends in vital signs and hemodynamic readings
- Presence of complete heart block, ventricular dysrhythmia, or sustained supraventricular tachycardia as evidenced by ECG
- Oxygen saturation < 90 percent

Appropriate nursing diagnoses for a patient experiencing a perfusion disorder include:

- Fluid volume deficit
- Fluid volume excess
- Altered tissue perfusion
- Decreased cardiac output
- Ineffective breathing patterns
- Pain

SECTION SIXTEEN REVIEW

Mary Foster, age 84, is admitted to your unit with a diagnosis of acute myocardial infarction (AMI). Questions 1 through 4 relate to Ms. Foster.

1. During the examination, you note that Ms. Foster has 3+ pitting edema of both legs. You should
   A. ask if Ms. Foster had the edema prior to today's events
   B. recognize this as a common symptom of AMI
   C. assess whether Ms. Foster has evidence of decreased plasma proteins (e.g., ascites)
   D. elevate her legs
2. Ms. Foster has been taking a diuretic, sleeping pill, nonsteroidal anti-inflammatory drug (NSAID), and stool softener. Which of these are important to note in the perfusion history?
   A. sleeping pill
   B. stool softener
   C. NSAID
   D. diuretic
3. You assess Ms. Foster's heart sounds and auscultate an S_4. Which of the following interpretations is NOT correct?
   A. S_4 is a normal finding
   B. S_4 is indicative of heart failure
   C. S_4 is possibly a normal finding in an 84-year-old woman
   D. S_4 is indicative of AMI

4. Based on the data available, which nursing diagnosis is most appropriate for Ms. Foster?
   A. altered tissue perfusion
   B. decreased cardiac output
   C. fluid volume excess
   D. impaired skin integrity

Answers: 1. A, 2. D, 3. A, 4. B

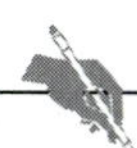

POSTTEST

1. Depolarization is precipitated by
   A. potassium moving into the cell
   B. calcium moving out of the cell
   C. sodium moving into the cell
   D. sodium moving out of the cell
2. When the SA node is pacing the heart, the heart rate will be
   A. irregular
   B. less than 50 bpm
   C. less than 100 bpm
   D. regular
3. The ST segment should be
   A. less than 0.20 second
   B. isoelectric
   C. positively deflected
   D. peaked
4. The length of the QT interval may vary in relation to
   A. blood pressure
   B. age
   C. heart rate
   D. sex
5. QRS complexes should be
   A. preceded by a T wave
   B. isoelectric
   C. positively deflected
   D. less than 0.12 second
6. Which of the following knobs may need to be turned if the complex is too small to view on the screen?
   A. capture knob
   B. volume knob
   C. alarm knob
   D. sensitivity knob
7. Time is represented by the
   A. vertical axis of the ECG paper
   B. color of ink on the ECG paper
   C. horizontal axis on the ECG paper
   D. asterisk at the bottom of the ECG paper
8. Fluid volume deficit primarily produces
   A. tachydysrhythmias
   B. cardiac conduction blocks
   C. bradydysrhythmias
   D. wide QRS complexes
9. Hypercalcemia results in
   A. increased automaticity
   B. premature atrial contractions (PACs)
   C. bradydysrhythmias
   D. tall, peaked T waves
10. Sinus bradycardia may be normal in
    A. athletes
    B. persons experiencing stressful situations
    C. elderly patients
    D. persons with hypertension
11. Atrial fibrillation is characterized by
    A. sawtoothed P waves
    B. regular QRS intervals
    C. absent P waves
    D. atrial rate less than 250 bpm
12. Verapamil may be used to treat
    A. sinus dysrhythmias
    B. conduction blocks
    C. ventricular dysrhythmias
    D. atrial dysrhythmias
13. Junctional tachycardia is differentiated from an accelerated junctional rhythm by
    A. presence of P wave
    B. length of PR interval
    C. rate of the rhythm
    D. QRS configuration
14. PACs are usually
    A. preceded by a hypoxic episode
    B. a signal of ventricular irritability
    C. harmless
    D. associated with digitalis toxicity
15. Type II second-degree heart block
    A. is associated with ventricular irritability
    B. is more ominous than type I second-degree heart block
    C. is less than 50 bpm
    D. requires treatment with verapamil
16. ST segment depression is characteristic of
    A. impaired ventricular repolarization
    B. hypokalemia
    C. digitalis toxicity
    D. atrial irritability
17. The coronary arteries are perfused during
    A. atrial diastole
    B. ventricular diastole
    C. ventricular systole
    D. ventricular depolarization

18. An anterior wall MI involves
    A. the right ventricle
    B. the SA node
    C. the left ventricle
    D. bundle of HIS
19. Streptokinase may produce which of the following side effects?
    A. anaphylaxis
    B. thrombophlebitis
    C. pulmonary emboli
    D. vomiting
20. Which of the following patients, based on their history, would NOT be suitable for thrombolytic therapy?
    A. motor vehicle crash 6 months ago
    B. reperfusion by t-PA 1 year ago
    C. right cerebrovascular attack 2 months ago
    D. delivered 6-pound daughter 6 months ago
21. The major difference between cardioversion and defibrillation is
    A. the number of times each can be repeated
    B. one method is synchronized to discharge with an ectopic impulse
    C. one method is used to treat delays in cardiac conduction
    D. one method requires the patient to be alert
22. Drugs that block beta receptors (i.e., propranolol, esmolol, and nadolol) will
    A. decrease automaticity
    B. increase contractility
    C. increase conduction
    D. stimulate the AV node
23. Failure to capture means the artificial pacing device
    A. is competing with the patient's own rhythm
    B. is not producing depolarization
    C. needs new batteries
    D. is causing PVCs
24. Balloon stents are used in patients undergoing PTCA to
    A. laser the lesion
    B. maintain artery patency
    C. collect microparticles
    D. introduce a rotating blade
25. Which of the following explains why a change in level of consciousness may indicate a perfusion problem?
    A. large protein molecules cannot penetrate the blood–brain barrier
    B. if the arterial pressure falls below 60 mm Hg, cerebral blood flow is reduced
    C. hyperglycemia may induce cerebral edema
    D. the brain receives blood flow from the carotid and vertebral arteries

POSTTEST ANSWERS

Question	Answer	Section	Question	Answer	Section
1	C	One	14	C	Nine
2	C	Two	15	B	Ten
3	B	Two	16	A	Eleven
4	C	Two	17	B	Eleven
5	D	Two	18	C	Eleven
6	D	Two	19	A	Twelve
7	C	Three	20	C	Twelve
8	A	Four	21	B	Thirteen
9	C	Four	22	A	Thirteen
10	A	Five	23	B	Fourteen
11	C	Six	24	B	Fifteen
12	D	Six	25	B	Sixteen
13	C	Seven			

REFERENCES

The ACC/AHA Task Force. (1999). 1999 Update: ACC/AHA guidelines for management of patients with acute myocardial infarction. *JACC* 34(3):890–911.

American Heart Association. (1997). *Textbook of Advanced Cardiac Life Support*. Dallas, TX: Author.

Braunwald, R. (ed). (1997). *Heart disease: A text of cardiovascular medicine*. Philadelphia: Saunders.

Dimengo, J. (1998). Surgical alternatives in the treatment of heart failure. *AACN Clin Issues* 9(2):192–207.

Doering, L. (1999). Pathophysiology of acute coronary syndromes leading to acute myocardial infarction. *J Cardiovasc Nurs* 13(3):1–20.

Dukovcic, A., Daleiden-Burns, A., & Shaul, F. (1998). Percutaneous cardiopulmonary support for high-risk angioplasty. *Crit Care Nurs Q 20*(4):16–28.

Finch, N., Sneed, N., Leman, R., & Watson, J. (1997). Driving with an internal defibrillator: Legal, ethical, and quality of life issues. *J Cardiovasc Nurs 11*(2):58–67.

Funkhouser, S.W. (1994). Cardiovascular anatomy and physiology. In L. Thelan, J. Davie, L. Urden, & M. Lough. (eds). *Critical care nursing: Diagnosis and management* (2nd ed.) (chapter 13). St. Louis: C.V. Mosby.

Guaglianone, D., & Tyndall, A. (1995). Comfort issues in patients undergoing radiofrequency catheter ablation. *Crit Care Nurse 15*(1):47–50.

Hoffman, R.L., & Reeder, S.J. (1998). Angiotensin-converting enzyme inhibitors and left ventricular remodeling: implications for nurses. *Dimensions Crit Care Nurs 17*(5):256–263.

Hudak, C., & Gallo, B. (1994). *Critical care nursing: A holistic approach* (6th ed.). Philadelphia: J.B. Lippincott.

Kayser, S. (1996). Antiarrhythmic drug therapy—part II: Atrial fibrillation. *Progress Cardiovasc Nurs 11*(4):35–43, 45.

Knight, L., Livingston, N., Gawlinski, A., & DeLurgio, D. (1997), Caring for patients with third generation implantable cardioverter defibrillator. *Crit Care Nurse 17*(5):46–61.

Kollisch, D., & Sloane, P. (1994). Chronic cardiac disease. In P. Sloane, L. Slatt, & P. Curtis. (eds). *Essentials of family medicine* (2nd ed.). Baltimore: Williams & Wilkins.

Konstam, M., & Remme, W. (1998). Treatment guidelines in heart failure. *Progress Cardiovasc Dis 411*(1 suppl):65–72.

Lefkovits, J., & Topol, E. (1997). Pharmacological approaches for prevention of restenosis after percutaneous coronary intervention. *Progress Cardiovasc Dis 40*(2):141–158.

Lipman, B., & Cascio, T. (1994). Markers of reperfusion after thrombolytic therapy for acute myocardial infarction. *J Emerg Nurs 21*:112–115.

Love, M. (1994). Cardiovascular diagnostic procedures. In L. Thelan, J. Davie, L. Urden, & M. Lough. (eds). *Critical care nursing: Diagnosis and management* (2nd ed.). St. Louis: C.V. Mosby.

Michael, K., & Parnell, K. (1998). Innovations in pharmacologic management of heart failure. *AACN Clin Issues* 9(2):172–191.

Moser, D. (1996). Maximizing therapy in the advanced heart failure patient. *J Cardiovasc Nurs 10*(2):29–46.

Moungey, S. (1994). Patients with sinus node dysfunction or atrio-ventricular blocks. *Crit Care Nurs Clin North Am* 6:55–68.

Ramsey, J.D., & Tisdale, L.A. (1995). Use of ventricular stroke work index and ventricular function curves. *Crit Care Nurse 15*(2):61–67.

Robert, C. (1999). Have we reached the therapeutic ceiling in acute myocardial infarction? *Crit Care Nurse 19*(5 suppl):7–11.

Sargent, D. (1999). Using ibutilide to convert atrial fibrillation and flutter. *Dimensions Crit Care Nurs 18*:2–7.

Schriger, D., & Baraff, L. (1991). Capillary refill—is it a useful predictor of hypovolemic states? *Ann Emerg Med 20*:601–605.

Schussheim, A., & Fuster, V. (1997). Thromobosis, antithrombotic agents and the thrombolytic. *Progress Cardiovasc Dis* 40(3):205–238.

Turner, D., & Turner, L. (1995). Right ventricular myocardial infarction: Detection, treatment and nursing implications. *Crit Care Nurs 15*:22–27.

Weitz, J.K. (1997). Low molecular weight heparins. *N Engl J Med 337*:688–698.

Williams, K., & Morton, P. (1995). Diagnosis and treatment of AMI. *AACN Clin Issues* 6(3):375–386.

Witherall, C.L. (1994). Cardiac rhythm control devices. *Crit Care Clin North Am* 6(1):85–101.

Module 16

Nursing Care of the Patient with Altered Tissue Perfusion

Pamela Stinson Kidd, Megan Switzer

This self-study module is designed to integrate the major points discussed in Modules 10, 13, 14, and 15 and summarizes relationships between key concepts, while assisting the learner in clustering information to facilitate clinical application. The module is divided into two case studies. Both case studies apply the content in an interactive learning style. The learner is encouraged to identify nursing actions based on assessment of a patient in a case study format. Nursing care of a patient with a fluid volume deficit is addressed in Case Study 1. Nursing care of a patient with a fluid volume excess condition is addressed in Case Study 2. Consequences of selecting a particular action are discussed, and the rationale for correct actions is presented. The module ends with a summary of nursing priorities in caring for a patient with altered tissue perfusion.

Objectives

Following completion of this module, the learner will be able to

1. Cluster assessment data to formulate perfusion patterns.
2. Appraise a patient's perfusion status based on a nursing assessment.
3. Identify priorities in nursing care for a patient experiencing an alteration in perfusion.
4. Explain rationale for nursing actions that support perfusion.

Abbreviations

AST. Aspartate aminotransferase, previously referred to as SGOT (serum glutamic oxaloacetic transaminase)

CO. Cardiac output

CI. Cardiac index

CPK. Creatinine phosphokinase

CVP. Central venous pressure

IABP. Intra-aortic balloon pump

LDH. Lactic dehydrogenase

LVSWI. Left ventricular stroke work index

MAST. Military antishock trousers, also known as pneumatic antishock garment

PAP. Pulmonary arterial pressure

PAWP. Pulmonary artery wedge pressure

SVR. Systemic vascular resistance

CASE STUDY 1

SUE S, A PATIENT WITH A FLUID VOLUME DEFICIT

Sue S is a 24-year-old, gravida 1 female who is 12 weeks pregnant. Her husband brought her to the emergency department when Sue passed out at home. Sue began vomiting en route and complaining of severe, continuous right lower quadrant pain that extended to her suprapubic area. She also complained of pain in the right shoulder area. Sue is admitted into your zone by the triage nurse.

The Initial Appraisal

On walking into Sue's patient care area, you note the following.

GENERAL APPEARANCE. Sue is diaphoretic. She is of moderate stature. Weight is appropriate for height. She is fully clothed.

SIGNS OF DISTRESS. Sue is moaning. She is lying on her left side with her knees drawn to her chest. She is clutching a man's hands.

OTHER. You do not note any IV lines or oxygen in use. The man identifies himself as her husband.

Focused Circulatory Assessment

You quickly place Sue in a hospital gown, noting her profuse diaphoresis and cool, clammy skin. Because Sue appears to be in acute distress, you immediately perform a rapid assessment, focusing on her perfusion status. The results are as follows.

Sue is restless but alert and oriented to person, place, time, and reason for being at the hospital. Her blood pressure is 90/70 (baseline according to her husband is 128/70), pulse is 126/min, respiratory rate is 28/min. Her respirations are shallow. Sue's radial pulse is regular. S_1 and S_2 are present without murmur. No extra heart sounds are auscultated. Breath sounds are clear bilaterally. Her capillary refill is 3 seconds. Her nailbeds are dusky. No bowel sounds are auscultated after 1 minute. Her abdomen is firm. Sue's pain increases dramatically on palpation of any part of her abdomen. She complains of increased pain unrelieved by change in position. Her oral temperature is 99°F (37.2°C).

After this initial assessment, you alert the emergency physician, Dr. P, who is busy examining a patient who is experiencing an acute myocardial infarction. Until she is able to examine Sue, Dr. P orders:

- 1,000 mL lactated Ringer's solution to be infused at 200 mL/hr through a large-bore IV line
- Stat complete blood cell count (CBC)
- Type and crossmatch for four units of blood
- Cardiac monitor
- Urinary catheter to straight drain
- Urinalysis and urine for pregnancy test
- Serum HCG
- Electrolyte panel
- CT scan of the abdomen
- Oxygen 2 L per nasal cannula

QUESTION

Considering Sue's presenting symptoms, prioritize the following orders. Which order should be implemented first?

A. computed tomographic (CT) scan of the abdomen
B. serum HCG
C. cardiac monitor
D. IV access

ANSWER

The correct answer is D. Because Sue's blood pressure is low compared with her normal value and she has had an episode of syncope at home, the IV line should be initiated first. IV access will provide a means of administering fluid boluses or volume expanders if necessary. Blood can be obtained at the same time for the laboratory tests. Oxygen should be administered next, since tachycardia increases myocardial demands for oxygenation. Next, Sue should be connected to the cardiac monitor because of her fast heart rate. The CT scan should be ordered to help determine the source of Sue's hypotension. Finally, the urinalysis should be obtained. The status of Sue's pregnancy can be determined by the serum HCG. The urine pregnancy test and urinalysis will provide supplemental data.

Stat Test Results

CBC

WBC = 15,000/mL	(Normal range 5,000–10,000/mL)
RBC = 5.0×10^6/mL	(Normal range 4.2–5.4 × 10^6/mL)
Hgb = 12 g/dL	(Normal range 12–16 g/dL in females)
Hct = 37%	(Normal range 28–47% in females)

Electrolytes

Sodium (Na) = 146 mEq/L	(Normal range 136–146 mEq/L)
Potassium (K) = 3.5 mEq/L	(Normal range 3.5–5.5 mEq/L)
Chloride (Cl) = 95 mEq/L	(Normal range 96–106 mEq/L)
Calcium (Ca) = 8.8 mg/dL	(Normal range 8.5–10.5 mg/dL)
Glucose = 140 mg/dL	(Normal range 80–120 mg/dL)

Serum HCG
  Pending
CT abdomen
  Scan positive for diffuse abdominal bleeding

QUESTION

What is the significance of the laboratory and radiographic data?

ANSWER

The WBC count is elevated, perhaps in response to abdominal infection secondary to bleeding. The CBC, Hgb, and Hct are on the low side of normal because of abdominal bleeding. It generally takes 6 hours after hemorrhage begins to detect a noticeable decrease in the Hct (Gawlinski, 1988). The high normal sodium is related to an increase in aldosterone secretion to maintain blood volume. Thus, renal excretion of sodium decreases. Renal excretion of potassium increases because of this same response as evidenced by Sue's low normal level. Her glucose is elevated due to sympathetic stimulation. The CT scan suggests a ruptured ectopic pregnancy originating in the right fallopian tube. This finding is consistent with Sue's history of being 3 months pregnant. Ectopic pregnancy is a life-threatening event because of associated internal bleeding. The results of the CT scan confirm that Sue requires surgical intervention.

Focused Nursing History

While Sue is in the radiology department with the emergency medicine resident, you speak with her husband to obtain the most critical historical data that may have an impact on Sue's present situation. The comprehensive nursing database will be completed within 24 hours postadmission. Her husband gives the following history.

Sue diagnosed her pregnancy using an over-the-counter pregnancy detection kit. Both she and her husband are excited about the pregnancy, since they have tried to conceive for over 2 years. Sue has not had any problems during the pregnancy. Before trying to conceive, Sue was using birth control pills. Her last menstrual period was 86 days ago. She has not had a previous pregnancy. For the past 2 days, she has complained of abdominal pain that has gradually increased in intensity. She has had nausea but did not begin vomiting until in the car on the way to the emergency department. Sue fainted when she got up to answer the phone after lying on the couch to try to relieve her abdominal pain. She has never fainted before. Sue does not have any medical conditions. She is not allergic to any medication. Her last meal was 6 hours ago. She has had two glasses of water since her last meal.

The Systematic Bedside Assessment

Sue returns from having a CT scan. You will complete a head-to-toe assessment, since you will be caring for Sue until the operating suite is ready and the general surgeon completes his present case. Sue signs a permit for an exploratory laparotomy.

HEAD AND NECK. Sue remains oriented, but she is restless. She is receiving 2 L of oxygen through a nasal cannula. Her neck veins are slightly filled at an angle of 30 degrees. No other abnormalities of the head and neck are noted.

CHEST. *Cardiac status*. As previously noted, apical heart rate is 138. The pattern that is present on the cardiac monitor is shown in Figure 16–1. Blood pressure is 88/70. Lactated Ringer's solution is being infused at 200 mL/hr

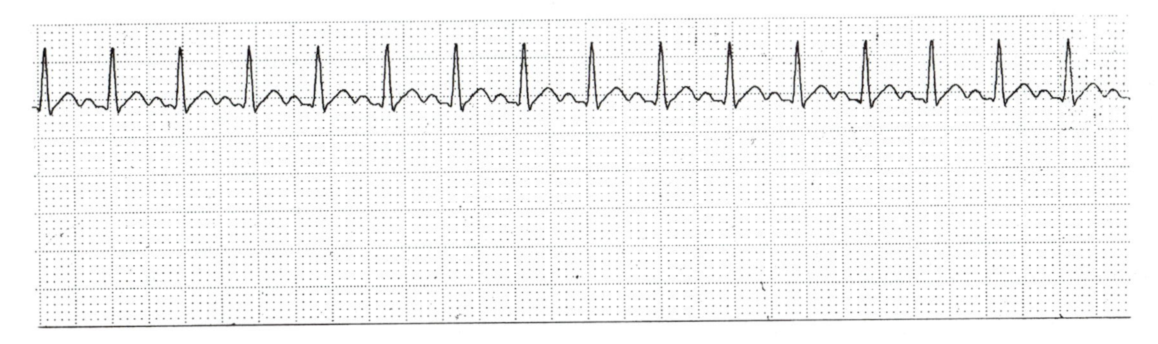

Figure 16–1.

via a No. 16 gauge IV catheter in the right forearm. The IV site is negative for edema and redness.

QUESTION

The pattern in Figure 16–1 is

- **A.** normal sinus rhythm
- **B.** sinus tachycardia
- **C.** supraventricular tachycardia
- **D.** atrial fibrillation

ANSWER

The correct answer is B. Sinus tachycardia is indicated because the rate is greater than 100 and P waves precede the QRS complex.

PULMONARY STATUS. As previously noted, the respiratory rate has increased to 32/min. Respirations remain shallow.

ABDOMEN. The abdomen is firm and tight. No bowel sounds are auscultated. Sue complains of increased pain in all quadrants and in her right shoulder on light palpation.

PELVIS. A No. 16 urinary catheter is in place draining light yellow urine, 40 mL in the first hour of placement. Reagent strip is negative for hematuria, ketones, and glucose.

EXTREMITIES. The skin is diaphoretic, cool, and clammy. The nailbeds are dusky. Capillary refill is sluggish. Peripheral pulses are palpable but faint (1+) in all extremities.

POSTERIOR. Posterior breath sounds are diminished in bilateral lower lung fields. No sacral edema is noted.

Development of Nursing Diagnoses

Clustering Data

You have just completed your head-to-toe assessment and are ready to list appropriate nursing diagnoses for Sue. To cluster the data, look for abnormal results found during the assessment. Sue's major symptoms at this time are her intense pain and hypotension. These primary symptoms can initiate your first cluster of critical cues.

CLUSTER 1

Subjective data: Sue complains of continuous abdominal pain unrelieved with change in position. Pain has increased over the past 2 days. The pain increased with abdominal palpation and radiates to all four quadrants and the right shoulder (Kehr's sign). Nausea and vomiting are present, and the patient fainted once at home.

Objective data: Blood pressure is 88–90/70. The heart rate is 126 to 138. Respirations are 28. Hgb and Hct are borderline low. Potassium is borderline low, and sodium is borderline high. Urine output low is at 40 mL/hr. The last menstrual period was 86 days ago, and she had a positive over-the-counter pregnancy test. The CT scan was positive for abdominal bleeding.

QUESTION

Based on these data, which of the following nursing diagnoses would you select as being appropriate in planning Sue's care?

- **A.** fluid volume deficit
- **B.** decreased cardiac output
- **C.** altered tissue perfusion: renal, peripheral
- **D.** all of the above

ANSWER

The correct answer is D. All three are present in Sue's case. However, the decreased cardiac output and tissue perfusion are directly related to the actual fluid volume deficit. Therefore, focusing your nursing interventions on addressing the fluid volume status will improve her cardiac output and tissue perfusion. The most appropriate of the three diagnoses is *Fluid volume deficit* related to abdominal bleeding.

Desired patient outcomes for Sue would include:

1. Systolic blood pressure > 90 mm Hg
2. Heart rate between 60 and 100 bpm
3. Respirations 12 to 16/min
4. Absence of abdominal pain
5. Urine output of at least 30 mL/hr
6. Absence of dizziness and syncope (Ulrich, Canale, & Wendell, 1999)

For the purposes of Sue's case study, only the perfusion-related nursing diagnosis will be developed further. In a true clinical situation, however, other clusters would be developed based on primary critical cues from the collected data. If data are insufficient, you should collect additional data to confirm or refute your hypotheses.

Based on Sue's available data, these additional nursing diagnoses also pertain to her case:

- *Infection* related to abdominal irritation as evidenced by elevated WBC count
- *Impaired gas exchange* related to decreased cellular oxygenation due to decreased perfusion
- *High risk for altered tissue perfusion: Renal,* related to decreased circulating blood volume
- *Alterated nutrition: Less than body requirements* related to increased metabolic rate
- *Acute pain* related to abdominal irritation
- *High risk for disturbance in self-concept, role performance, and body image* related to surgical incision, loss of pregnancy, and potential loss of reproductive abilities

Sue's fluid volume deficit is related to hemorrhage. Excessive diuresis and severe dehydration also may produce a fluid volume deficit. Sue's treatment goals will focus on stopping the source of her bleeding, restoring vascular volume, and optimizing perfusion. These general goals should be reflected in the nursing diagnoses and expected patient outcomes. For example, restoring vascular volume is addressed in the nursing diagnosis: *Fluid volume deficit*. Accomplishment of this goal will be measured in such criteria as systolic blood pressure > 90 mm Hg, heart rate between 60 and 100 bpm, and urine output of at least 30 mL/hr.

Development of the Plan of Care

Nursing interventions will be based on activities that will help Sue meet her expected patient outcomes. They will consist of collaborative interventions that are both multidisciplinary and interdisciplinary. Independent interventions are activities that are within the scope of nursing practice and do not require a physician's order.

Collaborative Interventions Related to Circulatory Status

The physician's orders may include the following:

1. *Volume replacement*. Crystalloids or colloids may be used to expand the vascular volume. Usually, lactated Ringer's solution is used initially because it contains potassium and calcium as well as lactate. Lactate is converted to bicarbonate to provide additional compensation for acidosis, which is encountered commonly in shock states. Packed red blood cells will be administered once the typing and crossmatching are performed. Whole blood is rarely given since the aim of the transfusion is to increase oxygen delivery to the tissue and not merely to increase circulating blood volume. In circumstances in which the patient has a history of heart or renal failure, packed red blood cells are given instead of whole blood to improve the oxygen-carrying capacity of the blood without reversing the volume deficit so quickly that a fluid overload condition may develop. Albumin and plasma may be administered in situations in which the fluid volume deficit is related to fluid shifting from the vascular space into the interstitial space. Synthetic volume expanders (Dextran and Hespan) may be used to rapidly expand volume until crossmatching is completed or blood is available. For additional information, refer to Module 10. This module further addresses fluid replacement.
2. *Vasopressor therapy*. Vasoconstrictors may be ordered to increase venous return and, ultimately, CO. The most commonly used vasoconstrictor is norepinephrine. The major problem associated with the use of vasoconstrictors is decreased renal perfusion, since the patient is already vasoconstricted due to sympathetic stimulation. Inotropes also may be administered. High-dose dopamine (greater than 10 mg/kg/min) may be given to produce peripheral vasoconstriction and increase venous return. Although in low doses dopamine has a dopaminergic action resulting in increased urinary output, high doses counteract this effect of increased renal circulation.
3. *Oxygen*. Oxygen is administered to ensure that the blood that reaches the tissues is adequately oxygenated. High-flow oxygen is preferred in hypovolemic states. A nonrebreather mask connected to 10 L of oxygen will promote hemoglobin saturation and help prevent respiratory acidosis. Since Sue's condition has not improved, the physician probably will change the route and amount of oxygen she is receiving.
4. *Military antishock trousers*. Although controversial, a MAST garment may be used to control internal bleeding. The exact mechanism by which MAST work is not known. Originally, it was thought that core circulation was promoted by redistributing peripheral blood flow. MAST are used also to tamponade bleeding in some situations. MAST may be used preoperatively to maintain a systolic blood pressure over 90 mm Hg. If Sue's blood pressure continues to drop, the trousers may be applied and inflated. The trousers are placed under Sue as a precautionary measure in anticipation of the need for inflation.
5. *Hemodynamic monitoring*. A central venous pressure line or a pulmonary arterial catheter may be inserted to provide direct measurements of CO and preload. Placement of a central line will provide another access route for IV fluid replacement and blood specimen removal as well as pressure monitoring.
6. *Laboratory and x-ray testing*. Serial Hgb and Hct levels will be obtained to monitor the degree of hemorrhage. A chest x-ray will be obtained preoperatively for baseline purposes or after placement of a central IV line to ensure proper placement. Arterial blood gases will be determined if Sue's level of responsiveness changes. A lactic acid level also would be obtained at that time to monitor acidosis.

Independent Nursing Interventions

1. Elevate Sue's legs to promote venous drainage from the legs.
2. Facilitate and maintain a position of comfort to decrease Sue's pain and anxiety and thus oxygen use.

3. Maintain accurate intake and output records.
4. Keep Sue NPO in anticipation of surgery.
5. Monitor vital signs continuously.
6. Monitor the effects of drug therapy and fluid replacement.
7. Monitor test results (report abnormal results).
8. Keep the patient and husband informed about the plan of care.
9. Assess for decreased perfusion (report abnormal results):
   - Systolic blood pressure less than 90 mm Hg
   - Narrowing of pulse pressure
   - Respirations less than 8 or greater than 30/min
   - Presence of bradycardia, tachycardia, or premature beats
   - Change in responsiveness
   - Urine output less than 30 mL/hr
   - Flat neck veins

Plan Evaluation and Revision

Sue's perfusion plan of care is now developed and ready to be executed. Her progress will be monitored at regular intervals to evaluate the effects of the various therapeutic actions. If progress is not being noted toward attainment of Sue's desired patient outcomes, her plan may need revisions, examining alternative interventions that may be more effective.

Sue's condition worsens. Her blood pressure is 66 mm Hg and obtainable only by Doppler. She is unresponsive. You call for the physician and adjust her IV fluids to a wide open rate. The runner from the blood bank has just arrived with four units of crossmatched packed red blood cells. Dr. P decides to insert a pulmonary artery catheter and a peripheral artery catheter. You assist her with the procedures while another nurse hangs the blood through the peripheral IV line. Dr. P gives an order to inflate the leg compartments of the MAST suit until the systolic blood pressure reaches 90 mm Hg.

Nursing Care of a Patient Being Monitored Hemodynamically

The goals and outcome criteria that are appropriate to the management of Sue while she is being hemodynamically monitored can be divided into two major groupings: support of her physiologic needs and support of her psychosocial needs.

Support of Physiologic Needs

Sue's physiologic needs will be met through nursing interventions that promote adequate fluid volume and distribution and prevent infection and hemodynamic monitoring complications. Sue's nursing management will be planned around interventions to attain these goals. These goals are addressed through the nursing diagnoses of *Decreased cardiac output, Fluid volume deficit, Altered tissue perfusion: Peripheral, Risk for infection*, and *Risk for injury*.

A pulmonary arterial catheter is inserted. Initial readings were CVP 2, RVP 16/0, PAP 17/6, PAP mean 8, PAWP 3. These readings are low, indicating a fluid volume deficit. Her cardiac output was 3.2 L/min. The mean arterial pressure reading was 65. Her SVR was 1,575 dynes $\cdot$ sec/cm^{-5}, indicating that her sympathetic nervous system is trying to compensate for the low venous return. Sue's CI was calculated to be 1.7 L/m^2 based on her surface area. Her LVSWI was 11.3g/m^2. The low PAWP and low LVSWI indicates a hypovolemia problem.

Decreased Cardiac Output

Obtaining Sue's CO, CI, and SVR measurements provides information about her response to fluid and medication administration. Sue's SVR reading will indicate the degree to which her sympathetic nervous system is trying to compensate for the low stroke volume. Her heart rate and pattern should be assessed to determine her hemodynamic response to changes in rate or rhythm. Dysrhythmias and tachycardia will further diminish her CO. Improvement in Sue's level of responsiveness would indicate improvement in her CO. Her urine output provides another parameter for monitoring CO, since 20 percent of the CO goes to the kidneys (Guyton, 1986).

Fluid Volume Deficit

Sue's preload will need to be monitored to determine her response to volume replacement. The impact of inotropes and vasopressors on Sue's preload can be examined by comparing CVP and PAWP readings after medication administration with baseline measures. Hemoglobin and hematocrit values will provide information regarding how much volume has been lost. Because Sue is being hemodynamically monitored, she is at risk for exsanguination if the tubing becomes disconnected or a stopcock is left open. To prevent this from occurring, keep all catheter connecting sites visible and reassess frequently. Keep monitor alarms on to detect changes in blood pressure. In addition, the assessment data that helped you evaluate Sue's cardiac output status will also help you evaluate her fluid volume status.

Altered Tissue Perfusion: Peripheral

Since Sue has a fluid volume deficit, her tissue perfusion is compromised. Because she also has pulmonary artery and peripheral artery catheters in place, she is at risk for further compromise in her peripheral perfusion. Thrombus formation or thrombophlebitis may occur. The insertion site should be examined at least every 8 hours for tenderness, redness, and skin temperature. A loss in arterial pulsation distal to the placement of the catheter may indicate arterial insufficiency related to thrombus formation.

Risk for Infection

The catheter dressing, tubing, stopcocks, and transducer should be changed according to institution protocol. Aseptic technique should be used when obtaining blood specimens and flushing the catheter. Ports should be cleansed of all blood after obtaining samples. Sue's WBC count is already elevated and should be monitored for further increases. Her temperature should be evaluated. If an infection is suspected related to the hemodynamic monitoring, the catheter may be removed or changed and cultures may be obtained from Sue's blood and the catheter.

Risk for Injury

If Sue becomes restless, she may pull out her pulmonary artery catheter. She may need to be restrained or sedated if a change occurs in her responsiveness level. If the pulmonary artery catheter tip falls into the right ventricle, Sue may experience life-threatening dysrhythmias. If you notice a right ventricular waveform pattern, the physician should be notified. The balloon will need to be inflated through the pulmonary artery balloon port by either the physician or nurse (depending on hospital policy). This should allow the catheter to float back into the pulmonary artery. If Sue has hemoptysis and abnormal ABGs and respirations, she may be experiencing a pulmonary infarction from permanent wedging of the balloon or lodging of the deflated balloon in the pulmonary capillary bed. Open the stopcock on the pulmonary artery balloon port and remove the syringe to allow for passive deflation of the balloon.

Support of Psychosocial Needs

Support of Sue's psychosocial needs will center around interventions that reduce anxiety and promote a balance between sleep and activity.

Anxiety Related to Equipment

Most patients identify that the monitoring of rhythms and patterns on oscilloscopes is equivalent to being critically ill. Hemodynamic monitoring is used most frequently in the unstable patient, but it can be used also for patients who require frequent blood specimens and multiple medications. Catheters may be left in place for fluid and medication administration after cardiac pressures are unable to be obtained due to catheter malfunction. Sue went from having one pattern monitored, her cardiac rhythm, to having four patterns monitored: cardiac rhythm, CVP, PAP, and arterial pressure. Family members may become alarmed when they notice the oscilloscope at the patient's bedside. Most individuals are accustomed to peripheral IV lines, but insertion of a catheter into the neck may be a foreign concept. Sue was unresponsive at the time the catheter was inserted. When she becomes responsive, the nurse will need to explain the purpose of the catheters and warn Sue not to touch any of the tubing or connections.

High Risk for Sleep Pattern Disturbance

Periodic assessment of hemodynamic readings may interrupt Sue's rest and sleep. Decreasing the light in her room at night while providing adequate lighting for obtaining measurements will foster Sue's rest. While Sue is in the emergency department, it will be difficult for her to rest because of the noise and constant patient flow. However, the priority in the emergency department is to improve Sue's fluid volume so her surgical procedure will be less stressful. After surgery, the nurse can obtain hemodynamic measurements in Sue's position of comfort (or sleep) as long as the nurse rezeros the transducer and maintains the transducer at the phlebostatic axis. Sue's position while the readings were obtained should be documented.

The operating suite is ready for Sue. Her hemodynamic lines are secured. Blood and lactated Ringer's are infusing through her CVP port and side port, respectively. The leg components of the MAST suit remain inflated, since her mean arterial pressure is 60. She is still receiving 10 L of oxygen through a nonrebreather mask. Sue remains in sinus tachycardia. The report is given to the operating room nurse. Sue's husband is escorted to the surgical waiting area.

CASE STUDY 2

DELORES GARCIA, A PATIENT EXPERIENCING FLUID VOLUME EXCESS

You are the nurse assigned to care for Mrs. Garcia. Mrs. Garcia was admitted to the telemetry floor with a diagnosis of *Angina: rule out myocardial infarction*. She was admitted through the emergency department 16 hours previously.

The Initial Appraisal

On walking into the room, you note the following.

GENERAL APPEARANCE. Mrs. Garcia is a Hispanic female of moderate stature. She is overweight and tidy in appearance.

SIGNS OF DISTRESS. Mrs. Garcia is diaphoretic. Her respirations are fast and shallow. She is sitting upright in bed.

OTHER. You note that she is receiving oxygen by nasal cannula. An IV solution of D_5W is infusing.

Focused Respiratory and Circulatory Assessment

Because Mrs. Garcia appears to be in acute distress, you immediately perform a rapid assessment, focusing on her cardiopulmonary status. The results are as follows.

Mrs. Garcia is restless but oriented to person, place, time, and reason for hospitalization. Her respiratory rate is 28/min, shallow and regular. On auscultation of her chest, you note bilateral medium crackles in the lower lung fields, left greater than right. S_1 and S_2 are present. No murmurs are noted, but an S_3 is auscultated. Her blood pressure is 156/106, and her pulse is 104 bpm. She is complaining of chest pain, sharp in nature, that is radiating down her left arm. She is in the cardiac rhythm shown in Figure 16–2.

QUESTION

The pattern in Figure 16–2 is

A. atrial flutter
B. complete heart block
C. atrial fibrillation
D. artifact

ANSWER

The correct answer is C. P waves are not distinguishable. The R–R interval is irregular.

Following this initial assessment, you check her admission orders. Mrs. Garcia has the following medications ordered.

- Nitroglycerin grain 1/150 SL PRN chest pain
- Morphine sulfate 4 mg IVP PRN q 2–3 hrs for chest pain

QUESTION

What effect will these medications have on Mrs. Garcia's perfusion status?

ANSWER

All the medications will help improve Mrs. Garcia's CO. Nitroglycerin is a fast-acting drug that will produce peripheral vasodilation, thus redistributing blood away from the congested pulmonary bed. Nitroglycerin also may increase collateral circulation to the myocardium. The vasodilation should decrease her pain. Morphine decreases preload by producing peripheral vasodilation. It decreases anxiety, which increases myocardial oxygen consumption. Morphine also relaxes airway smooth muscle, so it may decrease Mrs. Garcia's respiratory rate by improving gas exchange.

You administer both of the medications and place a call to her cardiologist. In the interim, Mrs. Garcia's morning laboratory results come back.

Electrolytes

Sodium (Na) = 142 mEq/L	(Normal range 136–146 mEq/L)
Potassium (K) = 3.5 mEq/L	(Normal range 3.5–5.5 mEq/L)
Chloride (Cl) = 104 mEq/L	(Normal range 96–106 mEq/L)
Calcium (Ca) = 9.0 mg/dL	(Normal range 8.5–10.5 mg/dL)

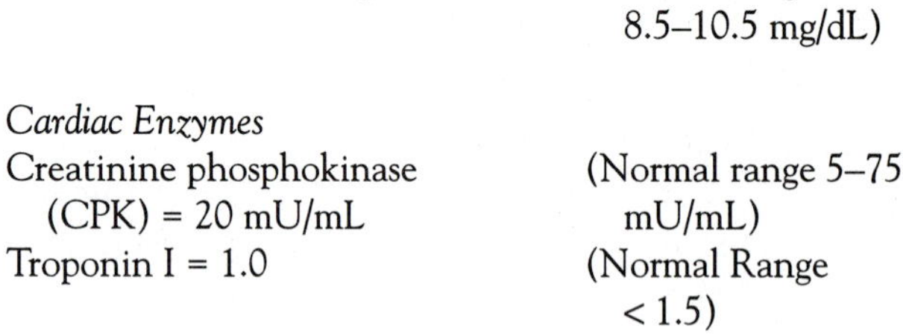

Cardiac Enzymes

Creatinine phosphokinase (CPK) = 20 mU/mL	(Normal range 5–75 mU/mL)
Troponin I = 1.0	(Normal Range < 1.5)

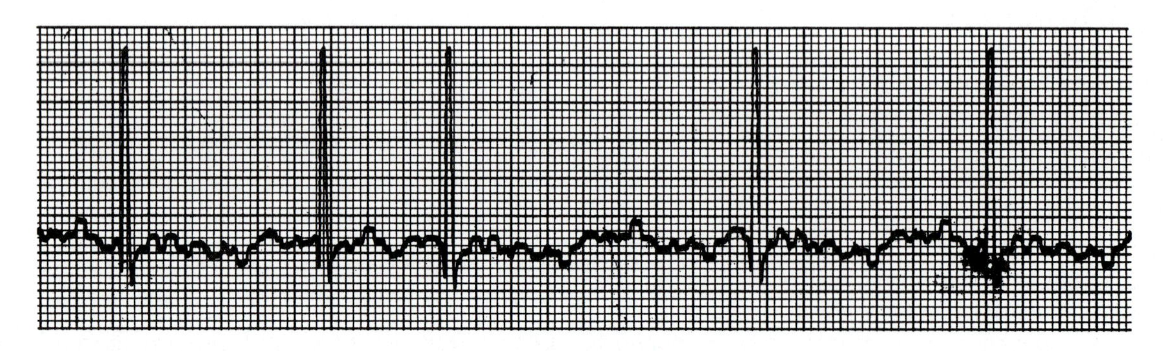

Figure 16–2.

QUESTION

What is the significance of these laboratory results?

ANSWER

Mrs. Garcia's electrolyte values are within normal limits. Thus, she should not be predisposed to cardiac dysrhythmias resulting from electrolyte disturbances. However, her potassium level is borderline low. You will need to check her chart to see if she has been taking diuretics at home for chronic medical conditions. If digitalis is prescribed because of her beginning pulmonary edema (as suspected based on the presence of crackles on pulmonary auscultation), Mrs. Garcia may be predisposed to digitalis toxicity. However, angiotensin-converting enzyme (ACE) inhibitors will be prescribed in most cases before digitalis.

The normal cardiac enzyme and marker levels indicate that Mrs. Garcia has not experienced a myocardial infarction. When the heart muscle is damaged, enzymes are released. The CPK level rises within 6 hours, peaks in 18 hours, and declines to normal 2 to 3 days postinfarction. If the CPK level was elevated, isoenzymes would be ordered to determine the cause of the elevation. CPK-MB is the isoenzyme associated with cardiac cells. The CPK-MB level will begin to rise 3 to 6 hours postinfarction. It does not rise during angina. Troponin I levels begin to increase 3 hours after myocardial ischemia occurs, peak at 14 to 18 hours, and remain elevated for 5 to 7 days. Detection of cardiac troponin I in serum is very specific for myocardial injury because this protein is found only on myocardial cells. Cardiac troponin I is the only biomarker that is 100% specific for myocardial necrosis (Murphy & Berding, 1999).

Mrs. Garcia's pain has not decreased. She is complaining of being short of breath. Her blood pressure has dropped to 114/72. Her heart rate is 92. Respirations remain at 28/min. Her daughter arrives in the room to see you administering a second grain 1/150 nitroglycerin tablet SL to her mother.

Focused Nursing History

Because Mrs. Garcia is still experiencing pain, you decide to speak with her daughter to obtain the most important critical historical data that may have an impact on Mrs. Garcia's present situation. The comprehensive nursing database has not yet been completed but will need to be finished within 24 hours of Mrs. Garcia's admission. Her daughter gives the following history.

Mrs. Garcia started experiencing chest pain the morning of her admission after she had moved a piece of bedroom furniture. She had been complaining of "heartburn" after eating heavy meals intermittently for the last 6 months. The pain yesterday would not go away after Mrs. Garcia rested. She called her daughter, who drove over to her house and convinced her to go to the hospital. Mrs. Garcia is not allergic to any medicine. She has a history of smoking one pack of cigarettes a day for 20 years. She is 47 years old and has a history of hypertension. She takes Lasix 10 mg orally daily for her blood pressure. She does not take potassium supplements, but her daughter states that Mrs. Garcia eats many bananas.

Even though most of this information should already be recorded in Mrs. Garcia's chart, you have not had time to read her chart. This information was important to obtain and will help you as you perform your systematic assessment.

The Systematic Bedside Assessment

HEAD AND NECK. Mrs. Garcia has an olive complexion. Perspiration is noted on her forehead. She remains oriented and alert. Oxygen is infusing through her nasal cannula at 2 L/min. She is in a semi-Fowler's position at 30 degrees. Her jugular veins are full but not distended.

CHEST.

Pulmonary status. Her crackles have increased since your initial assessment. Crackles in her right and left lung fields are equal in intensity. Respirations are 26/min.

Cardiac status. It is more difficult to hear her heart sounds because of the crackles. However, S_1, S_2, and S_3 are still audible. Her apical heart rate is irregular without a distinctive pattern. Her blood pressure is 92/70.

ABDOMEN. Her abdomen is soft and obese. Hypoactive bowel sounds are auscultated. No pain is elicited on palpation. Liver borders are nonpalpable.

PELVIS. Mrs. Garcia is voiding per bedpan and voided 100 mL in the last hour. Her urine has been yellow and clear. Reagent strips are negative for glucose, ketones, and blood.

EXTREMITIES. She has bilateral 2+ nonpitting pedal edema. Pedal pulses are faint (1+) but palpable. Capillary refill is 2 seconds in all extremities. Her skin is damp from perspiration.

POSTERIOR. No sacral edema is noted. Posterior breath sounds reveal bilateral coarse crackles lower to midlung fields.

Development of Nursing Diagnoses

Clustering Data

You are now ready to develop nursing diagnoses based on the available subjective and objective data. To cluster your data, look for abnormal values discovered during the assessment. Mrs. Garcia's major symptoms at this time are chest pain, decreasing blood pressure, and increasing pulmonary crackles. Thus, these primary symptoms can initiate your first cluster of critical cues.

CLUSTER 1

Subjective data. The patient is complaining of increasing chest pain not relieved with nitroglycerin SL × two or morphine sulfate 4 mg IVP. She also is complaining of shortness of breath despite oxygen administration at 2 L per nasal cannula. She has a previous history of hypertension and heartburn.

Objective data. Mrs. Garcia is diaphoretic with full neck veins, 2+ bilateral pedal edema. Crackles are auscultated in the bilateral posterior lung fields. S_3 is auscultated. Atrial fibrillation with rapid ventricular response is noted. On admission, cardiac enzymes were normal.

QUESTION

Based on the above data, which of the following nursing diagnoses is the priority diagnosis at this time for Mrs. Garcia?

A. decreased cardiac output
B. impaired gas exchange
C. altered tissue perfusion: peripheral
D. fluid volume excess

ANSWER

The correct answer is D. Although you might expect a decreased CO to be present, you lack data to confirm this diagnosis, since Mrs. Garcia is still voiding an appropriate amount and she remains alert. It is true that her blood pressure has decreased, but it may be decreased as a normal response to the vasodilating medications. Arterial blood gases have not been obtained, so impaired gas exchange cannot be supported. However, if Mrs. Garcia's tachypnea continues and her crackles continue to increase, impaired gas exchange probably will be present. Altered peripheral tissue perfusion cannot be supported adequately because even though her pedal pulses are faint (1+), they are present, and capillary refill is normal. Fluid volume excess is the most plausible diagnosis because of her increasing crackles and shortness of breath associated with increasing chest pain. She is also in atrial fibrillation, a pattern commonly associated with heart failure. Mrs. Garcia's admission diagnosis of angina and history of hypertension suggests that she is susceptible to congestive heart failure. Several factors can contribute to fluid overload: increased fluid intake, decreased fluid elimination, or decreased fluid distribution. Mrs. Garcia's fluid volume overload is related to distribution. The volume has remained unchanged. Her left ventricle has decreased contractility due to distention probably related to chronic hypertension.

The physician calls, and you inform him of Mrs. Garcia's present status. He orders a stat ECG, portable chest film, cardiac enzymes, and arterial blood gases. He wants you to initiate a nitroglycerin IV drip at 5 mg/min. He is coming to see Mrs. Garcia. She will be transferred to the coronary care unit as soon as a bed is available.

When you return to Mrs. Garcia's room, you notice that she is less responsive and responds to touch instead of verbal stimuli. Her daughter is crying and saying, "Momma don't die!" Mrs. Garcia's cardiac rhythm in lead II has changed to that shown in Figure 16–3.

QUESTION

The pattern in Figure 16–3 indicates which of the following?

A. ectopic pacemaker
B. infarction
C. conduction abnormality
D. ischemia

ANSWER

The correct answer is D. You recognize this pattern as indicating myocardial ischemia. The ST segment should be isoelectric. An alteration from isoelectric occurs from delayed repolarization.

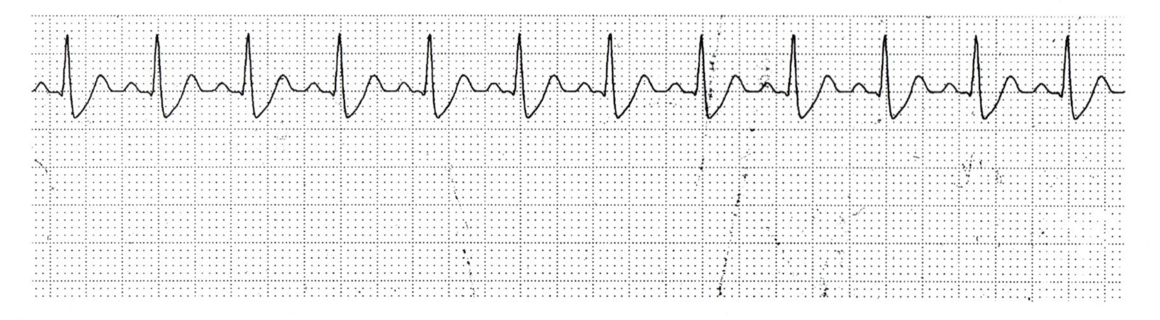

Figure 16–3.

You rush to start the IV nitroglycerin drip. You push the nurse call light to get extra help into the room. Another nurse enters and escorts Mrs. Garcia's daughter to the central waiting area. Fortunately, Mrs. Garcia's vital signs have not changed. The stat ECG and portable chest x-ray are completed. A blood specimen for enzyme analysis is obtained. An arterial stick is performed for blood gas analysis.

The physician arrives and reads the ECG and portable chest film. Based on her history and the ECG, Mrs. Garcia is diagnosed as having an acute anterolateral infarction. Cardiomegaly is present with bilateral infiltrates on the chest film. Congestive heart failure with acute pulmonary edema also is diagnosed. She is transferred immediately to the coronary care unit.

Quick Review

Mrs. Garcia's initial symptoms demonstrated compensatory efforts to maintain CO, which is determined by stroke volume and heart rate. The changes in the ECG indicate that myocardial oxygen supply is diminished, probably due to a blockage in the coronary arteries. Mrs. Garcia's pain is secondary to a decreased myocardial oxygen supply. Injured myocardial tissue cannot contract adequately, and blood remains in the left ventricle. As the left ventricle becomes stretched, contractility further decreases once the point of maximum elasticity is reached. Starling's law addresses the limits of cardiac compensation. The heart rate initially will increase in an effort to maintain CO. The sympathetic nervous system is stimulated, and peripheral vasoconstriction produces the symptoms of nausea and diaphoresis. Mrs. Garcia's CO has now decreased, as evidenced by her decreased responsiveness.

Because more data are available, it is time to reassess nursing diagnoses appropriate for Mrs. Garcia. Mrs. Garcia's perfusion problem is complex. Because the perfusion problem involves a fluid volume excess related to decreased fluid distribution and decreased CO related to decreased myocardial contractility, it is suggested that you join them together to address them.

Desired patient outcomes for Mrs. Garcia would include:

1. Absence of crackles on auscultation
2. Absence of dyspnea
3. Stable vital signs: systolic blood pressure > 90 and < 140
4. Absence of S_3
5. Absence of jugular venous distention
6. Absence of ascites and abdominal tenderness
7. Usual mental status
8. Urine output > 30 mL/hr
9. Arterial blood gases within normal limits (WNL) for Mrs. Garcia
10. Cardiac enzymes WNL
11. Absence of chest pain

For the purposes of Mrs. Garcia's case study, only the perfusion-related nursing diagnoses are further developed. However, in a true clinical situation, as the nurse creating Mrs. Garcia's plan of care, you would continue to develop other clusters based on assessment data. If data are insufficient, you should follow through on collecting the necessary data to confirm or refute your hypotheses.

Based on the preliminary data that has been collected on Mrs. Garcia, there is sufficient support to state the following nursing diagnoses:

- *Chest pain* related to myocardial ischemia
- *Altered tissue perfusion: Cerebral* related to decreased myocardial contractility
- *High risk for impaired gas exchange* related to pulmonary interstitial fluid
- *High risk for anxiety* related to impending transfer to coronary care unit
- *High risk for fear* related to severity of illness

Treatment goals for Mrs. Garcia will focus on increasing the blood supply to the heart, decreasing the demands placed on the heart, and improving the blood flow distribution. These general goals should be reflected in the nursing diagnoses and expected patient outcomes on the nursing care plan. For example, decreasing the demands placed on the heart is addressed in the nursing diagnosis of fluid volume overload. Accomplishment of the goal will be measured in such criteria as *Patient will be pain free*.

Development of the Plan of Care

Nursing interventions will be based on activities that will help Mrs. Garcia meet her desired patient outcomes. They will consist of collaborative interventions ordered by the physician but require nursing action and independent interventions that the nurse implements without a physician's order.

Collaborative Interventions Related to Perfusion Status

The physician's orders may include the following:

1. *Cardiovascular drug therapy*. Mrs. Garcia will be receiving several drugs while hospitalized. Thrombolytics may be ordered to dissolve a thrombus and thereby improve coronary artery perfusion, limit the extent of the myocardial ischemia, and improve left ventricular function.

Early reperfusion (within 12 hrs of onset of signs and symptoms of infarction) of the infarct-related artery is associated with better outcomes (Kline-Rogers, Martin, & Smith, 1999). Streptokinase and tissue plasminogen activator are commonly used thrombolytic agents. These drugs are contraindicated if the patient has a bleeding disorder, potential for bleeding, a recent surgery or cerebrovascular accident (brain attack), and uncontrolled hypertension (see Module 13, Section Twelve). The major nursing concern associated with administering thrombolytic agents is to monitor for complications. The most frequent complications are bleeding and allergic reaction (with streptokinase). Reperfusion dysrhythmias may occur with lysis of the thrombus and restoration of flow in the coronary artery but are self-limiting and should not be treated.

Inotropic agents, such as dopamine, dobutamine, and digitalis, may be administered. These agents will increase myocardial contractility and improve ventricular function. A negative effect of these agents is that they increase myocardial oxygen consumption.

Vasodilators may be ordered. Frequently used IV vasodilators are nitroprusside, nitroglycerin, and phentolamine. These drugs indirectly improve stroke volume and CO by decreasing afterload. The heart is able to eject against less resistance. Vasodilators should be used cautiously in right ventricular infarctions due to the decrease in preload that can occur and worsening of myocardial ischemia.

QUESTION

Which of the following may be an undesirable side effect of vasodilators?

- **A.** decreased systemic vascular resistance
- **B.** decreased CO
- **C.** increased PAWP
- **D.** increased CVP

ANSWER

The correct answer is B. Hypotension and a further decrease in CO may occur if preload is diminished due to venous pooling.

QUESTION

A diuretic is ordered for Mrs. Garcia to

- **A.** prevent renal failure
- **B.** increase the PAWP
- **C.** decrease vasoconstriction
- **D.** reduce preload

ANSWER

The correct answer is D. Diuretics may be given to reduce preload and pulmonary venous congestion.

Loop diuretics are the preferred drug of choice in cases of acute congestive heart failure. Furosemide has vasodilating and diuretic properties and thus has a greater potential of decreasing preload. The nurse must monitor for fluid volume deficit that may occur with other diuresis and electrolyte abnormalities.

Oxygen therapy is ordered to reduce myocardial workload and to meet cellular energy requirements.

2. *Mechanical support*. If Mrs. Garcia's heart failure worsens, she may need an intra-aortic balloon pump (IABP). This device improves coronary artery perfusion by inflating during diastole and increasing the coronary artery perfusion pressure. It deflates during systole, rapidly decreasing the coronary artery pressure and ventricular ejection resistance. The nurse caring for a patient with an IABP requires special preparation in order to adjust balloon inflation/deflation correctly.
3. *Dietary restrictions*. Mrs. Garcia may be placed on a sodium restricted diet. Use of table salt and salt in food preparation may need to be eliminated. She may also be placed on fluid restriction until her fluid distribution problem is under control. The nurse would need to monitor Mrs. Garcia's sodium level and intake and output record and ensure that she receives the correct meal tray. Family members need to be made aware of dietary restrictions so they do not bring food that would be detrimental to Mrs. Garcia's fluid volume status.
4. *Hemodynamic monitoring*. Mrs. Garcia may have a pulmonary artery catheter placed once she is in the coronary care unit. Nursing responsibilities associated with hemodynamic monitoring have been discussed earlier in this module. You would expect Mrs. Garcia's hemodynamic readings to be abnormal because of her fluid volume overload. Before initiation of drug therapy, Mrs. Garcia's CVP, PAP, and PAWP readings would be elevated due to increased volume. Her CO and CI would be decreased. Mrs. Garcia's LVSWI would be decreased due to diminished contractility. Mrs. Garcia's SVR would be elevated initially to try to compensate for her decreased stroke volume. However, her blood pressure has been decreasing, and a nitroglycerin IV drip was initiated. Her SVR should now be decreased. Medications will be administered and titrated to decrease her CVP, PAP, and PAWP while increasing her CO. The combination of inotropes and vasodilators can be confusing to a novice nurse, since they appear to

have opposite actions. However, the goal of using both of these agents is the same—improvement of CO.

5. *Laboratory and x-ray testing*. Cardiac enzymes and/or markers probably will be ordered at least every 6 hrs to determine the severity of Mrs. Garcia's myocardial infarction. ABGs will be ordered intermittently to monitor gas exchange. If a thrombolytic agent has been administered, ABGs may not be ordered to prevent repeated puncture or repeated arterial manipulation (via arterial line). Pulse oximetry may be used to monitor gas exchange noninvasively. Periodic chest x-rays will assist in determining the effects of interventions. The cardiomegaly and pulmonary infiltrates should diminish in size.

Independent Nursing Interventions Related to Perfusion Status

1. Assess for decreased perfusion
   - Systolic blood pressure < 90 mm Hg
   - Heart rate < 60 or > 100 bpm
   - Urine output < 30 mL/hr
   - Decreased responsiveness
   - Diminished peripheral pulses
   - Capillary refill > 2.9 seconds
   - Pedal edema
   - Dysrhythmias
2. Assess for fluid overload
   - Metabolic or respiratory acidosis
   - Dyspnea
   - Abnormal breath sounds
   - Extra heart sounds
   - Jugular venous distention
   - Ascites
   - Weight gain
   - Abnormal electrolyte levels
3. Implement measures to reduce cardiac workload
   - Place Mrs. Garcia in semi-Fowler's position
   - Allow for frequent rest periods
   - Monitor intake and output
   - Monitor for side effects of drug therapy
   - Keep oxygen device on patient
   - Administer pain medication as ordered and use imagery and other diversional activities
   - Decrease patient anxiety
     a. Refer to support services as necessary (e.g., chaplain, social services)
     b. Assist patient with identifying coping behaviors
     c. Explain procedures, environment, and equipment to degree of patient satisfaction

Plan Evaluation and Revision

Mrs. Garcia's plan of care is now ready to be executed by the coronary care unit nurse. Her progress will be monitored at regular intervals to evaluate the effects of various therapeutic actions. If progress is not being noted toward attainment of her expected patient outcomes, Mrs. Garcia's plan of care may need to be revised.

Summary

This module has addressed the nursing care of patients who are experiencing alterations in perfusion. Concepts from the perfusion-related modules (Modules 10, 13, 14, and 15) have been applied in a case study approach. It is impossible to address specifically each perfusion problem a nurse may encounter in the clinical setting. However, these problems can be managed by applying basic principles. These principles can be classified into fluid volume excess and fluid volume deficit situations. Two case studies were used to illustrate nursing care responsibilities in these situations. Review questions were integrated throughout the case study to encourage application of material in other modules and assimilation of content within this module. Nursing interventions for a patient being hemodynamically monitored were addressed specifically because of the frequency with which this intervention is used and its use in patients experiencing both fluid overload and fluid deficit.

REFERENCES

American College of Surgeons. (1993). *Advanced trauma life support course manual*. Chicago: Author.

American Heart Association (1997). *Advanced cardiac life support course manual*. Dallas: Author.

Bates, B. (1994). *A guide to physical examination* (4th ed.). Philadelphia: J.B. Lippincott.

Carpenito, L. (1987). *Nursing diagnosis: Application to clinical practice* (2nd ed.). Philadelphia: J.B. Lippincott.

Gawlinski, A. (1988). Cardiovascular physical assessment. In N. Holloway (ed). *Nursing the critically ill adult* (3rd ed.) (chapter 10). Menlo Park: Addison-Wesley.

Guyton, A. (1986). *Textbook of medical physiology* (3rd ed.). Philadelphia: W.B. Saunders.

Murphy, M., & Berding, C. (1999). Use of measurments of myoglobin and cardiac troponins in the diagnosis of acute myocardial infarction. *Crit Care Nurse 19*(1):58–66.

Rebenson-Piano, M., Holin, K., & Powers, M. (1987). An examination of the differences that occur between direct and indirect blood pressure measurement. *Heart Lung 16*:285–293.

Kline-Rogers, E., Martin, J., & Smith, D. (1999). New era of reperfusion in acute myocardial infarction. *Crit Care Nurse 19*(1): 21–33.

Schriger, D., & Baraff, L. (1991). Capillary refill—is it a useful predictor of hypovolemic states? *Ann Emerg Med 20*:601–605.

Ulrich, S., Canale, S., & Wendell, S. (1999). *Nursing care planning guide: A nursing diagnosis approach* (3rd ed.). Philadelphia: W.B. Saunders.

PART V

NEUROLOGIC

Module 17

Consciousness

Pamela Stinson Kidd, Robyn Cheung, Louise Jimm Zeeger

This self-study module was developed as a teaching guide for nurses caring for patients with alterations with a neurologic basis. Successful completion of this module will prepare you to care for these types of patients in a general care area. It will not prepare you to care for a patient in a neurologic intensive care unit.

This module is composed of fourteen sections, beginning with simple definitions of responsiveness and consciousness while moving into the concept of increased intracranial pressure as a contributing factor of impaired responsiveness. A more comprehensive discussion of etiologies affecting consciousness and responsiveness is provided. The module reviews common elements for assessment, in-depth assessment of impaired arousal, and how to document your assessment. The module then moves on to nursing interventions and medical and pharmacologic therapies for patients with alterations in responsiveness. The module ends with sections on seizure disorders and selected diagnostic procedures for patients with neurologic impairment. Each section includes a set of review questions to help the learner evaluate his or her understanding of the section's content before moving on to the next section. All Section Reviews and the module Pretest and Posttest include answers. It is suggested that the learner review those concepts answered incorrectly in the review questions before proceeding to the next section.

Objectives

Following completion of this module, the learner will be able to

1. Define consciousness and the components that make up consciousness.
2. Identify the anatomic bases that control arousal and content.
3. Explain the normal cerebrovascular anatomy and physiology and the cerebrospinal fluid dynamics related to cerebral perfusion.
4. Explain the autoregulation, chemoregulation, and metabolic regulation of cerebral perfusion.
5. Define cerebral perfusion pressure.
6. Discuss cerebral oxygenation and cerebral metabolism.
7. Discuss the measurement of cerebral oxygenation.
8. Discuss the relationship between intracranial volume and intracranial pressure.
9. Discuss compensatory mechanisms for increased intracranial volume.
10. Identify intracranial pressure monitoring types and systems and discuss nursing care for patients undergoing intracranial pressure monitoring.
11. Identify pathologies that can impair content and arousal.
12. Describe the outcome of uncompensated increased intracranial volume and state six contributing factors.
13. Describe common elements to be evaluated in the assessment of arousal and content.
14. Document assessment of arousal and content.
15. Identify nursing interventions and pharmacologic therapies for patients with an impaired level of responsiveness.
16. Briefly discuss seizure disorders, and identify nursing and pharmacologic management.
17. Identify selected diagnostic procedures and their clinical applications.

PRETEST

1. Consciousness includes the functions of the cerebral hemispheres and the
   A. cerebrum
   B. cerebellum
   C. sensorimotor fiber tracts
   D. reticular activating system (RAS)
2. Arousal is one component of consciousness. The other component is
   A. content
   B. intelligence
   C. wakefulness
   D. motor ability
3. The Monro–Kellie hypothesis states that volume increases in the adult intracranial vault
   A. are initially well tolerated through compensatory mechanisms
   B. are tolerated well because of the flexibility of the cranial vault
   C. can be compensated for only by cerebrospinal fluid buffering techniques
   D. usually result in death because the vault is unable to accommodate increases in volume
4. Cerebral blood vessels dilate in response to
   A. increased serum oxygen
   B. increased serum carbon dioxide
   C. decreased serum oxygen
   D. decreased serum carbon dioxide
5. Pressure regulation is an autoregulatory mechanism whereby cerebral blood vessels constrict in response to
   A. systemic hypertension
   B. hypercarbia
   C. systemic hypotension
   D. hypoxia
6. What is the cerebral perfusion pressure if mean arterial pressure (MAP) = 95 mm Hg and intracranial pressure (ICP) = 15 mm Hg?
   A. 65 mm Hg
   B. 80 mm Hg
   C. 110 mm Hg
   D. 125 mm Hg
7. Your patient responds appropriately to stimuli, and the Glasgow Coma Scale (GCS) score is 15. What would be your initial assessment and your next action?
   A. level of responsiveness is intact; vital signs would be the next logical step
   B. level of responsiveness most probably is not intact; an in-depth neurologic assessment is required
   C. you are unable to completely evaluate the level of responsiveness and need more clinical data
   D. the patient demonstrates no cognitive deficits; pupillary assessment would be the next logical step
8. The most important component of the neurologic assessment is
   A. the vital signs
   B. the level of responsiveness
   C. pupillary reactions
   D. the protective reflexes
9. A unilaterally dilated pupil is indicative of
   A. atropine or atropine-like drugs
   B. a brain stem lesion
   C. opiate overdose
   D. a cranial nerve lesion
10. The Glasgow Coma Scale assesses
    A. cognition
    B. speech patterns
    C. arousal
    D. problem-solving abilities
11. Your patient's intracranial pressure per monitor is 30 mm Hg. To assist your patient's compensatory mechanisms, your first action would be to
    A. hyperventilate the patient
    B. lower the head of the bed
    C. turn the patient to the left side
    D. drain the patient's ventricular catheter
12. Flexion of the neck may cause elevations in intracranial volume by
    A. causing a decrease in venous outflow
    B. causing an increase in venous return
    C. causing cerebral vasodilation
    D. increasing venous outflow
13. A seizure disorder that is considered a neurologic emergency is
    A. generalized seizures
    B. partial seizures
    C. complex seizures
    D. status epilepticus
14. A disadvantage of magnetic resonance imaging (MRI) over computed tomographic (CT) scanning is
    A. MRI is an invasive procedure
    B. MRI produces results that are less refined
    C. the time required for an MRI is longer
    D. MRI is not useful for imaging anatomic location of a lesion
15. Anaerobic metabolism manufactures adenosine triphosphate (ATP) by utilizing
    A. glucose
    B. protein
    C. calcium
    D. potassium
16. Which diagnostic procedure would be the best choice for an agitated, confused, head-injured patient?
    A. CT scan
    B. positron emission tomographic (PET) scan

C. MRI
D. evoked potentials

17. A jugular venous oxygen saturation measurement that is decreased or low indicates
A. cerebral perfusion is adequate
B. ICP is low
C. the cerebral metabolic rate is low
D. the brain is extracting higher amounts of oxygen from the cerebral circulation

18. The MOST accurate method of ICP monitoring is
A. epidural catheter monitoring
B. subarachnoid screw
C. ventricular catheter
D. Glasgow Coma Scale

19. Intracranial pressure monitoring cannot be used for
A. calculating cerebral perfusion pressure (CPP)
B. determining ICP
C. determining GCS
D. drainage of cerebrospinal fluid (CSF)

20. To decrease cerebral metabolic needs, a pharmacologic agent might be
A. mannitol
B. barbiturates
C. steroids
D. alkalinizing agents

21. Cranial nerve reflexes
A. can be tested only in the conscious patient
B. are the least sensitive indicators of central nervous system (CNS) injury
C. indicate integrity of the brain stem
D. are not useful in the neurologic evaluation

Pretest answers: 1. D, 2. A, 3. A, 4. B, 5. A, 6. B, 7. C, 8. B, 9. D, 10. C, 11. A, 12. A, 13. D, 14. C, 15. A, 16. D, 17. D, 18. D, 19. C, 20. B, 21. C

GLOSSARY

Arousal. The component of consciousness concerned with the ability of an individual simply to respond to environmental stimuli, such as opening the eyes to speech or turning the head toward a noise

Arteriovenous difference in oxygen content ($AVDO_2$). The difference in oxygen content between the arterial circulation and the jugular system; calculated as $AVDO_2 = (SaO_2 - SjVO_2) \times 1.34 \times Hgb/100$ mL/dL. Normal is 4 to 9 mL/dL

Autoregulation. A protective capacity of cerebral arterioles to alter their blood flow within an average systemic arterial pressure limit of 60 to 130 mm Hg in adults, thereby promoting a constant blood supply to the brain irrespective of systemic blood pressure fluctuations. When blood pressure increases, cerebral arterioles constrict; when blood pressure decreases, cerebral arterioles dilate, assuring adequate cerebral perfusion. Chemical regulation responds to blood levels of oxygen and, more strikingly, to levels of carbon dioxide; vessels dilate in response to elevated levels of carbon dioxide, less forcefully to decreased oxygen levels; vessels constrict in response to lowered levels of carbon dioxide

Battle's sign. Collection of CSF in the mastoid air cells

Blood–brain barrier. A protective vascular barrier found in brain capillaries that is impermeable to serum protein and large molecules, permitting only lipid-soluble substances to permeate it

Cerebral blood flow (CBF). Normally is maintained at a constant rate by vasodilation of the vessels to increase the flow or vasoconstriction to decrease the flow

Cerebral blood volume. The amount of blood in the cranial vault at any given point in time; occupies about 10 percent of the total intracranial volume

Cerebral perfusion pressure (CPP). An estimate of the adequacy of cerebral circulation. Perfusion pressure to the brain that is the difference between the mean systemic arterial pressure (arteries) and the mean intracranial pressure (reflecting veins). It is calculated as follows: CPP = MAP – ICP

Consciousness. State of general awareness of oneself and the environment; made up of the components of arousal and content

Content. The component of consciousness concerned with interpreting environmental stimuli; includes thinking, memory, problem solving, orientation, and speech

Elastance. A measure of stiffness, referring to the brain's ability to tolerate and compensate for volume increases; high elastance refers to small volume reserves in the cranial vault

Herniation. A protrusion of brain matter through a natural opening secondary to elevated intracranial pressure; carries a grave prognosis and is an ominous sign

Hydrocephalus. A clinical syndrome caused by an increased production of cerebrospinal fluid that exceeds the absorption rate

Hypercapnia. Abnormally elevated blood levels of carbon dioxide; results in vasodilation of the cerebral vessels

Hyperemia. A state in which cerebral blood flow is higher than cerebral metabolic needs; also known as "luxury perfusion"

Intracranial pressure. Pressure exerted by the cerebrospinal fluid within the ventricles of the brain; normal pressure is 0 to 15 mm Hg

Jugular venous oxygen saturation ($SjVO_2$). The percent of oxygenated blood exiting the cerebral circulation via the jugular system. Normal is 50 to 75 percent

Monro–Kellie hypothesis. A principle that states that the skull is a rigid vault filled with noncompressible contents: brain, blood, and cerebrospinal fluid; if any one component increases in volume, one or both remaining components must decrease in volume for overall volume to remain constant

Oligemia. A state in which cerebral blood flow is too low to support cerebral metabolic needs

Otorrhea. Drainage of fluid from the ear (usually CSF or blood)

Raccoon's eyes. Collection of CSF in the periorbital space

Responsiveness. A term synonymous with consciousness, which is a general state of awareness of oneself and the environment

Reticular activating system (RAS). A pathway of neurons and neuronal connections for transmission of sensory stimuli from the lower brain stem to the cerebral cortex; the anatomic basis of the arousal component of consciousness

Status epilepticus. A continuing series of seizures without a period of recovery or regaining of consciousness between attacks

ABBREVIATIONS

CBF. Cerebral blood flow

CPP. Cerebral perfusion pressure

CSF. Cerebrospinal fluid

CT. Computed tomography

EEG. Electroencephalography

EMG. Electromyelography

EOM. Extraocular eye movement

GCS. Glasgow Coma Scale

ICP. Intracranial pressure

IVC. Intraventricular catheter

LP. Lumbar puncture

MAP. Mean arterial pressure

MRI. Magnetic resonance imaging

PET. Positron emission tomography

RAS. Reticular activating system

SEP. Somatosensory evoked potential

TCD. Transcranial Doppler

THAM. Tromethamine

VEP. Visual evoked potential

SECTION ONE: Consciousness

At the completion of this section, the learner will be able to define consciousness and the components that make up consciousness.

Consciousness, or **responsiveness,** is defined as a state of general awareness of oneself and the environment and reflects the functional integrity of the brain as a whole. Consciousness is a dynamic state that is subject to change. Level of consciousness is the most important factor in the neurologic assessment.

Consciousness is divided into two components: content and arousal. **Arousal** is concerned with the appearance of wakefulness and stimuli necessary to wake an individual. **Content** includes the sum of cerebral mental functions and is concerned with interpretation of the internal and external environment or the thinking processes, known as cognition.

Content and arousal are independent but interrelated components. The arousal component must be functioning for content to be experienced. An individual who is not in a state of wakefulness, or arousal, would be unable to interpret internal and external stimuli.

The arousal component of consciousness is controlled by the **reticular activating system (RAS).** The RAS is a pathway of neurons and neuronal connections. It is located in the brain stem (midbrain and medulla) and projects into the cerebral hemispheres. The RAS receives impulses from the sense organs and transmits these impulses to the cerebral hemispheres. Thus, not only does the RAS control wakefulness or arousal, but it also has some control over content. Stimuli cannot be interpreted in the cerebral hemispheres unless they are received and transmitted to the cerebral cortex via the RAS.

The content component of consciousness includes all functions of the brain that add quality to the arousal component and is controlled by the cerebral hemispheres. Thus, content is dependent on intact, functioning cerebral hemispheres. Functions controlled by the cerebral hemispheres include thinking, imagining, and speech.

In summary, consciousness is a state of general awareness of oneself and the environment and is made up of two components: arousal and content. Arousal is controlled by the RAS, and content is controlled by the cerebral hemispheres. Content and arousal are two processes that are independent, but interrelated, and together comprise the state of consciousness.

SECTION ONE REVIEW

1. The ascending RAS is chiefly responsible for
   A. high-level cognitive skills
   B. recent and remote memory
   C. level of arousal
   D. affect and mood
2. A patient making inappropriate statements and appearing disoriented would be suspected of having an impairment of the
   A. cerebellum
   B. cerebral cortex
   C. occipital lobe
   D. brain stem

Answers: 1. C, 2. B

SECTION TWO: Selective Anatomy and Physiology of Cerebral Perfusion

This section describes the pertinent anatomy and physiology of the brain as related to understanding of brain attacks. At the completion of this section, the learner will be able to discuss cerebral blood flow and cerebrospinal fluid dynamics.

Arterial Circulation

The brain is supplied by two major pairs of arteries: the right and left internal carotid arteries (ICAs) and the right and left vertebral arteries (Fig. 17–1). Together their branches unite within the brain to form the circle of Willis, a connecting anastomosis that provides collateral blood flow to either side of the brain. The internal carotids supply the retinas and the anterior two thirds of the cerebral hemispheres via its branches, the middle cerebrals, the anterior cerebral, and the anterior and posterior communicating arteries. The middle cerebral arteries (MCAs) are the largest branches of the internal carotids. They supply almost the entire lateral surface of the frontal, parietal, and temporal lobes, the underlying white matter, and the basal ganglia. These arteries are most frequently involved in strokes. The anterior communicating artery (ACoA) connects the anterior cerebral arteries (ACAs); and the posterior communicating arteries (PCoAs) join the posterior cerebral arteries (PCAs) to complete the circle of Willis. The circle of Willis is protective because it is the primary collateral pathway when major cerebral vessels are occluded. For example, if the carotid artery is occluded, collateral flow may still be possible via the posterior communicating or anterior cerebral arteries to the ischemic brain areas supplied by the occluded ICA.

The vertebrobasilar system supplies the posterior portion of the cerebrum, cerebellum, and brain stem. The vertebral arteries originate from the subclavian arteries, enter the cranium, and at the pontine-medullary level, join to form the single basilar artery. The vertebral arteries (VAs) supply the lateral medulla and a portion of the cerebellum. The basilar artery supplies the pons and cerebellum. It divides at the junction of the pons and midbrain into the PCAs. The PCAs supply the midbrain, di-

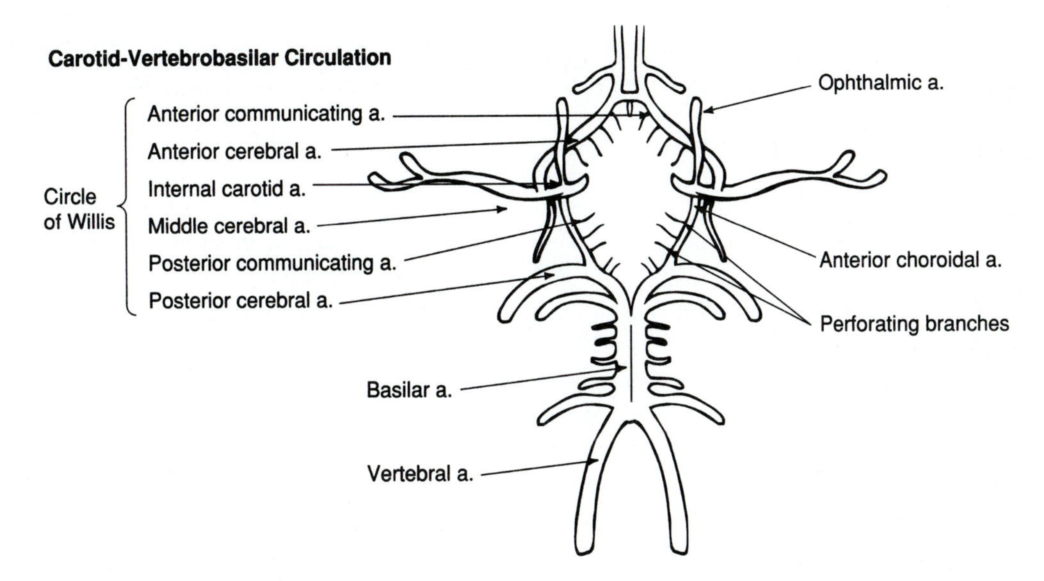

Figure 17–1. Carotid-vertebrobasilar circulation. (*Modified from Rhoton, A.L., Jackson, F.E., Gleave, J., & Rumbaugh, C.T. [1977]. Congenital and traumatic intracranial aneurysms.* Clin Symp *29(4):4.*)

encephalon (hypothalamus, subthalamus, thalamus), and inferior portion of the cerebrum. These major arteries are called conducting arteries and their small branches, which course at right angles into the depths of the brain, are called penetrating arteries. Penetrating arteries are frequently involved in small lacunar or mini-strokes.

A unique feature of the brain's vascular system is the protective **blood–brain barrier.** It permits only lipid-soluble substances to permeate its tight junctions formed by capillary endothelial cells. The blood–brain barrier is impermeable to serum protein and large molecules. When the blood–brain barrier is damaged, serum proteins and large molecules leak into the brain's interstitial spaces causing vasogenic brain edema and intracranial hypertension, a serious secondary effect of stroke. Cerebral arteries are thinner and more delicate than systemic arteries and more susceptible to rupture with severe hypertension, as can happen in stroke.

Venous Circulation

The venous circulation is a low-pressure capacitance system, as compared with the arterial circulation, which is a high-pressure, high-resistance system. Craniospinal veins are valveless and drain by gravity, an important characteristic to remember when positioning patients with increased **intracranial pressure (ICP).** The dura mater contains venous (dural) sinuses that collect blood from the cerebral, meningeal, and diploic veins of the cranium and empty it into the internal jugular veins (IJVs). The IJVs drain the cerebral hemispheres and to a lesser degree the brain stem and cerebellum. Venous pressures reflect ICP. When ICP becomes abnormally high, it may compromise venous outflow from the brain by compressing the low-pressure veins.

Cerebrospinal Fluid Dynamics

Most of the CSF is formed and secreted from the choroid plexuses in the ventricles, is absorbed from the arachnoid villi channels within the subarachnoid spaces, and flows into the sagittal sinus, thereby maintaining an equilibrium of CSF pressure. Absorption of CSF is pressure dependent. The amount of CSF secreted daily is about 0.35 mL/min, or about 500 mL, with about 25 mL remaining in the ventricles. There is approximately 125 to 150 mL of CSF circulating in the craniospinal subarachnoid spaces (Burt, 1993). The functions of CSF are to:

- Cushion and support the brain and spinal cord.
- Maintain a stable chemical milieu for the CNS.
- Excrete toxic wastes such as carbon dioxide, lactate, and hydrogen ions.

The normal adult CSF pressure in the supine position varies from 5 to 13 mm Hg, or 50 to 200 cm H_2O (Burt, 1993). Cerebrospinal fluid is similar to plasma content but has greater sodium, chloride, and magnesium levels. Potassium, glucose, and protein are lower in CSF than in plasma. This information can be used when interpreting CSF test results.

In summary, the anterior (carotid arteries) and the posterior (vertebrobasilar) arteries connect to form the circle of Willis, the major blood supply to the brain. The carotid system provides most of the brain's hemispheric circulation. The vertebrobasilar system provides circulation to undersurfaces of the hemispheres, the brain stem, and the cerebellum. The blood–brain barrier may be damaged in a stroke, leading to vasogenic brain edema. The venous circulation is valveless and drains by gravity, mostly through the internal jugular veins.

SECTION TWO REVIEW

1. Conducting arteries in the brain include all of the following EXCEPT
   A. lenticulostriate arteries
   B. anterior cerebral arteries
   C. middle cerebral arteries
   D. posterior cerebral arteries
2. The vertebrobasilar system supplies the entire
   A. frontal lobes
   B. occipital lobes
   C. brain stem
   D. basal ganglia
3. Craniospinal veins are characterized by which of the following?
   A. they are high-pressure vessels
   B. they are high-resistance vessels
   C. they are valveless vessels
   D. they control autoregulation
4. The blood–brain barrier is impermeable to
   A. water-soluble substances
   B. lipid-soluble substances
   C. serum protein
   D. small molecules
5. The absorption of CSF takes place in the
   A. lateral ventricles
   B. arachnoid villi
   C. choroid plexuses
   D. foramen of Monro

Answers: 1. A, 2. C, 3. C, 4. C, 5. B

SECTION THREE: Monro–Kellie Hypothesis

At the completion of this section, the learner will be able to define the Monro–Kellie hypothesis and state the three components of the intracranial vault.

The intracranial vault is a rigid container with limited space. The contents of the intracranial vault include the brain, cerebral blood volume, and cerebrospinal fluid. The volume of each component remains relatively stable. The **Monro–Kellie hypothesis** states that a change in volume of any one of these components must be accompanied by a reciprocal change in one or both of the other components (Davis & Briones, 1998). If this reciprocal change is not accomplished, the result is an increase in ICP (McNair, 1999).

Brain Volume

The brain is composed of neurons and glial cells. The brain volume is mainly water (80 percent), and the majority of the water is intracellular. The brain volume remains constant with the help of the blood–brain barrier.

The blood–brain barrier is a network of cells and membranes in the brain capillaries. This barrier is selective in terms of membrane permeability and molecular size of the substance attempting to enter the cerebral circulation. The blood–brain barrier is able to select which substances enter the cerebral circulation and which substances are prohibited from entering the cerebral vasculature. The blood–brain barrier is permeable to water, oxygen, lipid-soluble compounds, and carbon dioxide and slightly permeable to the electrolytes. Most drugs are prevented from crossing the blood–brain barrier, but it depends on their molecular composition. The blood–brain barrier can be physically disrupted by trauma or functionally impaired by metabolic abnormalities, such as drug overdoses. The result is an exit of fluid from the intravascular space into the extravascular space of the brain tissue.

Cerebral Blood Volume

Cerebral blood volume is the amount of blood in the cranial vault at any point in time. Cerebral blood volume is approximately 10 percent of the total intracranial volume and is maintained at a constant level through **cerebral blood flow (CBF).** The normal adult CBF averages 50 to 55 mL/100 g of brain tissue per minute, about 750 mL/min or 15 percent of the total resting cardiac output. CBF is normally controlled by autoregulation and chemoregulation such as carbon dioxide concentration, local hydrogen ion concentration, and oxygen concentration.

Cerebrospinal Fluid

CSF is the third component of intracranial volume and is produced in the choroid plexus of the lateral ventricles. CSF circulates in the subarachnoid spaces of the brain and spinal cord and is reabsorbed into the venous system by the arachnoid villi. Approximately 10 percent of the total intracranial volume is CSF, which accounts for about 150 mL of CSF at any given time. Of the three components, CSF can be displaced most easily and rapidly. Displaced CSF is eliminated into the external jugular veins. This explains why a flexed neck, tight endotracheal tube ties, and so on can increase ICP by obstructing CSF outflow.

In summary, the Monro–Kellie hypothesis states that the cranial vault is rigid and fixed and is made up of three compartments: the brain, the cerebral blood volume, and CSF. Brain volume is controlled by the blood–brain barrier, and cerebral blood volume is controlled by CBF. Of the three compartments, CSF is displaced most easily and rapidly and is the first reciprocal response to increase in intracranial volume.

SECTION THREE REVIEW

1. According to the Monro–Kellie hypothesis, an increase in one intracranial compartment must be accompanied by a reciprocal
   - **A.** decrease in another compartment
   - **B.** increase in the blood–brain barrier
   - **C.** decrease in the blood–brain barrier
   - **D.** increase in another compartment

2. Which mechanism controls brain volume?
   - **A.** cerebral blood flow
   - **B.** displacement of CSF
   - **C.** blood–brain barrier
   - **D.** vasoconstriction

Answers: 1. A, 2. C

SECTION FOUR: Relationship between Increased Intracranial Volume and Pressure

At the completion of this section, the learner will be able to describe the relationship between intracranial volume and ICP and how this relationship is balanced through use of compensatory mechanisms.

As was discussed in Section Three, volumes in the three intracranial compartments combine to form the total intracranial volume and, ideally, to produce a normal ICP. Although units of volume can be elevated in any compartment, ICP is measured in the CSF and is defined as the pressure exerted by the CSF within the ventricles of the brain. Normal ICP ranges from 0 to 15 mm Hg. ICP > 15 mm Hg for more than 5 minutes is considered abnormally elevated. Transient elevations in ICP > 15 mm Hg due to coughing or suctioning are normal if not sustained.

ICP is a dynamic process. It fluctuates constantly in response to changes in respiratory rate and body position and such activities as coughing and sneezing. Whereas ICP is a fluctuating phenomenon, intracranial volume is kept relatively stable and constant by reciprocal compensation, the principle outlined in the Monro–Kellie hypothesis. As this principle states, reciprocal compensation can occur in any one of the three compartments.

Cerebrospinal Fluid Volume

The first compensatory mechanism that occurs is displacement of CSF. As intracranial volume and pressure rise, CSF is shunted out of the cerebral subarachnoid space into the spinal subarachnoid space through natural openings called *foramina,* namely, the foramen of Magendie and foramen of Luschka. Second, as more CSF is shunted out of the subarachnoid space, the remaining CSF is absorbed at an increased rate by the arachnoid villi.

Cerebral Blood Volume

Cerebral blood volume is dependent on CBF. CBF is supplied by the internal carotid and vertebral arteries. If CBF is increased, so too is cerebral blood volume. Cerebral blood flow is dependent upon **cerebral perfusion pressure (CPP),** which is defined as the pressure gradient necessary to supply adequate amounts of blood to the brain. It is the difference between mean arterial pressure (MAP) and ICP. The MAP = $\frac{\text{systolic BP} + 2 \times \text{diastolic BP}}{3}$

$$\text{CPP} = \text{MAP} - \text{ICP}$$

The normal CPP is 80 to 100 mm Hg and must be at least 50 mm Hg to provide minimal blood flow to the brain. A CPP of ≤ 30 mm Hg is incompatible with life and results in neuronal hypoxia and cell death. For example, if the ICP is 10 mm Hg and the blood pressure is 120/80 mm Hg, the MAP is 93 ($120 + 2 \times 80 = 280/3 = 93$ MAP). The CPP in this situation would be 83 ($93 - 10 = 83$). CPP is within normal range. Cerebral perfusion is decreased with a high mean ICP or a low MAP or is increased with a lowered ICP or a higher MAP. If the mean ICP rises to the level of the MAP, brain perfusion ceases and brain death results.

Autoregulation is a compensatory mechanism that keeps CBF constant by maintaining an adequate CPP. Autoregulation works by automatic constriction or dilation of cerebral blood vessels in response to either changes in systemic arterial pressure or blood levels of carbon dioxide and oxygen. When systemic pressure rises, the vessels constrict to protect the brain from blood engorgement and to protect cerebral tissues from the full impact of the systemic pressure. When systemic pressure falls, the reverse occurs. Cerebral vessels dilate in an attempt to increase CBF. This compensatory mechanism is termed *pressure regulation*.

Constriction or dilation of cerebral vessels in response to blood levels of carbon dioxide and oxygen is termed *metabolic* or *chemical regulation* (Davis & Briones, 1998). Vessels dilate in response to **hypercapnia,** or elevated carbon dioxide levels > 45 mm Hg, and constrict in response to lowered levels of carbon dioxide (< 21 mm Hg will decrease CBF to one half of normal value) (Bouma & Muizelaar, 1992). Blood oxygen levels affect the diameter of cerebral vessels but are not as potent a stimulus as is carbon dioxide. Vessels dilate in response to decreased oxygen levels (< 50 mm Hg). Oxygen levels > 80 mm Hg will decrease CBF slightly.

Brain Volume

As was discussed in Section Three, the blood–brain barrier acts to control brain volume by controlling the solutes and water that attempt to cross it and enter the cerebral circulation. If this controlling mechanism is disrupted, either physically or functionally, an increase in brain volume will result secondary to an escape of fluid from the intravascular space to the extravascular space. Unless there is a reciprocal decrease in either cerebral blood volume or CSF volume, an overall increase in intracranial volume and ICP will result.

Obviously, the brain is limited in its compensatory abilities. It cannot decrease its size or displace itself. The brain possesses two properties called **elastance** and **compliance**. Elastance is a measure of stiffness. If the elastance value is high, the brain is considered tight, and the intracranial space has little volume reserve. On the other hand, compliance is a measure of slackness and is the inverse of elastance. For example, if elastance were low, compliance would be high; thus the brain would be able to tolerate increases in volume for a longer period than if elastance were high.

As with all compensatory mechanisms, these mechanisms operate only within specific parameters. Autoregulation is lost when a critical point is reached, either the ICP is > 30 to 35 mm Hg or systemic blood pressure is < 60 mm Hg or > 160 mm Hg. If a critical point is reached, CBF will vary passively with systemic blood pressure.

In summary, this section discussed how intracranial volume influences ICP. When intracranial volume is elevated, compensatory mechanisms are activated: displacement and increased absorption of CSF and autoregulation. The brain's ability to tolerate increases in volume depends on the degree of elastance and compliance. The outcomes of uncompensated volume increases are discussed in Section Six.

SECTION FOUR REVIEW

1. Hypercapnia causes
   A. cerebral vasodilation
   B. cerebral vasoconstriction
   C. decreased cerebral blood flow
   D. decreased cerebral blood volume
2. Cerebral blood flow is dependent on
   A. an intact blood–brain barrier
   B. cerebral perfusion pressure
   C. serum glucose levels
   D. cerebral blood volume
3. Your patient's MAP is 80 mm Hg and the ICP is 15 mm Hg. What is the cerebral perfusion pressure?
   A. 50 mm Hg
   B. 65 mm Hg
   C. 95 mm Hg
   D. 110 mm Hg
4. Autoregulation works by
   A. increasing or decreasing blood levels of oxygen and carbon dioxide
   B. displacing CSF into the spinal subarachnoid space
   C. altering elastance and compliance properties
   D. automatically constricting or dilating cerebral blood vessels
5. In terms of increased ICP, a high measure of elastance would indicate
   A. the autoregulatory mechanism will be lost
   B. the intracranial vault has little volume reserve
   C. the brain is able to tolerate additional increases in volume
   D. the compliance measure also is high

Answers: 1. A, 2. B, 3. B, 4. D, 5. B

SECTION FIVE: Cerebral Oxygenation

At the completion of this section, the learner will be able to describe the relationship between cerebral oxygenation and metabolism, anaerobic and aerobic metabolism, and factors that affect cerebral oxygenation.

The brain requires a continuous supply of glucose, oxygen, and substrates for energy because it has no way of storing oxygen reserves and brain glucose reserves last for only about 2 minutes. Cerebral metabolism varies regionally, with some areas of the brain being more metabolically active than others at any given time. CBF varies regionally as well. The brain attempts to match metabolism by locally increasing or decreasing CBF as needed. This localized matching of CBF with metabolism is achieved through the process of autoregulation, as described in Section Three. When CBF is inadequate to meet the brain's metabolic needs, a state of mismatching occurs, and ischemia results. Because the brain is unable to store oxygen or glucose, aerobic metabolism can no longer be supported and the brain is forced to switch to anaerobic metabolism. The normal cerebral metabolic rate of oxygen consumption ($CMRO_2$) is 3.5 mL of oxygen per 100 g of brain tissue per minute. When the $CMRO_2$ decreases to 3 mL/100 g/min, ischemic synaptic transmission failure occurs. When it decreases to 1.4 mL/100 g/min, infarction or cellular death occurs. The end product of anaerobic metabolism is only two molecules of ATP and lactate. Carbon dioxide, the end product of aerobic metabolism, readily crosses the blood–brain barrier and is reabsorbed. However, the lactate molecule does not cross the blood–brain barrier and accumulates, resulting in cerebral acidosis. As discussed in Section Three, cerebral acidosis causes cerebral vasodilation, which upsets the state of equilibrium in the cranial vault.

Because of the brain's attempt to match CBF with cerebral metabolism, CBF is a most important variable when addressing cerebral oxygenation. Oligemic cerebral hypoxia occurs when CBF is too low and unable to support cerebral metabolism; it may be secondary to anything that decreases CBF, such as cerebral edema, low cardiac output, or vasoconstriction. When CBF is higher than the metabolic needs of the brain, a state of hyperemia exists, also known as "luxury perfusion." Patients with this condition have progressive vasodilation, increased cerebral blood volume, and eventual loss of autoregulation, all of which contribute to increased ICP (Davis & Briones, 1998). Both **oligemia** and **hyperemia** have been described as pathophysiologic changes that occur following brain injury. Treatment of oligemia and hyperemia is aimed at maximizing cerebral oxygenation, by either increasing or decreasing CBF. Treatment modalities are discussed in Section Fourteen.

Maintaining adequate cerebral oxygenation is of the utmost importance to support aerobic metabolism. Every effort should be made to avoid episodes of hypoxia or hypotension. Studies demonstrate that even transient episodes of hypoxia or hypotension have a negative impact on patient outcome. To monitor the level of cerebral ischemia and the effect of interventions to promote cerebral oxygenation, **jugular venous oxygen saturation ($SjVO_2$)** can be measured.

Jugular Venous Oxygen Saturation

It is impossible to determine the type of CBF pattern by monitoring ICP or CPP alone. It is important to be able to determine which type of blood flow alteration exists because interventions differ for oligemia versus hyperemia. Although calculating CPP provides information about cerebral perfusion, neither CPP nor ICP measurements provide information about the other side of the equation—oxygen consumption.

Monitoring the saturation of venous blood leaving the brain and subtracting this measurement from the saturation of the arterial circulation gives information about the adequacy of CBF. Saturation of venous blood leaving the brain via the jugular vein can be continuously monitored by the placement of a fiber-optic catheter in the bulb of the dominant internal jugular vein. This reading, subtracted from the arterial oxygen saturation as determined by pulse oximetry, can assess the relationship between oxygen supply and demand of the brain. In effect, it is a method of determining the ability of the brain to maintain a matched state between CBF and cerebral metabolism.

Oxygen saturation of venous blood exiting the brain via the jugular vein is known as jugular venous oxygen saturation ($SjVO_2$). The $SjVO_2$ is 50 to 75 percent. If the brain is receiving less oxygen than it needs, it will extract more oxygen from the cerebral circulation and the saturation in the jugular vein will be lower. If CBF is higher than the brain requires, less oxygen will be extracted and the jugular bulb saturation will be higher. Saturation values < 50 percent reflect a state of oligemia; values > 75 percent reflect a state of hyperemia. Based on these measurements, interventions can be implemented that are specific to the blood flow alteration.

By comparing the difference between the oxygen saturation of arterial blood before it enters the brain (SaO_2) with the saturation of venous blood as it exits the brain ($SjVO_2$), one can calculate the amount of oxygen extracted from the cerebral circulation. The difference between arterial and venous oxygen content is known as the **arteriovenous difference in oxygen content ($AVDO_2$).** With this measurement, notice that the term "oxygen content" rather than "oxygen saturation" is used. Oxygen saturation reflects the amount of oxygen carried by hemoglobin, whereas oxygen content reflects the total amount of oxygen and includes oxygen carried by hemoglobin and oxygen dissolved in plasma. So oxygen content is a more complete measurement of the total amount of oxygen in the blood, venous or arterial. $AVDO_2$ is calculated by using the following formula:

$$AVDO_2 = (SaO_2 - SjVO_2) \times 1.34 \times Hgb/100 \text{ mL/dL}$$

The cofactor of 1.34 is used because that is the amount of oxygen that is bound by 1 g of hemoglobin; thus, each molecule of hemoglobin must be multiplied by 1.34. Normal $AVDO_2$ is 4 to 9 mL/dL and is inversely proportional to $SjVO_2$. As CBF decreases, the difference in oxygen content between the arterial and venous circulation will be higher because less oxygen is being extracted from a limited blood supply. In cases of hyperemia, the $AVDO_2$ will be lower and the $SjVO_2$ will be higher. Continuous monitoring of $SjVO_2$ and $AVDO_2$ provides valuable information in the detection of cerebral ischemia and dictates interventions used in the management of brain injury and their effect. If desaturation occurs following an intervention, the intervention has decreased CBF, resulting in blood with a lower oxygen saturation exiting the brain.

In summary, the brain relies on a continuous and constant supply of oxygen and glucose to support the metabolic needs of the cells. When the supply of oxygen and glucose is less than cellular demand, a state of mismatching occurs, ischemia ensues, and anaerobic metabolism is initiated. Hypoxia and hypotension are the primary causes of ischemia and must be avoided. Continuous monitoring of $SjVO_2$ and $AVDO_2$ can detect the presence of cerebral ischemia and monitor the effect of interventions on cerebral oxygenation.

SECTION FIVE REVIEW

1. Cerebral oxygenation is affected by all of the following EXCEPT

   A. cerebral metabolism
   B. cerebral blood flow
   C. serum sodium
   D. hypotension

2. Anaerobic metabolism
   A. is less efficient than aerobic metabolism
   B. results in carbon dioxide as an end product
   C. produces 38 molecules of ATP
   D. utilizes oxygen and glucose to manufacture ATP

3. $AVDO_2$
   A. assists in monitoring the effect of interventions on CBF
   B. decreases when CBF decreases
   C. increases when a state of hyperemia exists
   D. highly correlates with ICP

Answers: 1. C, 2. A, 3. A

SECTION SIX: Uncompensated Compartmental Volume Increases

At the completion of this section, the learner will be able to describe the outcome of uncompensated compartmental volume increases and the conditions that may contribute to these increases.

According to the Monro–Kellie hypothesis, any compartmental volume increase must be reciprocated by a volume decrease in one or both of the remaining compartments. If this reciprocity is not realized, total intracranial volume will increase, along with ICP. Primarily, intracranial volume is increased by any process that increases actual brain or blood volume or any process that interferes with CSF production or absorption.

Brain Volume

Space-occupying lesions and cerebral edema are the primary processes that increase brain volume. This type of lesion includes tumors, abscesses, hemorrhages, and hematomas. Cerebral edema may occur after any type of head trauma, including surgery, brain anoxia, or ischemia. The effect of increased brain volume depends on the rate of development. Slower-growing lesions, such as a chronic hematoma or slow-growing tumor, may remain asymptomatic and may be tolerated for a longer time period than an acute subdural hematoma, which develops at a faster rate. Postinjury cerebral edema is maximum at 72 hours.

A mass or edema that progresses and is uncompensated eventually will result in a shifting of brain tissue, or **herniation,** which carries a grave prognosis. This process causes displacement of brain tissue and pressure or traction on cerebral structures, which causes clinical symptoms. Herniation syndromes are described based on the end stage of the herniation. Four herniation syndromes are as follows:

- *Cingulate herniation.* Lateral shift of brain tissue, usually as the result of a lesion in one of the cerebral hemispheres
- *Central or transtentorial herniation.* Downward shift of one or both cerebral hemispheres, usually due to lesions in the frontal or parietal lobes
- *Uncal or lateral transtentorial herniation.* Lateral and downward shift of brain tissue, usually the temporal lobe, due to lesions located most laterally, such as the middle fossa in the temporal lobe. This type of herniation causes compression of the oculomotor nerve, or cranial nerve III, evidenced by the classic sign of a unilaterally dilated pupil
- *Tonsillar herniation.* Downward shift of brain tissue through the foramen magnum, which results in compression of the medulla and upper cervical spinal cord

Cerebral Blood Volume

Any systemic process that affects blood levels of carbon dioxide will affect CBF, CPP, and cerebral blood volume. Therefore, conditions that produce hypercapnia and hypoxemia will result in cerebral vasodilation and increased blood volume. These conditions may include chronic respiratory insufficiencies, inadequate ventilation, hypoventilation, sedation by drugs, and insufficient supplemental oxygen.

Cerebral blood volume may also be increased by any process that impedes venous outflow. This includes anything that may impede jugular circulation, such as head/neck rotation or flexion, Valsalva's maneuver, and use of positive end-expiratory pressure (PEEP).

A third cause of increased blood volume is loss of autoregulation. This regulatory mechanism may become ineffective in states of ischemia, sustained elevations in ICP, and sustained states of hyperemia. When autoregulation is lost, the cerebral blood vessels passively dilate, leading to further increases in cerebral blood volume and ICP.

Cerebrospinal Fluid

Volume increases in CSF result from increased production, obstructed circulation, or decreased absorption. This is a condition termed **hydrocephalus.** Obstruction to CSF can be caused by mass lesions or infection. Decreased absorption can result from a subarachnoid hemorrhage or meningitis.

Hydrocephalus is treated surgically or mechanically. If considered to be a permanent condition, a surgical shunt is placed; if considered temporary, a ventricular drain is inserted for intermittent or continuous drainage.

The following chart summarizes the causes and effects of increased intracranial volume. It must be kept in mind that any increase in brain volume, blood volume, or CSF that is unchecked will result in herniation.

Component	Cause	Effect
Brain volume	Space-occupying lesion	Herniation
	Cerebral edema	
Blood volume	Hypercapnia	Cerebral dilation
	Hypoxemia	
	Loss of autoregulation	Passive vessels
	Venous outflow obstruction	Increased cerebral blood volume
CSF	Obstruction	Hydrocephalus
	Decreased absorption	
	Increased production	

SECTION SIX REVIEW

1. Which of the following pathologies is NOT associated with increased intracranial volume?
   A. subdural hematoma
   B. hypotension
   C. subarachnoid hemorrhage
   D. meningioma
2. Which of the following is NOT a direct cause of increased CSF?
   A. meningitis
   B. hypoglycemia
   C. subarachnoid hemorrhage
   D. brain tumor
3. ICP can be increased by anything that
   A. increases intracranial volume
   B. results in high compliance
   C. results in low elastance
   D. decreases carbon dioxide levels
4. Chronic respiratory insufficiency may affect
   A. brain volume
   B. brain volume, cerebral blood volume, and CSF volume
   C. CSF volume
   D. cerebral blood volume

Answers: 1. B, 2. B, 3. A, 4. D

SECTION SEVEN: Impaired Arousal and Content

At the completion of this section, the learner will be able to identify pathologic conditions that impair the two components of consciousness—arousal and content—and discuss how these impairments occur.

Content and arousal are interdependent components. Various pathologies can affect each component or both components. Causes of decreased consciousness commonly fall into three categories: structural brain lesions, metabolic dysfunction, or psychiatric disorders. Conditions that impair content do so by widely affecting the cerebral hemispheres. Alterations in content are manifested by cognitive deficits such as memory impairment, disorientation, impaired problem-solving abilities, and attentional deficits. The degree of impairment of consciousness is related to the location and size of the lesion. Lesions that affect small areas of the hemispheres usually do not produce a significant depression in the level of consciousness. Hemispheric strokes and small intracerebral hematomas and contusions result in localized deficits. Conditions that affect the hemispheres diffusely can cause a significant depression in the level of consciousness and may result in coma. Anoxia, ischemia, metabolic alterations, poisons, drugs, and psychiatric disturbances can cause diffuse cerebral hemispheric dysfunction.

Conditions that affect arousal do so by directly or indirectly depressing the brain stem structures and the RAS. These conditions will result in immediate loss of consciousness and produce coma. Any condition that impairs arousal will naturally impair content as well. Processes that impair arousal include mass lesions that destroy the brain stem structures, compression of the brain stem by herniation, or any process that involves the brain stem and the cerebral hemispheres that is sufficient to produce a depressed level of consciousness.

The mnemonic *vowel tipps* is useful for remembering etiologies for impaired consciousness:

Alcohol	Trauma
Epilepsy	Infection
Insulin	Psych
Opiates	Poisons
Urates (renal failure)	Shock

In summary, various pathologies can impair content or arousal, either separately, as with impairments affecting content; or in combination, as in conditions affecting arousal.

SECTION SEVEN REVIEW

1. Findings from your initial assessment of your patient are as follows: patient is awake, eyes are open and focusing, patient responds appropriately to verbal commands. Based on these findings, you could determine that
   A. the state of arousal is intact, but not content
   B. the state of content is intact, but not arousal
   C. not enough data have been gathered to assess content completely, but arousal is intact
   D. not enough data have been gathered to assess arousal, but content is intact

Questions 2 and 3 pertain to the same patient.

2. Your patient exhibits memory and attentional deficits. This is an impairment of
   A. arousal
   B. the RAS
   C. the cerebral cortex
   D. the cerebellum
3. A possible etiology for this patient is
   A. depression of the RAS
   B. herniation
   C. alcohol intoxication
   D. massive intracranial bleed

Answers: 1. C, 2. C, 3. C

SECTION EIGHT: Clinical Assessment

At the completion of this section, the learner will be able to identify common components to be assessed for arousal and content.

Arousal

The level of consciousness is the most important factor in the neurologic assessment. The arousal component is assessed first. The first step is to determine what stimulus will arouse the patient, usually by calling his or her name. If the patient does not respond, shake the arm or shoulder gently. If no response is elicited, you must proceed from light pain to deeper pain to try to elicit a response. You should always start with the least noxious stimulus and then proceed to a more intense stimulus if necessary. An example of light pain to deeper pain is shaking the arm, to nailbed pressure, to applying pressure to the supraorbital notch. You are assessing two things: (1) Is the patient responsive to verbal stimuli?, and if not (2) Does the patient exhibit purposeful movement? Purposeful movement, such as removing the stimulus or withdrawing from the stimulus, indicates functioning of sensory pathways. Abnormal posturing in response to a noxious stimulus indicates a dysfunction of either the cerebral hemispheres or the brain stem. Decorticate posturing (abnormal flexion) indicates cerebral hemispheric dysfunction. Decerebrate posturing (abnormal extension) indicates brain stem dysfunction and is a more ominous sign. Patients whose extremities are restrained must be unrestrained when assessing their motor response.

Content

The content of consciousness is assessed by noting behavior. The patient should be assessed for orientation and should know his name, the date, and where he is. The patient is considered disoriented if unable to answer the questions correctly. Testing for orientation also assesses short-term memory. Orientation can be assessed only if the patient is able to respond verbally.

After assessing orientation, ability to follow commands is assessed. Ask the patient to perform such acts as sticking out the tongue or holding up two fingers. This not only tells you whether the patient is awake enough to respond but also whether he or she is aware enough to interpret and carry out the commands.

Behavioral changes are assessed next by noting any restlessness, irritability, or combativeness. Such behavioral indicators can be caused by many things, including hypoxia, hypoglycemia, drug use, pain, or increased ICP. As the nurse, your role is to pick up clues that may point to causes for changes in behavior. A more in-depth assessment of responsiveness is discussed in Section Nine.

The last component of content that is assessed is verbal response. Assessment of speech provides information about the function of the relationship between the speech centers in the cerebrum and the cranial nerves and can help localize the area of dysfunction. The patient's speech pattern should be assessed for clarity. Is it clear or slurred and garbled? This may indicate drug use, metabolic disturbance, or cranial nerve injuries. Content of speech should be assessed for use of appropriate or inappropriate words. Confused patients may use inappropriate words. Patients with cranial nerve dysfunction usually will not give inappropriate responses, although the speech pattern may be slurred. Patients may experience receptive, expressive, or global aphasia. Inability to understand written or spoken words is receptive aphasia. Inability to write or use language appropriately is expressive aphasia. Global aphasia includes both the inability to use or understand language.

In summary, the level of consciousness is the most important part of the neurologic assessment, of which arousal is assessed first. For patients who are not in a state of wakefulness, it would be pointless to start off by assessing content. Arousal is assessed by evaluating how much stimulus, if any, is needed for the patient to respond and what type of motor responses the patient exhibits. Content is assessed by evaluating behavior and behavioral changes, ability to follow commands, and verbal response.

SECTION EIGHT REVIEW

1. What is the first component to be assessed in the neurologic assessment?
   - **A.** content
   - **B.** arousal
   - **C.** behavior
   - **D.** speech
2. During evaluation of arousal, the two things being assessed are
   - **A.** stimuli required for the patient to respond and type of motor response
   - **B.** behavior and behavioral changes
   - **C.** presence of receptive and expressive aphasia
   - **D.** presence of confusion and state of orientation
3. A decorticate motor response indicates
   - **A.** brain stem dysfunction
   - **B.** the patient is close to death
   - **C.** cerebral hemispheric dysfunction
   - **D.** arousal is intact

Answers: 1. B, 2. A, 3. C

SECTION NINE: In-Depth Clinical Assessment

At the completion of this section, the learner will be able to identify and describe in-depth clinical assessment of patients with an alteration in arousal.

Beyond the clinical assessment of arousal and content, a more in-depth neurologic assessment includes pupillary reactions, vital signs, and assessment of cranial nerve reflexes.

Pupillary Reactions

Pupillary reactions provide information about the location of some lesions. Pupils should be assessed for size, symmetry, shape, and reaction to light.

A unilateral brain lesion can be ruled out if the pupils are equal in size. Nonreactive pupils in the midposition indicate damage to the midbrain (Fig. 17–2A). Pupils that are nonreactive to light and pinpoint indicate a pons lesion or opiate drug overdose (Fig. 17–2B). Pupils that are small but reactive to light may indicate a bilateral injury to the thalamus or hypothalamus or metabolic coma (Fig. 17–2C). A unilaterally dilated and fixed pupil may indicate compression of the oculomotor nerve (cranial nerve III) (Fig. 17–2D). Pupil changes are on the same side (ipsilateral) as the lesion.

When both pupils are dilated and nonreactive (fixed), emergency action is required. It may be caused by severe anoxia or ischemia. Remember that atropine-like drugs, as well as epinephrine, cause the pupils to dilate and this must be ruled out (Fig. 17–2E).

Vital Signs

Vital signs are important indicators, especially in the unresponsive patient. Vital signs should be assessed not only individually but also in relationship to each other. Unfortunately, changes in the vital signs occur in the late stages of increased ICP and neurologic deterioration. Cushing's triad is a specific change in the vital signs and is evidenced by (1) an increase in the systolic blood pressure, (2) a decrease in the diastolic blood pressure, and (3) bradycardia. Waiting until this triad of symptoms occurs before intervening can result in irreversible damage.

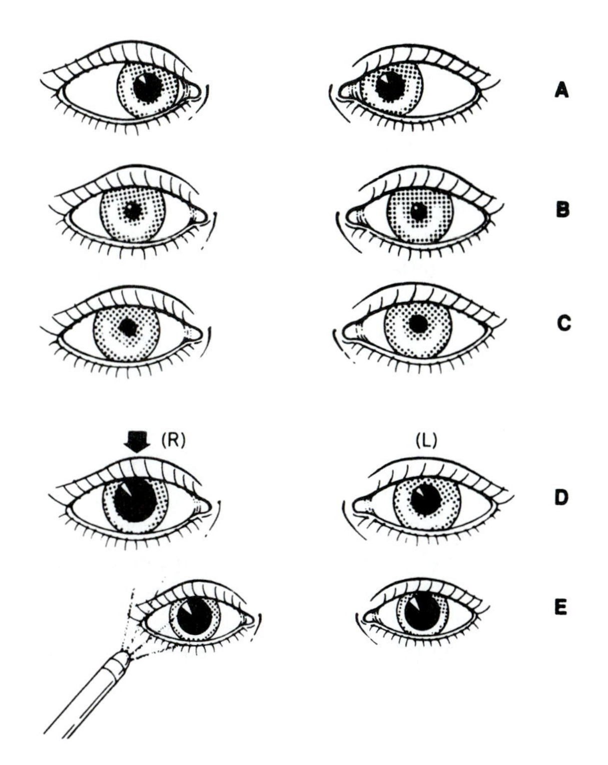

Figure 17–2. A. Unreactive pupils in midposition. B. Constricted unreactive pupils. C. Constricted reactive pupils. D. Unilateral dilated unreactive pupils. E. Dilated unreactive pupils. (*From Hickey, J. [1996].* The clinical practice of neurologic and neurosurgical nursing. *Philadelphia: J.B. Lippincott.*)

Respiration

The respiratory pattern provides the most valuable information because it can be correlated with the anatomic level of dysfunction. Respiratory rhythm and pattern are controlled by the medulla. Respirations should be assessed for rate and rhythm and should be counted for 1 full minute before stimulating the patient. Some of the more commonly described abnormal respiratory patterns found in the neurologically impaired patient are discussed in the following paragraphs. As a nurse, remember that it is more important to describe the pattern than to try to fit your patient's respiratory pattern into a category. If your patient is mechanically ventilated, it is difficult to observe these patterns, and it would be extremely detrimental to the patient to remove ventilatory support for the purpose of assessing abnormal patterns.

Cheyne–Stokes pattern indicates a bilateral lesion in the cerebral hemispheres, cerebellum, midbrain, or, in rare circumstances, upper pons and may be due to cerebral infarction or metabolic diseases. This respiratory pattern is evidenced by a rhythmic waxing and waning in the depth of the respiration, followed by a period of apnea (Fig. 17–3).

Central neurogenic hyperventilation indicates a lesion in the low midbrain or upper pons and may be due to infarction or ischemia of the midbrain or pons, anoxia, or tumors of the midbrain. This pattern is evidenced by respirations that have an increase in depth, are rapid (> 24), and are regular (Fig. 17–3).

Apneustic breathing indicates a lesion in the mid or low pons that may be due to infarction of the pons or severe meningitis. This pattern is evidenced by prolonged inspiration, with a pause at the point where the respiration is at its peak, lasting for 2 to 3 seconds. This may alternate with an expiratory pause (Fig. 17–3).

Cluster breathing indicates a lesion in the low pons or upper medulla that may be due to a tumor or infarction

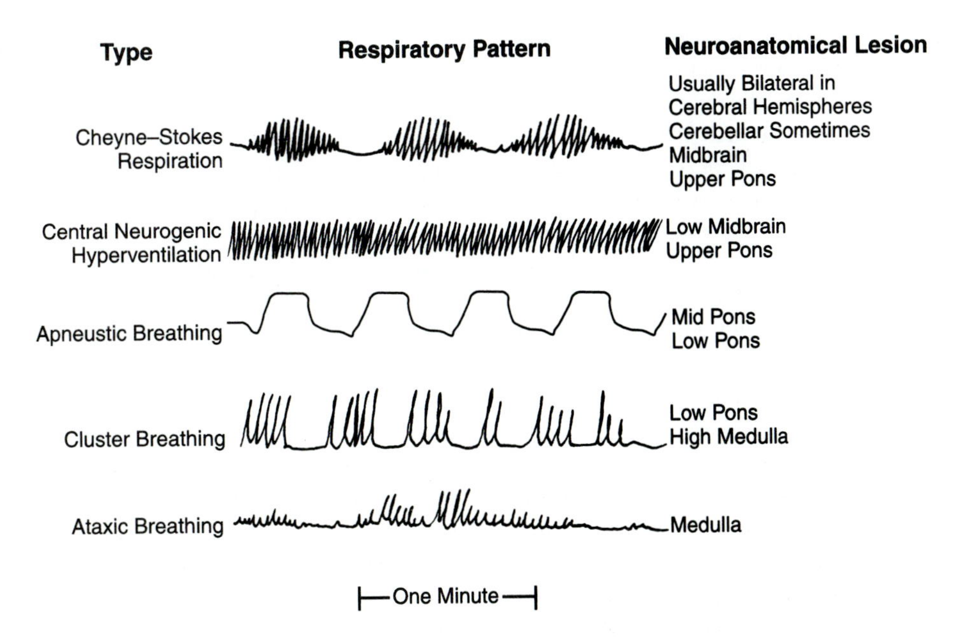

Figure 17–3. Abnormal respiratory patterns associated with coma.

of the medulla. This pattern is described as clusters of irregular breathing with periods of apnea that occur at irregular intervals (Fig. 17–3).

Ataxic breathing indicates a lesion in the medulla that may be due to a cerebellar or pons bleed, tumors of the cerebrum, or severe meningitis. These respirations are completely irregular, with deep and shallow random breaths and pauses (Hickey, 1996) (Fig. 17–3).

Remember that abnormal respiratory patterns also may be initiated by such factors as acidosis, respiratory alkalosis, electrolyte imbalances, anxiety, pulmonary processes, or drugs, especially narcotics and anesthetic agents that depress the respiratory center.

Heart Rate

The pulse should be assessed for rate, rhythm, and quality. Increased heart rate may indicate poor cerebral oxygenation. Decreased heart rate is present in the late stages of increased ICP, in which case the quality will be bounding.

Blood Pressure

The medulla regulates blood pressure based on input from chemoreceptors and pressor receptors. An important response to ischemia is known as the Cushing reflex. This response is activated when pressure in the CSF system rises to a point where it equals or exceeds arterial blood pressure. In response to this increase in pressure, the systolic blood pressure rises to a level slightly higher than that of the CSF, which permits CBF to continue.

Temperature

The center for temperature regulation is in the hypothalamus, which regulates body heat via afferent impulses. Hypothermia can occur as a result of spinal shock; metabolic coma; drug overdose, especially depressants; and destructive lesions of the brain stem or hypothalamus. Hyperthermia can occur as a result of CNS infection, subarachnoid hemorrhage, hypothalamic lesions, or hemorrhage of the hypothalamus or brain stem. Temperature may fluctuate widely and may exceed 106°F. Hyperthermia is treated vigorously because of the increased metabolic demands placed on the body and brain, resulting in an increase in carbon dioxide.

Cranial Nerve Reflexes

Protective reflexes are cranial nerve reflexes and indicate brain stem functioning. The unresponsive patient should be assessed for the presence of intact reflexes, and if reflexes are absent or decreased, measures should be taken to protect the patient from injury. The protective reflexes include (1) corneal reflex (blink), (2) gag reflex, (3) swallow reflex, and (4) cough reflex. Check the corneal reflex by touching the cornea, from the side, with a wisp of cotton. The eye will blink rapidly if the reflex is intact. The gag reflex is checked by touching the posterior tongue with a tongue blade. If intact, the patient will gag. The cough and gag reflexes can be checked also while suctioning the intubated patient.

Two other reflexes that are used to determine the integrity of the brain stem are the oculovestibular (caloric) and oculocephalic (doll's eyes) reflexes. Both reflexes involve cranial nerves III (oculomotor), IV (trochlear), VI (abducens), and VIII (acoustic). In the awake patient, it is easy to test these cranial nerves by asking the patient to perform a full range of eye movements. Asking the patient to look upward, downward, outward, inward, medially upward and outward, and laterally upward and outward will demonstrate full range of eye motion, also known as extraocular eye movements (EOMs). Deficits in eye movements usually indicate a cranial nerve dysfunction of one or more of the above cranial nerves. However, in the unresponsive patient, voluntary eye movement is lost and the patient is unable to perform EOMs. In this case, oculocephalic and oculovestibular responses are tested to evaluate eye movements.

The oculocephalic reflex is tested by holding the patient's eyes open and briskly turning the head from side to side, pausing at each end point. In the patient with an intact brain stem, the examiner will see conjugate eye movement opposite to the side the head is turned, known as "full doll's eyes." In cases of brain stem injury the eyes will remain stationary and doll's eyes are said to be absent. This test is contraindicated in patients whose cervical spine has not been cleared of injury.

The oculovestibular reflex is a more sensitive indicator of brain stem function and central nervous system injury. Patients with an absent oculocephalic reflex may have a normal oculovestibular reflex. Therefore, testing for the oculovestibular reflex must always follow testing for the oculocephalic reflex. The reflex is elicited by instilling cold water into the external auditory canal. This is known as *cold caloric testing*. The amount of water necessary to elicit a response varies depending on the patient's level of responsiveness, with 1 to 5 mL instilled initially. If there is no response, 20 mL up to 120 mL, may be instilled. The patient's head is raised to 30 degrees and cold water is slowly instilled into the external ear canal. The eyes are observed for direction of eye movements. In a normal response, the examiner will see the eyes deviate toward the ear with the irrigation flow. Nausea and vomiting are common occurrences. Abnormal responses, such as slow movement toward the instilled ear, dysconjugate eye movements, or absent eye movements, indicate brain stem impairment. Testing the oculovestibular reflex is contraindicated if there is leakage of CSF or purulent drainage from the ear, or perforation or tear of the tympanic membrane.

Results of oculocephalic or oculovestibular testing must be interpreted with caution. Many pharmacologic agents may depress these reflexes, such as ototoxic drugs, neuromuscular blockers, and ethyl alcohol.

In summary, clinical neurologic assessment is complex. In-depth areas commonly assessed include pupils, vital signs, and cranial nerve reflexes. Frequently, the location of some lesions or pathologies can be determined based on the clinical assessment.

SECTION NINE REVIEW

1. Which component of vital signs provides the most useful information for neurologic assessment?
   A. respiration
   B. blood pressure
   C. heart rate
   D. temperature
2. Pupils that are bilaterally pinpoint and nonreactive to light indicate
   A. unilateral brain lesion
   B. metabolic coma
   C. herniation
   D. lesion in the pons
3. The most important component of the neurologic assessment is
   A. level of consciousness
   B. pupil reactivity
   C. cranial nerve assessment
   D. vital sign assessment
4. Cranial nerve reflexes indicate
   A. level of lesion
   B. presence of increased ICP
   C. brain stem functioning
   D. intactness of the motor tracts

Answers: 1. A, 2. D, 3. A, 4. C

SECTION TEN: Documentation

At the completion of this section, the learner will be able to document his or her assessment of the arousal and content components of responsiveness.

It is important to document your assessment in a reliable and consistent manner to provide accurate transfer of information from clinician to clinician. Labels, such as comatose, lethargic, and stuporous, should be avoided because they lend themselves to subjective interpretation.

The Glasgow Coma Scale (GCS) is the most frequently used method to document neurologic assessment. The scale assesses eye opening responses and verbal and motor responses. Motor changes are contralateral or opposite the side of the lesion. The GCS assesses the arousal component of consciousness (Table 17–1).

The GCS was developed to provide a means for objective assessment of depth of coma. It provides a way to convey quantitatively a patient's neurologic status. It is an extremely useful scale for evaluating patients at lower levels of responsiveness because it evaluates reactivity-type patterns. Higher levels of responses require cortical functioning because of the interpretation of stimuli that is required. The GCS is not a complete and valid measure of content and often misses subtle changes in cognition, such as attentional deficits. For this reason, to identify and evaluate higher order responses, additional techniques are needed.

There are certain types of patients for whom the GCS is not usable. Patients with periorbital edema are unable to open their eyes and would receive an eye opening response score of 1, which may or may not be valid. Motor deficits, such as hemiparesis or paraplegia, may be overlooked, since the motor response scored is the best response elicited. Finally, it is impossible to evaluate a verbal response for patients who are intubated or have a tracheostomy.

To assess content, you must assess language, memory, and mood. This is possible only with the conscious patient. With an unconscious patient, you will be able to assess arousal only. Verbal response should be assessed not only for orientation but also for flow, clarity, spontaneity, and appropriateness. The patient's mood should be noted, and memory should be tested by asking the patient to name family members (if appropriate). Content can be assessed using a mental status examination.

TABLE 17–1. GLASGOW COMA SCALE

CATEGORY	SCORE	RESPONSE
Eye opening	4	Spontaneous—eyes open spontaneously without stimulation
	3	To speech—eyes open with verbal stimulation but not necessarily to command
	2	To pain—eyes open with noxious stimuli
	1	None—no eye opening regardless of stimulation
Verbal response	5	Oriented—accurate information about person, place, time, reason for hospitalization, and personal data
	4	Confused—answers not appropriate to question but correct use of language
	3	Inappropriate words—disorganized, random speech, no sustained conversation
	2	Incomprehensible sounds—moans, groans, and mumbles incomprehensibly
	1	None—no verbalization despite stimulation
Best motor response	6	Obeys commands—performs simple tasks on command; able to repeat performance
	5	Localizes to pain—organized attempt to localize and remove painful stimuli
	4	Withdraws from pain—withdraws extremity from source of painful stimuli
	3	Abnormal flexion—decorticate posturing spontaneously or in response to noxious stimuli
	2	Extension—decerebrate posturing spontaneously or in response to noxious stimuli
	1	None—no response to noxious stimuli; flaccid

Note: Total score = 15 in a neurologically intact person.

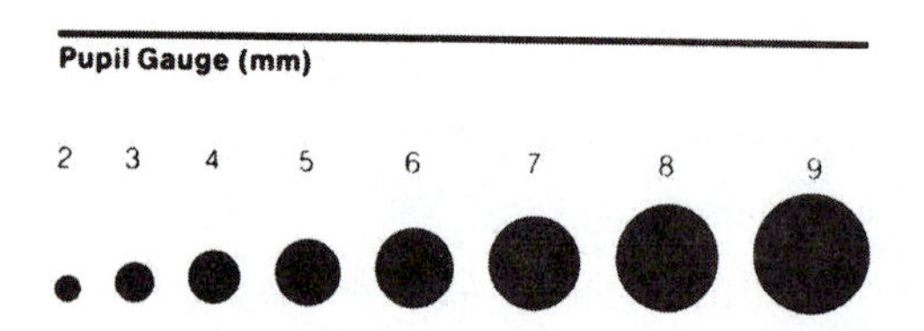

Figure 17–4. Pupil gauge in millimeters. (*From Hickey, J. [1996].* The clinical practice of neurologic and neurosurgical nursing. *Philadelphia: J.B. Lippincott.*)

Vital signs should be documented along with pupillary assessment. Pupil size should be assessed using a standard pupil gauge (Fig. 17–4).

In summary, the GCS is a standardized and well-accepted method of assessing the arousal component but is not a valid measure of cognitive abilities or content. To evaluate content, additional methods must be employed.

SECTION TEN REVIEW

1. The Glasgow Coma Scale assesses
   - **A.** cranial nerves
   - **B.** abstract thinking
   - **C.** arousal
   - **D.** awareness
2. The Glasgow Coma Scale is useful because it
   - **A.** is standardized
   - **B.** evaluates the ability to interpret stimuli
   - **C.** is subjective
   - **D.** evaluates vital signs and pupil reactivity
3. The Glasgow Coma Scale should not be used for
   - **A.** quantitative evaluation
   - **B.** evaluation of lower levels of consciousness
   - **C.** evaluation of attentional deficits
   - **D.** comatose patients

Answers: 1. C, 2. A, 3. C

SECTION ELEVEN: Diagnostic Procedures

At the completion of this section, the learner will be able to discuss selected diagnostic procedures and their clinical application, advantages, and limitations.

Until the latter half of the twentieth century, the neurodiagnostic tools were crude and yielded nonspecific results. Since the introduction of CT scanning in the 1970s, the diagnostic methods used in neuroscience have become more refined and accurate. This section discusses some of the most recent diagnostic developments, along with their clinical applications, advantages, and limitations.

Computed Tomographic Scanning

CT scanning occurs in a step-like process. The area is scanned in layers by x-ray beams that pass through the area and focus onto photographic film. This process is known as tomography. An x-ray tube is located around the area being scanned and rotates in a 180-degree arc. As the x-ray beams pass through the area, the radiation is either absorbed or transmitted onto an electronic detector. The density of the area determines whether the radiation is absorbed or transmitted, with bone absorbing the most, which will appear white on the scan, and air the least, which will appear black. Through a complex process, the radiation transmitted is converted to electric signals, which are digitized and stored in a computer. This information is reproduced as an image on a display monitor. The area can be scanned in various thicknesses, called slices, depending on the amount of detail desired.

CT scanning of the head is useful for detecting primary injuries, such as skull fractures, hematomas, and contusions; and such secondary injuries as herniation, edema, and shifting of brain tissue secondary to swelling; and abscesses and tumors.

The CT scan remains the initial procedure of choice in acute head injury because it is noninvasive, produces rapid results, is safe and painless, and has reduced the need for more invasive procedures, such as angiograms.

Magnetic Resonance Imaging

The MRI scanner is actually a large tube-shaped magnet that can create an extremely strong magnetic field. This magnetic field causes nuclei in the scanned area to line up in a uniform manner rather than spin in random directions, as is usual. Radiofrequency pulses are applied to various types of body tissue, causing body tissue nuclei to resonate. The nuclei emit energy signals, and by varying the radiofrequency pulses, different energy signals are produced. These signals are collected by a computer, which reproduces an image of the tissue scanned.

MRI is superior to CT scanning. As with CT scanning, MRI allows one to determine the anatomic location of a lesion. Additionally, MRI allows examination of the tissue itself, providing more anatomic detail than CT scanning. Therefore, detecting white matter shearing, infarction, and ischemic tissue is possible with the MRI. The MRI scan has the ability to detect pathologic processes at an earlier stage than is possible with the CT scan. Therefore, it is the procedure of choice for early diagnosis of cerebral infarction and brain tumors.

MRI carries limitations that the CT scan does not. The powerful magnetic field interferes with electrical devices. Thus, it is not an option for patients with pacemakers. Metal equipment cannot be introduced into the scanner because the magnetic field may dislodge the equipment. Patients with metal hip replacements, orthopedic pins, protheses, bullet fragments, and most ventilator equipment cannot be exposed to the MRI scanner. Obtaining an MRI takes longer than CT scanning, and MRI provides a poorer image of bone tissue. Therefore, CT scanning is the procedure of choice when time is a factor, as with the unstable trauma patient or in the detection of spinal fractures. Finally, the cost of MRI is 20 to 200 percent higher than a CT scan. The benefits of MRI must be weighed against the cost.

Positron Emission Tomography

PET is a technology used to study complex physiologic processes in different body systems and is useful in detecting biochemical and physiologic abnormalities. PET has the capacity of providing measurements of regional CBF, metabolism, and biochemistry. It may prove to be useful in the evaluation of cerebrovascular disorders because of the ability to measure changes in these variables.

The patient inhales or is injected with a biologically active radiolabeled compound. As these substances are metabolized they emit positrons, which are positively charged ions. These positrons emit gamma rays. The intensity of the gamma rays is measured by a computerized detector, which translates them to a tomographic image.

PET is used in clinical research for measurements of CBF and metabolism, protein synthesis, and drug kinetics. PET is impractical for clinical use because of the cost, the space required to house the unit, and the large staff required for its operation.

Transcranial Doppler

Transcranial Doppler (TCD) is a noninvasive tool for measuring blood velocity in branches of the circle of Willis, usually the middle cerebral artery. TCD is governed by the underlying principle that velocity depends on the pressure gradient between the two ends of a vessel, the radius of the vessel, and blood viscosity. Therefore, changes in velocity may reflect either changes in CBF or in the diameter of a vessel. Diameter and flow do not always change in concert, so interpretation must be cautious. Low velocity may reflect low flow or arterial dilation; high velocity may indicate high flow or vessel constriction. Hence, TCD may be used to differentiate hyperemia from vasospasm, or oligemia from failed autoregulation.

Evoked Potentials

Evoked potentials are recordings of the CNS response to visual, auditory, or somatosensory stimuli. Stimulation of the visual or auditory sensory organs or the peripheral nerves evokes an electrophysiologic response that is extracted from continuous EEG monitoring. Evoked potentials are used to detect lesions in the cerebral cortex or ascending pathways of the spinal cord, brain stem, and thalamus. This test is so sensitive that it can detect lesions that cannot be detected with other clinical or laboratory tests.

Visual evoked potentials (VEPs) are elicited by a flashing light or changing geometric pattern that stimulates the visual center in the occipital lobe. The delay, known as the degree of latency, correlates with disease severity. VEPs are used to diagnose multiple sclerosis, Parkinson's disease, and lesions of the optic nerve, optic tract visual center, and the eye.

Auditory evoked potentials are elicited by transmitting transient sounds such as clicking noises through earphones. They are useful in detecting lesions in the central auditory pathway of the brain stem, identifying lesions resulting in hearing disorders, and assisting in the diagnosis of acoustic tumors.

Somatosensory evoked potentials (SEPs) are elicited by the application of a peripheral stimulus. The response to this stimulus and the degree of latency is measured. SEPs are used in the evaluation of spinal cord injury, to monitor spinal cord function during surgery, and in the treatment of multiple sclerosis. SEPs also assist in evaluating the location and extent of brain dysfunction after a head injury.

Testing for evoked potentials does not require an alert cooperative patient and is not affected by anesthesia or sedation. Some literature suggests that evoked potentials may be useful in predicting coma outcome, although more research is needed.

Cerebral Angiography

Cerebral angiography involves injecting contrast material into arteries to visualize intra- and extracranial circulation. Results can help diagnosis AV malformations, vasospasm, and venous thrombosis. A major complication of the test is stroke caused by dislodging an atherosclerotic plaque.

Lumbar Puncture

A needle is placed into the subarachnoid space, usually at the L4–5 interspace. This allows removal of CSF for lab examination to reduce CSF pressure. Medications may also be administered by this route. This test is contraindicated in patients with increased ICP. Herniation of the brain stem, infection, and headache may be complications of the procedure.

Electroencephalography

Electroencephalography (EEG) allows recording of the electrical activity of the brain by recording electrodes being attached to the scalp. Abnormal voltage fluctuations indicate seizures or space-occupying lesions.

Electromyography (EMG)

Electrical activity from contracting muscle fibers is recorded by inserting needle electrodes into the muscle. Results help diagnose lower motor neuron disease or muscle disorders.

In summary, neuroscience technology is becoming more sophisticated. Not only do we now have the ability to determine the anatomic location of lesions, but with the advent of the CT scan, the MRI, and PET, we also are able to examine the tissues themselves and their metabolic and biochemical processes.

SECTION ELEVEN REVIEW

1. CT, rather than MRI, scanning would be the procedure of choice for detecting
   A. white matter shearing
   B. the early stages of brain tumors
   C. cerebral infarction
   D. spinal fractures
2. PET scanning is useful for detecting
   A. cellular metabolism
   B. spinal fractures
   C. skull fractures
   D. anatomic location of a brain tumor
3. Evoked potentials
   A. is an invasive procedure
   B. is useful for imaging cellular metabolism
   C. is used in clinical research only
   D. evaluates a sensory response to a stimulus
4. Which procedure could be useful in differentiating oligemia from arterial dilation?
   A. evoked potentials
   B. TCD
   C. PET scan
   D. auditory evoked potentials

Answers: 1. D, 2. A, 3. D, 4. B

SECTION TWELVE: Seizure Disorders

At the completion of this section, the learner will be able to relate seizure disorders as a sequela of head trauma and discuss the nursing and pharmacologic management of seizure disorders.

A seizure disorder, or epilepsy, has a variety of etiologies. Some individuals have a genetic predisposition to seizures. In others, seizures occur as the result of a pathologic process, such as infection, brain tumors, birth injuries, cerebral circulatory alterations, or head trauma. In this section, seizure disorders are discussed as a sequela of head trauma, known as *posttraumatic epilepsy*.

Epilepsy is considered a syndrome and is a result of CNS irritation, characterized by recurrent paroxysmal episodes in which there is a disturbance in skeletal motor function, sensation, autonomic visceral function, behavior, or consciousness. The dysfunction is produced by excessive and abnormal neuronal discharge.

Seizure activity may occur any time following a head injury. However, the onset of seizures appears to follow a definitive pattern. Seizure activity rarely appears before 2 months or later than 5 years after head trauma. The onset usually occurs between 6 months and 2 years posttrauma. As an acute care nurse, you probably will not witness seizure activity in the initial management stages of a head-injured patient. Therefore, teaching patients about the potential for seizures, symptoms, and management becomes a critical part of the nursing care and management of these patients.

Some seizure activity can be triggered by identifiable stimuli; others cannot. Precipitating factors include specific odors and noises, being startled, fatigue, hypoglycemia, emotional stress, lack of sleep, fever, alcohol consumption, constipation, menstruation, and hyperventilation. Teaching patients to avoid specific circumstances or to be aware of specific precipitating factors, if there are any, is one method of teaching patients to manage a seizure disorder.

In general, seizures are classified based on the clinical nature of the onset. There are four major categories: simple partial (focal), complex partial, generalized, and unclassified. An in-depth discussion of these categories is beyond the scope of this module.

Status Epilepticus

Status epilepticus is a neurologic emergency with potentially lethal consequences if untreated or if treatment is delayed. It is defined as a continuing series of seizures without a period of recovery or regaining of responsiveness between attacks. Status epilepticus may occur as a result of untreated or inadequately treated seizures and most commonly occurs from abrupt discontinuation of pharmacologic treatment. The continuous series of seizures can cause ischemic brain damage because of impaired respirations, producing systemic and cerebral anoxia. Therefore, immediate control of the seizures and maintaining a patent airway are critical interventions. For the patient with ICP problems, the implications are crucial. As discussed earlier, cerebral ischemia produces vasodilation, resulting in further increases in ICP. Controlling the seizure is urgent for these types of patients.

The drug of choice for status epilepticus is diazepam (Valium), given IV. Phenytoin (Dilantin) given IV also has been used as a drug for control of status epilepticus. After the seizure activity has been controlled, the patient may need to be intubated to ensure adequate oxygenation. At the least, a nasopharyngeal or oropharyngeal airway should be inserted to establish an airway. Frequent suctioning will maintain patency of the airway.

Pharmacologic Management

Anticonvulsant therapy reduces or controls seizure activity but does not cure a seizure disorder. Drug therapy is chosen based on the type of seizure and is introduced in gradually increasing doses until a therapeutic blood level is reached. Cessation of the drug is titrated in decreasing doses to prevent status epilepticus. Although many anticonvulsants currently are in use, either alone or in combination, some common drugs are phenytoin, phenobarbital (Luminal), and carbamazepine (Tegretol).

Nursing Management

The goals of nursing management of the patient with seizures are to protect the patient from injury, to control the seizure, and to provide patient/family teaching.

Any patient with the potential for seizure activity should be placed on seizure precautions. This includes padding the bedrails, keeping the bedrails up, placing suction equipment at the bedside, and keeping the bed in the lowest position.

Observation and documentation of the events surrounding the seizure are important to identify the type of seizure and the patient's response to the interventions and to select appropriate drug therapy. Level of consciousness immediately before, during, and after the seizure should be recorded. The time elapsed between the onset and cessation of seizure activity, the type of motor activity, and any complications, such as aspiration or apnea, should be noted also. The nurse has an important role in educating the patient and family in the management of seizure disorders. Teaching should include medication protocols, including side effects and adverse reactions, recognizing seizure activity, activity restrictions, and acute management.

In summary, seizure disorders are a common sequela of traumatic head injury. Acute management includes protection from injury, controlling the seizure, and patient/family teaching. Anticonvulsants are used for acute and long-term management.

SECTION TWELVE REVIEW

1. In teaching a patient recovering from a head injury, the nurse would include that the onset of a seizure most likely would occur
   A. within the first few weeks posttrauma
   B. within the first 6 months after head injury
   C. between 6 months and 2 years after head injury
   D. 3 to 5 years after head injury

2. An important nursing implication for patients experiencing seizure activity is
   A. the potential for aspiration
   B. restraining the patient until the seizure has abated
   C. the drug of choice for seizure control is mannitol
   D. checking the pupils for size, reactivity, and symmetry at 1-minute intervals until the seizure activity has stopped

Answers: 1. C, 2. A

SECTION THIRTEEN: Space-Occupying Lesions and SIADH

At the completion of this section, the learner will be able to describe the types of closed head injury (CHI). The complications of diabetes insipidus (DI) and syndrome of inappropriate antidiuretic hormone (SIADH) will also be addressed. Brain tumors will not specifically be discussed since the principles of management are the same as with other space-occupying lesions.

CHIs vary in their severity based on the site of injury and the forces applied to the skull. The least severe CHI is concussion.

Concussion

Concussion is a trauma-induced alteration in mental status that may or may not involve loss of consciousness (Kelly et al., 1991). It usually occurs from rotational forces applied to the head. The brain is shaken within the cranium. Symptoms may occur immediately, within the first hours following an event, or even weeks postevent. Initial symptoms are nausea, vomiting, headache, vertigo, inattentiveness, and problems with vision or speech. Later symptoms include fatigue, inability to concentrate, insomnia, and intolerance to bright lights or loud noises. Concussions are rated according to their severity. A more severe concussion involves posttraumatic amnesia and loss of consciousness. Neuroimaging studies (e.g., CT and/or MRI) should be performed in these cases (LeBlanc, 1999).

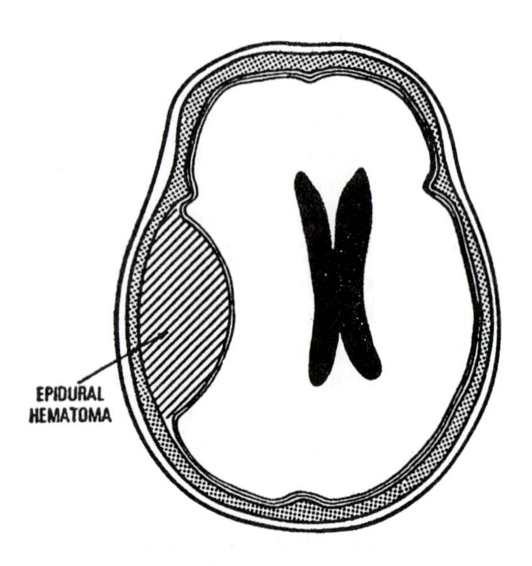

Figure 17–5. Epidural hematoma. *(From Marshall, S.B., Marshall, L.F., Vos, H.R., & Chestnut, R.M. [1990].* Neuroscience critical care. *Philadelphia: W.B. Saunders.)*

Epidural Hematoma

An epidural hematoma is a collection of blood in the space between the skull and the dura (outer meningeal layer) (Fig. 17–5). There is an associated skull fracture in the majority of cases. An artery or vein may be ruptured. In arterial bleeds, the hematoma increases rapidly in size and requires prompt surgical repair before ICP increases to the degree to produce herniation. Usually, the patient is lucid at the time of event but then experiences a decreased level of consciousness (LOC). The pupil may be fixed and dilated on the side of the lesion.

Subdural Hematoma

Subdural hematomas are due to nonarterial bleeding. The blood is accumulated between the dura and the arachnoid meningeal layer (Fig. 17–6). They may be acute (associated with major trauma, symptoms occur within 48 hours of event), subacute (associated with less severe contusions, symptoms occur from 2 days to 2 weeks postevent), and chronic (symptoms occur from 2 weeks to several months postevent). Eventually a change in LOC occurs. The patient may complain of a headache with slow onset and gradual increase in intensity. Eventually seizures may occur.

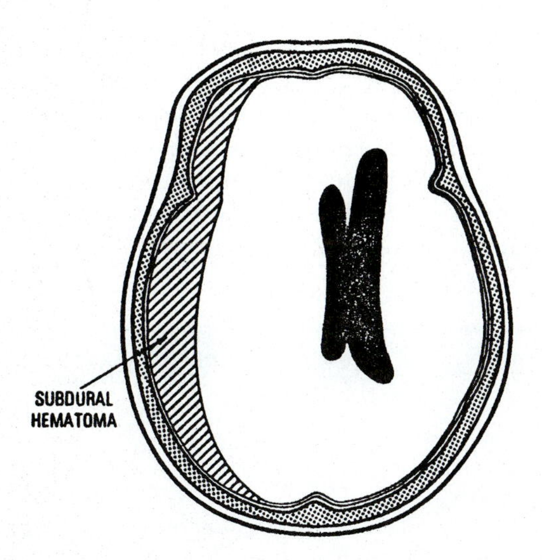

Figure 17–6. Subdural hematoma. (*From Marshall, S.B., Marshall, L.F., Vos, H.R., & Chestnut, R.M. [1990].* Neuroscience critical care. *Philadelphia: W.B. Saunders.)*

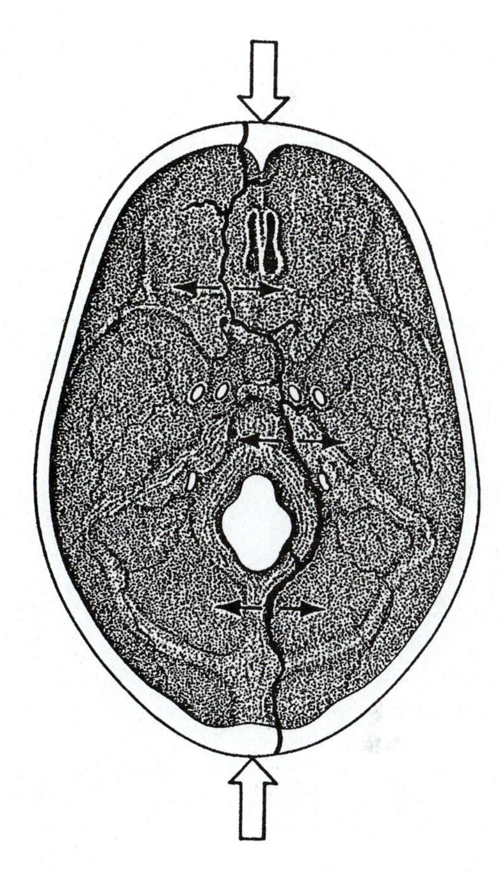

Figure 17–7. Fracture mechanism at base of skull. Bone is more resistant to compression than to tension. Impact forces compress outer skull and generate tension along fragile bones at base of skull. These tension forces result in linear fractures that may extend across entire skull base. (*Note: Open arrows,* compressive forces; *solid arrows,* tension.) (*Redrawn from Lingren, S. [1986]. Head injuries: Biomechanical principles,* Acta Neurochirurgica, Supplementum 36:*29.)*

Intracerebral Hemorrhage

An intercerebral hemorrhage is a large hemorrhage into brain tissue from severe trauma (such as a crush injury) that creates a mass lesion. It may occur anywhere in the brain. Thus, symptoms vary by location and size. There may be total loss of consciousness with decerebrate or decorticate posturing. In less severe cases, symptoms may be focal or unilateral in nature with sensory and motor deficits. Large, accessible hematomas are evacuated surgically.

Basilar Skull Fractures

A basilar skull fracture results from tension being placed on the fragile bones at the base of the skull. It is a linear fracture (Fig. 17–7). These fractures damage the dura, allowing CSF leakage, and can extend and damage the sinuses and cranial nerves. If the brain stem is lacerated or contused, immediate death can occur. The patient may have CSF leakage from the ear **(otorrhea).** Bleeding may occur behind the tympanic membrane *(hemotympanum)*, into the mastoid air cells **(Battle's sign),** or into the periorbital tissue **(raccoon's eyes).** Nursing care focuses on prevention of infection and increased ICP. CSF is allowed to flow freely and the patient is instructed not to blow his/her nose. Usually the leak will resolve in 2 to 10 days and no further treatment is necessary. Careful assessment of the cranial nerves is indicated.

Complications of CHI

Section Fourteen of this module will focus on prevention of increased ICP as a separate complication. Only DI and SIADH will be discussed in this section.

Central Diabetes Insipidus

Central DI (as compared with nephrogenic DI) usually occurs with damage to the hypothalamus or pituitary gland. It is a problem with production or release of ADH. Massive water loss occurs, increasing serum sodium and osmolality. Polyuria can be extreme with up to 15 L/day. The patient becomes hypovolemic and dehydrated. If alert, the patient will want to drink fluids. Treatment in the acute phase focuses on replacement of ADH, so vasopressin is administered.

SIADH

This condition results from too much ADH being produced or secreted. SIADH can occur from many causes, most frequently malignancies, CHI, and stroke. There is damage to the pituitary gland or hypothalamus, which causes failure of the feedback loop that regulates ADH. In contrast to DI, the patient retains water and serum sodium and osmolality decrease. The urine becomes concentrated. A change in LOC occurs due to electrolyte abnormalities. SIADH is treated by restricting water intake and administering 5% NaCl IV to correct hyponatremia (Heater, 1999). Furosemide (Lasix) may be administered to promote diuresis. Demeclocycline (Declomycin) and fludrocortisone (Florinef) may also be used to reduce renal response to ADH (Heater, 1999).

In summary, CHI varies in severity based on the forces applied and the tissues damaged. Arterial bleeding is more severe than venous bleeding. Sequelae from CHI can be non–life threatening, such as insomnia and difficulty concentrating as seen in concussion, to life threatening as in DI and SIADH resulting from cerebral-related hematomas or hemorrhage.

SECTION THIRTEEN REVIEW

1. The nurse should be MOST concerned about possible neurologic deterioration in a patient who is diagnosed with
   A. epidural hematoma
   B. subdural hematoma
   C. basilar skull fracture
   D. concussion
2. A patient has an intracerebral hemorrhage. Her urine osmolality is high. Her serum osmolality is low. All of the following should be assessed as a priority EXCEPT
   A. presence of edema
   B. LOC
   C. urine output
   D. glucose levels
3. A patient has raccoon's eyes and otorrhea. The nurse should assess
   A. gait
   B. urine output
   C. vision
   D. cranial nerves

Answers: 1. A, 2. D, 3. D

SECTION FOURTEEN: Nursing Interventions and Pharmacologic Therapies

At the completion of this section, the learner will be able to identify nursing interventions and pharmacologic therapies for patients with alterations in LOC.

Alterations in level of consciousness occur as impaired arousal or content. In general, impaired arousal is secondary to coma or a comalike state, such as occurs with increased ICP, fluid and electrolyte imbalances, fever, acidosis, hepatic coma, postsurgical delirium, and metabolic coma secondary to drug overdose. Impaired content generally is secondary to psychiatric illnesses and drug or alcohol abuse. The number one nursing intervention is to treat the primary problem.

Nursing interventions for patients with impaired arousal center around maintaining ventilation, controlling cerebral perfusion pressure (CPP), and instituting protective mechanisms and pharmacologic therapies. For impaired content, nursing interventions center around protecting the patient from injury.

Optimizing Cerebral Perfusion Pressure

Because CPP controls CBF and cerebral blood volume, efforts to optimize CPP are of primary importance and include blood pressure control, temperature control, and promoting venous return.

Optimally, the goal of blood pressure management is to keep it within normal limits so that CPP is between 60 mm Hg and 100 mm Hg. Pressures above or below this range will result in loss of autoregulation and inadequate CPP. Besides pharmacologic therapy to increase or decrease blood pressure, interventions include reducing noxious stimuli and volume replacement.

Temperature control is important because hyperthermia raises cerebral metabolism. The use of antipyretics and cooling blankets helps keep body temperature controlled. Therapeutic cooling may be initiated by means of a fluid-filled cooling blanket, air cooling device, ice water lavage, or a combination of methods. A target temperature of 34 to 35°C is the immediate goal while the ultimate goal is decreased ICP (Signorini & Alderson, 1999).

Promoting venous return is an area in which nursing has a large impact through body positioning and moving. Unless the patient has a cervical spine injury, the head of the bed should be elevated to at least 30 degrees. This position avoids jugular compression, promotes venous drainage, and decreases, or at least controls, ICP. However, recently this practice has been questioned. Others state that the patient should remain flat to avoid rebound edema from a decreased circulating cerebral blood volume (Simmons, 1997). Avoid neck flexion, lateral head rotation, and hip flexion of > 90 degrees. This positioning prevents increasing intra-abdominal or intrathoracic pressure, which can interfere with venous outflow and drainage. The body should be turned as a unit, with head, neck, trunk, and lower extremities turned in unison. This avoids head and neck rotation. Patients who are alert should be assisted in moving up in bed. Asking patients to help by pushing with their legs initiates Valsalva's maneuver, which increases intrathoracic pressure and impedes venous return.

Optimizing Cerebral Oxygenation

Cerebral blood flow is an important variable to monitor when addressing cerebral oxygenation, but more importantly, one must determine that CBF matches cerebral metabolism. This can be determined by calculating $AVDO_2$. By measuring $AVDO_2$, CBF patterns can be determined and interventions specific to the blood flow alteration can be implemented.

Maintaining Ventilation

Patients with a decreased level of arousal may be unable to maintain their own airway because of diminished protective reflexes, such as coughing, or may be unable to maintain an adequate respiratory pattern. Because hypoxia and hypercapnia can be better controlled with mechanical ventilation, patients may be intubated. Ventilatory rates may be set as high as 20 to blow off excess carbon dioxide and prevent cerebral vessels from vasodilating. The airway is kept patent by suctioning. Intubated patients are hyperventilated before and after suctioning with 100 percent oxygen for 60 seconds, and each suctioning pass is limited to 15 seconds (Parsons & Shogan, 1984). Keeping the patient pulled up in bed facilitates respiration, aids in keeping the patient oxygenated, and avoids carbon dioxide buildup.

Hyperventilation

Hyperventilation has been used to produce vasoconstriction of cerebral blood vessels. A second goal of hyperventilation is to produce systemic alkalosis to buffer cerebral acidosis.

Since it constricts cerebral blood vessels and thereby decreases CBF, hyperventilation is a treatment modality for hyperemia. Because it is possible to monitor $SjVO_2$ and $AVDO_2$, the practitioner is able to monitor the effects of hyperventilation on CBF and can titrate PCO_2 to cerebral metabolic needs. Oligemia, because it is a low-flow state, will be exacerbated by hyperventilation because this method will further decrease CBF. In this instance, to increase cerebral oxygenation, treatment modalities may include increasing PCO_2 to increase CBF. Because this may result in a concomitant increase in ICP, this treatment modality may be combined with osmotic diuretics, blood pressure elevation, volume expansion, or changing the position of the head of the bed.

In the face of failed autoregulation, the cerebral vasculature passively dilates, increasing the blood volume compartment in the cranial vault. The metabolic state of hypercapnia results in dilated cerebral blood vessels as well. Failed autoregulation and hypercapnia upset the delicate balance underlying the Monro–Kellie hypothesis. Therapeutic hyperventilation attempts to blow off excess carbon dioxide, thereby producing vasoconstriction, and acts as a buffer for cerebral acidosis.

In the past, ventilatory rates were set as high as 22/min to obtain a $PaCO_2$ as low as 23 mm Hg. Current literature suggests that a $PaCO_2$ of 27 to 33 mm Hg is sufficient to decrease cerebral blood volume effectively. Hyperventilating a patient to a $PaCO_2$ of < 27 mm Hg, while resulting in vasoconstriction, may induce or potentiate cerebral ischemia. The effectiveness of hyperventilation decreases over time and may result in a significant rebound effect with restoration of normocapnia, and may potentiate increased ICP. A predetermined $PaCO_2$ should never be used as the end point with hyperventilation. Variables such as ICP and CPP should be monitored to evaluate for ischemia and the effect of hyperventilation on ICP.

Pharmacologic Therapy

Drug therapy will be initiated for most patients with increased ICP. The goal is to decrease intracranial volume, either by decreasing brain volume, decreasing CSF production, or decreasing the metabolic rate. Drug therapy is classified into osmotic diuretics, sedatives and paralytics, alkalinizing agents, and barbiturates.

Osmotic Diuretics

Osmotic agents reduce brain volume by reducing extracellular fluid volume, and reduce cerebral blood volume by reducing blood viscosity. Mannitol, the osmotic diuretic of choice, removes water from both normal and edematous brain tissue. Mannitol is given as a bolus in doses ranging from 0.25 to 1.0 g/kg. Furosemide, a loop diuretic, is often given in conjunction with mannitol and is thought to have a synergistic effect. However, it is less reliable than mannitol in reducing ICP and will exacerbate the dehydrating effects of mannitol, possibly resulting in hypotension and hypokalemia.

Sedatives and Paralytics

Pain and agitation increase the metabolic rate, resulting in increased ICP. Therefore, controlling pain and agitation are important nursing interventions. Although the use of sedatives and paralytics obscure the neurologic evaluation, the control of ICP outweighs the loss of the neurologic evaluation. Chemical paralysis should never be used without the addition of a sedative. Agents such as pancuronium bromide or vecuronium have no analgesic or sedating effect. Used alone, these agents will not blunt noxious stimuli that may cause agitation and certainly will not block pain sensations. Paralytic agents are short acting and the sedative of choice should be short acting as well, to allow the nurse to assess periodically the neurologic status.

Barbiturates

Barbiturates are not a first-line therapy and generally are used to treat uncontrollable ICP in severe head injury that is not responsive to more conventional therapies. Barbiturates work by decreasing the metabolic rate, thereby reducing CBF and possibly reducing cerebral edema. Barbiturate coma decreases cerebral energy metabolism and blood flow to about 50 percent of normal (Schalen, Messeter, & Nordstrom, 1992). The aims of barbiturate therapy are to reduce cerebral energy metabolism and blood flow and increase intracellular pH, thereby promoting an alkalotic rather than acidic environment. This type of drug therapy produces a drug-induced coma, which makes the neurologic evaluation difficult and unreliable.

Barbiturates also depress cardiac function, which decreases cardiac output and blood pressure. It is essential that fluid status and blood pressure be monitored with the use of a pulmonary artery catheter to ensure normovolemia. Before inducing barbiturate therapy, patient preparation includes:

1. Intubation and mechanical ventilation
2. Placement of an arterial catheter for continuous blood pressure monitoring
3. Placement of a pulmonary artery catheter
4. Continuous heart monitoring

Reported complications associated with barbiturate therapy include pneumonia, urinary tract infection, line sepsis, sinusitis, hypotension, hypovolemia, sepsis, myocardial depression, hypokalemia, and hepatic and renal dysfunction.

Intracranial Pressure Monitoring

Intracranial pressure monitoring provides continuous data regarding the pressure exerted within the cranial vault. Since the 1960s, when direct cannulization of the ventricles was described, technologic advances have provided us with many different monitoring systems and techniques.

Data derived from ICP monitoring includes the ICP, CPP, and cerebral response to interventions or stimuli. Continuous monitoring of ICP also enables the clinician to identify impending brain herniation secondary to escalating ICP, determine the need for and impact of therapies, and predict outcome.

Patient selection is an important decision for the physician, as not all brain injuries require or are appropriate for ICP monitoring. Although the decision is individually based, there are a few generally accepted criteria for ICP monitoring:

- Glasgow Coma Scale score of ≤ 8
- Patients in whom neurologic assessment is unattainable, such as neurologic blockade or barbiturate therapy

Monitoring Types

ICP monitoring is classified by the anatomic placement of the device and the type of system (Figs. 17–8 and 17–9). Sites for anatomic placement will be discussed first (Table 17–2), followed by system types.

Intraventricular monitoring remains the gold standard against which all other monitoring types are compared. It is used for both diagnostic and therapeutic purposes. This type of monitoring involves placing an intraventricular catheter (IVC) into the anterior horn of the lateral ventricle, preferably in the nondominant hemisphere. The IVC is then connected to a monitoring system that converts impulses from the CSF into a waveform, which is displayed on a monitor. Diagnostically, it is the most reliable of the monitoring devices and provides the most precise and consistent waveform. Therapeutically, CSF can be drained from the intraventricular cavity, thereby decreasing the CSF compartment and reducing ICP. Drainage of CSF can be continuous or intermittent. Continuous drainage is an open system whereby CSF automatically drains when the ICP exceeds a certain point. This point is determined by how high or low the drainage bag is placed above the foramen of Munro, which is the anatomic landmark for the lateral ventricle. Usually, this landmark is at the top of the outer ear. Intermittent drainage is a closed system that is

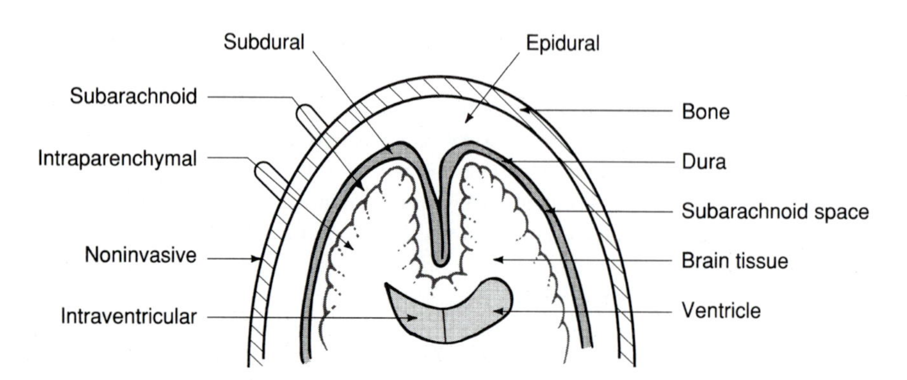

Figure 17–8. Location of intracranial pressure monitors.

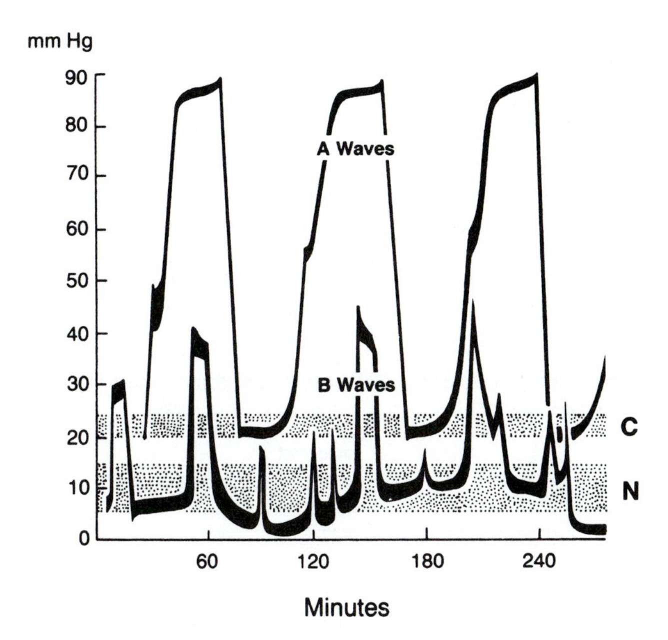

Figure 17–9. Intracranial pressure waveforms. Waveforms reflect pressure in mm Hg and time in minutes. Two abnormal waveforms are depicted, including A waves and B waves. A waves reflect intracranial pressure in the range of 50 to 100 mm Hg. They have a duration of 5 to 20 minutes or longer. Their waveforms have a distinctive plateau, and they are referred to as plateau waves. B waves occur as sharp, peaked (sawtooth pattern), rhythmic oscillations, which may reach a peak pressure of 50 mm Hg. They have a duration of ½ to 2 minutes. N, normal intracranial pressure waveforms, reflecting a pressure within the range of 0 to 15 mm Hg. C, pressure waveform for C waves. C waves usually are rapid, rhythmic waves with a amplitude of about 20 mm Hg. They occur every 4 to 8 minutes. (*From Dolan, J. [1991].* Critical care nursing: Clinical management through the nursing process. *Philadelphia: F.A. Davis.*)

opened for periodic drainage when the ICP exceeds a certain point, to be stipulated by the physician, but usually in the range of 15 to 20 mm Hg.

The IVC has several advantages. Because it is placed directly into the ventricle, it provides direct measurement of ICP and allows for drainage of CSF. However, the IVC is not risk free. It is the most invasive of the monitoring types and therefore carries the risk of infection. Because it is introduced directly into brain tissue, the risk of bleeding and destruction of neurons are factors that must be considered. Contraindications for placement of an IVC include patients with coagulopathies, small or collapsed ventricles, or severe generalized cerebral edema.

An alternative to the IVC is the subarachnoid bolt or screw. This type of monitoring device is used in patients whose ventricles are too small or have collapsed or shifted. The device is placed into the subdural or subarachnoid space and provides some of the same monitoring capabilities as the IVC, such as measurement of ICP and evaluation of waveforms, although the waveform easily becomes dampened due to bits of bone and brain tissue obstructing the tip of the bolt. Unlike the IVC, drainage of CSF is not possible because the ventricle is not cannulated.

Intraparenchymal monitoring devices are placed directly into the brain tissue via a bolt device, usually 1 cm below the subarachnoid space. These devices are easy to place, provide sharp and distinct waveforms, transmit accurate measurement of ICP, and carry a lower risk of infection. For these reasons, they are a desirable alternative to subarachnoid monitors. However, they are more costly, require a separate monitoring system, and do not have CSF drainage capabilities.

Types of Systems

Two systems used for ICP monitoring are fluid-filled and non–fluid-filled (Table 17–3). The fluid-filled system is the oldest and has been used exclusively in the past for all types of monitoring purposes—cardiac, pulmonary, and hemodynamic. Zero referencing and calibration of the system is done externally, similar to hemodynamic monitoring. However, the use of a fluid-filled system in ICP monitoring does not utilize the flush mechanism. The 3 mL/hr of fluid that is dispensed to maintain system patency would never be tolerated by the confining nature of the cranial vault and the Monro–Kellie hypothesis. This type of system is used with a subarachnoid or intraventricular device.

TABLE 17–2. COMPARISON OF ICP MONITORING SITES

SITE	ADVANTAGES	DISADVANTAGES
Intraventricular	"Gold standard" Allows for therapeutic intervention by drainage of CSF Direct measurement of CSF pressure	Most invasive—carries the highest risk for infection and bleeding Contraindicated with coagulopathies, ventricles that are small, collapsed, or misshaped Requires constant supervision
Subarachnoid	Less invasive than IVC Placement easier than IVC Lower risk of infection than with IVC Useful if ventricles cannot be cannulated Ability to sample CSF	Unable to drain CSF May become obstructed with bone or brain tissue Not as accurate or stable over time as IVC Risk of infection
Intraparenchymal	Easy placement Lower risk of infection Transmits accurate and precise waveforms	Unable to drain CSF Requires separate monitoring system

TABLE 17–3. COMPARISON OF ICP MONITORING SYSTEMS

	FLUID-FILLED	FIBER-OPTIC	NON–FLUID-FILLED PRESSURE SENSOR
Placement site	Intraventricular, subarachnoid	Intraventricular, subarachnoid, intraparenchymal	Intraventricular, subarachnoid, intraparenchymal
CSF drainage	Possible with intraventricular placement	Possible with intraventricular placement	Possible with intraventricular placement
Risk of infection	Highest	Lower than fluid-filled	Lower than fluid-filled
Waveform monitoring	Interfaces with patient monitor Prone to mechanical problems that may dampen or distort waveform	Requires dedicated monitor	Interfaces with patient monitor or may use a separate monitor
Zero referencing	Repeated zero referencing required with patient position changes	Zero referencing done at time of insertion and cannot be rechecked	Zero referencing done at time of insertion and cannot be rechecked
Transducer calibration	Required before insertion Able to recheck after insertion Transducer is external	Factory set Unable to recheck once inserted Transducer is internal	Factory set Unable to recheck once inserted Transducer is internal

Non–fluid-filled systems measure ICP by utilizing a pressure-sensitive diaphragm or fiber-optic device. With both of these non–fluid-filled systems, the transducer is internal and precalibrated. Zero referencing is done before insertion. For these systems, a major concern has been the accuracy and stability of ICP readings secondary to drift and the fragility of devices with fiber-optic cables. In addition, the fiber-optic devices require separate monitors, so there is a concern related to cost. Advantages with non–fluid-filled systems are a lower risk of infection, ease of insertion, and the lack of dampening or loss of waveform issues that frequently are problems with fluid-filled systems.

Studies comparing the fiber-optic system with the gold standard IVC demonstrate variable results. Some studies demonstrate a high correlation of ICP measurement with minimal drift. Other studies demonstrate ICP as measured by the fiber-optic system to exceed ICP as measured by the IVC by a mean difference of 9.2 mm Hg (Schickner & Young, 1992).

Non–fluid-filled systems are able to monitor pressures in the ventricular, subarachnoid, or intraparenchymal spaces. Drainage of CSF is possible with ventricular placement only.

Nursing Care

The focus of nursing care of the patient with an ICP monitoring device is on prevention of complications and maintenance of system integrity. Complications include those related to insertion, such as hemorrhage or hematoma formation; overdrainage of CSF; and infection, particularly with the IVC device.

Patients with coagulopathies are at higher risk for hemorrhage or hematoma formation. Because a hemorrhage or hematoma is a space-occupying lesion, the patient's neurologic status must be carefully monitored before, during, and after insertion of the ICP monitoring device to detect neurologic deterioration. If an intraventricular device is inserted, the color of the CSF must be carefully observed. Pink-tinged or bloody CSF is an indication that bleeding has occurred.

Overdrainage of CSF is a major complication of an intraventricular device, particularly an open system. Nursing prevention includes observing unit standards for CSF drainage; accurately measuring and positioning the CSF drainage bag using the correct landmarks; and securely fastening the drainage bag at the level determined by the physician. Systems that are closed and periodically opened for therapeutic drainage require nursing interventions that are sound and clinically based. For this type of system, drainage is instituted when the ICP is consistently elevated, usually > 15 mm Hg. The key word is consistent, rather than transient. Many things can result in transient ICP elevations, such as environmental stimuli, patient positioning, or nursing care activities. Once these stimuli are eliminated, the ICP may decrease to an acceptable level. If the ICP remains elevated for several minutes, the appropriate nursing action would be to institute CSF drainage.

There are three waveforms seen in ICP monitoring. C waves (16 to 20 mm Hg) fluctuate with blood pressure and respirations. They are not clinically significant. B waves are usually considered as warning waves that ICP may be increasing. They are between 20 and 50 mm Hg. A waves are waves between 50 and 100 mm Hg. They indicate increased ICP and the need for treatment (Fig. 17–8). Sustained pressures > 20 mm Hg are associated with poor outcome (Stewert-Amidei, 1998).

The risk of infection is the greatest concern. Factors associated with infection are duration of ICP monitoring and type of device and system used. Sterile technique must be absolutely observed during insertion of the ICP monitoring device. For fluid-filled systems, system integrity must be maintained. All connection points should be checked to ensure that they are tightly connected. Because fluid-filled systems require routine zero referencing and calibration, the risk of introducing pathogens into the system is increased. Care must be taken to rezero and recalibrate as aseptically as possible. The insertion site is inspected for signs of infection according to unit standards. The appearance of the insertion site and duration (in days) of the monitoring device placement is documented.

Troubleshooting and Maintenance of System Integrity

One of the most important nursing interventions is to gather, document, and report data that are accurate. Medical and nursing interventions are based on reported data. Instituting interventions for data that are inaccurate can negatively impact patient outcome. It is the nurse's responsibility to ensure that ICP monitoring systems are intact and that generated data are accurate (Table 17–4). Fluid-filled systems are the most prone to developing mechanical problems. The most common problem is a dampened, absent, or distorted waveform. Any interference, such as air bubbles within the system, kinked tubing, loose connections, or catheter occlusion from blood, brain, or bone tissue, can result in a dampened waveform and inaccurate ICP readings. Technical malfunction within the external system may also result in inaccurate data.

With a non–fluid-filled system, the transducer is internal and the need for a fluid-filled system to carry pressure waves to an external transducer is eliminated. However, the fiber-optic cables are delicate and can easily be broken. If this occurs, the device must be removed and a new device inserted. Additionally, with the non–fluid-filled systems, the internal transducer cannot be recalibrated. If significant drift is suspected and the data are suspect, the device must be replaced.

Providing a Safe and Protective Environment

The following nursing interventions are for patients with impaired content and are directed at protecting the patient from injury, reorienting, and creating a calm, safe environment. Patients with cognitive deficits become confused easily from external stimuli. Noise should be kept to a minimum, information should be presented simply and calmly, and the number of visitors at one time should be limited. Keeping a dim light on at night and frequent checking by the nurse will help to control confusion secondary to misperception of stimuli.

Patients with cognitive deficits often attempt to get out of bed and may pull out IV lines and catheters. Interventions such as keeping the bed in a low position, using siderails, and frequent checks will help keep the patient safe from harm. Frequent reorienting by the nurse will help decrease confusion and disorientation.

Trying to pick up clues that may point to the etiologies of deficits in level of consciousness is not an easy task, especially if the cause is unrelated to increased ICP. Identifying focal injuries, such as brain tumors or hematomas, as contributing factors of altered consciousness is a more straightforward process than identifying extracranial causes.

In summary, this section has discussed nursing interventions for patients with impaired arousal and content and has listed some of the pharmacologic therapies for patients with increased ICP.

In addition, ICP monitoring has been discussed. Intracranial pressure monitoring is an extremely useful adjunct in the care of the unresponsive patient but requires high-acuity, diligent nursing care. Various ICP monitoring devices and systems are available. The clinician must be familiar with the advantages and disadvantages specific to each device and system and should be aware of the potential complications associated with ICP monitoring. The nurse should have a working knowledge of each system and be able to recognize system inaccuracies.

TABLE 17—4. TROUBLESHOOTING SYSTEM INTEGRITY WITH ICP MONITORS

PROBLEM	POTENTIAL SOURCE	ACTION
Dampened, absent, or distorted waveform	Catheter occlusion by blood, brain, or bone tissue	Systematically assess for problems
	Air bubbles in system	Remove air from system
	Loose connections	Tighten all connections
	Recalibration and zero referencing needed	Recalibrate and zero
	Kinked catheter or tubing	Examine tubing for kinks
	Technical problem with transducer/pressure module	Replace transducer or pressure module
	Fiber-optic cables broken	Replace fiber-optic device
	Dislodgement of catheter	Replace monitoring device
ICP values suspect	Recalibration and zero referencing needed	Recalibrate and zero if fluid-filled system, replace device if fiber-optic
	Incorrect placement of catheter or transducer	Verify correct placement of external transducer
	Technical malfunction of system	
Leakage of fluid from tubing	Loosened connections	Tighten all connections

SECTION FOURTEEN REVIEW

1. Mannitol acts to decrease ICP primarily by
   A. decreasing CSF production
   B. preventing fluid absorption by cerebral cells
   C. reducing the amount of brain volume
   D. decreasing the blood–brain barrier
2. Which nursing intervention would be appropriate for a patient with intracranial hypertension?
   A. manual hyperventilation
   B. increasing the frequency of suctioning
   C. encouraging coughing and deep-breathing exercises
   D. keeping the head of the bed flat
3. Nursing interventions for patients with impaired content center around
   A. protection from injury
   B. maintaining the airway
   C. control of cerebral perfusion pressure
   D. drug therapy
4. One of the first pharmacologic agents that will be used for control of ICP likely will be
   A. steroids
   B. vasodilators
   C. barbiturates
   D. osmotic diuretics
5. A treatment modality for oligemia might be
   A. hyperventilation
   B. promoting a state of hypercarbia
   C. barbiturate therapy
   D. fluid restriction
6. Your patient's ICP reading per IVC is 22 mm Hg for over 5 minutes. Your first action would be to
   A. recalibrate and zero the internal transducer
   B. immediately drain CSF until the desired ICP is obtained
   C. notify the physician immediately
   D. eliminate all stimuli and reposition the patient

Answers: 1. C, 2. A, 3. A, 4. D, 5. B, 6. D

POSTTEST

1. The principle that explains reciprocal mechanisms involved in increased ICP is
   A. Monro–Kellie hypothesis
   B. cerebral perfusion formula
   C. autoregulation
   D. chemical regulation
2. As a compensatory mechanism, pressure regulation acts by constricting cerebral blood vessels in response to
   A. elevated blood levels of oxygen
   B. decreased blood levels of oxygen
   C. elevated systemic blood pressure
   D. decreased systemic blood pressure
3. Your patient's MAP is 100 mm Hg and ICP is 10 mm Hg. What is the CPP?
   A. 80 mm Hg
   B. 90 mm Hg
   C. 110 mm Hg
   D. 120 mm Hg
4. Elastance refers to the
   A. blood vessels' ability to accommodate increased volume
   B. measure of slackness in the brain
   C. ability of blood vessels to dilate and constrict
   D. amount of volume reserve in the intracranial vault
5. Aerobic metabolism is more efficient than anaerobic metabolism because the end product is
   A. lactate
   B. 38 molecules of ATP
   C. 2 molecules of ATP
   D. carbon dioxide
6. Jugular venous oxygen saturation
   A. indirectly measures ICP
   B. monitors saturation of cerebral arterial blood entering the brain
   C. monitors saturation of cerebral venous blood exiting the brain
   D. can be determined only in patients in a barbiturate coma
7. Arteriovenous difference in oxygen content can provide information about the
   A. extent of systemic hypertension
   B. volume status
   C. presence of intracranial hypertension
   D. relationship between cerebral oxygen supply and demand

8. Hypoxemia and hypercapnia cause
   A. cerebral vasodilation
   B. decreased ICP
   C. cerebral vasoconstriction
   D. decreased CBF
9. Keeping the head and neck in alignment results in
   A. decreased venous outflow
   B. increased venous outflow
   C. increased intrathoracic pressure
   D. increased intra-abdominal pressure
10. Conditions that impair content or the cerebral hemispheres
    A. usually result in cognitive deficits such as memory or attentional deficits
    B. result in immediate coma
    C. result from destruction of the RAS
    D. always occur in combination with impairments in arousal
11. The component of arousal is assessed by
    A. evaluating the patient's behavior
    B. evaluating the patient's ability to follow commands
    C. evaluating the type and amount of stimulus required to elicit a response
    D. asking the patient orientation questions
12. The earliest indicator of deteriorating neurologic status is
    A. level of consciousness
    B. motor response
    C. pupillary response
    D. vital signs
13. Your neurologic assessment reveals the following: verbal response is disorganized words and incomplete sentences, eyes open to verbal stimuli, patient pulls her hand away when nailbed pressure is applied to the same hand. What is this patient's GCS?
    A. 10
    B. 9
    C. 12
    D. 13
14. Hyperventilating a patient results in
    A. increased CBF
    B. decreased cerebral blood volume
    C. increased elastance
    D. increased compliance
15. Which of the following may increase ICP?
    A. Valsalva's maneuver
    B. raising the head of the bed
    C. manual hyperventilation
    D. use of osmotic diuretics
16. Barbiturate therapy for treatment of intracranial hypertension works by
    A. paralyzing the skeletal muscles
    B. acting as a diuretic
    C. decreasing the metabolic rate
    D. sedation, thereby promoting a calm response to environmental stimuli
17. An advantage of a fiber-optic ICP monitoring system is that
    A. fiber-optic cables are fragile
    B. the transducer is external
    C. the system is fluid-filled
    D. the risk for infection is lower
18. The gold standard for monitoring ICP is
    A. a subarachnoid device
    B. an intraparenchymal device
    C. noninvasive devices
    D. an intraventricular device
19. Before inducing a barbiturate coma, patient preparation should include
    A. continuous oxygen via nasal cannula or face mask
    B. noninvasive blood pressure monitoring
    C. placement of at least one large-bore peripheral IV line
    D. continuous monitoring of volume status via a pulmonary artery catheter
20. A critical nursing intervention for a patient with status epilepticus is
    A. protecting the airway
    B. padding the bedrails
    C. restraining the patient
    D. providing for privacy
21. MRI scanning, rather than CT scanning, is the procedure of choice for detecting
    A. white matter shearing
    B. hematomas
    C. bullet fragments
    D. spinal fractures
22. The internal carotid arterial system supplies the entire
    A. frontal lobes
    B. occipital lobes
    C. brain stem
    D. cerebellum
23. Mrs. O'Toole's blood pressure is 160/100 mm Hg and her ICP is 25 mm Hg. What is her cerebral perfusion pressure?
    A. 100 mm Hg
    B. 95 mm Hg
    C. 75 mm Hg
    D. 50 mm Hg
24. A patient is exhibiting a change in LOC and motor function 2 weeks after a fall injury. If the symptom is due to a CHI, the most likely CHI that would produce these symptoms 2 weeks later is
    A. epidural hematoma
    B. basilar skull fracture
    C. subdural hematoma
    D. intercerebral hemorrhage

POSTTEST ANSWERS

Question	Answer	Section	Question	Answer	Section
1	A	Three	13	A	Ten
2	C	Four	14	B	Fourteen
3	B	Two	15	A	Fourteen
4	D	Four	16	C	Fourteen
5	B	Two	17	D	Fourteen
6	C	Five	18	D	Fourteen
7	D	Five	19	D	Fourteen
8	A	Fourteen	20	A	Twelve
9	B	Fourteen	21	A	Ten
10	A	Eight	22	A	Two
11	C	One	23	B	Two
12	A	Eight	24	C	Thirteen

REFERENCES

Bouma, G.J., & Muizelaar, H. (1992). Cerebral circulation and metabolism after severe traumatic brain injury: The elusive role of ischemia. *J Neuros 75*:685–693.

Burt, A.M. (1993). *Textbook of neuroanatomy*. Philadelphia: Saunders.

Davis, A., & Briones, T. (1998). Neurological clinical physiology: Intracranial disorders. In M.R. Kinney et al. (eds). *AACN's clinical reference for critical care nursing* (4th ed.) (pp. 637–709). St. Louis: C.V. Mosby.

Heater, D.W. (1999). If ADH goes out of balance: SIADH. *RN 62*(7):47–49.

Hickey, J. (1996). *The clinical practice of neurologic and neurosurgical nursing* (4th ed.). Philadelphia: J.B. Lippincott.

Kelly, J.P. et al. (1991). Concussion in sports: Guidelines for the prevention of catastrophic outcome. *JAMA 266*:2867–2869.

LeBlanc, K.E. (1999). Concussion in sport: Diagnosis, management, return to competition. *COMP Ther 25*(1):39–44.

McNair, N. (1999). Traumatic brain injury. *Nurs Clin North Am 34*(3):637–659.

Parsons, L.C., & Shogan, J.S.O. (1984). The effects of the endotracheal tube suctioning/manual hyperventilation procedure on patients with severe closed head injuries. *Heart Lung 13*:37–80.

Schalen, W., Messeter, K., & Nordstrom, C.H. (1992). Complications and side effects during thiopentone therapy in patients with severe head injury. *Acta Anaesthesiol Scand 36*:369–399.

Shickner, D.T., & Young, R.F. (1992). Intracranial pressure monitoring: Fiberoptic monitor compared with the ventricular catheter. *Surg Neurol 37*:251–254.

Signorini, D.F., & Alderson, P. (1999). Therapeutic hypothermia for head injury. Cochrane Library Document. CD001048.

Simmons, B.J. (1997). Management of intracranial hemodynamics in the adult: A research analysis of head positioning and recommendations for clinical practice and future research. *J Neurosci Nurs 29*(1):44–49.

Stewert-Amidei, C. (1998). Neurologic monitoring in the ICY. *Crit Care Nurs Q 21*(3):47–60.

Module 18

Acute Cerebral Dysfunction

Louise Jimm Zegeer, Pamela Stinson Kidd

This self-study module is composed of sixteen sections. Section One defines stroke and explains its etiology and epidemiologic aspects. The major classification of brain attacks (ischemic and hemorrhagic) and their common subtypes are differentiated. Section Two presents the modifiable and nonmodifiable risk factors for stroke and preventive nursing measures. Section Three discusses the pathophysiology of stroke, including abnormal cerebral blood flow states and the cellular ischemic cascade that leads to focal ischemia and infarction. Section Four describes diagnostic testing used to discriminate ischemic from hemorrhagic strokes. Section Five presents the collaborative management of patients with ischemic stroke and explains the theory of thrombogenesis and medications designed to interrupt this process. Section Six discusses the surgical management of patients with stroke. Section Seven discusses a focused assessment of the acute stroke patient and priority nursing diagnoses that are potentially life threatening for acute patients. The significance of obtaining a pertinent history and clinical examination are discussed as they contribute to diagnosing the patient's stroke subtype and prioritizing nursing care. Section Eight describes systemic complications associated with stroke with implications for nursing interventions. Section Nine discusses motor and visual deficits in the acute stroke patient. Traditional (compensation) and neurodevelopmental (Bobath) (bilateral stimulation) principles of rehabilitation are introduced. Pattern of motor recovery following a stroke is described. Section Ten examines undernutrition secondary to dysphagia, impaired gag and swallowing reflexes, and perceptual and motor deficits that may occur in poststroke patients. Alteration in elimination is discussed in Section Eleven, which explains neurogenic bladder types and some types of incontinence. The focus of Section Twelve is on the effects of altered sensations following stroke and nursing interventions to protect the patient from injury. Section Thirteen discusses hemianopsia, the neglect syndrome, impaired right/left discrimination, agnosias, apraxias, and the spatial relations syndrome. Section Fourteen examines the dysphasias commonly observed in left hemispheric (dominant) stroke patients and includes Broca's, Wernicke's, and global dysphasias. Dysarthrias are differentiated from dysphasias in terms of lesion site, effects, and nursing care. Section Fifteen identifies stressors that can lead to ineffective patient and family coping, and describes the effects of stroke on sexual roles and body image. Section Sixteen identifies predictors of outcome poststroke and common causes of mortality in acute stroke patients. Each section includes a set of review questions to help the learner evaluate his or her understanding of the section's content before moving on to the next section. All Section Reviews and the module Pretest and Posttest include answers. It is suggested that the learner review those concepts answered incorrectly in the review questions before proceeding to the next section.

OBJECTIVES

Following completion of this module, the learner will be able to

1. Define stroke and its subtypes and cite its significance to society.
2. Identify preventive measures related to the risk factors of stroke (brain attack).
3. Explain the modifiable and nonmodifiable risk factors for stroke (brain attack).

4. Contrast "heart attacks" with "brain attacks."
5. Compare and contrast ischemic and hemorrhagic strokes.
6. Explain the pathophysiology of the cellular ischemic cascade that occurs in stroke.
7. Explain the therapeutic management of stroke and selective nursing implications of therapy.
8. Explain the focused assessment for acute stroke patients and its significance for nursing care.
9. Elicit from assessment findings those that are life threatening and prioritize nursing care accordingly.
10. Apply principles of rehabilitation in the nursing care of acute stroke patients.
11. Promote independence in activities of daily living (ADLs).
12. Describe nursing interventions that prevent aspiration.
13. Describe nursing interventions that promote adequate nutrition for the patient.
14. Describe nursing interventions that will promote urinary continence and normal bowel elimination.
15. Protect the acute stroke patient from injury.
16. Maintain skin integrity in the acute stroke patient.
17. Explain the effects of visual–spatial–perceptual deficits and their implications for nursing care.
18. Describe nursing interventions that enhance communication of aphasic and dysarthric stroke patients.
19. Identify stressors that can lead to ineffective coping for the stroke patient and family and nursing implications for care.
20. Identify the most common cause of death in acute stroke patients.

PRETEST

1. Assessment findings that suggest life-threatening signs or symptoms include all of the following EXCEPT
   A. hypotension
   B. sluggishly dilating pupil
   C. severe headache
   D. hypocarbia (decreased P_{CO_2})
2. Mrs. Green, age 45, was admitted with a severe explosive headache, a stiff neck, and photophobia. She was diagnosed with a subarachnoid hemorrhage from a ruptured aneurysm. While awaiting surgery, the nurse can provide a therapeutic environment by
   A. allowing her family unrestricted visiting privileges
   B. placing her bed near a window
   C. honoring her request for a television
   D. dimming the lights in her room
3. Jeffrey Porter, age 38, was brought to the emergency department with a hemorrhagic stroke and was drowsy and difficult to arouse. His left pupil was sluggish and dilating. (Questions 3 and 4 pertain to this situation.) Which of the following nursing measures would be performed first?
   A. perform a neurologic check
   B. listen to lung sounds
   C. assess airway patency
   D. get blood samples for ABGs
4. With a hemorrhagic stroke, Jeffrey is at high risk for which of the following complications during the first few days?
   A. increased intracranial pressure (ICP)
   B. vasospasms
   C. deep vein thrombosis
   D. pneumonia
5. In the acute stage of a stroke, the nurse promotes independence by
   A. anticipating needs for the patient
   B. providing opportunities for decision making when possible
   C. encouraging the patient to listen to the television or radio
   D. avoiding assistance at meal times
6. The typical hemiparetic posture of the stroke patient includes
   A. flexion of the knee
   B. extension of the arm
   C. flexion of the arm
   D. adduction of the arm
7. When assisting a stroke patient to remove his shirt, the nurse correctly teaches him to
   A. slide it over his head
   B. remove the shirt from the affected side first
   C. remove the shirt from the unaffected side first
   D. seek assistance from the nurse
8. When feeding a dysphagic person, the nurse would correctly
   A. ask him or her to flex the chin
   B. place the food on the affected side to stimulate chewing
   C. use liquids initially to feed the patient
   D. raise the head of the bed to 30 degrees before feeding
9. When assessing a stroke patient, all of the following are significant clues to potential swallowing problems EXCEPT

A. impaired phonation
B. impaired corneal reflex
C. drooling
D. aphasia

10. Detrusor hyperreflexia is best managed by
A. establishing a voiding schedule
B. intermittent catheterization
C. antispasmodic drugs
D. indwelling catheter

11. Nursing measures to assist patients with detrusor–sphincter dyssynergy include all of the following EXCEPT
A. establishing a timed voiding schedule
B. intermittent catheterization
C. checking postvoid residuals within 5 minutes of voiding
D. restricting fluids after dinner

12. To prevent pressure sores, the stroke patient can be taught to
A. lie only on the unaffected side and back
B. inspect the skin with a mirror
C. turn at least every 4 hours
D. eat a diet high in carbohydrates

13. When teaching a patient with a left hemispheric stroke, the astute nurse
A. uses visual aids to enhance teaching
B. uses audio aids to enhance teaching
C. expects impulsive behavior
D. expects euphoria

14. Mary Davis, age 30, had an embolic stroke with right hemiparesis. To promote a positive body image, the nurse correctly
A. teaches her to apply her lipstick on the affected side first
B. teaches her to focus on her disabilities and not her abilities
C. explains that her menstrual cycles will become normal soon
D. encourages her to wear her own clothes as soon as possible

15. To enhance communication for the patient with Wernicke's aphasia, the nurse can
A. use concrete words and short sentences
B. have the patient listen to the radio or television
C. provide multiple choices to assist in decision making
D. provide language-learning tape recordings

16. Sophie Sanders, age 40, had a brain stem stroke. Her speech was slurred and hard to understand. Upon nursing assessment, she followed directions well and was able to name objects correctly. Her communication impairment was most likely a
A. Broca's aphasia
B. Wernicke's aphasia
C. dysarthria
D. global aphasia

17. Which of the following regarding brain energy and reserves is true?
A. the brain has only 5 to 10 minutes of oxygen reserves
B. the brain has no glucose reserves
C. the white matter consumes more energy than the gray matter
D. increased brain activity will trigger more blood flow in normal brain

18. A transient ischemic attack (TIA) is a
A. completed stroke
B. stroke that extends beyond 24 hours but is reversible
C. reversible brain attack that lasts usually 2 to 15 minutes
D. stroke that evolves over several days

19. Stroke is an important cerebrovascular disorder because it
A. is the second leading cause of adult disability in North America
B. is the third leading cause of adult death in North America
C. claims approximately 100,000 new victims each year in the United States
D. is responsible for approximately 500,000 deaths in the United States each year

20. The most important modifiable risk factor for stroke is
A. diabetes mellitus
B. cardiac disease
C. hypertension
D. drug abuse

21. All of the following are preventive nursing measures for stroke patients EXCEPT
A. screening adults for hypertension
B. avoiding and reporting hypotensive episodes in hospitalized elders
C. identifying risk populations and referring them for treatment
D. teaching hypertensive patients to eat a low-potassium diet

22. Mr. Dixon, age 65, is a black man who has a history of atrial fibrillation. His blood pressure is 180/100 mm Hg. He weighs 200 pounds and is 5′5″. His blood cholesterol is 290 mg/dL; he has drinking binges on weekends, and he has smoked one pack of cigarettes per day for 30 years. How many modifiable stroke risk factors does Mr. Dixon have?
A. 2
B. 4
C. 6
D. 8

23. The highest incidence of stroke is caused by
A. atherothrombosis
B. emboli
C. primary intracerebral hemorrhage
D. subarachnoid hemorrhage

24. The most common cause of subarachnoid hemorrhage is a(n)
    A. lacunar infarct
    B. intracerebral bleeding
    C. vasospasm
    D. cerebral aneurysm
25. In the ischemic cascade, which electrolyte is believed to generate the greatest cellular damage when there is an ionic imbalance?
    A. potassium
    B. calcium
    C. sodium
    D. magnesium
26. The cerebral perfusion range, or "therapeutic window," for reversing focal cerebral ischemia within the first 6 hours is
    A. 50 to 40 mL/100 g/min
    B. 40 to 30 mL/100 g/min
    C. 30 to 20 mL/100 g/min
    D. 20 to 10 mL/100 g/min
27. Brain attacks are similar to heart attacks in all of the following EXCEPT they
    A. are managed with similar drugs
    B. warrant a 911 call
    C. have similar warning signs and symptoms
    D. have similar cellular pathophysiology
28. The diagnostic test used to distinguish cerebral hemorrhage from ischemic strokes during the first 6 hours of stroke onset is
    A. duplex ultrasound study
    B. transcranial Doppler study
    C. noncontrast CT scan
    D. magnetic resonance imaging
29. Mr. Jenkins, age 60, had a right parietal brain attack. He may have all of the following effects EXCEPT
    A. Wernicke's aphasia
    B. left homonymous hemianopsia
    C. neglect of half of his body or space
    D. denial of his illness

Pretest answers: 1. D, 2. D, 3. C, 4. A, 5. B, 6. C, 7. C, 8. A, 9. D, 10. A, 11. D, 12. B, 13. A, 14. D, 15. A, 16. C, 17. D, 18. C, 19. B, 20. C, 21. D, 22. C, 23. A, 24. D, 25. B, 26. D, 27. C, 28. C, 29. A

GLOSSARY

Agnosia. A perceptual impairment resulting in the failure to recognize familiar objects by the senses even though sensation is intact; types include

- *Tactile agnosia:* inability to recognize an object by touch (lesion site: parietal lobes)
- *Visual agnosia:* inability to recognize familiar sights (lesion site: occipitotemporoparietal lobes)
- *Auditory agnosia:* inability to recognize familiar sounds (lesion site: dominant temporal lobe)
- *Somatosognosia:* awareness of one's own body and its parts (lesion site: usually dominant parietal lobe)
- *Visual–spatial agnosia:* impaired understanding of relationships between objects and self (lesion site: parietal and frontal lobes)

Anosognosia. A severe form of neglect in which the patient fails to recognize his or her illness or paralysis

Apraxia. A perceptual and cognitive impairment resulting in an inability to perform movements voluntarily in the presence of intact motor power, sensation, or coordination. May move automatically but not purposefully. Types include dressing, ideational, ideomotor, motor, and constructional

Ataxia. Impaired gait characterized by unsteadiness, poor balance, and incoordination (lesion site: cerebellum)

Body schema. The perceptual ability to identify the position of the body parts and the relationship of body parts to each other

Cerebrovascular disease (CBVD). A pathologic process that chronically or progressively restricts the circulation in the brain

Diaschisis. Decrease in cerebral perfusion not only in the focal ischemic zone but also in distant unaffected areas of the brain. It is believed that the ischemic lesion interrupts afferent connections to the remote healthy sites resulting in less stimuli and less cerebral perfusion

Dysphasia/aphasia. Impaired capacity to interpret, formulate, or express meaningful language by speaking, writing, or gesturing (expressive or Broca's dysphasia); the inability to understand the written or spoken language (receptive or Wernicke's dysphasia). There are mild to severe degrees of aphasia (literally no speech) as opposed to dysphasia (difficulty with speech) (lesion site: left dominant hemisphere)

Dysphagia. Impaired swallowing

Flaccidity. Absence of muscle tone resulting in floppy, limp, flabby, hyporeflexic, nonfunctional limbs

Hemiparesis. Weakness of one side of the body

Hemiplegia. Paralysis or loss of voluntary movement of one side of the body

Homonymous hemianopsia. Damage to the postchiasmal optic pathways that results in blindness in the nasal half of one eye and the temporal half of the other eye. The person with left hemianopsia cannot see objects in the left visual field

Intracerebral steal. The shunting away of blood from focal ischemic zones with autoregulatory loss to healthy brain areas, providing excess perfusion in these areas and worsening the ischemia

Ipsilateral. Same side

Ischemia (focal). Inadequate cerebral perfusion (hypoperfusion) to localized areas of the brain

Luxury perfusion. Hyperperfusion in healthy tissue surrounding the penumbra. Cerebral blood flow is in excess of tissue demands in healthy tissue

Occupational therapist (OT). A health care provider specializing in assisting disabled persons regain occupations, roles, and ADLs through perceptual and cognitive skill training, leading to improved self-esteem and quality of life

Oligemia. A compensatory hypoperfusion state characterized by reduced cerebral blood flow

Paresthesias. Abnormal sensations such as burning or tingling of the skin, often occurring during stroke recovery

Penumbra. An ischemic zone of viable, threatened tissue surrounding the brain infarct. The tissue may be salvaged if treated within the first 6 hours of onset of the attack. Tissue in this zone has been referred to as the *sleeping beauty*

Physiatrist. Physician specialist in rehabilitation medicine

Pocketing. Food that is caught between the cheek and gum on the paralyzed side of the face, resulting in food not being chewed, swallowed, or digested properly

Pronation. Movement of the forearm with the palm facing down; after a stroke, spasticity of the upper arms often causes pronation

Proprioception. Sensory awareness of the position of body and its parts

Reverse steal. A therapeutic shunting by controlled hyperventilation of blood from healthy brain areas with intact carbon dioxide responsiveness to vasoparalytic areas, which lack autoregulation and carbon dioxide responsiveness, in focal ischemic zones, thereby improving perfusion to those areas

Spasticity. A state of increased tone of a muscle resulting in a stiff muscle and continuous resistance to stretching

Stroke. A brain attack; an interruption in the brain's blood supply usually caused by thrombosis or hemorrhage and resulting in a sudden loss of bodily function

Subluxation. Incomplete dislocation, most often seen in the shoulder joint following stroke

Synergy. A pattern of movement seen with high levels of spasticity in which muscles move together; voluntary movement of one joint by itself is not possible (e.g., attempts to flex the wrist would result in a mass flexion movement of the entire upper extremity)

Abbreviations

ACA. Anterior cerebral artery

ACoA. Anterior communicating artery

ADLs. Activities of daily living

AVM. Arteriovenous malformation

BBB. Blood–brain barrier

CBF. Cerebral blood flow

CBVD. Cerebrovascular disease

CI. Cerebral infarct

$CMRO_2$. Cerebral metabolic rate of oxygen consumption or brain metabolic energy demands

CPP. Cerebral perfusion pressure

CSF. Cerebrospinal fluid

CT. Computed tomography

DVT. Deep vein thrombosis

ECF. Extracellular fluid

ECG. Electrocardiogram

ECS. Extracellular space

FFAs. Free fatty acids

GCS. Glasgow Coma Scale

ICA. Internal carotid artery

ICF. Intracellular fluid

ICP. Intracranial pressure

IJV. Internal jugular vein

LMN. Lower motor neuron

MAP. Mean arterial pressure

MCA. Middle cerebral artery

Mean SAP. Average systemic arterial pressure

NSA. National Stroke Association

OEF. Oxygen extraction fraction

OT. Occupational therapist

PCA. Posterior cerebral artery

PCoA. Posterior communicating artery

PICH. Primary intracerebral hemorrhage

PNS. Parasympathetic nervous system

PT. Physical therapist

RIND. Reversible ischemic neurologic deficit

ROM. Range of motion

SAH. Subarachnoid hemorrhage

SIE. Stroke-in-evolution

SNS. Sympathetic nervous system

TCD. Transcranial Doppler

TIA. Transient ischemic attack

t-PA. Tissue plasminogen activator

UMN. Upper motor neuron

VA. Vertebral artery

SECTION ONE: Definition, Etiology, Epidemiology, and Classifications of Strokes (Brain Attacks)

This section discusses the etiology and epidemiology of stroke and differentiates the temporal categories of stroke. At the completion of this section, the learner will be able to describe the epidemiologic and etiologic aspects of brain attack and its various subtypes.

Definition and Etiology of Strokes

Stroke is a sudden disturbance in a person's brain perfusion associated with a neurologic deficit. It is caused by either focal brain ischemia or hemorrhage (McDowell, Brott, & Goldstein, 1993). Jennett and Lindsay (1994) define ischemic stroke as inadequate perfusion of a brain area with functional failure. Stroke is a form of **cerebrovascular disease (CBVD).** If it is severe or prolonged, infarction (neuronal death) develops. Ischemic strokes are produced by either vascular occlusion (thrombi, emboli) or perfusion failure (conditions producing a decreased cardiac output) (Jennett & Lindsay, 1994).

Hemorrhagic strokes can result from ruptured aneurysms, hypertensive hemorrhages, or arteriovenous malformations (AVMs), a congenital tangled coiling and mixing of arterial and venous blood that affects the brain's arterial perfusion.

Epidemiology of Stroke

Stroke is the third leading cause of death in the United States and Canada and a leading cause of adult disability (Joint National Committee on Detection, Evaluation, and Treatment of High Blood Pressure, 1993; McDowell, Brott, & Goldstein, 1993). Each year approximately 730,000 Americans have a new or recurrent stroke. Every 45 seconds in the United States, someone experiences a stroke. Stroke costs the United States $30 billion annually (National Stroke Association, http://www.stroke.org, 1998). Geographically, there is a high incidence of stroke in the southeastern region of the United States (the stroke belt) (Fig. 18–1).

Stroke mortality in the United States has declined 50 percent over the past 20 years. Still, nearly 160,000 Americans die each year from stroke (National Stroke

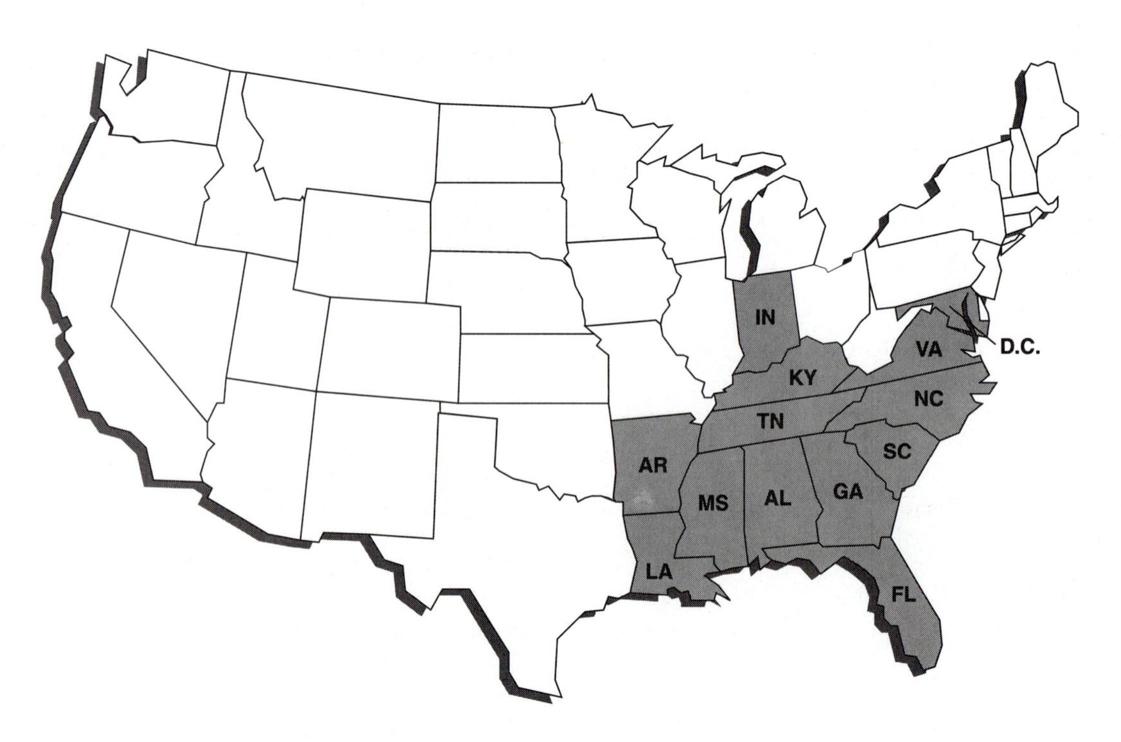

Figure 18–1. The stroke belt. *(Source: National Stroke Association.)*

Association, 1998). This decline has been attributed, particularly, to hypertension control, atherosclerosis prevention, therapy for cardiac disease, and lifestyle changes. Lifestyle changes include a decline in cigarette smoking, modification of diet, and increased exercise. Recently, the long decline in stroke morbidity and mortality has plateaued and there have been reports of a trend toward an increase in stroke incidence in the 1990s, attributed to better methods of detecting strokes, an increase in the elderly population, and patient noncompliance in taking antihypertensives. Approximately one third of all stroke survivors will have another stroke within 5 years (National Stroke Association, 1998). Consequently, stroke is and will be a major health problem in the future with the growing numbers of elders in our society.

Transient Ischemic Attacks

A stroke may be preceded by a transient ischemic attack (TIA) similar to angina in a heart attack. Transient ischemic attacks are acute reversible fleeting episodes of focal or localized neurologic deficits that usually last 2 to 15 minutes but may persist for up to 24 hours (Yatsu, Grotta, & Pettigrew, 1995). Clinically, the patient may present with sudden unilateral dimness or partial loss of vision (amaurosis fugax) in one eye, weakness, numbness, tingling, severe headache, speechlessness, or unexplained dizziness, depending on the artery involved. Carotid stenosis, which is related to atherosclerotic disease; microemboli from atherosclerotic plaques in major extracranial vessels; or, less frequently, a decrease in cardiac output can cause inadequate perfusion to the brain, which produces these symptoms. TIAs are warnings of an impending stroke and require immediate referral for treatment. Table 18–1 lists the warning signs of stroke that constitute a medical emergency and warrant a 911 call.

The greater the frequency of TIAs, the greater the likelihood of a future stroke. Whether TIAs are completed cerebral infarctions with no clinical symptoms or merely episodes of cerebral ischemia without infarction is an unresolved issue. Some patients with clinical TIAs have infarcts shown on CT scan, which account for their symptoms. Transient ischemic attacks lasting longer than 6 hours may produce infarcts.

Temporal Categories of Stroke

Strokes can be described on a temporal progression; some authors believe these to be stages of the same pathophysiologic processes. There are several categories of strokes:

- Reversible ischemic neurologic deficit
- Stroke-in-evolution
- Stable or completed stroke

Reversible ischemic neurologic deficit (RIND) is a stroke whose effects are reversible but the time frame extends beyond 24 hours and patient symptoms usually resolve in 1 to 3 weeks. This term is inaccurate because MRI reveals small deep lesions, suggesting that RIND represents a completed infarct (Yatsu, Grotta, & Pettigrew, 1995). A stroke-in-evolution (SIE) is an unstable, stuttering, and progressive stroke that may worsen with time. It is believed to result from an expanding intra-arterial thrombus that can cause further occlusion. These acute strokes require early management to arrest their devastating effects. A stable or completed stroke is one in which the patient has a fixed neurologic deficit lasting longer than 24 hours (Yatsu, Grotta, & Pettigrew, 1995).

The term *cerebrovascular accident* is a misnomer because strokes are not accidents but rather the outcome of a process often evolving over years. More recently, the term *brain attack*, which parallels the catastrophic event of a heart attack, has been endorsed because timing is critical to stroke therapy to avoid irreversible deficits. Many commonalities exist with brain attacks and heart attacks. They both require emergency treatment; may have warning signs; have similar pathologic processes; are treated with similar medications; and are life threatening.

Major Classifications of Stroke

It is important to differentiate the type of stroke within the first 6 hours of onset because each hour of ischemia and tissue injury increases the degree of irreversible neurologic damage and because effective emergency care is contingent on determining the type of stroke (Adams, Bendixen, & Kappelle, 1993; McDowell, Brott, & Goldstein, 1993). The major classifications of stroke are:

- *Ischemic:* atherothrombotic, embolic, hypoxic, and lacunar
- *Hemorrhagic:* subarachnoid hemorrhage, primary intracerebral hemorrhage, and arteriovenous malformations

Figure 18–2 illustrates some of the subtypes of ischemic and hemorrhagic strokes.

Ischemic Strokes

Approximately 84 percent of the strokes are ischemic and are usually thrombotic or embolic (Mitiguy, 1991). Atherosclerosis leading to atherothrombotic brain infarction accounts for most strokes, particularly in elders; while emboli account for most strokes in younger and middle-aged adults and the very old.

ATHEROTHROMBOTIC STROKES. Atherothrombosis produces a gradual, progressive stenosis with eventual arterial occlusion. This results from a buildup of fatty deposits (atherosclerotic plaques) that enlarge with superimposed thrombi over years in the carotid and other cerebral vessels, compromising cerebral perfusion. During this time, collateral circulation may develop in the vessels distal to

TABLE 18–1. MAJOR STROKES COMPARED

TYPE OF STROKE	AGE	RISK FACTORS	INCIDENCE	CHARACTERISTICS	MANAGEMENT
Ischemic Stroke					
Thrombotic	Elders	Hypertension, smoking, high cholesterol, diabetes mellitus, atherosclerosis	53%	May have TIAs Development during sleep or upon awakening May have mild headache Predictable locations and symptoms Intermittent attacks and progression	For SIE, emergency carotid endarterectomy for awake patients with minimal deficits if surgery can be done within first 6 hours. Do not treat blood pressure unless ≥ 230 mm Hg systolic or ≥ 120 mm Hg diastolic on repeated measurements at 20-minute intervals within the first 6 hours. Bed rest and close monitoring of blood pressure. Thrombolytic agents: t-PA, streptokinase, urokinase. May use calcium channel blockers or HHH therapy. Anticoagulant therapy: heparin and warfarin. Cerebral angioplasty.
Embolic	Young and middle-aged adults and very old	Cardiac abnormalities: arrhythmias (atrial fibrillation), valvular heart disease Carotid plaque or thrombosis	31%	No warning—sudden attack Maximal deficit at onset Symptoms and location vary with attack Usually daytime	Prevention: Antiplatelet therapy (aspirin and ticlopidine), Plavix. Treat source of emboli.
Hemorrhagic Stroke					
Nontraumatic subarachnoid hemorrhage (SAH)	Young and middle-aged adults	Nontraumatic ruptured aneurysms (most common) Arteriovenous malformations (AVMs), brain tumors, blood dyscrasias (less common)	6%	Usually no warning Sudden attack Possible reversal Very severe headache, bloody CSF, stiff neck, seizures, nausea/vomiting, photophobia, fever Hypertension: often Decreasing LOC	Early surgery for clipping aneurysms. Calcium channel blockers and cerebral angioplasty for vasospasms. AVMs: obliterative surgery.
Primary intracranial hemorrhage (PICH)	Elders	Chronic hypertension (most common) Microaneurysms, anticoagulant therapy, drug abuse (cocaine, amphetamines, alcohol), blood dyscrasias, amyloid angiopathy (less common)	10%	Usually no warning Gradual development No reversal Headache, nausea, and vomiting Bloody CSF, nuchal rigidity, photophobia Decreased LOC Motor–sensory deficit of face, arm, and leg Chronic hypertension: usual cause	Surgery for awake patients with hematomas > 3 cm. Strict control of blood pressure within first 6 hours. Systolic treated if ≥ 180/105 mm Hg on two repeated checks at 20-minute intervals. Restore blood pressure to prehemorrhagic levels. PICH > 30 mL are treated surgically.

the occlusion. These patients commonly have multiple stroke risk factors. Carotid occlusion is responsible for 75 percent of all strokes. Thrombotic strokes may be preceded by TIAs. Should headache or decreased level of consciousness occur after 24 hours following the brain attack, the cause is usually increased ICP (Jennett & Lindsay, 1994).

EMBOLIC STROKES. Emboli may break off from the carotid plaque or thrombus and occlude distal cerebral

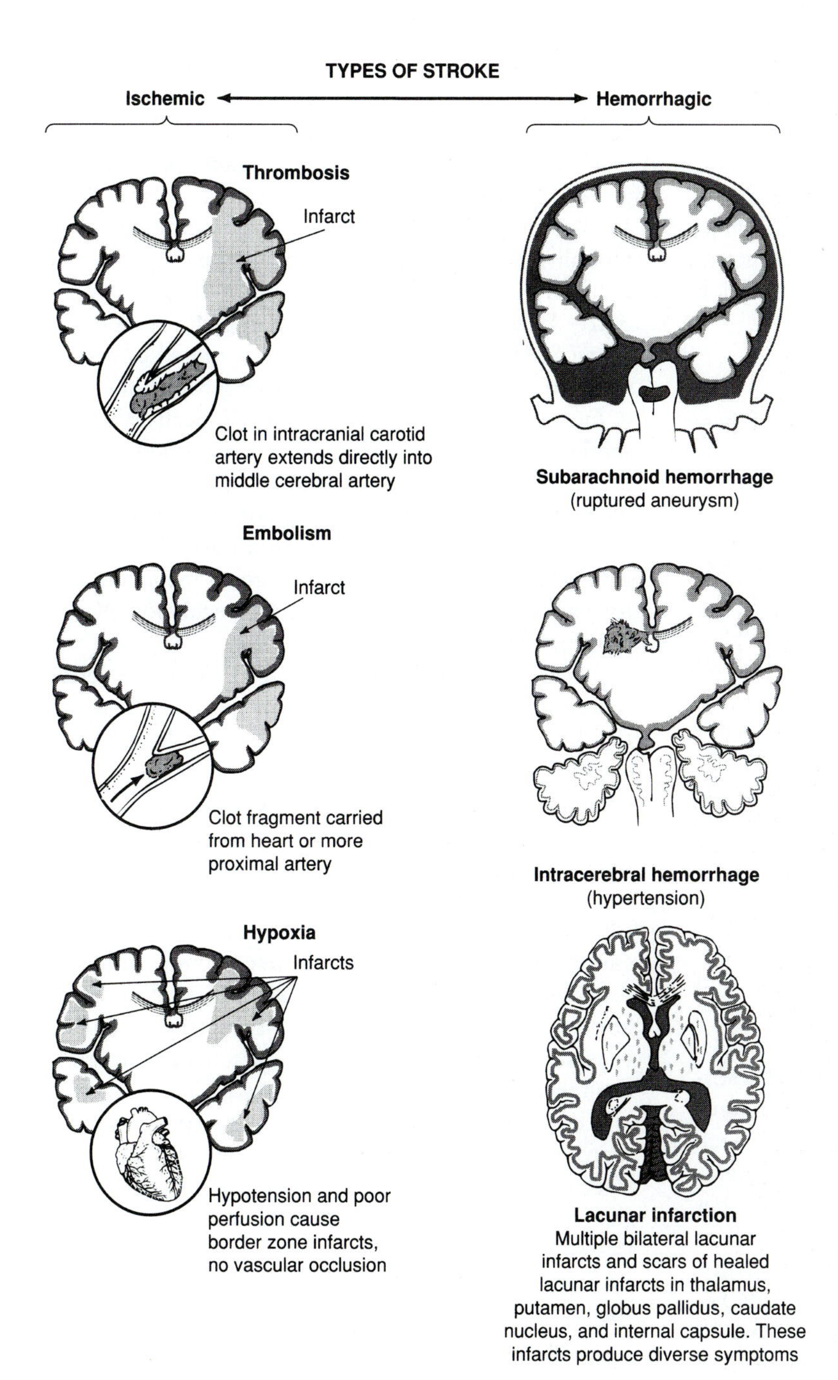

Figure 18–2. Types of stroke. *(From Caplan, L.R. [1988]. Stroke.* Clin Symp 40*(4):6, 25.)*

vessels without any warning. Sources of emboli may also be cardiogenic, one of the most common causes being atrial fibrillation.

HYPOXIC STROKES. Hypotension and low cardiac output related to cardiac disease can cause hypoperfusion to border zone areas lying between major arteries in the distal areas of the brain.

LACUNAR STROKES. Lacunar strokes may be ischemic or hemorrhagic strokes. About 10 to 15 percent of ischemic strokes are due to lacunar infarcts, which are ministrokes that commonly involve the deep, small, penetrating arteries of the brain such as the lenticulostriate arteries branching from the MCA. These arteries branch at 90 degrees from the major conducting arteries of the circle of Willis and are usually end arteries with poor collateral circulation. Chronic hypertension is believed to produce degenerative changes in the cerebral microvasculature and small lesions in the deep subcortical white and gray matter of the brain. Approximately two thirds of patients with lacunae are hypertensive, and many of these are diabetic. A subintimal accumulation of hyalin and fatlike material called *lipohyalinosis* occludes arteries. In addition, small atherosclerotic plaques occlude and weaken the vessel walls of the arteries, producing aneurysmal dilation with eventual rupture into the brain, causing small areas of "microinfarction" (Babikian, Kase, & Wolf, 1994; Kilpatrick et al., 1993). The infarcted area eventually becomes cystic and fills with a fluidlike lake, or "lacuna." Lacunar stroke patients may present with purely motor and/or sensory strokes; ataxic hemiparesis; the dysarthria–clumsy hand syndrome; or no apparent symptoms if they occur in "silent" areas of the brain. Most patients will experience a partial recovery of function (Yatsu, Grotta, & Pettigrew, 1995).

Hemorrhagic Strokes

Hemorrhagic strokes account for approximately 15 percent of acute strokes, with primary intracerebral hemorrhage being more than twice as common as subarachnoid hemorrhage (Broderick et al., 1993b).

SUBARACHNOID HEMORRHAGE. Subarachnoid hemorrhage (SAH) can result from degenerative changes that damage the elastic layer of the artery; developmental defects, which cause a poorly developed arterial wall; high blood flow areas, which cause hemodynamic stress; and hypertension, which accentuates any vascular weakness (Jennett & Lindsay, 1994). With SAH, blood extravasates into the subarachnoid spaces; SAH accounts for 5 to 10 percent of all strokes (Yatsu, Grotta, & Pettigrew, 1995). Leakage of blood from aneurysms (thin-walled balloonlike outpouchings of the arterial intima) is usually found at arterial bifurcations (branchings) where blood velocity is higher and can be lethal with rupture. Aneurysms can be saccular (with a neck) or fusiform (without a neck). Approximately 20 percent of patients have more than one aneurysm (Jennett & Lindsay, 1994). Clinically, these strokes develop suddenly without warning. The patient often complains of a sudden, severe unilateral headache—"the worst headache of my life"; neck pain or stiffness (nuchal rigidity); and vomiting (King & Martin, 1994). Meningeal irritation by blood produces the severe headache and other meningeal signs such as photophobia (intolerance to light) and nuchal rigidity. Hypertension is common. The CSF is usually bloody because the aneurysm commonly ruptures in the subarachnoid space. When ambulant, the patient may complain of leg pain, an irritant effect of blood around the lumbosacral roots in the spinal subarachnoid space (Jennett & Lindsay, 1994). Diplopia and fever may accompany SAH. Following the SAH, a decrease in CBF and transient loss of consciousness secondary to increased ICP may occur.

Mortality in patients with ruptured aneurysms is approximately 36.2 percent and is usually related to the delayed complications of aneurysmal rupture, such as:

- Rebleeding
- Vasospasm (cerebral arterial spasm)
- Delayed ischemic deficits
- Communicating hydrocephalus
- Increased ICP (Keith & Forsting, 1995)

Rebleeding occurs most commonly within the first 2 weeks in about 20 percent of untreated patients following aneurysm rupture, with the highest risk being within the first 24 hours. Mortality from rebleeding approaches 70 percent (Jennett & Lindsay, 1994; King & Martin, 1994). Vasospasm is the most frequent cause of morbidity and mortality in hospitalized patients with aneurysmal SAH. It usually occurs between the third and tenth day after SAH, with a peak in severity during the second week (King & Martin, 1994). Vasospasm is caused by periarterial blood degradation; the amount of subarachnoid blood is the best predictor of vasospasm. Clinically, there is a subtle and progressive loss of consciousness or focal deficit over the course of minutes to hours. Cerebral blood flow is dependent not only on the severity of the vasospasm, but also on blood pressure, ICP, blood viscosity, $PaCO_2$, collateral pathways, neuronal metabolic activity, and the presence of cerebral autoregulation (King & Martin, 1994).

Delayed ischemic deficits (DIDs) can cause deterioration in up to one third of patients who survive the initial hemorrhage. Symptoms usually develop within 3 weeks after the initial bleed, with peak incidence occurring in about 8 days. Some of the causes of DIDs are believed to be vasospasm, impaired autoregulation, excessive renal excretion of sodium, or hydrocephalus leading to raised ICP and reduced cerebral perfusion (Jennett & Lindsay, 1994). In over 20 percent of patients, communicating hydrocephalus occurs either acutely within the first few days or during the second week after the aneurysm rupture and results from subarachnoid blood or edematous tissue blocking the arachnoid absorption channels. This blockage leads to raised ICP.

Less common causes of hemorrhagic strokes are coagulopathies (e.g., hemophilia, sickle cell anemia), excessive anticoagulant therapy, trauma, tumors, drug abuse (amphetamines and cocaine), and congenital abnormalities such as AVMs, the abnormal collections of vessels with poorly developed muscle layers near the surface of the brain that look like coiled tangles of blood vessels.

Table 18–1 differentiates ischemic from hemorrhagic stroke on the basis of age, etiology, incidence, characteristics, and management.

PRIMARY INTRACEREBRAL HEMORRHAGE. Primary intracerebral hemorrhage (PICH) usually involves bleeding directly into the brain parenchyma; it may occur as small (< 3 cm) or larger (> 3 cm) hemorrhages. Large lobar hemorrhages greater than 6 cm in diameter have a high mortality rate. The brain does not tolerate large volumes of blood, and hemorrhages greater than 30 mL were found to have a mortality rate of 44 percent in one study (Broderick et al., 1993a; Brott & Broderick, 1993). Chronic hypertension, the major cause of PICH, produces gradual, degenerative changes in the small penetrating arteries, causing micro-aneurysms that burst with sudden increases in blood pressure. Approximately 50 percent of the patients survive, but two thirds remain disabled (Jennett & Lindsay, 1994).

In summary, strokes or brain attacks are the third leading cause of death in the United States and are medical emergencies that warrant a 911 call. A disruption in cerebral perfusion provides warning signs and symptoms that are reversible in some cases (TIAs and RIND) or irreversible in others (completed stroke). The public and health care providers must be educated to respond to these warning signs because effective therapy within the first 6 hours can prevent severe morbidity or mortality. In one study, only 42 percent of patients with acute strokes arrived at tertiary medical centers within 24 hours (Alberts, Bertels, & Dawson, 1990). Public education and education of health care providers decreases the mean elapsed time for seeking care after stroke onset from 19.4 to 1.5 hours (Barsan et al., 1988). Ischemic strokes are the most common type of stroke and are classified as atherothrombotic, embolic, hypoxic, or lacunar. Hemorrhagic strokes are less common and more lethal than ischemic strokes, particularly if the lesion is large and the location is in the brain stem. Hemorrhagic strokes include subarachnoid hemorrhages, primary intracerebral hemorrhages within brain tissue, and arteriovenous malformations.

Section One Review

1. Mrs. Davis, age 33, had a brief (3-minute) attack of heaviness in her right arm and leg and could not utter a word during this period. Her function returned to normal after this episode. The category of brain attack she has experienced is most probably a(n)
   A. SIE
   B. TIA
   C. stroke
   D. RIND
2. Which of the following statements concerning stroke epidemiology is true?
   A. it is the third leading cause of death in North America
   B. there are about 1 million new stroke victims each year in the United States
   C. stroke mortality has increased during the past 30 years
   D. stroke trends in the 1990s indicate a continuous decline in stroke mortality
3. Brain attacks are similar to heart attacks in all of the following options EXCEPT
   A. their warning signs
   B. their life-threatening nature
   C. pharmaceutical management
   D. their symptoms
4. Abnormal blood in the subarachnoid spaces, as occurs in hemorrhagic strokes, can be life threatening for the patient because of
   A. vasospasms
   B. an allergic reaction
   C. hemorrhagic shock
   D. a noncommunicating hydrocephalus
5. Which of the following is true of atherothrombotic strokes?
   A. they usually occur in young and middle-aged adults
   B. they are the most common type of strokes
   C. the brain attack usually occurs with activity
   D. the deficit is maximal at onset
6. Which of the following is true of an embolic stroke?
   A. it probably occurred while sleeping or upon awakening
   B. the deficit was maximal and sudden at onset
   C. it is usually found in persons in their sixth or seventh decade of life
   D. it is usually preceded by a TIA
7. All of the following are true regarding lacunar infarcts EXCEPT they
   A. involve conducting arteries
   B. can produce occlusion or bleeding
   C. may present with pure motor or sensory or no apparent deficits
   D. are ministrokes usually caused by lipohyalinosis
8. Which of the following is true of primary intracerebral hemorrhages (PICH)?
   A. they are not as common as subarachnoid hemorrhages
   B. the major cause of PICH is chronic hypertension
   C. they usually produce a communicating hydrocephalus
   D. with hemorrhages less than 50 mL, the mortality rate is low
9. Subarachnoid hemorrhages are usually caused by
   A. chronic hypertension
   B. vasospasms
   C. aneurysms
   D. cardiogenic problems

Answers: 1. B, 2. A, 3. D, 4. A, 5. B, 6. B, 7. A, 8. B, 9. C

SECTION TWO: Risk Factors for Stroke

This section discusses the modifiable and nonmodifiable risk factors that place a person at risk for stroke and stroke preventive measures. At the completion of this section, the reader will be able to:

- Identify four cardiovascular risk factors that are implicated in strokes
- Explain the modifiable and nonmodifiable risk factors for stroke
- Identify stroke preventive nursing measures related to these risk factors

Stroke prevention is a prime concern to nurses and can be accomplished by recognition and reduction of modifiable risk factors. Stroke risk factors can be related to alterations in cardiovascular components of blood flow such as blood pressure, blood vessels, blood constituents, or the heart (Mulley, 1985). Table 18–2 provides examples of cardiovascular risk factors for stroke.

Risk Factors

Stroke risk factors can also be categorized as established or not well-established, modifiable or nonmodifiable. Table 18–3 summarizes major established risk factors. Established modifiable risk factors for stroke are blood pressure extremes, cardiac disease, coagulopathies, diabetes mellitus, and drug abuse.

Blood pressure is the most important modifiable risk factor for stroke and is implicated in both ischemic and hemorrhagic strokes. Both systolic and diastolic hypertension (greater than 160/95) are risk factors.

TABLE 18–2. CARDIOVASCULAR RISK FACTORS FOR STROKE

1. Blood pressure
   a. Hypertension: the most important risk factor
   b. Hypotension: low blood volume
2. Blood vessels
   a. Atherosclerosis: arteriosclerosis
   b. Arteritis, vasculitis, aneurysms
   c. Blood vessel rupture; lipohyalinosis
   d. Congenital arteriovenous malformations
3. Blood constituents
   a. Red blood cells: polycythemia vera, sickle cell anemia
   b. White blood cells
   c. Platelets: thrombocytosis
   d. Proteins: hyperviscosity, high hematocrit
   e. Fibrinogen: hyperviscosity
4. Heart
   a. Arrhythmias producing emboli and low cardiac output
   b. Valvular disorders and artificial prostheses
   c. Left ventricular hypertrophy
   d. Ventricular mural thrombi

Adapted from Mulley, G.P. (1985). Practical management of Stroke. *Oradell, NJ: Medical Economics Books.*

TABLE 18–3. ESTABLISHED RISK FACTORS

MODIFIABLE	NONMODIFIABLE
Hypertension and hypotension	Age
Cardiac disease	Gender
Coagulopathies	Race
Diabetes mellitus	Genetic factors
Drug abuse	
Cigarette smoking	
Excessive alcohol consumption	
Cocaine	

Hypotension, particularly in the elderly, may be a significant risk factor if the episode is sudden and profound as may happen with the use of powerful antihypertensive agents, myocardial infarction, or bleeding. Dehydration also may dangerously lower blood pressure levels and perfusion to distal branches of cerebral vessels of elders who already have an age-related decline in CBF. Caplan (1993) uses the analogy of ". . . watering the grass (brain) . . . with the hose (cerebral blood flow). . . ." If the water pressure (arterial flow) diminishes, the distal yard (border zone areas) gets no water, and the grass (neurons) dies.

Conditions that create a decrease in cardiac output, stasis of blood, or emboli formation are all risk factors for stroke. Examples of these conditions are rheumatic valvular disease, cardiac dysrhythmias, left ventricular hypertrophy, and myocardial infarction. When cardiac output decreases, perfusion to the brain is reduced, leading to ischemia, particularly in the distal brain vessels and border zones between major cerebral arteries. Other cardiac sources of stroke are emboli that break off from diseased and artificial valves or from an atrial fibrillating heart, which promotes stasis and clotting of blood in the atria.

Elevated hematocrit, red blood cell content, and serum fibrinogen levels contribute to high blood viscosity and diminished blood flow and may increase the size of brain infarcts by altering collateral blood flow to the brain (Yatsu, Grotta, & Pettigrew, 1995). Hematocrit values above 50 percent place a person at risk for stroke. Excessive anticoagulation also may lead to brain hemorrhages.

Diabetes mellitus is a risk factor for ischemic stroke in large and small vessel disease, but its role in hemorrhagic stroke needs further study. Control of diabetes does not decrease stroke incidence, but control of hyperglycemia can diminish the severity of brain damage if an acute stroke occurs.

Abuse of alcohol, cocaine, heroin, and amphetamines and cigarette smoking increase the risk of stroke. Excess alcohol consumption and cigarette smoking increase blood viscosity. With narcotic abuse, stroke may be produced by either the direct effect of the drug or by infection or emboli produced with faulty intravenous injection. Amphetamines and cocaine are usually associated with hemorrhagic strokes in the younger adult. Noncompliance with antihypertensive medications is another risk factor for stroke.

Less established modifiable risk factors include elevated blood lipid levels, high-fat and -salt diets, obesity, high stress levels, cerebral infection, and hyperuricemia. Frequently, an interaction of multiple risk factors increases the risk of stroke. The risk of ischemic stroke is particularly enhanced in cigarette-smoking, childbearing-age women who use high-estrogen contraceptives; the risk increases if they also are hypertensive, hyperlipidemic, or diabetic.

Nonmodifiable factors for stroke are age, gender, race, and genetic factors. Age is the single most important nonmodifiable risk factor for stroke; for each successive decade after 55 years, the stroke rate more than doubles. Men have a greater stroke risk than women. African Americans, particularly males, have more hypertensive disease and more strokes than other races. Obesity, smoking, and diabetes mellitus are more prevalent among African Americans, which may account for their higher incidence of strokes (Kittner, McCarter, & Sherwin, 1993).

There is also a higher incidence of stroke and stroke mortality among the Japanese and Chinese as compared with Caucasians, which may be related to hypertension and a diet high in salt and low in animal fat. Congenital aneurysms account for more than 75 percent of subarachnoid hemorrhages (Yatsu, Grotta, & Pettigrew, 1995), and AVMs also are genetic sources of stroke. Persons with sickle cell anemia or who have maternal histories of a fatal stroke are at risk for stroke (Wolf et al., 1992). The risk of recurrent stroke increases 10 to 20 times in persons who have had a previous stroke.

Prevention

Stroke prevention includes:

1. Screening for hypertension (Table 18–4) and providing follow-up when blood pressure is higher than 140/90 mm Hg.
2. Assisting in control of hypertension by instituting lifestyle changes and antihypertensives, if indicated.
3. Preventing hypertensive and hypotensive episodes in the perioperative patient by avoiding preoperative dehydration in elders, bladder distention, fluid volume excess, excessive pain, and medication withdrawal.
4. Monitoring the client in the proper use of antihypertensives and determining reasons for noncompliance.
5. Attempting to maintain patient compliance by education or modification of drug regimen with the physician.
6. Collaborating with the physician in treating cardiac disease and conditions that produce low cardiac output states.
7. Identifying elders with multiple risk factors and minimizing these risks.
8. Monitoring lab results of patients who are on anticoagulant therapy to avoid excessive or ineffective anticoagulation.
9. Teaching patients to maintain good control of diabetes mellitus.
10. Teaching lifestyle changes to those who are at high risk for stroke.
11. Identifying drug abusers and educating and encouraging these persons to enroll in drug abuse treatment programs.
12. Encouraging smokers to stop smoking or to seek assistance in smoking cessation programs.
13. Identifying obesity and encouraging weight control by changes in lifestyle.
14. Monitoring patients with hyperlipidemia and teaching methods for controlling hyperlipidemia.

In summary, the past 50 years have seen a dramatic decline of strokes and stroke mortality. Treatment of blood pressure reduces stroke mortality at all ages, including persons in their eighties and nineties (Babikian, Kase, & Wolf, 1994). Nurses can assist in stroke prevention by being aware of definite and less well-established risk factors

TABLE 18–4. RECOMMENDATIONS FOR FOLLOW-UP BASED ON INITIAL SET OF BLOOD PRESSURE MEASUREMENTS FOR ADULTS[a]

SYSTOLIC	DIASTOLIC	FOLLOW-UP RECOMMENDED[b]
< 130	< 85	Recheck in 2 years
130–139	85–89	Recheck in 1 year
140–159	90–99	Confirm within 2 months; provide advance advice about lifestyle modifications
160–179	100–109	Evaluate or refer to source of care within 1 month
≥ 180	≥ 110	Evaluate or refer to source of care within 1 week, depending on clinical situation

[a]If the systolic and diastolic categories are different, follow the recommendation for the shorter follow-up.

[b]Modify the scheduling of follow-up according to reliable information about past blood pressure, other cardiovascular risk factors, or TOD.

From The Joint National Committee on Detection, Evaluation, and Treatment of High Blood Pressure. The sixth report of the Joint National Committee on Detection, Evaluation, and Treatment of High Blood Pressure, *Bethesda, MD, 1997, National Institutes of Health, U.S. Department of Health and Human Services.*

for stroke and the means to prevent them. Hypertension and advancing age are the most important risk factors for stroke. Hypotension, drug abuse, hyperlipidemia, cardiac disease, diabetes mellitus, TIAs, and obesity are all modifiable to some degree, many with effective teaching toward healthier lifestyle changes.

SECTION TWO REVIEW

1. The most important modifiable risk factor for stroke is
   A. hypotension
   B. hypertension
   C. atrial fibrillation
   D. diabetes mellitus
2. Cigarettes, as a risk factor in stroke, produce pathophysiologic effects on all of the following EXCEPT
   A. blood pressure
   B. blood vessels
   C. blood constituents
   D. blood urea nitrogen
3. Which of the nonmodifiable risk factor statements is true?
   A. race is the single most important nonmodifiable risk factor
   B. females have more strokes than males because they live longer
   C. African Americans have more hypertensive disease and strokes than Caucasians
   D. the Japanese have a low incidence of strokes
4. Preventive measures for stroke reduction include all of the following EXCEPT
   A. screening for systolic hypertension
   B. maintaining serum cholesterol levels between 120 and 180 mg/dL
   C. educating the public regarding the consequences of smoking, alcoholism, and other drug abuse
   D. teaching that TIAs are likely not to recur if they last less than 10 minutes

Answers: 1. B, 2. D, 3. C, 4. D

SECTION THREE: Pathophysiology of Stroke

This section discusses the pathogenesis of cerebral blood flow (CBF) in stroke and the cellular ischemic cascade. At the completion of this section, the reader will be able to explain the pathophysiology of stroke.

Cerebral Blood Flow in Focal Ischemia (Stroke)

Cerebral ischemia can be induced by systemic or intracranial causes (McNair, 1999). Systemic causes include hypoxemia, hypotension, anemia, or anything that reduces cardiac output and CBF. Intracranial causes include cerebrovascular occlusions and hemorrhage, trauma, brain edema, increased ICP, and vasospasms.

Oligemia is a compensatory hypoperfusion state characterized by reduced CBF (< 50 mL/100 g/min to 23 to 20 mL/100 g/min) that is still above the threshold for ischemia (Fig. 18–3). Recall that normal CBF is about 50 to 55 mL/100 g/min and that the brain uses only about one half of the oxygen carried by the blood. When CBF is in this oligemic range, the brain compensates by increasing oxygen extraction from the blood, and the patient is free of neurologic signs or symptoms (Lenzi et al., 1990). The OEF (oxygen extraction fraction) increases in oligemia and can be measured by arteriovenous oxygen difference ($AVDO_2$) or jugular venous saturation of oxygen ($SjVO_2$). The average resting value of OEF is 30 to 40 percent, and it can rise to over 90 percent to maintain normal brain metabolism. Consequently, compensated "low flow" states may be associated with increased OEF to sustain aerobic metabolism, normal $CMRO_2$, and neurological function (Paczynski, Hsu, & Diringer, 1995). This state has been labeled misery perfusion (Lenzi et al., 1990). It is important for nurses to recognize that patients may have significant impairment of CBF without any clinically detectable sign of cerebral hypoperfusion and they must be adequately ventilated and perfused to avoid the more severe low cerebral perfusion state of ischemia.

Ischemia occurs when CBF is too low to supply enough oxygen to support cellular function. As CBF decreases further, a mismatch between oxygen supply and tissue demands occurs. There is an increase in oxygen extraction, and the patient becomes symptomatic. The ischemic threshold (a threshold below which the brain's tissue function fails) is in a CBF range of 23 to 10 mL/100 g/min. When CBF falls to about 20 mL/100 g/min, the EEG flattens; at about 15 mL/100 g/min, cellular edema occurs and electrical activity fails; and below about 10 mL/100 g/min, infarction or irreversible cellular death oc-

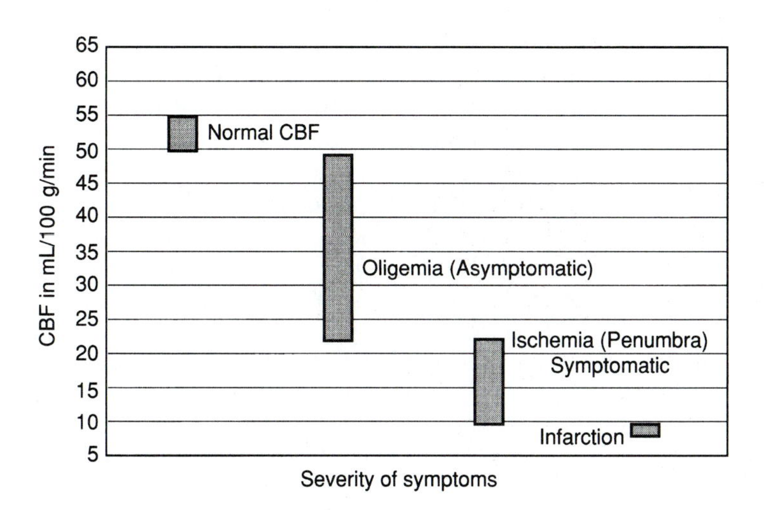

Figure 18–3. Cerebral blood flow thresholds in focal ischemia.

curs, with efflux of potassium into the extracellular spaces and depletion of ATP cellular energy. Within this ischemic range, a therapeutic window exists for reversing ischemia if appropriate therapy is initiated within the first 6 hours (Lenzi et al., 1990). The zone of threatened, collaterally perfused, ischemic brain tissue surrounding the infarct in stroke lesions is called the ischemic **penumbra** (Fig. 18–4). The brain cells in the penumbra remain viable and are capable of responding to therapy within a certain time frame but are functionally depressed due to inadequate perfusion. The ischemic cells within the penumbra can recover function if blood flow is increased above the critical threshold of 15 mL/100 g/min. This would require only small supplements in CBF to the penumbra to prevent infarction and irreversible cellular damage, such as what would be achieved by clearing the airway or improving CPP and avoiding hypotensive episodes during acute stroke. Outside the collaterally perfused areas, a zone of hyperperfusion or perifocal hyperemia may be found where the CBF is in excess of the metabolic needs of the tissue **(luxury perfusion).** Blood flow to reperfused brain often greatly exceeds demands of

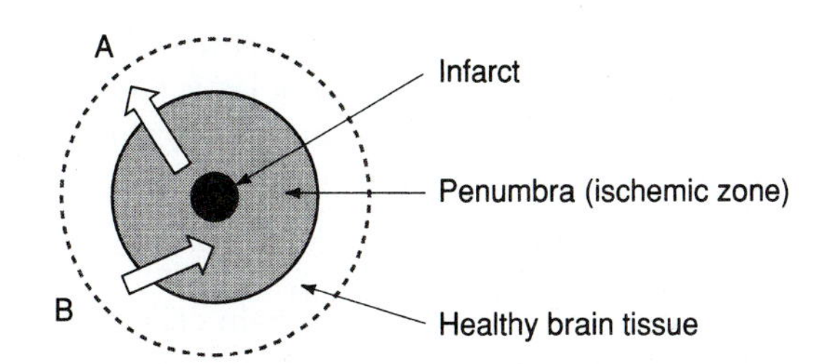

1. Effects of carbon dioxide. Response on cerebral blood flow in the penumbra.
   A. Intracerebral steal. ↑ PCO_2 healthy brain vessels vasodilate and produce shunting of blood away from the penumbra.
   B. Reverse steal. ↓ PCO_2 (hyperventilation) constricts vessels in healthy brain and ↑ cerebral blood flow into penumbra.

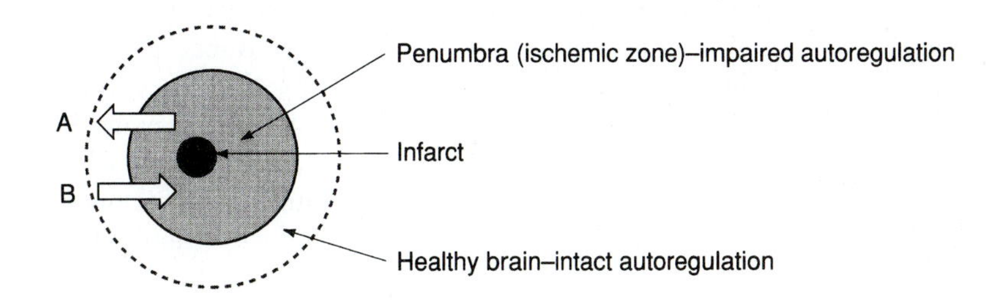

1. Effects of autoregulation on cerebral blood flow to ischemic penumbra.
   A. Decreased blood pressure → vasodilation in healthy brain → ↓ cerebral blood flow to collaterals supplying penumbra.
   B. Increased blood pressure → vasoconstriction in healthy brain → ↑ cerebral blood flow to collaterals supplying penumbra.

Figure 18–4. Effects of autoregulation and carbon dioxide response on cerebral blood flow to the penumbra.

tissue. Reperfusion hyperemia may be beneficial by bringing nutrients to and removing wastes from marginally perfused tissues and deleterious by delivering large amounts of oxygen which may produce potentially damaging free radicals (Paczynski, Hsu, & Diringer, 1995; Davis & Briones, 1998). Luxury perfusion is characterized by impaired autoregulation and a high CBF state owing to the uncoupling of CBF and metabolism. In this state, hypertension would cause further increases in CBF, blood–brain barrier damage, and vasogenic edema.

Diaschisis is a concept used to describe decreased CBF, not only in the ischemic area but also in remote or distant nonischemic brain areas that are functionally depressed. It is believed that the ischemic or infarcted lesion interrupts the afferent impulses connected to the unaffected distant site, decreasing metabolic demand and blood supply in the remote area. Thus, ischemic lesions may decrease CBF in remote areas.

Autoregulation

Autoregulation can be impaired or abolished by extremes in blood pressure, as may occur in strokes, hypoxia, hypercapnia, or trauma. In ischemic brain tissue, autoregulation of brain arterioles is often lost, causing CBF to follow passively the MAP. If the MAP exceeds the autoregulatory limits (MAP of 160 mm Hg) (Davis & Briones, 1998) in adults, overstretching of the delicate cerebral vessels may lead to hemorrhage or rupture of the blood–brain barrier with extravasation of serum proteins (vasogenic brain edema). If blood pressure falls below the lower limits, hypoperfusion leads to brain ischemia, particularly in the collateral circulation of the border zone areas located between the distal boundaries of the major cerebral arteries. In addition, the autoregulatory curve is shifted upward in hypertensive patients so that CBF falls at a higher MAP than normal. It is believed that increasing blood pressure will cause vasoconstriction in healthy brain surrounding the penumbra, thereby increasing CBF to collaterals supplying the penumbra. Conversely, hypotensive episodes will cause vasodilation in healthy brain surrounding the penumbra and reduce blood flow in the collateral vessels supplying the penumbra because autoregulation is impaired in collaterally perfused areas surrounding the ischemic zone as well as in the ischemic zone.

Chemoregulation

In the absence of autoregulation, the cerebral blood vessels may continue to respond to changes in Pa_{CO_2} by maintaining their vasoconstrictor resting tone. When Pa_{CO_2} increases, the normal reactive vessels dilate in healthy brain areas surrounding the ischemic zone and shunt the blood away from the ischemic vasoparalytic areas that have lost both autoregulation and carbon dioxide regulation and are maximally dilated. This is called an **intracerebral steal.** Hypocapnia is achieved through controlled hyperventilation. By lowering Pa_{CO_2}, reactive healthy vessels constrict and enhance CBF into the ischemic, edematous, and acidotic areas of brain, **a reverse steal.** A reverse steal tends to restore pH and normal vasomotion in these areas. This is the basis for mechanically hyperventilating patients with increased ICP. Cerebral blood flow changes by 4 percent for each 1 mm Hg change in Pa_{CO_2} (Wahl & Schilling, 1993). Acute increases in CBF occur when Pa_{CO_2} is less than 40 mm Hg (Davis & Briones, 1998).

Cellular Ischemic Cascade

In focal ischemia (Fig. 18–5), neurons are probably damaged by a cascade of chemical events that begin at the cellular level (Siesjo, 1992a). There are four major cellular ischemic events leading to infarction:

1. Energy pump failure
2. Ionic imbalances
3. Intracellular accumulation of calcium and excessive glutamate release
4. Cellular degradation with irreversible damage

Energy Pump Failure

When the brain's perfusion is impaired, it converts to energy-depleting anaerobic metabolism, and excessive amounts of lactic and pyruvic acids are produced. Any increase in acidity will increase the local tissue hydrogen ion concentration (acidosis) and increase CBF. Brain tissue acidosis results in depressed neuronal function. Consequently, the brain must receive adequate oxygenated blood or brain cells will die within 5 to 10 minutes. The ischemic events that trigger this lethal cascade in strokes are frequently occluded blood vessels that deprive the neurons of oxygen, glucose, and other nutrients. Without oxygen, the cells convert to anaerobic glycolysis, which provides only 2 ATP molecules rather than the 38 ATP molecules that result from normal aerobic metabolism (Ritter & Robertson, 1994). Thus, the high energy reserves for the mitochondrial pump are rapidly depleted leading to cellular pump and energy failure, an increase in lactic acid, and brain acidosis. Adults with hyperglycemia preceding anaerobic metabolism have increased lactic acid production and consequently more brain damage.

Ionic Imbalances

Without ATP energy, the normal ionic gradients (sodium, potassium, calcium, and chloride) and equilibrium across the cell membrane are disrupted between the extracellu-

A. Pump failure, leading to anerobic metabolism, leading to cellular acidosis.

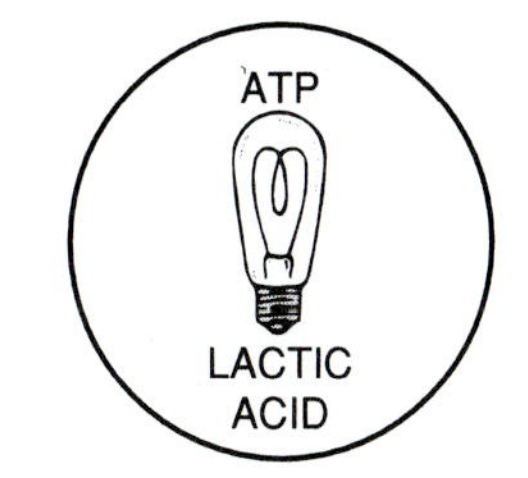

B. Ionic imbalances: cellular edema.

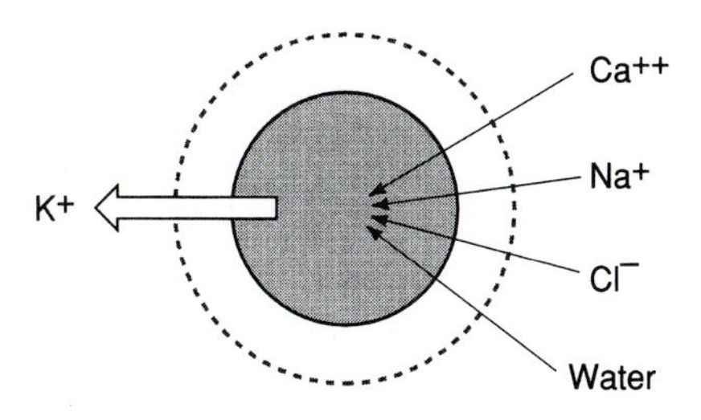

C. Intracellular accumulation of calcium and glutamate's role.

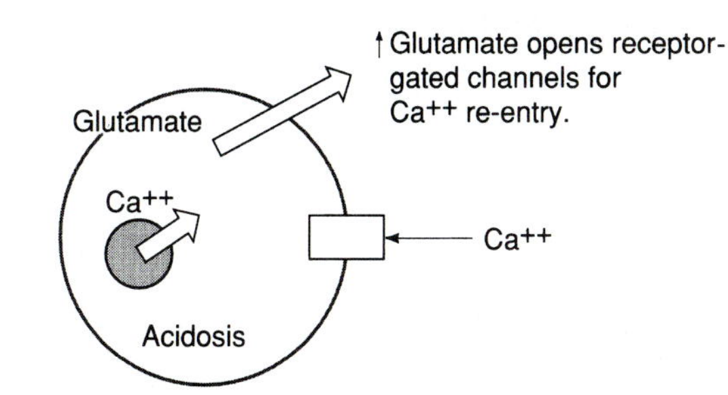

D. Cellular degradation.

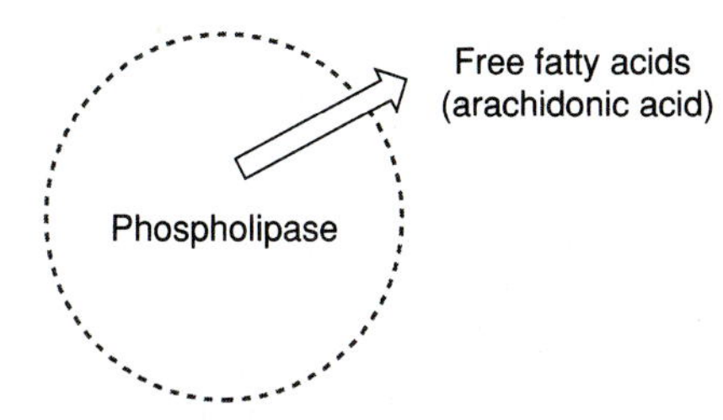

Figure 18–5. The ischemic cascade.

lar fluid (ECF) and intracellular fluid (ICF) spaces. Depolarization follows; the cellular membrane gates open and ionic imbalances result (see Fig. 18–5). Sodium, water, chloride, and calcium move into the cell as potassium moves out into the extracellular space (ECS), causing an ECF volume deficit and hyperkalemia. Intracellularly, the sodium and water accumulate, causing cellular edema; and intracellular free calcium increases. In addition, the acidotic cell facilitates the release of stored calcium ion from its protein-bound state, adding to the intracellular free calcium load. The intracellular accumulation of the free calcium ion is the major culprit in promoting ischemic cell death because it causes vasospasm in the microcirculation, reduces the tissue oxygen supply, and initiates cellular destruction. The ischemic threshold for cellular edema is about 15 mL/100 g/min. At this stage, the ischemia is still reversible.

Intracellular Accumulation of Calcium and Glutamate's Role

As CBF falls below 20 mL/100 g/min, ischemic neurons release excessive amounts of the excitatory neurotransmitter glutamate into the interstitial spaces (see Fig. 18–5) (Zivin & Choi, 1991). Normally, the neurons and glial cells would remove this excess glutamate. The reuptake of glutamate and the other excitatory neurotransmitters released requires energy; because energy is lacking in ischemic cells, the excess remains producing an excitatory toxic effect on the cell (Siesjo, 1992a). Glutamate opens receptor channels located on the cell membrane and triggers the influx of sodium and calcium, providing another route for entry of large amounts of free calcium into the cell. The excess glutamate excites and depolarizes neurons exhausting the reduced energy supply of the ischemic cells in the penumbra and then binds to receptors on neighboring neurons, recruiting them into the ischemic pathway of death if sufficient time elapses (Siesjo, 1992a).

Expression Stage: Cellular Degradation with Irreversible Damage

Finally, irreversible damage occurs when CBF falls below 10 mL/100 g/min (Zivin & Choi, 1991). The excess calcium accelerates cellular degradation by activating the phospholipase and other enzymes, which promote the breakdown of cellular membrane phospholipids releasing free fatty acids (FFAs) (Fig. 18–6) and degrading cellular DNA and its proteins. Free fatty acids have highly toxic metabolites (e.g., arachidonic acid), which accumulate in ischemic tissue and destroy lipids and proteins, major components of the cell membranes.

With cellular membrane destruction, more ECF calcium enters the cell and the deadly cycle continues. Arachidonic acid is catabolized by cyclooxygenase to form endoperoxides (prostaglandins and thromboxane A). It is also catabolized by 5-lipoxygenase to form leukotrienes, compounds that increase membrane permeability and cause edema, potent vasoconstriction of ves-

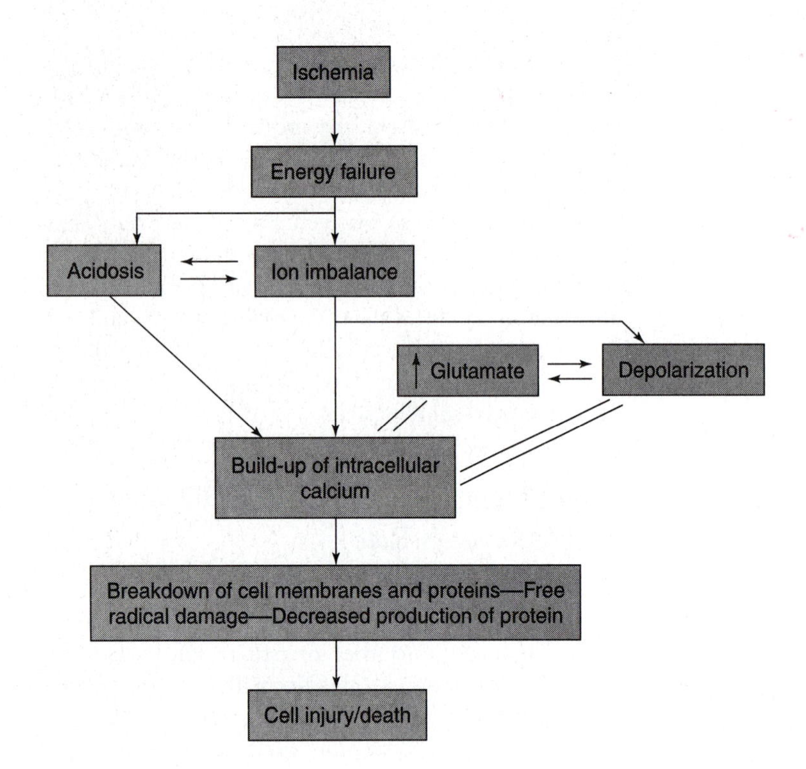

Figure 18–6. Processes contributing to ischemic brain cell injury. *(Source:* Med Strategy—Stroke: Focus on Opportunity, *Evan Dick, Ph.D.)*

sels, and toxic free radical injury. A normal by-product of prostaglandin biosynthesis is the toxic free oxygen radical, which causes direct tissue damage and inhibits the formation of the good prostaglandin, prostacyclin (PGI_2), a potent vasodilator that also protects brain vessels from platelet aggregation. Free radicals populate the unstable penumbra and participate in patterns of injury in reperfused tissues. Under acidic conditions, the release of iron from organic stores greatly enhances free radical production (Paczynski, Hsu, & Diringer, 1995). Normally, the body protects us from free oxygen radicals with endogenous free radical scavengers and enzymes that degrade free radicals such as superoxide dismutase catalase. Thromboxane A_2, a bad prostaglandin, is formed primarily from platelets in the microvessels; it promotes platelet aggregation and vasoconstriction, opposing the action of the protective prostacyclin. A balance normally exists between the two, but in ischemia, an imbalance occurs in favor of thromboxane A_2, allowing it to exert its devastating effects. The net effect of the arachidonic metabolism is an excess generation of superoxide or toxic free radicals, vasoconstriction, platelet aggregation, increased membrane permeability, and edema leading to cellular death (Heiss, 1992). The ischemic threshold of blood flow to induce membrane failure and potassium efflux from the cell is a CBF of about 6 to 8 mL/100 g/min; irreversible cellular death is believed to occur at this perfusion level.

In summary, the ischemic zone (penumbra) lacks autoregulation and, at times, carbon dioxide reactivity. Thus, a state of vasomotor paralysis exists. The penumbra's CBF varies with systemic blood pressure. The effects of vasomotor paralysis are serious in focal ischemia and if untreated lead to acidosis and infarction. The ischemic cascade is triggered by anaerobic metabolism, which leads to energy failure, ionic imbalances between the ECS and ICS, cellular edema, and cellular acidosis. Calcium, sodium, chloride, and water enter the cells and cause cellular edema, a reversible event. Intracellular free calcium levels increase and the calcium overload is exacerbated by the release of the excitatory neurotransmitter glutamate from the ischemic cell. Glutamate not only facilitates more calcium entry into the cell, but also exhausts the limited supply of oxygen from the ischemic cells in the penumbra. Excess glutamate binds to receptors on neighboring healthy neurons, recruiting them into the ischemic pathway and thereby extending the ischemic process (McHugh & Cheek, 1998). Finally, the accumulation of excess free calcium in the cell releases enzymes that destroy the cellular membrane and architecture. A by-product of this degradation is the highly toxic arachidonic acid, which initiates a cascade of lethal cellular events producing toxic free oxygen radicals, platelet aggregators, vasoconstriction, and, ultimately, infarction. Figure 18–6 summarizes this process.

SECTION THREE REVIEW

1. When the brain converts to anaerobic metabolism, which of the following happens?
   A. brain cells become alkalotic
   B. neuronal function becomes excitable
   C. bicarbonate accumulates in the brain
   D. there is excessive production of lactic and pyruvic acid
2. When CBF is subnormal, what compensatory mechanisms occur to maintain normal cerebral oxidative metabolism?
   A. the hemoglobin is increased
   B. there is an increase in the oxygen extraction fraction from the blood
   C. cerebral metabolic demand increases
   D. there is no compensatory mechanism
3. The penumbra in stroke victims
   A. is a zone of viable but nonfunctioning tissue surrounding the infarct zone
   B. is composed of dead brain tissue
   C. is described as having "luxury perfusion"
   D. has a high oxygen extraction ratio
4. Which of the following BEST describes brain cellular ischemia?
   A. it is a CBF between 30 and 50 mL/100 g/min
   B. it is a mismatch between oxygen supply and brain tissue demands
   C. it is a reduction in CBF of 25 percent of normal
   D. its causes are only intracranial
5. Which of the following lists ischemic events from the early to the late stages of focal ischemia?
   A. expression stage, ionic imbalances, energy failure, intracellular calcium accumulation
   B. ionic imbalances, expression stage, energy failure, intracellular calcium accumulation
   C. intracellular calcium accumulation, expression stage, energy failure, ionic imbalances
   D. energy failure, ionic imbalances, intracellular calcium accumulation, expression stage
6. If cerebral autoregulation is impaired in focal brain ischemia (stroke), cerebral perfusion in the penumbra is
   A. increased
   B. oligemic
   C. dependent on systemic blood pressure
   D. the same as in other brain vessels
7. Mrs. Selby, age 40, had an embolic stroke. Her breathing is shallow and her $PaCO_2$ is elevated at 55 mm Hg. This is detrimental to her cerebral perfusion because the
   A. healthy cerebral vessels will dilate and rob the ischemic zones of blood
   B. ischemic zone will get increased perfusion and increased ICP
   C. neurons will become excitable
   D. healthy cerebral vessels will increase CBF into the ischemic zone
8. In the ischemic cascade, which electrolyte is believed to generate the greatest cellular damage when there is an ionic imbalance?
   A. potassium
   B. calcium
   C. sodium
   D. magnesium
9. The cerebral perfusion range, or "therapeutic window," for reversing focal cerebral ischemia within the first 6 hours is
   A. 50 to 40 mL/100 g/min
   B. 40 to 30 mL/100 g/min
   C. 30 to 20 mL/100 g/min
   D. 20 to 10 mL/100 g/min

Answers: 1. D, 2. B, 3. A, 4. B, 5. D, 6. C, 7. A, 8. B, 9. D

SECTION FOUR: Diagnostic Testing

This section discusses the diagnostic methods used for a patient with strokelike symptoms in the high-acuity phase. At the completion of this section, the learner will be able to explain the rationale of the diagnostic tests in the high-acuity phase.

The goals of acute stroke management are to salvage the penumbral zone and prevent the extension of the infarct by improving cerebral perfusion to the ischemic brain area within the first 6 hours of onset of the stroke. Ultimate goals are to enable the patient with a neurologic deficit to achieve his or her highest potential for functional recovery. The management of stroke depends on its cause; therefore, the diagnosis must precede effective therapy during this critical time window. Questions to be resolved prior to treatment are:

- Is it an ischemic or hemorrhagic stroke? If ischemic, is the subtype embolic, evolving, completed, or lacunar?
- Is it a brain stem or hemispheric stroke?
- Is the ischemic arterial occlusion extracranial or intracranial?
- Is the ischemia caused by a carotid atherothrombotic source or a cardiogenic source?

The following tests or procedures should be performed as soon as possible after arrival of the patient. These tests are frequently performed in the emergency department.

- *Urgent noncontrast CT scan:* A CT scan detects acute hemorrhagic stroke in more than 95 percent of patients but is frequently normal in the early hours (24 to 48 hours) after an ischemic stroke (Yatsu, Grotta, & Pettigrew, 1995). Ultrafast MRI technology detects the fresh infarct within 1 hour of stroke onset but is more time consuming.

CT scanning is helpful in diagnosing cerebral hemorrhage. The diagnosis of subarachnoid hemorrhage (SAH) is made by evaluation of the patient's history and presenting symptoms, CT scan, lumbar puncture, and cerebral angiography. A CT scan can detect blood in the subarachnoid space in 96 percent of patients with aneurysm rupture when performed within 48 hours after the rupture but in only 50 percent of patients if performed 7 days after the bleed (Jennett & Lindsay, 1994). If a CT scan is normal but an SAH is suspected, a lumbar puncture is performed to detect any blood in the CSF. Lumbar punctures carry the risk for aneurysmal bleeding and brain herniation in the presence of elevated ICP. When the CT scan is positive, a four-vessel cerebral angiography is done to identify the site of bleeding, to confirm the presence or absence of multiple aneurysms, to detect vasospasm, and to grade the patient clinically (Broderick et al., 1999). Once an aneurysm has been diagnosed, surgery is usually performed within 24 hours unless contraindicated by severe vasospasm, cerebral edema, or medical problems. Magnetic resonance imaging and angiography may replace cerebral angiography in normotensive patients (Broderick et al., 1999).

Additional Tests

- *Lumbar puncture* may be done to detect blood in the CSF if SAH is suspected but not confirmed by CT scan.
- *12-Lead* ECG to detect any arrhythmias or cardiogenic sources of stroke. Precordial echocardiography is done in all stroke patients younger than 45 years (Yatsu, Grotta, & Pettigrew, 1995).
- *Chest x-ray* to rule out cardiogenic sources of stroke.
- *Complete blood count, coagulation profile (platelets, prothrombin time, partial thromboplastin time), fibrinogen, cardiac isoenzymes (CK-MB, troponin)* to detect any cardiovascular abnormalities and establish baselines for therapy.
- *Serum electrolytes and blood glucose levels* to rule out other causes for cerebral deficits. Electrolyte imbalances may be a source of cardiac arrhythmias, whereas a high or low glucose may produce impaired consciousness.
- *ABG levels, drug screen, sedimentation rate, and a serum alcohol level* may be done if indicated by history to detect possible causes of stroke.
- *Cervical Doppler ultrasonography* and *duplex imaging* are emergency noninvasive tests that, if available, are done when carotid disease is suspected.
- *Cerebral angiography* demonstrates stenoses and occlusions of vessels in the head and neck. It is definitive for confirming the cause of aneurysmal SAH and AVMs.

Transcranial Doppler Ultrasonography (TCD)
A noninvasive diagnostic tool, transcranial Doppler (TCD) sonography, has been used to detect the onset and monitor the degree of intracranial vasospasms. Intracranial vasospasms correlate with the amount of blood in the subarachnoid spaces. Mean blood flow velocities in the cerebral arteries are monitored. The narrowed diameter of the spastic artery increases cerebral vascular resistance and blood flow velocity in the affected segment, decreases CBF, and may produce focal cerebral ischemia. Impending ischemia may be predicted by a marked increase in blood flow velocity.

Xenon Clearance
The xenon clearance test is used intermittently to measure regional CBF in patients at risk for vasospasms and complements TCD data by measuring the effect of vasospasm on cerebral perfusion. Cerebral blood flow measurement is important because it detects a fall in CBF long before the development of ischemic symptoms.

Electroencephalography (EEG)
Continuous EEG has been proposed as a more sensitive test than angiogram for impending vasospasms since the presence of focal delta and theta waves appears to correlate with developing vasospasm in patients with SAH. More data are necessary to confirm these findings.

In summary, emergency management for stroke is dependent on the diagnosis of the type of stroke.

SECTION FOUR REVIEW

1. Acute stroke management goals include all of the following EXCEPT

   A. reverse the damage in the infarcted zone
   B. prevent extension of the infarct

C. salvage the penumbral zone
D. restore the patient to his or her potential for functional recovery

2. The critical therapeutic time window to institute care following a stroke according to the National Stroke Association guidelines is
A. 2 hours
B. 6 hours
C. 10 hours
D. 24 hours

3. During the emergency phase, all of the following tests are routinely ordered for all acute stroke patients EXCEPT
A. noncontrast CT scan
B. electrocardiogram (ECG)
C. complete blood count
D. duplex ultrasound

4. The diagnostic test that can distinguish cerebral hemorrhage from infarction during the first hours of stroke onset is
A. duplex ultrasound
B. transcranial Doppler study
C. noncontrast CT scan
D. EEG

Answers: 1. A, 2. B, 3. D, 4. C

SECTION FIVE: Pharmacologic Management of Patients with Ischemic Stroke

This section discusses the pharmacologic management of ischemic stroke patients. At the completion of this section, the learner will be able to describe medications used and their implications for ischemic stroke patients. To understand the physiologic basis of therapy, the learner may need to review the thrombogenesis theory.

The Thrombogenesis Theory

The thrombotic process differs in arteries and veins. Red thrombi usually form in veins with sluggish flow areas and are composed primarily of fibrin, platelets, and red blood cells. They are usually treated with anticoagulants such as heparin and warfarin. White thrombi usually form in damaged arteries with fast-moving streams and irregular surfaces and are composed primarily of platelets. They are usually treated with antiplatelet drugs such as aspirin and ticlopidine (Ticlid) (Benevente & Hart, 1999). Both types of thrombi are treated with newer thrombolytic drugs in emergencies.

In healthy arteries, the endothelium or intima (the inner lining of blood vessels) continuously secretes a protective prostaglandin—prostacyclin (PGI_2)—a powerful vasodilator that helps to prevent clotting in normal blood flow by inhibiting platelet aggregation in the intact vessel. Under this endothelial lining, collagen is normally present. When endothelial injury of the blood vessel occurs, as can happen in hypertensive, high-flow turbulent areas, especially at bifurcations (branchings) of blood vessels, the irregular surfaces of the subendothelium are exposed to circulating blood and attract circulating platelets, which adhere to the damaged intima. These platelets release adenosine phosphate, which causes platelets to aggregate and plug the diseased or damaged endothelium. A white, unstable platelet thrombus forms and may occlude the vessel lumen in areas. Thromboxane A_2, a harmful prostaglandin, powerful vasoconstrictor, and promoter of platelet aggregation, is released primarily by the aggregating platelets, which activate the clotting cascade by converting prothrombin to thrombin. Thrombin stimulates more platelet aggregation and catalyzes reactions that convert fibrinogen to fibrin. Strands of fibrin act to trap platelets, red blood cells, and circulating plasma proteins, resulting in clot formation in this calcium-dependent process. A red thrombus forms around the white thrombus stabilized by a few fibrin threads. Mixed white and red thrombi have been found at occluded arterial sites in stroke patients (Macabasco & Hickman, 1995).

Transient Ischemic Attacks and Ischemic Stroke

Treatment options available for patients with TIAs and ischemic strokes include anticoagulant and antiplatelet drug therapy and carotid endarterectomy. The aims of acute stroke therapy are to improve perfusion of ischemic tissue and to ameliorate ischemic injury with neuroprotective therapy (Fisher, 1995).

Anticoagulant Therapy

Tissue Plasminogen Activator

Use of t-PA within 3 hours of symptoms improves long-term functional outcome. However, 1 in 15 patients suffer brain hemorrhage as a side effect. Strict criteria must be followed to determine patient eligibility (Table 18–5).

Streptokinase

Streptokinase has not been shown to be as effective as t-PA. This agent is still being investigated in research trials.

TABLE 18–5. CRITERIA FOR THROMBOLYSIS OF PATIENTS WITH ACUTE ISCHEMIC STROKE USING TISSUE PLASMINOGEN ACTIVATOR

Inclusion criteria
Age > 18 years
Clinical diagnosis of ischemic stroke, with onset of symptoms within 3 hours of initiation of treatment
Noncontrast CT scan with no evidence of hemorrhage

Exclusion criteria
History
- Stroke or head trauma in previous 3 months
- History of intracranial hemorrhage that may increase risk of recurrent hemorrhage
- Major surgery or other serious trauma in previous 14 days
- Gastrointestinal or genitourinary bleeding in previous 21 days
- Arterial puncture in previous 7 days
- Pregnant or lactating patient

Clinical findings
- Rapidly improving stroke symptoms
- Seizure at onset of stroke
- Symptoms suggestive of subarachnoid hemorrhage, even if CT scan is normal
- Persistent systolic pressure > 185 mm Hg or diastolic pressure > 110 mm Hg, or patient is requiring aggressive therapy to control blood pressure
- Clinical presentation consistent with acute myocardial infarction or postmyocardial infarction pericarditis requires cardiologic evaluation before treatment

Imaging results
- CT scan with evidence of hemorrhage
- CT scan with evidence of hypodensity and/or effacement of cerebral sulci in more than one third of middle cerebral artery territory

Laboratory findings
- Glucose level < 50 mg/dL (2.8 mmol/L) or > 400 mg/dL (22.2 mmol/L)
- Platelet count < 100,000/mm^3 (100 × 10^9/L)
- Patient is taking warfarin and has abnormal international normalized ratio
- Patient has received heparin within 48 hours, and partial thromboplastin time is elevated

Information from Adams, H.P., Brott, T.G., Furlan, A.I., Gomez, C.R., et al. (1996). Guidelines for thrombolytic therapy for acute stroke: a supplement to the guidelines for the management of patients with acute ischemic stroke. A statement for healthcare professionals from a Special Writing Group of the Stroke Council, American Heart Association. Circulation *94:1167–1174.*

Heparin

Patients with TIAs within the past few hours have a high risk for recurrence if they have: a high-grade stenosis; an intra-arterial thrombus; been receiving antiplatelet therapy; a cardioembolic source; or increasingly frequent attacks. For these patients, anticoagulation may be initiated with short-term heparin therapy followed by warfarin (Coumadin) therapy. Heparin is used acutely in neurologically unstable patients (with large-vessel thrombosis) to limit damage; in patients at high risk for recurrent stroke (those with multiple TIAs, high-grade carotid stenosis, and cardiac disease); and in cardioembolic stroke patients, provided the anticoagulant therapy is withheld for 3 to 4 days after a major infarct (these infarcts often develop spontaneous hemorrhagic changes that can be worsened by heparin therapy). Recently the use of heparin has become controversial. Heparin has not been shown to improve neurologic outcome and increases the risk of bleeding (Benevente & Hart, 1999).

Heparin potentiates the effects of antithrombin and interrupts the clotting process by preventing platelet aggregation and thrombus formation. It does not dissolve existing clots because it does not have fibrinolytic action. Heparin is given intravenously or subcutaneously.

Coumadin (Warfarin)

Warfarin is a long-term anticoagulant and vitamin K antagonist and requires 4 to 6 days to achieve a steady state for prothrombin time (PT) values. As heparin therapy is being tapered, warfarin (Coumadin) is gradually administered in doses that maintain the prothrombin time between 1.2 and 1.5 times the patient's control value or an INR of 2 to 3 (Kistler, Ropper, & Martin, 1994). Anticoagulant therapy is avoided in patients with intraparenchymal bleeding, uncontrolled hypertension, and embolic infarctions that show hemorrhagic changes on an early CT scan (McDowell, Brott, & Goldstein, 1993).

Antiplatelet Therapy

Antiplatelet therapy commonly includes aspirin, ticlopidine (Ticlid), and clopidogrel (Plavix). Aspirin and ticlopidine (Ticlid) are believed to reduce stroke risk by only 20 to 30 percent following TIAs. Aspirin in low doses inhibits vitamin K–dependent clotting factors; platelet formation of thromboxane A_2; and the formation of the protective prostaglandin, prostacyclin, a vasodilator. Aspirin is prescribed in low doses of 300 mg or less daily, and the effects are almost immediate. The optimal dose for aspirin is yet to be firmly established (Schretzman, 1999). In acute stroke, administration of aspirin between 12 and 24 hours after symptom onset resulted in less mortality and disability (Benevente & Hart, 1999). Aspirin and ticlopidine (Ticlid) are used in preventive therapy of TIAs and ischemic strokes. Ticlopidine (Ticlid) is a platelet antagonist that does not inhibit the protective prostaglandin, prostacyclin, so it prolongs bleeding time. Ticlopidine (Ticlid) is more effective than aspirin, but its full effects may take several days. It also has more severe side effects than aspirin, including reversible leukopenia, diarrhea, skin rash, thrombocytopenia, and hypercholesterolemia (Yatsu, Grotta, & Pettigrew, 1995; Kistler, Ropper, & Martin, 1994). When aspirin is contraindicated or fails, ticlopidine (Ticlid) may be prescribed, particularly for persons who have had either a previous stroke or a TIA. Plavix, a new antiplatelet agent, has been effective in patients with a history of atherosclerotic heart disease. Plavix has demonstrated the same ability as aspirin to prevent strokes and myocardial infarction. However, it is more expensive than aspirin. Plavix may perform better than aspirin if the patient has peripheral arterial disease (Gorelick, Born, & D'Agostino, 1999).

When administering these anticoagulants and antiplatelet aggregating drugs, nurses must monitor the patient's PT, PTT, and INR for therapeutic levels and be alert for any occult bleeding such as bruising, petechiae, hematuria, gastrointestinal bleeding, delayed clotting, and any drug interactions that alter PT. For example, PT can be prolonged by cimetidine, amiodarone, and, possibly, phenytoin (Dilantin) or shortened by carbamazepine, barbiturates, cholestyramine, and penicillin (Yatsu, Grotta, & Pettigrew, 1995). In addition, the nurse must avoid unnecessary trauma such as pumping blood pressure cuffs too high or needle sticks. When the latter is unavoidable, the use of smaller needles as well as gentle handling of the patient is indicated. Should bleeding occur while the patient is taking anticoagulants, protamine sulfate may be given to reverse the effects of heparin, or vitamin K to reverse the effects of warfarin (Coumadin).

In the event of seizures, a full loading dose of phenytoin (Dilantin) is initiated and serum levels are kept within 10 to 20 mg/dL for control. The increased metabolic demands for oxygen created by seizures would be disastrous and further compromise the ischemic brain of its energy needs.

Blood Pressure

For ischemic strokes, elevations in blood pressure in the absence of low cardiac output or myocardial infarction are not treated unless the systolic pressure is > 230 mm Hg or the diastolic pressure is > 120 mm Hg on repeated measurements obtained 20 minutes apart (Benevente & Hart, 1999). Sodium nitroprusside (Nipride) 3 mg/kg/min may be used with diastolic pressure > 140 mm Hg (Benevente & Hart, 1999). The increased blood pressure may be needed to perfuse the brain because of loss of autoregulation poststroke. Elevated blood pressure may prevent ischemic areas from becoming infarcted. If marked hypertension exists, labetalol (Normodyne) 10 mg IV is used every 10 minutes up to the 160 mg maximum dose to reduce the blood pressure.

Anticonvulsants

Compared with ischemic strokes, hemorrhage-related seizures usually occur very early, are multiple, and are more likely to recur (Bladin & Willmore, 1994). Seizure prophylaxis is necessary to avoid seizure-induced hypertension and ischemia. A loading dose of 15 to 18 mg/kg of phenytoin followed by a maintenance dose of approximately 300 to 400 mg daily is usually prescribed to maintain serum levels between 14 and 23 mg/mL. Anticonvulsant therapy may be continued for up to 1 month and then tapered if there is no evidence of seizures (Broderick et al., 1999).

Osmotic Agents and Diuretics

Mannitol and Lasix improve cerebral perfusion and are given, when the blood–brain barrier is intact, to combat cellular edema. Avoidance of hyperglycemia (which in the absence of oxygen increases acidosis) has been recommended with the use of nondextrose IV solutions. Hyperglycemia > 150 mg/dL should be treated (Benevente & Hart, 1999).

Neuroprotective Therapy

Neuroprotective therapy, a new concept in stroke management, is aimed at protecting vulnerable brain tissue from further injury. The goal is to increase the tolerance of neurons to ischemia. It may be used as short-term, prolonged, or concomitant therapy. Neuroprotective agents include calcium antagonists, glutamate antagonists, and antioxidants (Fisher, 1995). Other neuroprotective agents such as Dilantin, Decadron, mannitol, and barbiturates stabilize cellular membranes, improve CBF, or decrease metabolic need for oxygen (Weaver, 1995).

Hypothermia and barbiturates may be neuroprotective by reducing metabolic rate and oxygen consumption, thus lowering oxygen demands to match the diminished blood supply. Barbiturates also increase vascular resistance in healthy areas of brain and shunt blood to the ischemic areas. To date, none of these agents have been shown to be beneficial but are still under investigation.

Experimental Therapies

Experimental therapies were derived because of evidence that widespread neuronal loss is progressive and continues in vulnerable brain regions for months to years after the precipitating event. These therapies modify postevent neurochemical and cellular processes to promote functional recovery.

The use of anticholinergic drugs (e.g., scopolamine) immediately postevent may restore reflexive and motor function while cholinomimetic therapy (e.g., suritozole) improves cognitive function. Because these agents diametrically oppose each other, research is being conducted to determine timing of administration (McIntosh, Juhler, & Wieloch, 1998).

Anti-inflammatory drugs may also be useful in stopping the infiltration of polymorphonuclear leukocytes and release of inflammatory mediators (e.g., cytokines). Both leukocytes and cytokines contribute to post- stroke brain swelling.

Calpain inhibitors may be useful in decreasing intracellular calcium levels and protein breakdown. Calpain is a protease located throughout the brain.

High-dose methylprednisolone and other 21-amino steroid compounds that lack glucocorticoid activity while maintaining the ability to protect cell membranes from breakdown may be used more frequently in the future.

The increased extracellular glutamate that occurs postbrain injury increases intracellular calcium and ultimately cell membrane breakdown and cell death. Glutamate antagonists to date have not been effective in improving functional outcome. Neurotrophic or growth factor has promise in accelerating motor recovery and decreasing cognitive deficits postbrain injury (McIntosh, Juhler, & Wieloch, 1998).

In summary, cerebral perfusion can be improved by decreasing platelet aggregation and removing arterial obstruction (thrombolytic therapy). Aspirin and t-PA should be given early in the management of stroke patients. Moderately elevated blood pressure assists in perfusion and prevents infarction.

SECTION FIVE REVIEW

1. Which of the following is NOT true about heparin?
   A. it is an anticoagulant
   B. its use improves functional outcome in stroke patients
   C. it may be used in conjunction with Coumadin (warfarin)
   D. it may cause bleeding
2. Mrs. Georgina Bledsoe, age 70, was placed on warfarin therapy for stroke prevention. She is admitted to the emergency department with tarry black stools and multiple petechiae. The drug most likely to be prescribed is
   A. protamine sulfate
   B. IV plasmanate
   C. vitamin K
   D. vitamin C
3. Mrs. Jasper, age 82, was admitted with the diagnosis of an ischemic stroke. Her blood pressure was 190/100 mm Hg 2 hours after onset of her stroke. Management would be to
   A. give her labetalol 10 mg to reduce the blood pressure
   B. do nothing, monitor the blood pressure every 2 hours, and place her on bed rest
   C. treat the blood pressure to reduce it below 140/100 mm Hg and place her on bed rest
   D. place her on a Nipride drip to maintain her blood pressure between 140/90 and 160/95 mm Hg
4. The protective substance in healthy blood vessels that prevents clotting and is a potent vasodilator is
   A. prostaglandin F (PGF)
   B. thromboxane A_2
   C. platelet-activating factor
   D. leukotrienes
5. Mr. Sallee is admitted with acute onset of seizures, change in level of consciousness (LOC), and numbness of his right leg. Mr. Sallee is NOT a candidate for t-PA because of
   A. his age
   B. seizures
   C. his LOC
   D. numbness of his right leg
6. Ms. Baxter was started on Ticlid 250 mg bid PO to reduce her chance of a recurrent stroke. The nurse should stress in Ms. Baxter's discharge instructions that she should
   A. take Ticlid with milk
   B. have weekly monitoring of her PT and INR
   C. have a CBC done in about 3 weeks
   D. take it at the same time each day

Answers: 1. B, 2. A, 3. B, 4. A, 5. B, 6. C

SECTION SIX: Surgical Management of Stroke

At the completion of this section, the learner will be able to explain when surgery is indicated for a stroke patient.

The goals of surgical management are to (1) remove as much blood clot as possible with the least amount of brain injury; (2) treat the underlying cause of hemorrhage such as aneurysm, AV malformation, ruptured vessel; and (3) prevent complications of intracerebral hemorrhage, such as hydrocephalus, and mass effect due to ischemic swelling secondary to a clot.

Carotid Endarterectomy

There is great debate about the effectiveness of carotid endarterectomy. Data from the North American Symptomatic Carotid Endarterectomy Trial over 10 years indicate that only a small number of patients benefit from this procedure (Barnett et al., 2000). Even with major blockages of the carotid arteries (70 to 99 percent), when a stroke occurs it is frequently due to blockage in a different artery than the carotids or from nonvalvular atrial fibrillation. Strokes arising from these other sources are not likely to be prevented with carotid endarterectomy. Before surgery is attempted, the patient should be examined for other potential causes of stroke that can be treated with different means.

Cerebral Angioplasty

Angioplasty has been successfully used to reverse neurologic deficits due to atherosclerotic lesions of the cerebral arteries and vasospasm (Davis, 1998). Indications for angioplasty are angiographic evidence of severe vasospasms that cause more than 50 percent luminal narrowing; a progressive neurologic ischemic deficit; and no evidence of recent cerebral infarction on CT scan. Angioplasty utilizes a balloon catheter endovascularly to mechanically dilate vasospastic vessels. Microballoon catheters are introduced via the femoral artery and directed to the major arteries at the base of the brain. Endovascular dilations using intra-arterial papaverine infusions have also been used to treat vasospasm successfully and are promising experimental therapies. Cerebral angioplasty carries the risks of intracerebral hemorrhage, injury to the vessel wall, and distal embolization. Results from this therapy are encouraging.

Following cerebral angioplasty, the patient is returned to the intensive care unit (ICU), and continuous nursing assessments for neurologic and vital sign changes are done at least every hour or more frequently until the patient is neurovascularly stable.

Evacuation of Hematomas: Primary Intracerebral Hemorrhage

Surgical removal of the hematoma is promising if done early, but there is no definitive evidence of the value of early evacuation of deep PICH. The patient's level of consciousness and the size of the hematoma are critical for appropriate management. Surgery is not usually done for awake patients with small hematomas (< 3 cm in diameter) because these patients usually recover with conservative management. Awake patients with hematomas > 3 cm are the best candidates for surgery (McDowell, Brott, & Goldstein, 1993). More trials are needed to support these approaches. Hematomas > 3 cm in patients with a decrease in levels of consciousness are surgically evacuated (Minematsu & Yamaguchi, 1995). Endoscopic evacuation of smaller hematomas can be conducted with no change in outcomes as compared with open surgical removal (Broderick et al., 1999).

As with other emergency bleeding, correcting airway, breathing, and circulation problems are priorities. If signs of acute bleeding are detected in the form of increased ICP, a prompt neurosurgical consultation is obtained. Careful blood pressure control is critical for patients with PICH. Unlike with ischemic stroke, patients with PICH are treated to maintain MAP of 130 mm Hg and CPP > 70 mm Hg. Blood pressure should not be reduced unless the systolic pressure is > 180 mm Hg or the diastolic pressure is > 105 mm Hg on two repeated checks made at 20-minute intervals. Labetalol, esmolol, enalapril, diltiazem, or verapamil may be given.

Cerebellar Hemorrhage and Infarction

Cerebellar lesions are critical because a hemorrhage or infarction can rapidly become life threatening by compromising the brain stem. Emergency surgery is indicated for cerebellar infarction or hemorrhage with clinical evidence of brain stem compression and increased ICP such as decreasing level of consciousness, restlessness, or cranial nerve palsies. The size of the hemorrhage or infarction is a critical variable in management. Patients with large hemorrhages or infarctions are more likely to have brain stem compression and urgent need for surgery. Patients with small cerebellar hemorrhages or infarctions, with no signs of increased ICP, can be managed with careful observation (McDowell, Brott, & Goldstein, 1993). Patients who are in the Hunt and Hess Grades 1, 2, or 3 are candidates for immediate surgery if they have SAH with surgically accessible aneurysms and no contraindications to surgery (i.e., no swollen brain or minimal or absent vasospasms) (Table 18–6). Many neurosurgeons are opting for early surgery (within the first 72 hours) for good-risk patients to remove periarterial blood, which produces vasospasms; to prevent aneurysm rebleeding; to eliminate the need for antihypertensive or antifibrinolytic therapy; and to avoid the risks of prolonged bed rest and hospitalization (Laumer et al., 1993). Patients with a Hunt and Hess Grade of 4 or 5 are poor risks for surgery unless they have hydrocephalus or an intracerebral hematoma, which would warrant decompressive surgery. Aneurysm clipping, trapping, or reinforcement by wrapping is the surgical therapy. If the risk of surgery is high, endovascular occlusion or obliteration of the aneurysm is attempted. Patients with a GCS score of ≤ 4 may be treated medically with massive PICH since they usually do not benefit from surgery and have extremely poor functional outcome if they live.

TABLE 18–6. CLINICAL GRADES FOR SAH

Grade 1	Asymptomatic or minimum headache or stiff neck
Grade 2	More severe headache, stiff neck, photophobia, cranial nerve involvement
Grade 3	Drowsy or confused, may have mild hemiparesis
Grade 4	Deeply stuporous, may have moderate to severe hemiparesis, early decerebrate signs
Grade 5	Deeply comatose

Adapted from Hunt, W.E., & Hess, R.M. (1968). Surgical risk as related to time of intervention in the repair of intracranial aneurysms. J Neurosurg *28:14–20.*

Ventricular CSF Drainage or Shunting

If hydrocephalus is accompanied by a decrease in level of consciousness or progressive neurologic deficit, ventricular CSF drainage or shunting is indicated. In the presence of raised ICP, the CPP is maintained at 70 or above. Diuretics are avoided because they lower intravascular volume and CPP. Placing a ventricular drain may allow for drainage and aspiration of a hematoma. Urokinase (6,000 U) is administered into the catheter. In cases of acute closed head injury, a single dose of t-PA has been injected with good results. The t-PA dissolves the clot, allows for drainage of blood, and reduces hydrocephalus and ischemia by preventing obstruction of drainage (Grabb, 1998).

In summary, surgery may be indicated for stroke patients to remove a blood clot, to treat the underlying cause of the hemorrhage, or to prevent complications of a hemorrhage.

SECTION SIX REVIEW

1. The two criteria used to determine if primary intercerebral hematomas are managed surgically are
   - **A.** pupil size and presence of seizures
   - **B.** hemiparesis and incontinence
   - **C.** LOC and size of the hematoma
   - **D.** hypertension and breathing patterns
2. Cerebral angioplasties are usually performed on patients with
   - **A.** angiographic evidence of severe vasospasms
   - **B.** a stable stroke
   - **C.** recent evidence of cerebral infarction on CT scan
   - **D.** lacunar stroke
3. All of the following may be used to treat hydrocephalus secondary to cerebral edema EXCEPT
   - **A.** t-PA
   - **B.** ventricular device
   - **C.** ventricular shunt
   - **D.** diuretics

Answers: 1. C, 2. A, 3. D

SECTION SEVEN: The Focused Assessment for Acute Stroke Patients

This section discusses the focused nursing assessment for acute stroke patients. At the completion of this section, the reader will be able to explain the focused clinical assessment of the acute stroke patient and identify from the assessment findings those that are life threatening and require nursing interventions.

Past Medical History

The past medical history is important in identifying the cause of stroke and establishing an early diagnosis. A brief history, preferably obtained from an eyewitness of the attack, can establish the time and mode of symptom onset. Questions to ask are:

1. When and how did the onset of the brain attack occur?
2. Was it during sleep, upon awakening, or during activity? Strokes that occur early in the morning or upon awakening suggest an ischemic origin.
3. Was it sudden or gradual? A sudden stroke suggests an embolic source or subarachnoid hemorrhage.
4. Is the stroke progressive and have the symptoms intensified (stroke-in-evolution [SIE])?
5. Is there a history of similar attacks (thrombotic) or different attacks (embolic)?
6. How long did they last (a transient ischemic attack [TIA] or reversible ischemic neurologic deficit [RIND])?
7. Does the patient have any cardiac disease, chest pain, or palpitations (cardiogenic origin)?
8. Is there a history of seizures, head trauma, previous strokes, or vomiting (National Stroke Association, 1995)?
9. Is the patient hypertensive and compliant with medications?

Risk factors such as hypotension or hypertension, diabetes mellitus, infection, smoking, and cardiac diseases usually support the diagnosis of ischemic stroke. Hypertension, severe headaches, neck stiffness or nuchal rigidity, and photophobia suggest a hemorrhagic stroke and the threat of increasing intracranial pressure (ICP). Clues to intracranial hemorrhage are based on the presence of at least one of the following: coma on arrival (a poor prognostic sign), vomiting, severe headache, warfarin therapy, systolic blood pressure greater than 220 mm Hg, and blood glucose level greater than 170 mg/dL in a nondiabetic patient (Goldstein & Matcher, 1994). The illicit use of drugs, excessive alcohol consumption, noncompliance with anticonvulsant medications, poor control of diabetes, and use of over-the-counter medications such as aspirin (hemorrhagic) are all useful data to assist in the diagnosis of the stroke subtype. Hyperglycemia and hypoglycemia can cause decreased LOCs that mimic stroke symptoms.

Focused Physical Examination

A focused clinical assessment of the patient is important to establish a baseline and to assist in diagnosis and prognosis in terms of survival and functional recovery. When a stroke is suspected, the ABCs (airway, breathing, and circulation) are assessed. Impaired airway clearance may result from hemiplegia, dysphagia, a weak cough reflex, and immobility. This places the stroke patient at high risk for hypoxemia, pneumonia, and aspiration, major concerns in the care of the acute stroke patient. Adequate ventilation is necessary to prevent further focal ischemia in the penumbral zone of the brain. At the time of initial contact, the patient is examined for airway patency, clear breath sounds, and adequacy of breathing. Obstructed airways must be identified and corrected by suctioning or positioning, or with intubation. Supplemental oxygen, 2 to 3 L nasally, is given during transport and continued to protect the ischemic neurons. Patients with pneumonia, pulmonary edema, or chronic obstructive pulmonary disease in addition to their strokes require the supplemental oxygen and close monitoring of ABGs. Continuous monitoring of breath sounds, breathing patterns, oxygen saturation, color, and ABGs is important. The patient should be assessed for the ability to handle secretions. Suction equipment should be available at the bedside for the patient who is comatose with brain edema, increased ICP, and respiratory compromise and may require intubation and controlled mechanical hyperventilation.

The acute stroke patient may present with an ineffective breathing pattern because of decreased level of responsiveness, aspiration, loss of protective reflexes, or a decrease in respiratory movements on the affected side. With inadequate ventilation, a buildup in carbon dioxide (hypercapnia) occurs, causing cerebral vasodilation in healthy brain areas, thus robbing blood from the penumbra and contributing to brain acidosis and extension of the infarct. In addition, vasodilation contributes to an increase in ICP, which can be detected with abnormal patterns of breathing such as Cheyne–Stokes. To prevent hypercapnia, the nurse should observe the rate and rhythm of breathing, the color of mucous membranes, and the level of consciousness and monitor the ABG results and oxygen saturation.

Cardiovascular assessment includes monitoring vital signs (particularly the blood pressure and heart rate) hourly or more frequently until the patient is stable. The heart is auscultated for dysrhythmias. Peripheral and carotid pulses are monitored. The nurse should examine the patient's head for signs of trauma, infection, or neck stiffness, and inquire about photophobia.

When the patient is neurologically unstable, neurologic checks, consisting of the Glasgow Coma Scale and selective cranial nerve assessment, may be used. Eye opening reflects wakefulness and level of responsiveness. If the patient is awake, the probability of a hemispheric stroke is high. If there is lid ptosis and cranial nerve III (oculomotor) is involved, a posterior stroke may have occurred. **Contralateral** hemiparesis involving the face and limbs is usually indicative of a hemispheric (anterior or carotid) stroke. The nurse should note extremity position and assess hand grips, arm drifts, or leg pushes for strength. The tone **(flaccidity or spasticity)** of the extremities should be noted. The nurse should detect incoherency, impropriety of speech content, and fluency of speech as well as orientation and the ability to follow commands. Loss of consciousness should raise suspicion of a posterior (vertebrobasilar) stroke or a bilateral hemispheric stroke. During the rapid physical assessment, the nurse must be sensitive to cognitive and perceptual–visual–spatial deficits. Confrontation testing of the eyes can expose a **homonymous hemianopsia.** Sensitivity to patient behavior manifesting neglect of the left body and space or poor judgment choices can be detected when the nurse is alerted to the possibility. Unusual patient behavior can be verified by the family's report of the patient's premorbid behavior, education, and occupation.

Cranial nerve abnormalities (III to XII) usually mean brain stem involvement or a vertebrobasilar stroke (Table 18–7). Cranial nerve assessment will assist the nurse to establish a baseline against which to compare the patient's progress and alert the nurse to potential problems of eating or aspiration. For example, should a problem occur with impaired corneal reflexes or dysarthria (slurred speech), the nurse should be alerted to a high risk for swallowing problems because of the proximity of cranial nerves IX (glossopharyngeal) and X (vagus) in the medulla (Bates, Bickley, & Hoekelman, 1995).

A 15-item neurologic scale was developed for assessment of acute stroke patients in clinical trials by Brott and colleagues in 1989 (Table 18–8). This scale tests for the presence of neurologic signs in the distribution of each of the major arteries of the brain. Using this scale, nurses can complete an assessment in about 7 minutes, thus rapidly monitoring acutely ill stroke patients. A value of zero is normal for all parameters; the higher the score, the greater the patient's neurologic deficits. Each item is rated independently. The examiner must use his or her judgment for items 14 and 15. Item 14 has three options: same (a change of 0–1 scale points); better (an improvement of 2 or more scale points); and worse (a deterioration of 2 or more scale points) (Brott, Adams, & Olinger, 1989). The National Institutes of Health assessment scale is a modification of this scale (Wityk et al., 1994).

TABLE 18–7. THE CRANIAL NERVES

NERVE	NUCLEI	TYPE	SITE	FUNCTION	TEST
I	Olfactory	Sensory	Anterior temporal cortex	Smell Perception/interpretation of smell	Test each nare for smell with soap
II	Optic	Sensory	Occipital lobes	Visual acuity Peripheral vision Perception/interpretation of visual objects Pupillary light and consensual (afferent limb of reflex arc)	Jaeger card; newspaper at 14" Confrontation testing Ask to identify familiar objects Pupillary light (afferent limb)
III	Oculomotor	Motor and autonomic	Midbrain	Eye movements; elevation of upper eyelid Superior, inferior, medial recti, and inferior oblique eye muscles Pupillary constriction; accommodation	III, IV, and VI tested together: test eye movements in all directions of gaze Observe for ptosis Pupillary light reflex (efferent limb)
IV	Trochlear	Motor	Midbrain	Superior oblique eye muscle; downward and lateral eye movements	III, IV, and VI tested together in all directions of gaze
V	Trigeminal	Sensory/motor	Pons	General sensation to face via three branches: Ophthalmic: cornea Maxillary: mucosa of nose Mandibular: mucosa of mouth Mastication: jaw clenching and lateral jaw movements	Pin, cotton for light touch to face along three branch sites Check corneal reflex (afferent limb) with wisp of cotton Palpate jaw muscles when jaws are clamped together; push jaws against resistance of hand
VI	Abducens	Motor	Pons	Lateral rectus eye muscle Involved in horizontal gaze	III, IV, and VI tested together in all directions of gaze
VII	Facial	Motor/sensory/ autonomic	Pons	Facial expression Taste (sweet and salty) on anterior two thirds of tongue Secretion of saliva and tears	Ask to wrinkle forehead, frown, smile; note asymmetry Blink reflex (efferent limb) Place sugar or salt on anterior two thirds of tongue Note excessive secretions
VIII	Vestibulocochlear (acoustic)	Sensory	Pons/medulla	Hearing Equilibrium	Whisper test or fingers rubbing near ears Special equipment needed; note balance
IX	Glossopharyngeal	Sensory/motor/ autonomic	Medulla	Taste (sour and bitter) posterior third of tongue General sensations from external ear and surrounding area Mucosa of pharynx and soft palate Pain and temperature involved in reflex control of blood pressure and respirations Swallowing and gag reflex (afferent limb) Phonation Salivary secretions	IX and X are tested together Touch each side of pharynx: gag reflex Palatal reflex: stroke each side of uvula—side touched rises Note speech Note drooling
X	Vagus	Sensory/motor/ autonomic	Medulla	General sensations from skin surrounding ear; pain and temperature Sensory from pharynx, larynx, thoracic, and abdominal visceral Swallowing, cough, and gag reflexes (efferent limb) Regulation of smooth and cardiac muscle and glands; carotid reflex	IX and X are tested together; see above for testing gag and swallowing reflexes Note effectiveness of cough
XI	Accessory	Motor	Medulla/cervical cord	Swallowing and control of larynx Movement of head and shoulders	Involved in swallowing reflex (see above) Have patient shrug shoulders against resistance and turn head against resistance. Note strength of trapezius and sternocleidomastoid muscles
XII	Hypoglossal	Motor	Medulla	Movement of tongue necessary for swallowing and phonation	With tongue protrusion, note any lateral deviation, tremor, or atrophy

From Bates, B., Bickley, L.S., & Hoekelman, R.A. (1995). A guide to physical examination and history taking, *6th ed. Philadelphia: J.B. Lippincott; and Fitzgerald, M.J.T. (1992).* Neuroanatomy: Basic and clinical, *2nd ed. Philadelphia: Bailliere-Tindall.*

TABLE 18–8. STROKE SCALE

1. a. Level of consciousness	Alert	0
	Drowsy	1
	Stuporous	2
	Coma	3
b. LOC questions	Answers both correctly	0
	Answers one correctly	1
	Incorrect	2
c. LOC commands	Obeys both correctly	0
	Obeys one correctly	1
	Incorrect	2
2. Pupillary response	Both reactive	0
	One reactive	1
	Neither reactive	2
3. Best gaze	Normal	0
	Partial gaze palsy	1
	Forced deviation	2
4. Best visual	No visual loss	0
	Partial hemianopia	1
	Complete hemianopia	2
5. Facial palsy	Normal	0
	Minor	1
	Partial	2
	Complete	3
6. Best motor arm	No drift	0
	Drift	1
	Can't resist gravity	2
	No effort against gravity	3
7. Best motor leg	No drift	0
	Drift	1
	Can't resist gravity	2
	No effort against gravity	3
8. Plantar reflex	Normal	0
	Equivocal	1
	Extensor	2
	Bilateral extensor	3
9. Limb ataxia	Absent	0
	Present in upper or lower	1
	Present in both	2
10. Sensory	Normal	0
	Partial loss	1
	Dense loss	2
11. Neglect	No neglect	0
	Partial neglect	1
	Complete neglect	2
12. Dysarthria	Normal articulation	0
	Mild to moderate dysarthria	1
	Near unintelligible or worse	2
13. Best language	No aphasia	0
	Mild to moderate aphasia	1
	Severe aphasia	2
	Mute	3
14. Change from previous exam	Same	S
	Better	B
	Worse	W
15. Change from baseline	Same	S
	Better	B
	Worse	W

From Brott, T., Adams, H.P., Jr., Olinger, C.P., et al. (1989). Measurements of acute cerebral infarction: A clinical examination scale. Stroke *20:865.*

Focused Assessment Findings and Nursing Diagnoses

SIE can produce characteristic life-threatening symptoms. The following findings strongly suggest the presence of a life-threatening stroke:

- Ineffective breathing patterns with hypoxia and hypercarbia
- Unacceptable hypertension or hypotension
- Decreased responsiveness
- Abnormal limb movements: decreasing strength, abnormal flexion (decorticate), and abnormal extension (decerebrate)
- Loss of cranial nerve reflexes
- Severe headache, neck stiffness, photophobia
- Elevated blood glucose level in nondiabetic patients (> 170 mg/dL)

In summary, the therapeutic window for reversal of focal ischemia is 3 hours after the brain attack. Therefore, the nurse must perform a rapid history and focused assessment and report significant findings to the physician. Understanding the rationale for the history and focused assessment helps the nurse prioritize nursing interventions to deliver effective therapy in a timely manner. The prioritization of nursing care for acute stroke patients is focused on the ABCs. Impaired airway clearance related to hemiplegia and weak cough reflexes may lead to life-threatening aspiration and hypoxemia. Ineffective breathing patterns related to decreased responsiveness pose another threat to the ischemic brain. The nurse also must facilitate the performance of laboratory and diagnostic tests to avoid delays in diagnosing and effectively managing the acute stroke patient.

SECTION SEVEN REVIEW

1. A focused nursing assessment for the acute stroke patient would include all of the following EXCEPT
   A. Glasgow Coma Scale check
   B. selective cranial nerve assessment
   C. heart sounds
   D. superficial and deep tendon reflexes
2. Pertinent data for a focused assessment of the acute stroke patient include all of the following EXCEPT
   A. urine color and consistency
   B. seizure history
   C. dysrhythmias
   D. time of the brain attack
3. Assessment findings that suggest life-threatening symptoms or signs in stroke patients include
   A. decreased level of consciousness
   B. left homonymous hemianopsia
   C. expressive aphasia
   D. left hemiparesis
4. Mrs. Phillips, age 24, had an embolic stroke and is drowsy and lethargic when she arrives in the emergency department. The nurse would initially assess her
   A. neurologic status
   B. airway patency
   C. breathing patterns
   D. vital signs

Answers: 1. D, 2. A, 3. A, 4. B

SECTION EIGHT: Nursing Interventions

At the completion of this section, the learner will be able to describe systemic complications of hemorrhagic stroke including cardiac, pulmonary, gastrointestinal, or fluid and electrolyte disorders.

Cardiac Complications

In approximately 60 percent of patients with SAH, ECG abnormalities occur commonly during the first 48 hours following the SAH. Prolonged QT interval, T wave inversion, prominent U waves, and ST segment elevation or depression may occur. Elevated levels of catecholamines are believed to produce supraventricular tachycardia, atrial or ventricular flutter or fibrillation, premature atrial and ventricular contractions, and torsades de pointes. Beta-adrenergic blockers (e.g., propranolol) have been effective in the management of these arrhythmias, and defibrillation has been effective for ventricular flutter or fibrillation.

Pulmonary Complications

Excessive catecholamine stimulation resulting from raised ICP produces high pressure and flow in the pulmonary vasculature with extravasation of fluid causing neurogenic pulmonary edema. Management includes oxygenation by intubation and mechanical ventilation using positive end-expiratory pressure (PEEP). Monitoring pulmonary artery pressures with a pulmonary arterial catheter can prevent the iatrogenic complication. Deep vein thrombosis (DVT) occurs in about 2 percent of patients with SAH and results in pulmonary edema in approximately 1 percent. Patients with DVT perioperatively should be treated with placement of a vena caval filter. Preventive measures for DVT include passive exercises, elastic and intermittent pneumatic compression stockings, early mobilization, and low-dose heparin in high-risk patients (King & Martin, 1994).

Gastrointestinal Complications

Gastrointestinal complications such as bleeding secondary to stress ulcers occurs in about 4 percent of patients post SAH. Prophylactic antacids and H_2 antagonists are usually prescribed for all patients with SAH.

Fluid and Electrolyte Complications

Hyponatremia (serum sodium < 135 mmol/L) occurs in about 4 percent of patients with ruptured aneurysms. The majority of patients with SAH develop salt-wasting hyponatremia with contraction of the patient's intravascular volume. With excessive catecholamine stimulation, atrial natriuretic factor is elevated, leading to increased renal excretion of sodium and water, hypovolemia, increased blood viscosity, and decreased cerebral perfusion. Another less common form of hyponatremia, the syndrome of inappropriate antidiuretic hormone (SIADH), is characterized by a dilutional hyponatremia with expansion of the intravascular volume (Heater, 1999). Symptoms of both forms of hyponatremia include anorexia, nausea and vomiting, irritability, lethargy, seizures, and coma. It is important to determine the cause of hyponatremia because the therapy is different for salt-wasting and SIADH. Patients with salt-wasting hyponatremia require volume replacement and cautious infusions of 3 percent sodium chloride, not fluid restriction, which is the therapy for SIADH. Fluid restriction in patients with salt-wasting hyponatremia can produce further hypovolemia, cerebral hypoperfusion, and infarction (King & Martin, 1994).

Perfusion Complications

Another serious threat to the hemiplegic stroke patient is DVT, which may lead to pulmonary embolus. Stroke patients are at high risk for DVT because of hemiplegia with loss of vasomotor tone, venous stasis, edema in the paralyzed, flaccid limbs, and immobility. Dehydration also places the patient at high risk for DVT. **Hemiplegia** or **hemiparesis** decreases muscle pump action for return of venous blood to the heart. Poor positioning (one extremity lying on another) or sitting for long periods in a chair can precipitate or exacerbate DVT. To detect DVT, the nurse must observe for leg edema, warmth, discoloration, and increased size. Assessment for Homan's sign in the unaffected leg can be done. Measurements of calf and thigh girths can confirm edema when it is suspected. To aid in venous return of blood to the heart, passive and active measures for preventing DVT are utilized. Passive measures include:

- Extremity elevation by raising the foot of the bed (promotes venous return to the heart)
- Intermittent pneumatic compression stockings (increase blood flow velocity, reduce venous stasis, and stimulate fibrinolytic activity)
- Continuous passive motion devices (increase muscle and venous valvular action)
- Elastic support hose (increase blood flow velocity and reduce edema and venous distention) (Hickey, 1996)

Dorsiflexion exercises will also help to prevent DVT. Active measures to prevent DVT include deep breathing, active ROM exercises of unaffected limbs, and early ambulation (Hickey, 1996). Acute flexion of the hips, legs, trunk, and neck should be avoided, particularly sitting for long periods in a wheelchair. This latter precaution helps to prevent not only DVT but also contractures. Minidose heparin (3,000 to 5,000 U) subcutaneously may be prescribed for patients with ischemic strokes to prevent DVT. Positioning should be done at least every 2 hours. The skin should be reassessed for redness and pallor after each turn, with adjustment of the turning schedule based on the assessment. Finally, hydration should be adequate ($\geq$ 2 L), unless contraindicated, to maintain a daily output of 1,500 mL and to avoid increased blood viscosity states.

Potential for Injury

Potential for injury is related to seizure activity. Hemorrhagic stroke patients present with seizures more often than those with ischemic strokes. Seizures create a hypermetabolic state: cerebral metabolic oxygen demands become greater than the oxygen supply to the ischemic brain, which may precipitate rebleeding and worsen ischemia. Nurses must be alert for seizures, report them, provide anticonvulsants at prescribed times to maintain therapeutic serum levels, and institute seizure precautions (bed in low position, padded siderails, available oral suction) to protect the patient from injury.

In summary, the management of patients with stroke is complex. Prevention of patient deterioration warrants frequent neurologic and cardiovascular monitoring and prompt correction of inadequate pulmonary artery wedge pressure (PAWP). Salt-wasting hyponatremia is more commonly observed in aneurysmal SAH patients than SIADH, and necessitates close monitoring of serum and urine electrolytes. Prophylactic anticonvulsants are administered for seizures. Prophylaxis for systemic complications are managed with beta blockers and defibrillation (cardiac); oxygenation and mechanical ventilation (pulmonary); vena caval filters and preventive measures for DVT; and prophylactic medications for stress ulcers.

Section Eight Review

1. Catecholamines are released at stroke onset; therefore, the nurse should monitor the patient for
   - **A.** Cheyne–Stokes respiration
   - **B.** cardiac dysrhythmias
   - **C.** rhonchi
   - **D.** venous stasis
2. Cerebrally induced cardiac arrhythmias are life threatening and are often treated with
   - **A.** vasodilators
   - **B.** alpha blockers
   - **C.** beta blockers
   - **D.** dopamine
3. Jacob Ash had an ischemic hemispheric stroke with aphasia and right hemiplegia. He is at risk for which life-threatening condition?
   - **A.** cardiac arrest
   - **B.** vasospasms
   - **C.** deep vein thrombosis
   - **D.** pneumonia

4. Interventions for preventing deep vein thrombosis in stroke patients include all of the following EXCEPT
   A. pneumatic compression stockings
   B. ROM exercises
   C. at least 2 L of fluid a day unless contraindicated
   D. out of bed and sitting in a chair for at least 3 hours a day

Answers: 1. B, 2. C, 3. C, 4. D

SECTION NINE: Impaired Physical Mobility

Impaired physical mobility is related to motor and sensory deficits in the acute stroke patient, particularly hemiplegia and impaired balance, changes in postural tone, and disinhibition of primitive reflex activity. This section introduces two principles of rehabilitation: traditional (compensation) and neurodevelopmental approach (bilateral stimulation). These principles are applied to nursing interventions throughout the remaining sections. At the completion of this section, the reader will be able to explain two principles of rehabilitation used in the care of acute stroke patients; describe the effects of stroke on mobility; and discuss interventions that nurses and other health care providers use to promote functional independence.

To increase independence, rehabilitation begins as early as possible following the onset of a stroke and is a multidisciplinary effort. Physical therapists assist with assessments of motor function, plan an exercise program, and provide splints to prevent contractures. The occupational therapist assesses, provides a plan of therapy, and evaluates sensory and cognitive problems that interfere with functional independence. The **physiatrist** is the physician responsible for diagnosing and treating rehabilitative problems such as spasticity and subluxations.

Two principles of rehabilitation are frequently used in the care of the stroke patient: compensation and neurodevelopmental (NDT) approach (stimulation). Traditionally, nurses used the compensation principle when they encouraged patients to ". . . use your strong side to make up for loss of function on the affected side . . ." or to do unilateral ADLs (Camp et al., 1995). This approach is still used and it assumes that the brain is irreversibly damaged and healthy neurons must be recruited to take over the lost functions. For example, the nurse places the bedside table and personal items on the patient's unaffected side and works with the patient from that side. NDT approach assumes that new pathways may be established in latent brain areas, or that the affected brain area may be viable and merely "idling." The affected brain must be developed from the primitive to the more sophisticated levels of human function, much like a newborn with primitive, uninhibited reflexes learning simple and complex movements. Thus, the damaged brain can relearn or restore its functions, if bilaterally stimulated. This approach is only successful if the exercises use and maintain inhibiting patterns to decrease tone and increase sensory input (Johnstone, 1995). Activity is divided into steps and repeated starting from simple to more complex tasks (Camp et al., 1995). The NDT approach inhibits abnormal reflex mechanisms, provides a sensory experience of movement, prevents overuse of the normal side, and facilitates normal movement. With this philosophy, nurses would encourage the patient to use his or her affected side and to function bilaterally so as to incorporate both sides of the body into movements. In practice, nurses may utilize either or both of these principles.

Motor Deficits

Following a stroke, cerebral shock usually occurs, causing hypotonicity or a flaccid hemiplegia. During the period of cerebral shock, a state of temporary disruption of neural transmission and integration processes **(diaschisis)** occurs (Phipps, 1991). When a stroke causes hemiplegia, initially the patient is flaccid; later, tone is palpated in the body of affected limb muscles and spasticity begins with some resistance to movement. Spasticity results when reflex activity is released from cerebral inhibition after damage to the motor system. This spasticity is associated with an upper motor neuron lesion since the frontal cortex (motor centers) and/or corticospinal (voluntary motor) tracts are interrupted. Upper motor neuron (UMN) lesions are characterized by muscle spasticity, hypertonicity, resistance to passive stretch in joints, and abnormally brisk reflexes. The increased tone is palpable in the affected limb muscles. A positive Babinski can be elicited (Fitzgerald, 1992). Deep tendon reflexes become brisk with increased abnormal muscle tone. Normal sensation must be restored with stimulation of the affected limb (Johnstone, 1995). Weight bearing on the affected side may achieve more normal muscle tone. Reduction of anxiety and pain and avoiding fatigue may also achieve more normal muscle tone. To assist the patient, emphasis is placed on establishing normal lying, sitting, and standing postures during rest and activity. The acute stroke patient can present with mild hemiparesis to severe hemiplegia, quadriplegia, **ataxia,** or involuntary movements depending on the stroke site.

Poststroke spasticity (excessive muscle tone) affects

the antigravity muscles. In the lower limbs, these are the knee extensors and plantar flexors of the foot. In the upper limbs, these are the elbow flexors and wrist and finger flexors. The patient assumes a spastic "hemiparetic posture," with the neck and trunk tilted toward the hemiparetic side; the shoulder pulled down and back; the elbow, wrist, and fingers flexed; and the arm adducted (Fig. 18–7). The lower limb is extended with the hip internally rotated and adducted, and the foot plantar flexed with supination, inversion, and flexed toes. Because flexor muscles are stronger in the arms and extensors stronger in the legs, the patient is prone to flexion contractures in the upper extremity and extension contractures in the lower extremities.

Motor Pattern of Recovery

With the passage of time, abnormal mass pattern movements (synergy) appear and the patient may lift the limbs against gravity. **Synergy** is observed with high levels of spasticity in which muscle groups move together, restricting isolated voluntary movements of one joint. Eventually, if recovery is not arrested at the flaccid, spastic, or synergy levels, the patient may be able to lift limbs against resistance and exhibit isolated voluntary muscle movements, such as pincer movements of the thumb and index fingers, which are so important in performing ADLs.

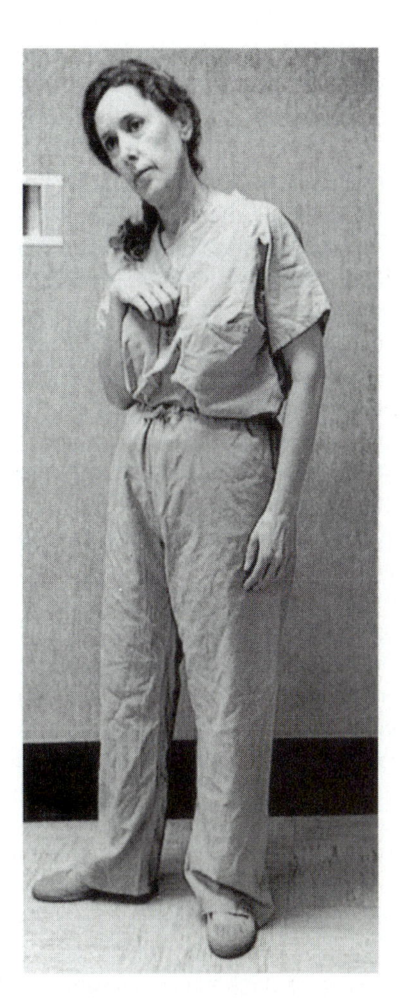

Figure 18–7. The hemiparetic posture.

Patients with stroke may experience balance and coordination impairments. The components for normal balance are vision, **proprioception,** and vestibular function, and at least two of these must be intact to adequately maintain balance. Imbalances occur with hemiparesis because of abnormal posture and in posterior strokes when there is involvement of the brain stem and cerebellum. The patient with impaired balance is at high risk for injury because of postural asymmetry, leaning or falling to the hemiparetic side, and the inability to use protective righting reflexes when the center of gravity is displaced. Physical therapists may assist patients to overcome these problems with therapeutic stimulation exercises (rolling from side to side on mats, scooting up in bed) to reestablish normal postural reflexes.

Patients with strokes affecting the extrapyramidal system (basal ganglia, cerebellum, and connecting pathways) may experience rigidity and involuntary movements such as tics, tremors, chorea, and hemiballismus. Rigidity differs from spasticity in that there is resistance throughout the full range of motion ("lead pipe rigidity"), or it may be ratchety during passive stretching of the limb ("cogwheel rigidity"). Awkward intended movements (intention tremor and ataxia) are produced by cerebellar stroke lesions or involvement of their connecting pathways. Involuntary movements (tremor-at-rest, chorea, etc.) are produced by basal ganglia lesions.

Assessment

Nurses can assess patient mobility, muscle strength, and tone during bathing. They can observe postural instability and involuntary movements and note rigidity or spasticity as the passive ROM exercises are done. Coordination and balance is assessed by asking the patient to touch his or her nose and then the nurse's finger several times or asking the patient to run his or her heel down the shin bone of the opposite leg. Proprioception is assessed by asking the patient to indicate the up or down position of his or her fingers or toes with the eyes closed. Normal position sense indicates intact proprioceptive pathways within the brain and spinal cord. Difficulty maintaining balance while sitting, standing, or walking creates safety problems. Reflexes also require intact sensory and motor function. The nurse can assess for a Babinski reflex by stroking the sole of the foot and observing for an upgoing big toe and fanning of the other toes. Clonus, a rhythmic contraction of flexor muscles 5 to 10 times per second, can be elicited at the ankle or wrist with sudden passive dorsiflexion (Fitzgerald, 1992). Muscle stretch reflexes are elicited by tapping the tendon of specific muscle groups with a reflex hammer and observing for a contraction of the muscles being tested. Reflexes are graded on a scale of 0 to 4, with 0 being areflexic, 2 normal, and 4 hyperreflexic. Motor strength can also be graded on a scale of 0 to 5 as follows (Bates, Brickey, & Hoekelman, 1995):

0 No muscular contraction detected
1 Barely detectable trace of contraction
2 Active movement of body part with gravity eliminated
3 Active movement of body part against gravity
4 Active movement of body part against gravity and some resistance
5 Active movement of body part against full resistance without fatigue—normal

Nursing Interventions

Exercises and Positioning

Maintaining functional abilities in the acute phase after stroke is important. Active and/or passive ROM exercises performed at least three or four times a day will prevent contractures. These exercises are important because muscle strength can deteriorate at a rate of 3 percent per day and rebuilds only half as fast (Yatsu, Grotta, & Pettigrew, 1995). The patient can be taught to exercise the shoulder, elbow, wrist, and hand by using the unaffected arm to move the affected arm. Leg mobility is maintained by exercising the hip, knee, and ankle. Nurses can encourage the patient to use the affected arm and leg in bilateral activities such as bathing, eating, and grooming. This increases afferent stimulation and perhaps efferent responses, and decreases the risk of contractures by maintaining functional mobility. Initially, care can be delivered from the unaffected side, but later, to encourage stimulation, it should be shifted to the affected side.

Proper body alignment is important to prevent contractures. The patient should be evaluated and positioned functionally and in positions to neutralize the abnormal hemiparetic posture. When lying supine, the head and spine should be straight and the entire affected arm should be elevated on pillows with the hand and fingers extended in a functional position, preferably with the palm up. A folded towel is placed under the affected shoulder so that both shoulders are symmetrical. A firm roll along the lateral aspect of the hip and thigh will neutralize the tendency of the affected leg to rotate externally. If positioned on the affected side, the patient's body is rotated slightly less than 90 degrees to rest on the shoulder blade rather than directly on the shoulder, to avoid the body's weight on the paralyzed arm or leg. The affected arm is extended perpendicular to the body, and the leg slightly flexed (Fig. 18–8). When positioned on the unaffected side, the patient's body is rotated more than 90 degrees with the affected shoulder forward, extremities beyond midline, the affected arm extended and elevated on pillows, and the affected leg functionally flexed and elevated on pillows. When eating in the upright position, the affected arm should be elevated on a pillow to maintain proper body alignment. During turning, avoid pulling on the affected arm as this may produce subluxation of the shoulder joint. Tennis shoes may help to avoid contractures in the flaccid stage but tend to stimulate more spasticity in the hyperreflexic stages. Hard rolls or inflatable splints are used to maintain functional hand and arm position and may be applied, particularly at night. Correct positioning by abduction and external rotation of the shoulder may prevent shoulder pain (Yatsu, Grotta, & Pettigrew, 1995). Abnormal tone may increase when fear, pain, lack of weight bearing, excessive effort, or abnormal posture or movement patterns exist. Weight bearing on the affected side is encouraged to achieve more normal muscle tone. Nurses can identify stressors, alleviate anxiety, minimize pain with proper positioning and prescribed medications, and provide rest periods to avoid fatigue when caring for these patients. Physicians may prescribe anti- spasmodic medications (dantrolene sodium, baclofen, diazepam) to reduce excessive tone and spasticity, which interfere with functional movements or cause pain. These medications are continued only if they are clearly beneficial. Alcohol and nerve injections decrease spastic tone with effects lasting 3 to 6 months (Katz, 1994).

Ambulation and Activities of Daily Living

The patient is ready to ambulate when there is evidence of strength in his or her legs, some balance, and proprioception. Muscle tone should be assessed regularly, and the patient should not be asked to do an activity with the disabled limb until muscle tone is restored. Traditional slings are avoided because they reinforce the abnormal posture of the spastic flexed arm and adduction and promote shoulder contractures. The affected arm must be handled gently to avoid subluxation of the shoulder joint and should be supported with pillows. The patient should not use the hand in any way without forearm support until he or she is able to hold the arm in space. Physical therapists will teach the patient exercises such as going up and down stairs, leading with the strong foot going up and the weaker foot going down with bannister support. They also will provide quad canes to assist with ambulation. Occupational therapists provide exercises that strengthen limbs for ADLs and provide assistive devices as needed. Nurses must be included in the plans to maintain continuity in the progress of the patient and to avoid confusing the patient. For example, the patient is taught to put on a shirt or blouse from the affected limb first and initially remove it from the unaffected limb. Occupational therapists will also adapt procedures and provide discharge evaluation of the home, suggesting environmental modifications that will promote independent living of the

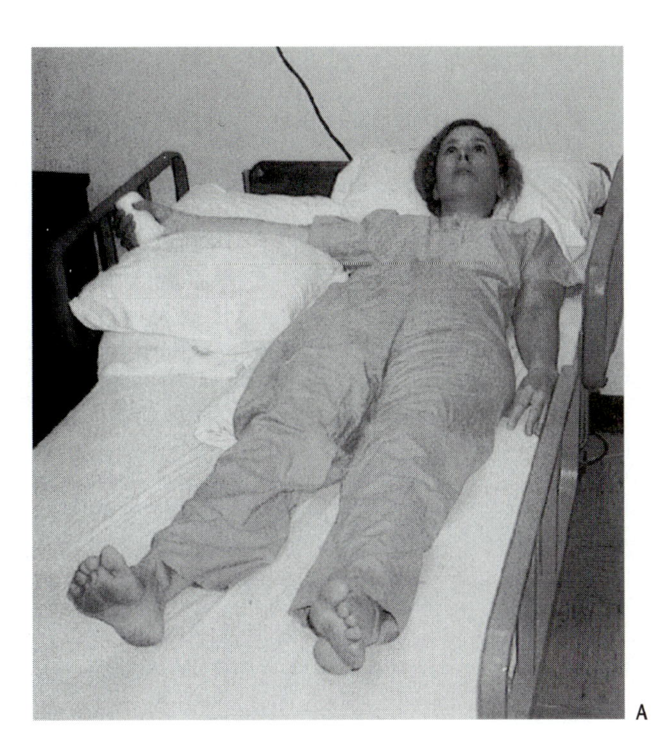

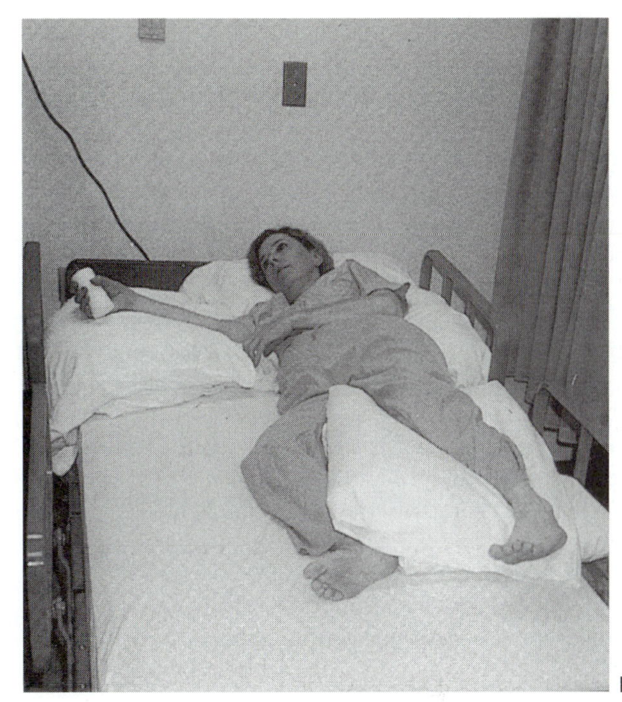

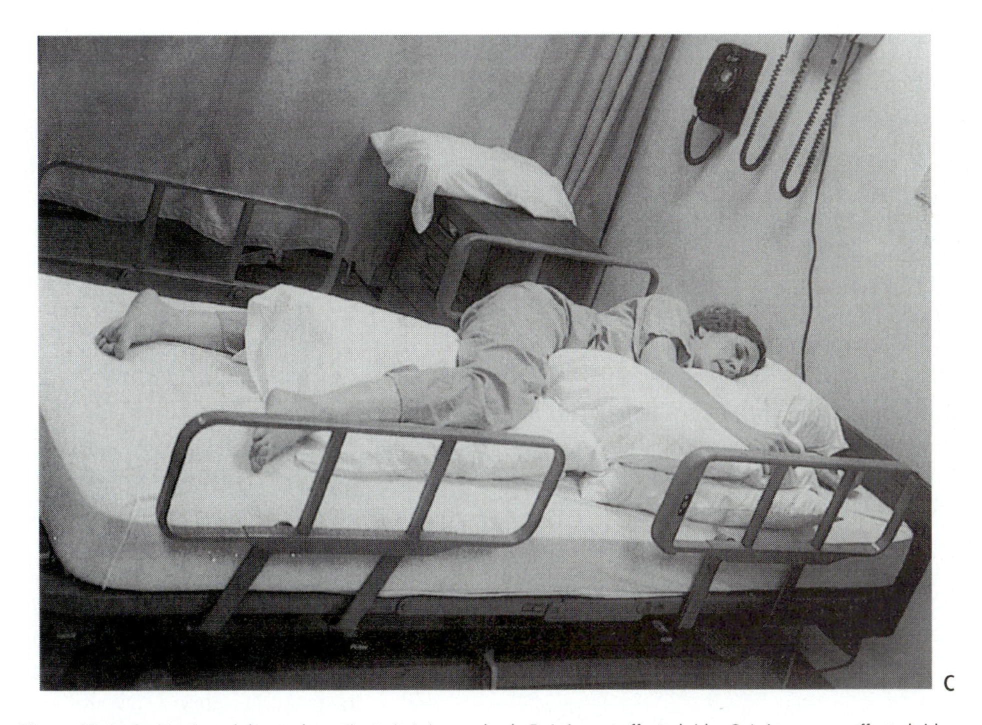

Figure 18–8. Positioning of the stroke patient. **A.** Lying on back. **B.** Lying on affected side. **C.** Lying on nonaffected side.

patient. Initially, these therapists assist the patient to compensate by adapting procedures; then, if necessary, adapting the environment; and finally, if necessary, adapting the patient's lifestyle to promote a functional recovery. Regular multidisciplinary conferences including the social worker, patient, and family are invaluable for maintaining continuity of care, effective management of patient problems, and patient and family satisfaction.

In summary, two principles of rehabilitation are used in the care of the stroke patient: compensation and neurodevelopmental approach (bilateral stimulation). A hemispheric stroke produces an upper motor neuron lesion when the frontal cortex (motor centers) and corticospinal (voluntary movement) tracts are interrupted. Cerebral shock initially produces a flaccid hemiplegia followed within days or a few weeks by a spastic hemiparesis. Upper motor neuron lesions are characterized by muscle hypertonicity, spasticity, and abnormally brisk reflexes, which are released from cortical inhibition. The reflex arcs are intact but disinhibited. These lesions involve any of the descending pathways that drive the lower motor neuron (LMN) or final common motor pathway. Conversely, LMN lesions involve the cell body of the LMN or its peripheral pathway, producing a flaccid paralysis, hypotonicity of muscles, and hyporeflexia because the reflex arc is broken and CNS motor commands cannot reach the muscles. Patient motor deficits following a stroke vary from mild to severe and usually follow a sequence of recovery from flaccidity to spasticity to mass pattern or synergy movement to voluntary movements. This sequence may be arrested at any level depending on the amount of brain damage incurred by the stroke. Nurses play a critical role in assessing mobility and in positioning, compensating, and stimulating the acute stroke patient to promote independence. The nurse must collaborate with the other health care providers by encouraging or performing prescribed patient exercises; maintaining proper positioning; encouraging the correct performance of ADLs; and adapting procedures, the environment, or lifestyles to promote independence and a functional recovery.

SECTION NINE REVIEW

1. The theory of rehabilitation that aims to restore the highest of humanistic functions is
   A. compensation
   B. idling
   C. neurodevelopmental
   D. inhibition
2. Which of the following is the general motor pattern of stroke recovery?
   A. spasticity, synergy, isolated voluntary movements, flaccidity
   B. synergy, isolated voluntary movements, flaccidity, spasticity
   C. isolated voluntary movements, flaccidity, spasticity, synergy
   D. flaccidity, spasticity, synergy, isolated voluntary movements
3. Correct positioning of the hemiplegic patient is described in which of the following?
   A. unaffected side: the patient's body is at 90 degrees with the affected arm flexed and elevated on a pillow
   B. supine: the head is midline and in neutral position with the arms at the side
   C. affected side: the patient's body is rotated laterally less than 90 degrees with the affected arm extended and elevated on pillows and the affected leg slightly flexed on pillows
   D. affected side: the patient's body is at 90 degrees with a pillow between the legs and the arm extended and elevated on pillows
4. When teaching a hemiplegic man to put on his shirt, the nurse correctly tells him to
   A. put his shirt on the unaffected arm first
   B. put his shirt on the affected arm first
   C. button his shirt and slip it over his head
   D. slip his shirt over his head and the unaffected arm first
5. Which of the following is true of hyperreflexic movements in stroke patients. They are
   A. usually seen in the acute early stages of stroke
   B. produced by lower motor neuron lesions
   C. characterized by involuntary tics and tremors
   D. associated with lesions of the corticospinal tracts

Answers: 1. C, 2. D, 3. C, 4. A, 5. D

SECTION TEN: Potential Alteration in Nutrition

The potential alteration in nutrition (less than body requirements) is related to dysphagia, impaired gag reflexes, and perceptual and motor deficits. At the completion of this section, the learner will be able to identify causes and effects of undernutrition in the acute stroke patient; perform a nutritional assessment; describe nursing interventions that prevent aspiration; and describe nursing interventions that promote adequate nutrition for the acute stroke patient.

Causes of Undernutrition

Stroke patients are at risk for undernutrition because of a decrease in intake and a hypermetabolic state produced by the brain attack. Dysphagia, absent or diminished gag reflexes, facial paralysis, perceptual and cognitive deficits, **hemiplegia** (particularly affecting the dominant hand), an inability to perform bilateral hand tasks, and immobility all contribute to undernutrition. A dominant hemiplegia requires the patient to use the nondominant hand, making eating awkward and cumbersome. Sensory and motor loss in one half of the mouth makes it difficult to move food to the back of the mouth for swallowing and can cause **pocketing** of food in the mouth, without patient awareness, setting up a source for infection. Absent gag reflexes and facial paralysis limit chewing and swallowing movements and increase the risk for aspiration. Perceptual deficits such as impaired depth perception, **agnosias, apraxias,** hemianopsia, or neglect may produce injury during eating. Patients with these deficits are unable to see all the food on the tray and therefore ignore it, or they are unable to recognize or properly use utensils. For the hemiparetic patient who may be unable to perform hand to mouth movements or bilateral hand tasks, the nurse must provide assistance in cutting food, opening containers, and placing the food within reach of the patient's uninvolved hand. Before self-feeding, the patient needs adequate sitting balance. A physical therapy referral is indicated to promote balance, coordination, and range of motion with selective exercises. The occupational therapist may provide assistive devices such as suction cups for stabilizing dishes and combination knife–fork utensils to promote more success in eating independently. In addition, cognitive deficits such as aphasia limit communicative ability to express needs or preferences at meals. Depression may further limit food and fluid intake.

The hypermetabolic stress response initiated by the brain attack results in hyperglycemia as well as decreased intake. Thus, metabolic demands become greater at a time when oral intake is often acutely restricted. Clinically, the patient may manifest a decrease in serum protein leading to a compromised immune state, weight loss, muscle weakness and atrophy, increased rate of pressure sores, higher morbidity and mortality, and a prolonged hospital stay.

If a nutritional deficit exists, the patient should be weighed at least weekly. In addition, serum protein, albumin, transferrin, complete blood count (for total lymphocyte count), and urinary urea nitrogen should be monitored weekly when these are available. Decreased laboratory values in blood work and a negative urinary urea nitrogen value are indicative of negative nitrogen balance. Nurses also need to monitor serum electrolytes, particularly potassium and sodium.

Assessment

The presence of hemiplegia, neglect, confusion, attention deficits, or incoordination should be noted. The nurse should assess the following as indicators of feeding potential: visual field deficits; the ability to chew and swallow; lip closure; the strength of the masseter muscles when the jaw is clenched together; tongue deviation upon protrusion; the presence of teeth or dentures; symmetry of the uvula; and presence of the gag reflex. Skin turgor, dry mucous membranes, and urine color are assessed as indicators of fluid status. Height and weight are obtained to provide baseline data.

The patient should be assessed for the ability to bring food to the mouth, handle utensils, see all the food on the tray, and successfully chew and swallow food and liquids, with no pocketing in the affected cheek.

In addition, the patient should be assessed for:

- Cognitive ability to feed self
- Drooling (a clue to swallowing problems) or difficulty swallowing liquids or foods
- Continuous clearing of the throat or coughing while eating
- Appropriate positioning during eating

The nurse can assess specific muscle movements for swallowing by asking the patient to say "me-me-me" for the lips; "la-la-la" for the tongue; and "ga-ga-ga" for the soft palate and pharynx. Normal movements of the tongue, hyoid bone, and thyroid cartilage can be detected by placing the index finger in the submandibular region and the middle and ring fingers on the hyoid bone and thyroid cartilage and noting elevation of these structures. If the swallowing reflex is impaired, no movements will be detected (Gauwitz, 1995). Prior to oral feeding and particularly in patients with vertebrobasilar strokes, the nurse should also assess for facial paresis or weakness such as asymmetry, flattened nasal folds, unequal eye opening, or an inability to whistle, smile, or frown. A weak hoarse voice or tongue deviation may be noted with brain stem lesions. During assessment, ask the patient to push out each cheek with the tongue; to move the protruded tongue from side to side; and to say "ah" while you listen for crackles and wheezes, which indicate possible aspiration. The nurse should assess the patient for a cough reflex because this reflex prevents food from entering the upper respiratory tract. Coughing at least twice in rapid succession will provide this information. For most persons, to complete a swallow requires an intact cortex (voluntary) and brain stem (reflexive) swallowing centers, but these tests are not always reliable. If the patient's cough and swallowing reflexes are intact, the gag reflex is tested. If intact, the palatal muscles will contract, but the presence of a gag reflex is no guarantee against aspiration because elderly patients may have a decreased reflex or small amounts of food or fluid may not always stimulate a gag (Gauwitz, 1995). The quality of the patient's voice is noted because cranial nerves VII (facial), X (vagus), and XII (hypoglossal) are involved in the motor control of speech (Phipps, 1991). If these reflexes are impaired, patients should be referred to a speech pathologist for videofluoroscopy and evaluation of swallowing ability before attempts at oral feeding are made (Buelow & Jamieson, 1990). During videofluoroscopy, the patient ingests barium orally in a sequence of four increasing consistencies: a thin liquid, a thick liquid, a pasty food, and a barium-coated cookie that requires chewing before swallowing. The barium coats the oral cavity, pharynx, and larynx, revealing the phases of swallowing, the speed of swallowing, motility problems, and the etiology of aspiration (Gauwitz, 1995).

Nursing Interventions

During the first 48 hours after an acute stroke, the patient is usually given intravenous fluids with potassium chloride. Glucose solutions are avoided because anaerobic metabolism produces excess lactate in the penumbra or ischemic zone (Siesjo, 1992b; McDowell, Brott, & Goldstein, 1993). When there is dysphagia and a risk for aspiration, a small-bore nasogastric tube, gastrostomy, or enteral tube feedings may be prescribed.

Dysphagia

Dysphagia, or difficulty in swallowing, is usually caused by lesions involving cranial nerves V (trigeminal), VII (facial), IX (glossopharyngeal), X (vagus), XI (accessory), and XII (hypoglossal) (see Table 18–7). There are three phases of swallowing: oral, pharyngeal, and esophageal; only the oral phase is under voluntary control. Dysphagia can be suspected when these signs appear: In the oral phase, choking, drooling, poor lip closure, food pocketing, asymmetry of the mouth or protruded tongue; in the pharyngeal phase, choking, aspiration or nasal regurgitation, weak, hoarse voice; and in the esophageal phase, regurgitation. Strokes may affect each of these swallowing phases and produce nutritional and other problems for the patient.

When patients have difficulty chewing or moving food to the back of the mouth or "pocket" food on the affected side, semisolid foods are best because they stimulate sensation and chewing and facilitate swallowing. Examples of these foods are oatmeal, casseroles, strained fruits and vegetables, rice, Jello, or puddings. Milk and most milk products, dry foods, pureed foods, and bananas are avoided because they can produce mucus or are viscid. Yogurt and cottage cheese are good alternate choices for calcium. Straws can be dangerous when the patient lacks lip closure because they can deposit liquid too far back in the mouth, increasing the risk of aspiration. To avoid fatigue and mealtime disruptions, half-hour rest periods are planned before eating, and oral care and toileting are completed before mealtime. The patient should be sitting and supported in a high-Fowler's position when eating. To prevent aspiration, one teaspoon of food at a time is placed in the intact side of the mouth and the patient is instructed to swallow twice after each bite while keeping the head flexed forward and downward and the chin at midline. Allow 30 to 45 minutes for meals to avoid rushing. Nonstimulatory bland foods and very hot or cold foods, which may cause injury to the desensitized mucous membranes of the mouth, are avoided. Solid foods and liquids are offered at different times to avoid sweeping the inadequately chewed solids down the throat by liquids. After eating, the nurse checks for pocketing and provides mouth care. The patient remains upright for 45 to 60 minutes after meals to minimize the risk of aspiration. Suction equipment should be available at the bedside for those at risk for aspiration (Gauwitz, 1995).

In summary, stroke patients are at high risk for undernutrition because of hemiplegia, dysphagia, and perceptual/cognitive deficits. Significant findings for predicting eating problems include drooling, tongue deviation, nasal regurgitation of fluids, choking, weak hoarse voice, facial asymmetry, and weak cough and gag reflexes. Patients with swallowing problems should be referred to a speech language pathologist to determine the nature of the swallowing problem. Nurses should monitor dietary intake, weight, hydration status, serum protein, prealbumin, albumin, transferrin, total lymphocyte counts, and urinary urea nitrogen for patients with eating problems. When orally feeding patients, the nurse can prevent aspiration by feeding them in the high-Fowler's position with the head and chin flexed downward and by using foods that facilitate swallowing (e.g., oatmeal, puddings, Jello). Food is placed in the nonaffected side of the mouth, and after eating, the patient's mouth is checked for pocketing of food. Oral hygiene should be provided after each meal. Suction equipment should be available at the bedside of stroke patients at risk for aspiration.

SECTION TEN REVIEW

1. All of the following are causes of undernutrition in stroke patients EXCEPT
   A. dysphagia
   B. hemiplegia
   C. perceptual deficits
   D. hypometabolic state
2. The effects of undernutrition in the stroke patient include all of the following EXCEPT
   A. positive urinary urea nitrogen
   B. hypoalbuminemia
   C. high risk for infections
   D. loss of motor tone
3. When assisting a stroke patient to eat, aspiration may be prevented by
   A. positioning the patient's head at 30 degrees while eating
   B. teaching the patient to flex the head downward while swallowing
   C. placing the food on the affected side of the mouth
   D. lowering the patient's bed to a supine position after eating
4. Significant clues to swallowing problems in a stroke patient include all of the following EXCEPT
   A. difficulty using a straw
   B. facial asymmetry
   C. voice quality changes
   D. loss of appetite
5. Dysphagia usually involves cranial nerves
   A. I (olfactory), II (optic), III (oculomotor), IV (trochlear), V (trigeminal), VI (abducens)
   B. III (oculomotor), IV (trochlear), V (trigeminal), VI (abducens), VII (facial), VIII (vestibulocochlear/acoustic)
   C. V (trigeminal), VII (facial), IX (glossopharyngeal), X (vagus), XI (accessory), XII (hypoglossal)
   D. II (optic), III (oculomotor), V (trigeminal), VII (facial), IX (glossopharyngeal), X (vagus)

Answers: 1. D, 2. A, 3. B, 4. D, 5. C

SECTION ELEVEN: Alteration in Elimination

Alteration in elimination may be related to impaired mobility, cognitive impairment, aphasia, and preexisting elimination problems. At the completion of this section, the learner will be able to differentiate the types of urinary and bowel incontinence found in acute stroke patients and describe nursing interventions that will promote urinary continence and normal bowel elimination.

Acute stroke patients may have detrusor impairments that cause urinary incontinence, constipation, impaired mobility, cognitive impairment, aphasia, perceptual deficits, and preexisting problems.

Elimination problems most frequently encountered in the stroke patient are:

- Detrusor hyporeflexia (flaccid bladder)
- Detrusor hyperreflexia (uninhibited or spastic bladder)
- Detrusor–sphincter dyssynergy (unsynchronized detrusor and sphincter muscles producing urinary retention)
- Constipation

The inhibition of bowel and bladder external sphincters is under voluntary control and is a learned function of the frontal lobe. During the period of cerebral shock, reflex activity is released from cerebral inhibition following damage to the motor system, producing a transient detrusor hyporeflexia which causes a flaccid distention of the bladder and overflow incontinence. Following this stage of cerebral shock, which lasts several days or weeks, the detrusor muscle becomes hyperreflexic, hypertonic, and spastic in patients with stroke lesions above the pons. The patient develops a spastic, small reservoir capacity bladder with urgency incontinence. Other effects include urinary frequency (voiding more often than every 2 hours), bladder contractions/spasms, nocturia, voiding in small amounts, and urgency incontinence. Patients with lesions involving the pons, below the pons, but above the sacral micturition reflex center may develop a detrusor–sphincter dyssynergy or a lack of synchronization between contractions of the detrusor muscle and the external sphincter (Table 18–9).

Normally, when the detrusor muscle contracts the bladder, the external urethral sphincter relaxes. In detrusor–sphincter dyssynergy, both muscles contract simultaneously, producing urinary retention and an obstructed outflow. Incontinence is common in hemispheric strokes and is usually transient, decreasing as mobility improves. In one study, functional incontinence was due to stroke-related cognitive and language deficits in patients with normal bladder function (Gelber et al., 1993). Functional urinary incontinence results when the hemiplegic patient has difficulty getting to the bathroom and performing toileting in a timely manner. Manipulating clothing with one functioning hand makes toileting and hygiene difficult. Mental confusion also contributes to incontinence even in the mobile patient. Altered bladder and bowel sensations and visual field deficits also contribute to incontinence. The inability to communicate the need to

TABLE 18–9. NEUROGENIC BLADDER TYPES IN THE ACUTE STROKE PATIENT

BLADDER TYPE	FEATURES	LESION SITE	EFFECTS ON PATIENT	NURSING APPROACH
Detrusor hyporeflexia	Flaccid (large capacity)	Above the pons (cerebral shock)	Overflow incontinence Distended bladder High urine residual volumes	Monitor intake and output (I&O) Observe for overdistention Intemittent catheterization Keep voidings > 400 mL
Detrusor hyperreflexia (uninhibited)	Spastic (small capacity)	Cerebral cortex, internal capsule, basal ganglia	Urinary frequency, urgency Bladder contractions/spasms Nocturia Low-volume voidings Incontinence (unable to reach toilet in time)	Voiding schedule every 2 hours or longer Monitor I&O Encourage fluids Limit caffeine and evening fluids Upright position to void Antispasmodics may be prescribed
Detrusor–sphincter dyssynergy (noncoordinated)	Spastic bladder and external sphincter that contract simultaneously (small capacity)	Pons, and pathways between pons and above sacral spinal cord	Small, frequent, or no voidings Sensation of bladder fullness Dribbling; overflow incontinence High urine residual volumes Dysuria	Consistent fluid intake Time voiding schedule Possibly intermittent catheterization within 5 minutes of voidings Observe for overdistention symptoms Keep residual < 75 mL Monitor I&O (output > 1,500 mL)

eliminate, as well as the inadequate ingestion of food or fluids, may result in incontinence, urinary tract infections, and/or constipation. Since many stroke patients are elderly, preexisting problems such as stress incontinence and benign prostatic hypertrophy aggravate effects of stroke that interfere with elimination.

Constipation is more common than bowel incontinence after stroke, probably because of age-related hypotonicity of the bowel, a decrease in roughage and fluid intake, immobility, the inability to communicate the need to defecate, and medications such as diuretics. Among the effects on the patient are straining at stool, which can elevate the blood pressure.

Assessment

To promote adequate elimination, the nurse should:

1. Assess the patient's prestroke and current voiding and bowel patterns
2. Inquire about past voiding problems and self-care practices
3. Determine current medications and their effect on elimination
4. Assess for other stroke deficits that result in functional incontinence
5. Determine the need for assistance or assistive devices to toilet
6. Assess fluid and dietary intake for several days
7. Observe urinary output, color, amount, and frequency in relation to the patient's intake; incontinence episodes; and awareness to void.

Assessing the abdomen for bladder distention and bowel sounds, and checking the rectum for fecal impaction, may be necessary if the patient has urinary retention or is constipated. A urinalysis, serum creatinine, and blood urea nitrogen can provide baseline information on the patient's urinary status at the time of onset of stroke. If there are problems, postvoid residuals and urodynamic tests may be done to determine the type of bladder problem. Finally, the nurse should assess for stroke deficits that result in functional incontinence.

Nursing Interventions

Patients with detrusor hyporeflexia have large-capacity, flaccid bladders with overflow incontinence. Nurses should monitor intake and output and participate in an intermittent catheterization program beginning every 4 hours to ensure that the urine volume does not exceed 400 mL. For patients with bladder hyperreflexia, a voiding schedule is established with the patient and family based on the previous patterns of voiding. When possible, diapers should be avoided. With urgency incontinence or dribbling, perineal pads may be an acceptable alternative for females, and leg bags for men. Methods to stimulate voiding can be employed. The program is initiated by offering the patient the opportunity to void every 2 hours, and, depending on the success rate, increasing the time intervals as needed. An intake and output (I&O) record should be maintained. Fluids are encouraged if there is cardiovascular stability and no fluid restrictions. The patient should be positioned upright for voiding whenever possible. A bedside commode or urinal should be available for easy access. Caffeine drinks and evening drinks are avoided or limited. Anticholinergics may be prescribed to reduce the spasticity of the bladder. The patient's ability to ask for help, reach for the urinal, use the call button, or use the commode are factors that must be assessed. Avoiding continuous indwelling catheters is important to prevent urinary tract infections and to improve bladder function. A catheter decompresses the bladder, which, like other muscles, needs exercise with filling and release of urine to maintain tone and an adequate reservoir capacity.

For stroke patients with detrusor–sphincter dyssynergy, a consistent fluid intake prevents large amounts of fluid buildup in the bladder at one time, particularly in the evening. A voiding schedule can be established; intermittent catheterization may be necessary to prevent retention or urinary tract infections. Catheterizations are done within 5 minutes after voiding to determine postvoid residuals. Postvoid residuals greater than 75 mL should be avoided when possible. Overdistention produces symptoms of restlessness, pallor, perspiration, headache, and chills. Overdistention may increase blood pressure, cause urinary reflux into the ureter, and produce urinary tract infection.

The desired outcomes for these bladder programs are continence, low postvoid residuals (< 75 mL), adequate voiding (1,500 mL/day), and normal urinalysis, BUN, and serum creatinine.

To promote adequate bowel elimination, a convenient pattern can be established after assessing former and current bowel patterns. Information related to fluids and foods that normally elicit bowel movements and patient preferences in roughage foods should be elicited. Stool softeners and suppositories are utilized to establish a regular pattern, as well as gastrointestinal reflexes when establishing an optimal toileting time (e.g., after meals). Daily assessment and outcome criteria should be established for bowel elimination based on the individual's pattern.

In summary, the elimination problems that stroke patients commonly encounter are detrusor hyporeflexia (flaccidity), detrusor hyperreflexia (spasticity), detrusor–sphincter dyssynergy, and constipation. Superimposed on these problems are the neurologic deficits produced by the stroke, which may cause a functional urinary incontinence. Age-related effects on elimination add to the problems. Detrusor hyporeflexia is characterized by a large-capacity bladder with overflow incontinence and high residual urine volumes. Strict intake and output monitoring, observations for overdistention, and intermittent catheterizations are done to keep urine volumes less than 400 mL. Detrusor hyperreflexia is characterized by a small-capacity bladder with urinary frequency, urgency, bladder contractions/spasms, nocturia, low-volume voidings, and incontinence. Establishing a voiding schedule of every 2 hours or longer, limiting caffeine and evening fluid intake, and administering antispasmodics may help ameliorate this problem. Detrusor–sphincter dyssynergy is characterized by a spastic bladder and external sphincter with small capacity. The patient has small, frequent, or no voidings; sensation of bladder fullness; dribbling; overflow incontinence; dysuria; and high urine residual volumes. To assist the patient with this problem, the nurse can provide a consistent and adequate fluid intake, establish a voiding schedule, and possibly perform intermittent catheterization within 5 minutes of voiding to check residuals. Constipation is to be avoided because of the effects of straining on blood pressure and other patient discomfort. A bowel elimination program can be established with patient preferences in roughage foods and adequate fluids. Stool softeners, suppositories, and the use of gastrointestinal reflexes are employed to establish a regular bowel pattern.

Section Eleven Review

1. The most common type of incontinence in acute stroke patients is produced by
   - A. bladder hyperreflexia (spasticity)
   - B. bladder hyporeflexia (flaccidity)
   - C. detrusor–sphincter dyssynergy
   - D. stress

2. Which of the following is true of elimination problems in acute stroke patients?
   - A. bowel incontinence is common
   - B. indwelling urinary catheters are useful for patients with hyperreflexic bladders
   - C. incontinence is usually stress related
   - D. scheduled voiding programs can promote continence

3. Mrs. Jackson had a pontine hemorrhagic stroke. She has a bladder that is described as detrusor–sphincter dyssynergia on the chart. What effects will Mrs. Jackson manifest?
   A. urgency to void
   B. urinary frequency
   C. large voidings
   D. overflow incontinence
4. For patients with detrusor hyperreflexia, all of the following are effective measures to promote continence EXCEPT
   A. establishing a voiding schedule
   B. avoiding caffeinated and evening fluids
   C. positioning upright to void
   D. insertion of an indwelling catheter
5. Mrs. Travis, age 60, has detrusor–sphincter dyssynergy following her stroke. Nursing interventions to promote continence include
   A. restricting fluids after the evening meal
   B. establishing a voiding schedule
   C. catheterizing 30 minutes postvoid to determine residual volumes
   D. encouraging fluids so that an acceptable urinary output is 1,000 mL

Answers: 1. A, 2. D, 3. D, 4. D, 5. B

SECTION TWELVE: Alteration in Sensation

Sensation and skin integrity may be altered in the stroke patient, related to loss of touch, pressure, temperature and sensation proprioception, motor, or vascular tone loss. At the completion of this section, the learner will be able to identify sensory hazards for the acute stroke patient, protect the patient from injury, and maintain the patient's skin integrity.

Alteration in sensation is related to loss of the primary sensations of touch, pressure, temperature, and proprioception. The primary sensation center is located in the parietal cortex and is responsible for localization and interpretation. Impaired sensation distorts information from the environment to the person. Lesions in the parietal cortex or its afferent pathways produce a loss of primary sensations or paresthesias, placing the patient at risk for burns, bruises, and other forms of skin injury. Impaired tactile sensation affects motor activity since sensory feedback is limited. It also affects perception because sensory information needed for interpretation and integration is limited. Loss of proprioception or position sense may lead to falls. Loss of vision and hearing can cause injury, social isolation, and impaired learning. A loss of the corneal reflex (cranial nerves V [trigeminal] and VII [facial]) may occur with brain stem strokes. Extraocular muscle impairments (cranial nerves III [oculomotor], IV [trochlear], and VI [abducens]) reflect brain stem injury and may produce double vision. The goal is to protect the patient from injury.

Assessment

The nurse can rapidly assess for light touch and proprioception by asking the patient to close the eyes and then checking the patient's ability to localize and discriminate touch and position with a wisp of cotton or tissue and positioning of the fingers up or down. The blink reflex can be stimulated with a wisp of cotton over the cornea. In addition, hypersensitivity, which is found with thalamic lesions, should be assessed.

Nursing Interventions

The nurse can protect the cornea by taping the eyelid shut and administering prescribed artificial tears or lubricants to prevent drying and corneal ulceration. For the diplopic patient, an eyepatch applied to one eye and alternated every 3 to 4 hours while awake permits a clear image. Avoiding extremes in heat and cold to desensitized areas is also important to prevent injury. Gentle handling of patients when transferring from bed to wheelchair and teaching the patient and family environmental hazards to avoid in the home are an essential aspect of care for patients with altered sensations. The patient should be taught to care for the neglected part and stimulate it whenever possible. Stimulation with warm water, a variety of textured fabrics, and tapping may be used. When transferring from bed to wheelchair, the neglected or hemiplegic part must be supported and protected.

In the acute stages of stroke, the patient is prone to pressure sores because of sensory, motor, or vascular tone loss as well as incontinence, parietal neglect, and spasticity in later stages. The stroke patient with a hemisensory deficit or hemiplegia cannot change positions and lacks the muscular pump action for return of venous flow from the extremities. Consequently, venous stasis occurs. In addition, if nutrition is poor, the skin tissue is likely to break down in the immobile patient. Perceptual deficits compound the problem, particularly parietal neglect, when portions of the body are ignored.

To protect the patient from injury and to maintain skin integrity in hemiplegics or those who are experiencing neglect or denial, the nurse must alert the patient and family to the deficit and hazards. This includes teaching them to inspect the skin with mirrors; to observe the skin for adequate capillary refill, pallor, and hyperemia; and to avoid pressure on the area should these appear. Nurses can turn the patient at least every 2 hours and inspect the skin before and after each turn, revising the turning schedule based on individual skin tolerance.

In summary, the acute stroke patient with motor and sensory deficits is at risk for injury and pressure sores. Assessment for these risk factors permits appropriate interventions to prevent injury and skin breakdown.

SECTION TWELVE REVIEW

1. Jerry Jones had a vertebrobasilar stroke and is experiencing double vision (diplopia). The nurse can assist him by
   A. applying an eyepatch to the right eye while awake
   B. administering prescribed artificial tears
   C. teaching him to remain in bed to prevent injury
   D. alternating patches on one eye every 4 hours while awake
2. Acute stroke patients are prone to pressure sores secondary to all of the following EXCEPT
   A. hemiplegia
   B. hemisensory deficits
   C. apraxia
   D. vascular tone loss
3. The center for primary sensations of touch, pressure, proprioception, and vibration is located in the
   A. frontal lobe
   B. parietal lobe
   C. temporal lobe
   D. occipital lobe
4. Mrs. Jefferson, age 40, is an acute stroke patient with hemiplegia and parietal neglect following a stroke. She is at risk for pressure sores for all of the following reasons EXCEPT that she
   A. has a loss of vasomotor tone
   B. ignores her left side
   C. has venous stasis of her affected limbs
   D. has dysphasia
5. The nurse assists Mrs. Jefferson by
   A. teaching her to inspect her skin for pallor or redness with a mirror
   B. turning her every 4 hours
   C. avoiding reference to her neglected side
   D. massaging her legs every 4 hours

Answers: 1. D, 2. C, 3. B, 4. D, 5. A

SECTION THIRTEEN: Visual–Spatial–Perceptual Alterations

This section discusses the effects, lesion site, assessment and nursing interventions for hemineglect syndrome (anosognosia and hemianopsia), body schema disturbances (including impaired right/left discrimination), agnosias, apraxias, and spatial relations disturbances. Many of these alterations are frequently found in right nondominant, hemispheric stroke patients. The objectives of nursing interventions are to protect the patient from injury and to promote independence. At the completion of this section, the learner will be able to explain the effects and lesion sites of visual–spatial–perceptual deficits found in stroke patients and describe the assessment of and nursing interventions for these deficits.

The stroke patient may present with a variety of visual–spatial–perceptual deficits, particularly if the stroke is in the right hemisphere. Perceptual deficits have a more detrimental effect on functional recovery than motor deficits and often go unrecognized in the stroke patient. Therefore, it is important for nurses to be alerted to these deficits when the stroke lesion site has been diagnosed.

Hemineglect and Denial Syndrome

Perceptual hemineglect is a disorder of attention causing an inability to integrate and use perceptions in the contralateral side or space (Quintana, 1995). The patient fails to respond to stimuli presented to the side contralateral to the brain lesion; therefore, that side is ignored but can be used if attention is drawn to it (Fitzgerald, 1992). Right brain damage produces the syndrome (Ferguson, 1991). Hemineglect can be seen alone or in combination with anosognosia and left homonymous hemianopsia (neglect syndrome) (Table 18–10). Patients with neglect will ignore the left half of their bodies, fail to dress or groom the left side of their bodies, neglect food on the left side of the plate, or bump into things in the left side of the environment. Anosognosia is a severe form of neglect whereby the individual denies the illness or ownership of his or her body. Denial of hemiplegia reportedly has occurred in 58 percent of patients with an acute right hemispheric stroke (Ellis & Small, 1994). The patient may rationalize the paralysis by saying that the affected arm is not moving because it is tired or lazy or is the body part of a cadaver or another person in bed with him or her. Neglect patients may also exhibit a "gaze preference," looking away from

TABLE 18–10. HEMINEGLECT SYNDROME

ALTERATION	PATIENT EFFECTS	LESION SITE	NURSING INTERVENTIONS
Hemineglect	Ignores opposite side of body	Usually nondominant posterior parietal cortex, brain stem reticular formation, limbic system, and frontal cortex	INITIALLY, COMPENSATE by approaching from unaffected side, positioning unimpaired side toward the action, arranging personal items within visual field, and teaching to scan head up and down, left to right
Denial (severe hemineglect)	Denies ownership of left side of body Inattention to left side and body space		
Anosognosia	Denial of illness		LATER, STIMULATE by placing personal items on the affected side, teaching the patient to handle, bathe, exercise, position, and dress the affected limbs, and position facing the impaired side
Homonymous hemianopsia	Visual field cut: half nasal field of one eye and half temporal field of other eye Usually left visual field deficit	Postchiasmal optic radiations to occipital lobe	

the affected side. When neglect or denial is present, the patient is at high risk for injury when transferring from bed to chair, from bumping into objects or persons in the left environmental space, or because of impaired judgment. The patient may manifest extinction to double simultaneous stimulation when identification of a single stimulus presented to the affected side is made but not when both sides receive the stimulus simultaneously. Only the stimulus presented to the unaffected side is identified correctly with this disorder.

Figure 18–9 illustrates how a stroke can result in a loss of visual fields in each eye. Homonymous hemianopsia, a visual field deficit with impaired vision in the nasal half of one eye and the temporal half of the other, can occur in either hemisphere but is more commonly found in persons with nondominant hemispheric strokes. These persons are frequently unaware of their deficit until it is brought to their attention. It occurs when the visual pathways (optic radiations) posterior to the optic chiasm (postchiasmal optic pathways) are involved in the stroke. Recall that once the optic nerve crosses at the optic chiasm, the medial half of the fibers of each eye cross and the lateral half of the fibers do not. Consequently, if the postchiasmal fibers in the right cerebral hemisphere are involved in a stroke, the patient will lose vision in the temporal half of the left eye and the nasal half of the

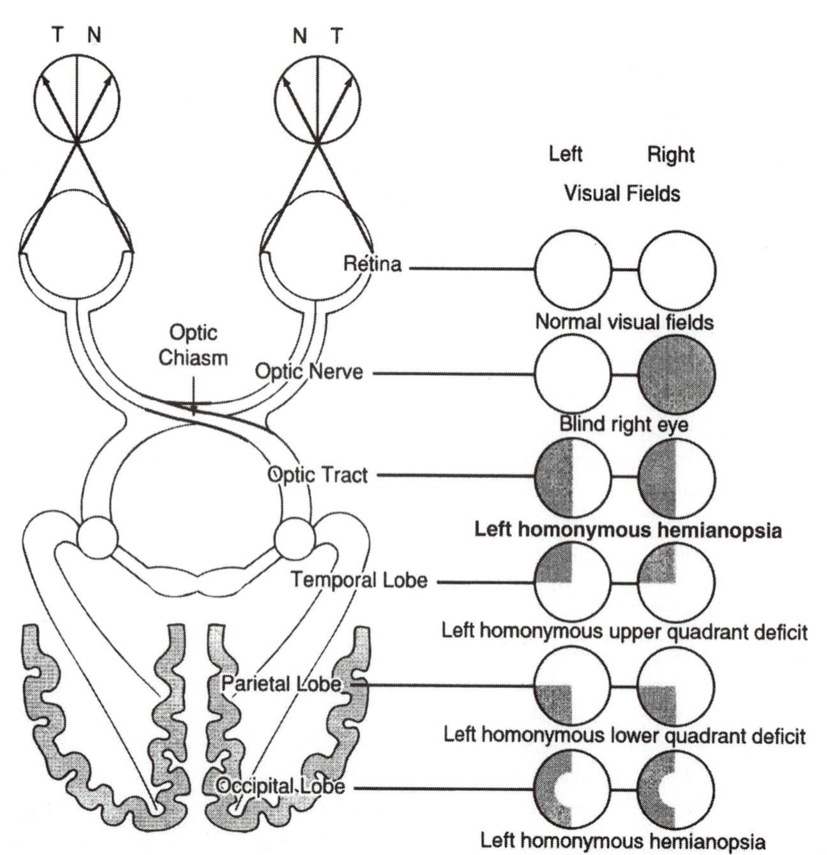

Figure 18–9. The visual fields. N = nasal; T = temporal. *(Adapted from Vazuka, F.A. [1968].* Essentials of the neurological examination, *p. 11. Philadelphia: Smith, Kline & French Laboratories.)*

right eye, which is the left visual field. Left homonymous hemianopsia often accompanies parietal neglect, resulting in a left visual field loss that usually improves several weeks after onset. Homonymous hemianopsia interferes with the patient's ability to eat and dress and is a potential hazard for the ambulating patient. Unilateral neglect is most pronounced immediately following the stroke and may be mild or severe. Recovery is usually slow and often incomplete (Quintana, 1995).

Assessment

Assessment for these deficits is done by performing confrontational testing for each visual field in the conscious patient or simply by having the patient draw a man or clock, read a page, or bisect a line (Fig. 18–10). With confrontational testing, the patient will not track an object into the affected field although full extraocular movements can be demonstrated by passive head turning. Only one half of the figure will be drawn in the presence of hemineglect, or one half of the page will be read. The line is bisected to the right of midpoint. Anosognosia is assessed by observing how the patient positions the hemiplegic limbs, how the patient refers to his or her limbs, and whether there is recognition of the loss of function of one side. The patient ignores the affected side and does not claim ownership of that side. The nurse can ask the patient to name and point to his or her body parts. Patients with homonymous hemianopsia may deviate their eyes away from the affected side and toward the normal side. Other clues to homonymous hemianopsia are unresponsiveness to visual stimuli in the affected field of vision, such as not eating food on one side of the tray, reading only half of a page, bumping into people or walls on the affected side, being unaware of environmental activities on the affected side, and apprehension. There is often a lack of insight into the problem; therefore, the patient should be asked whether he or she is aware of any peripheral vision loss. When assessment reveals deficits, these patients should be referred to occupational therapists for further testing and therapy.

Nursing Interventions

Nurses can assist a person with hemineglect syndrome by increasing the patient's awareness of the surroundings and by alleviating apprehension as to the source of the problem. When homonymous hemianopsia is present, initially the nurse compensates for the patient by approaching the patient from the unaffected side, positioning the patient so that the intact visual field is toward the action, arranging personal items within the field of vision, and teaching the patient to scan the environment by turning the head vertically and horizontally. As the patient's apprehension decreases, the nurse stimulates the patient by placing personal items toward the affected side to encourage awareness of and attention to that side. This may be accomplished by positioning so that the eyes are facing the affected side and by teaching the patient to handle, position, exercise, bathe, and dress the affected extremities with the patient's unaffected arm. **Anosognosia** (denial of illness) usually resolves as the patient recovers.

Body Schema Disturbances

Impaired body schema is the inability to identify body parts on self and others (Fig. 18–11). The lesion is usually in the left hemisphere. A related deficit includes right/left disorientation, or the inability to understand the concepts of right and left. Patients with right brain damage have difficulty in identifying the body parts of a confronting person (a visual spatial deficit) (Quintana, 1995).

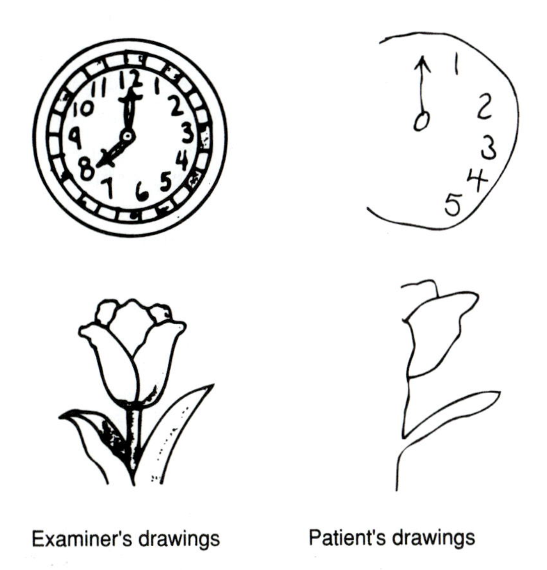

Figure 18–10. Examples of impaired performance on "copy clock, flower" test for unilateral neglect.

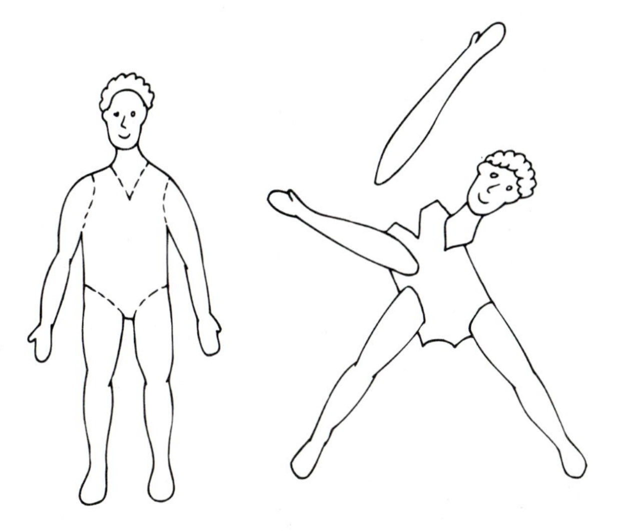

Figure 18–11. Impaired body schema. **Left:** human figure puzzle. **Right:** example of a severely impaired performance.

Assessment

To assess right/left disorientation, the nurse issues commands related to the right and left side, such as "Touch your right ear. Show me your right foot . . . your right eye . . . your left wrist."

Nursing Interventions

Cognitive cues can be provided by having the patient consistently wear a watch on either the left or right side and by color-coding clothing with one color for left and another for right. Stimulation can be used with quizzes on right/left discrimination.

Agnosias

Agnosia is the inability to recognize or interpret familiar sensory information although there is no impairment of sensory input or dementia. The agnosias can be tactile, visual, or auditory (Table 18–11); they are cortical impairments. Tactile agnosia (astereognosia) is the inability to recognize objects by touch although tactile sensation is present. Visual agnosia is the inability to recognize or name familiar objects or faces although visual acuity is intact (e.g., the patient is unable to recognize utensils, toothbrush, clothes, or photographs). Auditory agnosia is the inability to recognize familiar sounds such as the doorbell, telephone, horns, guns, or sirens.

Assessment

When assessing for agnosias, ask the patient to name objects and cite their purpose. Ask the patient to identify objects in the hands or to identify sounds, music, or songs with his or her eyes closed.

Interventions

When deficits are found, an occupational therapy referral is made and an **occupational therapist (OT)** evaluates and establishes a rehabilitative program that nurses will assist in implementing.

Apraxia

Apraxia is the inability to carry out a purposeful movement although movement, coordination, and sensation are intact (Quintana, 1995). There are several types of apraxias: motor, ideomotor, ideational, constructional, and dressing (Table 18–12). The lesion site varies with the type of apraxia. Motor apraxia may be related to a memory deficit, which results in the inability to follow a command although motor–sensory function is intact. It is similar to ideomotor apraxia except that the lesion site is in the frontal lobes. Ideomotor apraxia is the inability to perform a motor act on command even though the patient clearly understands the act. The lesion site is in the left dominant parietal lobe. The patient may have difficulty with eating, not knowing which utensils to use or how to use them because of loss of memory for the sequence of movements. Simple isolated acts can be performed but there is difficulty in sequencing motor acts. When asked to write with a pencil, the patient knows what to do but is unable to do it on command, although he or she may do it spontaneously at another time (Quintana, 1995). Ideational apraxia is the inability to perform activities automatically or on command because the patient no longer understands the activity. Simple isolated (but not complex) acts may be performed. Constructional apraxia is the inability to copy, draw, or construct designs in two or three dimensions on command or spontaneously (Zoltan, Siev, & Freishtat, 1991). The patient with dressing apraxia is unable to dress himself or herself because of a disorder in body schema, unilateral neglect, or constructional apraxia. Apraxias create problems for patients in performing ADLs, social interactions, and job performances because of their impaired ability to follow requests. The lesion site is hemispheric, with more frequency and severity in the right hemisphere. Patients with these deficits need referral to occupational therapy.

Assessment

To assess for motor and ideomotor apraxias, the nurse can observe responses to motor commands such as "Brush your teeth . . . comb your hair . . . put on your gown." Observation of spontaneous motor acts may differentiate ideomotor apraxic patients who are usually able to perform them from the ideational apraxic patient who cannot perform spontaneous acts or acts on command. These patients are evaluated by a speech language pathologist. Constructional apraxia can be assessed by asking patients to copy or draw a clock or daisy or build three-dimensional designs such as a house or a block. Dressing apraxia is assessed by asking the patient to put on or remove a shirt, gown, or robe. Observation of the patient's abilities in these areas will unmask an apraxia.

TABLE 18–11. AGNOSIAS

TYPE	LESION SITE	ASSESSMENT
Tactile (astereognosia)	Either parietal lobe	Ask patient to identify objects by touch with eyes closed (keys, coins, etc.)
Visual	Temporoparietal–occipital lobe of either hemisphere	Ask patient to identify safety pin, pen, or wristwatch (visual object recognition)
Auditory	Temporal lobe in dominant hemisphere	Ask patient to identify familiar sounds (tunes, telephone, etc.)

TABLE 18–12. APRAXIAS

TYPE	LESION SITE	ASSESSMENT
Motor: Memory deficit for motor sequences affecting only upper limbs, although muscle and sensory function are intact	Frontal lobes (premotor areas)	Observe ability to initiate responses to motor commands
Ideomotor: Inability to perform a motor act on command even though patient understands act and has muscle and sensory function. Can perform spontaneous, simple, isolated acts but not complex acts such as writing or dressing	Left dominant parietal lobe	Ask the patient to do a complex command such as writing, drinking from a cup Note ability to do spontaneous simple acts
Ideational: Inability to perform activities automatically or on command	Left dominant parietal lobe	Ask the patient to write. Is unable to conceptualize act, and cannot do a complex or spontaneous simple act
Constructional: Inability to copy, draw, or construct designs in two or three dimensions on command or spontaneously	Occipitoparietal cortices	Occupational therapy referral. Ask the patient to draw a cube, house
Dressing: Inability to dress self because of a disorder in body schema, unilateral neglect, and/or spatial relations	Usually nondominant (right) parietal–occipital area	Ask the patient to put on a gown, sweater, or robe

Nursing Interventions

The effectiveness of therapy for ideomotor and ideational apraxia is uncertain. For ideomotor and ideational apraxia, the components of a motor sequence leading up to the entire activity need to be broken down and taught in simple terms, speaking slowly with clear directions. The patient with dressing apraxia can be assisted by using labels to distinguish right and left, back from front, right and wrong side, or by color-coding garments. For all apraxic patients, repetition, consistency, avoidance of distractions, and visual motor coordination exercises are useful.

Spatial Relations and Position-in-Space Disturbances

The stroke patient with spatial relations disturbances may have perceptual deficits of figure ground, form constancy, topographical disorientation, depth–distance deficits, and position-in-space deficits. The patient with a figure-ground deficit is unable to differentiate the foreground from the background and has difficulty finding things such as a sleeve in a monocolored shirt or a comb in a cluttered drawer. The lesion site is usually in the nondominant parietal lobe or may involve a large hemispheric lesion or many small lesions anywhere in the brain. The patient with a form-constancy deficit is unable to attend to subtle variations in forms or shapes and may confuse a water glass or pitcher for the urinal. The lesion site is usually in the nondominant parietal lobe. Patients with topographical disorientation have difficulty understanding and remembering relationships of places to one another and get easily lost. The lesion site is in the occipitoparietal lobe more often in the nondominant hemisphere. The patient with depth and distance deficits is unable to judge depth and distance safely and may fall going up or down stairs, overreach or underreach a target, bump into doors or other objects, or continue pouring tea or coffee after a cup has been filled. The lesion site is the parietal lobe of either hemisphere. The patient with position-in-space deficits has problems with concepts such as over, under, front, back, inside, and outside. The lesion site is usually the nondominant parietal lobe. These deficits are potential risks for injury and create obstacles in achieving ADLs and independence (Quintana, 1995).

Skilled nurses caring for patients diagnosed with lesions in these sites can observe the patient for behavioral cues that alert them to spatial disturbances such as problems dressing, bathing, or eating. Nurses can refer patients with spatial-relations deficits to occupational therapy. Discriminating shapes such as blocks and letters, and encouraging the use of other senses by utilizing full-length mirrors for reorientation to the vertical plane, is also helpful. Nurses can adapt the environment by removing obstacles and clutter and keeping the furniture in the same place. With a physical therapy referral, the patient can practice walking up and down stairs and through furniture without injury. The bed should be in a low position.

In summary, patients with visual–spatial–perceptual alterations need careful assessment for subtle deficits, many of which the patient is unaware of. With knowledge of the deficit and lesion site, the nurse can actively assess for these deficits and refer the patient to OT or PT for further evaluation and a plan of therapy. The nurse can monitor and encourage the patient to implement the plan by either compensation, stimulation of the affected parts, or both, to prevent injury and achieve a functional recovery.

SECTION THIRTEEN REVIEW

1. Which of the following is true regarding the hemineglect syndrome seen in stroke patients?
   - **A.** it usually occurs in dominant strokes
   - **B.** it may be accompanied with left homonymous hemianopsia
   - **C.** the patient is paralyzed on one side of his or her body
   - **D.** the patient has insight into the cause of the impairment
2. Mrs. Anderson, age 50, had a right hemispheric stroke. She is unable to follow commands although she can automatically use both hands. Her problem is called
   - **A.** agnosia
   - **B.** apraxia
   - **C.** denial
   - **D.** neglect
3. All of the following interventions can assist stroke patients with agnosias EXCEPT
   - **A.** exercises in identifying pictures, objects, and places
   - **B.** referral to physical therapy
   - **C.** compensating with the use of intact senses
   - **D.** discriminating different cloth textures and objects with eyes closed
4. Assessment of Mary Carnes, age 30, for visual–perceptual deficits following an acute stroke would include all of the following EXCEPT
   - **A.** asking her to draw a clock
   - **B.** observing her dietary tray after meals
   - **C.** asking her to read a page or bisect a line
   - **D.** asking her to sing a song
5. All of the following are visual–spatial relations deficits EXCEPT the inability to
   - **A.** judge depth or distance
   - **B.** differentiate foreground from background
   - **C.** grasp an object when requested to do it
   - **D.** discriminate among various shapes and forms

Answers: 1. B, 2. B, 3. B, 4. D, 5. C

SECTION FOURTEEN: Impaired Communication

Language and speech are important humanistic functions that allow us to communicate our needs, maintain social interactions, and remain gainfully employed. Language is a broad term encompassing verbal and nonverbal means of communicating thoughts and feelings. It is learned and involves oral and written expression, auditory and reading comprehension, and emotional forms of communication. Speech, one component of language, is the sensory integration and motor act of verbally expressing our thoughts and feelings. This section discusses three forms of aphasia/dysphasia (Broca's, Wernicke's, and global) found in acute stroke patients with left hemispheric damage. At the completion of this section, the learner will be able to differentiate dysphasic/aphasias from dysarthrias, and describe nursing interventions to enhance the communication of dysphasic/aphasic and dysarthric stroke patients.

Stroke patients with left hemispheric damage caused by middle cerebral artery damage experience **dysphasia/aphasia** if the speech centers or their pathways are involved in the lesion. When one hears speech, the auditory impulses are transmitted via cranial nerve VIII to the primary auditory center in the dominant temporal lobe. From there, the impulses travel to Wernicke's area (temporal lobe) where the sensory impulses are integrated and interpreted. Once interpreted, the impulses travel through a bundle of nerve fibers (the arcuate fasciculus) to Broca's expressive speech area in the dominant frontal lobe. From Broca's area, the motor command for speech is issued to the speech muscles in the primary motor area, and we speak (Fig. 18–12).

Dominance for speech and language is in the left hemisphere for approximately 95 percent of the population. The right hemisphere has a role in the nonverbal component of communication—prosody. Prosody involves voice intonation, accent, timing, and emotions.

Aphasia/dysphasia is a disorder of linguistic processing in which a disruption of translating thought to language has occurred. Literally, aphasia means a total inability to understand or formulate language. Language comprehension, speech expression, or writing ability may be lost. Dysphasia is difficulty with comprehending, speaking, or writing. For purposes of this discussion, aphasia will be defined as a mild to severe disturbance in understanding or formulating language. It must be differentiated from dysarthria (impairment of the muscles that control speech). Two aphasias (Broca's and Wernicke's) will be compared and contrasted in terms of lesion site, speech characteristics, comprehension, capacity for repetition, and related stroke deficits (Table 18–13).

In Wernicke's aphasia, the patient receives auditory speech impulses but is unable to comprehend them. It is a receptive aphasia characterized by fluent, well-articulated speech with intact tone but inappropriate speech content that is unintelligible because of poor word choices. The patient makes up new words (neologisms) in his or her

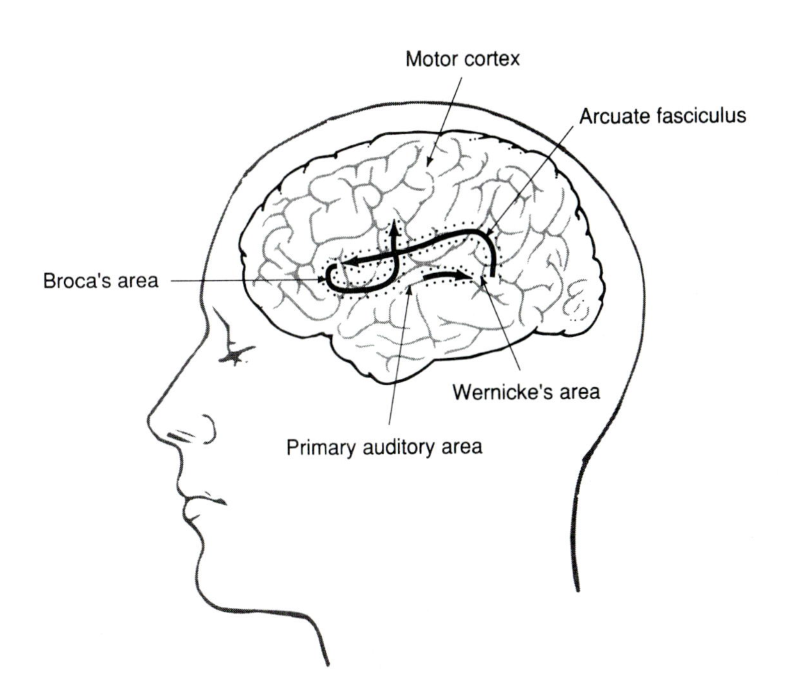

Figure 18–12. Pathways for motor speech: speaking a heard word. *(Adapted from Geschwind, N. [September, 1979]. Specializations of the human brain.* Scientific American. *Illustration by Carol Donner.)*

speech content. Reading and speech comprehension, repetition of speech, and naming of objects is impaired. The patient is unable to write coherently. Motor deficits are seldom seen in these patients because the lesion site is in the left temporal lobe (Damasio, 1992). The goal of therapy for acute stroke patients with Wernicke's aphasia is to develop an awareness of the language problem and to increase comprehension. Compensating with meaningful auditory and tactile stimuli may help. Touch and modulating voice tone can provide a calming effect on the patient. The removal of extraneous sounds and distractions such as the television or radio can assist in getting the person's attention. The use of repetition and naming drills may help. The patient and nurse can use nonverbal behavior to enhance communication. Keeping the conversation on one defined subject with one question at a time and avoiding multiple choices when communicating is helpful. Broca's aphasia is an expressive aphasia characterized by nonfluent, telegraphic speech with outbursts of profanity, uninhibited speech, and word-finding difficulty, which may reflect impaired memory for language. The patient uses nouns or phrases with pauses between words, and lacks grammar. An awareness of speech errors is present and speech production is labored and frustrating. A poor capacity for repetition and difficulty naming objects exists although recognition of objects is present. Oddly, these patients can sing fluently because musical ability is intact in the nondominant hemisphere. Comprehension is usually intact and responses are appropriate. Reading comprehension is variable and writing ability is impaired, possibly because an associated right hemiparesis or hemiplegia is often found in these patients since Broca's area is located adjacent to the primary motor centers in the frontal lobe. The goal for the patient with Broca's aphasia is to establish reliable language output to express needs. This may be accomplished initially by asking the patient "yes–no" questions. In addition, repetition drills, reading out loud, sentence completion drills, and the use of visual cues have been employed to stimulate speech. Singing, which is a function of the nondominant hemisphere, is fluent and may be used as therapy (Wallhagen, 1979).

Global aphasia is a combination of Broca's and Wernicke's aphasia with an almost complete loss of compre-

TABLE 18–13. BROCA'S AND WERNICKE'S APHASIAS COMPARED

TYPE	LESION SITE	SPEECH CHARACTERISTICS	COMPREHENSION	REPETITION	NAMING	WRITING
Wernicke's (receptive, sensory)	Temporal lobe	Fluent, well-articulated speech Intact tone, unintelligible; neologisms	Impaired verbal and reading comprehension	Impaired	Impaired	Impaired
Broca's (expressive, motor)	Frontal lobe	Nonfluent, telegraphic, uninhibited speech; word-finding difficulty; lacks grammar	Verbal usually intact; reading varies	Impaired	Impaired	Impaired (may be due to hemiparesis)

Adapted from Damasio, A.R. (1992). Aphasia. N Eng J Med *326:531–539.*

hension and expression of speech. The lesion involves the frontal and temporal lobes. The patient has nonfluent speech and an inability to express his or her ideas in speech or writing. The goal for the patient with global aphasia, a mixed sensory and motor aphasia, is to improve the ability to communicate. The patient is taught to enhance communication with nonverbal gestures and facial expressions and the measures cited for both Wernicke's and Broca's aphasias.

Dysarthria is an impairment of the muscles that control speech. Hemispheric or brain stem strokes can produce dysarthria, which is characterized by slurred, muffled, or indistinct speech. If the basal ganglia or cerebellum are involved, uncoordinated, slow, monotonal speech results. Language comprehension and formulation are intact unless the patient also has an aphasia. For the dysarthric patient, the goal of therapy is to strengthen the speech muscles in order to speak more clearly and fluently. Encouraging the person to enunciate one word at a time, particularly consonants, and increasing voice volume when it is low, helps.

Assessment and Nursing Interventions

When assessing the acute stroke patient for language dysfunction, the nurse should elicit the following:

- *History:* Is there a history of mental dysfunction, or visual or hearing impairments? Is the patient depressed? Is the attention span short? Are hearing and visual deficits evident?
- *Speech characteristics:* Is the speech fluent and coherent, or nonfluent, inappropriate, and with grammatical errors? Is the speech uninhibited, with outbursts of profanity? Does the patient use neologisms? Is there word-finding difficulty? Is the speech rhythmic or is it slurred and indistinct? Does the patient speak in words, phrases, or sentences?
- *Comprehension:* Is the patient able to comprehend what is said or read? Does the patient follow simple verbal or written instructions without the benefit of nonverbal cues?
- *Naming ability:* Can the patient name objects?
- *Repetition:* Is the patient able to repeat words or phrases?
- *Writing ability:* Is the patient able to write what is dictated?

When handedness cannot be established, observe the thumb nailbeds. Usually the dominant hand has a wider nailbed (Mulley, 1985). Any speech deficits identified in the assessment warrant referral to a speech language pathologist for further evaluation and language therapy. Nurses can collaborate with the speech language pathologist to monitor and assist in the prescribed speech therapy tailored for the patient's deficit. Spontaneous recovery from aphasia usually occurs in 6 to 12 weeks from onset, but additional improvement may occur for ≥ 2 years. The nurse can promote language stimulation by (Table 18–14):

- Having the patient name objects and repeat names as the nurse points to objects
- Encouraging the stable patient to listen to the radio and television when alone
- Practicing speech and teaching the family to encourage the patient to speak

In summary, patients who experience dominant hemispheric strokes may develop expressive (Broca's), receptive (Wernicke's), or global (both expressive and receptive) aphasias. Broca's aphasia, with the lesion site in the frontal lobe, is often accompanied by motor deficits, whereas Wernicke's aphasia, with a lesion site in the temporal lobe, is not. Patients with Broca's aphasia are usually aware of their deficit and have word-finding difficulty and nonfluent speech, but they comprehend speech. Those with Wernicke's aphasia are usually unaware of their deficit, have fluent, inappropriate speech, and do not comprehend speech. Those with global aphasia can neither understand nor express speech. Dysarthric patients have slurred but appropriate speech and comprehension since their deficit is a speech muscle problem. Speech muscle exercises will assist the dysarthric stroke patient. To assist all aphasic patients with communication, the nurse should speak slowly; praise communication progress; compensate with gestures, facial expressions, and visual and tactile communication boards; and keep verbal instructions simple and concise.

TABLE 18–14. IMPROVING COMMUNICATION FOR ALL APHASIC PATIENTS

Reinforce progress in communication with praise
Stimulate language by having the patient name objects and repeat names as you point to objects
Compensate with nonverbal communication such as gestures and facial expressions and supplement with visual and tactile aids such as digitized electronic device (palm pilot), computer
Pace questions
Ask for clarification, do not pretend to understand
Keep verbal instructions simple and concise

Source: Adapted from Wallhagen, M.I. (1979). The split brain. Implications for care and rehabilitation. AJN *79:2116–2125.*

SECTION FOURTEEN REVIEW

1. Dominance for language is located in the left cerebral hemisphere for approximately what percentage of the population?
   A. 95 percent
   B. 85 percent
   C. 75 percent
   D. 65 percent
2. Which of the following is true of prosody? It is
   A. the inability to express speech
   B. the inability to understand speech
   C. a function of the dominant hemisphere
   D. the emotional component of speech
3. Mrs. Beaumont, age 30, had an embolic stroke involving her left frontal and parietal lobes. She follows commands, has difficulty naming objects, blurts out profanities on occasion, and speaks in words and phrases in nonfluent speech. Her communication impairment most likely is
   A. Wernicke's aphasia
   B. global aphasia
   C. Broca's aphasia
   D. dysarthria
4. To assist Mrs. Beaumont to enhance her communication, the nurse would appropriately do all of the following EXCEPT
   A. avoid gestures when speaking
   B. speak more slowly and not loudly
   C. provide flash cards with pictures and words
   D. allow time for delayed processing when speaking
5. Mrs. Jericho, age 60, had a brain attack involving her left temporal lobe. She has difficulty following verbal directions. Her speech is fluent and well articulated, but inappropriate in content. Her communication impairment is most likely
   A. Broca's aphasia
   B. dysarthria
   C. Wernicke's aphasia
   D. global aphasia
6. To assist dysarthric patients to enhance their communication, the nurse can encourage
   A. singing
   B. listening to radio and television
   C. word drills enunciating consonants
   D. whistling and lowering voice volume

Answers: 1. A, 2. D, 3. C, 4. A, 5. C, 6. C

SECTION FIFTEEN: High Risk for Ineffective Patient and Family Coping

The potential for ineffective coping is related to abrupt change in lifestyle, loss of roles, dependency, and economic insecurity. This section discusses psychosocial stressors that acute stroke patients and their families frequently encounter and nursing interventions to assist them to cope more effectively with these problems. Referrals and resources are an important aspect of client and family coping during the acute as well as the chronic stages of the illness. At the completion of this section, the learner will be able to:

1. Identify stressors that can lead to ineffective patient and family coping
2. Identify the effects of stroke on sexual roles and body image
3. Promote a positive body image and positive coping mechanisms
4. Provide assistance including referrals and resources to assist the patient and family to cope more effectively with their deficits

The inability to cope with abrupt and severe changes in body function or image, lifestyle changes, fears of becoming a burden on the family, dependency, and economic insecurity with loss of the breadwinner role provide ample and valid reasons for ineffective coping. In addition, the family may have to assume new roles as care providers and relinquish jobs and salaries. They may be overwhelmed with medical bills or faced with nursing home placement of their loved one and subsequent guilt. Fears of another stroke as well as inability to care for the patient at home create more stress. Dominant hemispheric stroke patients, in addition, are prone to severe depression because of their awareness of their deficits. Depression may be manifested by decreased motivation, hopelessness, insomnia, feelings of low self-esteem, worthlessness, and lack of energy. Premorbid successful coping behaviors assist these patients in rehabilitation. Other causes for ineffective coping are the emotional and cognitive impairments following a stroke. Emotional lability with inappropriate crying, laughter, or euphoria, or socially inappropriate behavior with an inability to interpret social cues of communication, create stress for both the patient and family. Uninhibited behavior with outbursts of profanities or abrupt or impulsive behavior provide additional sources of stress. Confusion and bewilderment may compound the problem. In terms of impaired cognition, there may be delayed processing, diminished learning and reasoning ability, and a short attention span. Memory deficits vary with the hemispheric involvement. If the nondominant hemisphere is involved, a memory deficit for performance may be seen; if the dominant hemisphere is involved, a memory deficit for language, word-finding difficulty, and naming problems surface. In addition, there are hemispheric differences in judgment. Patients with lesions in the left hemisphere are slow, cautious, and underestimate their abilities. In contrast, patients with right hemispheric lesions may be prone to injury because they overestimate their abilities.

Stroke patients are threatened in their roles of parent, spouse, breadwinner, and homemaker. Body image is further assaulted with dependency in grooming, eating, toileting, and sexual activity. One study of 35 stroke survivors found that men experience a significant decrease in their ability to achieve erection and ejaculate, although libido was present. The five premenopausal women experienced major alterations in menses and decreased orgasms after stroke (Bray, DeFrank, & Wolfe, 1981). The good news is that libido returns about 6 weeks following a stroke, and erectile capacity returns in 7 weeks (Bronstein, Popovich, & Stewart-Amidei, 1991). The level of prestroke activity is the most important indicator for potential poststroke sexual activity. Compensatory adaptations for physical deficits can be made by altering the positions of the couple.

Assessment of premorbid personality, particularly coping behaviors, is important. The nurse must explore the patient's and family's concerns and fears related to the stroke experience and determine whether there is a realistic basis for these fears. Patient and family roles should be assessed. What stage of grieving is the patient experiencing? How is he or she coping now? Is the patient depressed, anxious, hopeless, angry, impulsive? What is the patient expressing verbally and nonverbally? Who is the patient's significant other? Are there any support systems that would assist the patient now? Differentiate confusion from inappropriate responses by assessing orientation, insight, or doing a mini-mental state assessment (Folstein, Folstein, & McHugh, 1975).

To assist the stroke patient in coping effectively, the nurse can provide appropriate information to alleviate fears and strengthen support systems. Clergy, friends, and stroke family support groups may be utilized to assist the patient to cope and may provide comfort for both the patient and the family. The nurse can maximize independency to the patient's potential and teach the family to do the same. This can begin with involvement in decision making and ADLs. Informing the patient that most recovery takes up to 6 months and some recovery of function even longer may be helpful in preventing unrealistic expectations for recovery.

If inappropriate crying or laughter occurs, the behavior may be stopped by diverting the patient's attention from the behavior. Provide feedback in a matter-of-fact way when behavior is inappropriate. Avoid nagging, angry, punitive responses. Be patient and gently slow down impulsive behavior. For judgmental impairments, the nondominant stroke patient must be supervised closely for safety. Do not rely on what patients with nondominant hemispheric strokes say they can do; rather, supervise their performance. Encourage the left hemispheric patient to perform those abilities he or she is capable of doing and reinforce success to instill confidence in these abilities. Setting short-term attainable goals will often reduce frustration during rehabilitation.

To promote a positive body image and maintain an adequate self-concept in stroke patients, nurses can promote grooming. Unilateral ADLs that a patient can initiate early are hair combing or shaving with an electric razor in front of a mirror. Brushing teeth may require assistance in squeezing toothpaste from the tube. To insert dentures into the mouth, teach the patient to place them toward the affected side first, where sensation is absent, and then the unaffected side, where sensation is present. To clean dentures over a basin, teach the patient to place a cloth and water in the basin or sink to prevent breakage should the dentures fall. To apply makeup, women are taught to begin on the unaffected side first because it provides a model for application to the affected side. Encourage the patient to dress in street clothes as early as possible. The nurse can assist the patient and family to resume or modify or adapt to new roles when this is indicated.

A positive body image is reinforced when one focuses on the function that is left and not on that which is lost. Speak positively about the remainder of body functions. Use terms such as *affected* and *unaffected* rather than *good* and *bad* side. Reinforce independence early by involving the patient in decisions in care. Teach the family to do the same related to family roles and care. The nurse may explain the sexual problems when the patient asks, or refer the questions to a physician or sexual counselor.

For the patient and family, multidisciplinary referrals may be necessary. Social workers, home health nurses, dieticians, occupational therapists, physiatrists, stroke support groups, and voluntary and governmental agencies (e.g., Medicare) that provide assistance are all multidisciplinary players on the patient's road to recovery. The American Heart Association and the National Stroke Association provide free and low-cost literature on stroke care developed by experts in the field. These referral groups and services are essential for the functional recovery of the stroke patient and provide invaluable assistance in restoring the stroke victim to a functional or complete recovery.

In summary, the stroke patient and family are faced with many stressors as a result of an abrupt change in lifestyle, loss of roles, dependency, guilt, and economic insecurity. Assessment of the client's premorbid personality, coping behaviors, and significant others will assist the nurse to mobilize support systems for both the patient and the family. Managing behavioral effects of stroke can be accomplished by diverting the patient's attention from inappropriate laughter or crying and avoiding angry punitive responses. A positive body image is promoted by sensitivity to body terminology used and by encouraging independence and grooming as early as possible after stroke onset. Finally, a variety of community support services should be utilized to promote a functional recovery of the stroke patient and assist the family.

Stroke can be a devastating multisystemic disorder that leads to depression, dysfunction, decreased quality of life, and death; with early treatment and rehabilitative care, however, the patient can be restored to a purposeful, functional recovery with an enhanced quality of life. Robert Louis Stevenson, G. Frederick Handel, and Louis Pasteur all suffered strokes and recovered sufficiently to continue their life's work without the benefit of today's technologies. Handel wrote the *Messiah*, and Pasteur accomplished 90 percent of his research after having his stroke (Graham, 1976). These remarkable achievements demonstrate that functional recoveries and productive lives are realistic goals for many stroke patients, particularly with the advantages of new knowledge and therapies, early treatment, motivation, support, and effective nursing care.

SECTION FIFTEEN REVIEW

1. All of the following are potential stressors for patients with acute brain attacks EXCEPT
   A. changes in body image
   B. independence
   C. fears of becoming a burden on the family
   D. role modification
2. Mrs. Della Hess, age 55, had a dominant hemispheric stroke. The nurse should be alerted to which of the following behavioral effects?
   A. depression
   B. impulsivity
   C. euphoria
   D. hyperactivity
3. When assisting Mrs. Foster, age 84, a left hemiparetic to perform ADLs, the nurse would appropriately teach her to
   A. insert her dentures first toward the unaffected side
   B. clean her dentures over a basin full of water
   C. clean her dentures over the empty sink
   D. put her makeup on the impaired side of her face first
4. Mrs. Beauchamp asks the nurse if her left hemiplegic arm and leg will ever be normal again. Which of the following responses would be most accurate?
   A. some function may return if the damaged nerve cells get an adequate blood flow
   B. nerve cells do regenerate in the brain, so function will be restored within 6 months
   C. once your blood pressure is controlled, your legs will move again
   D. when the brain swelling subsides, your function will return
5. When teaching a patient with a right hemispheric deficit, the effective nurse will
   A. use verbal aids in instruction
   B. use visual aids in instruction
   C. expect slow, cautious behavior
   D. expect depression

Answers: 1. B, 2. A, 3. B, 4. A, 5. A

SECTION SIXTEEN: Predictors of Outcome and Causes of Mortality

This section discusses clinical signs and symptoms associated with outcomes poststroke. The causes of mortality are addressed. At the completion of this section, the learner will be able to explain predictors of poor outcomes as well as the most frequent causes of death in the acute stroke patient.

Predictors of Outcome

Alteration in level of consciousness is the single strongest predictor of short-term survival. Altered level of consciousness indicates damage to the reticular activating system or involvement of both cerebral hemispheres. Other poor prognostic signs indicative of large areas of hemispheric damage are incontinence, conjugate gaze palsy, and gross hemiplegia (Case & Crowell, 1994). High serum glucose and ferritin levels in acute stroke patients are believed to promote more ischemic damage because of the increase in lactate and oxygen free radicals, respectively (Davalos, Fernandez-Real, & Ricart, 1994). Impaired cognition, language, visual function, and depression result in more dependency (Grotta, 1993a, b).

Other poor prognosticators for rehabilitation (McDowell, Brott, & Goldstein, 1993) include:

- Persistent flaccid hemiplegia
- Sensory loss on the left side
- Marked receptive dysphasia
- No family support
- Preexistent systemic disease, especially hypertension
- Depression
- Impaired interest and short attention span

Positive factors affecting recovery are motivation, acceptance, and understanding of the disability and a strong family support system. Gross motor performance at onset of stroke is one of the most important predictors of independence in the activities of daily living. The earlier the recovery of function, the more functional the recovery. The ability to form isolated movements voluntarily without eliciting movement synergy (all muscles moving together) is a good prognostic sign.

Many scales have been devised to assess the outcomes and progress of the patient toward recovery following a stroke. The Barthel Index assesses the functional recovery of nine categories (feeding, transfers, grooming, toileting, bathing, walking, climbing stairs, bowel and bladder control) and assigns and weights scores ranging from independence to total dependency (Mahoney & Barthel, 1965; Bronstein, Popovich, & Stewart-Amidei, 1991). The NIH Stroke Scale is a clinical assessment scale of neurologic function for acute stroke patients. It measures neurologic functions such as levels of responsiveness, gaze, movements, and sensation (Wityk et al., 1994).

Causes of Mortality

Most deaths following acute stroke occur within the first 30 days. Cerebral edema leading to transtentorial herniation is the most common cause of death in stroke patients during the first week after onset. Mortality during the first week may also be due to acute myocardial infarction or fatal arrhythmias. Deaths in the second and third weeks following acute stroke onset are caused by complications such as pneumonia, sepsis, and deep vein thrombosis leading to pulmonary emboli. Patients who are unable to swallow and aspirate succumb to pneumonia; while those who are immobile develop deep vein thrombosis leading to pulmonary emboli (Yatsu, Grotta, & Pettigrew, 1995). Nurses have an important role in preventing these secondary intracranial and systemic complications.

In summary, predictors of poor outcome in stroke are symptoms and signs that reflect diffuse hemispheric damage or upper brain stem damage. The most important predictor of poor outcome is altered level of consciousness. Positive factors affecting recovery are motivation, acceptance, and a strong family support system. Good prognosticators are gross motor performance at the onset of stroke and early recovery of function. Mortality following acute stroke during the first week is usually due to cerebral edema and herniation. Death during the second or third week is usually a result of systemic complications such as aspiration pneumonia, deep vein thrombosis, or pulmonary emboli.

SECTION SIXTEEN REVIEW

1. The single strongest predictor of poor outcome in stroke patients is
   A. incontinence
   B. decreased level of consciousness
   C. spasticity
   D. dysphasia
2. The lethal event for acute stroke patients during the first week after the attack is most frequently
   A. secondary pneumonia
   B. cerebral emboli
   C. congestive heart failure
   D. increased ICP and herniation

Answers: 1. B, 2. D

POSTTEST

1. All of the following assessment findings suggest life-threatening symptoms or signs in stroke patients EXCEPT
   A. decreased level of consciousness
   B. sluggishly dilating pupil
   C. decerebration
   D. body neglect
2. Mrs. Phillips, age 60, had a hemorrhagic stroke and was unresponsive on admission. The nurse correctly prioritized her care by initially
   A. taking her blood pressure
   B. assessing her airway and breathing
   C. taking her temperature
   D. doing a neurologic assessment
3. Cerebrally induced cardiac arrhythmias are life threatening and are often treated with
   A. vasodilators
   B. alpha blockers
   C. beta blockers
   D. dopamine

4. Mrs. Jones is in the flaccid stage of her stroke. She is at high risk for which life-threatening condition?
   A. deep vein thrombosis
   B. pressure sores
   C. septicemia
   D. seizure
5. Jackie Harris, age 50, had an embolic stroke. She was taught to exercise her affected arm with her unaffected arm. Which principle of rehabilitation is she using?
   A. compensation
   B. idling
   C. inhibition
   D. neurodevelopmental
6. The highest level of movement in functional recovery of stroke patients is
   A. flaccidity
   B. voluntary movements
   C. mass pattern movements
   D. spastic movements
7. The effects of undernutrition in the stroke patient include which of the following?
   A. high risk for infections
   B. increased motor tone
   C. hyperalbuminemia
   D. positive urinary urea nitrogen
8. When assisting a stroke patient to eat, aspiration may be prevented by
   A. placing the patient in a low semi-Fowler's position
   B. teaching the patient to flex the chin downward while swallowing
   C. placing the food on the affected side of the mouth
   D. giving the patient liquids with the food
9. Which of the following is true of elimination problems in acute stroke patients?
   A. bowel incontinence is common
   B. indwelling urinary catheters are useful for patients with hyperreflexic bladders
   C. incontinence is usually the stress type incontinence
   D. scheduled voiding programs can promote continence
10. Incontinent stroke patients can be assisted toward continence at night by
    A. limiting fluid intake to 1,200 mL/day
    B. restricting caffeinated and evening fluids
    C. teaching the patient to wear Attend pads
    D. attaching a leg bag to an indwelling catheter at night
11. Mrs. Derma has a left hemiplegia and hemisensory loss following a hemispheric stroke. All of the following place her at risk for pressure sores EXCEPT
    A. her inability to feel pressure
    B. her loss of vasomotor tone
    C. constipation
    D. her hemiparesis
12. Robert Reddy, age 50, had a primary intracerebral hemorrhage in his right parietal lobe and a left homonymous hemianopsia. Which of the following would be appropriate nursing interventions for Robert?
    A. initially, touching him from the left side before speaking
    B. placing an eyepatch on the left eye
    C. instilling artificial tears in his left eye
    D. initially placing personal items on his right side
13. With this deficit (see Question 12), Robert
    A. is totally blind in the left eye
    B. has a nasal loss of vision in his left and right eye fields
    C. has a loss of his peripheral vision
    D. has a nasal loss of vision in his right eye and a temporal loss in his left eye
14. To enhance communication for the patient with Wernicke's aphasia, the nurse can
    A. have the patient practice naming objects
    B. have the patient listen to the radio or television
    C. provide multiple choices to assist in decision making
    D. provide language-learning tape recordings
15. Mr. Williams, age 69, was taken to the emergency department within an hour of his brain attack. He was a reserved, respectable professor of engineering. In the emergency department, he began cursing the aide and nurse and shocked his embarrassed wife, who had never heard him speak with this foul language. During the nursing assessment, his speech was nonfluent, predominantly nouns and phrases, and telegraphic. His communication impairment is most probably a
    A. Broca's aphasia
    B. Wernicke's aphasia
    C. dysarthria
    D. global aphasia
16. Normal cerebral blood flow is about
    A. 90 to 100 mL/100 g/min
    B. 60 to 80 mL/100 g/min
    C. 50 to 60 mL/100 g/min
    D. 30 to 50 mL/100 g/min
17. Which of the following characterizes atherothrombotic strokes?
    A. they usually involve the carotid and middle cerebral arteries
    B. they usually occur with activity
    C. the strokes they produce usually have no warnings
    D. the deficit is maximal at onset
18. Which of the following individuals is at greatest risk for stroke according to current data?
    A. 65-year-old Japanese man
    B. 60-year-old Caucasian American woman
    C. 55-year-old African-American woman
    D. 65-year-old African-American man

19. Risk factors for stroke include all of the following EXCEPT
    A. low hematocrit
    B. hypertension
    C. cardiac valvular disease
    D. diabetes mellitus
20. In the ischemic cascade, which electrolyte is believed to generate the greatest cellular damage when there is an ionic imbalance?
    A. potassium
    B. calcium
    C. sodium
    D. magnesium
21. The cerebral perfusion range for oligemia is about
    A. 80 to 55 mL/100 g/min
    B. 60 to 43 mL/100 g/min
    C. 49 to 23 mL/100 g/min
    D. 22 to 10 mL/100 g/min
22. Mr. Dixon had a brain attack. By the time he arrived at the hospital, his blood pressure was 200/110 mm Hg. He was diagnosed as having an ischemic stroke of the middle cerebral artery. Guidelines for treating acute stroke victims would indicate that he should be given
    A. calcium channel blockers to bring the blood pressure down to 160/95 mm Hg
    B. a titrated IV solution of Nipride to reduce the blood pressure to his prestroke level
    C. angiotensin-converting enzyme (ACE) inhibitors to reduce his elevated blood pressure
    D. no treatment for his blood pressure at this time
23. Which of the following is true of heparin therapy in the management of stroke patients?
    A. it can be given orally
    B. the prothrombin time is monitored
    C. it acts by dissolving existing clots in arteries
    D. it is used for short-term therapy
24. For patients with chronic TIAs, which of the following drug therapies is usually prescribed to prevent strokes?
    A. aspirin and warfarin
    B. ticlopidine and heparin
    C. acetaminophen and aspirin
    D. aspirin and ticlopidine
25. Based on research trials, current management recommended for patients with TIAs who have 75 percent extracranial internal carotid artery occlusion is
    A. ticlopidine therapy
    B. carotid endarterectomy
    C. carotid angioplasty
    D. heparin therapy
26. The lethal event for acute stroke patients during the first week after stroke onset is usually
    A. pneumonia
    B. cerebral emboli
    C. septicemia
    D. brain edema and herniation

POSTTEST ANSWERS

Question	Answer	Section	Question	Answer	Section
1	D	Seven	14	A	Fourteen
2	B	Seven	15	A	Fourteen
3	C	Eight	16	C	Three
4	A	Eight	17	A	One
5	D	Nine	18	D	Two
6	B	Nine	19	A	Two
7	A	Ten	20	B	Three
8	B	Ten	21	C	Three
9	D	Eleven	22	D	Five
10	B	Eleven	23	D	Five
11	C	Tweleve	24	D	Five
12	D	Thirteen	25	B	Six
13	D	Thirteen	26	D	Sixteen

REFERENCES

Adams, H.P., Bendixen, B.H., Kappelle, L.J., et al. (1993). Classification of subtype of acute ischemic stroke: Definitions for use in a multicenter trial. *Stroke 24*:35–44.

Alberts, M.J., Bertels, C., & Dawson, D.V. (1990). An analysis of time of presentation after stroke. *JAMA 263*:65–68.

Babikian, V.K., Kase, C.S., & Wolf, P.A. (1994). Cerebrovascular disease in the elderly. In M.I. Albert & J.E. Knoefel (eds). *Clinical neurology of aging* (2nd ed.) (pp. 548–568). New York: Oxford University Press.

Barnett, H., Gunton, R., Eliasziw, M., Flemming, L., Sharpe, B., Gates, P., & Meldrum, H. (2000). Causes and severity of ischemic stroke in patients with internal carotid artery stenosis. *JAMA 283*(11):1429–1436.

Barsan, W.G., Brott, T.G., Olinger, C.P., et al. (1988). Identification and entry of the patient with acute cerebral infarction. *Ann Emerg Med 17*:1192–1195.

Bates, B., Bickley, L.S., & Hoekelman, R.A. (1995). *A guide to physical examination and history taking* (6th ed.) (pp. 505–512). Philadelphia: J.B. Lippincott.

Benavente, O., & Hart, R. (1999). Stroke: Part II. Management of acute ischemic stroke. *Am Fam Phys 59*:2828–2834.

Bladin, C., & Willmore, J. (1994). Seizures after stroke. *Stroke Clin Updates 5*(2):5–8.

Bray, G.P., DeFrank, M.A., & Wolfe, T.L. (1981). Sexual functioning in stroke survivors. *Arch Phys Med Rehab 62*: 286–288.

Broderick, J.P., et al. (1999). Guidelines for management of spontaneous intracerebral hemorrhage. *Stroke 30*:905–915.

Broderick, J.P., Brott, T.G., Duldner, J.E., et al. (1993a). Volume of intracerebral hemorrhage: A powerful and easy-to-use predictor of 30-day mortality. *Stroke 24*:987–993.

Broderick, J., Brott, T., Barsan, W., Haley, E.C., et al. (1993b). Blood pressure during the first minutes of focal cerebral ischemia. *Ann Emerg Med 22*:1438–1443.

Bronstein, K.S., Popovich, J.M., & Stewart-Amidei, C. (1991). *Promoting stroke recovery: A research-based approach for nurses.* St. Louis: Mosby-Year Book.

Brott, T., & Broderick, J.P. (1993). Intacerebral hemorrhage. *Heart Dis Stroke 2*(1), 59–63.

Brott, T.G., Adams, H.P., Jr., Olinger, C.P., et al. (1989). Measurements of acute cerebral infarction: A clinical examination scale. *Stroke 20*:864–870.

Buelow, J.M., & Jamieson, D. (1990). Potential for altered nutrition status in the stroke patient. *Rehab Nurs 15*:260–263.

Camp, Y.G., Davis, T.M., Salter, J.P., & Pierce, L.L. (1995). Stop and look: Two approaches to manage stroke patients. *J Neuro Nurs 27*:24–28.

Caplan, L.R. (1993). Stroke 1993: A new ballgame. Paper presented at the National Stroke Association Symposium, Lexington, KY, October 8, 1993.

Case, C.S., & Crowell, R.M. (1994). Prognosis and treatment of patients with intracerebral hemorrhage. In C.S. Kase & R.L. Kaplan (eds). *Intracerebral hemorrhage* (pp. 467–489). Boston: Butterworth-Heinemann.

Damasio, A.R. (1992). Aphasia. *N Engl J Med 326*:531–539.

Davalos, A., Fernandez-Real, J.M., Ricart, W., et al. (1994). Iron-related damage in acute ischemic stroke. *Stroke 25*: 1543–1546.

Davis, A.E. (1998). Neurological patient assessment. In M. Kinney, S. Dunbar, J. Brooks-Brunn, N. Molter, & J. Vitello-Cicciu (eds). *AACN's clinical reference for critical care nursing* (4th ed.). St. Louis: C.V. Mosby.

Davis, A., & Briones, T. (1998). Neurological clinical physiology: Intracranial disorders. In M.R. Kinney et al. (eds). *AACN's clinical reference for critical care nursing* (4th ed.) (pp. 637–709). St. Louis: C.V. Mosby.

Ellis, S.J., & Small, M. (1994). Denial of eye closure in acute stroke. *Stroke 25*:1958–1962.

Ferguson, K. (1991). Alterations in sensation and perception. In K.S. Bronstein, J.M. Popovich, C. Stewart-Amidei (eds). *Promoting stroke recovery: A research-based approach for nurses.* St. Louis: Mosby-Year Book.

Fisher, M. (1995). Prophylactic neuroprotection. In M. Fisher (ed). *Stroke therapy* (pp. 233–245). Boston: Butterworth-Heinemann.

Fitzgerald, M.J.T. (1992). *Neuroanatomy: Basic and clinical* (2nd ed.). Philadelphia: Baillere-Tindall.

Folstein, M.F., Folstein, S.E., & McHugh, P.R. (1975). Mini-mental state: A practical method for grading the cognitive state of patients for the clinician. *J Psych Res 12*:189–198.

Gauwitz, D. (1995). How to protect the dysphagic stroke patient. *Am J Nurs 95*:34–38.

Gelber, D.A., Good, D.C., Laven, L.J., & Verhulst, S.J. (1993). Causes of urinary incontinence after acute hemispheric stroke. *Stroke 24*:378–382.

Goldstein, L.B., & Matcher, D.B. (1994). Clinical assessment of stroke. *JAMA 271*:1114–1120.

Gorelick, P.B., Born, G.V.R., & D'Agostino, R.B, Hanley Jr., F., Moye, L., & Pepine, C.J. (1999). Therapeutic Benefit: Aspirin revisited in light of the introduction of Clopidogrel. *Stroke 30*, 1716–1721.

Grabb, P.A. (1998). Traumatic intraventricular hemorrhage treated with intraventricular recombinant-tissue plasminogen activator: A case report. *Neurosurgery 43*:966–969.

Graham, L. (1976). Stroke rehabilitation—a creative process. *The Canadian Nurse 10*(2):22–25.

Grotta, J.C. (1993a). Acute stroke management: Diagnosis: Part I. *Stroke Clin Updates 3*:17–20.

Grotta, J.C. (1993b). Acute stroke management: Part II. *Stroke Clin Updates 3*:21–24.

Heater, D.W. (1999). If ADH goes out of balance: SIADH. *RN 62*(7):47–49.

Heiss, W.D. (1992). Experimental evidence of ischemic thresholds and functional recovery. *Stroke 23*:1668–1672.

Hickey, A. (1996). Catching deep vein thrombosis in time. *Nursing 94 24*:34–41.

Jennett, B., & Lindsay, K.W. (1994). *An introduction to neurosurgery* (5th ed.) (pp. 142–171). London: Butterworth-Heinemann.

Johnstone, M. (1995). *Restoration of normal movement after stroke*. New York: Churchill Livingstone.

Joint National Committee on Detection, Evaluation, and Treatment of High Blood Pressure. (1993). The fifth report of the Joint National Committee on Detection, Evaluation, and Treatment of High Blood Pressure (JNC V). *Arch Intern Med 153*:154–183.

Katz, R.T. (1994). Spasticity—Part II: How is it treated. Be Stroke Smart. *NSA Newsletter 11*:7–8.

Keith, W., & Forsting, M. (1995). Endovascular therapy. In M. Fisher (ed). *Stroke therapy* (pp. 373–392). Boston: Butterworth-Heinemann.

Kilpatrick, T.J., et al. (1993). Hematologic abnormalities occur in both cortical and lacunar infarction. *Stroke 24*:1945–1950.

King, W.A., & Martin, N.A. (1994). Critical care of patients with subarachnoid hemorrhage. *Neurosurg Clin North Am* 6:767–787.

Kistler, J.P., Ropper, A.H., & Martin, J.B. (1994). Cerebrovascular diseases. In K.J. Isselbacher, E. Braunwald, J. Wilson, J.B. Martin, A.S. Fauci, & D.L. Kasper (eds). *Harrison's principles of internal medicine*, vol. 2 (pp. 2235–2255). New York: McGraw-Hill.

Kittner, S.J., McCarter, R.J., Sherwin, R.W., et al. (1993). Black–white differences in stroke risk among young adults. *Stroke 24*(suppl. I):I13–I15.

Laumer, R., Steinmeier, R., Gonner, F., Vogtmann, T., et al. (1993). Cerebral hemodynamics in subarachnoid hemorrhage evaluated by transcranial Doppler sonography. Part I: Reliability of flow velocities in clinical management. *Neurosurgery 33*:1–9.

Lenzi, G.L., DiPiero, V., Pantano, P., & Ricci, M. (1990). Pathophysiology of ischemic brain disease. In A. Scriabne, G.M. Teasdale, D. Tettenborn, & W. Young (eds). *Nimodipine: Pharmacological and clinical results in cerebral ischemia* (pp. 125–129). New York: Springer-Verlag.

Macabasco, A.C., & Hickman, J.L. (1995). Thrombolytic therapy for brain attack. *J Neurosci Nurs 27*:138–149.

Mahoney, F.I., & Barthel, D.W. (1965). Functional evaluation: The Barthel index. *Maryland State Med J 14*:61–65.

McDowell, F.H., Brott, T.G., Goldstein, M., et al. (1993). Stroke: The first six hours: Emergency evaluation and treatment. National Stroke Association Consensus Statement. *Stroke Clin Updates 4*(1):1–12.

McHugh, J., & Cheek, D. (1998). Nitric oxide and regulation of vascular tone: Pharmacological and physiological considerations. *Am J Crit Care 7*(2):131–142.

McIntosh, T., Juhler, M., & Wieloch, T. (1998). Novel pharmacologic strategies in the treatment of experimental traumatic brain injury: 1998. *J Neurotrauma 15*:731–769.

McNair, N. (1999). Traumatic brain injury. *Nurs Clin North Am 34*(3):637–659.

Minematsu, K., & Yamaguchi, T. (1995). Management of intracerebral hemorrhage. In M. Fisher (ed). *Stroke therapy*. (pp. 351–372). Boston: Butterworth-Heinemann.

Mitiguy, J. (1991). The brain under attack. *Headlines 2*:6.

Mulley, G.P. (1985). *Practical management of stroke*. Oradell, NJ: Medical Economics Books.

National Stroke Association. (1995). Know the warning signs of stroke. *Be Stroke Smart 11*(2):20.

National Stroke Association. (1998). *http://www.stroke.org*

Paczynski, R., Hsu, C.Y., & Diringer, M.N. (1995). Pathophysiology of ischemic injury. In M. Fisher (ed). *Stroke therapy*. (pp. 29–65). Boston: Butterworth-Heinemann.

Phipps, M.A. (1991). Assessment of neurologic deficits in stroke: Acute care and rehabilitation implications. *Nurs Clin North Am 26*:957–970.

Quintana, L.A. (1995). Evaluation of perception and cognition. In A.C. Trombly (ed). *Occupational therapy for physical dysfunction* (4th ed.) (pp. 201–204). Baltimore: Williams & Wilkins.

Ritter, A.M., & Robertson, C.S. (1994). Cerebral metabolism. *Neurosurg Clin North Am 5*:633–645.

Schretzman, D. (1999). Acute ischemic stroke. *Nurse Practitioner 24*(2):71–72, 75, 80, 82, 87–88.

Siesjo, B.K. (1992a). Pathophysiology and treatment of focal cerebral ischemia. Part 1. *J Neurosurg 77*:169–184.

Siesjo, B.K. (1992b). Mechanisms and treatment of focal cerebral ischemia. Part 2. *J Neurosurg 77*:337–354.

Wahl, M., & Schilling, L. (1993). Regulation of cerebral blood flow—A brief review. *Acta Neurochir 59*(suppl):3–10.

Wallhagen, M.I. (1979). The split brain: Implications for care and rehabilitation. *Am J Nurs 79*:2116–2165.

Weaver, J.P. (1995). Subarachnoid hemorrhage. In M. Fisher (ed). *Stroke therapy* (pp. 399–435). Boston: Butterworth-Heinemann.

Wityk, R.J., Pessin, M.S., Kaplan, R.F., & Caplan, L.R. (1994). Serial assessment of acute stroke using the NIH stroke scale. *Stroke 25*:362–365.

Wolf, P.A., D'Agostino, R.B., O'Neal, M.A., et al. (1992). Secular trends in stroke incidence and mortality: The Framingham Study. *Stroke 23*:1551–1555.

Yatsu, F.M., Grotta, C., & Pettigrew, L.C. (1995). *Stroke: 100 maxims in neurology*, vol. 3. Boston: Edward Arnold.

Zivin, J.A., & Choi, D.W. (1991). Stroke therapy. *Sci Am 265*:56–63.

Zoltan, B., Siev, E., & Freishtat, B. (1991). *The adult stroke patient: A manual for evaluation and treatment of perceptual and cognitive dysfunction* (2nd ed.). Thorofare, NJ: Slack Inc.

Module 19

Nursing Care of the Patient with Altered Cerebral Function

Pamela Stinson Kidd

Module 19 is designed to integrate the major points discussed in Modules 17 and 18. This module summarizes relationships between key concepts and assists the learner in clustering information to facilitate clinical application. The module is divided into parts. Content is applied in an interactive learning style. The learner is encouraged to identify nursing actions based on an assessment of a patient in a case study format. Consequences of selecting a particular action are discussed and the rationale for correct actions is presented. The last part focuses on nursing management of a brain attack patient in the nonacute phase. The module ends with a brief summary of nursing priorities.

If additional reinforcement of these principles and concepts is needed, refer to Module 35. This module describes the case of a patient with a closed head injury.

Objectives

Following completion of this module, the learner will be able to

1. Describe appropriate nursing assessment data to collect for a patient experiencing a change in consciousness.
2. Identify relationships among patient symptoms, clinical signs, and pathophysiology for a patient experiencing a brain attack.
3. Cluster assessment data to formulate nursing diagnoses associated with brain attack.
4. Identify priorities in care for a patient with brain attack.
5. Explain rationale for nursing actions that prevent complications associated with brain attack.

Glossary

Aphasia. Total inability to understand or formulate language

Cerebral angiography. Contrast medium is injected into an artery for the purpose of visualizing cerebral blood flow

Computed tomography (CT). Directed use of x-ray beams to determine the presence of normal versus abnormal anatomic structures through computerized measurement of the attenuation of the beams based upon density of structures

Dysarthria. Impairment of the muscles that control speech

Dysphasia. Difficulty comprehending, speaking, or writing

Palmar erythema. Red palms usually due to vasodilation from alcohol intake or fever

Penumbra. An ischemic zone of viable, threatened tissue surrounding a brain infarct. The tissue may be salvaged if treatment is initiated early

Spider angioma. Skin vascular lesion, with a red center and radiating legs, frequently occurs in liver disease and pregnancy, vitamin B deficiency

Transcranial Doppler study. The use of ultrasound waves to image intracerebral vessels and to measure blood velocity

ABBREVIATIONS

ADLs. Activities of daily living

aPTT. Activated partial thromboplastin time

CBC. Complete blood count

CHI. Closed head injury

CT. Computed tomography

DKA. Diabetic ketoacidosis

DVT. Deep vein thrombosis

ECG. Electrocardiogram

EEG. Electroencephalogram

GCS. Glasgow Coma Scale

IDDM. Insulin-dependent diabetes mellitus

KVO. Keep vein open

LOC. Level of consciousness

LP. Lumbar puncture

MVC. Motor vehicle crash

NIDDM. Non–insulin-dependent diabetes mellitus

PT. Prothrombin time

ROM. Range of motion

TCD. Transcranial Doppler

TIA. Transient ischemic attack

tPA. Tissue plasminogen activator

CASE STUDY

Ella C is brought to the emergency department (ED) after being involved in a minor motor vehicle crash (MVC). She was alert and oriented at the scene, according to the person who was involved in the crash with Ella, but as the police officer was completing the crash report, Ella became disoriented, her speech became slurred, and she was unable to walk due to "weakness in her legs." An ambulance was called and transported Ella to the ED.

Initial Appraisal

You are on duty in the ED when she arrives. Ella received oxygen in route through a nonrebreather mask. She has an intravenous line in place with lactated Ringer's infusing at a keep vein open (KVO) rate. Her vital signs are BP 164/100, pulse rate 76 (irregular), temperature 98°F. Spo_2 is 92 percent. The police officer is asking for a blood alcohol level to be drawn due to her behavior at the scene.

Focused Assessment

You proceed with your nursing assessment. Ella responds to questions, but you cannot always tell what she is saying due to her slurred speech. Ella denies chest or back pain. She can spontaneously move her left extremities but not her right extremities. Her pupils are unequal in dilation (L > R) but both are reactive to light. Her Glasgow Coma Scale (GCS) score is 14. You place Ella on the cardiac monitor and she is in atrial fibrillation. The oxygen is continued at 100% by way of nonrebreather mask. Her breath sounds are clear. There are no extra heart sounds but she does have a pulse deficit (apical rate is greater than peripheral pulse rate).

Focused Nursing History

Meanwhile, Ella's family arrives. They tell you that she has been in good health for her age. Ella is 74. She is overweight at 170 pounds. She has a history of hypertension and non–insulin-dependent diabetes (NIDDM). She has been recently treated for an irregular heartbeat. The family does not know the exact names of the medications Ella is on. They are hunting for her purse in hopes the medications are inside. As far as they know, she does not have any medication allergies. She has had what the family describes as "ministrokes" about two years ago without residual neurologic deficit. At this point, it may be necessary to place a call to Ella's primary physician to get an accurate medical history.

QUESTION

Based on the assessment data you have collected thus far, which of the following factors could be the source of Ella's neurological symptoms?

A. alcohol
B. closed head injury
C. irregular heartbeat
D. brain attack
E. hypoglycemia
F. hyperglycemia
G. stress
H. hypertension

ANSWER

The most likely factors that should be considered are: (A) closed head injury, (C) irregular heartbeat, (D) brain attack, (E) hypoglycemia, and (F) hyperglycemia.

Closed Head Injury (CHI)

You should check the prehospital run sheet, and/or speak with the police officer to see if Ella was wearing a seat belt, the estimated speed at the time of the crash, and damage to the vehicle. As discussed in Module 34, all of these factors interact in determining severity of injury. In this case, Ella was restrained, the crash occurred at an intersection at an estimated 30 mph, and the major damage was to the passenger side of Ella's vehicle. The windshield was not broken, Ella was not ejected. Therefore, the likelihood of a closed head injury (CHI) is lower. However, it would be helpful to determine the medications Ella is taking to see if she is taking any anticoagulants. You should also try to determine Ella's use of aspirin and nonsteroidal anti-inflammatory agents as over-the-counter drugs. Elderly patients are more likely to experience subdural hematomas as a form of CHI due to less pliable vessels and more space between the dura and the skull. This risk is greater if the patient is anticoagulated.

Irregular Heartbeat

Ella is currently in atrial fibrillation. This means her atria are not completely emptying with each contraction. Therefore, as blood pools in the atria, emboli can form and, if ejected, produce a brain attack. Again, her medication history is important. An irregular heartbeat may not be problematic if she is anticoagulated. Her family informed you that she was recently treated for this irregular heartbeat. Since the irregular rhythm is still occurring, you should question if Ella was taking the medication appropriately or if she is experiencing an acute cardiac event (such as a conduction disorder; conduction block, or myocardial ischemia). The fact that she has no chest or back pain, no extra heart sounds, breath sounds are clear, and a pulse deficit supports the atrial fibrillation rhythm and that left ventricular dysfunction has not occurred due to a primary cardiac event. However, to be certain, a 12-lead electrocardiogram (ECG) should be obtained.

Brain Attack

Ella has several modifiable risk factors for stroke. She is obese, has a history of NIDDM, hypertension, and irregular heartbeat. All of these factors contribute to a gradual, progressive, arterial stenosis with eventual arterial occlusion from a buildup of fatty deposits. The new appearance of the irregular heartbeat may have been the final precipitating factor to producing a thrombus. Her age is also a nonmodifiable risk factor for stroke. She may have experienced transient ischemic attacks (TIAs) based on her family's description. You should ask her family if either of Ella's parents or siblings had a stroke. Try to determine if Ella smokes or drinks alcohol. Nicotine and alcohol are additional modifiable risk factors. Genetic history is a nonmodifiable risk factor. This may also help you determine if a blood alcohol level should be obtained.

Hypoglycemia

The likelihood of hypo- or hyperglycemia to the degree that it produces a change in level of consciousness (LOC) is less in NIDDM than in IDDM. However, if Ella took her oral hypoglycemic drug inappropriately (assuming she is on this type of medication) and she did not eat prior to the MVC, these factors combined with the stress of being involved in an MVC may have produced hypoglycemia. However, Ella's sensory and motor symptoms are unilateral. She is alert. She is not diaphoretic. Therefore, hypoglycemia should be considered as a possible cause and a bedside glucose measurement obtained, but it is less likely than other precipitating causes already discussed.

Hyperglycemia

Ella is not flushed. She is not diaphoretic. She does not have symptoms of diabetic ketoacidosis (DKA) (Kussmaul respirations, uremia, loss of consciousness). Hyperglycemia is an unlikely cause of her symptoms but as stated above, because of her history of NIDDM, a bedside glucose measurement should be obtained.

The factors least likely to precipitate Ella's symptoms are alcohol, stress, and hypertension. There is a witness who describes Ella's behavior as changing from time of the MVC to police arrival. There is no mention of smelling alcohol on Ella's breath. Unless Ella's family tells you differently or you discover an enlarged liver on abdominal assessment and **spider angiomas** and/or **palmar erythema** on skin assessment, there is no reason to suspect alcohol abuse or acute intoxication. The stress of being involved in an MVC will release catecholamines that increases one's heart rate (which could contribute to dislodgement of a thrombus), and blood glucose levels. However, the stress alone will not produce Ella's symptoms. A psychogenic source of the problem would be more likely if she had a history of mental health problems and if her sensory and motor symptoms were not unilateral. Although Ella has a history of hypertension, her blood pressure is not high enough currently to produce a cerebral hemorrhage.

The following diagnostic tests are ordered:

- Noncontrast **computed tomography (CT)** of the brain
- Cerebral angiography
- Complete blood count (CBC)
- Chest x-ray
- Comprehensive metabolic profile
- Platelet count
- Prothrombin time (PT)
- Activated partial thromboplastin time (aPTT)
- International normalized ratio (INR)
- ECG

Quick Review

What is the rationale for ordering these tests in Ella?

Noncontrast CT of the Brain

This test will confirm the presence of an ischemic stroke and exclude the presence of cerebral hemorrhage. It should be performed prior to cerebral angiography since angiography is not necessary in a hemorrhagic stroke.

Cerebral Angiography

This procedure will confirm infarct size and location.

CBC

A CBC will provide baseline measurement of hemoglobin and hematocrit. Although Ella was restrained and appears to have no acute injuries from the MVC, it is possible, though not likely, that internal bleeding may be occurring. Hematocrit must also be determined in order to interpret **transcranial Doppler (TCD) study** results, if performed (see below). Infection can cause a change in LOC. Infection can be ruled out with this simple test.

Chest X-ray

This will help confirm that Ella does not have congestive heart failure, suspected aorta aneurysm, or pulmonary malignancy that could complicate treatment of her symptoms.

Comprehensive Metabolic Profile

This will assess her electrolyte levels, liver enzymes, glucose level, and renal function. Hypo- or hyperkalemia can contribute to an irregular heartbeat. Liver and renal function are important to assess prior to administration of anticoagulants. Hyperglycemia (if acute) can increase lactic acid production and contribute to greater brain damage with ischemia. Abnormal glucose levels are exclusion criteria for tissue plasminogen activator (tPA) administration (Benavente & Hart, 1999).

Platelet Count, PT, aPTT, and INR Levels

A platelet count $< 100{,}000/mm^3$ is an exclusion criteria for administration of tPA in brain attack. Elevated PT and aPTT levels may also influence course of therapy. The World Health Organization now recommends that the INR be used for interpreting PT results. Therapeutic INR levels are considered to be 2.0 to 3.5 in most facilities (Pagana & Pagana, 1999).

ECG

An ECG will help to assure there is no myocardial ischemia present. If present, this will need treatment simultaneously with treatment for the neurologic symptoms Ella is experiencing. A myocardial infarction may alter the tPA administration procedure (see Module 15).

QUESTION

Does Ella need an electroencephalogram (EEG), lumbar puncture (LP), or a TCD?

ANSWER

No. An LP helps diagnose increased intracranial pressure and subarachnoid bleeding. Ella's GCS score is 14. Her pupils are reactive to light. She has a history that supports a gradual onset of symptoms. Her sensory and motor symptoms are unilateral and more consistent with an ischemic rather than a hemorrhagic stroke. An EEG will not give you any additional information that will alter treatment. An EEG is helpful in diagnosing seizure activity. Ella did not experience a seizure today and has a negative history for seizures. Seizure activity is more consistent with a hemorrhagic stroke. A TCD test will determine narrowed or patent arteries. The velocity of blood flow is measured from sound waves reflecting from the red blood cells (RBCs) (Davis, 1998). The hematocrit level influences blood viscosity and thus flow so TCD results are interpreted based on hematocrit and RBC count. Anemia will also influence results. Findings from this test can best identify vasospasm and arteriovenous (AV) malformations. However, results can help determine if the patient would benefit from cartoid endarterectomy. This test can be performed at a later time. It will not provide immediate data from which to treat Ella.

The results of some of the diagnostic tests are back. Ella's CBC and platelets are normal. Her PT, aPTT, and

INR are at the high end of normal values. Her glucose is 140 mg/dL. Electrolytes are normal. Liver enzymes, BUN, and creatine are normal. The chest x-ray shows a slightly enlarged heart without pulmonary edema. Her ECG is negative for ischemia. She remains in an atrial rhythm and tachycardic. Her chest x-ray shows a slightly enlarged heart without pulmonary edema and ischemia.

The CT scan reveals an increased density on the left, indicating infarction. There is no evidence of hemorrhage.

QUESTION

It has now been 3 hours since the onset of Ella's symptoms. Is Ella a candidate for tPA administration?

ANSWER

This is a tough call. Ella's stroke could be the result of emboli (from atrial fibrillation) or thrombosis (from her history of TIAs, NIDDM, and obesity). Both are classified as ischemic in nature and technically eligible for treatment with tPA. Unlike with some patients, the exact onset of Ella's symptoms is known. Ella could be treated within the 3-hour timeline. However, we are not sure that Ella meets all of the screening criteria. Although her PT and aPTT are normal now, she may have taken large doses of nonsteroidal anti-inflammatory drugs or aspirin, which could precipitate bleeding post tPA administration. More importantly, the CT scan shows evidence of infarction or necrosis even though it was < 3 hours from the onset of symptoms. When tPA is given after infarction has occurred, reperfusion of infarcted tissue can cause new strokes and intracerebral hemorrhages (Schretzman, 1999). Because of these factors, the physician decides not to administer tPA.

Ella's vital signs are now BP 170/100 mm Hg, heart rate 92, and respiratory rate 20. Her temperature is 100°F; SpO_2 is 92.

QUESTION

Which of these vital signs should concern you the most?

- **A.** blood pressure
- **B.** heart rate
- **C.** temperature
- **D.** peripheral oxygen saturation

ANSWER

The correct answer is C. Mild elevations in temperature are associated with poorer neurologic outcomes from stroke. The exact mechanism for this relationship is not known. Treatment of Ella's fever is a priority. Ella's blood pressure is elevated, but an elevated blood pressure is necessary poststroke to perfuse the collateral vessels supplying blood to the **penumbra.** This ischemic area can infarct if increased cerebral blood flow is not maintained through vasoconstriction. Systolic pressure should exceed 180 mm Hg and diastolic pressure should exceed 120 mm Hg before treatment is initiated (Benavente & Hart, 1999). Ella's peripheral oxygen saturation is low but adequate. Digitalis or cardioversion may be ordered in an attempt to convert her atrial fibrillation to prevent embolization. Anticoagulation using low-molecular-weight heparin may be instituted although its benefits are questionable. However, this should be administered after treating her fever with aspirin. In this case, aspirin can serve as an antipyretic and an antiplatelet agent. The fever is not high enough to require a cooling blanket or apparatus. Early administration of aspirin has been associated with less death and disability poststroke.

Development of Nursing Diagnoses

Ella continues to receive 100 percent oxygen. She has received 325 mg of aspirin PO. Her IV fluids are changed to .45 NS at 60 cc/hr. A urinary catheter is placed, with 350 cc obtained on insertion. She receives a loading dose of digitalis IV. She is admitted to the intensive care unit (ICU) to monitor for poststroke complications. You are developing a plan of care for Ella based on the data you have collected during her ED stay.

CLUSTER 1

Subjective data. History of TIAs, NIDDM, obesity, acute onset of slurred speech, unilateral weakness; denies chest or back pain.

Objective data. GCS score on arrival = 14. Pupils unequal but reactive to light. Weakness in right extremities. CT scan shows left cerebral infarction. ECG shows atrial fibrillation. Hyperglycemic.

CLUSTER 2

Subjective data. History of irregular heartbeat. Denies chest or back pain.

Objective data. Pulse deficit, no extra heart sounds, breath sounds clear, chest x-ray and ECG consistent with slight cardiomegaly without acute cardiac ischemia or pulmonary edema. SpO_2 adequate.

CLUSTER 3

Subjective data. Currently on bedrest. History of irregular heartbeat.

Objective data. Ischemic stroke confirmed on CT scan of head. Left pupil dilated > right pupil. Right extremities weaker than left extremities. PT, aPTT, and INR are normal.

All of the following nursing diagnoses may apply to Ella:

Alteration in cerebral tissue perfusion
Alteration in urinary elimination

Impaired physical mobility
Impaired verbal communication
Risk for ineffective airway clearance
Risk for decreased cardiac output
Altered peripheral tissue perfusion
Risk for fluid volume imbalance
Risk for ineffective individual coping
Risk for ineffective family coping
Risk for injury
Unilateral neglect
Risk for impaired skin integrity
Risk for impaired swallowing
Bathing/hygiene self-care deficit
Dressing/grooming self-care deficit
Risk for altered nutrition

QUESTION

Based on the three clusters of assessment data, which nursing diagnoses should be the priority focus during the high acuity nursing phase?

Alteration in cerebral tissue perfusion (supported by cluster one)
Risk for ineffective airway clearance (supported by cluster one)
Risk for impaired swallowing (supported by cluster one)
Risk for decreased cardiac output (supported by cluster two)
Altered peripheral tissue perfusion (supported by cluster three)
Risk for altered nutrition

Independent nursing interventions in the high-acuity phase should focus on the above nursing diagnoses.

Altered Cerebral Tissue Perfusion

As you recall from the pathophysiology of a stroke, cerebral edema occurs secondary to cellular membrane destruction and intracellular contents moving into the interstitial space. Ischemia begins this process. It is critical to assess minor changes in neurological status in order to prevent additional ischemia. Changes in LOC, pupillary reaction, and sensory and motor function are signs of cerebral edema and increased intracranial pressure as well as damaged neurons. Enhancing cerebral oxygenation through maintenance of airway patency, supplemental oxygen, elevating the head of the bed all help cerebral perfusion. [*Note:* There is evidence that cerebral blood flow may be promoted by leaving the patient's head flat (Simmons, 1997). The nurse should look for new findings in the literature related to this procedure.]

Risk for Decreased Cardiac Output

The nurse can help promote an adequate cardiac output by maintaining blood pressure and heart rate in an acceptable range. Medications may be used to support these vital signs (i.e., calcium channel blocking agents like verapamil, cardiac glycosides such as digitalis; see collaborative interventions below). A change in LOC may also indicate a change in cardiac output and not a primary cerebral event. Promoting oxygenation will also decrease myocardial ischemia and prevent angina.

Risk for Ineffective Airway Clearance and Risk for Impaired Swallowing

When there is dysphagia, and risk for aspiration, a nasogastric or gastrostomy tube may be placed to support enteral feedings as a collaborative intervention. In Ella's case, she has slurred speech and most likely some facial paralysis. However, she was able to swallow the aspirin without difficulty. You should keep suction equipment close at hand and be prepared to initiate an oral airway if her LOC decreases and gag reflex diminishes secondary to intracranial pressure and brain edema. Monitor for aspiration and atelectasis.

Risk for Altered Nutrition

Stroke patients are at risk for undernutrition because of a decrease in intake and a hypermetabolic state. Dysphagia, absent or diminished gag reflexes, facial paralysis, perceptual and visual deficits, and dominant hand hemiplegia all contribute to decreased food intake. In the less acute phase, usually after 48 hours, the patient is assessed for the ability to feed self, drooling (as a sign of dysphagia), ability to maintain an upright position, ability to bring food to his or her mouth, and the ability to see all food items on the tray. In the interim it is important to maintain patency of the IV line because this is providing Ella with fluids.

Altered Peripheral Tissue Perfusion, Impaired Skin Integrity

Sensory changes in the affected extremities and altered mobility puts Ella at risk for pressure ulcers. Vascular tone is disrupted to the extremity, encouraging pooling of blood and supporting the development of deep vein thrombosis (DVT) and pressure ulcers. There is no muscular pump to return venous flow from the affected extremities. The nurse needs to turn Ella every two hours and alter her position frequently. Ella can be reminded to shift her weight with her unaffected arm once she is not on bedrest. The skin should be assessed for pallor, pulses, temperature, and capillary refill. Assess for the presence of Homan's sign in both lower extremities.

Later, when Ella is less acute and increased intracranial pressure is less of a threat and the threat of additional strokes is minimized, the nursing care will expand to address the following nursing diagnoses.

Risk for Injury

The components for normal balance are vision, proprioception, and vestibular function, and at least two of these must be intact to adequately maintain balance. Poststroke postural asymmetry, leaning or falling to the hemiparetic side, and the inability to use protective righting reflexes when the center of gravity is displaced contribute to injury.

Impaired Physical Mobility

Proper body alignment is important to prevent contractures. This would include supporting her shoulders to prevent adduction. Use trochanter rolls to prevent hip rotation as well as foot supports. Her fingers and hands should be placed in anatomical alignment.

Active or passive ROM exercises performed 3 to 4 times daily will prevent contractures and loss of muscle strength. The patient can be taught to exercise the affected extremities by using the unaffected arm to move the affected extremities. Nurses can encourage the use of the affective arms in bathing, eating, and grooming.

Risk for Ineffective Individual Coping and Ineffective Family Coping

Depression frequently occurs poststroke. Provide appropriate information so the patient understands treatment goals and probabilities of outcomes. Clergy, friends, family members, and support groups may provide comfort to both patient and family. Try to maximize Ella's independence by involving her in decision making and activities of daily living.

Impaired Verbal Communication

Ella's stroke involves her left hemisphere, the center for speech and language in 95% of people. Thus, she may experience **aphasia** and **dysphasia.** She is already experiencing **dysarthria** as evidenced by her slurred speech. You should speak slowly, praise any attempt Ella makes to communicate, and help her to use gestures, facial expressions, and visual/tactile communication boards.

Risk for Altered Urinary Elimination

Without a more definitive description of the type of stroke Ella has experienced, it is impossible to anticipate the exact voiding problems she may have. However, once the urinary catheter is removed, she may experience functional incontinence due to difficulty getting to the bathroom and performing toileting in a timely manner because of her change in mobility and balance. She may not be able to verbally convey the need to go to the bathroom. Developing a schedule wherein the nurse consistently assesses Ella's need to void and provides her with an opportunity to void will help Ella regain bladder control.

Collaborative Nursing Interventions

Fever Control

The physician will order 160 to 300 mg aspirin daily as an antiplatelet agent. This dose may be increased in an attempt to control fever. Anticipate more aggressive cooling measures if Ella's fever increases greater than 100°F.

Hyperglycemia Control

Insulin may be ordered if Ella's blood sugar continues to rise. Generally, levels > 150 mg/dL are treated. Oral hypoglycemic agents may also be used.

Atrial Fibrillation Control and DVT Prevention

Beta blockers may be administered in addition to digitalis. Low-molecular-weight heparin may be ordered to prevent DVT and to inhibit clot propagation. Coumadin will be started prior to hospital discharge.

Administration of IV Fluids

The IV fluid Ella is receiving is her only nutritional source at the present time. If secondary damage to the pituitary gland or hypothalamus occurs due to cerebral edema or extension of the stroke, syndrome of inappropriate antidiuretic hormone (SIADH) may result. If SIADH would occur, fluids would need to be restricted. At the present time Ella's stroke is ischemic in nature and relatively confined according to the CT scan. Thus, the probability of SIADH is low. In her case, prevention of dehydration is paramount because dehydration promotes increased blood viscosity and greater likelihood of thrombosis.

Desired Patient Outcomes in the High-Acuity Phase

Intracranial pressure within normal limits as evidenced by no change in neurological status, no vomiting, no headache. Blood pressure and heart rate in expected range, no new dysrhythmia, no angina. Peripheral pulses remain strong and symmetrical, no peripheral edema, skin color normal without streaks, temperature of extremities warm (not hot) and symmetrical.

Summary

In summary, this module has focused on the nursing care of the brain attack patient during the high-acuity phase. For the purposes of the case presented, potential injuries from the MVC were not explored because injury is the focus of other modules. Rather, assessment of the patient with a suspected brain attack, diagnostic tests, and nursing diagnoses and interventions were presented.

REFERENCES

Benavente, O., & Hart, R. (1999). Stroke: Part II. Management of acute ischemic stroke. *Am Fam Phys* 59:2828–2834.

Davis, A.E. (1998). *AACN's clinical reference for critical care nursing*. (pp. 663–683). M. Kinney, S. Dunbar, J. Brooks-Brunn, N. Molter, J. Vitello-Cicciu (4th ed.). St. Louis: C.V. Mosby.

Pagana, K., & Pagana, T. (1999). *Diagnostic testing and nursing implications: A case study approach*. St. Louis: C.V. Mosby.

Schretzman, D. (1999). Acute ischemic stroke. *Nurse Practitioner* 24(2):71–88.

Simmons, B.J. (1997). Management of intracranial hemodynamics in the adult: A research analysis of head positioning and recommendations for clinical practice and future research. *J Neurosci Nurs* 29(1):44–49.

Module 20

Spinal Cord Injury

Pamela Stinson Kidd

Approximately 10,000 individuals in the United States sustain a permanent spinal cord injury (SCI) each year (Hudak & Gallo, 1994). The most frequent sites are the cervical region (more than 54 percent of all cases) and thoracic region (more than 30 percent of all cases) (Nobunaga, Go, & Karunas, 1999). In the past decade, the percentage of women and nonwhites who received an SCI increased. Violence and fall-related SCIs have increased, whereas SCIs from motor vehicle crashes and sports have decreased. Ninety percent of SCI persons return home and use rehabilitative services (Zejdlik, 1992). Twelve-year survival rates are good (85 percent), especially for persons < 25 years of age at the time of injury and for individuals with incomplete lesions (DeVivo, Stover, & Black, 1992). Respiratory complications are the most frequent cause of death. Prognosis is poorest for individuals over the age of 50 with complete lesions at the time of injury (DeVivo, Stover, & Black, 1992).

This self-study module is composed of 12 sections. Sections One and Two review the principles of spinal cord anatomy and function. Section Three describes common mechanisms of SCI. Section Four examines diagnostic testing of SCI patients. In Section Five, secondary injury of the spinal cord is discussed. Section Six explains pharmacologic therapy used to treat SCI patients. Section Seven addresses the relationship between pathophysiology and neuroassessment. Sections Eight and Nine explain pathophysiologic events associated with SCI. Nursing care based on these events is discussed. Stabilization strategies are addressed in Section Ten. Section Eleven discusses psychosocial sequelae of SCI and issues surrounding life-support decisions. Section Twelve describes SCI prevention strategies. Each section includes a set of review questions to help the learner evaluate his or her understanding of the section's content before moving on to the next section. All Section Reviews and the module Pretest and Posttest include answers. It is suggested that the learner review those concepts answered incorrectly in the review questions before proceeding to the next section.

Objectives

Following completion of this module, the learner will be able to

1. Describe the anatomy of the spinal cord region.
2. Describe the neural functions of the spinal cord.
3. Explain the relationship between mechanism of injury and pathology.
4. Examine secondary injury associated with a primary spinal cord injury.
5. Identify tests used in diagnosing spinal cord injury.
6. Discuss stabilization of spinal cord injuries.
7. Describe physiologic effects associated with spinal cord injury.
8. Assess a spinal cord–injured patient for movement, sensation, and reflex activity.
9. Describe spinal cord injury prevention strategies.
10. Analyze the relationship between pathology associated with spinal cord injury and nursing care priorities.
11. Discuss psychosocial issues following spinal cord injury.
12. Identify medications used in treating acute and nonacute spinal cord injury.

PRETEST

1. Mark White has been diagnosed with a cauda equina spinal cord syndrome. Which of the following is correct?
   A. he will be a quadriplegic
   B. he has a good prognosis of recovery of function
   C. he will require surgical stabilization
   D. he is at high risk for autonomic dysreflexia
2. Interference with sympathetic nervous system most frequently occurs with an SCI in which region?
   A. thoracic
   B. lumbar
   C. lumbosacral
   D. sacral
3. Which of the following physiologic effects occur in the acute phase post-SCI?
   A. peripheral vasoconstriction
   B. hyperthermia
   C. bradycardia
   D. hypocapnia
4. Which region of the spinal cord is most susceptible to injury?
   A. cervical
   B. thoracic
   C. lumbar
   D. sacral
5. Degenerative changes in a person's spine may increase their susceptibility to what type of spinal injury?
   A. cervical
   B. thoracic
   C. lumbar
   D. sacral
6. Spinal cord injury should be suspected in a patient with
   A. pelvic fracture
   B. maxillofacial injury
   C. kyphosis
   D. tibia fracture
7. Secondary injury to the spinal cord occurs from
   A. improper movement of the patient
   B. the forces producing a closed head injury
   C. cellular membrane destruction of neurons
   D. small hemorrhages in spinal gray matter
8. A myelogram of the spine is ordered for a patient with a C6 injury. To prepare the patient for this test, the nurse should tell the patient the contrast dye is injected
   A. by a peripheral IV
   B. by a lumbar puncture
   C. intramuscularly
   D. through a central IV line
9. A somatosensory evoked potential (SEP) test is ordered for a patient. There are no SEPs during the test. This means the patient has
   A. an incomplete lesion
   B. a stable lesion
   C. a complete lesion
   D. an uppermotor neuron lesion
10. A patient is to have Gardner–Wells tongs inserted to stabilize his cervical spine. This device requires all of the following EXCEPT
    A. screws implanted in the skull
    B. weights
    C. part of the head to be shaved
    D. bone grafting
11. Methylprednisolone is ordered for a patient with an SCI. Before administering this medication, the nurse should get the patient's
    A. weight
    B. current medications being taken
    C. prior history of steroid use
    D. age
12. To be effective, methylprednisolone must be administered within how many hours of injury?
    A. 1
    B. 4
    C. 8
    D. 24
13. The rehabilitation potential of a person with an L1–L5 injury is
    A. independent eating, independent bathing, independent mobility with the use of knee, ankle, and foot orthoses
    B. independent eating, independent bathing, electric wheelchair
    C. independent eating, minor assistance with bathing, manual wheelchair
    D. independent eating, independent bathing, manual wheelchair
14. Diving-related SCI may be prevented by all of the following EXCEPT
    A. checking the depth of the pool prior to diving
    B. checking the contour of the pool prior to diving
    C. marking the bottom of the pool
    D. using a diving board
15. Autonomic dysreflexia is a health emergency because
    A. airway spasm occurs
    B. severe vasoconstriction occurs
    C. spasticity produces joint immobility
    D. hypoxia results from regurgitation
16. Suctioning may produce which of the following in the SCI patient?
    A. airway spasm
    B. bradycardia
    C. hypertension
    D. vomiting

17. Severe hypotension in the SCI patient is initially treated with
    A. vasopressors
    B. changing the patient's position
    C. intravenous fluids
    D. methylprednisolone

18. The SCI patient is at greatest risk for suicide
    A. within 4 years postinjury
    B. within 1 month postinjury
    C. while hospitalized
    D. during rehabilitation

Pretest answers: 1. B, 2. A, 3. C, 4. A, 5. A, 6. B, 7. C, 8. B, 9. C, 10. D, 11. A, 12. C, 13. A, 14. D, 15. B, 16. B, 17. C, 18. A

GLOSSARY

Actual hypovolemia. Decreased circulating blood volume related to extravasation

Analgesia. Decreased sensation of pain

Anesthesia. Absence of normal sensation

Arch. Posterior section of the vertebra

Autonomic dysreflexia. A condition that occurs in SCI at the T6 level and above after the resolution of spinal shock. It is due to excessive sympathetic nervous system stimulation that produces extreme vasoconstriction and hypertension

Body. Anterior section of the vertebra

Bulbocavernosus reflex. Reflex tested by inserting a gloved finger into the rectum while tugging on the penis or clitoris. The external anal sphincter will contract, indicating an intact reflex arc. The absence of this reflex indicates a poor prognosis for bowel, bladder, and sexual function

Cauda equina. The end of the spinal cord that houses nerve roots L2–S5

Complete spinal cord injury. Traumatic disruption that completely transects the spinal cord resulting in loss of sensation and motor transmission to areas below the region of injury

Conus medullaris. Lower section of the spinal cord that houses nerve roots T11–L1

Dermatome. A cutaneous section of the body innervated by a cranial or spinal nerve

Dysesthetic pain. Central pain arising from the spinal cord

Hypoesthesia. Reduced sensation

Hyperesthesia. Exaggerated sensation

Incomplete spinal cord injury. Traumatic disruption of part of the spinal cord with some motor and sensory transmission below the level of injury

Lower motor neuron injury. Lesion or injury that damages cell bodies or axons (or both) of lower motor neurons located in the anterior horn cells of the spinal cord and the spinal and peripheral nerves; flaccid paralysis results

Micturition. Sequence of events leading to voiding. Involves sensory input from the bladder, activation of the spinal voiding center, and cerebral control

Plexus. Complex network of spinal nerves outside the spinal cord that innervates a section of the body

Poikilothermia. Loss of internal temperature control whereby the patient assumes the temperature of the environment

Priapism. Persistent penile erection produced by reflex activity

Proprioception. The ability to determine spatial position; knowing where the body or a body part is positioned in space

Relative hypovolemia. Reduced circulating blood volume produced by shifting of volume from the vascular to the interstitial space

Somatosensory evoked potentials (SEPs). Stimulation of pain and touch peripheral nerves to determine whether a response is elicited by the cerebral cortex

Spinal shock. A condition that occurs within 60 minutes of transection of the spinal cord. Bradycardia and vasodilation occur due to unopposed parasympathetic stimulation. Paralysis, anesthesia, and areflexia occur below the level of injury

Unstable spinal injury. An injury to two or more of the spinal columns, exposing the spinal cord to additional damage due to lack of support

Upper motor neuron injury. Damage to neurons that originate in the brain and terminate at each segment of the spinal cord, resulting in spastic paralysis

ABBREVIATIONS

BPM. Beats per minute

SCI. Spinal cord injury

SEPs. Somatosensory evoked potentials

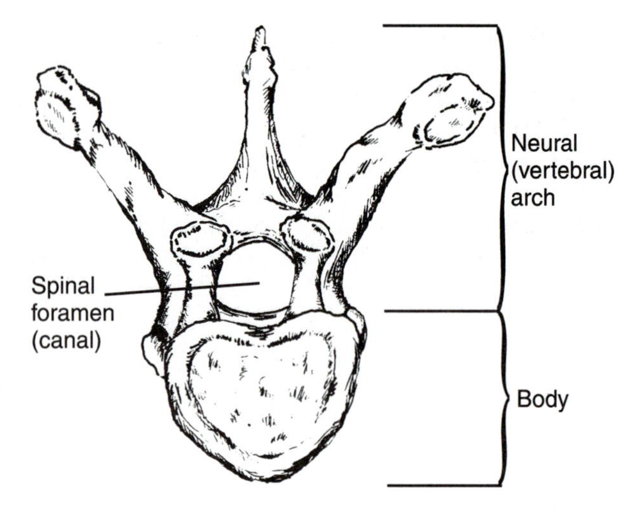

Figure 20–1. A simple cross-section of a vertebra.

SECTION ONE: Spinal Anatomy

At the completion of this section, the learner will be able to explain anatomic features of the spinal cord and vertebrae.

The spine is composed of 33 individual and fused vertebrae. There are 7 cervical, 12 thoracic, and 5 lumbar vertebrae. The sacral and coccygeal vertebrae are fused in the adult. Each vertebrae consists of a **body** (anterior) and an **arch** (posterior). The arch section is composed of two pedicles that attach the arch to the body and two laminae that form the roof of the arch. Seven bony protrusions from the arch help it articulate with other vertebrae. The two superior facets are located at the top, two inferior facets are located below, two transverse processes are located at the sides, and the spinous process is located at the rear of the vertebrae (Figs. 20–1 and 20–2). In order to bear additional weight, vertebral bodies increase in size as they descend.

The main blood supply to the spinal cord is provided by the anterior spinal artery and the posterior spinal arteries. Any disruption in this vascular supply may damage the cord without direct physical trauma.

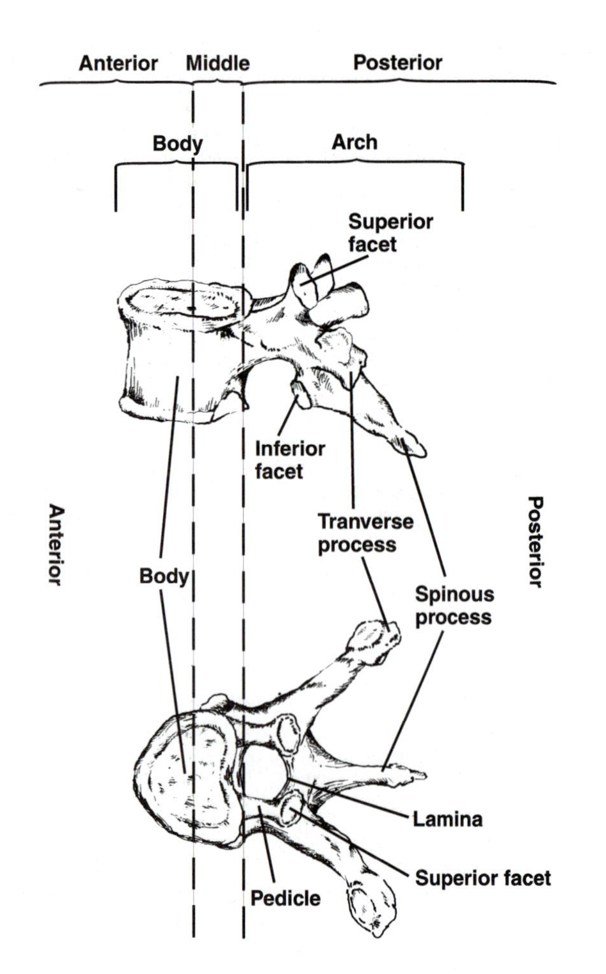

Figure 20–2. A lateral view and cross-section of a vertebra detailing the vertebral arch.

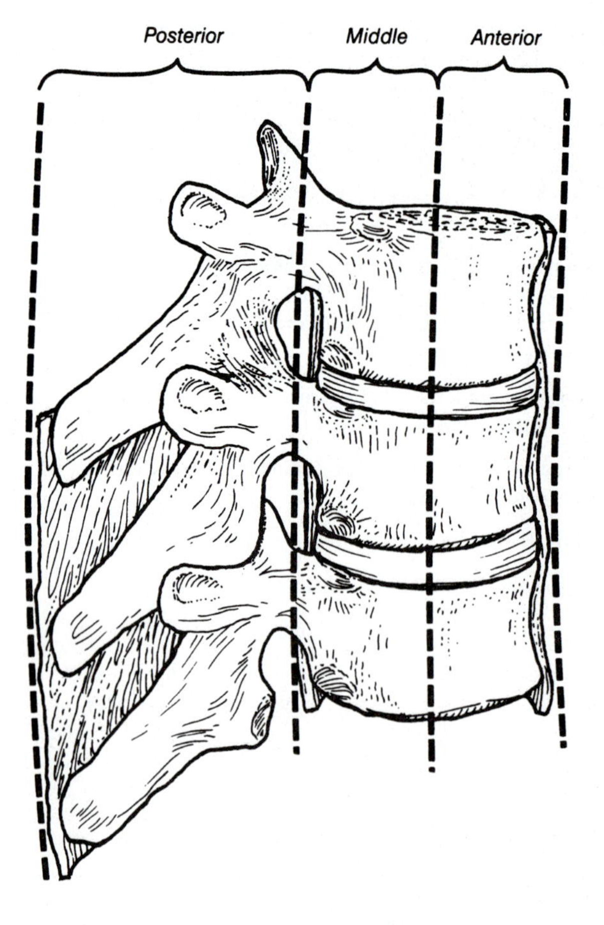

Figure 20–3. Three-column model of the spine. *(Reproduced with permission from Galli, R., Spaite, D., & Simon, R. [1989].* Emergency orthopedics: The spine *[p. 162]. Norwalk, CT: Appleton & Lange.)*

The spine is conceptualized as having three columns: an anterior column that includes the anterior part of the vertebral body; a middle column that houses the posterior wall of the vertebral body; and a posterior column that includes the vertebral arch (Fig. 20–3). If two or more of these columns are damaged, the injury is considered unstable (Somers, 1992). **Unstable spinal injury** exists when the vertebral and ligamentous structures are unable to support and protect the injured area (Zejdlik, 1992).

The spinal cord runs through the center of the vertebral column. It starts at the foramen magnum of the brain and ends at the first or second lumbar vertebra. In the cervical region, the cord receives afferent impulses from the upper and lower extremities. The end of the cord **(conus medullaris)** contains reflex centers for bowel, bladder, and sexual function. Figure 20–4 on page 488 illustrates the relationship between the spinal cord and the spinal nerves and between the spinal nerves and innervated sites. An SCI is usually defined by the level of the lowest uninvolved segment of the cord.

The C1–7 spinal nerves exit above the correspondingly numbered vertebrae. The C8 spinal nerve exits below the C7 vertebrae. There are seven cervical vertebrae and eight cervical spinal nerves. The spinal nerves of T1 and below, exit below the correspondingly numbered vertebrae. The spinal nerves join complex networks **(plexus)** after leaving the cord to innervate parts of the body. The **cauda equina** is formed from the lowest spinal nerve roots. Injuries in this area have a better prognosis of recovery of function. They are not classified as a true SCI since the spinal cord ends at L1–2.

In summary, the vertebrae are designed to articulate with one another and to protect the spinal cord. The severity of an SCI may be influenced by the degree of stability of the injured region and the type of spinal nerves disrupted and their target sites.

SECTION ONE REVIEW

1. Mary Smith has been diagnosed with an unstable SCI. This means
   - **A.** she has injured the reflex center for bowel function
   - **B.** the vertebral structures are unable to support the injured area
   - **C.** multiple spinal fractures are present
   - **D.** the main blood supply to the spinal cord is disrupted
2. Ms. Smith is able to contract her bicep but unable to contract her tricep (see Fig. 20–4). Her spinal cord lesion would be classified as
   - **A.** C5
   - **B.** C4
   - **C.** C6
   - **D.** C7
3. Spinal nerve injuries in which of the following areas have the best prognosis for recovery of function?
   - **A.** cauda equina
   - **B.** conus medullaris
   - **C.** anterior column
   - **D.** posterior column

Answers: 1. B, 2. A, 3. A

SECTION TWO: Neural Function

At the completion of this section, the learner will be able to explain the relationship between neural transmission and manifestations of injury.

The spinal cord contains gray matter (cell bodies of neurons). The gray matter helps in transmitting motor activity from the brain to the body. It also serves as a "relay" station for sensory messages from the body to the brain. In the first thoracic through the second lumbar section of the cord, the gray matter gives rise to the sympathetic nervous system. Activation of the thoracic section gray matter will stimulate the sympathetic nervous system to increase perfusion and ventilation, decrease elimination and digestion, and stimulate greater release of epinephrine from the adrenal gland.

The white matter of the spinal cord consists of insulated nerve fibers that function as transmission cables (tracts). The three major tracts are the corticospinal, spinothalamic, and posterior column tracts for touch, vibration, and position sense, respectively. The corticospinal tract originates in the brain and crosses over in the brain stem to innervate the opposite side of the body. It transmits motor activity. The spinothalamic tract originates in the spinal cord, where it crosses over within two segments of entry into the cord, and ascends to the thalamus in the brain. It transmits pain and temperature. The posterior horn contains axons from the peripheral sensory neurons.

The parasympathetic nervous system originates in a group of neurons located in the brain stem and in a group located between the second and fourth sacral segments of the cord. Parasympathetic stimulation produces specific responses that assist elimination and digestion, among other functions.

Damage to specific regions of the cord may produce alterations in either sympathetic or parasympathetic func-

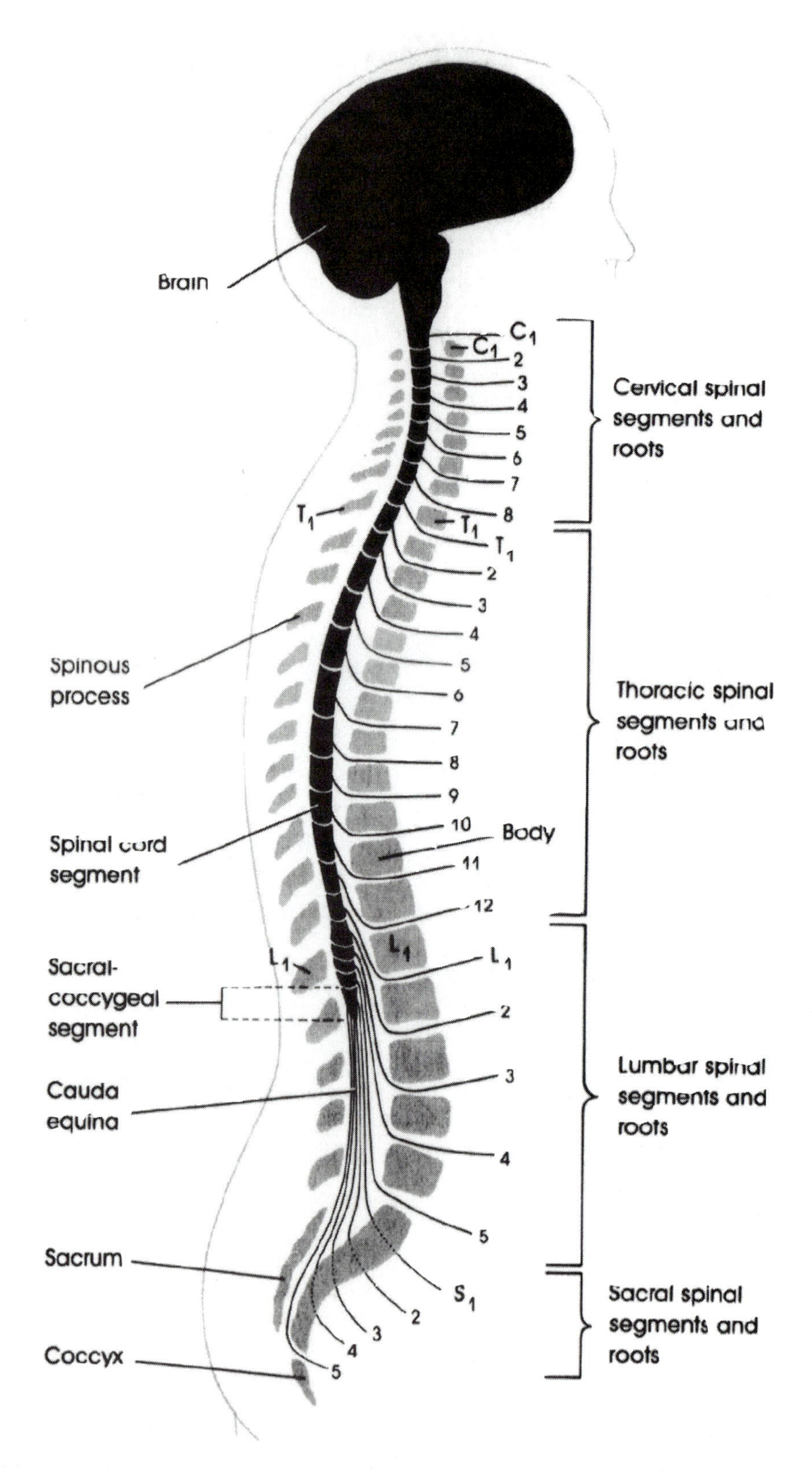

Figure 20–4. The spinal cord and spinal nerves. (*From Zejdlik, C.:* Management of Spinal Cord Injury, *© 1992. Boston: Jones & Bartlett Publisher. Reprinted with permission.)*

tion. The physiologic effects of these alterations are the foundation of nursing care for the SCI patient. The balance between sympathetic and parasympathetic function can be managed by increasing the stimuli to either system or by blocking the amount of discharge from either system (Zejdlik, 1992).

Spinal cord injury may be described as **complete** (loss of all conscious motor and sensory function below the level of injury) due to transection of the spinal cord or **incomplete** (preservation of some sensory and/or motor function below the level of injury due to partial transection of the spinal cord). Several types of incomplete injuries are described in Table 20–1. Of these injuries, recovery from central cord syndrome is the most promising (Bissonette, 1988). For nursing care purposes, it may be helpful to use the American Spinal Injury Association (ASIA, 1996) Impairment Scale (Table 20–2).

Spinal cord injury can damage upper and/or lower motor neurons. **Upper motor neurons** originate in the brain and synapse with **lower motor neurons,** which arise in the spinal cord. Damage to an upper motor neuron pathway results in loss of cerebral control over reflex activity below the lesion level. Upper motor neurons may become hyperactive to local stimuli, producing a spastic form of paralysis. Lower motor neurons originate in the spinal cord and form spinal nerves outside the cord. They transmit from target organs/sites to the spinal cord, where they synapse with another lower motor neuron to transmit back to the same target/site. Lower motor neurons create reflex arcs and involuntary responses. Flaccid paralysis results from damage to lower motor neurons.

TABLE 20–2. ASIA IMPAIRMENT SCALE

- ❑ A = **Complete:** No motor or sensory function is preserved in the sacral segments S4–5.
- ❑ B = **Incomplete:** Sensory but not motor function is preserved below the neurological level and includes the sacral segments S4–5.
- ❑ C = **Incomplete:** Motor function is preserved below the neurological level, and more than half of key muscles below the neurological level have a muscle grade less than 3.
- ❑ D = **Incomplete:** Motor function is preserved below the neurological level, and at least half of key muscles below the neurological level have a muscle grade of 3 or more.
- ❑ E = **Normal:** Motor and sensory function is normal.

CLINICAL SYNDROMES

- ❑ Central Cord
- ❑ Brown-Séquard
- ❑ Anterior Cord
- ❑ Conus Medullaris
- ❑ Cauda Equina

From ASIA (1996). See reference.

In summary, spinal cord injury can be classified as complete or incomplete as well as an upper or lower motor neuron lesion. Incomplete injuries are one of six types (Table 20–1). The location of injury along the cord influences parasympathetic/sympathetic nervous system balance. Destruction of white and/or gray matter will determine the degree of sensory and motor involvement.

TABLE 20–1. COMMON CORD SYNDROMES

			FUNCTION	
SYNDROME	MECHANISM	REGION	Lost	Present
Anterior cord	Flexion	Cervical	Motor; pain, temperature, and touch sensations	Proprioception, vibration
Brown-Séquard	Penetrating missile	Cervical	Ipsilateral motor; ipsilateral proprioception and vibration; contralateral pain, temperature, and touch sensation	Contralateral motor; contralateral proprioception and vibration; ipsilateral pain, temperature, and touch sensation
Central cord	Hyperextension	Cervical	Arm movement	Leg movement
Posterior cord	Hyperextension	Cervical	Vibration, proprioception, and line touch	Motor, temperature, and pain
Cauda equina	Compression	Lumbosacral	Motor and/or sensory function from lumbar, sacral, and coccygeal spinal nerve roots	Motor and/or sensory function may recover with lower motor neuron regeneration
Sacral sparing	Compression	Sacral	All motor, and mostly all sensory function below level of lesion	Saddle area (upper inner thigh and groin) sensation

Section Two Review

1. Pat South is diagnosed with an upper motor neuron lesion. The nurse expects Ms. South to experience

   A. excessive parasympathetic stimulation
   B. flaccid paralysis
   C. spastic paralysis
   D. temporary paralysis

2. Doug Wade has been diagnosed with anterior cord syndrome (see Table 20–1). This syndrome represents
   A. an upper motor neuron problem
   B. a lower motor neuron problem
   C. the best prognosis for recovery
   D. an incomplete cord syndrome

3. Parasympathetic nervous system function will be most affected by an injury to which region?
   A. cervical
   B. thoracic
   C. lumbar
   D. sacral

Answers: 1. C, 2. D, 3. D

SECTION THREE: Mechanism of Injury

At the completion of this section, the learner will be able to define forces that contribute to spinal cord injury.

The spinal cord can be injured by blunt or penetrating forces. Injury is rarely caused by direct vertebral damage. Violent motions of the head and trunk are the most frequent causes of injury (Somers, 1992). As discussed in Module 32, associated factors such as the position of the person's head, neck, and trunk at the time of injury, and the magnitude and duration of the injuring force, affect vertebral injury.

Blunt Forces

Cervical Injuries

The cervical region is the most vulnerable region of the spine due to its poor stability. Complete cord injuries at the C1 or C2 level are often fatal. Flexion injuries of the cervical spine are associated with rapid deceleration. They have the greatest incidence of neurologic injury (Somers, 1992). Flexion can occur with axial compression, such as occurs in a fall onto the buttocks. Diving injuries produce a high-velocity blow to the head resulting in vertical compression and flexion (Fig. 20–5). C4 and C5 damage frequently occurs from diving accidents.

Flexion with rotation may occur from being expelled from a vehicle or other events in which the body is twisted and the upper half is propelled in one direction and the lower half is propelled in the opposite direction (Fig. 20–6).

Forced extension or hyperextension may occur when a person falls and strikes the chin on an object (Fig. 20–7). They also occur from being struck from behind when riding in a vehicle. Degenerative changes due to osteoarthritis in the spine predispose a person to hyperextension injuries. Damage usually occurs in the C4–5 region (Somers, 1992).

Cervical spine injuries are extremely rare in children. When they occur, C1 or C2 is the most frequent site of injury (Little, 1989). Because children have ligamentous and not bony injuries, injury is difficult to detect on x-ray. Soft-tissue swelling in the region along with motor and sensory deficits are clues to injury. Calculating the strength of the mechanical forces involved in an injury may increase the suspicion of cervical injury.

Thoracic Injuries

Great force is needed to produce T1 through T10 injuries due to the stability of the rib cage. The most common site of thoracic spinal injury is located at the T12–L1 junction (Somers, 1992). Flexion may occur with compression of the anterior aspects of the vertebrae. A fall onto the upper back can produce flexion along with rotation. Thoracic region injuries may result from vertical compression forces experienced during a fall onto the buttocks or feet. A patient with calcaneus fractures of the feet should be suspected of having thoracic damage.

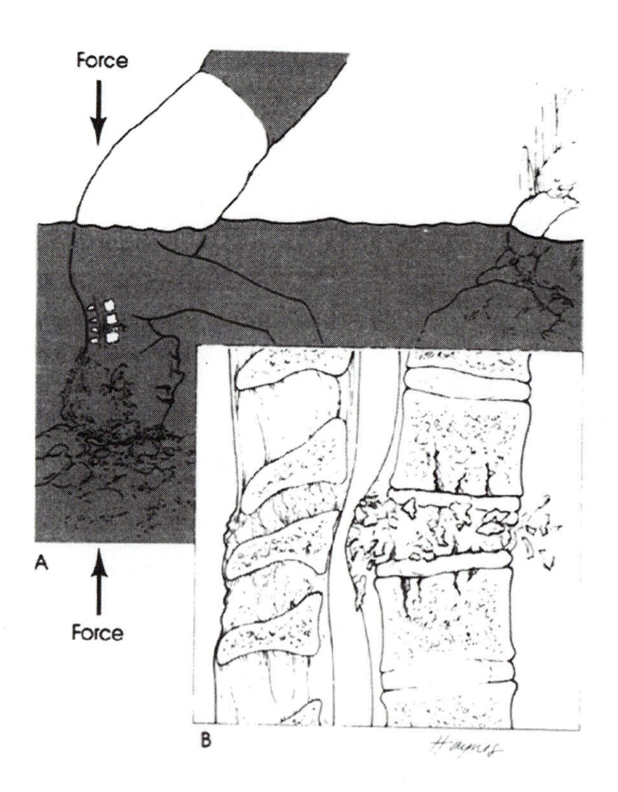

Figure 20–5. Vertical compression (flexion-axial compression). Fractures resulting from vertical compression typically occur at the cervical and sometimes thoracolumbar areas of the spine. A high-velocity blow to the top of the head can cause a shattered vertebral body to burst into the spinal cord. *(From Zejdlik, C.:* Management of Spinal Cord Injury, *© 1992. Boston: Jones & Bartlett Publisher. Reprinted with permission.)*

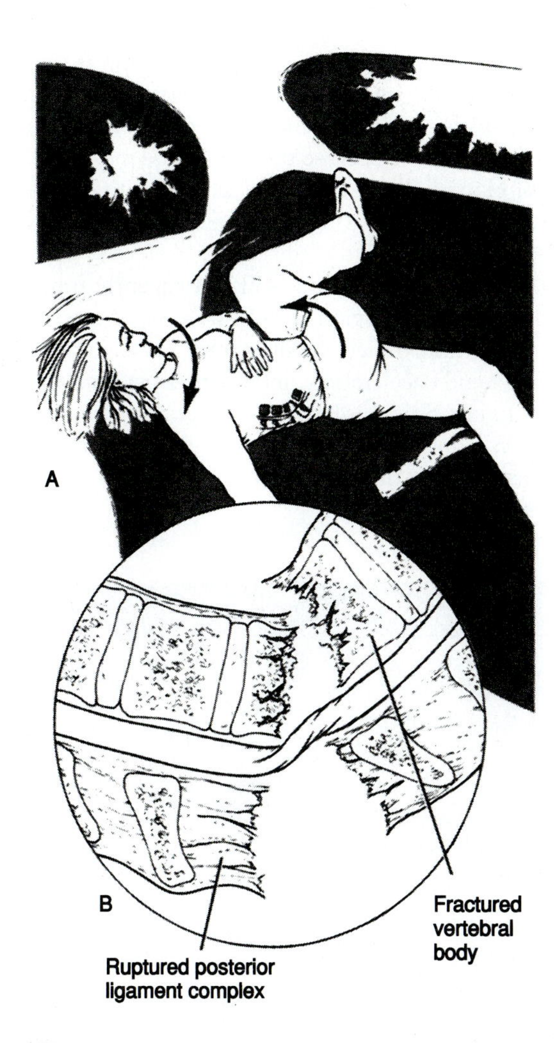

Figure 20–6. Flexion with rotation (distraction). Flexion and rotational forces occurring concurrently are particularly potent and are associated with fracture dislocations at any level of the spinal column. Typically the posterior ligamentous complex is ruptured, accompained by vertebral body fracture(s), rendering this injury highly unstable. (*From Zejdlik, C.:* Management of Spinal Cord Injury, *© 1992. Boston: Jones & Bartlett Publisher. Reprinted with permission.)*

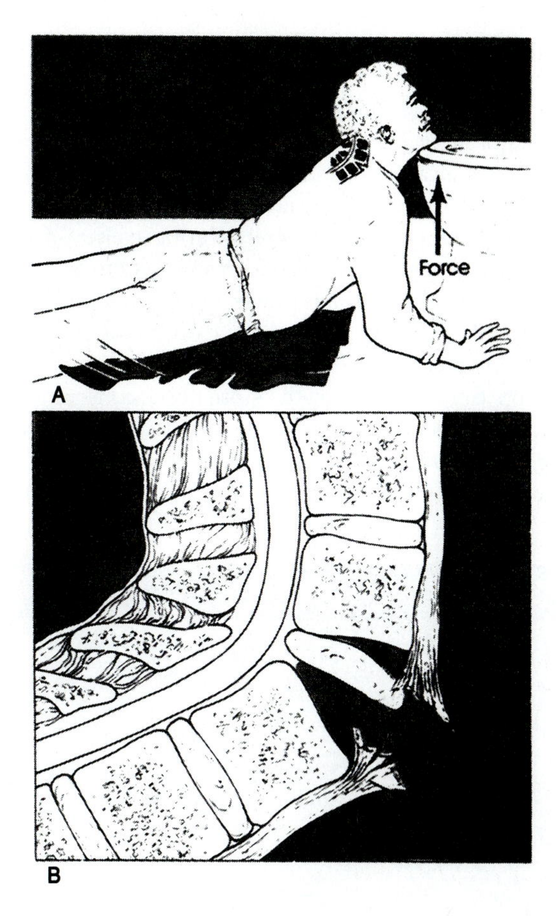

Figure 20–7. Forced extension (hyperextension). Forced extension injuries are typically seen in elderly persons, in whom degenerative changes have narrowed the spinal cord. Injuries, usually at the cervical level, are often related to falls in which the chin or face is struck, causing violent extension of the neck. (*From Zejdlik, C.:* Management of Spinal Cord Injury, *© 1992. Boston: Jones & Bartlett Publisher. Reprinted with permission.)*

Lumbar Injuries

The lumbar region of the spine is better protected than the cervical region but less protected than the thoracic region. The same forces producing thoracic injuries may be responsible for lumbar injuries. Violent flexion of the lumbar spine may occur with wearing a lap belt without a shoulder restraint (e.g., middle passenger in the rear seat) in a motor vehicle crash. Approximately 15 percent of these injuries result in neurologic damage (Cook, 1988; Somers, 1992).

Penetrating Forces

Regardless of the site of the penetrating object along the spine, surgery is not indicated unless the missile is impinging on the cord and creating progressive neurologic deficit (Ragnarsson & Lammertse, 1991). Penetrating trauma frequently results in damage to one side of the cord only (Brown–Sequard's syndrome) (see Table 20–1). There may be disruption in motor function on the side of the injury and sensory disruption on the contralateral side.

Associated Factors

Spinal cord injury is frequently associated with closed head injury. Therefore, the health care professional should assume that an unconscious patient has an SCI until it is ruled out. SCI should also be suspected in a patient with maxillofacial injury and clavicle or upper rib fractures. Likewise, a walking and talking patient who is admitted to your unit for a different problem may have an unstable spinal fracture. There is a 3 percent rate of SCI in these cases. Injury results from improper patient handling since an injury is not assumed to be present (Ball, 1990).

Nontraumatic Etiologies

Several conditions may produce narrowing of the spinal canal and subsequent SCI. Ankylosing spondylitis (calcification of ligaments and soft tissue) and rheumatoid arthritis (inflammation causing osteoporosis and decreased mobility) are two precipitating causes of SCI. Space-occupying lesions (abscesses and solid tumors) may produce spinal cord compression. Lymphoma and multiple myeloma are two oncologic conditions associated with bone metastases. The first sign of spinal cord compression from tumor growth is usually a constant, dull, back pain aggravated by coughing or sneezing. Leg weakness, urinary retention, and sexual dysfunction may also develop.

In some regions where deep sea diving is a recreational activity, spinal cord injury may result from gas bubbles in the vertebral venous system (a form of decompression sickness). Because the spinal cord receives a high rate of blood flow, venous stasis secondary to bubble formation obstructs flow (Gertsch-Lapcevic et al., 1991).

In summary, the spine is most frequently injured in the lower cervical region (C4–5) from blunt forces. Certain mechanisms, such as falls, motor vehicle crashes involving rapid deceleration, and diving are associated with spinal injury. Spinal injury from penetrating forces is less common. Illnesses associated with spinal injury include rheumatoid arthritis, ankylosing spondylitis, and secondary bony metastases.

SECTION THREE REVIEW

1. An associated SCI should be suspected in which of the following patients?
   A. pediatric patient with leukemia
   B. patient with chest trauma
   C. patient with a fractured femur
   D. unconscious trauma patient
2. A restrained passenger riding in the middle of the rear seat is susceptible for which of the following in a rear-ended crash?
   A. lumbar injury
   B. high cervical injury
   C. low cervical injury
   D. thoracic injury
3. Which of the following symptoms occurs initially in a spinal cord lesion resulting from bone metastasis?
   A. paralysis
   B. bowel incontinence
   C. back pain
   D. spasticity

Answers: 1. D, 2. A, 3. C

SECTION FOUR: Diagnostic Testing

At the completion of this section, the learner will be able to describe diagnostic tests frequently used to identify the type and severity of SCI.

Frequently, diagnostic testing of the SCI patient is completed in the emergency department prior to transfer to a critical care unit. In situations in which SCI is suspected later in the hospitalization, diagnostic testing may be initiated in a high-acuity setting. Therefore, the nurse should be aware of the type of tests ordered and the information they provide in order to prepare the patient and family. Radiographic assessment is used to document the level of injury and to provide information regarding the stability of the injury.

Radiographs

A lateral film of the cervical spine may be obtained initially, particularly if the patient's airway is becoming compromised and a decision will be needed regarding intubation technique. C1 to T1 (swimmer's view) must be visualized on this film before the cervical area can be deemed free of injury. In cases of cervical injury, blind nasotracheal or fiber-optic–assisted intubation technique should be used (Browner & Prendergast, 1991) if needed. Later, anterior–posterior and odontoid films will be obtained. The nurse can assist during filming by supplying in-line immobilization of the patient's neck. Thoracic, lumbar, and sacral films will be obtained frequently.

Computed Tomographic Scan

The advantage of a computed tomographic (CT) scan is that injuries to other organs can be demonstrated. The accuracy of detecting posterior injuries, the middle column of the spine, and cord impingement is greater with a CT scan than with standard radiographic films (Zejdlik, 1992). A CT scan is a painless, noninvasive procedure. If radiopaque contrast is used, the nurse must question the patient about dye and seafood allergies. Careful monitoring of vital signs is essential to detect quickly hypotension from a dye reaction. The patient may be hypotensive already owing to lack of sympathetic stimulation. Thus, any further decrease in blood pressure should be communicated to the physician. The patient's skin should be monitored for development of a rash. Increased fluid intake postprocedure may be necessary to promote dye dilution and excretion.

Magnetic Resonance Imaging

Magnetic resonance imaging (MRI) is useful in detecting tumors and vascular disruptions to the spinal cord. It is used more frequently in nontraumatic disorders. MRI may be more accurate in detecting the relationship between bone fragments and the spinal cord. The advantage of an MRI is that contrast dye is not needed. Skull tongs and halo devices have been developed to be compatible with MRI (Zejdlik, 1992).

Myelography

Myelography may be used if no further neurologic improvement has occurred or if the deficit progresses rapidly. It is an invasive procedure in which radiopaque dye is injected into the arachnoid space by way of a lumbar puncture. The nurse may assist by getting the proper trays available, prepping the area with povidone–iodine solution, and having local anesthetic available (if necessary). As with the CT scan using a contrast solution, an increased fluid intake postprocedure may be necessary to promote dye excretion.

Somatosensory Evoked Potentials

Somatosensory evoked potentials (SEPs) are used to help establish a functional prognosis after spinal cord edema has subsided (e.g., after spinal shock has resolved). A peripheral nerve in an extremity below the level of injury is stimulated. The response of the cerebral cortex to this stimulation (evoked potential) is recorded using scalp electrodes. In complete SCI, SEPs are absent since the stimulus is not transmitted to the cortex.

In summary, diagnostic testing may create a great deal of anxiety for the SCI patient. This anxiety may not originate from the test itself, since the tests are generally performed quickly with minimal body invasion. Waiting for the results of these tests, and ultimately a functional prognosis, is often the source of the anxiety. Explaining to the patient the sequence of events in test preparation, conduction, and interpretation may make the waiting easier.

SECTION FOUR REVIEW

Mr. French has been admitted with a diagnosis of a possible C7 compression injury. The following questions pertain to Mr. French.

1. A CT scan with contrast of the cervical spine is ordered for Mr. French. The nurse should
   - **A.** remove all metal objects
   - **B.** supply in-line mobilization of the neck
   - **C.** ask if he is allergic to seafood or radiopaque dye
   - **D.** prep his neck with povidone–iodine solution
2. After the CT scan, the decision is made to complete an MRI of the cervical area to assess the vascular supply. The advantage to this test is that it
   - **A.** requires a smaller amount of contrast dye
   - **B.** is faster than a CT scan
   - **C.** does not require in-line mobilization
   - **D.** does not require contrast dye
3. Two days later an SEP test is used to help establish a functional prognosis. Mr. French did not have any SEPs during the test. This means
   - **A.** his SCI is complete
   - **B.** his SCI is unstable
   - **C.** he has an upper motor neuron lesion
   - **D.** he has a lower motor neuron injury

Answers: 1. C, 2. D, 3. A

SECTION FIVE: Secondary Injury

At the completion of this section, the learner will be able to identify the sequence of pathophysiologic events associated with secondary injury of the spinal cord.

The 24-hour period immediately following SCI involves a series of events that contributes to the degree of neural function lost. These events can be placed into three categories: ischemia, electrolyte shifts, and inflammatory processes. These three simultaneous events lead to cellular membrane destruction. Once pathophysiology is understood, there is an appreciation of the rationale for immediate treatment strategies. These events are very similar to the events discussed in Module 11.

Ischemia

Blood flow to the gray matter of the spinal cord decreases immediately upon injury. There is up to an 8-hour delay in decreased blood flow to the white matter. Thrombi in the microcirculation impedes blood flow. Elevated interstitial pressure related to edema further slows the circulation. Vasoconstrictive substances, such as norepinephrine, histamine, and prostaglandins, are released postinjury, contributing to decreased circulation and cellular perfusion. **Relative hypovolemia** related to spinal shock, and **actual hypovolemia** secondary to hemorrhage from additional injuries, decrease circulating blood volume.

Electrolyte Shifts

Neurons require a normal sodium–potassium balance to generate action potentials. Post-SCI, extracellular concentrations of sodium and potassium increase. Potassium is released due to tissue damage. The increased sodium elevates the osmotic pressure in the injured area, contributing to edema. Tissue necrosis and loss of function occur when impulse transmission is lost.

Calcium ions accumulate in injured cells, causing breakdown of protein and phospholipids. Demyelination and destruction of the cell membrane occur when these substances are broken down. The breakdown of phospholipids releases fatty acids. The fatty acids produce arachadonic acid, which ultimately produces leukotrienes and prostaglandins. These are mediators in the inflammatory process. Prostaglandins are also produced. Both eicosanoids and prostaglandins, as well as mediators, contribute to cellular membrane damage. Once the cell membrane is damaged, neuronal death occurs (Nayduch, Lee, & Bulter, 1994). Refer to Module 11 for more information about how the inflammatory response creates cell death.

Inflammatory Processes

Polymorphonuclear (PMN) leukocytes infiltrate the injured area immediately postinjury. The inflammatory process is another factor in edema formation, further decreasing blood supply to the injured area. As the cord swells within the bony vertebrae, edema moves up and down the cord rather than laterally. A patient may exhibit symptoms due to the edema and not the initial injury. For example, a patient with a C4 injury may have edema up to the C2 level. The patient may require mechanical ventilation due to phrenic nerve paralysis.

Free radicals are generated by extravasation of hemoglobin and other ion complexes from blood. Injury activates neuronal excitatory amino acid receptors. This activation contributes to free radical production. Free radicals are neurotoxic because they damage cell membranes and disrupt the sodium–potassium pump.

In summary, primary injury to the spinal cord occurs immediately upon injury due to small hemorrhages in the central gray matter (Ragnarsson & Lammertse, 1991). Secondary injury is believed to occur over an 8-hour period and results from a series of events.

SECTION FIVE REVIEW

1. The events contributing to secondary injury of the spinal cord include all of the following EXCEPT
   A. ischemia
   B. electrolyte shifts
   C. hypertension
   D. inflammatory process
2. Damage from edema in SCI is related to
   A. increased extracellular concentrations of sodium and potassium
   B. vasodilation
   C. generation of free radicals
   D. decreased polymorphonuclear leukocyte function
3. Secondary injury to the spinal cord
   A. is a process that occurs in the first hour postinjury
   B. results from small hemorrhages in the gray matter
   C. is only present in complete cord syndromes
   D. occurs over an 8-hour period

Answers: 1. C, 2. A, 3. D

SECTION SIX: Stabilization of SCI

At the completion of this section, the learner will be able to discuss internal and external stabilization techniques used in SCI.

There is great controversy concerning the need for surgical stabilization of SCI. Even those who advocate surgical management debate the time at which surgery is conducted postinjury. Some favor waiting at least a week postinjury for swelling to subside. All agree that timely spinal alignment and stability maximizes cord recovery, minimizes additional damage, and prevents late deformity. Surgery may be reserved for patients not sufficiently aligned with manual means.

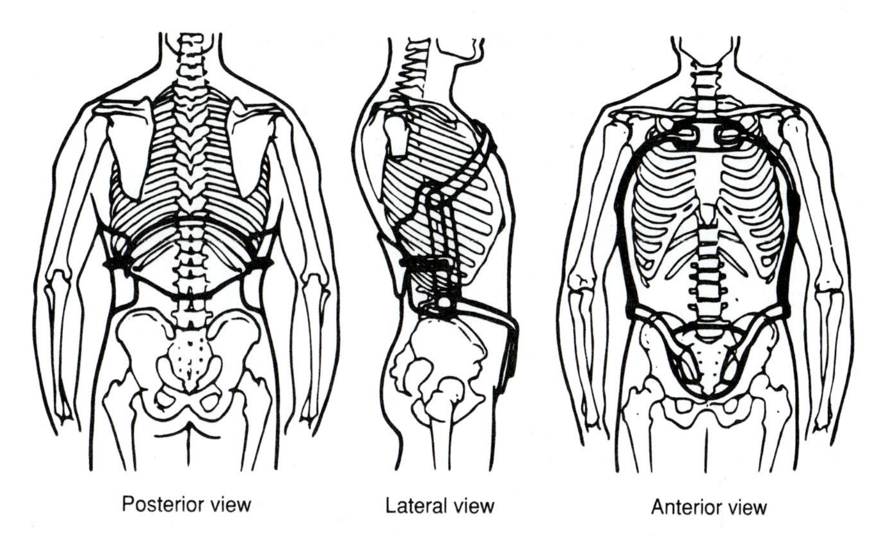

Figure 20–8. The Jewett orthosis. *(Reproduced with permission from* Spinal Orthotics: New York University Post-Graduate Medical School *[1983]).*

Surgical Stabilization

The best advantage to surgical stabilization is that it affords earlier mobilization and thus decreases complications attributed to immobility (e.g., pulmonary emboli) (Herman & Sonntag, 1991). Spinal segments may be fused during surgery. Spinal canal decompression may also be accomplished. Rods may be inserted to stabilize thoracic spinal injuries. Eventually the fusion, and not the rod, provides the major stability. Bone for grafting is harvested from the iliac crests if a posterior approach was used during surgery. Excised rib can be used for grafting in anterior approaches. An anterior approach is preferred when the fracture is older than 2 weeks since greater visibility of the spinal column can be achieved (McKenna & McCarthy, 1989). External traction may be required postoperatively. Special braces, such as the Jewett orthosis, may be used postoperatively to maintain hyperextension when the patient is not supine (Fig. 20–8).

Manual Stabilization/Traction

Traction is used to stabilize unstable cervical injuries. It may also be used when surgical intervention is not possible owing to the patient's hemodynamic instability. Traction is used to maintain alignment, prevent movement of unstable bones, reduce dislocations, and decompress the spinal cord and nerves (Nolan, 1994). Traction is rarely used with thoracolumbar or sacral injuries. Bedrest in the acute phase of these cases is the preferred treatment.

Halo Device

The halo device may be used initially to reduce fractures by adding sequential weights. Surgical stabilization may be necessary even after wearing a halo brace. The halo brace is generally worn for 6 to 8 weeks postinjury. It keeps the spine extended during ambulation. Wrenches should be taped to the vest in case the patient experiences cardiac arrest and rapid removal is necessary (Fig. 20–9).

Tongs

Tong devices, such as the Gardner-Wells apparatus, may also be used initially to reduce a fracture. Sequential weights can be added to this device. Ten pounds of traction is applied if an injury but no fracture is present. If a fracture is present, 5 pounds per interspace beginning

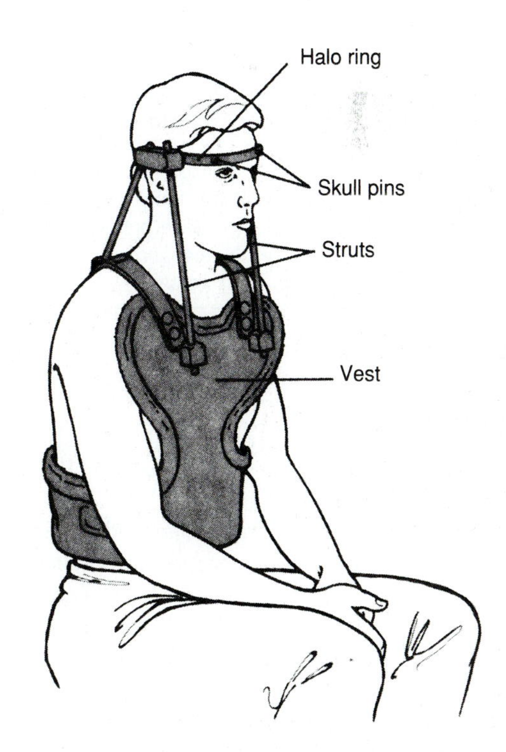

Figure 20–9. The halo vest. The halo traction brace immobilizes the cervical spine, which allows the patient to ambulate and participate in self-care. *(From Thelan, L. et al [1994].* Critical Care Nursing Diagnosis and Management, *2nd ed. [p. 744] St. Louis: Mosby.)*

TABLE 20–3. METHODS, INDICATIONS, LENGTH OF THERAPY, AND PRECAUTIONS OF VARIOUS SPINE IMMOBILIZATION TECHNIQUES

METHODS	INDICATIONS	GOAL OF THERAPY	LENGTH OF THERAPY	PRECAUTIONS
Cervical Spine				
Hard Cervical Collar (Short-Term) Philadelphia collar and Stif-neck collar	Prehospital immobilization Uncleared c-spine	Pre-evaluation, presumptive	< 48 hours	Ensure good collar fit Skin care Decubitus ulcers
Hard Cervical Collar (Long-Term) Miami-J collar and Aspen collar	Stable c-spine fracture Ligamentous injury	Hasten healing, diminish pain	8–12 weeks	Ensure good collar fit Worn continuously—provide second collar for washing Meticulous skin care
Soft Cervical Collar	Cervical strain, whiplash	Symptom management	Varies, dependent on symptom severity	Limit use to avoid dependence, e.g., nighttime, riding in car only
Cervical Traction				
Gardner-Wells tongs	Unstable maligned c-spine fracture, dislocation, or ligamentous injury	Cervical reduction Bridge to operative therapy	Varies	Pin site care and assessment Reposition patient every 2 hours
Halo vest	Unstable c-spine fracture, dislocation, or ligamentous injury	Definitive cervical immobilization	8–12 weeks	Pin site assessment and care Decubitus ulcers beneath vest
Four poster or Yale brace	Stable c-spine injuries or adjunct to surgery for unstable c-spine injuries	Hasten healing, diminish pain	8–12 weeks	
Thoracic or Lumbar Spine				
Hyperextension Cast and Thoraco–Lumbar Support Orthotic (Clam-Shell or Tortoise-Shell Brace)	Stable thoracic or lumbar spine column fractures; anterior compression fracture with <40% loss of height; burst fractures with no neurologic deficit, <50% vertebral body involvement, <30% canal compromise, angulation <20°	Hasten healing, diminish pain After spinal decompressive and stabilization surgery for support and comfort	8–12 weeks	Requires custom fit Meticulous skin care
Elastic Thoraco–Lumbar Supports	Minor compression fractures or transverse process fractures Lumbar strain	Symptom management	Varies, dependent on symptom severity	

From Logan © 1999, Principles of Practice for the Acute Care Nurse Practitioner, *reprinted by permission of Prentice Hall Inc., Upper Saddle River, NJ.*

with C1 to the level of the lesion is applied. A maximum of 10 pounds per interspace is added until reduction occurs. Weights greater than this have been used successfully but they remain controversial (Kidd, 1990). Muscle relaxants may promote the efficacy of the traction.

Screws are implanted into the patient's skull. The patient feels pressure but no pain. However, the patient may fear brain penetration. The nurse may assist by prepping the region (sides of the head) using povidone–iodine solution and shaving. Local anesthetic is needed. Antianxiety agents may be ordered for the patient.

Braces

A Philadelphia collar and a molded plastic body jacket (clam shell) brace may be sufficient for stabilization of some injuries (Fig. 20–10). Braces such as the Jewett orthosis are most frequently used with thoracic and lumbar spine injuries.

In summary, whether a manual or surgical stabilization is conducted, the goals are the same: to align and stabilize the spine, minimize additional damage, and prevent late deformity (See table 20–3.).

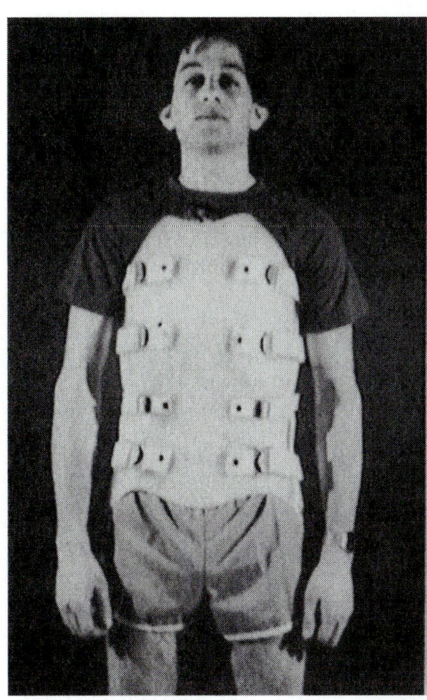
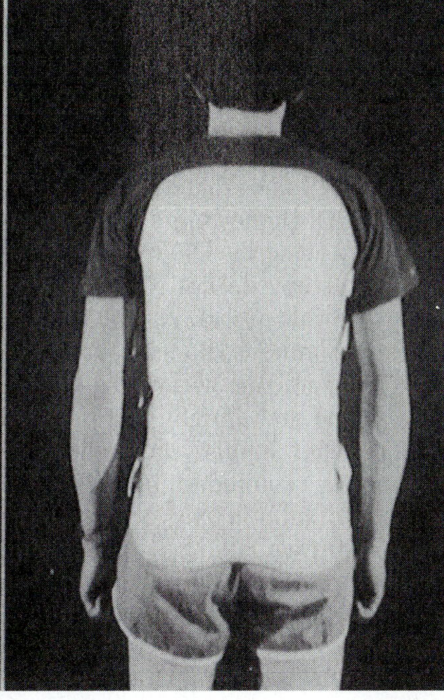

Figure 20–10. Molded plastic body jacket. *(Reproduced with permission from Fishman, S., Berger, N., Edelstein, J., & Springer, W. (1985).* Spinal Orthoses. *In: American Academy of Orthopedic Surgeons: Atlas of Orthotics: Biomechanical Principles and Application, 2nd ed., St. Louis: Mosby.)*

SECTION SIX REVIEW

1. Which of the following devices is used to manually stabilize a cervical injury?
   A. clam shell brace
   B. Jewett brace
   C. halo brace
   D. Rohandur brace

2. Mr. Lewis is going to have Gardner-Wells tongs inserted. The nurse should tell him that
   A. his head will be shaved completely
   B. the pain subsides as the screws are inserted
   C. he will feel pressure in his head
   D. he will hear a cracking noise from his head

Answers: 1. C, 2. C

SECTION SEVEN: Pharmaceutical Therapy in SCI

At the completion of this section, the learner will be able to describe drugs administered to SCI patients and the rationale for their use.

Acute Phase Drug Therapy

Drug therapy for SCI patients has two goals in the acute phase: (1) prevention of further injury to the spinal cord (methylprednisolone and lazaroids, experimental drugs), and (2) restoration of cellular membrane of the spinal cord cells (GM-1 ganglioside, an experimental drug).

Methylprednisolone sodium succinate is administered post-SCI for the following reasons:

- It decreases free fatty acid production
- It inhibits phospholipid breakdown
- It reduces infiltration of polymorphonuclear leukocytes (Anderson & Hall, 1993)

By these actions, secondary injury to the spinal cord is decreased because blood flow to the cord is improved and mediators of the inflammatory process (such as arachidonic acid and subsequently leukotrienes and prostaglandins) are not released. However, patients receiving high-dose steroids may have a greater infection rate and longer hospitalization than patients who do not receive steroids.

A bolus dose of 30 mg/kg IV over 15 minutes is given within 8 hours of injury. The bolus can be administered via syringe, in-line infusion chamber (e.g., Soluset), or piggyback device. This is followed by an infusion of 5.4 mg/kg/hr for 23 hours. Higher and lower doses have not been effective, nor have doses initiated later than 8 hours postinjury. An infusion pump should be used to administer the drip to ensure consistent administration and completion within 23 hours. When the infusion is completed, the tubing should be flushed with normal saline to ensure that the full dose was administered. Mortality and morbidity is not greater in patients who receive this dosage as compared with patients who do not receive steroids (Nayduch, Lee, & Butler, 1994). Since it is difficult to weigh an SCI patient, estimated weights are used. A baseline neurologic examination should be conducted prior to giving the bolus to document effectiveness of the medication.

The acetate form of methylprednisolone cannot be given intravenously. The succinate form is available in multiple concentrations. In patients in whom fluids must be restricted (e.g., those with a closed head injury), the drug should be mixed in more concentrated forms and administered in a smaller volume. Nurses must be extremely cautious when selecting a concentration and in the reconstitution of the medication. The following steps are recommended:

- Calculate the total dose in grams
- Reconstitute the methylprednisolone with sterile water
- Calculate the volume to be administered for the bolus and infusion doses (Hilton & Frei, 1991)

Methylprednisolone can be administered with most other medications using a Y-site connection. Normal saline or lactated Ringer's can be used for the infusion. Medications should not be mixed directly in the same container with the methylprednisolone.

Non-Acute Phase Drug Therapy

Drugs used in the non-acute phase of SCI address complications that arise due to improper neurologic functioning.

Perfusion

Autonomic dysreflexia is discussed in detail in Section Ten. The danger of this complication is the excessive sympathetic stimulation that produces vasoconstriction. While the search for the stimulus that has triggered the sympathetic response is being conducted, vasodilators may be administered simultaneously if the blood pressure is elevated greatly. Among the vasodilators commonly used are nifedipine (Procardia), phenoxybenzamine (Dibenzyline), and nitrates (e.g., nitroprusside [Nipride]). Nifedipine is a coronary and peripheral vasodilator. Phenoxybenzamine is an alpha-adrenergic receptor blocker; thus, it blocks the effects of catecholamines and produces vasodilation. It also relaxes bladder wall musculature. Bladder spasms frequently produce autonomic dysreflexia. Nitrates are direct-acting vasodilators.

Spasticity

Some degree of spasticity helps to promote movement. When spasticity is excessive, movement is inhibited and contracture formation is increased. Spasticity also effects the **micturition** reflexes, producing high bladder pressures and subsequently ureteral dilation and renal insufficiency. Administration of clonidine (Catapres) has been related to decreased urethral pressure and improved control of micturition. It has also been effective in treating general spasticity.

The relationship between anxiety and spasticity is well documented. As anxiety increases, so does spasticity. Baclofen (Lioresal) is used to treat spasticity because it is thought to reduce stimulation of receptors and inhibit reflex pathways. Research findings are contradictory concerning the effectiveness of baclofen in treating spasticity. Baclofen has demonstrated ability to decrease anxiety, which may contribute to less spasticity. Dantrolene (Dantrium) is also used to treat spasticity.

Pain

Dysesthetic pain (referred to as phantom or central pain) is frequently experienced by SCI patients. This pain is described as a burning, stabbing pain aggravated by movement. It occurs within one year of injury and is more prevalent in paraplegic patients. Amitriptyline (Elavil), carbamazepine (Tegretol), and gabapentin (Neurontin) are administered to relieve this pain. Tricyclic antidepressants (e.g., amitriptyline) increase the availability of serotonin. Anticonvulsants (e.g., carbamazepine) and gabapentin suppress abnormal neural discharge. The relationship between serotonin and pain has not been fully explored.

In summary, several medications may be used in the acute and non-acute phase of an SCI. The medications listed in this section are not all inclusive. As research continues in SCI, the medicines administered will change.

SECTION SEVEN REVIEW

1. Methylprednisolone is used in acute SCI patients to
   - **A.** increase free fatty acid production
   - **B.** transmit impulses from the periphery
   - **C.** maintain bladder function
   - **D.** prevent further injury to the spinal cord

2. Methylprednisolone therapy must be initiated within how many hours postinjury to be effective in SCI?
   - **A.** 1
   - **B.** 4
   - **C.** 8
   - **D.** 24

3. Phenoxybenzamine (Dibenzyline) may be used in cases of autonomic dysreflexia because in addition to vasodilation it
   - **A.** promotes cerebral blood flow
   - **B.** relaxes bladder wall musculature
   - **C.** has an analgesic effect
   - **D.** decreases anxiety

Answers: 1. D, 2. C, 3. B

SECTION EIGHT: Assessing Function in SCI Patients

At the completion of this section, the learner will be able to discuss techniques for assessing motor, sensory, and reflex activity in SCI patients.

Accurate assessment of motor, sensory, and reflex function is important for several reasons: to assist in diagnosis of the lesion; to provide a baseline with which to compare effectiveness of treatment; to determine realistic functional goals; and to detect the presence or absence of spinal shock. It is difficult to classify a spinal injury accurately until spinal shock has resolved. The ASIA Standard Neurological Classification of SCI assessment form allows recording of sensory and motor function (Fig. 20–11).

Motor Assessment

Motor strength may vary owing to preinjury characteristics such as gender, fitness level, and age. Voluntary movement requires both upper and lower motor neuron activity. Motor activity should be assessed for strength. Initially, the examiner starts with gravity being eliminated (for example, the wrist may be propped on a pillow and placed through flexion and extension). Next, movement against gravity is assessed (pillow is removed and the arm may be dangling off the bed while flexion and extension are performed). Finally, the patient's range of movement against resistance (examiner's hand) is noted. Each side is evaluated and compared. Flexion and extension of the joint are assessed.

Sensory Assessment

The most important data to collect in the sensory examination is the exact point on the patient where normal sensation is present. Sensation is tested along dermatomes. A **dermatome** is a section of the body innervated by a particular spinal (or cranial) nerve (Fig. 20–12). Several terms may be used in documenting sensation (e.g., **anesthesia, analgesia, hypoesthesia, hyperesthesia**). Usually, a cotton swab is used to assess sensation (spinothalamic tract function). A pin prick is used to assess pain (posterior column function). The patient's eyes should be closed. The examination should begin distal and move proximal (that is, up the neurologically intact area). Position sense **(proprioception)** can be tested by moving the big toes and thumbs up and down and asking the patient to confirm the direction. The areas where sensation and pain are present should be marked on the patient and dated. Table 20–4 shows the relationship between nerve root and innervated area.

Reflex Activity

The presence of deep tendon reflexes (Table 20–5) below the level of injury indicates an incomplete lesion or resolution of spinal shock. However, if spinal shock is present, the patient will be flaccid with depressed or absent reflex activity. The presence of perineal reflexes indicates that bowel and bladder training may be feasible. **Priapism** may be present in males. The anal wink reflex is initiated by a pin prick in the perianal area. A visual external anal sphincter contraction will occur if the reflex is present. The **bulbocavernosus reflex** is initiated by placing a gloved finger in the patient's rectum and tugging on the penis or the clitoris. The rectal sphincter will contract if the reflex is present. The presence of the anal wink and bulbocavernosus reflexes after spinal shock resolves indicate that the injury is an upper motor neuron injury.

Baseline and ongoing motor, sensory, and reflex assessment provide information about the patient's neurologic progress. Rehabilitative goals can be set and independence (to the degree possible) of the patient encouraged early. Bowel and bladder routines can be initiated and ambulation supported as necessary. Table 20–6 outlines functional goals appropriate for the patient, based on level of SCI.

In summary, nursing assessment focuses on motor, sensory, and reflex function. Motor ability is assessed through voluntary movements and movement against gravity and resistance. Sensation is assessed in the areas of touch, temperature, pain, and position (proprioception). Deep tendon and perineal reflex activity is also examined.

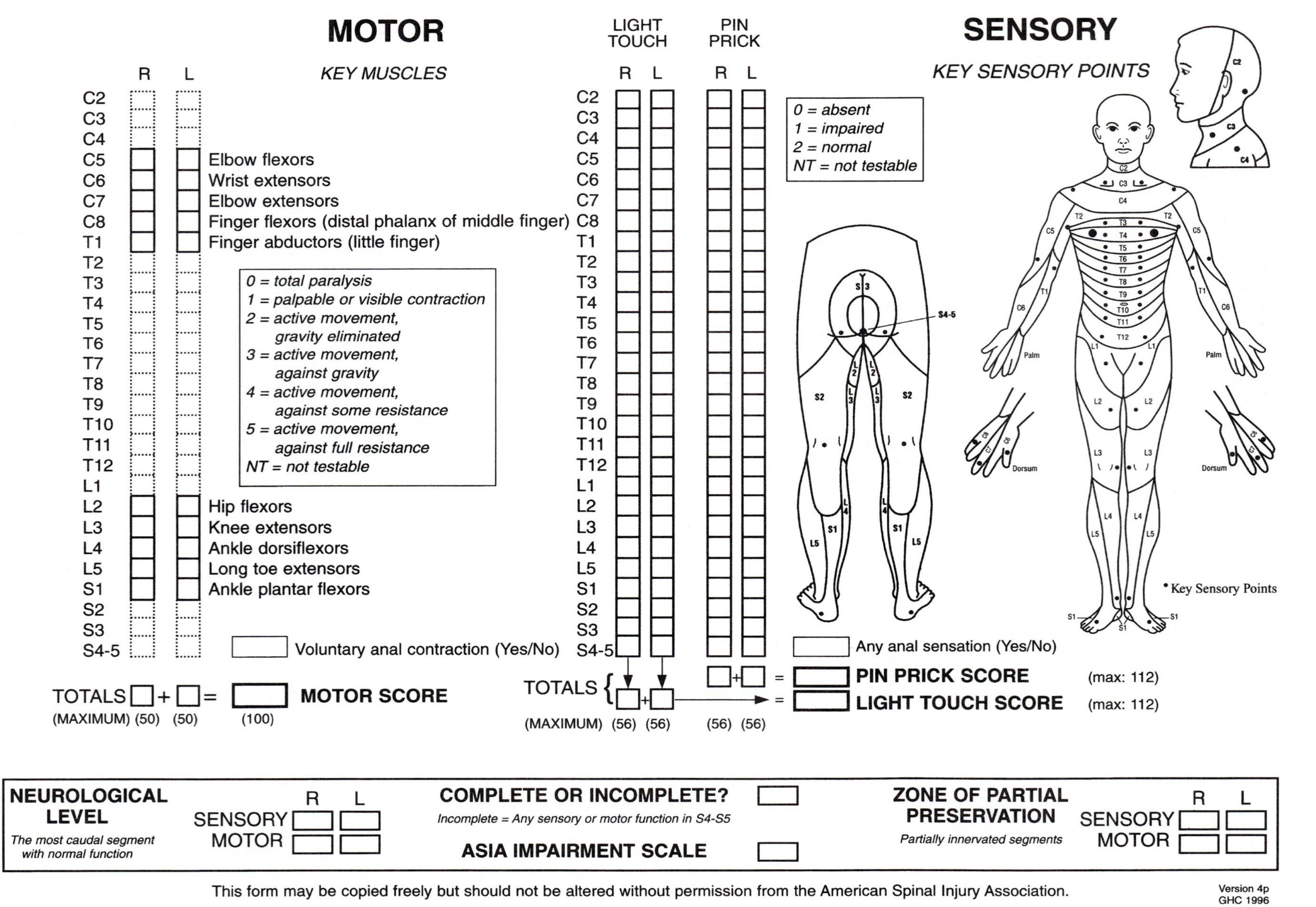

MOTOR

KEY MUSCLES

	R	L	
C2			
C3			
C4			
C5			Elbow flexors
C6			Wrist extensors
C7			Elbow extensors
C8			Finger flexors (distal phalanx of middle finger)
T1			Finger abductors (little finger)
T2			
T3			
T4			
T5			
T6			
T7			
T8			
T9			
T10			
T11			
T12			
L1			
L2			Hip flexors
L3			Knee extensors
L4			Ankle dorsiflexors
L5			Long toe extensors
S1			Ankle plantar flexors
S2			
S3			
S4-5			

0 = total paralysis
1 = palpable or visible contraction
2 = active movement, gravity eliminated
3 = active movement, against gravity
4 = active movement, against some resistance
5 = active movement, against full resistance
NT = not testable

☐ Voluntary anal contraction (Yes/No)

TOTALS ☐ + ☐ = ☐ **MOTOR SCORE**
(MAXIMUM) (50) (50) (100)

	LIGHT TOUCH R	LIGHT TOUCH L	PIN PRICK R	PIN PRICK L
C2				
C3				
C4				
C5				
C6				
C7				
C8				
T1				
T2				
T3				
T4				
T5				
T6				
T7				
T8				
T9				
T10				
T11				
T12				
L1				
L2				
L3				
L4				
L5				
S1				
S2				
S3				
S4-5				

TOTALS { ☐ + ☐ → = ☐ **LIGHT TOUCH SCORE** (max: 112)
☐ + ☐ = ☐ **PIN PRICK SCORE** (max: 112)
(MAXIMUM) (56) (56) (56) (56)

SENSORY

KEY SENSORY POINTS

0 = absent
1 = impaired
2 = normal
NT = not testable

☐ Any anal sensation (Yes/No)

NEUROLOGICAL LEVEL
The most caudal segment with normal function
SENSORY R ☐ L ☐
MOTOR R ☐ L ☐

COMPLETE OR INCOMPLETE? ☐
Incomplete = Any sensory or motor function in S4-S5

ASIA IMPAIRMENT SCALE ☐

ZONE OF PARTIAL PRESERVATION
Partially innervated segments
SENSORY R ☐ L ☐
MOTOR R ☐ L ☐

Version 4p
GHC 1996

Figure 20–11. Standard neurological classification of spinal cord injury.

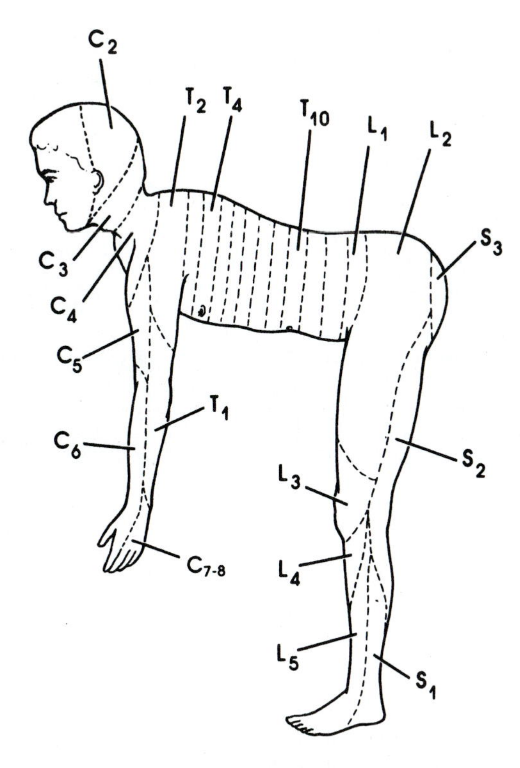

Figure 20–12. Arrangement of dermatomes is more easily understood when an individual is considered in the quadruped (crouched) position. (*From Zejdlik, C.:* Management of Spinal Cord Injury, *© 1992. Boston: Jones & Bartlett Publisher. Reprinted with permission.)*

TABLE 20–4. RELATIONSHIP BETWEEN NERVE ROOT AND INNERVATED AREA FOR SENSORY TESTING

NERVE ROOT	INNERVATED AREA
C5	Upper lateral arm
C6	Posterior aspect of thumb
C7	Posterior aspect of middle finger
C8	Posterior aspect of little finger
T4	Nipple line
T10	Umbilicus
L1	Groin
L2	Anterior thigh
S1	Sole of the foot
S3, S4, S5	Perianal

TABLE 20–5. DEEP TENDON REFLEXES AND THEIR NEURAL SOURCE OF ORIGIN

DEEP TENDON REFLEX	NEURAL ORIGIN
Biceps	C5
Supinator	C6
Triceps	C7
Knee (patellar)	L3
Ankle (Achilles)	S1

TABLE 20–6. FUNCTIONAL STATUS BASED ON LEVEL OF SCI

LEVEL	EATING	DRESSING	BATHING	BOWEL/BLADDER	MOBILITY
C1–4	Dependent	Dependent	Dependent	Dependent	Electric wheelchair with breath, head, or shoulder controls Requires ventilator, partial or full use
C5	Independent with aids	Major assistance with aids	Wheelchair shower with major assistance	Major assistance with aids	Electric wheelchair with adapted hand control
C6	Independent with aids	Minor assistance with aids	Independent in wheelchair shower	Independent with aids	Independent in manual wheelchair driving with hand controls Can use some manual wheelchair types
C7	Independent	Independent with aids	Independent wheelchair shower or tub with bath board	Independent with aids	Independent in manual wheelchair driving with hand controls
C8–T1	Independent	Independent	Independent in tub with bath boards	Independent with aids	Independent in manual wheelchair
T2–12	Independent	Independent	Independent	Independent with aids	Independent in manual wheelchair
L1–5	Independent	Independent	Independent	Independent	Optional use of knee–ankle–foot orthoses
S1–5	Independent	Independent	Independent	Independent	Independent with or without ankle–foot orthoses

SECTION EIGHT REVIEW

1. When assessing motor function, the nurse should consider all of the following EXCEPT
   A. gender
   B. fitness level
   C. age
   D. tremors
2. Sensation is assessed
   A. distal to proximal
   B. anterior to posterior
   C. ventral to dorsal
   D. thumbs to toes
3. Which of the following assessment findings indicates an upper motor lesion
   A. presence of anal wink reflex
   B. absence of bulbocavernosus reflex
   C. sensation above the umbilicus
   D. motor function of elbow with gravity eliminated

Answers: 1. D, 2. A, 3. A

SECTION NINE: Nursing the SCI Patient in the High-Acuity Phase

At the completion of this section, the learner will be able to explain changes in ventilation, perfusion, and elimination that occur immediately after SCI and discuss priorities in caring for the SCI patient in the acute phase.

Ventilation

Ventilation is severely impacted by SCI. The diaphragm requires C3–5 innervation to function. External and internal intercostal muscles are used to elevate the ribs during inspiration and assist in expiration and coughing. T1–12 innervate these muscles. The abdominal muscles (T5–12) are used for forceful expiration such as coughing. Tidal volume and vital capacity decrease post-SCI due to reduction in inspiratory and expiratory ability. Vital capacity may decrease to 1,200 mL (as compared with a normal vital capacity of 4,000 to 5,000 mL) although a level less than 15 mL/kg usually requires intubation (Hughes, 1990). Gradual improvements in these parameters occur as accessory muscles in the neck gain strength. Cardiac dysrhythmias may develop due to hypoxia.

Airway and Breathing Considerations

As with any patient, the nurse begins with assessing airway, breathing, and circulation. Airway and breathing may be compromised in the SCI patient. High-flow oxygen is usually administered via mask or nasal cannula until information regarding the site of the injury is available. Pulse oximetry is initiated. If data are available regarding the injury location, the nurse can anticipate complications. A lesion at the C4 level or above necessitates mechanical ventilation owing to the inability of the phrenic nerve to stimulate the diaphragm. A lesion at the T7 level or above necessitates assistance with secretions. The SCI patient must be suctioned carefully to prevent additional bradycardia. The patient should be preoxygenated with 100 percent oxygen and suctioned for < 15 seconds. Hypoxemia may occur secondary to retained secretions. A patient with a lesion at the T12 level or above is at risk for atelectasis and pneumonia owing to decreased support from the intercostal muscles. Aggressive respiratory therapy (pulmonary toilet) should be employed including "quad coughing" (assisted cough) and medical management of secretions. A patient with a medical history of cardiac disease and/or smoking will be at higher risk for respiratory complications. Aspiration also places the patient at greater risk. The signs below indicate ineffective breathing patterns and impending respiratory failure:

Patient is anxious; complains of not getting enough air
Weak cough
Shallow rapid breathing (respiratory rate > 30/min)
Oxygen desaturation by pulse oximeter (< 90%)

The goal is to anticipate respiratory problems so that intubation is nontraumatic to decrease potential for further cord injury. The patient may fatigue suddenly from spontaneous breathing. Intubation and oxygenation equipment should be at the bedside.

Perfusion

Sympathetic outflow arises from spinal segments T1–L2. When SCI occurs above T1, communication between this area and the brain stem is lost. The heart does not receive sympathetic input. Parasympathetic input remains (remember that parasympathetic outflow partially originates in the brain stem [Section Two]). Bradycardia (pulse < 60 bpm) develops and peripheral vasodilation occurs below the lesion. The resulting hypotension (systolic blood pressure 70 mm Hg or less) may produce a change in level of consciousness, particularly if the patient is hypovolemic due to actual blood loss from a concomitant injury. This series of events is frequently called **spinal shock.** Spinal shock usually occurs within 30 to 60 minutes of injury. It may last several months. Other symptoms accompanying this condition are sweating above the level of the lesion, flaccid paralysis, and venous pooling in the extremities (pink, warm, dry skin). The end of spinal shock is detected by the return of the anal reflex. It is difficult to classify a spinal injury accurately until spinal shock has resolved.

It is very easy to volume overload an SCI patient since they have lost the heart rate increase response to an increased fluid volume. The patient can enter congestive heart failure quickly. A heart rate and blood pressure low enough to produce a change in level of consciousness is treated initially with conservative amounts of intravenous fluid. Thus, a patent IV line is necessary. An indwelling urinary catheter is inserted to measure output as well as to treat urinary retention. The patient should be cardiac monitored for bradydysrhythmias. A pacemaker may be inserted to treat a bradydysrhythmia. Antiembolic stockings or compression hose are applied to prevent thrombi formation due to venous pooling.

Elimination

Voluntary control of bowel and bladder requires communication between the sacral cord region and the brain. Incontinence of stool and urine results from lack of voluntary control. Unopposed parasympathetic stimulation to the stomach increases gastrin production, contributing to stress ulcer formation. Gastric distention may be present due to paralytic ileus postinjury. Distention may further decrease diaphragmatic excursion and increase the likelihood of aspiration. Both aspiration and decreased diaphragmatic excursion further impair ventilation. A nasogastric tube is inserted to protect the airway from gastric reflux. Pepsin inhibitors (e.g., Carafate) may be given through the nasogastric tube to protect against ulcer formation and bleeding. Histamine blocking agents (e.g., Tagamet and Zantac) may be given intravenously.

Initial bladder management is with an indwelling urinary catheter. When urine output becomes < 2,000 cc/day, the urinary catheter will be removed and intermittent catheterization every 4–6h (maintaining bladder volumes < 400 cc) should be implemented to reduce risk of urinary tract infection. Formal bowel care should be employed including Ducolax suppositories and digital stimulation qod to prevent ileus and constipation.

Other Considerations

After airway, breathing, and circulation are stabilized, the nurse will perform a neurologic assessment as discussed in Section Eight. After getting these baseline data, medications (particularly methylprednisolone) will be administered (Section Seven). The nurse may assist with manual stabilization (skeletal traction and skull tongs) of the spine or the patient may be prepared for transfer to the operating suite.

Loss of Temperature Control

Interruption in communication between the spinal cord and the hypothalamus results in loss of temperature control **(poikilothermia).** Venous pooling also contributes to heat loss by promoting radiation of body heat to the environment. This problem resolves once spinal shock ends and peripheral reflex activity returns. Hyperthermia then becomes a problem because loss of sympathetic control of the sweat glands below the level of the lesion prohibits sweating as temperature rises. A cooling/warming blanket may be needed to treat temperature fluctuations.

Nutrition

Patients with SCI are hypermetabolic and require a high-protein, high-calorie diet. They are at risk for receiving less than their body requirements due to interruption of bowel innervation, limited ability to feed self, anorexia from lack of taste sensation, and depression. Nursing care includes daily weights and administering total parenteral nutrition and/or enteral feedings as scheduled (after ensuring patency of line and/or tube). In some cases, dysphagia will be problematic and food may need to be thickened to allow formation of a food bolus.

Skin Integrity

The SCI patient is at high risk for decubiti formation owing to loss of sensation, immobility, bowel and bladder incontinence, and altered nutrition. The patient and/or caregiver must be taught how to do weight shifts and skin checks. Numerous kinetic beds are available that provide continuous motion. The advantages of these beds are mobilization of pulmonary secretions, improved gas exchange, and decreased decubiti formation.

In summary, ventilation, perfusion, elimination, and temperature control are immediately affected by SCI. Physiologic effects in one system contribute to decreased efficiency in other systems. Nursing care focuses on supporting ventilatory efforts, maintaining an adequate cardiac output, preventing hypothermia, and administering medications as discussed in Section Seven. Although the patient will have elimination, mobility, and sexuality needs, these needs become the focus of nursing care in the non-acute phase and are beyond the scope of this book.

SECTION NINE REVIEW

1. Which of the following contributes to hypothermia immediately post SCI?
   A. venous pooling
   B. bradycardia
   C. hypoxia
   D. gastric distention
2. Hypoxia may result immediately after a complete cervical SCI owing to all of the following factors EXCEPT
   A. gastric distention
   B. decreased diaphragmatic excursion
   C. increased neck accessory muscle use
   D. decreased intercostal muscle use
3. The hypovolemia associated with spinal shock is due to
   A. increased sympathetic nervous system stimulation
   B. increased parasympathetic nervous system stimulation
   C. unopposed parasympathetic nervous system stimulation
   D. hemorrhage of the gray matter

Questions 4 and 5 pertain to Mr. Garrett.

4. Mr. Garrett has a C5 SCI. He complains of shortness of breath. Which of the following would provide more information concerning his ventilatory status?
   A. placing an automatic blood pressure cuff on his arm
   B. initiating cardiac monitoring
   C. suctioning his secretions
   D. initiating pulse oximetry
5. Mr. Garrett's blood pressure drops to 60/40 mm Hg. He is responsive when the nurse shakes his head. The nurse should anticipate
   A. starting vasopressors
   B. increasing his IV fluid rate
   C. administering a fluid bolus
   D. increasing environmental stimuli

Answers: 1. A, 2. C, 3. C, 4. D, 5. B

SECTION TEN: Physiologic Complications of SCI

At the completion of this section, the learner will be able to explain physiologic complications associated with SCI.

Complications associated with SCI (Fig. 20–13) can be classified into three broad categories, related to changes in mobility, perfusion, and reflex activity.

Complications Related to a Change in Mobility

Pneumonia and Atelectasis

Respiratory infection may result from compromised accessory muscle function and phrenic nerve involvement. Loss of abdominal muscle use decreases cough effectiveness. A decreased vital capacity leads to atelectasis. Decreased mobility also contributes to pneumonia and atelectasis.

Decubiti

Several factors contribute to skin breakdown in the SCI patient. Sensory and motor impairment results in areas of the skin being subjected to prolonged periods of pressure, with the patient being unable to feel the pain of the pressure and unable to change position independently. Venous pooling and chronic vasodilation decrease nutrient and oxygen transport to tissue. Moisture exposure due to bowel and bladder incontinence also contributes to decubiti formation.

Decreased Joint Mobility

This complication is preventable. The tendency to remain in one position for extended periods is greater when one is dependent on someone else to initiate movement. Spasticity may contribute to this problem by exaggerating responses to movement. The higher the level of the lesion, the greater the spasticity. Spasms can be used positively to enable use of some assistive devices. Deformity and contracture can develop if joint mobility is not maintained.

Deep Vein Thrombosis

Peripheral vasodilation in conjunction with decreased muscle function encourages venous stasis. Pulmonary emboli from dislodged clots may account for up to 16 percent of SCI deaths (Somers, 1992).

Heterotopic Ossification

Ectopic bone formation (overgrowth of bone) occurs below the SCI, further restricting joint mobility. The cause of this phenomenon is unknown.

Complications Related to Abnormal Perfusion

Autonomic Dysreflexia

Autonomic dysreflexia occurs when a stimulus triggers excessive sympathetic nervous system activation below the level of the SCI. Systemic vasoconstriction results, producing sweating, anxiety, headache, blurred vision,

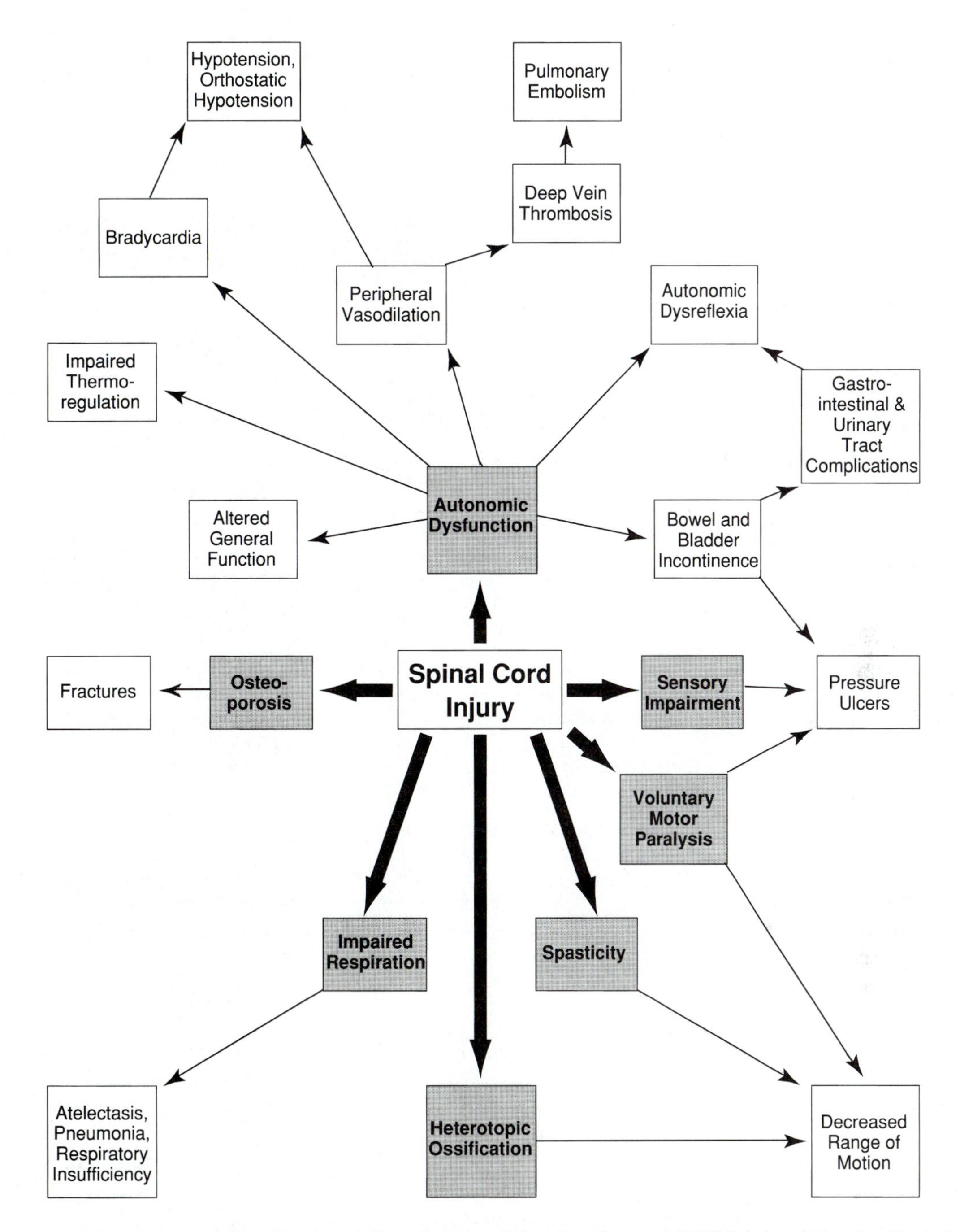

Figure 20–13. Schematic representation of the physical effects of spinal cord injury. (*From Somers, M. [1992].* Spinal cord injury: Functional rehabilitation. Norwalk, CT: *Appleton & Lange.*)

and hypertension. The parasympathetic nervous system tries to compensate for this reaction by producing massive vasodilation above the level of the lesion and bradycardia. However, this compensation is inadequate since it can affect only the neurologically intact section of the body, while the sympathetic reaction is affecting the total body. If left untreated, the sympathetic response results in cerebrovascular accidents, renal failure, atrial fibrillation, and seizures. This phenomenon occurs after spinal shock has ended, usually within the first 6 months of injury. However, autonomic dysreflexia remains a potential problem throughout the patient's life. Therefore, both family and patient must be taught how to recognize and treat the condition. It is more prevalent in lesions at and above T6. Numerous factors can produce autonomic dysreflexia; the most frequent factors are:

- Bladder distention/spasm
- Bowel impaction
- Stimulation of anal reflex
- Labor (in females)
- Temperature change

- Pain
- Decubiti
- Urinary tract infection
- Tight, irritating clothes
- Ingrown toenails

Orthostatic Hypotension

An SCI patient has low blood pressure related to chronic peripheral vasodilation. This factor in combination with a quick position change may result in a loss of consciousness.

Anemia

Anemia is common in the acute and non-acute phases of SCI. In the acute phase, anemia is contributed to blood loss from injury, gastrointestinal bleeding, and surgery. Because malnutrition is also present in the acute phase of SCI, erythropoiesis may be depressed owing to protein

TABLE 20–7. NURSING CARE OF THE SCI PATIENT

DIAGNOSIS	EVALUATIVE CRITERIA	INTERVENTIONS
High risk for injury R/T spinal cord deterioration	Absence of further motor/sensory impairment	Immobilize head and neck Assess motor/sensory status with every weight change or adjustment and every shift Log roll Decrease cord edema (steroids, oxygen)
Ineffective breathing patterns R/T diaphram muscle paralysis	Normal ABGs, Clear breath sounds Normal temperature Clear sputum Vital capacity 60–75 mL/kg	Assess RR, BS, respiratory pattern, chest expansion Quad assistive cough Glossopharyngeal breathing Suction Incentive spirometer Oxygen
Decreased cardiac output R/T impaired vasomotor tone	HR > 50 bpm systolic BP < 80 mm Hg UO > 30 mL/hr GCS score = 15	Antiembolic stockings/compression devices Elevate foot of bed to prevent thrombi, HOB to adapt to position changes I&O IV fluids and vasopressors
Impaired thermoregulation R/T loss of sympathetic simulation	Normal temperature	Use hypo/hyperthermia blanket No heating pad or lamp Modify drinks, clothing for weather Use sunblock
High risk for aspiration R/T paralytic ileus loss of protective reflexes	No emesis Clear breath sounds No fever	Abdominal assessment Maintain patency of NG tube (connect to low wall suction) Administer antacids, histamine blockers, sulcrafate Suction at bedside
Altered urinary elimination R/T impaired reflex function	UO 30 mL/hr, < 400 mL retained No urinary tract infection	I&O Check for bladder distention Begin intermittent catheterization when oral/IV intake is < 2,000 cc/day
Altered bowel elimination R/T impaired reflex function	No skin breakdown Soft stool Regular bowel elimination pattern	Record last BM Administer stool softener Encourage high-fiber foods Adhere to regular bowel elimination schedule
High risk for impaired skin integrity R/T decreased mobility, impaired bowel and bladder function	No impaired skin integrity	Use clock to time turns, turn Q 2° in acute setting Encourage/teach weight shifting when in chair or wheelchair Q 15 minutes Instruct patient to inspect skin using mirrors Lift arms while in wheelchair or instruct patient to do so

ABGs = arterial blood gases; RR = respiratory rate; BS = breath sounds; HR = heart rate; BP = blood pressure; UO = urine output; GCS = Glasgow Coma Scale; HOB = head of bed; I&O = intake and output; NG = nasogastric; BM = bowel movement deficiency. Plasma albumin, carotene, transferrin, ascorbate, thiamine, and folate levels are decreased (Laven et al., 1989). In the non-acute phase, anemia is related to the presence of a chronic infection (e.g., urinary tract infection) (Hirsch, Menard, & Anton, 1991).

Temperature Hypersensitivity

As mentioned in Section Nine, initially the patient is at risk for hypothermia. Even in the non-acute phase, frostbite can occur quickly due to lack of sensation and peripheral vasodilation and loss of heat to the atmosphere. The inability to dissipate heat owing to lack of ability to sweat contributes to heat stroke.

Complications Related to Abnormal Reflex Activity

Bowel and Bladder Dysfunction

The SCI patient may experience urinary retention and/or vesicourethral reflux, leading to urinary tract infection. Both patients with upper motor neuron injuries and those with lower motor neuron injuries eventually gain bladder control through intermittent catheterization.

Sexual Dysfunction

Fertility is usually affected in males. Erection is mediated by the parasympathetic nervous system in the S2–4 area. Ejaculation is mediated by the sympathetic nervous system in the T12–L2 area. Therefore, the lower the spinal cord injury, the greater the sexual dysfunction due to difficulty in maintaining an erection.

In the female, amenorrhea may occur for the first year postinjury. After this, the female may conceive. Labor may initiate autonomic dysreflexia.

In summary, several complications are associated with SCI. Some of these may occur in the acute phase of injury while others, like autonomic dysreflexia, occur in the non-acute phase.

The type of complication is influenced by the level of the lesion. Figure 20–13 illustrates the potential physical impact of an SCI. Table 20–7 summarizes nursing diagnoses appropriate for the SCI patient in the acute phase.

Section Ten Review

Questions 1 through 3 pertain to John Smith. Mr. Smith was diagnosed with a complete T1 injury 7 months ago. He is readmitted to your unit for a urinary tract infection.

1. Mr. Smith tells the nurse that he thinks he is having an "attack of his reflexes" (autonomic dysreflexia). Of the following data, which suggest that he is experiencing this disorder?
   - **A.** bradycardia
   - **B.** fever
   - **C.** hypertension
   - **D.** hypoxia
2. Because of the level of Mr. Smith's injury, the nurse realizes Mr. Smith will
   - **A.** not be able to control his bladder
   - **B.** require an indwelling catheter
   - **C.** be able to perform intermittent catheterization
   - **D.** require an external urine collection device
3. Mr. Smith asks the nurse about his potential sexual function. The nurse responds by saying most patients with this type of injury
   - **A.** are impotent
   - **B.** are not able to ejaculate
   - **C.** have unpredictable erections
   - **D.** are capable of erection and ejaculation

Answers: 1. C, 2. C, 3. D

SECTION ELEVEN: Psychosocial Issues in SCI

At the completion of this section, the learner will be able to describe responses of patients, family, and staff to SCI.

Spinal cord injury changes the independent individual into a more dependent person. Adaptation depends on personality, coping styles, and life experiences (Partridge, 1994). Several emotions have been described by SCI patients, including fear of death, fear of living, anger, denial, and hopelessness (Browner & Prendergast, 1991). Educational level, employment status, income, and social support systems are factors associated with the quality of life postinjury (Clayton & Chubon, 1994). Families adjust better to their situation when they perceive a high level of social support.

Patients with an SCI have a higher-than-average suicide rate. Suicide is usually accomplished within 4 years of injury. Those at greater risk for suicide are older at the time of injury; have a history of drug abuse pre- and post-SCI; and/or were actively involved in acquiring the injury. The nurse should assess SCI persons for their suicide potential. Open-ended questions such as "Have you ever thought about harming yourself?" or "Do you consider life worth living?" should communicate to the patient the nurse's willingness to discuss coping strategies. The nurse should be credible in answers and reliable in promises (Browner & Prendergast, 1991). The patient must be taught how to direct others to meet his or her needs effectively.

Health care providers may have biases toward SCI persons. Many believe that resuscitation efforts after SCI are too aggressive (Gerhart et al., 1994). Patients tend to be more optimistic about their quality of life than the health care providers (Gerhart et al., 1994). It is very difficult to make life-support decisions in the high-acuity setting, soon after injury, because communication with the patient may be impaired. Additional physiologic problems may be present (e.g., associated head injury) confounding the ability to make an informed decision. Patients usually do not have enough information on which to base a life-support decision. Patients need to know rehabilitation possibilities, what adaptive devices are available, and the consequences of their cord injury prior to making life-support decisions.

In summary, SCI is a major life event requiring special coping skills in order to have a good quality of life. Social support is vital to both patient and family coping. The nurse should assess each SCI person for their suicide potential. Nurses should be credible and honest when providing information about rehabilitation and the consequences of SCI to the patient.

SECTION ELEVEN REVIEW

1. Mr. Clark, age 20, is admitted to neuro ICU with a C4 SCI and a subdural hematoma. The ICU nurses believe that life-support measures should be minimal. As patient advocate, you should maintain life support measures for all of the following reasons EXCEPT
   A. the patient has a concomitant head injury
   B. his wishes are not known
   C. the patient does not have enough information on which to act
   D. rehabilitation at C4 level is not possible
2. Mr. Clark was injured while diving at a school swim party. He had alcohol on his breath when he was admitted. He is at risk for suicide because
   A. of his age
   B. the injury occurred at a school event
   C. his actions produced the injury
   D. he had alcohol on his breath

Answers: 1. D, 2. C

SECTION TWELVE: Preventing SCI

At the completion of this section, the learner will be able to discuss SCI prevention programs and strategies.

Prevention of SCI generally focuses on one of three items:

1. Persuading people at risk to alter their behavior
2. Requiring persons to change their behavior through legislation
3. Providing automatic protection

Host Factors

Spinal cord injury, like other forms of traumatic injury, is associated with excessive speed, alcohol use, and risk-taking behavior. Risk-taking behavior may take a variety of forms, such as failing to wear a seatbelt or engaging in an activity (racing) with a high injury risk. In motor vehicle crashes, the more severe SCIs are associated with not wearing a seatbelt. Diving-induced SCIs occur more frequently when the person does not check the depth and contour of the pool. Sports with a high frequency of personal contact (e.g., football) have a higher risk of SCI. Violence also contributes to SCI through penetrating trauma to the spinal cord.

Agent Factors

Losing control of an all-terrain vehicle (ATV) may produce SCI. Four-wheel ATVs are more stable than three-wheel ATVs in terms of control, but falling from the ATV can occur regardless of the wheel base. Pool design is an important factor in preventing SCIs. The bottom of the pool should be marked, as should points of depth transition. The development of high head rests in automobiles has decreased hyperextension injuries.

Environmental Factors

Signs should be posted warning of water depths at swimming pools and in natural environments. Docks and piers are frequent injury sites.

Standardized SCI prevention programs have been developed by several different agencies for use by schools, companies, and health care professionals. An extensive review of programs can be found in the document Resources: A National Directory of Spinal Cord Injury Prevention Programs (University of Alabama–Birmingham). "Feet First, the First Time" is an educational program designed to prevent SCIs. Information about this program can be obtained through the American Association of Neuroscience Nurses.

SECTION TWELVE REVIEW

1. The severity of an SCI in a motor vehicle crash is directly related to all of the following EXCEPT
   A. restraint status of the person
   B. gender
   C. speed of the vehicle
   D. type of terrain where crash occurred

Answer: 1. B

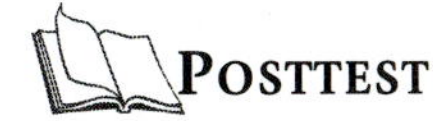

POSTTEST

1. A diagnosis of unstable SCI is made based on
   A. disruption of two or more of the spinal columns
   B. degree of sensory involvement
   C. presence of associated hemodynamic changes
   D. degree of flaccid paralysis present
2. An upper motor neuron lesion results in
   A. permanent loss of bladder function
   B. flaccid paralysis
   C. contralateral motor effects
   D. spastic paralysis
3. Diving is frequently associated with _____ spinal cord lesions.
   A. cervical
   B. cervical–thoracic
   C. thoracic
   D. lumbar
4. A patient with calcaneus fractures of the feet should be suspected of having damage to the _____ region of the spinal cord.
   A. cervical
   B. thoracic
   C. lumbar
   D. sacral
5. Which of the following chronic health conditions is associated with SCI?
   A. epilepsy
   B. rheumatoid arthritis
   C. Paget's disease
   D. renal disease
6. An SEP test is used to determine a patient's
   A. functional prognosis
   B. bowel and bladder function
   C. level of spinal cord injury
   D. potential for decubiti
7. Secondary injury to the spinal cord can be prevented during what time frame postinjury?
   A. first hour
   B. within the first 24 hours
   C. first 8 hours
   D. within the first 72 hours

Questions 8 and 9 pertain to Mary Wade.

8. Mary was admitted 1 hour ago with an unstable, incomplete C6 SCI. In order to administer methylprednisolone to her, what data must be obtained?
   A. prior steriod use
   B. past medical history
   C. time since injury
   D. age
9. The nurse had administered a methylprednisolone bolus to Ms. Wade. The remaining dose must be
   A. administered over 23 hours
   B. mixed with mannitol
   C. given in intermittent doses
   D. equivalent to 30 mg/kg
10. After spinal shock resides, a lower motor neuron injury is suggested by the assessment finding of
    A. priapism
    B. absence of bulbocavernosus reflex
    C. movement of elbow against gravity
    D. sensation above the groin

11. A person with a C7 injury has the following rehabilitation potential:
    A. dependent eating, dependent dressing, electric wheelchair mobility
    B. independent eating, dependent dressing, electric wheelchair mobility
    C. dependent eating, minor assistance with dressing, electric wheelchair mobility
    D. independent eating, independent with aid dressing, independent mobility in manual wheelchair
12. Spinal shock is characterized by
    A. peripheral vasoconstriction
    B. flaccid paralysis
    C. peripheral diaphoresis
    D. hyperthermia

Questions 13 and 14 pertain to Mr. Soap.

13. Mr. Soap, age 65, has a T7 SCI. His medical history is positive for diabetes. He smokes 2 packs of cigarettes a day. He is at risk for respiratory failure because of
    A. his diabetes
    B. the level of his SCI
    C. his smoking history
    D. his age
14. Mr. Soap develops a weak cough with crackles on auscultation. His heart rate and blood pressure remain unchanged. The nurse should seek a physician's order to
    A. decrease his IV fluid rate
    B. insert an indwelling urinary catheter
    C. place a nasogastric tube
    D. increase his oxygen
15. Which of the following statements accurately describes autonomic dysreflexia?
    A. it is a spastic disorder limiting mobility
    B. it is a cardiovascular problem produced by decreased cardiac output secondary to bradycardia
    C. it is a vasoconstrictive problem produced by excessive sympathetic nervous system stimulation
    D. it is a parasympathetic nervous system problem resulting from unopposed vasodilation
16. An advantage of surgical stabilization over manual stabilization of the spine is that it
    A. requires bone grafting
    B. promotes earlier mobilization
    C. prevents deformity
    D. can be completed immediately postinjury
17. When assessing a patient's ability to cope with an SCI, which of the following is the most important factor to assess?
    A. income
    B. education
    C. age
    D. social support system
18. Prevention of SCI focuses on all of the following EXCEPT
    A. establishing a comprehensive rehabilitation program
    B. persuading people at risk to alter their behavior
    C. requiring persons to change their behavior through legislation
    D. providing automatic protection

POSTTEST ANSWERS

Question	Answer	Section	Question	Answer	Section
1	A	One	10	B	Seven
2	D	Two	11	D	Seven
3	A	Three	12	B	Eight
4	B	Three	13	C	Eight
5	B	Three	14	A	Eight
6	A	Four	15	C	Nine
7	C	Five	16	B	Ten
8	C	Six	17	D	Eleven
9	A	Six	18	A	Twelve

REFERENCES

American Spinal Injury Association. (ASIA) (1996). *International standards for neurological and functional classification of spinal cord injury*. Chicago: Author.

Anderson, D.K., & Hall, E.D. (1993). Pathophysiology of spinal cord trauma. *Ann Emerg Med 22*(6):987-92.

Ball, R. (1990). Don't add insult to injury. *J Emerg Med Serv* 40:40–41, 43–46.

Bissonette, D. (1988). Sorting out spinal cord syndromes. *J Am Acad Phys Assist 1*:4–18.

Browner, C., & Prendergast, V. (1991). Spinal cord damage with diving injuries. *Crit Care Nurs Clin North Am 3*:339–352.

Clayton, K., & Chubon, R. (1994). Factors associated with the quality of life of long term spinal cord injured persons. *Arch Phys Med Rehabil 75*:633–638.

Cook, P. (1988). Radiology of the spine and spinal cord injury. In L. Illis (ed). *Spinal cord dysfunction: Assessment* (pp. 41–103). New York: Oxford University Press.

DeVivo, M., Stover, S., & Black, K. (1992). Prognostic factors for 12 year survival after spinal cord injury. *Arch Phys Med Rehabil 73*:156–162.

Gerhart, K., Koziol–McLain, J., Lowenstein, S., & Whiteneck, G. (1994). Quality of life following spinal cord injury: Knowledge and attitudes of emergency care providers. *Ann Emerg Med 23*:807–812.

Gertsch-Lapcevic, Y., Guin, P., Butler, J., & Ryan, S. (1991). Hyperbaric oxygen therapy: Treatment for spinal cord decompression sickness. *Spinal Cord Injury Nurs 8*:97–101.

Herman, J., & Sonntag, V. (1991). Diving accidents. *Crit Care Nurs Clin North Am 3*:331–337.

Hilton, G., & Frei, J. (1991). High-dose methylprednisolone in the treatment of spinal cord injuries. *Heart Lung, 20*(6):675–680.

Hirsch, G., Menard, M., & Anton, H. (1991). Anemia after traumatic spinal cord injury. *Arch Phys Med Rehabil 72*:195–205.

Hudak, C., & Gallo, B. (1994). *Critical care nursing: A holistic approach* (6th ed). Philadelphia: J.B. Lippincott.

Hughes, M. (1990). Critical care nursing for the patient with a spinal cord injury. *Crit Care Nurs Clin North Am 2*:33–40.

Kidd, P. (1990). Emergency management of spinal cord injuries. *Crit Care Nurs Clin North Am 2*:349–356.

Laven, G., Huang, C., DeVivo, M., Stover, S., Kuhlemeier, K., & Fine, P. (1989). Nutritional status during the acute stage of spinal cord injury. *Arch Phys Med Rehabil 70*:277–282.

Little, N. (1989, May 15). In case of a broken neck. *Emerg Med* pp. 22–32.

McKenna, M., & McCarthy, C. (1989). Acute care of the patient with spinal cord injury. *Can Orthop Nurs Assoc 11*:5–10.

Nayduch, D., Lee, A., & Butler, D. (1994, August). High-dose methylprednisolone after acute spinal cord injury. *Crit Care Nurse* pp. 69–78.

Nobunaga, A., Go, B., Karunas, R. (1999). Recent demographic and injury trends in people served by the Model Spinal Cord Injury Care Systems. *Arch Phys Med Rehabil* 80:1372–1382.

Nolan, S. (1994). Current trends in the management of acute spinal cord injury. *Crit Care Nurs Q 17*(1):64–78.

Partridge, C. (1994). Spinal cord injuries: Aspects of psychological care. *Br J Nurs 3*(1):12–15.

Ragnarsson, K., & Lammertse, D. (1991). Rehabilitation in spinal cord disorders. *Arch Phys Med Rehabil 72*:S295–S297.

Somers, M. (1992). *Spinal cord injury: Functional rehabilitation*. Norwalk, CT: Appleton & Lange.

Zejdlik, C. (1992). *Management of spinal cord injury*. Boston: Jones & Bartlett.

Module 21

Nursing Care of the Patient with Spinal Cord Injury

Pamela Stinson Kidd

This module is designed to integrate major points discussed in Modules 17 through 20, with a major emphasis on Module 20. This module summarizes key relationships between concepts and assists the learner in clustering information to facilitate clinical application. Content is presented in an interactive learning style. Using a case study format, the learner is encouraged to identify nursing actions based on the assessment of a patient with a spinal cord injury (SCI). The consequences of selecting a particular action are discussed. Rationale for all answers is presented. The module ends with a brief summary of major points.

Objectives

At the completion of this module, the learner will be able to

1. Describe an appropriate database for a patient with an SCI.
2. Explain the assessment of a patient with an SCI.
3. Discuss development of nursing diagnoses appropriate for a patient with an SCI.
4. Discuss development of a plan of care for the patient with an SCI.

Abbreviations

DTR. Deep tendon reflex

DVT. Deep vein thrombosis

GCS. Glasgow Coma Scale

MRI. Magnetic resonance imaging

SCI. Spinal cord injury

CASE STUDY

Jeff R, 16 years of age, is admitted to your neurosurgical floor. He was transferred from a rural emergency department after falling off a trampoline. You are told in report that he has a spinal cord injury. He has just arrived at your unit and is awaiting assessment. You will be his primary nurse for the shift.

Initial Appraisal

On walking into the room you quickly note the following:

GENERAL APPEARANCE. Jeff is of large stature, muscular, and well nourished. He has a Miami-J hard collar in place around his neck. He is lying flat in bed on a backboard to which he is strapped.

SIGNS OF DISTRESS. Jeff's extremities are flushed. He is breathing rapidly, with diaphragmatic movement present. His eyes are puffy from crying.

OTHER. You note that Jeff has one intravenous (IV) line in place in his right hand. There is a methylprednisolone drip infusing per IV pump. His parents are at the bedside. You overhear his Dad talking with another nurse about Jeff missing football season; he is the quarterback of his high school team.

Focused Respiratory Assessment

Because Jeff is breathing rapidly, you immediately perform a rapid assessment, focusing first on his pulmonary status, even though his clinical problem is neurologic in nature.

Jeff is scared but alert and oriented, with a Glasgow Coma Scale (GCS) score of 10. Jeff is restless. His respiratory rate is 40/min; breathing is shallow and regular. There is no intercostal muscle movement. Accessory muscles in his neck are contracting. Breath sounds are clear to auscultation bilaterally although diminished in the lower lung fields. His blood pressure is 82/60 mm Hg and his pulse is 58 bpm.

You scan his admission orders. An arterial blood gas (ABG), pulse oximetry, 40 percent oxygen per face mask, nasogastric (NG) tube, and urinary catheter have been ordered.

QUESTION

You decide that the NG tube and urinary catheter can wait. Which of the remaining orders would you implement first?

A. pulse oximetry
B. oxygen
C. ABG

ANSWER

The correct answer is B. You should administer the oxygen first even if Jeff may be reluctant to wear a mask due to the "smothering" feeling. It is true that oxygen administration may alter the ABG results; thus, you should notify the lab regarding how much oxygen Jeff is receiving and for how long he has been receiving it. Pulse oximetry is needed for you to monitor Jeff's response to the oxygen, but this can wait until you start the oxygen. If you delay with the oxygen administration, Jeff may go into respiratory arrest.

QUESTION

How would you interpret Jeff's blood pressure and pulse?

A. they are directly related to his athletic training
B. they reflect the beginning of autonomic dysreflexia
C. they are indicative of spinal shock
D. they are abnormal and indicate that he needs an IV fluid bolus

ANSWER

The correct answer is C. In spinal shock, vasomotor tone is lost and blood pools in the periphery owing to unopposed parasympathetic stimulation. Spinal shock may last weeks to months postinjury. It is true that Jeff's cardiovascular conditioning will produce a lower-than-average pulse and blood pressure; however, 82/60 mm Hg is too low for his surface area. Autonomic dysreflexia occurs later in the injury process after spinal shock subsides. It is heralded by a grossly elevated blood pressure that results from stimuli (e.g., distended bladder) that produce a sympathetic nervous system discharge below the level of injury. Uncontrolled vasoconstriction occurs. If Jeff becomes symptomatic (e.g., demonstrates a decreased level of responsiveness) with this blood pressure and pulse, then an IV fluid bolus would be necessary.

Jeff responds well to the oxygen. His respiratory rate has decreased to 32/min. You take time to scan his admission history and physical exam notes. You discover that

Jeff has a hyperflexion injury. He had an MRI performed on the way to the floor. Initial reading of the MRI revealed vertebral fractures of C5 and C6 with anterior subluxation of C4.

Focused Neurologic Assessment

Jeff's GCS score is still 10. You reassessed this because of the risk of associated head injury with an SCI. You assess his motor function next. Jeff is able to turn his head and move his shoulders. He has no extremity movement. He does have 2+ deep tendon reflex (DTR) responses of his biceps bilaterally. All other DTRs are absent. He has no rectal sphincter tone, indicating a complete cord lesion. Sensation is intact in his head, shoulders, and clavicle regions as well as the lateral aspect of his arms. He is incontinent of urine.

QUESTION

What respiratory needs or risks does Jeff have based on the location and extent of his injury? Select all correct options.

A. He will need mechanical ventilation for the rest of his life after spinal shock subsides.
B. He is at risk for respiratory muscle fatigue.
C. He is at risk for atelectasis.
D. He is at risk for respiratory failure.

ANSWER

The correct answers are B, C, and D. The diaphragm is innervated by the phrenic nerve, which travels through the third, fourth, and fifth cervical segments of the cord. His neck muscles may become fatigued from assisting the diaphragm. Fatigue may produce hypoventilation and respiratory failure even though he has function of the diaphragm. His ability to cough up secretions will be severely limited. This fact, in conjunction with his decreased mobility, increases his risk of atelectasis. He is at risk for aspiration until the NG tube is placed. Aspiration would increase Jeff's risk for pneumonia. Another factor not mentioned is his IV fluid rate. If Jeff receives too much fluid, he is at risk for pulmonary edema; thus, fluid boluses are administered cautiously. Jeff has a great number of respiratory risks. He will require frequent monitoring of tidal volume, oxygen saturation, and breath sounds.

Jeff's parents ask you to come out in the hall to discuss what is in store for Jeff. They ask you about his injury.

QUESTION

What are the characteristics of a hyperflexion injury and how does this affect Jeff's care?

ANSWER

Hyperflexion injuries are most common at C5–6 because this is the most mobile portion of the spine (Johnson, 1998). Injury occurs from compression of the cord as a result of fragments and from dislocation of the vertebral bodies. Instability of the spinal column is common because of tearing of the posterior muscles and ligaments. The implication for Jeff's care is that the stabilization process may take place in two steps. First, alignment of the vertebrae will be accomplished. Then the stability of the column will be addressed.

Focused Nursing History

Jeff is tired from breathing and is resting; you decide to talk with his parents to obtain the most critical historical data that may have an impact on Jeff's present situation. The total nursing database will need to be completed within 24 hours postadmission. Jeff's parents give you the following history.

Jeff's younger brother, Gary, age 12 years, was given a trampoline for his birthday. The family had just set up the trampoline in the back yard when the injury occurred. Gary had performed a double somersault and dared Jeff to "top that." Jeff had jumped several times prior to completing the somersault to get enough height. When he came out of the somersault, he landed on the "back of his neck" with his chin pulled into his chest. He went limp and could not move himself off the trampoline. Jeff's Dad and Gary pulled Jeff off the trampoline, thinking he had "knocked the wind out of him." When Jeff stated he could not move, they loaded him into the pick-up truck and went to the nearest hospital, 30 minutes away. They were told at the hospital that Jeff needed a neurosurgeon and that he would be transferred to this hospital (the regional trauma center) by ambulance.

Jeff has a negative past medical history. He does not use any medications or recreational drugs. He was not drinking alcohol at the time of injury. He has smoked since he was 10. His Dad doesn't really know how many cigarettes a day Jeff smokes, since Jeff works and pays for his own. Jeff has been on the football team since freshman year, at which time he was good enough to make varsity. His life goal is to play for the NFL.

Systematic Bedside Assessment

To develop appropriate nursing diagnoses for Jeff, you initiate a head-to-toe assessment.

HEAD AND NECK. Jeff has perspiration over his upper lip and on his forehead. His head is pale compared with the rest of his body. Jeff remains completely oriented (GCS score = 10). Nasal flaring is noted. Face mask is intact and connected to 40 percent oxygen. No other abnormalities of the head and neck are noted. Miami-J collar is still in place.

CHEST. Respiratory status remains unchanged since your last assessment except for some fine crackles auscultated in the lower lung fields bilaterally. S_1 and S_2 are present without rub or murmur. Rate is regular. He remains bradycardic.

ABDOMEN. Jeff's abdomen is slightly distended. Bowel sounds are absent. No sensation is noted on palpation.

PELVIS. Jeff has voided on the sheets. No priapism is noted. Rectal tone is still absent.

EXTREMITIES. Lower extremities are flushed and cool to touch. No edema is noted. Pulses are 2+. No motor or sensory function is noted except as stated in the focused neurologic assessment.

POSTERIOR. You defer assessment of this region until Jeff's spine is stabilized since there are not enough professionals available to log roll Jeff.

Development of Nursing Diagnoses

You have just completed your head-to-toe assessment and are ready to develop a problem list based on the subjective and objective data that you have collected thus far. To cluster your data, you look for abnormalities found during the assessment.

PRIORITY CLUSTER

Subjective data. Jeff complained of being tired from breathing. He has a history of smoking.

Objective data. Shallow, rapid respirations ranging from 30 to 40 per min. Perspiration on forehead and upper lip. Diminished breath sounds and fine crackles in lower lung fields bilaterally. Use of neck muscles to assist breathing. C5–6 fractures. Jeff is lying flat on a backboard restrained with straps. Abdomen is slightly distended. No bowel sounds auscultated. Jeff's injury is recent, thus the cord may continue to swell, paralyzing his diaphragm.

Based on these data, you make the following nursing diagnoses:

- *Ineffective breathing pattern: respiratory muscle paralysis and accessory muscle fatigue* related to disruption of nerves
- *High risk for impaired gas exchange* related to increased secretions and decreased mobilization of secretions
- *Ineffective airway clearance* related to diminished cough and flat position
- *High risk for aspiration* related to lack of peristalsis

Desired patient outcomes (DPOs) for Jeff (evaluative criteria) would include:

- Improved or clear breath sounds
- Oxygen saturation > 95 percent
- Respiratory rate > 12 but < 30/min
- No dyspnea
- Chest x-ray normal without infiltrates
- Temperature normal

QUESTION

Based on your knowledge of SCI, what other nursing diagnoses are appropriate for Jeff in the acute phase? Select all correct options.

A. altered tissue perfusion
B. hypothermia
C. altered nutrition: less than body requirements
D. altered urinary elimination

ANSWER

This is a tough question! All these nursing diagnoses are appropriate in the acute as well as the non-acute phase. Rehabilitation begins in the acute phase. Although airway, breathing, and circulation are always our primary concerns, care of the patient with an SCI involves multiple dimensions.

Altered tissue perfusion in the acute phase is usually related to hypotension from spinal shock. The goal is to provide adequate perfusion and oxygenation to prevent secondary injury from cord edema and the inflammatory process. Jeff is also at risk for deep vein thrombosis (DVT) secondary to decreased mobility, venous stasis, and potential fluid volume deficit from vasodilation.

Hypothermia results from vasodilation and heat loss. The patient becomes poikilothermic, taking on the temperature of the environment, which is several degrees below normal body temperature.

Patients with SCI tend to lose weight quickly owing to their hypermetabolic state in the acute phase. Testosterone levels also decrease, contributing to negative nitrogen balance and protein wasting (Poyner, 1992). Their caloric intake should be close to 2,000 calories per day through enteral or parenteral routes. If not fed quickly, the patient will have decreased muscular ability to use adaptive devices, experiences bone loss, and develop decubiti.

Jeff is at risk for skin breakdown if his urine is not collected. There is great controversy concerning whether indwelling urinary catheters should be used. Generally, intermittent catheterization is used for bladder management once spinal shock has resolved and urine output is < 2,000 cc/day. Until then, an external collection device can be used.

Developing the Plan of Care

Treatment goals for Jeff are:

- Optimizing his oxygenation status
- Promoting airway clearance
- Maintaining functional alveoli
- Promoting adequate perfusion
- Preventing infection
- Maximizing mobility

These general goals are reflected in the nursing diagnoses and DPOs on the nursing care plan or critical pathway.

Nursing interventions are based on activities to help Jeff meet his DPOs. They consist of collaborative interventions, which are activities ordered by the health care practitioner but require some actions by the nurse, and independent interventions, activities that are within the nursing scope of practice to write and carry out as nursing orders.

Collaborative Interventions Related to SCI in the Acute Phase

1. *Pulmonary therapy:* Intubation and mechanical ventilation may be used if the vital capacity drops below 1,200 mL. Postural drainage and percussion may be ordered. "Quad coughing" is used for secretion management. Bronchodilators and expectorants may be used to liquefy secretions and aid removal by suction. Hydration will be closely titrated to help mobilize secretions without producing a fluid volume excess since Jeff is unable to increase his heart rate to manage an increased stroke volume.
2. *Laboratory and x-ray testing:* Chest x-rays will be ordered intermittently, as will ABGs. Red cell and white cell counts will be ordered as needed to rule out infection and anemia. A repeat MRI will be conducted to check alignment once stabilization measures have been implemented.
3. *Mobility:* An oscillating bed or turning frame will be ordered once Jeff's spine is stabilized. A physical therapy consult will be initiated.
4. *Cardiovascular therapy:* Jeff will be started on low-molecular-weight heparin (Lovenox 30 mg bid) to prevent DVT. He may receive an IV fluid bolus of atropine if his heart rate continues to decrease and he becomes symptomatic.
5. *Steroid therapy:* Jeff received a loading dose of methylprednisolone at the first hospital. He will receive 5.4 mg/kg/hr for 23 hours postinjury. Steroids are thought to decrease further injury to the cord from the inflammatory process. Steroids decrease fatty acid production and the mediators produced by way of fatty acid breakdown (for more information, refer to Module 11). This prevents the breakdown of the cell membrane and further release of mediators that produce vasodilation.
6. *Stabilization:* Immobilization of the cervical spine is accomplished by skeletal traction. Cervical tongs (e.g., Crutchfield or Gardner–Wells tongs) and the halo apparatus are the most common forms of traction used.

Jeff was fitted with a halo device connected to 10 pounds of weights to achieve good alignment. Two weeks later, he underwent surgery for an anterior cervical cordectomy with placement of a fibula strip bone graft and plate placement. This fusion provided stability of the cervical region.

A rehabilitation medicine consult may be obtained in the first 24 hours postinjury to establish level of injury, ASIA classification, and assist with acute care issues.

Independent Nursing Interventions in the Acute Phase

1. Assess for decreased respiratory function:
   - Change in respiratory rate (< 12 or > 30/min)
   - Increasing dyspnea
   - Decreasing oxygen saturation level
   - Change in responsiveness
   - Abnormal breath sounds
   - Change in sputum
   - Increasing fatigue/perspiration
   - Nasal flaring
2. Suction secretions as necessary. Hyperoxygenate and ventilate prior to suctioning. Be prepared to administer atropine if Jeff's heart rate drops further during suctioning.
3. Prevent secondary cord injury:
   - Administer methylprednisolone as ordered
   - Administer oxygen as ordered
   - Administer IV fluids as ordered
4. Monitor fluid intake and output to maintain thin secretions and 1 mL/kg/hr urine output.
5. Maintain airway patency:
   - Insert NG tube and connect to low wall suction
   - Suction nasopharynx as needed
6. Apply thromboembolic devices, monitor peripheral perfusion status.
7. Promote nutrition:
   - Administer drugs to decrease gastric irritation as ordered
   - Initiate and monitor enteral and parenteral feedings as ordered
   - Weigh patient daily
   - Guaiac test stools

8. Prevent infection:
   - Hand washing
   - Sterile suctioning and tube insertion (as appropriate)
   - Cleanse tong insertion sites per policy
   - Monitor for signs of infection (temperature, urine, sputum)
9. Place Jeff on an oscillating bed.
10. Promote normothermia:
    - Increase room temperature as appropriate
    - Administer warmed IV fluid if necessary
    - Use external warming devices

Bowel and bladder training is initiated once spinal shock has subsided and peristalsis returns. Not addressed in this module are the psychosocial sequelae associated with SCI, which may include body image disturbance, hopelessness, and ineffective individual coping.

Plan Evaluation and Revision

Jeff's plan of care is now developed and ready to execute. His progress will be monitored at regular intervals to evaluate the effects of the various therapeutic actions. If progress is not being noted toward Jeff's expected outcomes, his plan of care may need revision, examining alternative interventions that may be more effective.

Jeff was discharged to a rehabilitation facility 1 month postinjury. His family attended caregiving sessions in order to care for Jeff at home. Jeff is now at home and has returned to school. He has a head-controlled wheelchair and writes with an adaptive tool held in his mouth.

REFERENCES

Johnson, K. (1998). Trauma. In L. Thelan, J. Davie, L. Urden, & M. Lough (eds.), *Critical care nursing: Diagnosis and management* (3rd ed.) (pp. 1051–1095). St. Louis: C.V. Mosby.

Poyner, M. (1996). Vertebral and spinal cord trauma. In J. Hickey (ed.), *The clinical practice of neurological and neurosurgical nursing* (3rd ed.) (Chapter 18). Philadelphia: J.B. Lippincott.

PART VI

Metabolic

MODULE 22

Metabolic Responses

Theresa Loan

This self-study module focuses on the metabolic responses that occur in the high-acuity or critically ill patient. The module is composed of seven sections. Section One provides an overview of normal metabolism. Section Two describes the purposes of nutrition and the metabolism of the specific macronutrients—carbohydrates, lipids, and proteins. Section Three explains the interpretation of physiologic and laboratory data pertinent to nutritional assessment of the high-acuity patient. Common metabolic alterations encountered in high-acuity patients are discussed in Section Four, while Section Five presents an overview of nutritional needs of patients with specific disease processes. The module concludes with a discussion of methods of nutrient delivery in Sections Six and Seven. Each section includes a set of review questions to help the learner evaluate his or her understanding of the section's content before moving on to the next section. All Section Reviews and the module Pretest and Posttest include answers. It is suggested that the learner review those concepts answered incorrectly in the review questions before proceeding to the next section.

OBJECTIVES

Following completion of this module, the learner will be able to

1. Explain basic normal metabolism.
2. Describe the primary functions of carbohydrates, lipids, and proteins, and the nutritional needs of the high-acuity patient.
3. Differentiate between patients with normal versus altered metabolism.
4. Recognize the typical metabolic alterations in the high-acuity/critically ill patient.
5. Describe the major nutritional alterations associated with refeeding syndrome, hepatic failure, pulmonary failure, acute and chronic renal failure, cardiac failure, gut failure, burns, and head injury.
6. Describe the enteral methods used to provide nutrition for the high-acuity/critically ill patient, including potential complications.
7. Discuss the parenteral methods used to provide nutrition for the high-acuity/critically ill patient, including potential complications.

PRETEST

1. The metabolic stress response is the result of
   A. psychologic stress
   B. overexertion from exercise
   C. injured tissue in the body
   D. hyperventilation

2. The two phases of the metabolic stress response are
   A. ebb phase and catabolic phase
   B. ebb phase and flow phase
   C. ebb phase and recovery phase
   D. flow phase and recovery phase

3. Hypermetabolism refers to
   A. an elevated metabolic rate
   B. the breakdown of total body protein
   C. elevated serum insulin levels
   D. increased immunoglobulins
4. Hypercatabolism refers to
   A. an elevated metabolic rate
   B. the breakdown of total body protein
   C. elevated serum insulin levels
   D. increased immunoglobulins
5. Enteral nutrition has many advantages over total parenteral nutrition (TPN), including each of the following EXCEPT
   A. less risk of bacterial translocation
   B. providing central venous access
   C. maintaining gut morphology and function
   D. less costly
6. Which nutrient is the body's preferred energy source?
   A. intact proteins
   B. amino acids
   C. carbohydrates
   D. lipids
7. Feeding tube occlusion is a potential mechanical complication of enteral feedings. All of the following are possible causes EXCEPT
   A. viscous formulas
   B. lack of proper flushing
   C. food coloring
   D. medications
8. Which of the following conditions is a complication associated with intragastric tube feeding?
   A. nosocomial pneumonia
   B. bacterial translocation
   C. stress ulcer
   D. metabolic acidosis
9. TPN is indicated when
   A. adequate amounts of nutrients cannot be delivered through the gastrointestinal tract
   B. the patient is hypermetabolic
   C. bowel sounds are not audible
   D. the hypercatabolic patient is not able to eat for 3 days
10. TPN with glucose concentration greater than 10 percent should be administered through a
   A. nasoenteric feeding tube
   B. peripheral vein
   C. surgically placed jejunal feeding tube
   D. central vein
11. Catheter-related sepsis (CRS) is a potentially lethal complication of TPN and is primarily caused by
   A. a malpositioned catheter or guidewire during the central line insertion
   B. lack of sterility during central line placement and inadequate maintenance of the line
   C. inadvertent puncture or laceration of the subclavian or carotid artery
   D. puncture or laceration of the vein on insertion of the needle/catheter
12. Mechanical complications of TPN consist of all of the following EXCEPT
   A. air embolism
   B. hydrothorax
   C. pneumothorax
   D. CRS
13. What nursing action would you undertake first when a patient receiving tube feeding develops diarrhea?
   A. stop the tube feeding
   B. send a stool specimen for *Clostridium difficile* cytotoxin analysis
   C. check liquid medications for sorbitol content
   D. dilute the tube feeding
14. Nutritional goals for the patient with pulmonary failure include all of the following EXCEPT
   A. higher sodium content
   B. lower protein content
   C. lower carbohydrate content
   D. higher fat content
15. A high-acuity patient with acute renal failure may experience abnormalities in each of the following EXCEPT
   A. protein catabolism
   B. fluid and electrolytes
   C. fat absorption and digestion
   D. increased carbon dioxide levels

Pretest answers: 1. C, 2. B, 3. A, 4. B, 5. B, 6. C, 7. C, 8. A, 9. A, 10. D, 11. B, 12. D, 13. C, 14. A, 15. D

GLOSSARY

Cachexia. Observable wasting of body mass caused by malnutrition

Catheter-related sepsis (CRS). A potentially lethal complication of total parenteral nutrition (TPN); microorganisms are introduced through the TPN catheter, eventually causing a systemic infection (sepsis)

Ebb phase. The first phase of the metabolic stress response, characterized by reduced systemic circulation, decreased metabolic rate, gluconeogenesis, glycogenolysis, and hyperglycemia, and persisting for 24 to 48 hours

Energy. Synonymous with calories; most common sources are carbohydrates and fats

Enteral nutrition. Nutrition delivered into the gastrointestinal tract through a feeding tube; it is a lactose-free, nutritionally complete formula composed of protein, carbohydrates, fats, electrolytes, vitamins, and minerals

Flow phase. The second phase of the metabolic stress response, characterized by hypermetabolism, hypercatabolism, increased nitrogen losses, gluconeogenesis, and hyperglycemia

Gluconeogenesis. Formation of glucose from protein and fat stores in the body; seen in the ebb phase and flow phase

Glycogenolysis. Conversion of glycogen into glucose in the body tissues; seen only in the ebb phase

Harris–Benedict equation. Estimates caloric requirements of a resting, fasting, unstressed individual based on the individual's height, weight, age, and sex; expressed in kilocalories

Hypercatabolism. Breakdown of total body protein; skeletal muscle protein is used initially for conversion to glucose through gluconeogenesis; visceral (organ) protein is used after skeletal muscle protein; occurs in the flow phase of the metabolic stress response

Hypermetabolism. An increased metabolic rate in response to a major bodily insult requiring increased quantities of oxygen and nutrients to meet the increased metabolic needs; occurs in the flow phase of the metabolic stress response

Indirect calorimetry. A technique of estimating an individual's metabolic or energy expenditure through the measurement of oxygen consumed ($\dot{V}O_2$) and carbon dioxide produced (VCO_2); can also calculate respiratory quotient (RQ)

Macronutrients. Carbohydrates, lipids (fats), and proteins

Metabolic stress response. A well-defined pattern of metabolic and physiologic responses that occur as the result of injured tissue in the body

Micronutrients. Electrolytes, vitamins, and trace elements

Nitrogen. A basic unit of protein (amino acid) breakdown; excreted primarily in urine in the form of urea; a 24-hour urinary urea nitrogen (UUN) measures nitrogen losses for a 24-hour period

Respiratory quotient (RQ). A ratio of carbon dioxide (VCO_2) to oxygen consumed ($\dot{V}O_2$); provides information about fuel composition used by the body; VCO_2 and $\dot{V}O_2$ are obtained from an indirect calorimetry study

Total parenteral nutrition (TPN). A nutritionally complete, IV-delivered solution composed of protein, carbohydrate, fat, electrolytes, vitamins, and trace elements; TPN with a glucose concentration of greater than 10 percent is administered through a central vein

ABBREVIATIONS

AAA. Aromatic amino acid

ATP. Adenosine triphosphate

BCAA. Branched-chain amino acid

BMR. Basal metabolic rate

BUN. Blood urea nitrogen

CRS. Catheter-related sepsis

CNS. Central nervous system

IDPN. Intradialytic parenteral nutrition

kcal. Kilocalories

MSOD. Multisystem organ dysfunction

NPO. Nothing by mouth

PEM. Protein-energy malnutrition

REE. Resting energy expenditure

RQ. Respiratory quotient

TLC. Total lymphocyte count

TPN. Total parenteral nutrition

VCO_2. Carbon dioxide produced

$\dot{V}O_2$. Oxygen consumed

SECTION ONE: Metabolism

At the completion of this section, the learner will be able to explain basic normal metabolism.

The energy required to maintain life is generated by chemical processes involving transformation of nutrients and occurring throughout the body. Collectively these processes are called metabolism, which means state of change. Metabolism is further described as anabolic, catabolic, aerobic, or anaerobic.

Anabolism and Catabolism

Anabolism is considered a constructive process since it involves synthesis of cell components and contributes to tissue building. Anabolic events require energy. The conversion of complex nutrients into more basic elements such as glucose, fatty acids, and amino acids is a catabolic process. Catabolism occurs when energy is needed. Both of these processes are ongoing and occur simultaneously to varying degrees under normal circumstances. However, when the individual is faced with acute or chronic illness, catabolism may exceed anabolism and threaten survival. Anabolic and catabolic processes both require enzyme catalysts. Substances acted on by enzymes are called *substrates*. Therefore, nutrients are called substrates since enzymatic processes are required for their utilization as fuel (Pleuss, 1998).

Aerobic and Anaerobic Metabolism

Production of energy is a highly organized process. Nutrients are transformed into energy for immediate use or for storage inside the cell mitochondria for later use. Energy is used or stored in the form of adenosine triphosphate (ATP). Energy is generated from two distinct physiologic pathways—aerobic and anaerobic.

The cell mitochondria is the site of aerobic metabolism. Oxidation of nutrients (carbohydrates, lipids, and proteins) in the mitochondria produces carbon dioxide and water, which are generally harmless and easily excreted from the body. However, excess retention of either of these substances has the potential to be problematic.

Not all cells contain mitochondria, so they are not capable of aerobic metabolism. Cells without mitochondria receive their energy by the oxidation of glucose to pyruvate, which is then converted to ATP. This oxidation of glucose occurring in the cytoplasm is called glycolysis. Decreased or delayed oxygen delivery to the cells (even those containing mitochondria) also initiates energy production in this manner, which is referred to as anaerobic metabolism.

Nicotinamide-adenine dinucleotide (NAD^+), an oxygen-reducing enzyme, is needed for glycolysis. Maintaining adequate levels of NAD^+ is dependent on oxygen. When the oxygen supply is adequate, the pyruvate produced by glycolysis is able to move into the mitochondria to be processed in the citric acid cycle. When the oxygen supply is not adequate, pyruvate produces lactic acid, which is released into the extracellular fluid. This action helps to rebuild levels of NAD^+ to reestablish normal glycolysis. Most body cells can use lactic acid as an energy source temporarily. However, the brain and nervous system have extremely limited capabilities to extract lactic acid as a fuel source.

The anaerobic metabolic pathway is very inefficient as an energy source, but is reversible with the reestablishment of an adequate oxygen supply. Anaerobic metabolism is partially a compensatory mechanism that allows for energy production to proceed in times when energy demands exceed oxygen supply, such as during exercise. However, this mechanism is intended only to be temporary and cannot sustain life indefinitely. High-acuity patients are at increased risk of developing anaerobic metabolism owing to periods of severe and/or sustained decreases in oxygen delivery to the tissues. Serum lactic acid levels serve as an indicator of the severity and duration of inadequate anaerobic metabolism (Pleuss, 1998).

Energy

The ability to do work is called **energy.** Heat is generated in the conversion of nutrients to energy. Energy is measured in units called *calories*, which is the amount of energy needed to raise the temperature of 1 gram of water by 1 degree Centigrade. Because a calorie is such a minute quantity, energy measurement within the body is usually described in terms of a kilocalorie (1,000 calories). A kilocalorie (kcal), then, is the amount of energy needed to increase the temperature of 1 kilogram (1,000 g) of water by 1 degree Centigrade (Ahrens & Rutherford, 1993).

The majority of energy needed by the body (about 40 percent) is utilized to maintain ion gradients across cell membranes. Synthesis of proteins and central nervous system functions each require about 20 percent of the energy expenditure. Other essential functions such as oxidation of nutrients, breathing, and cardiac pumping consume the rest of the energy expenditure. Physical activities require an even greater amount of energy above that required to maintain normal homeostatic mechanisms in a resting state.

In summary, normal metabolism requires an adequate supply of nutrients and oxygen. Inadequate oxygen intake such as may occur in high-acuity patients leads to anaerobic metabolism. Anaerobic metabolism has limited capabilities to sustain life; therefore, provision of an adequate oxygen supply is a priority in caring for such patients.

SECTION ONE REVIEW

1. Catabolism is best described as
   - **A.** metabolism occurring in the absence of oxygen
   - **B.** metabolism occurring in the presence of oxygen
   - **C.** breakdown of complex nutrients into more basic nutrients
   - **D.** building of cells and tissues from nutrients

2. Which of the following lab tests is frequently used as an indicator of anaerobic metabolism
   - **A.** total lymphocyte count
   - **B.** lactic acid
   - **C.** arterial blood gas (ABG)
   - **D.** blood urea nitrogen (BUN)

3. Which part of the cell is the site of aerobic metabolism?
   A. mitochondria
   B. cell membrane
   C. cytoplasm
   D. nucleus

4. High-acuity patients are at risk for significant anaerobic metabolism due to
   A. NPO status
   B. increased energy requirement
   C. severe and/or sustained decrease in oxygen delivery
   D. fluid volume overload

Answers: 1. C, 2. B, 3. A, 4. C

SECTION TWO: Nutrition in the High-Acuity Patient

At the completion of this section, the learner will be able to describe the primary functions of carbohydrates, lipids, and proteins and the nutritional needs of the high-acuity patient.

Intake of nutrients is necessary for two primary reasons:

1. Nutrients provide the energy source required for growth of all body structures and maintenance of all bodily functions.
2. Nutrients support the immune function of the bowel.

Nutrients as an Energy Source

Nutrients are divided into two basic categories. **Macronutrients** consist of carbohydrates, proteins, and lipids (fats). Vitamins (fat soluble and water soluble), minerals, and trace elements are called **micronutrients.** Adequate intake of both macronutrients and micronutrients is essential to restore health and to promote healing in the high-acuity/critically ill patient (Pleuss, 1998).

Carbohydrates

Carbohydrates are the desired fuel source for most tissues and are necessary to supply energy for the most basic cellular functions. Heat produced during the oxidation of carbohydrates is used to maintain body temperature. Carbohydrates are introduced into the body in various forms of sugars or starches, all of which are converted to glucose. Excess glucose not needed for cellular activities is stored as glycogen in the liver and muscle cells. This process is called **gluconeogenesis.** Stored glycogen can then be reconverted to glucose to maintain blood glucose levels within a relatively steady range. Also, during times of physiologic stress, glycogen can be metabolized into glucose to provide an immediate fuel source. This utilization of glycogen is called **glycogenolysis.**

Glucose metabolism is regulated by the two hormones, insulin and glucagon. Insulin is necessary for transport of glucose into cells. Under normal circumstances, ingestion or infusion of glucose causes an increase in insulin release from the beta cells of the pancreas. This process is altered during periods of physiologic stress, leading to hyperglycemia. Hyperglycemia typical of the body's stress response is discussed further in Section Four.

Glucagon, secreted by the alpha cells of the pancreas, is released in response to falling blood glucose levels. This event then stimulates conversion of stored glycogen into glucose. Stored glycogen is also released in response to increased levels of epinephrine, norepinephrine, vasopressin, and angiotensin II. These hormones are immediately released during physiologic stress. Glycogen stores are utilized rapidly in the high-acuity patient who experiences intense and/or prolonged physiologic stress, such as occurs with surgery, trauma, or infection. Excess glucose is converted to lipid and stored for later conversion back into glucose when energy is needed (Berry & Braunschweig, 1998).

Approximately 25 percent of the body's glucose supply is consumed by the brain and nervous system. The brain's capacity to store glucose is extremely limited, so maintenance of blood glucose levels within a narrow range is essential for preservation of central nervous system (CNS) functioning. Although the brain can use ketone bodies (derived from fat metabolism) as a fuel source, this does not supply enough energy for the brain to maintain its essential cellular functions (Heath & Vink, 1999).

Adequate carbohydrate intake prevents proteins from being utilized as a fuel source. Proteins can provide energy, but it is not beneficial to overall well-being since proteins are primarily needed for other cellular functions. Carbohydrates supply 4 kcal of energy for each gram ingested. About 50 percent of calories consumed should be in the form of carbohydrates (Bagley, 1996).

Proteins

Proteins are composed of various combinations of amino acids and contain nitrogen in addition to carbon, hydrogen, and oxygen. Formation of proteins requires metabolism of carbohydrates and lipids. Proteins serve many complex functions at the cell membrane and are essential for formation and maintenance of all cells, tissues, and organs. Proteins also play a role in many of the body's transport mechanisms, such as transmission of nerve impulses. Proteins can be considered building blocks since they contribute to the structure of muscles, organs, antibodies, enzymes, and hormones. Maintenance of osmotic pressure and appropriate blood pH are also dependent on an adequate protein supply.

Proteins are categorized according to their location in the body:

- Visceral proteins are found within internal organs. Prealbumin, albumin, and transferrin, which are plasma proteins, are frequently measured in laboratory tests as indicators of protein status as well as overall nutritional status.
- Somatic proteins are found in accessory and skeletal muscles.

Protein synthesis and degradation is an ongoing process. Under usual circumstances, the overall content of proteins in the body is relatively steady. However, under stress conditions, protein catabolism is increased. In the high-acuity patient, inadequate protein intake can quickly lead to malnutrition, prolonged wound healing, diminished resistance to infection, and even death (Brody, 1999).

Like carbohydrate metabolism, protein metabolism is influenced by hormones. Protein synthesis is enhanced by growth hormone. Conversely, synthesis is diminished when insulin levels decrease.

When carbohydrate availability is not adequate to meet the body's energy requirements, proteins are broken down into their amino acid components. Ketoacids, a byproduct of amino acid metabolism, can then be further metabolized in the Krebs' cycle to produce glucose needed for cellular energy (Lennie, 1997).

Proteins supply 4 kcal/g. Average, healthy adults require about 15 percent to 20 percent of their nutrient intake as proteins. This amount increases considerably under conditions of physiologic stress. Protein malnutrition leads to atrophy of the gut mucosa and is a factor in the development of bacterial translocation (discussed under the heading Alterations in the GI Tract). Impairment of skin integrity, delayed wound healing, and loss of skeletal muscle mass result from protein malnutrition (Bagley, 1996).

Lipids

Lipids are also referred to as fats. At the cellular level, lipids contribute to the structure of the membrane. Lipids are the primary source of fuel reserve and are readily stored as triglycerides, phospholipids, and cholesterol for later use as a fuel source. A portion of the triglyceride molecule can be utilized for glucose metabolism.

Lipids provide 9 kcal/g, more calories than any other nutrient. Functionally, lipids are similar to carbohydrates since their availability as a fuel source can save proteins from being broken down for energy.

As with the other macronutrients, insulin influences lipid synthesis and reserves. Insulin is needed for the transport of glucose into fat cells. Only small quantities of stored fat are found in the circulating blood. Most fat is stored in adipose tissue and the liver.

The liver can produce lipids from glucose or amino acids, a process called lipogenesis. This occurs when there is more carbohydrate present than needed for energy or for glycogen storage in the liver. Under normal conditions, lipogenesis predominates. During stress, lipolytic metabolism predominates. The end product is availability of fatty acids for ATP and energy (Bagley, 1996).

Lipids are a source of essential vitamins and aid the absorption of the fat-soluble vitamins A, D, E, and K. Stored lipids provide insulation for the body in the form of subcutaneous fat and provide structural protection for some organs such as the kidneys. The American Heart Association guidelines recommend consumption of no more than 30 percent of the total diet as fats. However, fat intake in the United States generally exceeds this recommendation (National Institutes of Health, 1998). Table 22–1 summarizes the caloric content of macronutrients.

Nutrients as Immune Function Support

The intake of nutrition via the gastrointestinal (GI) tract helps maintain tissue integrity and supports the bowel's immune function. In the high-acuity patient, concern for the proper functioning of the gut is often overlooked until there is an overt problem such as vomiting, bleeding, or diarrhea. The GI tract is primarily thought of as the body region involved with digestion and absorption of nutrients. Of equal importance are the significant immune functions served by the gut (Krenitsky, 1996).

The organs of the GI tract are basically hollow vessels that accept and process food. Specialized cells throughout the tract participate in secretion of digestive substances and absorption of nutrients. The GI tract is structured with four distinct cellular layers:

1. *Serosa*—the outermost layer, with a surface epithelial layer and connective tissue
2. *Muscularis propria*—contains perpendicular layers of smooth muscle responsible for peristalsis

TABLE 22–1. CALORIC VALUE OF NUTRIENTS

NUTRIENT	CALORIC VALUE
Fats (lipids)	9 kcal/g
Proteins	4 kcal/g
Carbohydrates	
Enteral	4 kcal/g
Intravenous	3.4 kcal/g

3. *Submucosa*—connective tissue and highly vascular with lymph system and nerves
4. *Mucosa*—the innermost layer is the site of intestinal immune activities, secretion of digestive substances, and nutrient absorption. The mucosa forms a barrier between highly contaminated GI contents and the sterile interior of the abdomen (Johnson, 1997)

Normal Digestion

Digestion begins with intake of food into the mouth and proceeds through the stomach where gastric juice (containing hydrochloric acid) mixes with the food. The acid medium of the stomach is one of the immune mechanisms that discourages bacterial growth in the area. The major activities of digestion, however, occur in the small intestine. The small intestine is about 20 feet long and consists of three sections: the duodenum, the jejunum, and the ileum. The surface area is more extensive due to fingerlike projections of the mucosal layer, called villi. Reabsorption of water and gastric juices occurs mainly in the large intestine (Cole, 1999).

Alterations in the GI Tract

When a patient has undergone surgical alteration of the GI tract, it is essential that the nurse knows the precise anatomic changes. Surgical intervention in the tract can alter the digestive and absorptive functions, which greatly affects the patient's clinical status and nutritional needs.

Mucosal cells have a high energy requirement, and thus are dependent on a steady supply of nutrients and oxygen to maintain proper functioning. This also means that the mucosa is highly susceptible to hypoxia and diminished tissue perfusion. Interruption of oxygen and nutrient supply can cause death of mucosal cells followed by mucosal atrophy (Stechmiller, Treloar, & Allen, 1997).

As mentioned earlier, the mucosal cells perform an important barrier function between the interior of the GI structures, with its many toxic substances, and the sterile environment of the peritoneal cavity. When this barrier is interrupted, microbes cross the mucosal layer into the lymphatics, blood vessels, or even into the free peritoneal cavity. This activity is called bacterial translocation, which is accepted as a major source of multisystem organ dysfunction (MSOD) (Cole, 1999).

Nutrition in the High-Acuity Patient

Characteristic alterations of metabolism occur in the individual who is experiencing starvation or stress. In the high-acuity patient, the presence of these conditions may coincide. Older adults or those with chronic illness may be in a starvation or semistarvation state at the time of an injury or acute illness. These patients need to be rapidly identified since their already compromised nutritional/metabolic state will only complicate any other health alteration they are experiencing. Starvation can develop in hospitalized patients. Most high-acuity patients have a greatly increased need for nutrients and calories due to the stress response. Patients who are kept with nothing by mouth (NPO) for several days can easily develop starvation. Since many high-acuity patients are unable to take nourishment by mouth owing to decreased consciousness or treatments such as intubation or sedation, provision of nutrition by alternate means is a nursing priority. Individuals who are experiencing some degree of starvation are at risk of developing serious, even life-threatening, electrolyte abnormalities during refeeding. Refeeding syndrome is discussed in Section Four.

In summary, nutrition serves as the body's energy source and plays an important role in maintaining overall immune function by discouraging bacterial translocation from the intestinal tract.

Section Two Review

1. Glucose metabolism is regulated by which two hormones
   A. epinephrine and norepinephrine
   B. glycogen and glucagon
   C. insulin and vasopressin
   D. glucagon and insulin
2. Which nutrient provides the greatest amount of calories per volume
   A. carbohydrates
   B. fats
   C. visceral proteins
   D. somatic proteins
3. Which organ is most dependent on maintenance of normal blood glucose levels
   A. heart
   B. lungs
   C. kidney
   D. brain
4. Maintenance of appropriate osmotic pressure is dependent upon which nutrient
   A. complex carbohydrates
   B. simple sugars
   C. proteins
   D. fats

Answers: 1. D, 2. B, 3. D, 4. C

SECTION THREE: Nutritional and Metabolic Assessment

At the completion of this section, the learner will be able to differentiate between patients with normal and altered metabolism.

Assessment of the patient's nutritional/metabolic status provides the nurse with information that is essential to development of a comprehensive nursing care plan. The nutritional/metabolic aspect of the nursing assessment allows identification of the patient's present status, provides a baseline with which to compare the effectiveness of therapies, and permits identification of patients who may be at risk for complications related to refeeding or patient's presenting with some degree of malnutrition.

Ideally, the nutritional assessment should begin with the individual's history relative to food and fluid intake, barriers to normal food consumption, alterations in gastrointestinal anatomy, and weight changes. When dealing with an individual who is acutely ill, the history may be difficult to obtain. Family members may need to be contacted to obtain pertinent data.

The nurse caring for high-acuity patients faces several challenges. Assessment of the patient's nutritional/metabolic condition is an integral part of the nursing care of the patient. The primary nurse, nutrition support clinical nurse specialist, physician, pharmacist, and clinical dietitian all have expertise to contribute to the patient's nutritional/metabolic assessment and therapies. Since the nurse is the caregiver most directly involved with the delivery of therapies, the nurse should be able to determine whether the patient is receiving nutritional support that is appropriately individualized.

The patient's metabolic status is pertinent to everything else that he or she may be experiencing. Therefore, an understanding of the laboratory and physiologic methods commonly used to assess the patient's overall metabolic/nutritional status is essential to providing safe, efficient nursing care.

Laboratory Data

Common laboratory tests used to assess nutritional/metabolic status include serum electrolytes, albumin, prealbumin, transferrin, and total lymphocyte count. Urine urea nitrogen obtained by 24-hour urine collection indicates the amount of nitrogen being excreted and permits calculation of the patient's nitrogen balance.

Albumin

Serum albumin, prealbumin, and transferrin are indicators of visceral protein status. Below-normal levels of these plasma proteins indicate that muscle has been utilized for energy. Breakdown of muscle for use as a fuel source is undesirable.

Albumin is a plasma protein and the major protein produced in the liver. Albumin is frequently measured in high-acuity patients, and is often used by clinicians as a primary indicator of overall nutritional status. Low albumin levels coincide with increased occurrence of clinical complications and poor patient outcomes. However, this value must be interpreted cautiously. Albumin has a 20-day half-life and is dispersed throughout many sites, factors that make it of little value for assessing nutritional status in an acute situation. Albumin therefore should not be used as an indicator to detect early malnutrition or effectiveness of nutrition support (Bernstein et al., 1995). Below-normal values of albumin may be detected in patients with liver or renal disease even when protein intake is adequate. In patients who receive fluid resuscitation, serum albumin values are likely to be dilutional and not an accurate indicator of the actual albumin level. The greatest utility of albumin is in tracking long-term changes in protein status (Berry & Braunschweig, 1998).

Prealbumin

Prealbumin aids transport of thyroxine in the plasma and is the carrier for retinol-binding protein. The half-life is 24 to 48 hours with a small body pool. The Prealbumin in Nutritional Care Consensus Group advocates that prealbumin is a more reliable indicator of acute changes in catabolism than serum albumin. Prealbumin is technically easy and inexpensive to measure in the laboratory. Prealbumin is not influenced by hydration, renal, or liver status to the same extent as albumin. Periodic monitoring of prealbumin provides an indication of the effectiveness of nutrition support and the overall catabolic state. Upward trending of prealbumin levels indicate improvement in the overall anabolism (Bernstein et al., 1995).

Transferrin

Transferrin is a plasma protein that binds with and transports iron to cells. Transferrin may be more useful than albumin for tracking responses to nutritional therapies since its half-life is 8 to 10 days. Accuracy of transferrin as a nutritional indicator depends on the patient's underlying iron level. Many high-acuity patients experience blood loss and transfusions so its usefulness in the high-acuity patient may be limited (Trujillo, Robinson, & Jacobs, 1999).

Nitrogen Balance

In the high-acuity patient, **nitrogen** balance is an accurate indicator of protein status. Simply defined, nitrogen balance is the difference between nitrogen output and nitrogen intake. Calculation of nitrogen balance first requires collection of a 24-hour urine specimen with an accurate account of urinary output during the collection time. Since nitrogen is a component of protein, it is necessary to also know the patient's protein intake during the time of the UUN collection. The major disadvantage of using the UUN level to assess protein need is that it is not valid in renal failure. Urinary nitrogen output is expected to be low in renal failure since the inability of the kidneys to excrete nitrogen is one of the primary characteristics of renal failure. Nitrogen balance is easy to calculate once the UUN is reported by the laboratory. Table 22–2 provides the equations needed to calculate nitrogen balance.

The UUN is used to calculate the amount of protein needed. The UUN value (plus 4 g for insensible nitrogen loss) is multiplied by the constant 6.25 (the number of grams of protein equal to 1 g of nitrogen) to provide the amount of protein needed to obtain zero nitrogen balance. For a patient who is stressed and catabolic, the goal of protein administration should be to provide a positive nitrogen balance (Trujillo, Robinson, & Jacobs, 1999).

Sample Calculation of Nitrogen Balance

The result of the 24-hour UUN collection is reported as 10 g. From the documented dietary consult, you find that the patient received 100 g of protein during the previous 24 hours (which coincided with the 24-hour urine collection). Divide 100 g by the constant 6.25 to determine the amount of nitrogen contained in the protein received by the patient. This yields 16 g of nitrogen received. Using the equations provided in Table 22–2, the nitrogen balance is +2, which is a desirable value.

Total Lymphocyte Count

Many cells of the immune system, such as antibodies and lymphocytes, contain a significant amount of protein. Proper functioning of the immune system depends on an adequate total protein level. Therefore, measurement of the total lymphocyte count (TLC) provides some quantification of the effect of protein loss on immune system functioning. The TLC is an easily obtained indicator of overall immune status and adequacy of protein. This indicator is considered most reliable when white blood cell and lymphocyte counts are relatively stable. Therefore, TLCs should be interpreted with caution in the high-acuity patient experiencing hypermetabolism or infections. The TLC should be about 20 percent to 40 percent of the total white blood cell (WBC) count. It can be calculated with the following equation (Krenitsky, 1996):

$$\text{TLC} = \text{WBC} \times \frac{\%\ \text{lymphocytes}}{100}$$

TABLE 22–2. CALCULATING NITROGEN BALANCE

Nitrogen balance = nitrogen in – (nitrogen out + 4 g/day)
Nitrogen in = g of protein received during the 24 hours of UUN collection, divided by the constant 6.25
Nitrogen out = g of protein excreted in the urine as measured by the UUN plus insensible loss, estimated at 4 g

Guidelines for interpreting the total lymphocyte count is as follows:

2,000/μL	Normal
1,200 to 2,000/μL	Mild malnutrition
800 to 1,199/μL	Moderate malnutrition
< 800/μL	Severe malnutrition

A summary of laboratory values pertinent to the nutritional/metabolic assessment of the high-acuity patient is provided in Table 22–3.

Anergy Screen

Cell-mediated immunity is one of the body's defense mechanisms that is most affected by malnutrition. Delayed cutaneous hypersensitivity screening, also referred to as skin testing, is a simple method for evaluating cell-mediated immunity status. A test dose of a known antigen such as tuberculin, *Candida*, mumps, or *Trichophyton* is administered intradermally. The individual's ability to respond to this immunologic challenge is evaluated 24 and 48 hours after administration. If cellular immunity is intact, an induration of 2 to 5 mm should be observed at the injection site. If no skin reaction occurs, the patient is considered to be anergic, which means that cellular immunity has been negatively effected by malnutrition (Lehmann, 1993).

Physiologic Data

Oxygen consumption ($\dot{V}O_2$) and energy expenditure are indicators of the metabolic state. Oxygen consumption is the amount of oxygen used by the tissues, measured in mL/m^2/min. Oxygen consumption in a healthy individual ranges from 150 to 300 mL/m^2/min. Consumption of oxygen by the tissues requires energy; therefore, oxygen consumption is associated with energy expenditure. Any situation that increases tissue's oxygen requirement also causes an increase in energy expenditure. Fever, shivering, pain, and increases in environmental temperature and physical activity are common sources of increased oxygen consumption and energy expenditure. The nurse should attempt to minimize these factors in the high-acuity patient.

TABLE 22–3. LABORATORY TESTS TO ASSESS NUTRITIONAL STATUS

TEST	NORMAL VALUE
Blood urea nitrogen (BUN)	8–23 mg/dL
Serum creatinine	0.6–1.6 mg/dL
Albumin	3.5–5.5 g/dL
Prealbumin	15.7–29.6 mg/mL
Transferrin	250–300 mg/dL

From Gianino, S., & St. John, R.E. (1993). Nutritional assessment of the patient in the intensive care unit. Crit Care Clin North Am 5:1–16

Energy expenditure is the amount of kilocalories being burned. Normal values are established based on gender, height, weight, age, and activity level. An average-sized adult with an estimated average oxygen consumption of 200 $mL/m^2/min$ is considered to have an energy expenditure of 1440 kcal/day (Ahrens, 1996).

Oxygen consumption and energy expenditure can be assessed by various methods. In-depth discussion of energy expenditure is beyond the scope of this text, but a basic understanding of the measurement is beneficial to the nurse caring for the high-acuity patient.

Normally, the body extracts about 25 percent of the oxygen available from arterial blood for consumption by the tissues. This equates to about 250 $mL/m^2/min$ of oxygen. After gas exchange occurs at the capillary bed, about 750 $mL/m^2/min$ of oxygen is returned to the venous blood. Normal oxygen saturation of venous blood (SvO_2) is therefore considered to be 75 percent. Continuous measurement of SvO_2 can be accomplished at the bedside by use of a thermodilution fiber-optic catheter (Ahrens, 1996).

Oxygen Consumption

Oxygen consumption can be measured by indirect calorimetry (discussed below) or calculated using the Fick equation. The Fick method (Table 22–4) requires blood gas analysis of arterial and venous blood.

The disadvantage of the Fick method is that it represents the oxygen consumption for only one moment in time. Indirect calorimetry provides a value obtained from a minute-to-minute value averaged over the length of the testing procedure, usually 15 to 20 minutes. Indirect calorimetry is not available in all facilities though, so the Fick method can offer an acceptable substitute when the nurse is attentive to drawing the blood over a 30-second time frame and avoiding introduction of air bubbles into the blood specimen. Error in calculation of the cardiac output is another factor that will alter the accuracy of the oxygen consumption value obtained with the Fick method (Berry & Braunschweig, 1998). A more detailed description of oxygen consumption is provided in Module 9.

Energy Expenditure

Similar to oxygen consumption, energy expenditure can be estimated, derived by calculation from arterial and venous blood gases or by measurement of gas exhalation. Several equations are in current use to estimate an individual's resting energy expenditure (REE), but the **Harris–Benedict equation** is one of the more commonly used formulas. This equation states that the REE should be the same for persons of the same gender, age, weight, and height with the same activity level. The Harris–Benedict equation for both genders is:

$$\text{Male: } 66 + (13.7 \times \text{weight [kg]}) + (5.0 \text{ (height [cm]}) - (6.8 \times \text{age})$$

$$\text{Female: } 655 + (9.6 \times \text{weight [kg]}) + (1.7 \times \text{height [cm]}) - (4.7 \times \text{age})$$

This formula was developed in 1919 using 100 normal resting subjects; therefore, the total must be multiplied by a stress factor for elevated body temperature, activity, disease processes, and trauma (Harris & Benedict, 1919). Some of the more commonly encountered conditions and their stress factors are listed in Table 22–5. The following is an example of use of the Harris–Benedict equation to estimate daily caloric need:

> If a patient with multiple trauma was estimated by the Harris–Benedict equation to have an energy expenditure of 2,000, this figure would be multiplied by 1.1 to 1.5 to obtain an energy expenditure of 2,200 to 3,000. This patient would require 2,200 to 3,000 non-protein kilocalories per day.

The Harris–Benedict equation assumes that the patient is within the range of ideal weight relative to their height. Ideal weight for adult males and females is 100 pounds for a height of five feet. For males, the weight al-

TABLE 22–4. FICK EQUATION FOR OXYGEN CONSUMPTION

$$\dot{V}o_2 = (Cao_2 - Cvo_2) \times CO \times 10$$

CO = Cardiac output
Cao_2 = hemoglobin × 1.34 × arterial oxygen saturation (in decimal value)
Cvo_2 = hemoglobin × 1.34 × venous oxygen saturation (in decimal value)

From Ahrens, T.S. (1996). Respiratory monitoring. In J. Clochesy, C. Breu, S. Cardin, A.A. Whittaker, & E.B. Rudy (eds.). Critical care nursing *(p. 250). Philadelphia: W.B. Saunders.*

TABLE 22–5. HARRIS–BENEDICT EQUATION AND STRESS FACTORS

CLINICAL CONDITION	STRESS FACTOR
Well-nourished, unstressed	1.0
Maintenance	1.0–1.2
Surgery	
Minor	1.2
Major	1.2–1.5
Cancer	1.0–1.5
Sepsis (acute phase)	
Hypotensive	0.5
Normotensive	1.2–1.7
Sepsis (recovery)	1.0
Multiple trauma (acute phase)	
Hypotensive	0.8–1.0
Normotensive	1.1–1.5
Multiple trauma (recovery)	1.0–1.2
Burned (before skin graft)	
0–20% BSA	1.2–1.5
20–40% BSA	1.5–2.0
> 40% BSA	1.8–2.5
Burned (after graft)	1.0–1.3

From Schlichtig, R., & Ayres, T.S. (1988). Nutritional support of the critically ill. *Chicago: Year Book Medical Publishers.*

lowance is six pounds for every inch above five feet. For females, the ideal weight allowance is five pounds for every inch above five feet. For patients above their ideal weight, a calculation is made for an adjusted weight to be used in the Harris–Benedict equation. Adjusted weight is obtained from the following calculation:

$$\text{Adjusted weight} = \text{Actual weight} - \text{Ideal weight} \times 0.25 + \text{Ideal weight}$$

Indirect Calorimetry

Measurement of energy expenditure can also be accomplished by direct or **indirect calorimetry.** Direct calorimetry measures whole body heat production while the individual is located in a chamber or a room specifically equipped for this purpose. Obviously, this is highly impractical for clinical application. Indirect calorimetry offers a practical approach to bedside measurement of energy expenditure, oxygen consumption, and nutrient oxidation. An indirect calorimeter is also called a 'metabolic cart.' This portable unit (about the size of a portable monitor) estimates the resting energy expenditure (REE) by measurement of respiratory gas exchange.

The procedure, which takes 15 to 20 minutes, can be performed on patients receiving mechanical ventilation or breathing room air. The metabolic cart estimates energy expenditure by comparing the amount of oxygen consumed with expired carbon dioxide. In the high-acuity patient, the energy expenditure obtained by indirect calorimetry may be multiplied by 1.1 to 1.2. Since the measurement of the energy expenditure occurs only over a relatively brief period, not a 24-hour day, this multiplication is done to account for possible changes in the patient's activity or body temperature during a 24-hour period.

The **respiratory quotient (RQ)** is another valuable parameter provided by indirect calorimetry. The RQ is the ratio of carbon dioxide produced to oxygen consumed. The normal value of 0.82 to 0.85 indicates that the individual is utilizing about an equal amount of carbohydrates, fats, and proteins for energy. The greater the amount of glucose being utilized, the higher the RQ. An RQ above 0.85 indicates that the patient is receiving too much carbohydrate. Since glucose breaks down to carbon dioxide, excess carbohydrate intake can be harmful to the high-acuity patient and can lead to carbon dioxide retention (Trujillo, Robinson, & Jacobs, 1999).

SECTION THREE REVIEW

1. Which lab value is the best indicator of current nutritional status?
   A. prealbumin
   B. albumin
   C. transferrin
   D. BUN
2. What information is obtained by indirect calorimetry?
   A. amount of protein needed
   B. kilocalories being utilized
   C. body fat composition
   D. condition of immune system
3. Which of the following is an indicator of the patient's daily protein need?
   A. UUN
   B. BUN
   C. hemoglobin
   D. albumin
4. Which one of the following conditions makes the 24-hour urine urea nitrogen test a nonvalid indicator of protein breakdown?
   A. diabetes mellitus
   B. liver failure
   C. renal failure
   D. hypercatabolism

Answers: 1. A, 2. B, 3. A, 4. C

SECTION FOUR: Metabolic Alterations in the High-Acuity Patient

At the completion of this section, the learner will be able to recognize the typical metabolic alterations occurring in the high-acuity/critically ill patient.

Before proceeding with this section, it is necessary to have an understanding of the following terms:

Starvation—a clinical condition that occurs when nutrient intake, particularly calories and protein, is unable to meet the body's energy demands

Hypometabolism—a clinical condition in which the basal metabolic rate (BMR) is less than expected in an individual relative to age, gender, weight, height, and activity

Hypermetabolism—a clinical condition in which nutrients are metabolized at an increasing rate to supply the energy needed to support immune functions and tissue repair

Hypercatabolism—the acceleration of protein breakdown for use as a fuel source. The degree of hypercatabolism can be assessed by measurement of urinary nitrogen loss (24-hour UUN)

Malnutrition

Malnutrition in hospitalized patients is associated with increased length of stay, complications, and increased morbidity and mortality. The incidence is as high as 30 to 50 percent (Berry & Braunschweig, 1998). Malnutrition that is severe and ongoing leads to a more advanced state of compromise called starvation.

Starvation

Starvation is a continuum along which clinical severity progresses until the patient receives adequate intake. Starvation occurs when the individual does not receive adequate nutrition. The nurse should be aware that starvation can occur in as little as a week. This makes provision of sufficient nutrition a priority in the high-acuity patient. Starvation, a severe condition of malnutrition, is generally described as two types—marasmus and kwashiorkor.

Marasmus occurs when there is inadequate intake of calories and protein. Generalized body wasting is evident. Adult marasmus can progress until there are severe losses of fat and protein stores. Marasmus is often associated with altered GI functioning or prolonged periods of anorexia. Immune system integrity often remains intact at this stage.

Adult marasmus coupled with the occurrence of a physiologic insult such as surgery, injury, or infection leads to a more severe hypoalbuminemic malnutrition. Skeletal and visceral protein mass deteriorates further. At this stage immune function is impaired. With passage of time, the patient progresses to an adult kwashiorkor-like syndrome.

Prolonged deficiency or absence of protein, in the presence of adequate carbohydrate intake, leads to kwashiorkor. In this condition, stores of fat and skeletal muscle protein are preserved. However, there is ongoing breakdown of visceral proteins such as serum albumin and immunoglobulins (antibodies). Edema is an easily recognizable symptom of kwashiorkor. A decrease in the serum albumin lowers osmotic pressure, which allows water to leak from the circulating blood volume into the extracellular spaces. Marasmus and kwashiorkor occur in varying intensities. Both conditions are also referred to as protein-energy malnutrition (Brody, 1999).

One of the first responses to inadequate nutrient intake is the individual's voluntary limitation of physical activity. In the hospitalized high-acuity patient, physical activity may already be minimal relative to the clinical condition. The body attempts to compensate for the inadequate intake by decreasing release of catecholamines and thyroid hormone. The result is an involuntary decrease in the BMR, which is the same as resting energy expenditure.

Stored carbohydrate is an insignificant factor during starvation since only about 1,200 kcal of energy is stored as carbohydrate at any given time. For the average-sized adult, at rest, 1,200 kcal is less than one day's caloric need.

As previously described, protein is metabolized to provide a fuel source when carbohydrate intake is inadequate, but the rate of protein turnover is also diminished during starvation. When a fasting situation exists, the amount of protein in the muscles is usually only about enough to meet the brain's energy requirements for 2 weeks.

After about 2 weeks of starvation, the body switches to using fat as the main fuel source. Ketone bodies, which are by-products of fatty acid metabolism, replace glucose as the fuel source for the brain. However, the brain cannot extract enough energy from ketone bodies to meet its energy needs, and an undesirable state of anaerobic metabolism is established in the brain (Robertson, Clifton, & Grossman, 1984).

As energy requirements continue to exceed nutrient supply, fat stores are utilized. Survival is linked to the amount of stored fat. Theoretically, an obese person should survive longer than a nonobese person during starvation. Fat stores will last about 60 to 75 days in an adult with ideal body weight.

Weight loss accompanies inadequate nutrient supply. Weight loss reaches a plateau, however, as physical activity and BMR decline. As protein is burned for energy, cell death occurs due to inadequate protein for cellular repair and synthesis. Cell death also contributes to potassium losses. The fluid constituents of the destroyed cells are shifted to the extracellular volume, thus edema may be evident. Edema also occurs as a result of water and sodium conservation. Volume losses, most prominent during the first 2 weeks of fasting, facilitate hemodynamic instability. Loss of bone mass occurs only in the most severe starvation conditions (Bagley, 1996).

Metabolic Stress Response

The **metabolic responses** to physiologic stress such as surgery, trauma, or infection are fairly predictable. Two distinct phases of this response have been identified. The initial phase is called the **ebb phase,** which lasts about 24 hours after the occurrence of tissue injury. The ebb phase is followed by the **flow phase.** The duration of the flow phase can be highly variable and is associated with the patient's clinical condition (Shuster, 1996).

Ebb Phase

The individual's metabolic rate is likely to be initially unchanged or slightly decreased during the first 24 hours after injury. Exceptions to this are patients with burns and severe head injury (Glasgow Coma Scale score ≤ 8). Body temperature that is slightly hypothermic may be observed secondary to decreased oxygen consumption. Increases in blood glucose and lactate levels are common.

Alterations in both carbohydrate and lipid metabolism are observed in the ebb phase. Glucose production is increased after injury in an attempt to provide energy for wound healing. Increased release of hormones such as epinephrine, glucagon, and cortisol stimulates conversion of glycogen stores to glucose. Decreased production of insulin along with insulin resistance in peripheral tissues contributes to hyperglycemia following injury.

Controversy exists regarding the utility of providing nutrition during the ebb phase. Arguments that the instillation of nutrients into the GI tract immediately after injury could divert blood flow from the major organs, thereby promoting hemodynamic instability, have not been well supported. Recent studies have observed beneficial effects such as decreases in the hypermetabolic response when enteral feeding is initiated within the first 24 hours after injury.

Fat stores are mobilized to contribute to energy needs. As fats are oxidized, fatty acids are produced and contribute to increases in lactate levels. Lactate levels increase as anaerobic metabolism occurs in injured, ischemic tissues. The increasing quantity of lactate is converted to glucose in the liver, thereby increasing hyperglycemia (Shuster, 1996).

Flow Phase

Symptoms of the flow phase such as tachycardia, tachypnea, increased cardiac output, and fever are typically first observed about 24 to 36 hours following the physiologic insult. The flow phase is characterized by increased demands for oxygen and calories to provide for wound healing. **Hypercatabolism** is prominent as stored protein is metabolized to help meet the sudden increased oxygen consumption and energy expenditure. Increased oxygen consumption and energy expenditure along with hypercatabolism comprise the clinical condition known as **hypermetabolism.**

Hyperglycemia is frequently observed after tissue injury. Glucose production is increased in response to increased energy demands. The immediate release of catecholamines upon injury stimulates the liver to increase glucose production. Insulin production and utilization are altered following injury. Resistance to insulin in the peripheral tissues also contributes to higher levels of blood glucose, but the primary cause of hyperglycemia is increased gluconeogenesis. Administration of insulin is often ineffective in controlling elevated glucose levels during the metabolic stress response.

Patient prognosis worsens as hypermetabolism persists. Individuals experiencing tissue trauma (from any etiology) usually have a decreased capacity to take nutrition. Therefore, they are dependent upon their caregivers to provide appropriate nutrient intake. Normal utilization of carbohydrates, proteins, and lipids is altered following tissue trauma, another factor that contributes to malnutrition in the high-acuity patient.

The peak of the hypermetabolic response is reported as 3 to 4 days following the initiating event (surgery, trauma, infection). In the patient without complications, the hypermetabolic stress response usually lasts 7 to 10 days. However, the high-acuity patient experiencing hypermetabolism is rarely without complications. Exacerbation of the hypermetabolic response occurs with repeated episodes of tissue ischemia, localized infections, or septicemia. The metabolic alterations occurring with hypermetabolism and hypercatabolism can be a vicious cycle leading to further clinical deterioration if the patient does not receive adequate metabolic/nutritional support within the first few days of the precipitating event. The risks of multisystem organ failure and death become greater as hypermetabolism continues (Shuster, 1996). Table 22–6 provides a synopsis of the metabolic differences between starvation and the hypermetabolic stress response.

Refeeding Syndrome

Lean body mass is progressively decreased during starvation. Urinary losses of electrolytes such as sodium, potassium, and phosphorus begin as soon as 48 hours without nutrient intake. Cell death is primarily responsible for diminished potassium levels.

During acute starvation, fluid volume decreases are also attributable to cell death. However, during prolonged

TABLE 22–6. COMPARISON BETWEEN STARVATION AND HYPERMETABOLISM

	STARVATION	HYPERMETABOLISM
Metabolic goal	Preservation of lean body mass	Repair of injured tissue
Metabolic rate	Decreased	Increased
Energy needs	Decreased	Increased
Fuel source	Primarily fat (Stored glycogen depleted within 24 hours)	Mixed
Protein metabolism	Decreased synthesis	Decreased synthesis
	Decreased catabolism	Increased catabolism
	Decreased ureagenesis	Increased ureagenesis
	Decreased UUN	Increased UUN
Carbohydrate	Decreased gluconeogenesis	Increased gluconeogenesis
Metabolism	(Stored glycogen depleted within 24 hours)	Hyperglycemia
Fat metabolism	Increased ketones	Increased compared to normal; ketones decreased compared to starvation

starvation, fluid volume increases owing to sodium retention. Edema is then an observable sign.

Stored fat becomes the body's primary fuel source during periods of starvation, rather than the glucose that is normally the major fuel source. When refeeding of starving individuals occurs, the introduction of carbohydrates and proteins causes an increase in blood insulin levels. This increase then stimulates a change in preferred energy source from stored fat back to carbohydrate, and then to protein. When refeeding begins, there is a sudden influx of glucose, phosphorus, potassium, and magnesium into the cells. These changes are observed in individuals who have been in a fasting state for as little as 3 days. As carbohydrate intake continues, phosphorus levels drop dramatically below normal since it is needed for glucose uptake by the cells. One of the primary indications that the patient is experiencing refeeding syndrome is this sudden decrease in the blood phosphorus level. The patient will require intravenous phosphorus replacement as well as scheduled doses of phosphorus via the GI tract (if access is available). When refeeding syndrome is present, the patient is at great risk for cardiac dysrhythmias and respiratory muscle dysfunction owing to decreased electrolyte levels and should be monitored closely.

Decreases in blood insulin levels during starvation produce a hyperglycemic response with the initiation of refeeding. Glucose levels must be monitored frequently and treated with insulin administration. Higher than usual levels of insulin may be required since insulin resistance is likely. Subcutaneous insulin should be avoided in the patient in a shock state. The insulin will not be absorbed (or will be absorbed in unknown quantities) when subcutaneous tissue perfusion is diminished. With reestablishment of perfusion, though, absorption of subcutaneous insulin may be rapid, causing hypoglycemia (Atkin et al., 1991). Hyperglycemia should be treated promptly since it is a factor in the development of sepsis.

Identification of individuals at risk for refeeding syndrome is the main preventive step. In patients with the potential to develop refeeding syndrome, feeding should begin slowly. Caloric intake should not be more than 1.2 times the patient's resting energy expenditure (as calculated by the Harris–Benedict equation or measured by indirect calorimetry). Increases of feeding to the target level may need to occur over several days to minimize the sudden and severe electrolyte changes attributable to rapid refeeding in the starved patient. Individuals at high risk for refeeding include those with NPO status for 7 to 10 days, chronic alcoholism, anorexia nervosa, and cardiac or cancer cachexia (Jolly & Blank, 1994).

In summary, patients who experience tissue injury will experience alterations in their metabolic processes to some extent. In some circumstances, the patient succumbs not to the initial traumatic event, but to the metabolic sequelae. The nurse's ability to identify accurately those patients with alterations in metabolism is essential to achievement of positive patient outcomes. The nurse has two primary objectives in caring for the patient with altered metabolism: (1) delivery of optimal nutrition and (2) provision of optimal oxygenation.

SECTION FOUR REVIEW

1. Which of the following conditions is characteristic of the flow phase of the metabolic stress response?
   A. conservation of protein
   B. hypothermia
   C. increased energy expenditure
   D. hypoglycemia
2. Which of the following conditions places an individual at risk for refeeding syndrome?
   A. diabetes
   B. NPO status for 7 days
   C. excess fat intake
   D. obesity
3. The metabolic rate would be expected to decrease in
   A. flow phase metabolic stress response
   B. starvation
   C. hyperglycemic stress response
   D. hyperthermia
4. During NPO status, the average-sized adult has enough stored carbohydrate to supply energy needs for
   A. 1 day
   B. 1 week
   C. 48 hours
   D. 3 days

Answers: 1. C, 2. B, 3. B, 4. A

SECTION FIVE: Nutritional Alterations in Specific Disease States

At the completion of this section, the learner will be able to describe the major nutritional alterations associated with specific disease states.

Specific nutritional alterations occur in hepatic failure, pulmonary failure, acute and chronic renal failure, cardiac failure, gut failure, burns, and head injury, all of which require more specialized nutritional regimens.

Hepatic Failure

Hepatic failure can be caused by cirrhosis, hepatitis, acetaminophen toxicity, or total parenteral nutrition. The liver plays a vital role in nutrition and metabolism. Major metabolic functions of the liver include synthesis and excretion of plasma proteins, synthesis of bile acids, conversion of ammonia to urea, storage of fat-soluble vitamins, maintenance of adequate coagulation, and metabolism of carbohydrates, proteins, and lipids.

The liver plays a key role in metabolism of carbohydrates, the body's preferred energy source. The liver converts complex carbohydrates to simple sugars (glucose) that can be used for immediate energy needs or stored for later use. Excess carbohydrate converted to glycogen is then stored for later use. Excess carbohydrate converted to glycogen is then stored in the liver as an energy reserve. During times of physiologic stress, when energy needs rapidly accelerate, the liver converts stored glycogen back to glucose. When glycogen stores are depleted, the liver then converts protein and stored fat (triglycerides) to glucose as an energy source.

All the plasma proteins, except gammaglobulins and immunoglobulins are produced in the liver. Most of the circulating plasma proteins are also secreted by the liver, including albumin, prealbumin, and transferrin. Decreased serum albumin is a major indicator of severe liver dysfunction. However, with a long half-life of 14 to 21 days, decreased albumin is not immediately evident.

The liver is the primary site for lipid synthesis and degradation. Excess carbohydrate is converted to triglycerides by the liver. Triglycerides are then stored in adipose tissue deposits as a reserve energy source. Cholesterol, phospholipids, and lipoproteins, which are also produced by the liver are necessary for cell wall integrity and transmission of nerve impulses.

Nutritional alterations of hepatic failure include hyperglycemia, hypercatabolism, hyponatremia, and impaired fat metabolism. Hyperglycemia is caused by decreased pancreatic production of insulin and insulin resistance in the peripheral muscles. Reduced nutrient intake due to general malaise, nausea, vomiting, and/or diarrhea leads to hypercatabolism. Coagulopathy and gastrointestinal varices often complicate feeding tube placement. Progressive malnutrition leads to increased breakdown of skeletal muscle with release of branched-chain amino acids (BCAAs) and aromatic amino acids (AAAs). In some patients, excessive uptake of AAA by the central nervous system may contribute to encephalopathy, which is characteristic of later stages of hepatic failure.

Impaired fat metabolism is also a factor in hypercatabolism. Lipids stored as triglycerides in adipose deposits are not metabolized normally due to diminished production of ketone bodies. Increasing triglyceride levels are associated with hepatic failure.

Hyponatremia is usually dilutional secondary to declining water excretion by the kidneys. Renal failure combined with hepatic failure is often an indicator of poor outcome. Patients need adequate protein intake due to hypercatabolism. With renal failure, dialysis is often indicated to treat elevated BUN levels, which can be worsened by excessive protein intake or accumulation of free blood within the gastrointestinal tract.

Energy expenditure is typically increased in high-acuity patients with hepatic failure, therefore they need high carbohydrate intake, normal to moderate protein intake, but low fat intake. Excessive fat intake can contribute to progressive liver dysfunction with accumulation of fatty deposits in the liver cells. Due to the numerous metabolic alterations associated with hepatic failure, overfeeding is just as detrimental as underfeeding. This category of patients would benefit from having their energy expenditure measured by indirect calorimetry.

The amount and type of protein intake appropriate for patients with hepatic failure remains somewhat controversial. Since hypermetabolism and hypercatabolism are often present, protein may be provided in amounts of about 1 to 1.4 g/kg. However, when the patient is experiencing hepatic encephalopathy, protein intake may be slightly more restricted. Higher than needed protein dosing contributes to accumulation of serum ammonia and aromatic amino acids, which lead to hepatic encephalopathy. Ammonia, which crosses the blood–brain barrier, is toxic to brain cells. Aromatic amino acids are hypothesized to interfere with normal neurotransmitter activity in the central nervous system, causing sedation. Nutritional products, which contain about 50 percent of their protein source as branched-chain amino acids may be beneficial to mental status in some patients. Fluid and electrolyte imbalance and infection are causes of hepatic encephalopathy, which should be corrected before initiating feeding with significant amounts of branched-chain amino acids (Smith, 1996).

Pulmonary Failure

Malnutrition is common among high-acuity patients with pulmonary failure. Energy expenditure increases with work of breathing, yet food intake declines due to fatigue and dyspnea. In the absence of adequate calorie and protein intake, the respiratory muscles are catabolized to meet acute energy requirements. As protein deficiency progresses, decreased oncotic pressure leads to pulmonary edema.

Carbon dioxide is produced when carbohydrates, lipids, and proteins are metabolized for energy. The largest quantity of carbon dioxide is released by carbohydrates. Excessive carbohydrate intake is associated with elevated carbon dioxide values in some patients. Respiratory rate increases in an attempt to compensate for carbon dioxide accumulation.

Phosphorus levels should be closely monitored in patients with impaired gas exchange. Phosphorus is a component of 2,3-diphosphoglycerate (2,3-DPG), which facilitates oxygen transport. Low levels of 2,3-DPG diminishes hemoglobin's ability to release oxygen to the tissues. Elevated levels of 2,3-DPG lowers hemoglobin's affinity for oxygen thereby contributing to impaired gas exchange. Low phosphorus causes decreased contractility of the diaphragmatic muscles and promotes abnormal breathing patterns. Ventilator weaning should not be attempted in patients with low phosphorus.

Nutritional needs of pulmonary failure patients are similar to other hypermetabolic, hypercatabolic patients. Excessive carbohydrate and overall calorie intake may contribute to increased carbon dioxide levels in some patients. Carbohydrate intake of about 50 percent of total calories is generally recommended for patients with carbon dioxide retention with the remaining 50 percent divided between proteins and lipids (Malone, 1997).

Excessive protein intake increases minute ventilation, respiratory rate, and oxygen demand. Nitrogen balance, blood urea nitrogen, and creatinine should be monitored frequently to individualize protein dosing (see Section Three for details). Sodium and fluid restriction may be indicated for patients with pulmonary edema.

Acute Renal Failure

Metabolic alterations of acute renal failure include hypercatabolism, hypermetabolism, volume overload, and abnormal electrolytes and trace elements. Inadequate nutritional intake, loss of nutrients in dialysate, and underlying comorbid conditions contribute to hypermetabolic and hypercatabolic responses. Serum levels of potassium, phosphorus, and magnesium are usually elevated due to catabolism of lean body mass and decreased electrolyte excretion by the kidneys. Volume overload is a major concern during the oliguric phase of acute renal failure.

When acute renal failure is due to fluid volume deficit, kidney function may return without dialysis. In this situation, nutrition support, especially protein intake may be withheld due to elevated BUN. Acute renal failure often accompanies other physiologic conditions that produce significant increases in energy expenditure. Provision of nutrition support may contribute to volume overload and accumulation of metabolic waste, such as BUN. In some patients, dialysis may need to be performed to permit adequate nutrition support.

Protein dosing varies dependent upon whether or not the patient is receiving some form of dialysis. In the absence of dialysis, daily protein intake will be restricted to about 0.75 to 0.90 g/kg of protein. When dialysis is used, protein intake can be liberalized to about 1.2 to 1.5 g/kg.

Specialty renal formulas are available, which contain little or no electrolytes and low protein. The protein content is low in most of these formulas that protein needs to be added to the formula even when the patient is protein-restricted. Many patients can be maintained on regular enteral formulas that have lower protein content. Specialty renal formulas may be reserved for use in patients who have elevated electrolytes. Patients with acute renal failure require close monitoring of their fluid and electrolyte status. Nutritional goals will fluctuate relative to changes in their underlying condition and dialysis therapy.

Chronic Renal Failure

In patients undergoing long-term hemodialysis, morbidity and mortality are higher among those who are malnourished. Until very recently the trend in nutrition care in this population has been to treat malnutrition if it developed rather than focusing on prevention.

Chronic renal failure predisposes the individual to anorexia, nausea, and delayed gastric emptying, attributable to uremia. Weight loss with resultant decrease in lean body mass is common. Serum albumin levels are inversely correlated with morbidity and mortality. Anorexia may be related to unappetizing and restricted diets. Nutrients are also lost into the dialysate bath.

During the past 20 years, an ongoing debate has questioned the benefit of parenteral nutrition administered during the typical 3- to 4-hour dialysis period. Intradialytic parenteral nutrition (IDPN) is easy to deliver via the dialysis machine, but research has not validated its usefulness in the acute-care setting. The studies devoted to IDPN have been hampered by small sample sizes, inconsistent methods and analyses, and a lack of nutritional assessment prior to initiation of IDPN. Therefore, the research has not produced a consensus opinion regarding the benefit of this costly and potentially risky nutritional therapy.

One of the most serious risks of IDPN is the large glucose load delivered in a short period. Generally, a liter of IDPN, containing 250 g of glucose, is administered over 3 to 4 hours. Blood glucose levels can rise dramatically during this interval. Usually, this amount of glucose in a TPN solution is delivered over nearly a 24-hour period. Patients receiving IDPN need to have their blood glucose monitored frequently during the dialysis period as well as for a few hours after therapy. Extremely high values of blood glucose have been observed in patients within the first few hours after receiving IDPN.

Studies have observed increases in levels of serum albumin or transferrin with administration of IDPN. This finding is suggestive of improved visceral protein stores and sparing of lean body mass. Across studies, however, flaws in research design make comparisons difficult (Foulks, 1999).

Cardiac Failure

Protein-energy malnutrition (PEM) is relatively common in hospitalized patients, with an incidence as high as 25 to 50 percent. While it was once believed that the heart was spared from the muscle-wasting effects of malnutrition, this has been negated. Loss of muscle mass results in decreased pumping effectiveness. Cardiac cachexia is a specific type of PEM that develops with persistent circulatory failure. As cardiac failure continues, tissues become increasingly deprived of oxygen. This is essentially a form of tissue injury and hypermetabolism is observed. The patient experiences the scope of the hypermetabolic response as described in Section Four. Muscle proteins and stored fat are utilized for energy with resultant loss of lean body mass. With a vicious cycle effect, cachexia contributes to the progression of cardiac failure.

Nosocomial cardiac **cachexia** develops postoperatively in adequately nourished patients when surgical complications prevent them from consuming oral intake. Malnutrition develops in days or weeks in patients who are not receiving appropriate nutritional support. For surgical patients with cardiac disease, nutrition support should be started within 3 to 5 days if they do not have optimal intake.

Nutritional needs of all high-acuity patients with cardiac disease should be closely monitored. Nutritional intake can have a negative effect on hemodynamics in some patients. Oxygen consumption increases with food intake. For patients who have meals, the postprandial elevation of oxygen consumption can be significant enough to cause hemodynamic instability. The presence of food in the gastrointestinal tract results in greater blood flow through the splanchnic circulation. This increased blood volume is obtained by shunting blood from other vital organs such as the myocardium, kidneys, and/or brain. Therefore, among patients who can eat, intake should be limited to frequent, small amounts of food. For patients who require enteral or parenteral nutrition support, continuous infusion of the formula is more beneficial than intermittent intake to regulate the thermogenic effect of the nutrients (Katz, Wiese, & Gay, 1996).

Anorexia is a frequently observed characteristic in patients with cardiac failure. Dyspnea, fatigue, and unappetizing restricted oral diets contribute to lack of appetite. Cardiac contractility is impaired by low levels of many of the electrolytes. Thiamine deficiency leads to vasodilation of the peripheral blood vessels, producing high-output failure. Cardiomyopathy can be attributed to selenium deficiency in patients receiving long-term total parenteral nutrition.

Balanced nutrient intake is important for anyone, but particularly so for patients with potential or actual alterations of oxygenation. Hospitalized patients receiving only intravenous glucose will have a significant increase in their respiratory quotient. An RQ value near 1.00 is indicative of significantly increased carbon dioxide production.

Gut Failure

Inadequate intestinal perfusion produces increased gut permeability and facilitates bacterial translocation from the bowel into the peritoneal cavity, lymph, and portal circulations. Bacterial translocation is now accepted as a major etiology of sepsis in hospitalized patients (Stechmiller, 1997). Intestinal ischemia is a recognized adverse effect of cardiopulmonary bypass (CPB). Although the incidence of ischemia related to CPB is only 0.6 percent to 2 percent, mortality is as high as 15 percent to 63 percent (Ohri et al., 1993).

Regional assessment of splanchnic circulation can be performed indirectly by gastric tonometry, which measures the pH of the gastric mucosa. The value of the gastric intramucosal P_{CO_2} is obtained by aspiration of a fluid sample via a specially designed nasogastric tube (gastric tonometer). An arterial blood gas supply is obtained at the same time as the gastric sample. The bicarbonate value of the blood and the P_{CO_2} value of the gastric sample are placed into the Henderson–Hasselbach equation. The final value is called the intramucosal pH (pHi). If the result is acidic, the assumption is that circulation to the splanchnic organs is compromised. Values of gastric intramucosal pH have been observed to change prior to changes in more traditional assessments of tissue oxygenation such as oxygen delivery, oxygen consumption, and mixed venous P_{O_2} (Ruffolo, 1998).

Burns

Burn patients are among those with the highest expected energy, protein, and fluid needs. The extent of the hypermetabolic response is related to the severity of the burn. Energy expenditure typically increases from 2 to 2.5 times above the individual's resting value. However, energy demands seem to reach a peak with a 50 percent burn. Burns greater than 50 percent severity are observed to have less intense energy expenditure. The exact nature of this decrease in the hypermetabolic alterations is thought to be due to the body's inability to respond to such a dramatic insult as a greater than 50 percent burn injury.

Elevated energy expenditure may persist longer in the burn patient than in other types of tissue injuries. Alteration of the temperature-regulation mechanism increases core temperature, which is responsible for the dramatic elevation of energy expenditure. Blunting of the hypermetabolic response is observed when nutrient intake is initiated within the first few hours after injury.

Decreases in the patient's energy needs will be noticed when skin grafting is done or when there is regeneration of epithelium. As with other types of injuries, hypermetabolism reoccurs with repeated infections or additional insults such as multisystem organ failure (Rieg, 1993).

As with any extensive wounds, vitamin supplementation is beneficial for healing and maintenance of overall immune function. Vitamins A, B complex, and C, along with zinc, support wound healing. Dosage recommendations vary, but the general intent for supplementation is to treat or prevent micronutrient deficiencies (Whitney & Heitkemper, 1999).

Burn patients are expected to have massive fluid losses since the skin serves as a barrier against evaporative water loss. Protocols for calculating fluid resuscitation are found in various sources including Advanced Trauma Life Support guidelines for the burn patient.

The body's temperature-regulation mechanism is altered in the burn patient. Increased skin cooling due to accelerated evaporation was once considered to be the cause of the extreme elevation of energy expenditure, but this was not supported experimentally. Increase in the core temperature is viewed as the causative factor of the dramatic elevation of energy expenditure in burn patients. Blunting of the hypermetabolic response is observed when nutrient intake is initiated within the first few hours after injury (De-Souza & Greene, 1998).

Traumatic Brain Injury

Second only to burns, traumatic brain (TBI) injury causes the most extreme hypermetabolic and hypercatabolic responses. Energy expenditure is highest in patients with decerebrate/decorticate activity (Klein, 1999). As with any tissue injury, the sympathetic nervous system stimulates release of corticosteroids from the adrenal medulla, catecholamines, and glucagon. Increases of these hormones are responsible for conversion of glycogen to glucose for energy. Glucagon acts on the liver to convert amino acids into glucose while stored fat is also converted into glucose (Lennie, 1997).

As described previously, insulin release from the pancreas is decreased. Combined with the rapid conversion of stored nutrients into glucose, hyperglycemia occurs. Hyperglycemia has been identified as a significant predictor of outcome from head injury (Merguerian et al., 1981; Young et al., 1989).

The extent of hypermetabolism in head-injured patients is inversely correlated with the Glasgow Coma Score (Robertson et al., 1984). With head trauma, energy expenditure increases by 1.4 to 2 times above that normally expended by an individual of the same gender, age, height, and weight at rest (Young et al., 1992).

Hypercatabolism is prominent with TBI. The exact mechanism of significant urinary nitrogen losses is unclear. Immobility, decreased nitrogen efficiency, steroid administration, and decreased nutrient intake have all been suggested as causative factors (Ott & Young, 1994).

The brain is the organ with the highest oxygen consumption. When oxygen demand exceeds supply, cardiac output is increased along with the amount of oxygen that the brain extracts from the blood. When oxygen demand surpasses supply, hypoxemia occurs. The brain tries to compensate for the hypoxemia by increasing blood flow and therefore oxygen delivery to the brain. However, this compensatory response contributes to the increased intracranial pressure that is the hallmark of head injury. Hypoxemia leads to anaerobic metabolism in the brain tissue. Lactic acid, an end product of anaerobic metabolism, cannot adequately supply the brain's energy needs (Heath & Vink, 1999).

Treatment for refractory intracranial hypertension sometimes includes pentobarbital-induced coma, which lowers overall oxygen consumption. Clinicians are sometimes hesitant to attempt enteral feeding in these patients due to gastroparesis and the belief that enteral feeding will not be absorbed due to the effects of pentobarbital. Even though gastrointestinal motility is greatly diminished, absorption of nutrients by the small bowel is usually maintained.

Transpyloric placement of a small-bore feeding tube using a blind approach is possible, but success seems to be related to clinician experience. Endoscopic feeding tube placement may be necessary. Enteral feeding during pentobarbital-induced coma is efficacious and well tolerated by many patients, thus limiting the need for parenteral nutrition (Magnuson et al., 1999)

In summary, nutrition plays a major role in the care of the high-acuity patient. Specific disease states or clinical conditions produce alterations in normal metabolism. The nurse should be familiar with the nutritional/metabolic alterations that may occur with common disease states to permit early intervention. Nutritional/metabolic therapies should be appropriately individualized to avoid potential metabolic complications.

Section Five Review

1. A high-acuity patient with hepatic failure may typically experience all of the following EXCEPT
   A. breakdown of skeletal muscle protein
   B. diminished fat use
   C. hyponatremia
   D. increased carbon dioxide levels
2. Nutritional goals for the patient experiencing pulmonary failure include all of the following EXCEPT
   A. higher sodium content
   B. lower protein content
   C. lower carbohydrate content
   D. higher fat content
3. A high-acuity patient with acute renal failure may typically experience abnormalities in each of the following EXCEPT
   A. protein catabolism
   B. fluid and electrolyte levels
   C. metabolic rate
   D. glucose levels
4. The purpose for supplementing nutritional intake with vitamins A, B complex, and C as well as zinc is to
   A. promote red blood cell count
   B. promote wound healing
   C. lower BUN level
   D. lower cholesterol

Answers: 1. D, 2. A, 3. D, 4. B

SECTION SIX: Methods of Enteral Nutrition

At the completion of this section, the learner will be able to describe the benefits and potential complications of enteral nutrition, explain the rationale for gastric versus postpyloric feeding, and identify barriers to providing optimal enteral nutrition to the high-acuity patient.

Criteria for Selection of Enteral Nutrition

Nutrition support should be provided via the enteral route in patients with a functional GI tract. Unless there is known traumatic disruption or chronic malabsorptive disease, it is generally assumed that the GI tract is capable of absorption of nutrients, fluids, and electrolytes. Patients with a high-acuity illness or injury, who are unable to consume oral nutrition will require a feeding tube. Selection of the specific type of enteral feeding is based on the following criteria: (1) GI integrity and function, (2) baseline nutritional status, and (3) illness severity and possible duration.

Gastrointestinal Integrity and Function

When assessing a patient's GI function, first consider if the patient will be able to eat within 3 to 5 days. If so, nutritional support may not be indicated. If the patient is expected to be unable to eat for this time period or longer, he or she will require placement of a feeding tube. The specific type of feeding tube placed is related to the anticipated time of recovery, the patient's level of consciousness, comfort, and cost-effectiveness.

Illness Severity and Possible Duration

Energy expenditure, and therefore calorie and protein requirements, increases with the severity of illness. The hypermetabolism of the metabolic stress response can persist for extended periods in the presence of physiologic complications such as extensive wounds or sepsis. Advances in the understanding of the metabolic stress response and the immunologic functions of the gut have led to a greater appreciation for the need to provide nutrition support to the high-acuity patient early during the course of illness or injury (Cole, 1999).

Timing of Nutrition Support

Providing nutrition early in the course of illness or injury is a treatment priority. Numerous randomized clinical trials (RCTs) among general surgical patients indicate that early provision of **enteral nutrition** facilitates wound healing. RCTs examining the effect of early versus delayed enteral feeding on infectious morbidity in trauma patients have produced contradictory findings. No studies have yet reported a significant difference in mortality among critically ill patients given early enteral nutrition compared to delayed feeding (Heyland, 1998).

Readiness for enteral feeding should not be determined by the presence of bowel sounds. Active bowel sounds has been used as a criteria to initiate feeding, but there is no scientific evidence to support this practice. Bowel sounds are a poor indicator of small bowel motility and nutrient absorption. Bowel sounds result from air being taken into the stomach and passing through the intestinal tract. Many interventions such as nasogastric suctioning, sedation, and NPO status prevent the normal passage of air through the GI tract. Therefore, waiting for bowel sounds places the patient at undue risk for malnutrition (Loan, Magnuson, & Williams, 1998).

Benefits of Enteral Nutrition

1. Maintenance of gut immunologic function
2. More physiologic than parenteral nutrition
3. Possible decrease in severity of metabolic stress response
4. More cost-effective than parenteral nutrition
5. Decreased risks of infectious complications
6. Enhancement of wound healing

A major benefit of enteral nutrition is that it may maintain gut barrier function. Reductions in gut barrier function are associated with increased bacterial translocation, systemic inflammatory response syndrome (SIRS), and multisystem organ dysfunction. In animal models, fasting is associated with increased translocation of bacteria from the GI tract into mesenteric lymph nodes, portal circulation, and the peritoneal cavity (Cole, 1999).

Enteral formulas are more calorie-dense than total parenteral nutrition and can provide higher nutrient intake in patients who are fluid restricted. Although invasive, feeding tube insertion has less inherent risk of mechanical and infectious complications than central venous line insertion for TPN administration. The cost of enteral formulas is about 10 to 20 percent of the daily cost of TPN. Even the most expensive specialty enteral formulas do not equal the cost of providing TPN.

Contraindications to Enteral Nutrition

1. Gastrointestinal hemorrhage
2. Distal gastrointestinal fistula
3. Severe malabsorption
4. Total small bowel obstruction
5. Inability to place a feeding tube due to mechanical obstruction (such as a tumor)

Contraindications to enteral nutrition have diminished as its safety and efficacy has been demonstrated in many types of high-acuity patients. Many patients who were once thought to require TPN are now often successfully fed via the enteral route. Enteral nutrition can be provided to patients with GI fistulas if the tube can be positioned distal to the site of the fistula.

Criteria for Selection of Nutritional Support

Selection of the type of nutritional support is based on the following criteria: (1) GI function, (2) baseline nutritional status, and (3) present catabolic state and possible duration.

Gastrointestinal Function

When determining a patient's GI function, first consider whether the patient will be able to eat solid food within 2 to 3 days. If so, nutritional support may not be instituted.

If the patient is unable or unwilling to ingest sufficient nutrients normally by mouth and has a relatively functional GI tract, the preferred route of nutritional support is enteral.

Baseline Nutritional Status

Baseline nutritional status is an important determinant for deciding when and what type of nutritional support to initiate. Clinical studies indicate that severely malnourished patients have a greater risk of developing complications and eventually dying. High-acuity patients should be fed as early as possible, particularly if they are in a malnourished state.

Present Catabolic State and Possible Duration

For the high-acuity patient who is highly catabolic (nitrogen loss greater than 15 to 20 g/day), nutritional support should be initiated as soon as possible after arrival in the critical care unit. The goal is to minimize further breakdown of the skeletal muscle and visceral protein stores.

Numerous enteral formulas are available. Choosing the appropriate formula for the high-acuity patient is based on the energy and protein requirements of the patient, the underlying disease state or organ function, intestinal absorptive and digestive function, and fluid requirements. Commonly used are the lactose-free, nutritionally complete formulas that contain a mixture of carbohydrates, fats, protein, trace elements, and vitamins. Feedings are supplied in varying osmolalities and range in caloric density from 1 to 2 kcal/mL.

A number of Silastic or polyurethane, weighted, or nonweighted small-bore (8 to 12 Fr) feeding tubes are available for enteral patients; endoscopic or surgical placement of a gastric or jejunal feeding tube may be preferable.

Feeding Tube Placement

Enteral feeding access can be achieved by a variety of methods that include blind placement of a small-bore feeding tube, percutaneous placement of a gastrostomy and/or jejunostomy, or surgical placement of a gastrostomy or jejunostomy. The small-bore feeding tube is the least invasive and most economical device for delivery of enteral nutrition. This polyurethane weighted or nonweighted tube can be used for gastric or transpyloric feeding.

Transpyloric placement of the feeding tube via the nasal or oral cavity has a low success rate and requires consideration of technique, tube design, and/or prokinetic medications (Ahmed et al., 1999). Passage of the feeding tube from the stomach into the small bowel is associated with upper GI motility. Motor function of the upper GI tract is known to be altered in patients with critical illness, receiving mechanical ventilation (Dive et al., 1994), or in chronic conditions such as diabetes mellitus (Janssens et al., 1990; Tack et al., 1992), vagotomy, and intestinal pseudo-obstruction.

Repeated attempts to position the feeding tube transpyloric can cause patient discomfort and delay of feeding. Repeated abdominal x-rays to verify tube position and clinician time contribute to increased cost (Clevenger & Rodriguez, 1995).

Gastric versus Transpyloric Feeding

One of the ongoing controversies of nutrition support is whether high-acuity patients should be fed by means of intragastric or transpyloric feeding. In situations when repeated blind attempts to place the feeding tube transpyloric delays onset of feeding, it may be beneficial to initiate gastric feeding with a more concentrated formula at a low hourly rate in some patients. Delayed gastric emptying (gastroparesis) associated with critical illness is a primary reason for preference of feeding into the small bowel instead of the stomach. Some clinicians believe that transpyloric feeding decreases the risk of aspiration, but that belief is not supported by the literature. The documented benefits of transpyloric feeding include less interruption of feeding and therefore higher nutritional intake and lower incidence of pneumonia in some groups (Heyland, 1998). Recent studies report tolerance of intragastric feeding among patients with traumatic brain injury (Spain et al., 1995) and those with diverse critical illness receiving mechanical ventilation (Heyland et al., 1999).

Increased gastric colonization of gram-negative bacilli has been reported in mechanically ventilated critically ill patients receiving intragastric feeding. The normal high acidity of gastric contents protects against gastric colonization. Histamine type 2 blockers and enteral formulas both elevate the intragastric pH, reducing the protection usually provided by higher gastric acid against gram-negative colonization (Montecalvo et al., 1992; Heyland & Mandell, 1992). Colonization of gastric gram-negative bacilli leads to nosocomial pneumonia.

Aspiration is the major mechanism for entry of bacteria into the lungs and contributes to development of noscomial pneumonia. The risk of pulmonary aspiration of tube feeding is increased by medications such as theophylline, dopamine, anticholinergics, calcium channel blockers, and meperidine that cause relaxation of the lower esophageal sphincter (Farmer, Rolandelli, & Smith, 1997).

Patients with transpyloric feeding tube placement are likely to receive more of their prescribed nutritional intake compared to gastric feeding (Montecalvo et al., 1992). Gastric feedings are interrupted for instillation of medications, vomiting, formula retention, and abdominal distention. Transpyloric tube feedings do not need to be interrupted when medications are delivered into the stomach via a nasogastric tube. Enteral feeding is held for an hour before and after phenytoin (Dilantin) as a precaution against drug–nutrient interaction, regardless of site of administration (Gilbert, Hatton, & Magnuson, 1996).

Complications of Enteral Nutrition

Complications of enteral feedings are classified under five categories: gastrointestinal, nutritional, mechanical, metabolic, and infectious. Table 22–7 lists potential enteral complications, possible causes, and suggested treatment.

In summary, enteral feedings are the preferred route of nutritional support in the high-acuity patient who cannot or will not ingest sufficient nutrients by mouth but has a functioning gastrointestinal tract. Enteral feedings have many advantages over parenteral feedings. Commonly used enteral feedings are lactose-free, nutritionally complete formulas that contain a mixture of carbohydrates, fats, protein, trace elements, and vitamins. Enteral feedings are delivered preferably to the small bowel via a nasoenteric feeding tube. Potential complications of enteral feedings are categorized under gastrointestinal, nutritional, mechanical, metabolic, and infectious complications. There are various causes for these potential complications. Diagnostic, pharmacologic, and dietary treatments are suggested for these potential complications.

TABLE 22–7. COMPLICATIONS OF ENTERAL NUTRITION

COMPLICATION	POSSIBLE CAUSE	SUGGESTED TREATMENT
Gastrointestinal		
Nausea/vomiting	Hyperosmolar feeding	Start isotonic feeding
	Rapid infusion rate	Start feedings slowly and advance as tolerated
	Obstruction	Reassess gastrointestinal function
	Delayed gastric emptying	Prokinetic agent (metoclopramide, erythromycin) to increase gastric emptying: feed distal to pylorus
	Contaminated solution or infusion set	Hang canned formula for no longer than manufacturer's recommendation; hang prepared formulas no longer than 4 hours; change container and infusion set every 24 hours; use good handwashing technique before handling formulas
Diarrhea	Antibiotics may alter intestinal flora causing bacteria overgrowth: *Clostridium difficile* infection and pseudomembranous colitis	Send stool specimens for culture and sensitivity, white blood cell count, ova, parasites, and *Clostridium difficile* cytotoxin. Flexible sigmoidoscopy provides a faster and more reliable diagnosis than stool studies; treatment of choice for *Clostridium difficile* toxin is IV/PO metronidazole (Flagyl) or IV vancomycin; hold any antidiarrheal agents until infectious source is ruled out
	Liquid medications containing sorbitol or other concentrated sugar base have a laxative effect (common cause of diarrhea in patients receiving liquid medications)	Crush tablet form of medication if possible
Nutritional		
Malnutrition	Malnutrition associated with loss of microvilli, villous brush border enzymes, and subsequent reduction in intestinal absorptive surface area	Supply elemental diet to improve absorption; elemental diets are for digestive disorders requiring a more easily digested, absorbed diet
Hypoalbuminemia	Hypoalbuminemia is associated with lack of intravascular osmotic pressure required to draw nutrients across intestinal epithelium, thus compromising absorption	Poor tolerance is evident in patients with serum albumin < 2.5 mg/dL; benefit of albumin administration should outweigh cost and potential complications
	Protein-losing enteropathy	Semi-elemental formula
Mechanical		
Feeding tube occlusion	Medications lack of proper flushing; viscous formulas	Irrigate feeding tube with 30–50 mL warm water every 4 hours, after medication administration, after checking residuals (gastric) Alternate positive/negative pressure with syringe to dislodge clot Warm water, juices, or colas have been cited as agents to dissolve clots Do not attempt to dislodge clots with stylet; may cause esophageal/gastric mucosal perforations; *prevention* is key
Metabolic		
Hypoglycemia	Sudden cessation of feeding	Provide supplemental glucose
Hyperglycemia	Stress response, diabetic or glucose intolerance	Usually resolves as stress is alleviated; initiate feedings slowly; monitor blood glucose every 6 hours
Electrolyte imbalance	Dilutional states (dehydration or fluid overload)	Monitor fluid status; monitor electrolytes and replace as needed Replace fluid and electrolytes as needed
	Excess losses (diarrhea, fistula, nasogastric drainage, ascites)	
	Disease states (renal/liver failure)	Provide appropriate organ failure formula
Infectious		
Aspiration pneumonia	High-risk patients include comatose, weak, debilitated	Elevate head of bed at least 30 degrees; feed into small bowel distal to pylorus
	Patients with tracheostomies or intubated patients; patients with neuromuscular disorders	Add food coloring to feeding to detect for aspiration Check residuals every 4 hours if feeding into stomach

SECTION SIX REVIEW

1. Which of the following conditions is associated with intragastric feeding?

   A. nosocomial pneumonia
   B. stress ulcer
   C. accelerated gastric emptying
   D. diarrhea

2. The severely malnourished patient has a greater risk of developing complications and eventual death. These severely malnourished patients should be fed
   A. whenever oral intake is possible
   B. after recovery from the acute illness
   C. as early as possible
   D. never
3. A patient has a relatively functioning gastrointestinal tract but is unable to take adequate nutrients by mouth. What is the best method for administering nutritional support to this patient?
   A. nasoenteric feedings
   B. oral diet
   C. withhold nutrition
   D. TPN
4. Enteral nutrition has many advantages over TPN, including all of the following EXCEPT
   A. less risk of bacterial translocation
   B. providing central venous access
   C. maintaining gut morphology and function
   D. less costly
5. Enteral feedings are preferably delivered to the ___ via a nasoenteric feeding tube.
   A. oral cavity
   B. gastric mucosa
   C. small bowel
   D. large bowel
6. The categories of potential complications of enteral feedings include all of the following EXCEPT
   A. gastrointestinal
   B. mechanical
   C. metabolic
   D. intravenous
7. Diarrhea may occur from enteral feedings, but the more common cause is antibiotics. Antibiotics can alter intestinal flora, causing bacterial overgrowth (*Clostridium difficile* infection and pseudomembranous colitis). The suggested treatment includes all of the following EXCEPT
   A. send stool specimens for testing
   B. perform flexible sigmoidoscopy
   C. administer IV/PO metronidazole (Flagyl) or IV vancomycin
   D. administer antidiarrheal agents
8. Possible causes of an occluded feeding include all of the following EXCEPT
   A. lack of proper flushing
   B. elemental diet
   C. medications
   D. viscous formulas
9. Which one of the following factors is an advantage of transpyloric feeding?
   A. less likely to cause diarrhea
   B. prevents tube feeding aspiration
   C. prevents stress ulcers
   D. patients receive more tube feeding compared to intragastric route

Answers: 1. A, 2. C, 3. A, 4. B, 5. C, 6. D, 7. D, 8. B, 9. D

SECTION SEVEN: Methods of Total Parenteral Nutrition

At the completion of this section, the learner will be able to discuss the parenteral methods used to provide nutrition for the high-acuity/critically ill patient, including potential complications.

Total parenteral nutrition (TPN) is a nutritionally complete, IV-delivered solution composed of amino acids (protein), dextrose (carbohydrate), fats, electrolytes, vitamins, and trace elements. TPN with > 10 percent glucose must be delivered via a central line. Glucose concentrations of ≤ 10 percent can be delivered via a peripheral vein, as peripheral parenteral nutrition (PPN). Solutions are designed to meet the individual energy and protein needs of a patient based on the clinical condition, underlying disease states, and organ function.

TPN is indicated when nutrition cannot be delivered through the GI tract. Conditions appropriate for TPN include total bowel obstruction, mechanical obstruction, gut versus host disease of the gut, some cases of severe acute pancreatitis, acute bowel inflammation producing persistent diarrhea, or some cases of short bowel syndrome. Patient refusal to have a feeding tube placed does not necessitate nutrition support with TPN.

TPN is contraindicated in those patients with a functioning, usable GI tract capable of absorption of adequate nutrients, when sole dependence is anticipated to be less than 5 days, when aggressive support is not warranted, and when the risks of TPN outweigh the potential benefits.

Catheters commonly used are multilumen. These catheters allow for one central venous access, with multiple ports for hemodynamic monitoring and fluid/medication delivery without risk of drug incompatibility. To minimize the risk of line infections, one part of multilumen catheters should be dedicated for TPN administration.

Complications of Total Parenteral Nutrition

Complications from TPN fall under three classifications: septic, metabolic, and mechanical.

Septic Complications

Catheter-related sepsis (CRS) is a potentially lethal complication, particularly in the high-acuity population. Review of the literature reveals that the primary causes of CRS are:

1. Lack of sterility during placement of central lines
2. Inadequate precautions taken with maintenance of the central line (i.e., changing tubings, dressings, bags)

Clinical signs and symptoms of CRS are

- Bacteremia/septicemia/septic shock
- Leukocytosis
- Sudden temperature elevation that should resolve upon catheter removal
- Sudden glucose intolerance that may occur up to 12 hours before temperature elevation
- Erythema, swelling, tenderness, and purulent drainage from the catheter site

Prompt evaluation and identification of the source of septicemia is important. Pancultures (urine, sputum, and two sets of peripheral blood cultures) should be sent. If a catheter tip culture results in growth of more than 15 colonies, the catheter should be removed, since this most likely indicates migration of bacteria from a contaminated solution, administration set, catheter, or infected skin tract. Antimicrobial therapy should be initiated.

Prevention is the key. To avoid contamination of the catheter, maintain dry, sterile, and intact dressings at all times, prepare the junction of administration sets with povidone–iodine, minimize the number of entries into the system, and always use meticulous technique with all aspects of catheter care (Rombeau, 1993).

Metabolic Complications

Metabolic complications of TPN are similar to those of enteral nutrition. Refer to Section Six for metabolic complications, possible causes, and suggested treatment.

Other possible metabolic derangements of TPN are prerenal azotemia and hepatic dysfunction.

Prerenal azotemia is caused by overaggressive protein administration and is aggravated by underlying dehydration. Presenting signs and symptoms include an elevated serum BUN, serum sodium, and clinical signs of dehydration. If the condition is not corrected, the patient may develop progressive lethargy and possibly coma. Close monitoring of body weight, fluid balance, and adequate protein intake is important in preventing this complication.

Hepatic dysfunction can occur secondary to long-term TPN administration. Serum liver function tests (including SGOT, SGPT, alkaline phosphatase, and, rarely, bilirubin levels) become elevated during the course of TPN and usually return to normal spontaneously when the infusion is stopped. Almost all components of the TPN solution have been implicated as the cause of hepatic dysfunction. Excessive glucose administration has been mentioned most frequently as the culprit (Farmer, Rolandelli, & Smith, 1997).

Mechanical Complications

Mechanical complications include pneumothorax, hydrothorax, subclavian/carotid artery puncture, air embolism, and dysrhythmias. All may be a result of the central venous catheter insertion.

Pneumothorax, the most common mechanical complication, is caused by the puncture or laceration of the pleura on insertion of the needle/catheter. Air enters into the pleural space, with partial or complete collapse of the lung. Most pneumothoraces produce symptoms, although some are totally asymptomatic. In general, the larger the collapse, the more pronounced the symptoms. Commonly seen are shortness of breath, restlessness, dyspnea, hypoxia, and chest pain radiating to the back. Treatment depends on the severity of the collapse and respiratory compromise. Moderate to large collapse will require a chest tube to restore negative pressure within the chest cavity.

Hydrothorax occurs when fluid is introduced into the pleural space. Symptoms are similar to those of pneumothorax. A diagnostic tap (thoracentesis) should be performed; a chest tube may be required if reaccumulation of fluid occurs.

Inadvertent puncture or laceration of the subclavian or carotid arteries is indicated by a flashback of arterial blood in the syringe, pulsatile blood flow, bleeding from the catheter site or development of a large hematoma, and hypotension. Treatment involves withdrawing the syringe/catheter and applying direct pressure to the site until bleeding ceases.

Air embolism may occur whenever the central venous system is open to air. Signs and symptoms vary with the amount of air pulled into the venous system but may include respiratory distress, tachycardia, hypotension, sudden cardiovascular collapse, neurologic deficits, or cardiac arrest. Immediate action is required. Occlude the catheter nearest to the entry site of the skin. Place the patient on the left side and in the Trendelenburg position. Prevention is the key. Always use Luer-Lock connectors and air-eliminating filters on central line tubings.

Dysrhythmias during central venous insertions are the result of a malpositioned catheter or guidewire. The result may be atrial, nodal, or ventricular dysrhythmias, which may cause decreased cardiac output, decreased blood pressure, or loss of consciousness. Appropriate intervention is to withdraw the catheter or guidewire partially. If the dysrhythmia continues, an antiarrhythmic may be required.

In conclusion, the nurse, as the member of the health care team who is in constant contact with the patient, is in a significant position to manage individual nutritional/metabolic therapies, support energy and oxygen needs, and prevent complications related to the numerous metabolic complications that occur with tissue injury. With an increasing emphasis on providing therapies that are beneficial yet cost-saving, the nurse is in a pivotal position to evaluate the appropriateness and effectiveness of nutritional therapies in the high-acuity patient. Nurses are ideally suited to design and implement research protocols related to the metabolic needs of the high-acuity patient.

SECTION SEVEN REVIEW

1. TPN is indicated when
   A. adequate amounts of nutrients can be delivered through the GI tract
   B. adequate amounts of nutrients cannot be delivered through the GI tract
   C. a functioning, usable gastrointestinal tract is capable of absorption of adequate nutrients
   D. aggressive nutritional support is not warranted
2. TPN with a > 10 percent glucose should be administered through a
   A. nasoenteric feeding tube
   B. peripheral vein
   C. surgically placed jejunal feeding tube
   D. central vein
3. Which of the following factors can lead to prerenal azotemia in the patient receiving TPN?
   A. excessive protein administration
   B. excessive carbohydrate administration
   C. excessive fluid administration
   D. excessive lipid administration
4. CRS is a potentially lethal complication of TPN and is caused primarily by
   A. a malpositioned catheter or guidewire during the central line insertion
   B. lack of sterility during central line placement and inadequate maintenance of the line
   C. inadvertent puncture or laceration of the subclavian or carotid artery
   D. puncture or laceration of the vein on insertion of the needle/catheter
5. Hypoglycemia is a potential metabolic complication of TPN and results from
   A. gluconeogenesis
   B. glucose intolerance
   C. sudden cessation of feeding
   D. insulin resistance
6. Mechanical complications of TPN consist of all of the following EXCEPT
   A. air embolism
   B. hydrothorax
   C. pneumothorax
   D. CRS

Answers: 1. B, 2. D, 3. A, 4. B, 5. C, 6. D

POSTTEST

1. Which organ plays a major role in lipogenesis?
   A. spleen
   B. pancreas
   C. liver
   D. gallbladder
2. Which one of the following substances is the body's preferred energy source?
   A. proteins
   B. lipids
   C. carbohydrates
   D. amino acids
3. A high-acuity patient with hepatic failure may experience all of the following EXCEPT
   A. breakdown of skeletal muscle protein
   B. diminished fat use
   C. hyponatremia
   D. increased carbon dioxide levels
4. Nutritional goals for the pulmonary failure patient are the following EXCEPT
   A. higher sodium content
   B. lower protein content
   C. lower carbohydrate content
   D. higher fat content
5. For the high-acuity patient with acute renal failure, which of the following nutritional therapies is appropriate for the patient undergoing hemodialysis?
   A. protein intake should be restricted to about .75 to .90 g/kg/day
   B. protein intake should be liberalized to about 1.2 to 1.5 g/kg/day
   C. carbohydrate intake should be limited to less than 50 percent of total nutrition
   D. lipid intake should not exceed 20 percent of total nutrition

6. A patient has a functioning GI tract but is unable to take adequate nutrients by mouth. What is the BEST method for administering nutritional support to this patient?
   A. nasoenteric feedings
   B. oral diet
   C. withhold nutrition
   D. TPN
7. The absence of a skin reaction after cutaneous administration of an anergy screen indicates
   A. the normal response
   B. that the patient's cellular immunity has been negatively effected by malnutrition
   C. that the patient is adequately nourished
   D. that the patient's cellular immunity is intact
8. The primary rationale for transpyloric feeding is that it
   A. prevents aspiration of tube feeding
   B. negates the need for a nasogastric tube
   C. promotes greater amount of nutritional intake in patients likely to have delayed gastric emptying
   D. facilitates bolus feeding
9. TPN is appropriate for use in which one of the following types of patients?
   A. liver failure patient with nausea
   B. nonresectable gastric tumor which prevents passage of enteral feeding tube
   C. chronic pancreatitis
   D. hyperemesis gravidarum
10. Which one of the laboratory findings below is indicative of refeeding syndrome?
   A. hypophosphatemia
   B. hypoglycemia
   C. hyperkalemia
   D. hypernatremia

POSTTEST ANSWERS

Question	Answer	Section	Question	Answer	Section
1	C	Two	6	A	Six
2	C	Two	7	B	Three
3	D	Five	8	C	Six
4	A	Five	9	B	Seven
5	B	Five	10	A	Four

REFERENCES

Ahmed, W., Levy, H., Kudsk, K., et al. (1999). The rates of spontaneous transpyloric passage of three enteral feeding tubes. *Nutrition in Clinical Practice*, *14*:107–110.

Ahrens, T. (1996). Respiratory Monitoring. In J.M. Clochesy, C. Breu, S. Cardin, A.A. Whittikar, & E.B. Rudy (eds.). *Critical care nursing* (p. 250). Philadelphia: W.B. Saunders.

Ahrens, T.S., & Rutherford, K. (1993). *Essentials of oxygenation*. Boston: Jones & Bartlett.

Atkin, S.H., Dasmahapatra, A., Jaker, MA., Cohorost, M.I., & Reddy, S. (1991). Fingerstick glucose determination in shock. *Ann Int Med 114*:1020–1024.

Bagley, S.M. (1996). Nutritional needs of the acutely ill with acute wounds. *Crit Care Nurs Clin of North Am 2*:159–167.

Bernstein, L., Meguid, M., Ament, M., et al. (1995). Measurement of visceral protein status in assessing protein and energy malnutrition: Standard of care. *Nutrition 11*:169–171.

Berry, J.K., & Braunschweig, C.A. (1998). Nutritional assessment of the critically ill patient. *Crit Care Nurs Q 21*:33–46.

Brody, T. (1999). *Nutritional biochemistry*. San Diego: Academic Press.

Clevenger, F.W., & Rodriguez, D.J. (1995). Decision-making for enteral feeding administration: The why behind where and how. *Nutr Clin Pract 10*:104–113.

Cole, L. (1999). Early enteral feeding after surgery. *Crit Care Nurs Clin of North Am 11*:227–231.

De-Souza, D.A., & Greene, L.J. (1998). Pharmacological nutrition after burn injury. *J Nutrition 128*:797–803.

Dive, A., Moulart, M., Jonard, P., Jamart, J., & Mahieu, P. (1994). Gastroduodenal motility in mechanically ventilated critically ill patients: A manometric study. *Crit Care Med 22*:441–447.

Farmer, D.G., Rolandelli, R.H., & Smith, E.L. (1997). The role of enteral nutrition in organ and cellular transplantation. In J.L. Rombeau & R.A. Rolandelli (eds.). Clinical nutrition—Enteral and tube feeding (3rd ed.) (p. 492). Philadelphia: Saunders.

Foulks, C.J. (1999). An evidence-based evaluation of intradialytic parenteral nutrition. *AJKD 33*:186–192.

Gilbert, S., Hatton, J., & Magnuson, B. (1996). How to minimize interaction between phenytoin and enteral feedings: Two approaches. *Nutr Clin Pract 11*:28–31.

Harris, J.A., & Benedict, F.G. (1919). *A biometric study of basal metabolism in man*. Washington, DC: Carnegie Institute of Washington, Publ. no. 279.

Heath, D.L., & Vink, R. (1999). Secondary mechanisms in

traumatic brain injury: A nurse's perspective. *J Neurosci Nurs 31*:97–105.

Heyland, D.K. (1998). Nutritional support in the critically ill patient. *Crit Care Clin 14*:423–440.

Heyland, D.K., Konopad, E., Alberda, C., et al. (1999). How well do critically ill patients tolerate early, intragastric enteral feeding? Results of a prospective, multicenter trial. *Nutr Clin Pract 14*:23–28.

Heyland, D., & Mandell, L.A. (1992). Gastric colonization by gram-negative bacilli and nosocomial pneumonia in the intensive care unit patient: Evidence for causation. *Chest 101*:187–193.

Janssens, J., Peeters, T.L., Vantrappen, G., et al. (1990). Improvement of gastric emptying in diabetic gastroparesis by erythromycin. *N Engl J Med 322*:1028–1031.

Johnson, L.R. (1997). *Gastrointestinal physiology*. St. Louis: Mosby.

Jolly, A.F., & Blank, R. (1994). Refeeding syndrome. In G.P. Zaloga (ed.). *Nutrition in critical care* (pp. 765–782). St. Louis: C.V. Mosby.

Katz, D.P., Wiese, S., & Gay, W.A. (1996). Cardiac metabolism and nutrition support. In V. Kvetan & D.R. Dantzker, (eds.). *The critically ill cardiac patient*. Philadelphia: Lippincott-Raven.

Klein, D.G. (1999). Management strategies for improving outcome following severe head injury. *Crit Care Nurs Clin North Am 11*:209–225.

Krenitsky, J. (1996). Nutrition and the immune system. *AACN Clin Issues 7*:359–369.

Lehmann, S. (1993). Nutritional support in the hypermetabolic patient. *Crit Care Nurs Clin North Am 5*:97–103.

Lennie, T.A. (1997). The metabolic response to injury: Current perspectives and nursing implications. *Dimensions Crit Care Nurs 16*:79–87.

Loan, T.D., Magnuson, B., & Williams, S. (1998, August). Debunking six myths about enteral feeding. *Nursing 98*:43–48.

Magnuson, B., Hatton, J., Williams, S., & Loan, T. (1999). Tolerance and efficacy of enteral nutrition for neurosurgical patients in pentobarbital coma. *Nutr Clin Pract 14*: 131–134.

Malone, A.M. (1997). Is a pulmonary enteral formula warranted for patients with pulmonary dysfunction? *Nutr Clin Pract 12*:168–171.

Merguerian, P., Perel, A., Wald, U., Feinsod, M., & Cotev, S. (1981). Persistent nonketotic hyperglycemia as a grave prognostic sign in head-injured patients. *Crit Care Med* 9:838–840.

Montecalvo, M.A., Steger, K.A., Farber, H.W., et al. (1992). Nutritional outcome and pneumonia in critical care patients randomized to gastric versus jejunal tube feedings. *Crit Care Med 20*:1377–1387.

National Institutes of Health. (1998). *Clinical guidelines on the identification, evaluation, and treatment of overweight and obesity in adults*. Rockville, MD.

Ohri, S.K., Bjarnason, I., Pathi, I., et al. (1993). Cardiopulmonary bypass impairs small intestinal transport and increases gut permeability. *Annals of Thoracic Surgery* 55:1080–1086.

Ott, L., & Young, B. (1994). Neurosurgery. In G.P. Zaloga (ed.). *Nutrition in critical care* (pp. 691–706). St. Louis: C.V. Mosby.

Pleuss, J. (1998). Alterations in nutritional status. In C.M. Porth (ed.). Pathophysiology: Concepts of altered health status (5th ed.) (pp. 1243–1263). Philadelphia: Lippincott.

Rieg, L.S. (1993). Metabolic alterations and nutritional management. *AACN Clin Issues 4*:388–398.

Robertson, C.S., Clifton, G.L., & Grossman, R.G. (1984). Oxygen utilization and cardiovascular function in head-injured patients. *Neurosurgery 15*:307–313.

Rombeau, J. (1993). *Clinical nutrition: Parenteral nutrition* (2nd ed.). Philadelphia: W.B. Saunders.

Ruffolo, D.C., (1998). Gastric tonometry: Early warning of tissue hypoperfusion. *Crit Care Nurs Q 21*:26–32.

Shuster, M.H. (1996). Nutrition in the critically ill. In J.M. Clochesy, C. Breu, S. Cardin, A.A. Whittaker, & E.B. Rudy (eds.). *Critical care nursing* (p. 250). Philadelphia: W.B. Saunders.

Smith, S.L. (1996). Patients with liver dysfunction. In J.M. Clochesy, C. Breu, S. Cardin, A.A. Whittaker, & E.B. Rudy (eds.). *Critical care nursing* (p. 250). Philadelphia: W.B. Saunders.

Spain, D.A., DeWeese, C., Reynolds, M.A., & Richardson, J.D. (1995). Transpyloric passage of feeding tubes in patients with head injureis does not decrease complications. *J Trauma: Injury, Infection, and Critical Care* 39:1100–1102.

Stechmiller, J.K., Treloar, D., & Allen, N. (1997). Gut dysfunction in critically ill patients: A review of the literature. *Am J Crit Care* 6:204–209.

Tack, J., Janssens, J., Vantrappen, G., et al. (1992). Effect of erythromycin on gastric motility in controls and in diabetic gastroparesis, *Gastroenterology 103*:72–79.

Trujillo, E.B., Robinson, M.K., & Jacobs, D.O. (1999). Nutritional assessment in the critically ill. *Critical Care Nurse 19*:67–78.

Whitney, J.D., & Heitkemper, M.M. (1999). Modifying perfusion, nutrition, and stess to promote wound healing in patients with acute wounds. *Heart & Lung* 28:123–133.

Young, B., Ott, L., Dempsey, R., Haack, D., & Tibbs, P. (1989). Relationship between admission hyperglycemia and neurological outcome of severe brain-injured patients. *Ann Surg 210*:466–473.

Young, B., Ott, L., Yingling, B., & McClain, C.J. (1992). Nutrition and brain injury. *J Neurotrauma* 9(suppl. 1):S375–S383.

ADDITIONAL READINGS

Bass, M. (1998). Fluid and electrolyte management of ascites in patients with cirrhosis. *Crit Care Nurs Clin North Am* 4:459–467.

Cobean, R.A., Gentilello, L.M., Parker, A., Jurkovich, G.L., & Maier, R.V. (1992). Nutritional assesment using a pulmonary artery catheter. *J Trauma 33*:452–456.

Kaminski, M.V., & Blumeyer, T.J. (1994). Albumin supplementation: Starling's law as a guide to therapy and literature review. In G.P. Zaloga (ed.). *Nutrition in critical care* (pp. 143–165). St. Louis: C.V. Mosby.

Keithley, J.P., & Eisenberg, P. (1993). The significance of enteral nutrition in the intensive care unit patient. *Crit Care Nurs Clin North Am* 5:23–29.

Long, C.L. (1984). The energy and protein requirements of the critically ill patient. In R.A. Wright & S. Heymsfield (eds.). *Nutritional assessment*. St. Louis: C.V. Mosby.

Metheny, N.A., Aud, M.A., & Wunderlich, R.J. (1999). Survey of bedside methods used to detect pulmonary aspiration of enteral formula in intubated tube-fed patients. *Am J Crit Care* 8:160–167.

Metheny, N., McSweeney, M., Wehrle, M.A., & Wiersema, L. (1990). Effectiveness of the auscultatory method in predicting feeding tube location. *Nursing Research* 39:262–267.

Saffle, J.R., Wiebke, G., Jennings, K., Morris, S.E., & Barton, R.G. (1997). Randomized trial of immune-enhancing enteral nutrition in burn patients. *J Trauma: Injury, Infection, and Critical Care* 42:793–802.

Sabol, V.K., & Friedenberg, F.K. (1990). Diarrhea. *AACN Clin Issues* 8:425–436.

Zaloga, G.P., & MacGregor, D.A. (1990). What to consider when choosing enteral or parenteral nutrition. *J Crit Ill* 11:1180–1200.

Module 23

Acute Hematologic Dysfunction

Kathleen D. Wagner

This self-study module presents the physiologic and pathophysiologic processes involved in acute hematologic dysfunction and management of the patient who is experiencing one or several blood cell abnormalities. The module is composed of six sections. Section One is a review of the anatomy and physiology of the blood. Section Two provides an overview of the assessment and diagnosis of hematologic problems. Sections Three through Five describe specific hematologic disorders, including disorders of red cells, white cells, and platelets (hemostasis). Finally, Section Six provides a brief discussion of the nursing implications that commonly apply to patients with hematologic problems. Each section includes a set of review questions to help the learner evaluate her or his understanding of the section's content before moving on to the next section. All Section Reviews and module Pretest and Posttest include answers. It is suggested that the learner review those concepts answered incorrectly in the review questions before proceeding to the next section.

Objectives

Following completion of this module, the learner will be able to

1. Describe the anatomic components and physiologic functions of the blood.
2. Discuss the assessment and diagnosis of hematologic disorders.
3. Describe the etiology, pathophysiology, clinical manifestations, and management of red cell disorders.
4. Discuss the etiology, pathophysiology, clinical manifestations, and management of white cell disorders.
5. Describe the etiology, pathophysiology, clinical manifestations, and management of thrombocytopenia and disseminated intravascular coagulation (DIC).
6. Discuss the nursing implications appropriate to managing the care of patients experiencing acute hematologic dysfunction.

Pretest

1. An inadequate amount of vitamins B_{12} and/or folic acid in the body causes
   A. bone marrow failure
   B. slower reproduction of red blood cells (RBCs)
   C. uncontrolled proliferation of RBCs
   D. overstimulation of bone marrow cells
2. Adequate iron is a crucial part of hemoglobin because
   A. it cements the hemoglobin chain together
   B. it facilitates the release of oxygen to the tissues
   C. the heme molecule attaches to it to make a chain
   D. the oxygen molecule attaches to it

3. The process by which circulating neutrophils and macrophages squeeze out of a capillary to migrate to the site of injury is called
   A. diapedesis
   B. chemotaxis
   C. margination
   D. translocation
4. Platelets are not actually cells—they are _________ from __________ in the bone marrow.
   A. granules; leukocytes
   B. lysosomes; erythrocytes
   C. cell fragments; megakaryocytes
   D. secretions; plasma cells
5. An elevated reticulocyte count in the presence of anemia indicates that the
   A. RBCs are being destroyed prematurely
   B. bone marrow is depressed
   C. RBCs are be sequestered in the spleen
   D. bone marrow is functioning correctly
6. Hematocrit is best defined as a measurement of
   A. weight
   B. concentration
   C. volume
   D. dehydration
7. When a shift to the left occurs in the neutrophil count, it refers to a(n)
   A. elevated band level
   B. decreased band level
   C. elevated seg level
   D. decreased seg level
8. The bone discomfort associated with anemia is usually caused by
   A. inflammation of the bone
   B. decreased oxygen in the bone marrow
   C. irritation of nerves in the bone marrow
   D. increased hematopoietic activity in bone marrow
9. The most common form of anemia found worldwide is
   A. megaloblastic anemias
   B. iron-deficiency anemia
   C. aplastic anemia
   D. blood loss anemia
10. The definitive treatment for aplastic anemia is
    A. blood transfusions
    B. antibiotic therapy
    C. immunosuppressant therapy
    D. bone marrow transplant
11. The most common cause of blood loss anemia is
    A. alcohol abuse
    B. menorrhagia
    C. trauma
    D. gastrointestinal bleeding
12. When severe neutropenia is present, the primary symptom of infection may be
    A. pus formation
    B. fever
    C. local edema
    D. local erythema
13. About 70 percent of acute lymphocytic leukemia (ALL) cases involves proliferation of immature
    A. B cells
    B. T cells
    C. plasma cells
    D. megakaryocytes
14. The major characteristic of chronic lymphocytic leukemia (CLL) is the presence of ___________ mature lymphocytes.
    A. larger-than-normal
    B. fewer-than-normal
    C. irregularly shaped
    D. abnormally small
15. The MOST common cause of death in adults with acute leukemia is
    A. hemorrhage
    B. infection
    C. tissue hypoxia
    D. brain infiltration
16. A "complete remission" is obtained when there are no leukemic cells in the
    A. lymph nodes and bone marrow
    B. lymph nodes and peripheral blood
    C. bone marrow and brain
    D. bone marrow and peripheral blood
17. The initial treatment of the acute leukemias is
    A. surgery
    B. chemotherapy
    C. radiation therapy
    D. bone marrow transplant
18. Treatment of CLL is usually initiated
    A. when the WBC count is > 100,000
    B. when the hemoglobin is < 6
    C. at stage III or IV of disease
    D. at the time of diagnosis
19. The typical bleeding pattern of thrombocytopenia involves bleeding into the
    A. joints
    B. peritoneum
    C. internal organs
    D. skin and mucous membranes
20. The major treatment of idiopathic thrombocytopenia purpura is
    A. alkylating chemotherapy
    B. platelet transfusions
    C. corticosteroid therapy
    D. bone marrow transplant
21. The activity intolerance created by some of the hematologic disorders is specifically related to a(n)
    A. intravascular fluid volume loss
    B. O_2 supply-and-demand imbalance
    C. decreased systemic blood flow
    D. inadequate secondary defenses

22. A nursing diagnosis that commonly addresses tissue hypoxia associated with hematologic disorders includes
    A. fatigue
    B. pain
    C. risk for infection
    D. decreased cardiac output

Pretest answers: 1. B, 2. D, 3. A, 4. C, 5. D, 6. B, 7. A, 8. D, 9. B, 10. D, 11. C, 12. B, 13. A, 14. D, 15. B, 16. D, 17. B, 18. C, 19. D, 20. C, 21. B, 22. A

Glossary

Anemia. A condition in which there is decreased numbers of RBCs, decreased hemoglobin, and/or decreased hematocrit

Band (stab). An immature neutrophil

Bandemia. Elevated serum band (immature neutrophil) level

Cell differentiation. Development of specific cell functions through a maturation process

Chemotaxis. Directional migration of leukocytes to the site of injury

Committed stem cell. A pluripotential stem cell that has committed its development to either the myeloid or lymphoid cell line

Diapedesis. The movement of WBCs through an intact vessel wall through ameboid movement

Erythrocytes. Red blood cells; part of the myeloid stem cell line; produced in the bone marrow

Granulocyte. A type of blood cell with granules located in the cytoplasm

Hemolytic anemia. Breakdown of red blood cells

Hemostasis. Stoppage of bleeding; stagnation of blood flow

Hypochromic. The abnormal pale coloring of RBCs, indicating reduced hemoglobin content

Macrocytic. Abnormally large RBC

Macrophages. Mature monocytes, large phagocytes

Margination. The movement and adhering of circulating WBCs to the capillary wall in preparation for shifting out of the vessel to move to the site of injury

Mean corpuscular volume (MCV). A measurement of the size (volume) of RBCs

Mean corpuscular hemoglobin (MCH). A measurement of the average weight (concentration) of hemoglobin in red blood cells

Mean corpuscular hemoglobin concentration (MCHC). The ratio of the weight of hemoglobin to the volume of erythrocytes (Turgeon, 1999, p. 76)

Microcytic. Abnormally small cell

Neutropenia. Abnormally low number of neutrophils

Neutrophils. Polymorphonuclear granulocytes of the myeloid cell line

Normochromic. The normal coloring of RBCs, indicating normal hemoglobin content

Platelet factor 4. A protein located in the platelet alpha granules

Polycythemia. Abnormally elevated red blood cell mass

Polymorphonuclear. The presence of multiple nuclei in a cell (e.g., neutrophils)

Normocytic. Normal-sized cells

Reticulocytes. Immature RBCs

Reticuloendothelial system. A group of cells found throughout the body that are capable of ingesting particles; cells include macrophages, reticular cells, and other tissue macrophages

Segmented cells (segs). Mature neutrophils

Thrombosis. Intravascular aggregation of cells creating a blood clot

Abbreviations

ALL. Acute lymphocytic leukemia

AML. Acute myelocytic leukemia

ATG. Antithrombocyte globulin

CBC. Complete blood count

CLL. Chronic lymphocytic leukemia

CML. Chronic myelocytic leukemia

DIC. Disseminated intravascular coagulation

EBV. Epstein–Barr virus

G-SCF. Granulocyte-colony stimulating factor

Hgb. Hemoglobin

Hct. Hematocrit

HLA. Histocompatibility antigen

HTLV-1. Human T cell leukemia virus type 1

IF. Intrinsic factor

IgG. Immunoglobulin G

ITP. Idiopathic thrombocytopenic purpura

MCH. Mean corpuscular hemoglobin

MCHC. Mean corpuscular hemoglobin concentration

MCV. Mean corpuscular volume

Ph[1]. Philadelphia chromosome

PHSC. Pluripotential hematopoietic stem cell

PMN. Polymorphonuclear neutrophil

RBC. Red blood cell

SLE. Systemic lupus erythematosus

WBC. White blood cell

SECTION ONE: Anatomy and Physiology of the Blood

At the completion of this section, the learner will be able to describe the anatomic components and physiologic functions of the blood.

Blood is composed of plasma, plasma proteins, and blood cells. Blood cells include **erythrocytes** (red blood cells), leukocytes (white blood cells), and thrombocytes (platelets). All three types of blood cells develop from the same stem cells, called *pluripotential hematopoietic stem cells (PHSCs)*, which reside in the bone marrow. Once appropriately induced to reproduce a particular type of blood cell, the pluripotential stem cell divides. During PHSC division, one cell may remain as a PHSC while the other becomes a *committed stem cell* of either the myeloid or lymphoid cell line (Fig. 23–1). This means that the newly committed cell begins to mature down a particular cell development pathway of cell growth and differentiation. The term *cell differentiation* refers to the maturation process that a cell undergoes. It begins as an immature, undifferentiated cell with no specific functions and ultimately becomes a mature, well-differentiated cell with specific cell functions. The cell maturation process requires special proteins, called growth inducers and differentiation inducers. Factors external to the bone marrow trigger the formation of these special proteins. For example, chronic hypoxia induces increased production of erythrocytes (Guyton & Hall, 1997).

Erythrocytes

When compared to the total numbers of white cells and platelets (Table 23–1), it is readily apparent that red blood cells (RBCs) or erythrocytes are by far the most plentiful of the blood cells. There are six stages of erythrocyte development (Table 23–2). Maturation from stage one to stage six requires about 1 week.

The Roles of Erythropoietin and Vitamins B_{12} and Folic Acid

Erythrocyte production is tightly regulated. The purpose of erythrocytes is oxygen transport; thus, regulation is based on the level of tissue oxygenation, which is a function of tissue demand and oxygen transport. Erythrocyte production is regulated by *erythropoietin*, a circulating hormone that is primarily produced by the kidneys (about 90 percent). It is believed that erythropoietin may be produced in the renal tubular cells. The renal tubular cells are major consumers of oxygen that are particularly sensitive to lowering oxygen levels. Erythropoietin is a critical part of an erythrocyte production feedback loop (Fig. 23–2). Two vitamins, B_{12} and folic acid, are essential to the maturation of erythrocytes for normal development of deoxyribonucleic acid (DNA). When an inadequate amount of either vitamin exists, it interferes with normal cell nucleus development and reproduction. As a result, erythrocytes mature and reproduce more slowly. They are misshapen, more fragile, and have a shorter life span than normal erythrocytes.

Hemoglobin

Hemoglobin is sometimes referred to as the respiratory protein since its function is to transport oxygen. As its name suggests, hemoglobin has two components—heme (nonprotein) and globin (protein). One heme molecule contains one iron atom and one oxygen molecule. The oxygen molecule (O_2) located in hemoglobin is attached only to the single iron atom in the molecule; thus, when there is deficient iron in the body (e.g., iron-deficiency anemia), the oxygen-carrying capacity is significantly reduced. A heme molecule joins with a polypeptide chain to form a hemoglobin chain. It takes four hemoglobin chains, linked together, to form one hemoglobin molecule. In a normal person, there are about 15 g of hemoglobin in every 100 mL of blood. Each gram of hemoglobin can bind with a maximum of about 1.34 mL of oxygen. Normally, the hemoglobin in 100 mL of blood (if fully saturated with oxygen) can bind with 20 mL of oxygen. Oxygen combines with hemoglobin loosely and reversibly. This means that oxygen can be loaded up on the hemoglobin, transported to the tissues, and then released from the hemoglobin to diffuse across the capillary membrane into the tissues.

Leukocytes

The environment in which we live is not a sterile one. We are exposed to potentially disease-producing organisms (pathogens) on a daily basis. It is through the strong

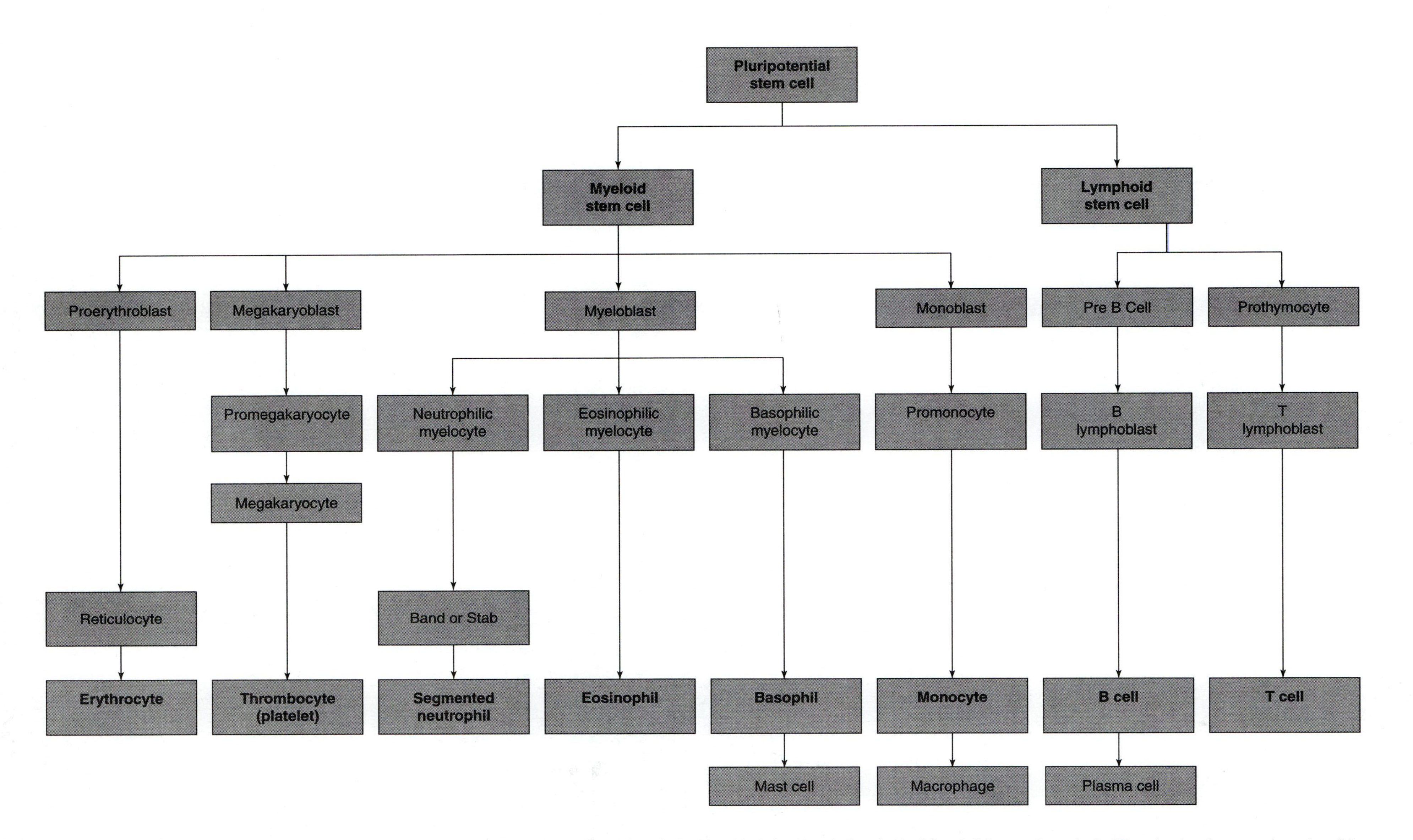

Figure 23–1. Simplified illustration of blood cell lineage. Committed cell proliferation follows either the myeloid cell line (shaded area) or the lymphoid cell line. Cells become increasingly differentiated as they move down the cell line toward maturity. *(Adapted From Guyton, A.C., & Hall, J.E. [1997].* Human physiology and mechanisms of disease, *6th ed. Philadelphia: W.B. Saunders; and Turgeon, M.L. [1999].* Clinical hematology: Theory and procedures, *3rd ed. Philadelphia: Lippincott-Williams & Wilkins.)*

TABLE 23–1. BLOOD CELL COUNT (ADULT)

CELL TYPE	NORMAL RANGE
Red blood cells (million/μL × 10^{12}/L)	Male: 4.6–6.0 Female: 4.0–5.0
Reticulocyte count (%)	0.5–1.5
RDW (%)	11.5–14.5%
White blood cells (cells/μL)	4,500–10,000
Differential counts (% of total WBC count)	
Neutrophils	50–70%
Segs	50–65%
Bands	0–5%
Basophils	0.4–1.0%
Eosinophils	1–3%
Monocytes	4–6%
Lymphocytes	25–35%
Platelets (cells/μL)	150,000–400,000

Sources: Kee, J.L. (1999). Laboratory & diagnostic tests with nursing implications, *5th ed. Stanford, CT: Appleton & Lange; and Turgeon, M.L. (1999).* Clinical hematology: Theory and procedures, *3rd ed. Philadelphia: Lippincott-Williams & Wilkins.*

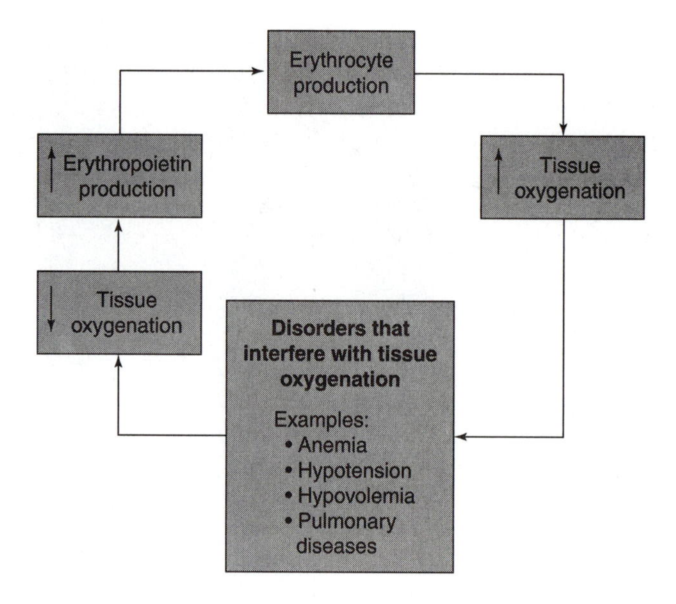

Figure 23–2. Erythrocyte production feedback loop.

protective mechanisms of the immune system that we are able to survive such constant pathogen exposure. The leukocytes (white blood cells) are the circulating cells of the immune system. There are five types of leukocytes, including neutrophils, monocytes, lymphocytes, eosinophils, and basophils. The leukocytes are produced in the bone marrow, with the exception of lymphocytes, which are primarily produced in the lymph tissue. Leukocytes comprise only about 1 percent of the total blood volume (Sommers, 1998). While their quantities are limited, they are an extremely quick and powerful defense system. This section focuses on neutrophils and briefly discusses monocytes. Lymphocytes are presented in detail in Sections Four and Five of Module 24.

TABLE 23–2. ERYTHROCYTE DEVELOPMENT

STAGE	CELL NAME	COMMENTS
1	Proerythroblast	• Iron is taken in at this stage
2	Basophil erythroblast	
3	Polychromatophil erythroblast	• Hemoglobin begins to appear
4	Orthochromatic erythroblast	• Significant increase in amount of hemoglobin present • Nucleus disappears • Last stage where mitosis occurs
5	Reticulocyte	• Matures in bone marrow initially and moves to circulating blood • No nucleus present
6	Erythrocyte	• Approximately one-half the size of the proerythroblast • Life span: approximately 120 days

Sources: Guyton, A.C., & Hall, J.E. (1997). Human physiology and mechanisms of disease, *6th ed. Philadelphia: W.B. Saunders; and Turgeon, M.L. (1999).* Clinical hematology: Theory and procedures, *3rd ed. Philadelphia: Lippincott-Williams & Wilkins.*

Neutrophils

Neutrophils, eosinophils, basophils, and monocytes have a common origin, the myelocyte. Neutrophils, eosinophils, and basophils are all *polymorphonuclear granulocytes*. The term **polymorphonuclear** refers to the presence of multiple nuclei, and explains why they are commonly referred to as *polys* or *polymorphonuclear neutrophils (PMNs)*. Neutrophils significantly outnumber all of the other types of leukocytes, comprising 50 to 70 percent of the total leukocyte (WBC) count (Kee, 1999). The myelocyte cell lineage is illustrated in Figure 23–1.

The term **granulocyte** refers to cells with granules located within the cytoplasm. The granules contain special enzymes that break down foreign substances. According to Parslow (1994), neutrophils mature in the bone marrow and are held there for about 5 days in reserve before being sent into the general circulation. At any one time, there are approximately 50 billion mature neutrophils in the circulation. Once released from the bone marrow, they have a brief life span of only 24 to 48 hours; thus, they must be reproduced at an extremely fast rate to keep up with the rapid turnover, accounting for about 60 percent of the bone marrow's total activity.

Neutrophils are the immune system's first line of defense in the presence of an acute infection or inflammation. They are first at the scene, within 90 minutes of the injury event (Sommers, 1998). Neutrophils are responsible for the formation of pus. As neutrophils die, their degrading enzymes are released, causing breakdown and liquefaction of local cells as well as foreign substances (Parslow, 1994). This forms pus, a thin liquid residue. Pus is an important indicator of inflammation. This becomes important in the presence of neutropenia and will be discussed in more detail later in the module.

Monocytes

Monocytes are large, single-nucleus phagocytes that provide the second line of defense. They act as long-term backup for **neutrophils,** arriving at the scene within about 5 hours of the event. Monocytes and neutrophils become the predominant cell types at the site of injury within 48 hours of the precipitating event (Sommers, 1998). Monocytes live much longer than neutrophils, with a life span of 4 to 5 days. Monocytes circulate in the blood for about a day before taking up residence in a tissue, becoming tissue macrophages (histiocytes) (Parslow, 1994). Tissue macrophages can remain in a fixed position within the tissue for months or years until they are required to protect the tissue through their phagocytic functions.

Circulating monocytes are immature immune cells that do not actively participate in defense. Guyton and Hall (1997) explain that monocytes undergo maturational changes once they move into the tissues. During the maturation process, they enlarge by up to fivefold and develop a very large number of lysosomes in their cytoplasm. Lysosomes provide a digestive system that can digest nutrients, bacteria, or other particles that are brought into the cell. Once they have matured, the monocytes are called **macrophages,** which are powerful phagocytes.

Migration Properties of Neutrophils and Macrophages

Circulating neutrophils and macrophages require some means to recognize where they are needed, and then they must be able to transfer from the circulation to the site of injury. The process by which they do this involves multiple steps, including margination, diapedesis, migration, and chemotaxis. Soon after initiation of the inflammatory response, the capillary endothelium becomes more permeable, allowing fluid to escape into the inflamed or injured area. The loss of fluid locally results in increased blood viscosity and increased concentration of cells in the local capillaries. Sommers (1998) explains that when tissue becomes inflamed, a variety of chemicals, including chemical mediators and cytokines, are released at the site of injury. These chemical substances cause alterations of local capillary endothelial cells and stimulate leukocytes to increase their release of adhesion molecules. **Margination** occurs as circulating leukocytes begin to accumulate and adhere to the capillary wall. Once the cells have adhered to the capillary wall, they develop pseudopods and squeeze out of the capillary using ameboid movement, a process called **diapedesis.** Once the leukocyte is outside the capillary, it must have guidance to move to the correct location. This is accomplished through **chemotaxis,** which is defined by Lewis (2000) as "the directional migration of white blood cells (WBCs) along a concentration gradient of chemotactic factors, which are substances that attract leukocytes to the site of inflammation" (p. 191). The leukocytes then follow the signal, traveling by ameboid action to move to the site. Figure 23–3 illustrates this concept.

Thrombocytes

The hematologic system is sometimes referred to as a fluid organ. Correct functioning of an organ requires that its borders remain intact. The blood vessel walls constitute the hematologic system's borders. Vascular integrity is maintained through two closely interwoven mechanisms, hemostasis and blood coagulation. Discussion here will focus on the cellular component of hemostasis, the thrombocytes (platelets).

Platelets are not actually cells. They are tiny cell fragments composed of cytoplasm that are shed from megakaryocytes in the bone marrow. Mazur (1998) suggests that the mechanism by which shedding occurs is not well understood. One theory suggests that mature megakaryocytes may transform in response to some unknown signal, forming spiderlike projections called *proplatelets*. These tiny proplatelets break off from the megakaryocyte due to shearing force when they come into contact with blood flow in the bone marrow sinusoids. The normal platelet count in an adult is 150,000 to 400,000/μL (Kee, 1999). Platelet production is closely regulated by thrombopoietin, which is primarily produced by the liver. Certain cytokines (e.g., interleukin-3) are also known to stimulate the production of platelets using different mechanisms (Mazur, 1998). Mature platelets survive for 8 to 10 days, with about two-thirds being in the circulation at all times and the remaining one-third being

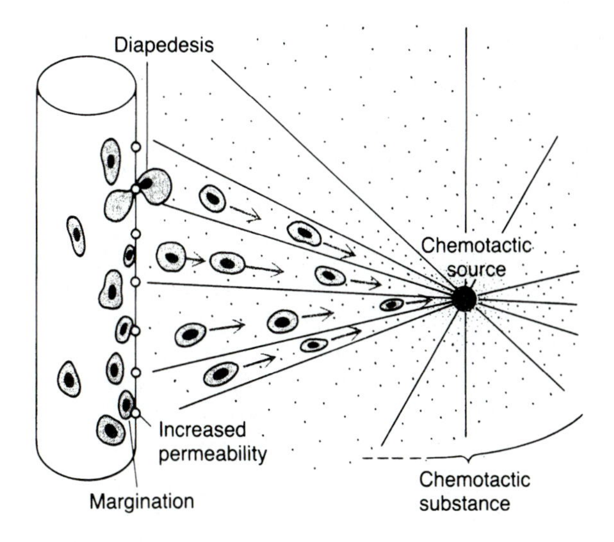

Figure 23–3. Movement of leukocytes to injury site. Movement of neutrophils by the process of chemotaxis toward an area of tissue damage. *(From Guyton, A.C., & Hall, J.E. [1997].* Human physiology and mechanisms of disease, *6th ed. [p. 282]. Philadelphia: W.B. Saunders.)*

stored in the spleen. The stored platelets are continuously exchanging with circulating platelets (Turgeon, 1999).

The Hemostatic Function of Platelets

Guyton and Hall (1997) define **hemostasis** as "prevention of blood loss." Platelets play a crucial role in hemostasis by creating a platelet plug to seal off leaking vessels. Their internal structures also contain a variety of coagulation-related proteins and enzymes that all interact with the coagulation process. Under normal circumstances, platelets circulate freely throughout the vascular system as smooth, disk-shaped particles. When vessel endothelial injury occurs, special activating factors, such as thrombin and platelet-activating factor, stimulate platelet hemostatic activities. Upon activation, the platelets undergo significant changes including adhesion and aggregation. According to Turgeon (1999), within 1 to 2 minutes after vascular integrity is lost, platelets begin to adhere to the collagen fibers of the damaged subendothelium. To do this, they rapidly reshape themselves, developing fingerlike projections (pseudopods) along the vessel's endothelial surface. As the platelets accumulate, they begin to aggregate or clump together and eventually form a cohesive mass, called a *platelet plug*. Once the platelet plug is formed, it is stabilized and consolidated by fibrinogen, eventually forming a fibrin clot. Platelet plugs are particularly effective in rapid repair of small vascular leaks.

In summary, the major solid components of the blood include erythrocytes, leukocytes, and thrombocytes. All of these cells come from the same pluripotential stem cell but take different committed pathways to maturation. Erythrocytes provide an effective oxygen transport system. Adequate production of healthy erythrocytes requires erythropoietin and vitamins B_{12} and folic acid. Hemoglobin, the major component of the erythrocyte, is the actual oxygen carrier. Hemoglobin requires iron as an integral part of its molecular structure. Leukocytes are the circulating cells of the immune system. There are five different types of leukocytes: neutrophils, monocytes, lymphocytes, eosinophils, and basophils. Each one plays a somewhat unique role in providing immune defense. Neutrophils are small, powerful, granulated polymorphonuclear cells that are the first line of defense. Monocytes, upon activation as macrophages, provide the second line of defense. Neutrophils and monocytes are able to leave the vascular system and move to a site of inflammation or infection through the mechanisms of margination, diapedesis, migration, and chemotaxis. Thrombocytes are tiny cell fragments that protect the body's vascular integrity. They are an integral part of the hemostatic and coagulation functions. Their major activity is the sealing of tears in the blood vessels, thus stopping bleeding. Table 23–1 provides a summary of the normal serum values of the blood cells.

SECTION ONE REVIEW

1. Upon appropriate stimulation, pluripotential hematopoietic stem cells divide and create a
   A. RBC
   B. WBC
   C. committed stem cell
   D. megakaryocyte
2. The purpose of the erythrocyte is
   A. oxygen transport
   B. nutrient transport
   C. hemostasis
   D. protection
3. An inadequate amount of vitamins B_{12} and/or folic acid in the body causes
   A. bone marrow failure
   B. slower reproduction of RBCs
   C. uncontrolled proliferation of RBCs
   D. overstimulation of bone marrow cells
4. Adequate iron is a crucial part of hemoglobin because
   A. it cements the hemoglobin chain together
   B. it facilitates the release of oxygen to the tissues
   C. the heme molecule attaches to it to make a chain
   D. the oxygen molecule attaches to it
5. The primary purpose of granules located in the granulocyte, such as neutrophils, is to
   A. detect the presence of infection
   B. breakdown foreign substances
   C. stimulate production of monocytes
   D. initiate ameboid cell movement
6. To actively participate in phagocytic activities, monocytes must mature into
   A. neutrophils
   B. lysosomes
   C. cytokines
   D. macrophages
7. The process by which circulating neutrophils and macrophages are able to squeeze out of a capillary to go to the site of injury is called
   A. diapedesis
   B. chemotaxis
   C. margination
   D. translocation

8. Platelets are not actually cells, they are ________ from ________ in the bone marrow.
   A. granules; leukocytes
   B. lysosomes; erythrocytes
   C. cell fragments; megakaryocytes
   D. secretions; plasma cells

Answers: 1. C, 2. A, 3. B, 4. D, 5. B, 6. D, 7. A, 8. C, 9. B

SECTION TWO: Assessment and Diagnosis

At the completion of this section, the learner will be able to discuss the assessment and diagnosis of hematologic disorders.

Learning some basic information about laboratory tests that evaluate blood cells can assist the nurse in gaining a better understanding of the patient's condition and cause of clinical manifestations. It can also assist the nurse in developing an effective plan of care based on this understanding. A proactive knowledge of such tests may alert the nurse to potential complications so that preventative measures can be taken in a timely manner.

Evaluation of Erythrocytes

Basic information about the size, shape, and concentration of erythrocytes is easily obtained through performing peripheral blood smears. Tests that are commonly used to evaluate erythrocytes include reticulocyte count, mean corpuscular volume (MCV), total RBC count, hemoglobin and hematocrit, and evaluation of erythrocyte color. Table 23–1 provides a summary of normal values of these tests.

Reticulocyte Count

Reticulocytes are immature erythrocytes that are easily detected and measured. Under normal circumstances, only about 1 percent of circulating erythrocytes are reticulocytes that have entered the circulation to replace dying mature erythrocytes. There are two general reasons why the reticulocyte count rises: (1) due to an increase in circulating reticulocytes, or (2) due to a reduction in circulating red cells. A common type of reticulocyte count is the "corrected" count that corrects for the presence of anemia. The corrected reticulocyte count is calculated as:

$$\% \text{ Reticulocytes} \times \frac{\text{Hct (patient)}}{\text{Hct (normal)}}$$

Obtaining a corrected reticulocyte count helps differentiate between types of anemia. An elevation (> 1.5 percent) occurs when the bone marrow is stimulated by erythropoietin to produce more reticulocytes. As a result of erythropoietin stimulation, reticulocytes are produced and released from the bone marrow at a faster rate. An elevated reticulocyte count is present in types of anemia where the bone marrow is functioning normally (e.g., blood loss and extrinsic hemolytic anemias). A reduced reticulocyte count suggests that the bone marrow is unable to respond to the increased demand (e.g., aplastic anemia, bone marrow depression or failure).

Mean Corpuscular Volume

Rose and Berliner (1998) explain that measurement of **mean corpuscular volume (MCV)** evaluates the size (volume) of the RBCs. Using MCV criteria, anemias can be divided into three categories: microcytic, normocytic, and macrocytic. A low MCV value indicates the presence of *microcytic* RBCs, which are smaller than normal in size and are present in such conditions as iron deficiency anemia and thalassemia. Normocytic RBCs are normal in size and are present in blood loss anemia, aplastic anemia, and early iron-deficiency anemia. *Macrocytic* RBCs are larger than normal in size and are found in conditions such as vitamin B_{12} deficiency and drug-induced anemias. Anemias associated with chronic illness are generally either microcytic or normocytic.

Mean corpuscular hemoglobin (MCH) and **mean corpuscular hemoglobin concentration (MCHC)** are frequently measured with MCV; however, they provide little additional information that is not found in the MCV since MCH values parallel MCV values (Rose & Berliner, 1998). The MCH measures the average weight (concentration) of hemoglobin in red blood cells. The MCHC is "the ratio of the weight of hemoglobin to the volume of erythrocytes." (Turgeon, 1999, p. 76).

Total RBC Count

The healthy adult has between 4 to 6 million/µL x 10^{12} red blood cells (Kee, 1999). Men normally have a higher RBC count than women or children. Abnormally low levels are associated with specific anemias (e.g., blood loss, chronic renal failure), alcoholic cirrhosis, and other conditions. Abnormally high levels may be seen in posthemorrhage states, leukemias, *hemolytic* and sickle cell anemias, and other conditions.

Hemoglobin and Hematocrit

HEMOGLOBIN (HGB). Hemoglobin has been discussed in the previous section. Higher-than-normal Hgb levels may result from hemoconcentration (e.g., dehydration), polycythemia, severe burns, and others. Lower than normal levels may result from certain anemias (e.g., aplastic, iron deficiency), hemorrhage, hepatic cirrhosis, leukemias, and many other conditions (Kee, 1999). Hemoglobin and the RBC count do not maintain a completely parallel relationship with each other. As an example, Kee explains that when iron deficiency anemia is present, a person could have a normal RBC count with a decreased hemoglobin level. Table 23–3 summarizes the severity of anemia based on hemoglobin levels.

HEMATOCRIT (HCT). The hematocrit is a concentration measurement. It is the volume (in milliliters) of packed red blood cells in 100 mL of blood and is stated as a percentage. A higher-than-normal hematocrit suggests dehydration situations, such as severe diarrhea or hypovolemia, polycythemia vera, secondary polycythemia (as seen with late chronic obstructive pulmonary disease [COPD]), and other problems. A lower-than-normal hematocrit is most commonly associated with leukemias and anemias (Kee, 1999).

Evaluation of Erythrocyte Color

Laboratory descriptions of erythrocytes as well as descriptions of erythrocytes in anemias usually include the descriptive terms, hypochromic or normochromic. Normally, the color of the biconcave disk-shaped RBC is pinkish-red in color in the outer two-thirds of the disk and very pale in the center third (called the *central pallor*). This 2:1 (dark-to-light) ratio gives the RBC its "healthy" appearance, reflecting the presence of adequate levels of hemoglobin. The normal color appearance is called **normochromic.** In certain anemia types, the 2:1 ratio is lost, and the central pallor extends beyond its one-third border. This extended pallor gives the RBC a pale, or **hypochromic** appearance. Hypochromic RBCs are most commonly seen in iron-deficiency anemia. Color alterations can also reflect cell immaturity, if the immature RBC has not yet taken in all of its hemoglobin.

Red Cell Mass

Red cell mass, also called red cell volume, is used to make a differential diagnosis of polycythemia. To perform this serum test, the patient has about 25 mL of blood drawn. This blood sample is radiolabeled with chromium (Cr-51) and then a known quantity of the labeled blood is reinjected into the patient's bloodstream. After about one hour, a second blood specimen is obtained. The second sample is then appropriately prepared and the circulating blood volume can be calculated. Patients with polycythemia have abnormally high circulating red cell volumes.

Red Cell Density Weight

The red cell density weight (RDW) is a recent addition to erythrocyte laboratory tests. According to Turgeon (1999), it is an index of RBC size variation and is calculated using a histogram. The normal RDW range is 11.5 percent to 14.5 percent. An elevated level (> 14.5 percent) has been associated with anemias caused by deficiencies in folic acid, B_{12}, and iron. Although it maintains an independent relationship with MCV, the RDW is often used in comparison with MCV values. The RDW value is an earlier indicator of nutritional deficiencies than the MCV value. Comparisons of the two tests can also help distinguish between types of anemia. For example, iron-deficiency anemia results in a high RDW and a normal to low MCV, and anemia associated with chronic disease results in a normal RDW and a normal to low MCV.

Evaluation of Leukocytes

While a simple WBC count is often adequate for general screening purposes, it is insufficient for gaining an in-depth understanding of the patient's infectious or inflammatory status. This information is obtained through the WBC differential count. The differential cell count breaks out the constituent cells of the WBCs: neutrophils (immature and mature), monocytes, eosinophils, and basophils. Table 23–1 summarizes the normal serum values.

Neutrophils

Neutrophils are measured in the serum as being mature or immature. The mature neutrophils, called **segmented cells,** or **segs** (referring to a segmented nucleus) normally constitute about 50 to 65 percent of the total WBC count (Kee, 1999). Immature neutrophils, called **bands** or **stabs**

TABLE 23–3. SEVERITY OF ANEMIA BASED ON HEMOGLOBIN LEVEL

SEVERITY	HEMOGLOBIN LEVEL	COMMON MANIFESTATIONS
Mild	10–14 g/dL	Asymptomatic usually *Cardiopulmonary:* None, or may have mild palpitations and/or dyspnea on exertion
Moderate	6–10 g/dL	May be asymptomatic if slow onset and/or patient is sedentary *Cardiopulmonary:* Dyspnea, increased palpitations *Other:* Fatigue
Severe	< 6 g/dL	Symptomatic at rest or with activity *Cardiopulmonary:* Tachycardia, increased blood pressure, tachypnea, dyspnea, orthopnea, congestive heart failure, myocardial infarction *Other:* Bone pain, pallor, vertigo, headache, and decreased activity tolerance

Source: O'Mara, A.M., & Whedon, M.B. (2000). Nursing management: Hematologic problems. In S.M. Lewis, M.M. Heitkemper, & S.R. Dirksen (eds.), Medical-surgical nursing, *5th ed. St. Louis: C.V. Mosby.*

(referring to the band- or horseshoe-shaped nucleus), normally makes up only 0 to 5 percent of the total WBC count (Kee). When called into action, neutrophils are produced at a faster rate by the bone marrow to meet the new demand. During periods of extremely high neutrophil production (e.g., severe infection), the bone marrow releases immature neutrophils, causing elevated band serum levels. The elevated band level **(bandemia)** is referred to as a "shift to the left." The neutrophil count increases (neutrophilia) in response to inflammatory disorders, bacterial infections, and tissue necrosis (Sommers, 1998). An abnormally low neutrophil count (neutropenia) can occur under several circumstances, including increased destruction, excessive demand, and decreased production. Neutropenia is discussed in detail in Section Four.

Monocytes

Monocytes comprise about 4 to 6 percent of the total WBC count (Kee, 1999). Elevated levels of monocytes (monocytosis) are associated with chronic infections (e.g., bacterial endocarditis and tuberculosis), rickettsial diseases (e.g., malaria), and inflammatory bowel disease. Monocytosis is also seen in Hodgkin's disease and monocytic leukemia (Sommers, 1998; Rosmarin, 1999).

Bone Marrow Biopsy

The bone marrow biopsy is used to rule out, confirm, or make a differential diagnosis of a hematologic disorder involving the bone marrow. It is often performed after suspicious cells are found in the peripheral blood. The biopsy is usually performed by needle aspiration and is usually taken from the sternum or iliac crest in an adult. The cells are examined for the presence, number, and type of abnormal cells and/or the absence of normal cells.

In summary, a variety of measurements are used to evaluate blood cells. This section provided an overview of some of the major tests used to evaluate the bone marrow, erythrocytes, and leukocytes. Tests that evaluate erythrocytes include the reticulocyte count, MCV, MCH, MCHC, total red cell count, hemoglobin, and hematocrit. Tests that evaluate leukocytes include the WBC count with or without the differential cell count. The differential is a more valuable test since it separates out and measures the relative values of each of the WBC component cells, including neutrophils, monocytes, lymphocytes, eosinophils, and basophils. The bone marrow biopsy is performed to confirm a diagnosis or to evaluate the severity of a hematologic problem.

SECTION TWO REVIEW

1. An elevated reticulocyte count in the presence of anemia indicates that the
   A. red blood cells are being destroyed prematurely
   B. bone marrow is depressed
   C. red blood cells are be sequestered in the spleen
   D. bone marrow is functioning correctly
2. An example of a condition that is associated with microcytic red blood cells (a low MCV) is
   A. aplastic anemia
   B. vitamin B_{12} deficiency anemia
   C. iron-deficiency anemia
   D. blood loss anemia
3. A higher-than-normal hemoglobin level can result from
   A. dehydration
   B. aplastic anemia
   C. hepatic cirrhosis
   D. leukemia
4. Hematocrit is best defined as a measurement of
   A. weight
   B. concentration
   C. volume
   D. dehydration
5. Segmented neutrophils normally make up ____ percent of the total WBC count.
   A. 20 to 35
   B. 35 to 50
   C. 50 to 65
   D. 65 to 80
6. When a shift to the left occurs in the neutrophil count, it refers to a(n)
   A. elevated band level
   B. decreased band level
   C. elevated seg level
   D. decreased seg level
7. An elevated monocyte (monocytosis) level is associated with
   A. early bacterial infection
   B. aplastic anemia
   C. hemolytic anemia
   D. chronic infections

Answers: 1. D, 2. C, 3. A, 4. B, 5. C, 6. A, 7. D

SECTION THREE: Red Blood Cell Disorders

At the completion of this section, the learner will be able to describe the etiology, pathophysiology, clinical manifestations, and management of red cell disorders.

Red blood cell disorders can be divided into two general groups: problems of too few RBCs (anemia) and problems of too many RBCs (polycythemia).

Anemia

The term **anemia** literally means "without blood." Its definition, however, refers to a reduction of or dysfunction in erythrocytes (RBCs). It can be clinically expressed in terms of a reduced RBC, hematocrit, or hemoglobin count. Anemia is not a disease; rather, it is an important symptom of some underlying disorder.

Clinical Manifestations

Regardless of the cause, the clinical manifestations of anemia are primarily attributable to one dysfunction—*impaired oxygen transport.* Additional manifestations may be present, related to the rate of onset of the anemia, the hematocrit level, and the underlying cause (Rose & Berliner, 1998).

Tissue Hypoxia Manifestations

Impaired oxygen transport causes tissue hypoxia. Compensatory mechanisms in response to tissue hypoxia result in tachycardia and tachypnea, and contribute to bone pain that may develop owing to increased hematopoietic activity in the bone marrow. Other hypoxia-related manifestations include easy fatigability, exercise intolerance, dyspnea, orthopnea, inability to concentrate, vertigo, irritability, anorexia, and others.

Rate of Onset

The speed with which the anemia occurs is an important factor in determining the severity of symptoms. When a mild-to-moderate anemia develops slowly the person often remains asymptomatic as long as the body is not taxed (increasing oxygen demand). Given a slow enough onset, a person may remain relatively asymptomatic (if sedentary) with a hemoglobin as low as 6 or 7 (Turgeon, 1999). When the onset of anemia is rapid (e.g., severe hemorrhage) there is not sufficient time for adequate compensatory mechanisms to set in, leading to potentially lethal consequences.

Underlying Cause

Because anemia is a symptom, not a disease, the patient's clinical manifestations usually reflect both the underlying disorder and the anemia. For example, a person with end-stage renal failure will have symptoms related to anemia plus symptoms resulting from severe renal dysfunction. Some of the anemias also have their own unique manifestations. For example, sickle cell anemia (sickle cell disease) has many unique symptoms related to microvascular occlusion. One type of anemia (aplastic) is part of a pancytopenia problem (involving two or more blood cell types). If pancytopenia is present, the patient will develop the clinical manifestations of deficiencies in the other cell types.

Categories of Anemias

There are different ways that the experts categorize anemias. The mechanism by which the anemia occurs is a particularly useful category system. There are three mechanisms: decreased RBC production, increased destruction, and increased blood loss (Fig. 23–4). This section focuses on acute anemias that are particularly found in the high-acuity patient.

Decreased RBC Production

In Section One, RBC proliferation was presented as a tightly regulated and sequential maturation process in the bone marrow. Under certain circumstances, however, RBC proliferation becomes depressed. This can result from inadequate intake or absorption of certain vitamins

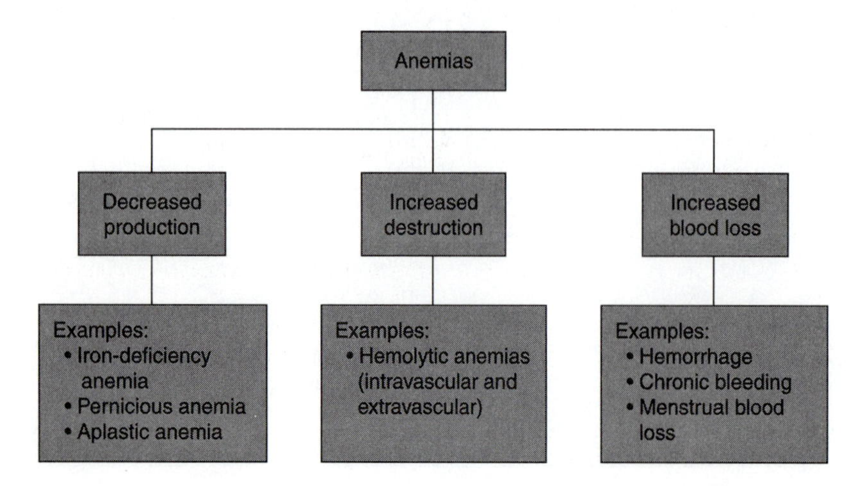

Figure 23–4. Classification of anemias.

or minerals, particularly iron (iron-deficiency anemia), vitamin B_{12}, and folic acid (both are megaloblastic anemias). It can also result from bone marrow depression or failure (aplastic anemia).

Iron-Deficiency Anemia

Iron-deficiency anemia is the most common form of anemia found worldwide. Iron-deficiency is caused by inadequate dietary intake, increased demand for iron, or increased loss (e.g., acute or chronic bleeding or menstrual blood loss). Because iron is the atom that oxygen attaches to on the hemoglobin molecule, its lack directly alters the oxygen-carrying capacity of the hemoglobin. Laboratory analysis of RBCs in iron-deficiency anemia shows microcytic and hypochromic RBCs and a decreased MCV and MCHC. The RBC membrane often becomes more fragile, making it more susceptible to damage (Gaspard, 1998).

Megaloblastic Anemias

The term *megaloblastic* refers to the large size of the RBCs. These cells typically have large, immature nuclei with fairly mature cytoplasm (Rose & Berliner, 1998). Vitamins B_{12} (cobalamin) and folic acid are essential components of RBC development. Vitamin B_{12} deficiency most commonly occurs under two circumstances: (1) through inadequate dietary intake, and (2) through malabsorption, such as seen with loss of intrinsic factor (IF), a glycoprotein that is produced by the parietal cells in the fundus of the stomach. When vitamin B_{12} enters the stomach, it forms a stable *IF–cobalamin complex*. In this form, it travels through the gastrointestinal system to the ileum, where it is reabsorbed (Turgeon, 1999). Loss of intrinsic factor from any cause (e.g., autoantibodies) leads to vitamin B_{12}–deficiency anemia (pernicious anemia). Folic acid is also necessary in RBC development. Folic acid deficiency is most commonly caused by inadequate intake and alcohol abuse. Laboratory analysis of RBCs associated with megaloblastic anemias shows the presence of megaloblastic RBCs and an extremely low RBC count and Hgb. The Hct, however, may be normal because of the large size of the RBCs. Megaloblastic anemias are most commonly seen as a chronic form of anemia.

Acquired Aplastic Anemia

Aplastic anemia, a hypoproliferative form of anemia, is characterized by a decrease in production or growth of the blood cells (Turgeon, 1999). It has two peak incidence periods: A major peak in young adults (20 to 25) and a lesser peak in the elderly (60 to 65) (Andreoli et al., 1997). In the high-acuity patient, it may be seen as part of bone marrow depression or failure secondary to some acquired (extrinsic) mechanism, such as viral, drug, radiation, or autoimmunity. Most often, however, the etiology remains unknown, and is referred to as *idiopathic* aplastic anemia. Because the entire bone marrow is usually compromised, it results in a pancytopenia. Fatty tissue replaces the normal hematopoietic tissue in the bone marrow.

ETIOLOGY. In cases in which causation has been adequately established, aplastic anemia has been associated with:

- Benzene
- Drugs (e.g., chloramphenicol and cytotoxic chemotherapeutic agents)
- Infections (rare; e.g., Epstein–Barr virus, hepatitis B and C)
- Ionizing radiation

PATHOPHYSIOLOGY. Turgeon (1999) suggests that immune-mediated bone marrow destruction is the most common known etiology, which frequently goes through three phases (Table 23–4). Aplastic anemia varies widely in severity, from mild to severe. The prognosis is based on the severity of the disease (Andreoli et al., 1997). Severe aplastic anemia is a relentless disease with rare spontaneous remissions. If left untreated, the prognosis is poor, with most patients dying within 6 months of onset. Even with effective treatment, life expectancy is often only a few years.

Treatment

Andreoli et al. (1997) state that treatment for aplastic anemia focuses on three general areas: supportive, immunosuppressive, and bone marrow replacement. Supportive therapy includes blood transfusions to replace RBCs

TABLE 23–4. PHASES OF IMMUNE-MEDIATED APLASTIC ANEMIA

PHASE	DESCRIPTION
1—Onset of Disease	• Initiating event → immune system attack of bone marrow hematopoietic elements → cell destruction → remaining stem cells continue to reproduce blood cells to the extent that they are able. • Circulating blood cells die off according to normal life span. • As circulating cells die, they cannot be replaced adequately, resulting in decreasing blood cell counts.
2—Recovery	• A response occurs, partial or full, without initial increase in stem cell numbers • In small percentage, some repopulation of primitive cells may occur over time due to stem cell self-renewal
3—Late Disease	• May develop relapse of pancytopenia, even years following initial recovery • Abnormal stem cell clone may develop, causing other blood disorders (e.g., acute myelogenous leukemia or myelodysplasia)

Source: Turgeon, M.L. (1999). Clinical hematology: Theory and procedures, *3rd ed. Philadelphia: Lippincott-Williams & Wilkins.*

and platelets, and antibiotic therapy to protect from infection. If the patient is a candidate for bone marrow transplantation, blood transfusions will be limited with no transfusions coming from potential marrow donors. This helps reduce the risk of hypersensitivity reactions and potential bone marrow rejection. Immunosuppressive therapy frequently consists of antithymocyte globulin (ATG) or antilymphocyte globulin and/or cyclosporine. These drugs are used when bone marrow transplantation is not planned. Bone marrow transplantation is the definitive treatment for aplastic anemia. The best results come from an identical twin transplant, but there has been some success (to a significantly lesser degree) with nonidentical HLA matches. The survival rate is about 60 percent when this treatment plan is performed; however, about 15 to 30 percent of those who are treated successfully develop other blood disorders, such as myelodysplasia.

Increased Destruction of RBCs

The term **hemolytic anemia** refers to anemias that are caused by premature destruction of red blood cells, either intravascularly or within the **reticuloendothelial system** (Rose & Berliner, 1999). Hemolytic anemia can result from intrinsic (e.g., congenital) problems or, more commonly, from extrinsic problems. The high-acuity patient is much more at risk for acquired (extrinsic) problems. Acquired hemolytic anemia is often categorized by the condition or agent that causes the destruction, including immune disorders, infections, physical agents, and conditions associated with microangiopathy.

Immune Disorders

Premature destruction of RBCs by the immune system is a major cause of hemolytic anemia. Antibodies or complement (or sometimes both) coat the red cell membrane, causing premature death of the cell. The antibodies can be autoimmune induced, isoimmune induced, or drug induced (e.g., sulfonamides, insulin). Autoimmune-induced hemolytic anemia (AIHA) results from production of autoantibodies against the person's own red blood cells. The cause is unknown, but it is theorized that the autoimmune reaction may at times result from an infectious agent such as infectious mononucleosis (Turgeon, 1999). Isoimmune-induced hemolytic anemia is primarily seen in two situations. It most commonly results from ABO incompatibility between mother and baby. It can also result from Rh incompatibility in newborn infants. Drug-induced immune hemolytic anemia can damage and prematurely destroy RBCs by several mechanisms:

- Attachment of the drug or immune complexes to RBC membrane
- Production of autoantibodies (usually IgM) (Turgeon, 1999)

Examples of drugs that are known to cause drug-induced hemolytic anemia include alpha-methyldopa and sulfonamides. Fortunately, RBC destruction caused by drugs is often transient, ending when the agent is removed; thus, rapid recognition of the offending agent with rapid withdrawal is the priority action in initiating treatment.

Infectious Agents

Infectious agents have a variety of mechanisms by which they destroy RBCs. Some bacteria produce toxins and other substances that hemolyze cells, for example, *Clostridium perfringens* infections. Malaria is a protozoan infectious disease in which the protozoa enters the RBC and begins reproducing. Eventually, the RBC ruptures, and the disease spreads to other RBCs.

Physical Agents

RBCs are exposed to high temperatures in severe burn injury. Heat is a physical agent that makes RBCs fragile and causes them to fragment. The fragmented cells are filtered out by the spleen and serum RBC levels drop significantly (Turgeon, 1999).

Conditions Associated with Microangiopathy

Rose and Berliner (1999) explain that microangiopathic hemolytic anemia involves the fragmentation of RBCs as they move through damaged small blood vessels. Microangiopathy occurs in such conditions as disseminated intravascular coagulation (DIC), HELLP syndrome (hemolysis, elevated liver enzymes, and low platelet count), eclampsia, and others. It can also result from damage caused by administration of certain drugs (e.g., cyclosporine). The fragmented cells, known as *schistocytes*, are easily found on peripheral blood smears. RBC fragmentation caused by artificial heart valve trauma is also sometimes classified under this category.

Blood Loss

Anemia caused by blood loss is a common problem. Blood loss can be acute (rapid onset) or chronic (slow, insidious onset), and can involve gross or occult bleeding. These two sets of factors largely determine the patient's clinical presentation.

Acute Blood Loss Anemia

Trauma is a major cause of acute blood loss. It is also associated with surgery and acute gastrointestinal (GI) bleeding. The clinical manifestations of acute blood loss are usually more severe than those associated with chronic blood loss due to the inability of the body to muster sufficient compensatory mechanisms in an acute situation. Turgeon (1999) suggests that a less than 20 percent of total blood volume loss (< 1 L in an adult) often remains asymptomatic. Blood loss of over 20 percent significantly reduces total blood volume, producing cardiovascular changes. A blood loss of over 30 percent (> 1.5 L) is associated with decreased blood pressure at rest and increased restlessness; and a loss of over 40 percent (> 2 L) produces hypovolemic shock (discussed in detail in Module 10). Acute GI bleeding is presented in detail in Module 28.

During acute bleeding, early laboratory studies are deceptive. Hemoglobin and hematocrit do not initially reflect anemia, since plasma as well as cells are equally lost. As bleeding continues, fluid begins to shift from the extravascular spaces into the intravascular space. This fluid shift causes dilution of the remaining blood cells. In addition, as fluid resuscitation is initiated, the intravascular space is loaded with fluids, which further extends the dilutional effect. The end result is a significant reduction in serum hemoglobin and hematocrit. The full extent of the bleed cannot be evaluated using Hgb and Hct values until 48 to 72 hours after the acute bleed. There is an elevation of the reticulocyte count within several days of the bleeding event as the bone marrow begins to produce and release the immature RBCs at a rapid rate. The anemia resulting from acute bleeding is usually described as normocytic and normochromic with a normal MCV.

Sickle Cell Anemia

Sickle cell disease is a recessive inherited hemoglobinopathy. It is most commonly found in persons of African descent but is also present in other populations that are native to areas where malaria is prevalent (e.g., Middle East, the Mediterranean). Sickle cell disease is caused by a defect in the beta chain of the hemoglobin molecule, which is referred to as *Hb S*. Sickle cell anemia is the homozygote form of the disease (inherited from both parents). The person with sickle cell anemia has almost all Hb S hemoglobin, which is referred to as *Hb SS*. When deoxygenated, Hb S radically alters its shape. The usual normal smooth, oval shape of the RBC takes on an elongated "sickled" appearance, which is readily noted on a blood smear. Initially, the sickled cells regain their normal shape when adequate oxygenation is reestablished. After repeated sickling episodes, however, the affected RBCs remain permanently sickled and are hemolyzed through normal body mechanisms, which results in anemia. Sickling episodes are particularly precipitated by hypoxia and acidosis conditions.

The term *sickle cell crisis* (or vaso-occlusive crisis) refers to a major vaso-occlusive event associated with sickle cell anemia. Sickled cells can clump and obstruct blood flow in the small arterioles. The resulting hypoxia triggers more sickling activity, which further worsens the hypoxia. Vascular occlusion results in tissue or organ ischemia distal to the obstruction. In addition to the intense pain associated with sickle cell crisis, the affected tissues and organs become increasingly damaged with repeated hypoxic episodes. Common complications associated with sickle cell crisis include organ failure (e.g., heart, renal, and hepatic), stroke, arthritis, acute chest syndrome, leg ulcers, and autosplenectomy (Turgeon, 1999). The life expectancy of a person with sickle cell anemia has improved dramatically, owing to earlier and more effective treatment. The current median age at death is 48 years (women) and 42 years (men) (Turgeon, 1999).

Management of the patient with sickle cell disease primarily focuses on treating complications and supporting the patient. The patient's tissue status, organ function, degree of anemia, and PaO_2 all require monitoring, with increased attention being given to these assessments during a sickle cell crisis episode. Oxygen therapy may be ordered to increase tissue oxygenation and reduce sickling. Hydration helps to reduce pain and decrease clumping by adding fluid volume to the intravascular space. The pain associated with sickle cell crisis is often difficult to manage and may require large doses of opioids on a continuous basis (e.g., patient-controlled analgesia) to reduce the pain to a level that is acceptable to the patient. Development of significant organ dysfunction or failure is treated accordingly. Blood transfusions are usually reserved for times of extreme need, such as severe anemia, stroke, multiple organ damage, or prolonged surgery (Andreoli et al., 1997).

Polycythemia

Polycythemia refers to the production and presence of an abnormally high number of red blood cells. There are two major forms of polycythemia: primary and secondary. This section provides a brief overview of primary polycythemia and focuses on secondary polycythemia, which is more commonly seen in the high-acuity patient.

Primary Polycythemia

Primary polycythemia, called *polycythemia vera*, is a rare, clonal myeloproliferative disease involving the pluripotent hematopoietic stem cell (PHSC). All cells in the myeloid cell line are usually affected, including erythrocytes, leukocytes, and thrombocytes. It involves excessive production of all three cell types but the degree of RBC proliferation is particularly striking. Polycythemia vera is a chronic disease that exists on a continuum from mild to severe but tends to worsen over many years. It is a disorder of older age and affects more men than women. The cause is unknown but certain risk factors have been identified, such as chemical exposure and unclear genetic influences. The disease is characterized by a significant increase in the RBC mass, an elevated hematocrit, hypervolemia, increased viscosity of the blood, and splenomegaly from pooling of RBCs. Since RBC proliferation is the most extreme, the major clinical manifestations revolve around this characteristic. In general, the clinical manifestations associated with the erythrocytosis aspect of polycythemia vera are the same as seen with secondary polycythemia.

TABLE 23–5. CLINICAL MANIFESTATIONS AND LABORATORY FINDINGS OF SECONDARY POLYCYTHEMIA

	MANIFESTATIONS/FINDINGS	UNDERLYING PROBLEM
Neurologic system	Headache, tinnitus, and dizziness	Sluggish cerebral blood flow; hypertension
Cardiovascular system	Hypertension	Increased blood volume; increased blood viscosity
Integumentary system	Ruddy skin appearance; may have a dusky or cyanotic cast to skin	Increased RBCs; stagnant blood flow in microvasculature
Laboratory findings	*Hct:* > 54% (males); > 46% (females) *Red cell mass:* > 36 mL/kg (males); > 32 mL/kg (females)	Increased RBC count

Sources: Turgeon, M.L. (1999). Clinical hematology: Theory and procedures, *3rd ed. Philadelphia: Lippincott-Williams & Wilkins; Andreoli, T.E., Carpenter, C.C., Bennett, J.C., & Plum, F. Disorders of the hematopoiet stem cell. In T.E. Andreoli et al. (eds.),* Cecil's essentials of medicine, *4th ed. Philadelphia: W.B. Saunders; and Gaspard, K.J. (1998). The red blood cell and alterations in oxygen transport. In C.M. Porth (ed.),* Pathophysiology: Concepts of altered health states, *5th ed. Philadelphia: J.B. Lippincott.*

Secondary Polycythemia

Secondary polycythemia, or *erythrocytosis*, is not a disease; rather, it is a symptom of some underlying pathology or environmental factor. In the high-acuity patient, secondary polycythemia frequently occurs as an appropriate compensatory response to chronic tissue hypoxia. Compensatory secondary polycythemia can result from environmental factors (e.g., living at a high altitude); from chronic cardiac or pulmonary diseases (e.g., congenital heart disease or COPD); and from smoking. In the presence of chronic tissue hypoxia, the kidneys produce more erythropoietin, which then stimulates the bone marrow to produce more RBCs (erythrocytosis). The elevated RBC count results in increased oxygen-carrying capacity of the blood and ultimately, increased oxygen to the tissues (Rose & Berliner, 1999; Turgeon, 1999).

Clinical Manifestations. The clinical manifestations of secondary polycythemia can be attributed to three underlying problems:

1. Increased red blood cell count
2. Increased viscosity of the blood
3. Increased blood volume

A significant increase in red blood cell mass increases the thickness (viscosity) of the blood as well as the blood volume. The end result of these events is sluggish or stagnant blood flow, particularly in the microcirculation. Laboratory studies reflect these events, as well. Table 23–5 summarizes the clinical manifestations and laboratory findings typically noted with secondary polycythemia. Complications result from blood hyperviscosity and include hypertension and thrombosis, which may be manifested as a stroke, peripheral vascular disease, or ischemic heart disease (Rose & Berliner, 1999). Treatment focuses on eliminating or reducing the underlying problem. Phlebotomy is frequently performed to maintain a hematocrit of < 45 percent, which reduces the risk of complications (Shulman, 1998).

In summary, anemias can be divided into three general categories based on the cause, including decreased RBC production, increased RBC destruction, and blood loss. Anemias that result from decreased RBC production include iron-deficiency and aplastic anemias. Iron-deficiency anemia is the most common type of anemia and is found worldwide. Aplastic anemia usually involves all blood cell types (pancytopenia) and, in severe cases, has a very high mortality rate. Acquired hemolytic anemias cause premature RBC destruction, which may be related to immune, infectious agents, physical agents, and microangiopathic conditions. Blood loss anemia cannot be accurately measured until 2 to 3 days following the bleed, when fluid shifts have stabilized. Acute bleeding is generally more symptomatic because of the inability to muster adequate compensatory mechanisms with rapid fluid volume loss. Polycythemia refers to excessive red blood cells. It can occur as a malignant disease called polycythemia vera, a rare myeloproliferative disease. This form involves hyperproliferation of all myeloid cell lines. More commonly, polycythemia occurs as simple erythrocytosis. In the high-acuity patient, it most frequently results from chronic tissue hypoxia. Clinical manifestations and complications develop from increased RBCs, increased blood viscosity, and increased blood volume.

Section Three Review

1. The clinical manifestations of the anemias are primarily attributable to
   A. decreased cardiac output
   B. impaired oxygen transport
   C. decreased blood volume
   D. impaired bone marrow function
2. The bone discomfort associated with anemia is usually caused by

A. inflammation of the bone
B. decreased oxygen in the bone marrow
C. irritation of nerves in the bone marrow
D. increased hematopoietic activity in bone marrow

3. The severity of symptoms associated with anemia is largely dependent on the
A. type of anemia
B. total blood volume
C. speed with which it develops
D. degree of bone marrow involvement

4. The most common form of anemia found worldwide is
A. megaloblastic anemias
B. iron-deficiency anemia
C. aplastic anemia
D. blood loss anemia

5. Loss of intrinsic factor (IF) causes development of which form of anemia?
A. megaloblastic
B. hemolytic
C. aplastic
D. iron-deficiency

6. The form of anemia that usually involves pancytopenia is
A. aplastic
B. hemolytic
C. megaloblastic
D. iron-deficiency

7. The definitive treatment for aplastic anemia is
A. blood transfusions
B. antibiotic therapy
C. immunosuppressant therapy
D. bone marrow transplant

8. The most common etiology of hemolytic anemia is
A. infectious agents
B. autoimmune reaction
C. physical agents
D. microangiopathy

9. The most common cause of blood loss anemia is
A. alcohol abuse
B. menorrhagia
C. trauma
D. GI bleeding

10. Sickle cell anemia is
A. inherited from only one parent
B. a defect of the myeloid stem cell
C. inherited from both parents
D. a defect of the plasma cell

11. A sickle cell crisis episode develops when
A. HbS begins to hemolyze
B. a person becomes too alkalotic
C. a person experiences intense pain
D. sickled cells obstruct blood flow

12. The *underlying* cause of secondary polycythemia is
A. chronic tissue hypoxia
B. myeloproliferative disease
C. depletion of erythropoiesis
D. chronic obstructive pulmonary disease

Answer: 1. B, 2. D, 3. C, 4. B, 5. A, 6. A, 7. D, 8. B, 9. C, 10. C, 11. D, 12. A

SECTION FOUR: White Cell Disorders

At the completion of this section, the learner will be able to discuss the etiology, pathophysiology, clinical manifestations, and management of white cell disorders.

Neutropenia

Neutropenia (granulocytopenia) refers to an abnormally low level of neutrophils. Neutropenia is not a disease; rather, it is an important symptom of some other underlying problem. High-acuity patients are at risk for developing neutropenia related to the severity of their illnesses. Neutropenia exists when the neutrophil count drops below 50 percent of the total WBC count. It is commonly defined as a neutrophil count of less than 1,500 cells/μL (Caudell, 1998). A neutrophil count below 1,000/μL places the neutropenic person at high risk for developing an infection and a count below 500/μL is considered life threatening (Andreoli et al., 1997)—the lower the neutrophil count, the higher the risk. Severe neutropenia, called **agranulocytosis,** exists when the neutrophil count falls below 200 cells/μL (Caudell, 1998). Neutropenia can be intrinsic (rare) or acquired. Acquired neutropenia is associated with three major mechanisms, including premature destruction, decreased production, and increased demand.

Premature Destruction

Premature death of neutrophils is most commonly associated with drugs. Certain drugs (e.g., cephalothin) can cause development of drug–antibody immune complexes, which then attach to the neutrophils. The resulting reaction, which is sometimes referred to as an "innocent bystander" reaction, destroys the neutrophils (Sommers, 1998). Neutropenia can also result from an isolated autoimmune process, or as a complication of another autoimmune disorder, such as systemic lupus erythematosus (SLE) (Sommers, 1998). In addition, the spleen is capable of entrapping neutrophils and destroying them; this sometimes occurs with disorders that includs splenomegaly.

Decreased Production

Decreased production of neutrophils can occur by direct injury to the bone marrow (e.g., aplastic anemia); by overcrowding of normal bone marrow components from infiltration of malignant cells (e.g., leukemia); or bone marrow suppression by cancer chemotherapy or irradiation. It can also result from severe nutritional deficits (e.g., starvation). Decreased production is sometimes desirable and is accomplished through immunosuppressant drug therapy; for example, as used for preventing graft rejection in organ transplantation.

Increased Demand

The body's available stores of blood cells is not infinite. In acute high-demand situations, such as septicemia, extremely large numbers of neutrophils are required in a short period of time. If the demand is too high, the numbers of available neutrophils becomes significantly depleted when the bone marrow is unable to produce new neutrophils at a sufficiently rapid rate to keep up with the demand.

Clinical Manifestations

Neutropenia causes altered responses to inflammation and infection, since neutrophils are the first line of internal defense against infection and play a crucial part in the inflammatory process. The patient who develops neutropenia is at risk for infection. The source of the infection is often from normal flora, since the body is host to a variety of pathogens, both externally and internally. Under normal circumstances, these pathogens remain harmless, but in conditions such as neutropenia, they can invade the body and cause serious, sometimes life-threatening infections.

The clinical manifestations associated with infection are altered to the degree that the neutrophil count is compromised. In mild cases of neutropenia, a fairly normal inflammatory response to infection occurs. The person may exhibit typical manifestations: fever, chills, malaise, and formation of exudate, adventitious breath sounds (e.g., pneumonia), but perhaps to a lesser degree. In more severe cases of neutropenia, however, the inflammatory response becomes significantly depressed. A moderate fever may become the primary symptom—often no higher than 100.5°F (38.1°C). Formation of pus may occur later in the infection or not at all if severe neutropenia is present.

Treatment

Early discovery and aggressive treatment of the underlying cause is imperative. Investigation of the cause may include antibody and/or bone marrow testing, or discontinuing drugs. Antibiotic therapy is often initiated, with close attention being placed on monitoring for secondary infections. G-CSF (granulocyte-colony stimulating factor) may be administered to try to stimulate the bone marrow to increase production of neutrophils. Nursing management of the immunosuppressed patient is discussed in Module 24, Section Ten.

Leukemia

Leukemia is a malignant process in which there is a transformation of hematopoietic cells, causing unregulated clonal growth (Shulman, 1998). Leukemias are categorized as being either acute or chronic. The acute leukemias are characterized by aggressive proliferation of immature lymphoid or myeloid blast cells. Examine Figure 23–1 to view the early stage of blast cells in cell development. Chronic leukemias, however, are characterized by production of mature, differentiated cells of either lymphoid or myeloid lineage. Chronic leukemias have a more insidious long-term clinical course than the acute leukemias. Chronic myelogenous leukemia (CML) is a myeloproliferative disease, which refers to a malignancy involving all of the cells in the myelocytic cell line. Examples of other myeloproliferative disorders include acute myelogenous leukemia (AML) and polycythemia vera.

The uncontrolled production of malignant cells in the bone marrow suppresses and replaces the normal cells leading to eventual pancytopenia. In untreated acute leukemia, the patient rapidly succumbs to complications of pancytopenia, particularly infection or hemorrhage (Shulman, 1998). The acute leukemias are also associated with infiltration into other tissues such as the gums, spleen, central nervous system, and lymph nodes creating clinical manifestations specific to each affected tissue. Diagnosis of the exact type of leukemia can be difficult. The blast cells are sometimes so primitive that it is difficult to initially determine whether the malignant cell clones are of myelocytic or lymphocytic origin.

Causes

The exact causes of leukemia are unknown. It is believed that there may be multiple factors involved in development of each of the different leukemias, including environmental and genetic factors. There is a higher incidence of leukemia in identical twins (Caudell, 1998). In several types of leukemia, a chromosomal abnormality has been isolated, called the Philadelphia chromosome (Ph^1), which is the translocation between the long arms of chromosomes 22 to 9 (Caudell, 1998; Shulman, 1998). Certain chemical and drug exposures are associated with development of leukemia (e.g., benzene, chloramphenicol, and some antineoplastic agents). Radiation exposure provides an environmental hazard such as occurs in nuclear disasters (bombings or accidents) or following radiation treatment for previous malignancies. While human viruses are suspected as a potential cause of leukemia, only one has been established: human T cell leukemia virus type I (HTLV-1) (O'Mara & Whedon, 2000).

Acute Leukemias

There are two forms of acute leukemia: acute lymphocytic (lymphoblastic) leukemia and acute myelocytic leukemia.

Acute Lymphocytic (Lymphoblastic) Leukemia. Acute lymphocytic leukemia (ALL) is primarily a disease of childhood. It is also the most common type of leukemia in children, accounting for 80 to 90 percent of all childhood leukemias (Caudell, 1998; Andreoli et al., 1997). ALL is associated with proliferation of immature lymphoblasts from the B cell (about 70 percent of ALL cases) or, less commonly, the T cell lineage (Shulman, 1998). The leukemic cells fail to mature or differentiate any further than the stage at which they are produced and therefore cannot carry on normal immune functions.

Laboratory findings typically found in ALL include leukocytosis that is usually not severe. According to Turgeon (1999), the peripheral blood contains almost all lymphoblasts and lymphocytes. Anemia and thrombocytopenia are common but the cells are normal mature erythrocytes and platelets to the extent that they are present at all. Somewhat immature neutrophils may be present in the peripheral blood but no Auer rods are present in their cytoplasm. Auer rods are pathological rod-shaped aggregations of myeloblast lysosomes present in some forms of leukemia (Turgeon, 1999).

Acute Myelocytic Leukemia. Acute myelocytic leukemia (AML) is most commonly seen in the adult population, with about one-half of cases occurring over the age of 60 (Caudell, 1998). AML is characterized by proliferation of malignant blast cells from the myeloid stem cell lineage (Shulman, 1998). The proliferation can involve any or all of the cells in the myeloid lineage (erythroblasts, megakaryoblasts, monoblasts, and/or myeloblasts). Blast cells are not programmed to die; thus, malignant blast clones can produce malignant cells indefinitely (Shulman, 1998). Cells rapidly accumulate in the bone marrow and then infiltrate into other tissues.

Laboratory findings consistent with AML include the presence of thrombocytopenia and anemia in about 85 percent of cases (Shulman, 1998; Turgeon, 1999). Leukocytosis is commonly noted, usually accompanied by neutropenia. An examination of peripheral blood and the bone marrow shows a predominance of myeloblastic cells. Auer rods may be present in the cytoplasm of the myeloblasts. A standard diagnostic criterion for AML is that over 30 percent of the hematopoietic cells must be myeloblasts (Shulman, 1998).

Chronic Lymphocytic Leukemia. According to Turgeon (1999), chronic lymphocytic leukemia (CLL) is primarily a disease of middle-aged to older adults (> 50 years old), and it is more commonly seen in males than females. It has a variable life expectancy, ranging from 2 to 10 years with some patients surviving for 30 years or more. Death commonly results from infection but many persons with CLL die of unrelated causes. About one-third of persons with CLL eventually develop hemolytic anemia of autoimmune etiology. The most common type of CLL is B cell type. The major characteristic of CLL is the presence of smaller-than-normal mature lymphocytes in the peripheral blood and bone marrow. These cells can often be found in the spleen and lymph nodes, causing splenomegaly and lymphadenopathy.

The small CLL lymphocytes often are not fully functional as immune cells, causing *hypogammaglobulinemia*, which means abnormally low levels of gamma globulin in the blood. When present, the person with CLL is immunodeficient and at increased risk for development of infection. A significant number of persons with CLL eventually develop autoimmune disease (Turgeon, 1999). Some of the common autoimmune blood cell disorders include autoimmune hemolytic anemia (about one-third of CLL patients), and autoimmune thrombocytopenia purpura (Andreoli et al., 1997; Turgeon, 1999).

Laboratory findings consistent with CLL include anemia and thrombocytopenia. These two conditions are further aggravated if autoantibodies develop, causing premature cell destruction. Existing granulocytes, thrombocytes, and erythrocytes appear normal. Diagnostic criteria for CLL include a lymphocyte count of ≥ 15,000 cells/μL and the presence of at least 40 percent lymphocytes in the bone marrow (Andreoli et al., 1997). About one-third of persons with CLL have a leukocyte count of > 100,000 cells/μL. A sample of the peripheral blood usually shows between 80 and 90 percent small leukocytes (Turgeon, 1999). Hypogammaglobulinemia is present on serum electrophoresis.

Chronic Myelogenous Leukemia. Like acute myelogenous leukemia, chronic myelocytic leukemia (CML) is a type of myeloproliferative disease. It is more common than CLL and is primarily a disease of adults (30 to 50 years of age) but occurs at all ages (Turgeon, 1999). More males than females are affected and in 5 to 10 percent of cases, there is a history of high radiation exposure (Turgeon, 1999). CML is directly linked to the Ph^1 chromosome abnormality. CML, like AML, involves hyperproliferation of myelocytic stem cells; thus, it involves all of the cell types in the myelocyte lineage. CML is characterized by the predominance of excessive numbers of mature and immature myelocytic cells. It is a slow-onset, slowly progressive disease. The course of CML typically runs in phases: chronic, accelerated, and acute.

During the *chronic phase*, the patient has leukocytosis, but the neutrophils and thrombocytes are usually normal. It is during this phase that the diagnosis is usually made. The patient typically presents with marked thrombocytosis and splenomegaly (Shulman, 1998; Turgeon, 1999). The chronic phase is usually treatable and the patient does well and remains asymptomatic. Without treatment, the chronic phase lasts from 2 to 4 years (O'Mara & Whedon, 2000). With treatment, this phase may last 5 or more years.

The *accelerated phase* begins with the onset of increased signs and symptoms. It usually occurs with or without treatment; however, treatment during the chronic phase can significantly delay onset of the accelerated phase. Eventually, most persons with CML develop resistance to therapy, heralding in the accelerated phase. The accelerated phase generally ends in an *acute (blast transformation) phase*, when the patient's leukemia changes from chronic to acute. The acute phase is characterized by the onset of a "blast crisis" in which the blast cells are no longer able to differentiate into their more mature forms, resulting in blast cell domination in the bone marrow and peripheral blood. In most cases, the blast crisis reflects a transformation that is similar to AML; however, in about 20 percent of cases, there is a transformation of lymphocytes, with subsequent ALL type findings (Shulman, 1998; Timmerman, 1998). The blast crisis is typically resistant to treatment and usually ends in death within a few months.

Laboratory findings consistent with CML are dependent on the phase of the disease. Overall, however, CML is characterized by extreme leukocytosis and the existence of any combination of mature and immature myelogenous cells in the bone marrow and blood. The total leukocyte count may exceed 300,000, placing the patient at high risk for leukostasis problems (Turgeon, 1999). Anemia and thrombocytosis are often present early in the disease, although thrombocytopenia is possible. The myeloblast count is usually 5 percent or less (Turgeon, 1999).

Clinical Manifestations

The initial clinical presentation of a person at the onset of acute leukemia is often dramatic, with complaints of fevers and headache. Other common presenting symptoms include infection, bleeding, and malaise (Andreoli et al., 1997; Turgeon, 1999). The major clinical manifestations of the leukemias can be categorized into two groups: those that are caused by pancytopenia and those that are caused by expansion and infiltration of malignant cells into other tissues.

PANCYTOPENIA MANIFESTATIONS. As the red blood cell count decreases, the person with leukemia becomes increasingly anemic, demonstrating all of the manifestations of that problem. As the normal leukocyte count decreases, the patient becomes immunodeficient and becomes increasingly at risk for infections; however, the typical clinical picture associated with infection may be diminished or absent. Infection is the most common cause of death (about 70 percent) in adults with acute leukemia (Turgeon, 1999). Fever is commonly noted related to infection and increased metabolism of the malignant cells (Caudell, 1998). Finally, as thrombocyte numbers decrease, the patient develops bleeding problems, particularly petechiae and ecchymosis on the skin, as well as epistaxis and bleeding gums.

MALIGNANT CELL EXPANSION AND INFILTRATION MANIFESTATIONS. As the malignant cells proliferate and infiltrate in the bone marrow, their expanding volume increases the pressure inside the bone. The increased pressure causes bone tenderness or pain. Malignant cells tend to infiltrate into the central nervous system, leading to multiple central nervous system (CNS)-related manifestations, such as nausea and vomiting, headache, seizures, coma, papilledema, and possible cranial nerve palsies (Caudell, 1998). Infiltration of malignant cells into the spleen and liver gives rise to splenomegaly and hepatomegaly, which can cause general abdominal discomfort (Caudell, 1998). According to Turgeon (1999) the extreme degree of leukocytosis (> 100,000) associated with some types of leukemia (e.g., ALL, CML) can precipitate a severe complication called *leukostasis*. Small, thin-walled capillaries become dilated and congested with rigid leukemic (blast) cells, causing impaired circulation. Two organs are most commonly involved—the lungs and the brain. The primary pulmonary manifestation is dyspnea. CNS manifestations include confusion, visual problems, and/or headache.

Diagnosis and Treatment

Diagnosis of leukemia requires bone marrow aspiration with analysis of the cells. It is critical that the leukemic cells be identified and characterized for planning of correct treatment. When either AML or ALL is diagnosed, or if the leukocyte count is > 100,000, the situation is considered to be a medical emergency. Once identified, leukostasis is quickly treated using leukocyte electrophoresis followed by chemotherapy (Andreoli et al., 1997). Leukemias are classified and/or staged to aid in diagnosis and treatment. A variety of classification and staging systems have been developed over the years to aid in diagnosis and treatment. For example, the French–American–British (FAB) classification system was developed to differentiate acute leukemias by morphology (see Table 23–6); and chronic leukemias have been staged by degree of risk (see Table 23–7).

ACUTE LEUKEMIA TREATMENT. According to Andreoli et al. (1997), there are two major goals underlying the treatment plan for the acute leukemias: to destroy the malignant cells and to produce complete remission. This is achieved through aggressive chemotherapy, which may require multiple courses of treatment that possibly last for two or more years of treatment (Andreoli et al., 1997). The initial phase of chemotherapy is referred to as *induction*, which lasts for approximately 1 week. Induction in the AML patient may include cytosine arabinoside, and a drug from the anthracycline group. Induction in the ALL patient usually requires a more complex combination chemotherapy approach and may include prednisone,

TABLE 23–6. FRENCH–AMERICAN–BRITISH (FAB) CLASSIFICATION OF ACUTE LEUKEMIA

Acute myelocytic leukemia (AML)	M_1: AML, undifferentiated
	M_2: AML, differentiated (myeloblasts and promyelocytes predominate)
	M_3: Acute promyelocytic leukemia; promyelocytes
	M_4: Acute myelomonocytic leukemia; monocytes and myelogenous cells predominate
	M_5: Acute monocytic leukemia; monocytes predominate
	M_6: Erythroleukemia; predominance of erythroid and granulocyte precursors
	M_7: Megakaryotic leukemia; predominance of megakaryoblasts (large and small)
Acute lymphocytic leukemia (ALL)	L_1: Homogeneous; predominance of one cell type, primarily small cells; childhood type
	L_2: Heterogeneous; cells larger than L_1, adult type
	L_3: Large cells (Burkitt-like); homogenous, large cells

Sources: Turgeon, M.L. (1999). Clinical hematology: Theory and procedures, *3rd ed. Philadelphia: Lippincott-Williams & Wilkins; Andreoli, T.E., Carpenter, C.C., Bennett, J.C., & Plum, F. Disorders of the hematopoietic stem cell. In T.E. Andreoli et al. (eds.),* Cecil's essentials of medicine, *4th ed. Philadelphia: W.B. Saunders.*

L-asparaginase, vincristine, and others. Induction therapy aims at creating a state of complete remission—no leukemic cells in the bone marrow or peripheral blood. Induction therapy produces complete remission in about 75 percent of AML patients less than 60 years of age. Long-term remission is less common in adults than in children. In children with ALL, induction is associated with complete remission for over 5 years in about 90 percent of cases. Induction therapy may be followed by *consolidation* chemotherapy, which aims to solidify the remission and eliminate any remaining leukemic cells. It frequently includes the same chemotherapeutic agents used during induction, which are included as part of a combination therapy. The final phase of chemotherapy is called *maintenance* chemotherapy, which is primarily required for treatment of ALL. During this phase, the patient with ALL may have intrathecal prophylactic treatment of the CNS and possibly brain radiation. Bone marrow transplant may be the curative treatment of choice, particularly in patients with AML. The best results come from a well-matched family donor.

TABLE 23–7. CHRONIC LYMPHOCYTIC LEUKEMIA (CLL) CLINICAL STAGING

STAGE/LEVEL OF RISK	COMMENTS
0/Low	Lymphocytosis limited to bone marrow and peripheral circulation
I/Low	Lymphocytosis in bone marrow, peripheral circulation with infiltration into lymph nodes
II/Intermediate	Lymphocytosis in peripheral circulation, bone marrow; plus splenomegaly or hepatomegaly (with or without lymph node enlargement)
III/Intermediate	Lymphocytosis with non–immune-related anemia (with or without splenomegaly, hepatomegaly, or lymph node enlargement)
IV/High	Lymphocytosis with non–immune-related thrombocytopenia (with or without anemia, splenomegaly, hepatomegaly, or lymph node enlargement)

Adapted from Turgeon, M.L. (1999). Clinical hematology: Theory and procedures, *3rd ed. Philadelphia: Lippincott-Williams & Wilkins.*

CHRONIC LEUKEMIA TREATMENT. Treatment of CLL may be reserved until the person moves into the advanced stages (III and IV) of the disease, develops pancytopenia, and/or becomes symptomatic (Andreoli et al., 1997; Salmon & Sartorelli, 1998). Chemotherapy is the usual initial form of therapy, often using a combination of an alkylating agent (e.g., chlorambucil) and corticosteroids (e.g., prednisone) (Salmon & Sartorelli, 1998). A newer chemotherapeutic agent, fludarabine, may be used as initial therapy in the presence of advanced stage CLL. Fludarabine has been shown to significantly reduce tumor size and possibly induce a complete remission in cases in which more traditional chemotherapeutic regimens have only brought about partial remission (Andreoli et al., 1997). Partial remission exists when no malignant cells are found in the peripheral blood but some can be found on examination of the bone marrow. Radiation therapy may be used to reduce the size of bulky masses in the lymph nodes or spleen. Splenectomy may be performed if autoimmunity develops. Antibiotic therapy is ordered as necessary to treat infections.

Andreoli et al. (1997) explains that treatment of CML typically begins during the chronic phase and focuses on reduction of the leukocyte count and splenomegaly. Antimetabolite therapy (e.g., hydroxyurea and busulfan) is frequently ordered to accomplish these tasks. While antimetabolite therapy can prolong the chronic phase, it does not prevent the acceleration phase. A newer therapy, alpha-interferon, has improved the prognosis associated with CML. Alpha-interferon, administered intravenously, has been found to decrease the number of bone marrow cells with the Ph^1 chromosome and increase the number of normal clone cells. Bone marrow transplant is the only curative therapy, with a cure rate up to 50 percent under ideal conditions (Salmon & Sartorelli, 1998). The best results come from a sibling donor who is HLA matched.

In summary, this section has presented major disorders of the white blood cells. Neutropenia, abnormally low levels of neutrophils can be caused by decreased production (e.g., aplastic anemia, leukemia), premature destruction (e.g., immune reaction), or increased demand (e.g., overwhelming infection). Neutropenia causes an altered response to inflammation and infection. The leukemias consist of a group of disorders that are characterized by uncontrolled growth of malignantly transformed blood cells in the bone marrow. There are types of leukemias, including acute lymphocytic leukemia (ALL), acute myelogenous leukemia (AML), chronic lymphocytic leukemia (CLL), and chronic myelogenous leukemia (CML). AML and CML are both myeloproliferative disorders that involve all of the blood cells in the myeloid stem cell lineage. The clinical manifestations of the leukemias are divided into two general groups: those resulting from pancytopenia (anemia, leukopenia, and thrombocytopenia) and those resulting from malignant cell expansion and infiltration. Diagnosis of leukemia requires bone marrow aspiration followed by careful analysis of the blood cells.

SECTION FOUR REVIEW

1. A neutrophil count of less than _______ cells/μL places the patient at high risk for development of an acute infection.
   A. 1,500
   B. 2,000
   C. 2,500
   D. 3,000
2. The most common cause of premature destruction of neutrophils is
   A. environmental toxins
   B. autoimmune disorder
   C. drug–antibody reaction
   D. bacterial infection
3. When severe neutropenia is present, the primary symptom of infection may be
   A. pus formation
   B. fever
   C. local edema
   D. local erythema
4. The myelocytic leukemias differ from lymphocytic leukemias in that both forms of myelocytic leukemias involve
   A. more than one type of blood cell
   B. a predominance of mature blood cells
   C. all blood cell lines
   D. plasma cell proliferation
5. In general, the cause of death in the patient who has untreated acute leukemia is
   A. infection
   B. tissue hypoxia
   C. pancytopenia
   D. hemorrhage
6. About 70 percent of ALL cases involves proliferation of immature
   A. B cells
   B. T cells
   C. plasma cells
   D. megakaryocytes
7. The presence of Auer rods in the cytoplasm is primarily found in which type of leukemia?
   A. ALL
   B. AML
   C. CLL
   D. CML
8. The major characteristic of CLL is the presence of ____________ mature lymphocytes.
   A. larger-than-normal
   B. fewer-than-normal
   C. irregularly shaped
   D. abnormally small
9. CML is associated with a *blast crisis*, which is best described as occurring when the
   A. disorder transforms into acute leukemia
   B. blast cells obstruct the circulation
   C. bone marrow completely fails
   D. blast cells infiltrate into the brain
10. The most common cause of death in adults with acute leukemia is
    A. hemorrhage
    B. infection
    C. tissue hypoxia
    D. brain infiltration
11. The term *leukostasis* refers to
    A. infiltration of brain and lungs by blast cells
    B. inability of leukocytes to move out of bone marrow
    C. loss of vision or stroke caused by stagnant blood flow
    D. impaired circulation due to capillary congestion by blast cells
12. Diagnosis of leukemia requires analysis of
    A. peripheral blood
    B. leukocyte electrophoresis
    C. bone marrow
    D. lymph node cells
13. A "complete remission" is obtained when there are no leukemic cells in the
    A. lymph nodes and bone marrow
    B. lymph nodes and peripheral blood
    C. bone marrow and lymph nodes
    D. bone marrow and peripheral blood
14. The initial treatment of acute leukemias is
    A. surgery
    B. chemotherapy

C. radiation therapy
D. bone marrow transplant

15. Treatment of ALL may include "maintenance" therapy, which commonly includes
A. intrathecal chemotherapy
B. total body irradiation
C. bone marrow transplantation
D. corticosteroid therapy

16. Treatment of CLL is usually initiated
A. when the WBC count > 100,000
B. when the hemoglobin < 6
C. at stage III or IV of disease
D. at the time of diagnosis

17. Use of alpha-interferon in the treatment of CML has been found to
A. prolong the acceleration phase
B. put patients in complete remission
C. decrease number of normal clonal cells
D. decrease number of Ph[1] chromosome cells

Answers: 1. A, 2. C, 3. B, 4. A, 5. C, 6. A, 7. B, 8. D, 9. A, 10. B, 11. D, 12. C, 13. D, 14. B, 15. A, 16. C, 17. D

SECTION FIVE: Hemostasis Disorders

At the completion of this section, the learner will be able to describe the etiology, pathophysiology, clinical manifestations, and management of thrombocytopenia and disseminated intravascular coagulation (DIC).

This section focuses on thrombocytes (platelets), the cellular component of hemostasis. Discussion is specific to disorders associated with abnormally low levels of thrombocytes—thrombocytopenia. It also provides a brief overview of DIC.

Thrombocytopenia

Thrombocytopenia is clinically defined as a platelet count of < 100,000 cells/μL. The major complication of thrombocytopenia is bleeding. The bleeding associated with thrombocytopenia is different from bleeding caused by other coagulopathies. Thrombocytopenia typically manifests itself as petechiae and purpura on the skin and mucous membranes. Coagulopathies caused by missing or abnormal coagulation factors tend to cause internal bleeding. Thrombocytopenia is usually not a life-threatening condition; however, the underlying disorder that is causing it may be serious or life threatening. Thrombocytopenia can be intrinsic (e.g., hereditary disorder) or acquired. This section focuses on acquired types of thrombocytopenia.

Causes of Thrombocytopenia

There are three general conditions that cause thrombocytopenia, including decreased production, increased destruction or utilization, and problems with distribution (Turgeon, 1999).

Problems of Decreased Production. Any problem that injures the bone marrow can result in a temporary or permanent reduction in megakaryocytes, for example, chemicals, drugs, and irradiation. Production can also be decreased by problems with thrombopoiesis, as is seen with megaloblastic and iron-deficiency anemias. Both anemias cause alterations in the size or function of megakaryocytes, thus potentially altering thrombopoiesis.

Problems of Increased Destruction. Turgeon (1999) explains that destruction of platelets can result from several types of immune reactions. Certain drugs (e.g., quinidine, heroin, and morphine) and substances (e.g., snake venom) can destroy platelets. The mechanism of destruction is generally a drug antibody–platelet antigen response, or complement activation. Platelets can also be destroyed when they attach to antigen–antibody immune complexes. This is seen with certain types of bacterial sepsis. A second immune mechanism involves the attachment of a bacterial antigen to platelets, forming an antigen–platelet complex. The complex activates formation of antibodies, which then coat the complex, destroying the platelet. This has been shown to occur with a specific form of malaria (*Plasmodium falciparum*). A third immune mechanism is direct destruction of platelets by antibodies of autoimmune or isoimmune origin. The autoimmune problem can occur in the neonate due to maternal platelet autoantibodies. The isoimmune problem is rare and can result from blood transfusions or an inherited fetal platelet antigen.

Problems of Increased Utilization. Increased platelet consumption most commonly results from idiopathic (immunologic) thrombocytopenia purpura (ITP). ITP is more common in children than adults. In adults, it is most commonly found in young women as a chronic disorder of autoimmune origin, with formation of platelet autoantibodies (usually IgG), and it sometimes develops in conjunction with SLE. Characteristics of ITP include a normal bone marrow with a low platelet count, absence of spleno-megaly, and no identifiable cause of thrombocytopenia. Ruling out all other possible etiologies of thrombocytopenia is the major diagnostic criterion. The clinical manifestations of ITP are typical of any thrombocytopenia, including petechiae, purpura, bleeding gums, epistaxis, and **menorrhagia.** Less common findings include GI bleeding and hematuria, which are considered to be more serious symptoms. The bleeding associated with ITP is not usually serious. Treatment includes oral glucocorticoids (e.g., prednisone) and possibly immunoglobulin for acute bleeding management. The spleen is a major destroyer of the antibody-coated platelets, but splenectomy is usually reserved for patients who do not respond to corticosteroid therapy. Platelet transfusions are not generally required unless the patient is hemorrhaging. Complete remission is not common in severe ITP, regardless of the treatment regimen (Mazur, 1999; Turgeon, 1999).

PROBLEMS OF PLATELET DISTRIBUTION. In the presence of splenomegaly, the spleen can hold vast numbers of platelets, which significantly reduces the numbers in the circulating blood. The total number of platelets may increase by two to three times normal to compensate for those pooled in the spleen. Disorders associated with this problem include cirrhosis (posthepatic or alcoholic), leukemias, lymphomas, and others (Turgeon, 1999).

HEPARIN-INDUCED THROMBOCYTOPENIA. According to O'Reilly (1998) and Turgeon (1999), heparin is the major drug-related cause of thrombocytopenia. About 3 to 5 percent of patients receiving intravenous heparin develop a transient form of mild-to-moderate thrombocytopenia. In a small percentage of patients, however, the decreased platelet count can drop as low as 20,000/μL, causing a severe heparin-induced thrombocytopenia. It is theorized that antibodies (probably IgG) in the patient's serum bind to a complex formed by heparin and a component of platelets **(platelet factor 4).** These antibody–heparin/platelet complexes activate platelets, causing platelet aggregation and release of granular contents. Platelet aggregation can result in thromboembolism (*paradoxical thromboembolism*) or arterial thrombosis (*white clot syndrome*) (Owen & Webster, 1998). Platelet aggregation can also result in thrombocytopenia, rather than **thrombosis,** if the platelets are removed by the reticuloendothelial system. Patients who are receiving heparin therapy should have their platelet count monitored on a regular basis. Treatment usually consists of discontinuing the heparin and substituting oral anticoagulant therapy, as necessary. Heparin use is contraindicated in patients who have a history of severe heparin-induced thrombocytopenia.

Disseminated Intravascular Coagulation

DIC is a complication of some underlying condition rather than a disease in itself. General conditions that it has been associated with include shock, infection, obstetric conditions, tissue trauma, hematologic crises, and many others (Owen & Webster, 1998). DIC is a coagulation paradox—the blood is coagulating at the same time that clots are being dissolved, which results in bleeding. It is caused by overstimulation of the normal coagulation cascade (Owen & Webster, 1998). A summary of the pathologic events associated with DIC is presented in Figure 23–5. DIC causes multisystem problems. Bleeding can occur in multiple parts of the body such as the skin, cranium, lungs, GI tract, and kidneys (Owen & Webster, 1998). Actual clinical manifestations reflect the volume of blood being lost and organ-related manifestations. Management of DIC centers on treatment of the underlying condition, fluid volume replacement, support of the cardiovascular and other systems as they become damaged, and prevention of further complications. Nursing management focuses on protection of the patient, prevention of further injury, and pain management.

In summary, thrombocytopenia is an abnormally low platelet count. It results in bleeding problems, primarily of the skin and mucous membranes. Acquired thrombocytopenia is associated with five major underlying mechanisms:

1. Decreased production (e.g., bone marrow injury or decreased production of thrombopoiesis)
2. Increased platelet destruction, which usually involves an antigen–antibody immune reaction that destroys the platelets, but can also resultfrom an autoimmune or isoimmune problem

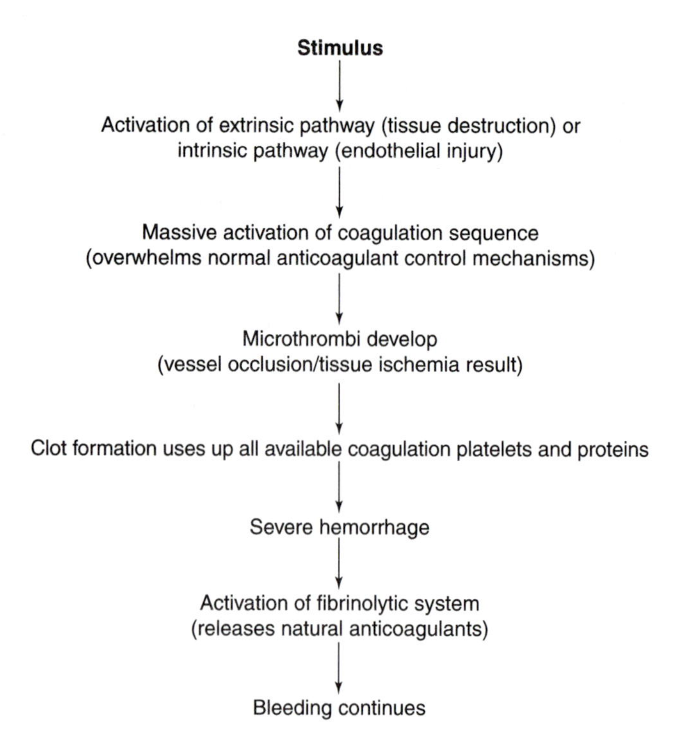

Figure 23–5. Disseminated intravascular coagulation sequence of events. *(From Gaspard, K.J. [1998]. The red blood cell and alterations in oxygen transport. In C.M. Porth [ed.],* Pathophysiology: Concepts of altered health states, *5th ed. Philadelphia: J.B. Lippincott.)*

3. Increased platelet utilization, which is associated with idiopathic thrombocytopenia purpura
4. Pooling of platelets in the spleen in the presence of splenomegaly
5. Heparin-induced thrombocytopenia, which is caused by antibody–heparin/platelet complex destruction

DIC is a rare paradoxical bleeding complication that can be triggered by many underlying problems. The triggering condition causes overstimulation of the extrinsic or intrinsic coagulation pathway. The result is consumption of coagulation factors at the same time that clots are being dissolved. DIC is a multiple system problem that can cause severe organ damage and death.

SECTION FIVE REVIEW

1. Thrombocytopenia is clinically defined as a platelet count of less than
   A. 50,000
   B. 100,000
   C. 150,000
   D. 200,000
2. The typical bleeding pattern of thrombocytopenia involves bleeding into the
   A. joints
   B. peritoneum
   C. internal organs
   D. skin and mucous membranes
3. An example of decreased platelet production caused by a reduction in thrombopoiesis is
   A. iron-deficiency anemia
   B. hemolytic anemia
   C. sequestration of platelets in spleen
   D. idiopathic thrombocytopenia purpura
4. The most common mechanism of platelet destruction by drugs is
   A. autoimmune reaction
   B. drug antibody–platelet antigen reaction
   C. antigen–antibody immune complex reaction
   D. direct toxic effect
5. Idiopathic thrombocytopenia purpura is believed to be
   A. of autoimmune origin
   B. caused by a drug reaction
   C. closely associated with splenomegaly
   D. antibody–antigen immune complex origin
6. The major treatment of idiopathic thrombocytopenia purpura is
   A. alkylating chemotherapy
   B. platelet transfusions
   C. corticosteroid therapy
   D. bone marrow transplant
7. The paradoxical thromboembolism associated with heparin-induced thrombocytopenia is caused by
   A. platelet aggregation
   B. heparin–platelet complexes
   C. accumulation of leukocytes
   D. red blood cell aggregation
8. Which of the following statements is correct regarding DIC?
   A. vessels become occluded due to vasospasm
   B. clot formation uses up all available platelets
   C. DIC is a disease that causes multiple organ hemorrhage
   D. DIC is caused only by activation of the intrinsic pathway

Answers: 1. B, 2. D, 3. A, 4. B, 5. A, 6. C, 7. A, 8. B

SECTION SIX: Nursing Implications

At the completion of this section, the learner will be able to describe the nursing implications appropriate to managing the care of patients experiencing acute hematologic dysfunction.

This section provides an overview of nursing considerations including a focused nursing history and assessment, as well as some of the more common nursing diagnoses that may apply to individuals experiencing the hematologic problems described in this module. Many of the nursing diagnoses included in this section are presented in more detail in other modules in the text.

The Focused Nursing Database

The Focused Nursing History

Obtaining a thorough nursing history is essential since many hematologic problems are linked to health conditions and behaviors, recent illnesses, environmental/occupational exposure, or heredity. The patient's family history may suggest possible hereditary problems, such as sickle cell anemia or hemophilia. Information on the patient's residential or occupational environment may give clues to possible exposures to toxic substances, such as benzene, that have been associated with aplastic anemia. A dietary history can indicate a risk for nutritional-related problems, such as iron-deficiency anemia. Obtaining information regarding the patient's medical history and prescription drug use may indicate a risk for such problems as hemolytic anemia.

The Focused Nursing Assessment

FOCUSED NEUROLOGIC ASSESSMENT. The neurologic status of the patient can change related to tissue hypoxia, bleeding, or leukemic cell infiltration. The nurse's neurologic assessment may include level of consciousness (LOC), pupillary checks, cranial nerve assessment, and monitoring for increased intracranial pressure. The patient's state of consciousness is a sensitive indicator of tissue oxygenation; thus, in the presence of severe anemia (an oxygen transport problem), LOC should be closely monitored. Cranial bleeding may manifest itself as headache, weakness, altered LOC, pupillary changes, altered cranial nerve functions, or symptoms of increased intracranial pressure. Patients suffering from leukemia may develop leukostasis, which is associated with impaired circulation caused by a massive circulating blast cell count (Caudell, 1998). CNS manifestations of leukostasis include severe headache and confusion.

FOCUSED CARDIOPULMONARY ASSESSMENT. Hematologic problems can cause significant alterations in the hemodynamic and oxygenation status of the high-acuity patient. In the presence of anemia, infection, or bleeding, the nurse can anticipate development of compensatory vital signs, such as tachycardia, tachypnea, and changes in blood pressure. Blood pressure may rise with oxygenation problems or may fall, associated with hypovolemia from bleeding. The patient may develop dyspnea or orthopnea associated with tissue hypoxia. Sputum should be checked for occult blood in patients with bleeding problems. If the hematologic problem causes increased risk for hemorrhage, vital signs and hemodynamic parameters should be monitored closely for hypovolemic shock.

FOCUSED GASTROINTESTINAL ASSESSMENT. Hepatomegaly and splenomegaly are associated with several hematologic disorders; thus, the nurse may want to palpate for their presence. Patients with bleeding disorders should have all GI secretions closely monitored for occult or gross bleeding. Intestinal bleeding is also associated with cramping, diarrhea, and melena.

FOCUSED RENAL ASSESSMENT. Patients with bleeding problems should have their urine routinely tested for occult blood. If hemoglobin is free in the urine, hemoglobinuria develops, which has a characteristic port wine coloring to it (Webster & Owen, 1998).

FOCUSED INTEGUMENTARY ASSESSMENT. In the patient with anemia, monitoring the skin, nailbeds, and mucous membranes for the presence and degree of cyanosis is important. If the patient develops thrombocytopenia, the skin and mucous membranes should be examined for petechiae, purpura, and ecchymoses. Patients experiencing hemolytic anemia should be monitored for jaundice, owing to excessive bilirubin from RBC destruction. The jaundice may also be accompanied by pruritus.

The Nursing Plan of Care

There are no North American Nursing Diagnosis Association (NANDA)-approved nursing diagnoses that directly address anemia, polycythemia, leukopenia, or thrombocytopenia. A plan of care is developed around the manifestations and complications associated with each disorder. These can be divided into five major underlying problems:

1. Tissue hypoxia
2. Hypertension
3. Stasis of blood flow
4. Infection
5. Bleeding

TISSUE HYPOXIA. Impaired oxygen transport associated with the anemias causes varying degree of tissue hypoxia, depending on the severity of the anemia. Many of the clinical manifestations associated with tissue hypoxia are addressed as nursing diagnoses, such as:

- *Fatigue* related to decreased energy production
- *Activity intolerance* related to oxygen supply and demand imbalance
- *Altered tissue perfusion* related to decreased oxygen-carrying capacity of the blood
- *Ineffective breathing pattern* related to decreased energy, fatigue
- *Risk for injury* related to tissue hypoxia
- *Pain* related to tissue hypoxia

Potential complications associated with tissue hypoxia include organ ischemia and infarction.

HYPERTENSION. Hypertension is a common finding in polycythemia related to increased intravascular volume and increased RBC mass. Ulrich, Canale, and Wendell (1998) suggest that three nursing diagnoses commonly apply to hypertension:

1. *Altered tissue perfusion* related to decreased systemic blood flow
2. *Pain: headache*, related to distention of cerebral blood vessels
3. *Activity intolerance* related to decreased tissue perfusion

Potential complications associated with hypertension include stroke, heart failure or myocardial infarction, renal dysfunction, and others.

STASIS OF BLOOD FLOW. Stagnant blood flow is particularly associated with polycythemia (extreme erythrocytosis) and leukemia (extreme leukocytosis). The major nursing diagnosis that addresses this problem is *altered tis-*

sue perfusion related to decreased systemic blood flow (venous stasis). Stasis of blood flow places the patient at risk for thrombus and thromboembolus complications.

INFECTION. Hematologic problems that particularly place the patient at risk for the complication of infection include aplastic anemia, polycythemia vera, neutropenia, and the leukemias. The collaborative nursing diagnosis that addresses infection is *risk for infection* related to inadequate secondary defenses. The degree of infection is largely dependent on the severity of the leukopenia.

BLEEDING. The bleeding related to decreased platelets is associated with aplastic anemia, polycythemia vera, leukemia, and thrombocytopenia. Although the bleeding caused by thrombocytopenia is not usually severe, it could potentially cause hemorrhage. Nursing diagnoses that apply to excessive bleeding include *fluid volume deficit* related to intravascular fluid volume loss and *decreased cardiac output* related to decreased intravascular volume.

In summary, this section provided a brief overview of some of the typical nursing diagnoses that might apply to patients with hematologic problems. The nursing diagnoses were categorized by five major underlying problems associated with the hematologic disorders discussed in this module, including tissue hypoxia, hypertension, stasis of blood flow, infection, and bleeding.

SECTION SIX REVIEW

1. Which of the following causes the neurologic manifestations associated with anemia?
   A. leukostasis
   B. bleeding
   C. tissue hypoxia
   D. increased intracranial pressure
2. The compensatory vital signs changes associated with anemia, infection, and bleeding result in
   A. elevated temperature
   B. increased heart rate
   C. decreased respiratory rate
   D. decreased blood pressure
3. A nursing diagnosis that commonly addresses tissue hypoxia associated with hematologic disorders includes
   A. fatigue
   B. pain
   C. risk for infection
   D. decreased cardiac output
4. Altered tissue perfusion related to decreased systemic blood flow is a nursing diagnosis that addresses which of the following underlying problems?
   A. tissue hypoxia
   B. infection
   C. bleeding
   D. hypertension
5. The activity intolerance created by some of the hematologic disorders is specifically related to a(n)
   A. intravascular fluid volume loss
   B. O_2 supply and demand imbalance
   C. decreased systemic blood flow
   D. inadequate secondary defenses

Answer: 1. C, 2. B, 3. A, 4. D, 5. B

POSTTEST

Questions 1 through 7 pertain to the following case: Robin T, a 24-year-old woman, is brought to a local walk-in clinic by her husband with complaints of severe fatigue, recurrent respiratory infections accompanied by high fevers, and intermittent episodes of epistaxis. Petechiae and purpura are noted on her trunk and arms. Her history is negative for exposure to toxins, and she takes no medications other than occasional nonsteroidal anti-inflammatory drugs (NSAIDs) for headache. Blood work is drawn and shows pancytopenia, with a reticulocyte count of 80,000/μL, neutrophil count of 1,000/μL, and platelet count of 60,000/μL. She is diagnosed as having idiopathic aplastic anemia.

1. Her low reticulocyte count suggests
   A. overproduction of RBCs in bone marrow
   B. microcytic, hypochromic RBCs
   C. bone marrow depression or failure
   D. RBCs are being rapidly hemolyzed
2. Her current hemoglobin is 5 g/dL. Which of the following descriptions is most consistent with this level of anemia?
   A. asymptomatic at rest
   B. dyspnea and palpitations
   C. spontaneous epistaxis
   D. intermittent high fevers

3. Robin's neutrophil count is most likely the cause of
   A. recurrent infections
   B. severe fatigue
   C. intermittent epistaxis
   D. petechiae and purpura

Robin complains of activity intolerance, an inability to concentrate, and orthopnea. Her heart rate is 106/min and respirations are 24 to 26/min.

4. Which of the following underlying problems best explains these manifestations?
   A. slow internal bleeding
   B. chronic infection
   C. tissue hypoxia
   D. increased bone marrow activity
5. An aspiration bone marrow biopsy is taken. In the presence of aplastic anemia, the bone marrow should consist of
   A. immature cells
   B. plasma cells
   C. normal tissue
   D. fatty tissue
6. The definitive treatment for aplastic anemia is
   A. transfusions of RBCs and platelets
   B. bone marrow transplant
   C. immunosuppressive therapy
   D. supportive therapy
7. If Robin is not a candidate for bone marrow transplantation, her supportive treatment regimen will include
   A. radiation therapy
   B. immunosuppressive therapy
   C. alpha-interferon
   D. vitamin B_{12} injections

Questions 8 through 11 pertain to the following case: Joey P, 3 years old, is brought into the pediatric clinic by his mother with a high fever associated with a persistent respiratory infection that has been treated multiple times with antibiotic therapy. His mother states that he is no longer able to play with his siblings but lies on the floor or in a chair for most of the day. The nurse notes petechiae on Joey's trunk and arms. He has had several episodes of epistaxis and bleeding gums that are difficult to control. A complete blood count (CBC) shows a pancytopenia present. Following further blood work, a diagnosis of acute lymphoblastic leukemia (ALL) is made.

8. The pancytopenia associated with Joey's leukemia is caused by which problem of the bone marrow?
   A. crowding out of normal cells
   B. bone marrow failure
   C. proliferation of fatty tissue
   D. hemolysis by antigen–antibody complexes
9. Which of the following statements best reflects leukemic cell maturation?
   A. they mature at an accelerated rate
   B. they differentiate slower than normal cells
   C. they differentiate in an unpredictable manner
   D. they do not mature beyond the stage at which they are produced
10. Joey's leukocyte count climbs to 105,000/μL. He develops dyspnea, confusion, and severe headache. These manifestations are most consistent with which complication of leukemia?
    A. leukostasis
    B. severe neutropenia
    C. CNS infiltration
    D. bone marrow failure
11. Joey is now receiving "consolidation" chemotherapy. The goal of this drug regimen is best described as
    A. production of a complete remission
    B. halting all bone marrow cell production
    C. elimination of leukemic cells from the CNS
    D. solidification of remission/elimination of remaining leukemic cells
12. Common clinical manifestations of thrombocytopenia include
    A. internal hemorrhage
    B. corneal hemorrhage
    C. purpura on mucous membranes
    D. altered level of consciousness, headache
13. Disseminated intravascular coagulation is said to be a coagulation paradox because
    A. coagulation and bleeding are occurring simultaneously
    B. the intrinsic and extrinsic coagulation pathways are both stimulated
    C. coagulation occurs throughout the vascular system
    D. a coagulation problem can result in multiple organ failure
14. When performing a cardiopulmonary assessment on a patient with a problem of hematologic function, the nurse should focus on the patient's
    A. urine output
    B. lung sounds
    C. vital signs
    D. level of consciousness
15. The nurse is developing a list of nursing diagnoses appropriate to a patient with aplastic anemia. The nursing diagnosis that best reflects impaired oxygen transport would be
    A. risk for infection
    B. activity intolerance
    C. fluid volume deficit
    D. decreased cardiac output

POSTTEST ANSWERS

Question	Answer	Section	Question	Answer	Section
1	C	Two	9	D	Four
2	B	Two	10	A	Four
3	A	Two	11	D	Four
4	C	Three	12	C	Five
5	D	Three	13	A	Five
6	B	Three	14	C	Six
7	B	Three	15	B	Six
8	A	Four			

REFERENCES

Andreoli, T.E., Carpenter, C.C., Bennett, J.C., & Plum, F. (1997). Disorders of the hematopoietic stem cell. In T.E. Andreoli, C.C. Carpenter, J.C. Bennett, & F. Plum (eds.), *Cecil's essentials of medicine* (4th ed.) (pp. 358–380). Philadelphia: W.B. Saunders.

Caudell, K.A. (1998). Disorders of white blood cells and lymphoid tissues. In C.M. Porth (ed.), *Pathophysiology: Concepts of altered health states* (5th ed.) (pp. 151–164). Philadelphia: J.B. Lippincott.

Gaspard, K.J. (1998). The red blood cell and alterations in oxygen transport. In C.M. Porth (ed.), *Pathophysiology: Concepts of altered health states* (5th ed.) (pp. 133–149). Philadelphia: J.B. Lippincott.

Guyton, A.C., & Hall, J.E. (1997). *Human physiology and mechanisms of disease* (6th ed.). Philadelphia: W.B. Saunders.

Kee, J.L. (1999). *Laboratory & diagnostic tests with nursing implications* (5th ed.). Stamford, CT: Appleton & Lange.

Lewis, S.M. (2000). Nursing management: Inflammation and infection. In S.M. Lewis, M.M Heitkemper, & S.R. Dirksen (eds.), *Medical–surgical nursing: Assessment and management of clinical problems* (5th ed.) (pp. 189–211). St. Louis: C.V. Mosby.

Mazur, E.M. (1998). Platelets. In F.J. Schiffman (ed.), *Hematologic pathophysiology* (pp. 123–160). Philadelphia: Lippincott-Raven.

O'Mara, A.M., & Whedon, M.B. (2000). Nursing management: Hematologic problems. In S.M. Lewis, M.M. Heitkemper, & S.R. Dirksen (eds.), *Medical–surgical nursing* (5th ed.) (pp. 736–789). St. Louis: C.V. Mosby.

O'Reilly, R.A. (1998). Drugs used in disorders of coagulation. In B.G. Katzung (ed.), Basic and clinical pharmacology (7th ed.) (pp. 547–562). Stamford, CT: Appleton & Lange.

Owen, D.C., & Webster, J.S. (1998). Hematology disorders. In M.R. Kinney, S.B. Dunbar, J.A. Brooks-Brunn, N. Molter, & J.M. Vitello-Cicciu, *AACN's clinical reference for critical care nursing* (4th ed.) (pp. 897–914). St. Louis: C.V. Mosby.

Parslow, T.G. (1994). The phagocytes: Neutrophils & macrophages. In D.P. Stites, A.I. Terr, T.G. Parslow, *Basic and clinical immunology* (8th ed.) (pp. 9–21). Norwalk, CT: Appleton & Lange.

Rose, M.G., & Berliner, N. (1998). Red blood cells. In F.J. Schiffman (ed.), *Hematologic pathophysiology* (pp. 49–96). Philadelphia: Lippincott-Raven.

Rosmarin, A.G. (1999). White blood cells. In F.J. Schiffman (ed.), *Hematologic pathophysiology* (pp. 97–120). Philadelphia: Lippincott-Raven.

Salmon, S.E., & Sartorelli, A.C. (1998). Cancer chemotherapy. In B.G. Katzung (ed.), *Basic and clinical pharmacology* (7th ed.) (pp. 881–915). Stamford, CT: Appleton & Lange.

Shulman, L.N. (1998). Hematologic malignancies. In F.J. Schiffman (ed.), *Hematologic pathophysiology* (pp. 291–317). Philadelphia: Lippincott-Raven.

Sommers, C. (1998). Immunity and inflammation. In C.M. Porth (ed.), *Pathophysiology: Concepts of altered health states* (5th ed.) (pp. 189–212). Philadelphia: Lippincott.

Timmerman, P. (1998). Common hematological disorder. In C.M. Hudak, B.M. Gallo, & P.G. Morton, *Critical Care Nursing: A Holistic Approach* (7th ed.) (pp. 933–949). Philadelphia: Lippincott.

Turgeon, M.L. (1999). *Clinical hematology: Theory and procedures* (3rd ed.). Philadelphia: Lippincott-Williams & Wilkins.

Ulrich, S.P., Canale, S.W., & Wendell, S.A. (1998). *Medical–surgical nursing care planning guides* (4th ed.). Philadelphia: W.B. Saunders.

Webster, J.S., & Owen, D.C. (1998). Hematological patient assessment. In M.R. Kinney, S.B. Dunbar, J.A. Brooks-Brunn, N. Molter, & J.M. Vitello-Cicciu, *AACN's clinical reference for critical care nursing* (4th ed.) (pp. 887–895). St. Louis: C.V. Mosby.

Module 24

Altered Immune Function

Helen F. Hodges

With respect to normal physiologic functioning, the immune system serves to protect the body from foreign invaders. These invaders might be disease-producing pathogenic microorganisms (also called pathogens) or abnormal cells, such as cancer cells. However, the immune system is actually the body's third and slowest line of defense against such invasion. An intact skin tissue provides the first line of defense, creating a physical barrier between the internal environment of the body and the external environment surrounding it. If, however, an invading organism or other foreign agent manages to get past this barrier, the inflammatory response is initiated, whereby invading agents are neutralized or destroyed. Failing that mechanism of protection, the immune system is alerted for action. This module is devoted to the structure and function of the immune system, with particular emphasis on the acutely ill adult.

Section One discusses the location and function of specialized cells and organs of the immune system. Particular organs and tissues are described in their relationship to immunity. The emphasis of Section Two is the primary characteristics of active and passive immunity. Section Three presents the learner with characteristics and outcomes of antigen–antibody activity. Section Four addresses with more detail the origin and function of the various cellular components of the immune system, including T cells, B cells, and macrophages. Section Five discusses the nature of immune mechanisms, including cell-mediated and humoral immunity, phagocytosis, and the role of interferon. Section Six explores the pathogenesis of hypersensitivity reactions and the notion of autoimmune disorders. Section Seven discusses manifestations of the autoimmune disorder systemic lupus erythematosus. Human immunodeficiency virus (HIV) is addressed in Section Eight with regard to the nature of the virus, its transmission and growth, and attempts toward treatment. Section Nine summarizes the impacts of aging, malnutrition, stress, and trauma on the immune system. Section Ten discusses nursing considerations pertinent to care of the immunocompromised patient.

Each section includes a set of review questions to help the learner evaluate his or her understanding of the section's content. All Section Reviews and the module Pretest and Posttest include answers. It is suggested that the learner review those concepts answered incorrectly in the review questions before proceeding to the next section.

Objectives

Following completion of this module, the learner will be able to

1. Cite the location and functional role of organs and tissues primarily involved in the immune response.
2. Contrast the nature of natural immunity and acquired (active and passive) immunity.
3. Describe the characteristics of antigens and antigen–antibody responses.
4. Discuss the nature and primary function of cellular components of the immune system.
5. Describe mechanisms of specific immunity (humoral and cell-mediated) and mechanisms of nonspecific immunity.
6. Explain the theoretical concepts for the occurrence of types I, II, III, and IV immunoglobulin hypersensitivity and autoimmune disorders.

7. Characterize the autoimmune dysfunction of systemic lupus erythematosus (SLE), including the pathophysiologic patterns, risks to the acutely ill patient, assessment and treatment approaches, and ultimate effects of the disease.
8. Characterize the immunodeficiency pattern of HIV, including the mechanism of transmission, viral invasion, growth, antibody formation, treatment approaches, and the ultimate effect of the disease.
9. Describe the pathogenesis of aging, malnutrition, trauma, and stress related to the functions of the adult immune system.
10. Discuss nursing considerations pertinent to care of the immunocompromised patient.

PRETEST

1. Which of the following is primarily responsible for T cell differentiation?
   A. bursa equivalent
   B. thymus
   C. stem cells
   D. lymph nodes
2. The bursa equivalent is thought to be located in the
   A. spleen
   B. Peyer's patches
   C. bone marrow
   D. thymus
3. Nonspecific immune response involves
   A. recognition of a particular antigen
   B. production of antibody
   C. recognition of nonself
   D. T cell differentiation
4. A child who first has chickenpox and then is immune from that disease in the future is said to have
   A. active acquired immunity
   B. passive acquired immunity
   C. natural immunity
   D. species-specific immunity
5. An individual whose antibody titer is greater than the preestablished level of immunity is said to
   A. demonstrate immunity from the disease in question
   B. require reimmunization
   C. demonstrate a specific antigen–antibody complex
   D. transmit the disease as a carrier
6. HLA antigen is located on which of the following sites?
   A. gamma globulin protein fraction
   B. erythrocytes
   C. chromosome 6
   D. RNA chains
7. Which of the following is responsible for direct antigen attack and destruction?
   A. helper T cell
   B. killer T cell
   C. suppressor B cell
   D. memory B cell
8. Macrophages are primarily responsible for
   A. interfering with the immune response
   B. protecting against local mucosal invasion of bacteria
   C. triggering the complement system
   D. carrying the antigen to B cells and T cells
9. Humoral immunity is best characterized by
   A. development of antibodies from B cells
   B. recognition of self and nonself
   C. specific recognition and memory of antigens
   D. differentiation of cellular function known as killer, helper, and suppressor cells
10. Which of the following immunoglobulins comprises about 75 percent of the total immunoglobulins in the healthy human body?
    A. IgA
    B. IgE
    C. IgG
    D. IgM
11. Which of the following immunoglobulins affords the body local protection at the mucosal level against invading organisms?
    A. IgA
    B. IgG
    C. IgD
    D. IgE
12. An example of therapeutically eliciting the primary and secondary response patterns of humoral immunity is
    A. exposure to chickenpox and subsequent immunity
    B. tetanus vaccine and booster vaccines
    C. interferon treatment for malignancy
    D. transference of killer T cells from donor to recipient
13. The results of a true type I hypersensitivity response are due to
    A. a histamine precursor causing anaphylaxis
    B. antigen–IgE–mast cell interaction
    C. antigen–antibody complexes deposited in vessel walls
    D. massive numbers of destroyed red blood cells (RBCs)

14. What characterizes the concept of autoimmune disease?
    A. recognition of self as foreign
    B. exacerbation and death
    C. accelerated production of killer T cells
    D. immunosuppression and altered cortisol levels
15. For which of the following reasons is SLE considered an added risk to the critically ill patient?
    A. exacerbation of symptoms creates complex assessment and treatment situations
    B. pituitary involvement poses a potential threat to the heart
    C. toxicity may occur with high levels of T cells
    D. severe fistula development is related to dermatologic involvement
16. Which of the following best characterizes HIV disease?
    A. symptoms result from opportunistic pathology
    B. clinical manifestation is of a characteristic and predictable sequence
    C. the HIV virus invades cells primarily through the bloodstream
    D. individuals who test positive for the HIV virus are carriers and considered contagious
17. Which of the following fluids is known to be a mode of transmission for the acquired immune deficiency syndrome (AIDS) virus?
    A. tears
    B. perspiration
    C. plasma
    D. saliva
18. What is the function of zinc in the competent immune system?
    A. it is required for normal function of lymphocytes
    B. zinc protects B cells from being destroyed by macrophages
    C. T cells require zinc for production of gamma globulin
    D. macrophages are composed primarily of zinc
19. What effect does the normal aging process have on the immune system?
    A. B cell function in general is particularly depressed
    B. the immune system becomes hypervigilant to invading organisms with increasing age
    C. autoantibodies begin to diminish with increasing age
    D. T cells begin to deteriorate in functioning
20. In the acutely ill adult, which of the following nutritional losses to the body is a critical factor in the immune system integrity?
    A. protein
    B. vitamin C
    C. complex carbohydrate chains
    D. iron
21. Decreased levels of neutrophils are associated with
    A. stress
    B. bone marrow depression
    C. infectious conditions
    D. tissue necrosis
22. The most important clinical manifestation associated with infection in an immunocompromised patient is
    A. elevated WBC
    B. local inflammation
    C. fever
    D. pain

Pretest answers: 1. B, 2. C, 3. C, 4. A, 5. A, 6. C, 7. B, 8. D, 9. A, 10. C, 11. A, 12. B, 13. B, 14. A, 15. A, 16. A, 17. C, 18. A, 19. D, 20. A, 21. B, 22. C

GLOSSARY

Acquired immunity, active. Immunity resulting from exposure to a specific antigen and subsequent formation and programming of antibodies; may be produced from having the disease or by injection of the weakened organism (vaccination)

Acquired immunity, passive. Temporary immunity provided by injection of sera containing antibodies, placental crossover, or mother's milk

Adaptive immunity. Immunologic activity that is highly antigen specific and has the capacity for long-term immunologic memory. Resistance following subsequent exposure is evident in competent adaptive immunity

Alpha-fetoprotein (AFP). An antigen produced normally during fetal development by the yolk sac and the liver. It is also found in serum of patients with cirrhosis, and testicular and some liver cancers. This antigen is an example of low immunogenicity and does not evoke an immune response

Allergic response. A hypersensitivity reaction of antigen–antibody activity in response to a specific substance that in nonsensitive people in similar amounts produces no effect

Antigens. Coded materials that allow the body to distinguish tissue as "nonself" or "self" and are generally capable of eliciting immune responses; antigens that do not evoke immune responses include tumor-associated antigens such as CEA, AFP, and PSA

Antigenic determinant site. Sites on antigens that interact with specific immune cells to bind in lock-and-key fashion; the binding elicits the immune response

Arthus vasculitis reaction. A severe local inflammatory reaction to an antigen; one example of a type III antigen–antibody hypersensitivity reaction

Autoimmunity. A destructive response in which the immune system recognizes self as foreign and begins to destroy the body's own cells and tissues

B lymphocytes (B cells). Lymphocytes primarily responsible for antibody formation on exposure to a specific antigen; the primary cells in humoral immunity

Bursa equivalent. Tissue thought to be located in the bone marrow, primarily responsible for differentiating lymphocytes into B cells for humoral immunity

Carcinoembryonic antigen (CEA). An antigen found in the bloodstream of patients with colon, lung, breast, and pancreatic tumors; this antigen is an example of an antigen that is not immunogenic

CD markers. Refers to "clusters of differentiation" cell surface antigen markings on lymphocytes. All T cells express the CD3 marker, and all B cells express the CD19 marker. Subsets of T cells and B cells are distinguished and recognizable by these markings (e.g., helper T cells, or T4 cells, are specifically marked as CD4)

Cell-mediated immunity. A type of protection against invading antigens characterized by surveillance and direct attack of foreign material; the primary effector cell is the T lymphocyte

Chemotaxis. Attraction of cells to a chemical stimulus (e.g., a mechanism of attracting neutrophils to site of injury is by an eosinophil chemotactic factor)

Complement system. A progressive, sequential cascade of events produced by substances found naturally in the circulating sera; components of the system must be triggered individually and cause cellular lysis of antigens

Cytokines. A collective term referring to chemical messengers primarily produced by leukocytes that activate other components of the immune system. Cytokines produced by B cell and T cell lymphocytes are called lymphokines; those produced by macrophages are called monokines. Examples include tumor necrosis factor (TNF), interferons (INF), and interleukin (IL)

Haptens. Substances with such a low molecular weight that they cannot act as antigens unless attached to a carrier, such as a protein; examples include dander, dust, and pollen

Histocompatibility antigens (HLA, human leukocyte antigens). Genetically determined surface antigens found in all nucleated cells in the body; one's own HLA antigens are substances that the body recognizes as self

Humoral immunity. The type of protection against foreign antigens provided by antibody formation from B lymphocytes

Hypersensitivity. An exaggerated response of the immune system to an antigen or antigens otherwise considered nonpathogenic; an allergy to a certain substance is an example of a hypersensitivity reaction

Immunity. A normal adaptive response to the external environment; it functions to protect the body from disease by means of both resistance to offending organisms and attack on offending organisms

Immunodeficiency. A general term referring to a state of deficient immune activity

Immunodeficiency, primary. Failure of either T cell or B cell function or both, resulting from embryonic or congenital lack of development of such organs as the thymus

Immunodeficiency, secondary. A deficiency of T cells or B cells or both resulting from illnesses, chemotherapy, radiation therapy, or a direct pathogenic attack on the immune system

Immunogenicity/immunogenic. Capable of evoking an immune response; in varying degrees, antigens are immunogenic; some antigens do not evoke an immune response (e.g., CEA, AFP)

Immunoglobulins. The product of plasma cells in the humoral immune response following exposure to a specific antigen; the five classes of immunoglobulins are IgG, IgA, IgE, IgM, and IgD

Innate immunity. Immunologic activity that is relatively nonspecific and generally prevents infection. Components include the skin and mucous membranes, chemical cytolytic substances produced by the body, and cellular types including monocytes, macrophages, eosinophils, neutrophils, and natural killer cells

Interferons. A family of lymphokines, originating from effector T cells, that are responsible for promoting nonspecific immunity against viruses and other intracellular pathogens

Lymphokines. Substances produced by T cells that influence the function of macrophages and inflammatory cells

Macrophage. A lymphocyte that ingests and digests antigens, then carries the antigen to the T cells and B cells; the link between the immune response and the inflammatory response

Major histocompatibility complex (MHC). A group of genes located on the sixth chromosome; responsible for coding histocompatibility antigens

Natural immunity. A type of species-specific immunity with which one is born

Natural killer (NK) cells. Leukocytes containing lethal substances that kill on contact when released. NK cells are neither T cells nor B cells in structure, but contribute to cell-mediated immunity through nonspecific attack. They are incapable of developing immunologic memory and are particularly effective against viruses

Opsonins. Provide binding sites for attachment of macrophages or neutrophils to the antigen; composed of IgG immunoglobulin and C3b, a fragment of the complement system

Pathogens. Disease-producing microorganisms

Plasma cells. The result of transformation of mature B cells in response to exposure to a specific antigen; primary cell to produce or secrete antibodies (immunoglobulins)

Primary response. The initial humoral response to antigen exposure; characterized by a latency period during which the antigen is recognized as nonself and identified specifically, and antibodies are formed in response to the antigen makeup

Rejection phenomenon. Attempted destruction of transplanted tissue at the cellular level by the host's immune system

Secondary response. The humoral response to subsequent exposure to the same antigen; immune response is heightened, and antibody formation is triggered more quickly than in the primary response

T lymphocytes (T cells). Lymphocytes primarily responsible for direct attack and destruction of invading antigens; for primary cell in cell-mediated immunity; killer T cells directly attack invading antigen; helper T cells enhance the action of B lymphocytes; suppressor T cells suppress or inhibit the action of B lymphocytes

Thymus. An organ in the mediastinum primarily responsible for differentiating lymphocytes into various types of T cells for cell-mediated immunity

ABBREVIATIONS

AFP. Alpha-fetoprotein

AIDS. Acquired immune deficiency syndrome

AZT. Azidothymidine

B cells. Bursa cells

CEA. Carcinoembryonic antigen

HIV. Human immunodeficiency virus

HLA. Human leukocyte antigen

HTLV. Human T cell lymphotropic virus

Ig. Immunoglobulin

IL-1. Interleukin-1

IL-2. Interleukin-2

INF. Interferon

MHC. Major histocompatibility complex

NK cells. Natural killer cells

SCID. Severe combined immune deficiencies

SLE. Systemic lupus erythematosus

T cells. Thymus cells

TNF. Tumor necrosis factor

SECTION ONE: Role of the Immune System in Body Defense

At the completion of this section, the learner will be able to cite the location and functional role of organs and tissues primarily involved in the immune response.

Acting much as a surveillance mechanism, the immune system monitors the internal environment for foreign agents. It is a complex system of organs and cells capable of distinguishing self from nonself, remembering previous invaders, and reacting according to needs as they arise. The primary organs of the immune system are the thymus, spleen, and specialized cells of the lymph nodes and tonsils. Contributing to the immune response are lymphoid tissues in nonlymphoid organs (such as the intestinal tissue), and circulating immune cells, such as T cells, B cells, and phagocytes. The circulating immune cells are discussed further in Section Four. Figure 24–1 shows primary organs and lymph tissue sites as well as the sites of T cell and B cell differentiation.

The Thymus

The **thymus** is a flat, lobed organ located in the neck below the thyroid and extending into the upper thorax behind the sternum. Reaching its peak size at puberty, it diminishes in size and composition steadily until it is hardly distinguishable in adulthood. Its lymphoid tissue is gradually replaced by adipose tissue over one's lifetime. The thymus produces a hormone called *thymosin*, thought to be active in the production of lymphocytes and also under investigation as an agent that stimulates the immune function in some immunodeficiency states.

The primary function of the thymus is the development of the immune system. During embryonic life, most lymphocytes develop from stem cells in the bone marrow and travel to the thymus after birth to be marked as T cells (T, of thymus origin). However, there is also evidence to suggest that some lymphocytes are actually in the thymus before birth and, along with other cells, migrate and become the spleen and the lymph nodes.

During extrauterine life, the role of the thymus is to differentiate lymphocytes into various types of T cells. In this process, the thymus alters the surface antigens of these cells, which gives them their identity as T cells, a specialized lymphocyte. Mature, differentiated lymphocytes are released into the bloodstream, and they relocate in peripheral lymph tissue, such as lymph nodes, tonsils, intestines, and spleen, where they await a call to action in body defense.

Bursa Equivalent

Much like the thymus in T cell maturation, the **bursa equivalent** in the bone marrow differentiates lympho-

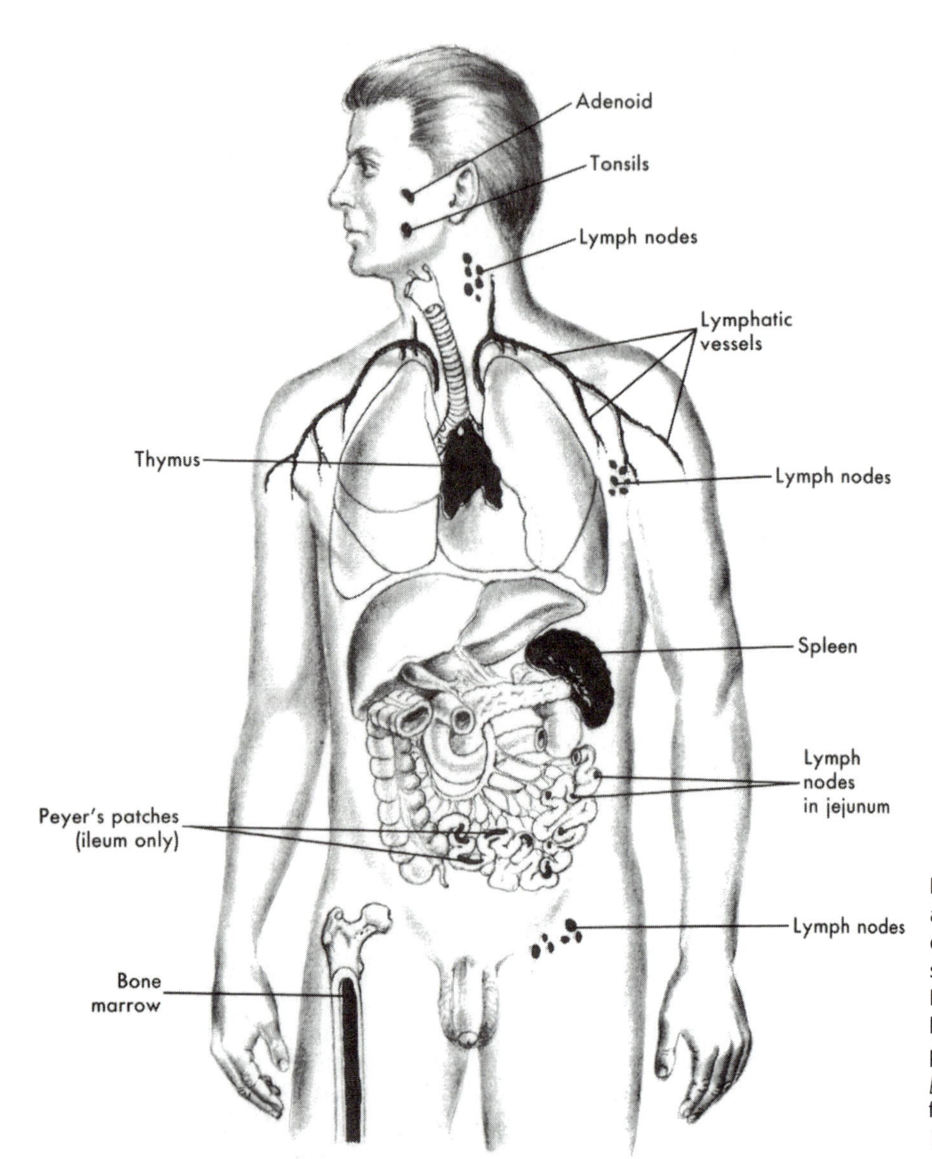

Figure 24–1. Lymphoid tissues: sites of B cell and T cell differentiation. Immature lymphocytes migrate through central lymphoid tissues, the bone marrow and the thymus. Mature lymphocytes later reside in the T and B lymphocyte-rich areas of the peripheral lymphoid tissues. *(From McCance, K., & Huether, S. [1990].* Pathophysiology: The biologic basis for disease in adults and children, *3rd ed [p. 178]. St. Louis: C.V. Mosby.)*

cytes into B cells (B, of bursa origin). Once released, these immature B cells migrate to the peripheral lymph tissue (lymph nodes, spleen, and tonsils), where they mature and await the body's need for defense against foreign agents.

Lymph System

The blood is filtered continuously by the lymph system. The lymph nodes actually serve two purposes for the body: They act as a filtering system for foreign materials, and they serve as a reservoir for the specialized immunologic T cells and B cells. Peripherally, the serous portion of the bloodstream (excluding platelets, red blood cells, and large proteins) diffuses from the capillaries into the peripheral lymph channels, where it is progressively filtered and then returned to the cardiovascular system. Lymph ducts carry this serous fluid through lymph nodes, where it is filtered. It may be useful to think of a lymph node much as a sponge, where the meshwork serves as a surface on which antigens and other foreign materials are arrested and destroyed or neutralized. Large clusters of lymph nodes are found in the axillae, groin, thorax, abdomen, and neck. With many infectious processes, these nodes become enlarged as their activity increases and defense cells proliferate. T cells are most abundant here, although B cells can be found also.

Spleen

The spleen is a small organ about the size of a fist in the left upper quadrant of the abdomen. It is protected by the 9th, 10th, and 11th ribs and, thus, usually is nonpalpable. The spleen serves three functions, only one of which is actually immune related. First, it is the site for the destruction of injured and worn-out red blood cells. Second, it is a reservoir for B cells, although T cells also are found there, and third, it serves as a storage site for blood, which it can release from its distended vessels in times of demand. The tonsils, Peyer's patches in the intestine, and the appendix are quite similar in function and structure to the lymph nodes and the spleen. The tonsils, like the thymus, diminish in size after childhood and, unless inflamed, are difficult to distinguish from surrounding tissue in the posterior pharynx.

In summary, the ability to produce and maintain an intact immune system requires the interaction of the thymus, bursa equivalent, lymph nodes, spleen, and tonsils as well as lymphoid tissue in nonlymphoid organs, such as the intestines. Although much of the immune system is well in place before birth, ongoing processes of marking and maturation of cells are critical to adequate functioning for nonspecific immune responses and specific antigen–antibody reactions to occur.

SECTION ONE REVIEW

1. Which of the following is primarily responsible for T cell differentiation?
   A. bursa equivalent
   B. thymus gland
   C. stem cells
   D. lymph nodes
2. As a person ages, thymus gland lymphoid tissue is slowly replaced by
   A. Peyer's patches
   B. stem cells
   C. bursa cells
   D. adipose tissue
3. The bursa equivalent is thought to be located in the
   A. spleen
   B. Peyer's patches
   C. bone marrow
   D. thymus
4. A major function of the lymph nodes is to
   A. filter foreign substances
   B. destroy worn-out red blood cells
   C. produce lymphocytes
   D. produce stem cells
5. Which of the following is correct regarding the spleen?
   A. it destroys worn-out white blood cells
   B. it filters out foreign materials
   C. it produces the hormone thymosin
   D. it is a reservoir for B cells

Answers: 1. B, 2. D, 3. C, 4. A, 5. D

SECTION TWO: Characteristics of the Immune System

At the completion of this section, the learner will be able to contrast the nature of natural immunity and acquired (active and passive) immunity.

Immunity is a normal adaptive response to the external environment. It functions to protect the body from disease by means of both resistance to offending organisms and attack on offending organisms. Immunity can be either natural or acquired.

Natural Immunity

Natural immunity is species-specific; that is, human beings are immune to a variety of diseases to which certain animals are susceptible, and vice versa. For example, human beings are not vulnerable to feline leukemia, and cats are not susceptible to human immunodeficiency virus (HIV).

Natural immunity is innate, in that human beings are born with specific immunities. This **innate immunity** is relatively nonspecific and provides primary protection against infection with cells that are incapable of developing long-term memory. Therefore, natural resistance to a particular infectious agent is not improved with repeated exposure to the agent. Natural immunity includes physical barriers to disease by means of the skin and mucous membranes, and natural chemical barriers found in the gastrointestinal tract, respiratory tract, and genitourinary structures. Specialized leukocyte cells that provide innate immunity include monocytes, macrophages, eosinophils, and **natural killer (NK) cells.** NK cells are instrumental in surveillance functions and provide antiviral activity on contact (Appelbaum, 1992; Imboden, 1994).

Acquired/Adaptive Immunity

Acquired immunity is a highly integrated adaptive process that is antigen-specific. Resistance to a particular infectious agent is significantly improved with repeated exposure to specialized cells that have been differentiated into long-term memory cells. This **adaptive immunity** includes certain monocytes and macrophages, and **T lymphocytes (T cells)** and **B lymphocytes (B cells)** (Appelbaum, 1992).

Acquired immunity can be either active or passive. **Active acquired immunity** is developed on exposure to an antigen, such as the chickenpox virus, during which time antibodies are programmed to protect the body from illness with future exposures. These antibodies are quite specific, often providing lifetime immunity against another attack of the same antigen. Active immunity also can be developed, again with lifetime protection, by exposure to a specific antigen through inoculation. Such vaccines as smallpox and polio vaccines provide a lifetime force of antibody protection without an actual illness occurring. Active immunity following exposure to a specific antigen does not provide immediate protection but develops over a period of days. However, the programming of specific antibodies provides heightened protection with subsequent exposures within a matter of minutes or hours.

Passive acquired immunity is a temporary immunity involving the transference of antibodies from one individual to another or from some other source (laboratory cultures, other animals) to an individual. An infant receives passive immunity both in utero and from breast milk. A neonate does not yet have a mature immune system capable of efficient development of antibodies in response to invading agents. Passive immunity can be transferred also through vaccination either of antiserum such as rabies, an antitoxin such as tetanus, or as gamma globulin, which contains a variety of antibodies.

Both passive and active immunity create levels of antibodies circulating in the body. Many of these levels can be monitored by venipuncture blood tests to determine full immunity to a particular disease. The result of testing the level of a particular antibody is called the antibody titer. The titer of the specific antibody is compared with a preestablished level thought to guarantee immunity. If the individual's titer is found to be lower than the preestablished norm, he or she may require reimmunization with the vaccine. An example of such a process is the increased scrutiny of individuals regarding their immune status to rubella.

In summary, there is ongoing interaction between the body and the environment as substances known as antigens come in contact with the immune system. The body has several avenues by which it might protect itself against foreign antigens. First, a natural immunity occurs normally and is species-specific. Second, the healthy body is able to respond to antigenic stimulation and produce its own antibodies that continue to circulate long after the antigen is destroyed, in some cases for a lifetime. Finally, antibodies may be transferred to the body by injection or through the common maternal–fetal circulation and breast milk.

SECTION TWO REVIEW

1. A child who first had chickenpox and then is immune from that disease in the future is said to have
   - A. active acquired immunity
   - B. passive acquired immunity
   - C. natural immunity
   - D. species-specific immunity
2. An infant who receives temporary immunity while being breastfed has
   - A. active acquired immunity
   - B. passive acquired immunity
   - C. natural innate immunity
   - D. species-specific immunity
3. An individual whose antibody titer is greater than the preestablished level of immunity is said to
   - A. require reimmunization
   - B. transmit the disease as a carrier
   - C. demonstrate a specific antigen–antibody complex
   - D. demonstrate immunity from the disease in question

Answers: 1. A, 2. B, 3. D

SECTION THREE: Antigens and Antigen–Antibody Response

At the completion of this section, the learner will be able to describe characteristics of antigens and antigen–antibody responses.

Antigens

Antigens are substances that are capable of triggering an immune response if they can be recognized by a B cell antibody or T cell (Goodman, 1994a, b). The immune response can involve either humoral or cellular components of the immune system, but commonly involves both. The degree to which an antigen stimulates an immune response is referred to as its **immunogenicity** or its **immunogenic** nature and is influenced by factors such as physical and chemical properties of the antigen, the relative foreignness of the antigen, and the person's genetic makeup. Antigens may be either foreign to the body or be important self-markers or tumor markers.

Foreign Antigens

Some foreign-body antigens are capable of causing disease and are called **pathogens** or **pathogenic antigens.** Many bacteria, viruses, parasites, and other microorganisms are pathogenic antigens, such as *Staphylococcus aureus*, *Mycobacterium tuberculosis*, herpes simplex, and human immunodeficiency virus (HIV). Other antigens, such as vaccines, are foreign to the body but are not pathogenic microorganisms. Vaccines induce a protective immunologic response by introducing either viruses or bacteria that are killed or treated, or those that are attenuated (selectively altered). Either type of vaccine presents a weak or killed antigen that is incapable of inducing a disease state, but effectively stimulates a mild immune response as a protective mechanism against similar live microorganisms.

Another example of a nonpathogenic antigen is a transplanted heart or kidney. The cells making up the tissues of these organs are not disease-producing but are recognized by the body as being nonself and, thus, can precipitate an immune reaction.

Although the immune system is certainly capable of distinguishing self from nonself in its natural state, it is not able to determine that a foreign material is acceptable even if that material is beneficial to the well-being of the body as a whole. This is the scenario that occurs in organ transplant rejection. The organ is viewed by the immune system as an invading antigen and is then attacked with the intent to destroy. Immunosuppressive drugs are administered to diminish the immune response. At the present time, there is no way to educate the system that an incoming heart, kidney, liver, lung, or other donor tissue must be accepted as self.

Histocompatibility Antigens

In addition to foreign materials being antigens, it is known that all nucleated cells in the body contain surface antigens, proteins found on the surface of a cell. These proteins distinguish an individual's tissue from tissue of other persons. Surface antigens are genetically determined and are referred to as **histocompatibility antigens** or **human leukocyte antigens (HLA).** They were first discovered on leukocytes, thus the label HLA. These surface antigens are similar to ABO antigens found on erythrocytes. Individuals with type A blood type have the A antigen on the surface of their red blood cells. Individuals with type B blood type have B antigens on their red blood cells. Type O blood type individuals have neither A nor B antigens, and type AB blood has both A and B antigens on the red blood cells. Like the ABO antigens, HLA antigens must be matched carefully before transplantation. The HLA antigens are genetically transmitted. The histocompatibility antigens are proteins that are coded by a group of genes called the **major histocompatibility complex (MHC)** located on the sixth chromosome. Five HLA antigen sites have been identified thus far and labeled: HLA-A, HLA-B, HLA-C, HLA-D, and HLA-DR. Each of these sites contains varying degrees of information that code the development of the surface antigen. For example, for HLA-A there are approximately 20 pairs of genes carrying information, for HLA-B there are approximately 30, for HLA-C there are approximately 6, and so on (McCance and Huether, 1994). Figure 24–2 represents the relationship of HLA sites to the major histocompatibility complex genes.

Since each offspring receives a pair of genes, one from each parent, the combination of the genes determines the HLA type. There are multiple possibilities of the coding of surface cell antigens for one individual. It is the surface cell antigens in most cases that the immune cells recognize as self. The closer in match of HLA surface cell antigens between two individuals, the less severe the immune response to a transplanted organ or graft.

It is thought that several pathologic disorders may be related to the presence of certain HLA antigens coded by the MHC genes. For example, ankylosing spondylitis appears to have a high correlation with HLA-B27, and rheumatoid arthritis is highly correlated with the presence of HLA-DR4 (Porth, 1998). Clinical interest continues to grow in research efforts in this area.

Tumor-Associated Antigens

Identification of tumor-associated antigens has progressed rapidly with technologic advances in tumor immunology.

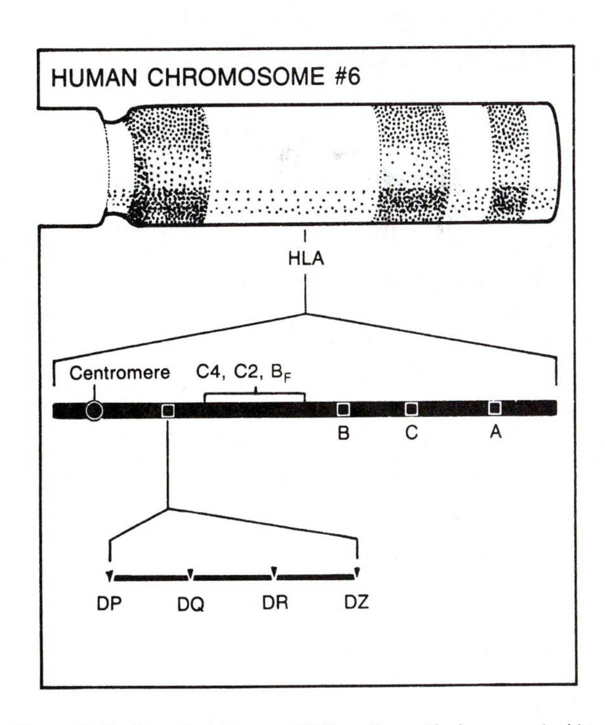

Figure 24–2. Genes for histocompatibility antigens. The human major histocompatibility complex (MHC) known as HLA (human leukocyte antigen) is found on chromosome 6. It consists of five regions. The D region is subdivided into four parts, which code for membrane 1a antigens. Between D and B, there are genes for three proteins of the complement system. B, C, and A (especially A and B) are genes for the serologically defined MHC class I antigens expressed on all nucleated cells and platelets. *(From Dolan, J.T. [1991]. Critical care nursing:* Clinical management through the nursing process *[p. 1163]. Philadelphia: F.A. Davis.)*

Some human tumors have been found to display particular antigens that distinguish normal cells from abnormally transformed cells. Tumor-associated antigens typically do not evoke an immune response (low immunogenicity), perhaps because they are recognized as self from early development during embryonic and fetal stages. Although many of these antigens occur naturally in small quantities, an elevation of the particular antigen type can be helpful in detecting potentially abnormal cells and tracking progression of disease or regression of disease following treatment (Appelbaum, 1992; Greenberg, 1994). For example, **carcinoembryonic antigen (CEA)** has been found to be elevated in a variety of adenocarcinomas of the colon, lung, breast, and pancreas; **alpha-fetoprotein (AFP)** is frequently elevated in patients with testicular and hepatic cancer; and serum elevations of prostate-specific antigen (PSA) has been found in occurrences of prostatic cancer (Appelbaum, 1992). Serum elevations of tumor-associated antigens are also possible with several nonmalignant disease states. Success in identifying and characterizing tumor-specific antigens that are not found in other disease states or on other host cells has been less successful to date.

Antigenic Determinants

Antigens have several specific sites, called **antigenic determinant sites,** which interact with immune cells to elicit the immune response. These sites are quite specific in configuration, requiring a specific structure of the immunoglobulin molecule or antibody. The binding of antigen to antibody occurs at specific receptor sites and is similar to the notion of a lock and key. Some molecules are so small that they cannot act as antigens until they attach to larger molecules or carriers. These substances are called **haptens.** Examples of haptens are house dust, animal hair particles, and pollen.

Immune Responsiveness

Immune responsiveness may be either specific or nonspecific. A specific response requires the recognition of a particular antigen and involves the production and action of a programmed antibody for that antigen. Normally, an antibody circulates in the bloodstream until it encounters an appropriate antigen to which it can bind. Such binding results in antigen–antibody complexes, or immune complexes. The process of binding is such that the antibody binds to particularly conformed antigenic determinant sites on the antigen, effectively preventing the antigen from binding with receptors on host cells (Fig. 24–3). The overall effect is protection of the host from antigen infection or penetration.

An antigen–antibody reaction can cause several consequences to the invading agent. The reaction can cause agglutination or clumping of the cells, neutralization of

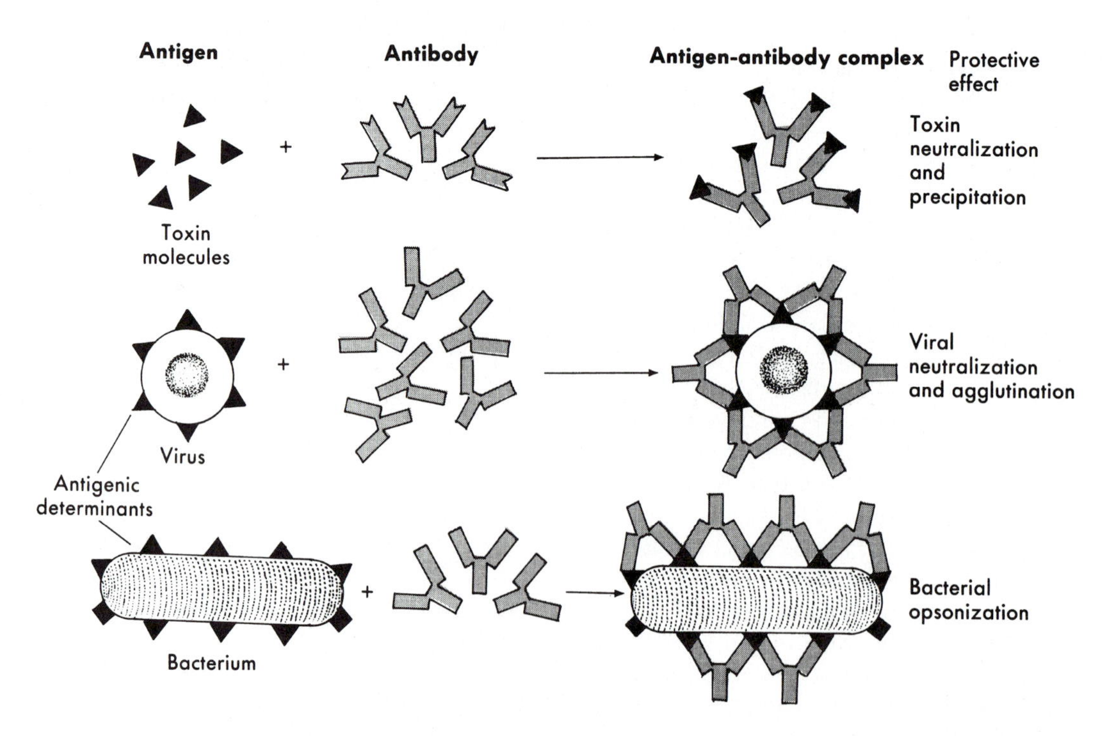

Figure 24–3. Antigen–antibody complex. Protective activities of antibodies: neutralization of bacterial exotoxins, neutralization of viruses and prevention of their interactions with cellular membranes, and opsonization of bacteria. All of these mechanisms are followed by removal of the antigen by phagocytosis, drainage along with body fluid, or both. *(From McCance, K., & Huether, S. [1998].* Pathophysiology: The biologic basis for disease in adults and children, *3rd ed [p. 188]. St. Louis: C.V. Mosby.)*

the antigen toxin, such as a bacterial toxin, cell lysis or destruction of the antigen, enhanced phagocytosis of the antigen by other cells, opsonization, or activation of the complement system.

A nonspecific response requires only the recognition of the invader being nonself, or foreign, but does not involve a particular antibody. A nonspecific immunologic response might involve the complement system, interferons, natural killer cells, and phagocytosis. These mechanisms of immunity are discussed in Section Five.

Antigen Entry Site

The entry site of an antigen is an important consideration. Many enzymes and other secretions are important components as defense mechanisms. Some antigens are destroyed before they cross into the bloodstream. For example, some antigens are readily destroyed or neutralized by salivary and other digestive enzymes in the gastrointestinal tract and are rendered incapable of causing disease. Other antigens are not affected by these enzymes and can proliferate rapidly, creating pathologic states. The site of entrance also determines the strength or virulence of the antigen. For example, an antigen that is neutralized by digestive enzymes in the gastrointestinal tract might be quite virulent if entering the body through the genitourinary tract or the respiratory tract, where digestive enzymes are not normally found.

In summary, the antigen–antibody phenomenon is the cornerstone for much of the body's protective immune system. Both antigens and antibodies have particular configurations that allow them to bind to one another. Once an antibody binds with an antigen, the antigen is no longer capable of binding with the host cell. The effect of binding may result in either neutralization, precipitation, lysis (destruction), enhanced phagocytosis, opsonization, or agglutination of the offending antigen. Which effect occurs depends on the class of antibody and the nature of the antigen.

SECTION THREE REVIEW

1. A nonspecific immune response involves
   - **A.** T cell differentiation
   - **B.** production of antibody
   - **C.** recognition of nonself
   - **D.** recognition of a particular antigen
2. HLA antigens are located on
   - **A.** RNA chains
   - **B.** erythrocytes
   - **C.** chromosome 6
   - **D.** gamma globulin protein fraction
3. Specific sites on antigens that interact with immune cells to elicit the immune response are called
   - **A.** antigenic determinants
   - **B.** surface cells
   - **C.** human leukocyte antigens
   - **D.** histocompatibility complexes
4. Antigens that precipitate disease states are called
   - **A.** immunoglobulins
   - **B.** pathogens
   - **C.** human leukocyte antigens
   - **D.** histocompatibility antigens
5. All of the following statements regarding the entry site of an antigen are correct EXCEPT
   - **A.** saliva in the mouth destroys many antigens
   - **B.** digestive enzymes neutralize many antigens
   - **C.** site of entry helps determine virulence of the antigen
   - **D.** entry location does not determine strength of the antigen

Answers: 1. C, 2. C, 3. A, 4. B, 5. D

SECTION FOUR: Cells of the Immune Response

At the completion of this section, the learner will be able to discuss the nature and primary function of cellular components of the immune system.

There are at least three types of cells involved in the immune response to foreign material: the T cell, the B cell, and the macrophage. Each cell carries a distinct responsibility and contributes to the integrity of the body as a whole. Each set of cells has effector cells and memory cells. The effector cells are those that are capable of attacking and destroying a particular antigen. The memory cells are those that are further imprinted with the antigenic code and are responsible for remembering and recognizing that antigen within minutes of a subsequent exposure.

T Lymphocytes (T Cells)

The T cells provide a type of immunity called cell-mediated immunity, which is discussed in a later section. T cells have a life expectancy of several years. They are marked by the thymus with specific surface antigens that characterize them and distinguish them from B cells. The T cells represent approximately 70 to 80 percent of the total lymphocytes.

Subsets of mature T cells are identified by a nomenclature referred to as *clusters of differentiation*. These clusters are actually surface antigens commonly known as **CD markers.** For example, helper T cells (T4 cells) bear a CD4 marker; suppressor T cells and killer/cytotoxic T cells (T8 cells) carry a CD8 marker. Approximately 70 percent of mature T cells carry the CD4 marker, and 30 percent carry the CD8 marker. Some central nervous system cells are thought to bear the CD4 marker, as are several types of gastrointestinal and skin cells (Stephens, 1997). This finding may help to explain the broad range of target tissues commonly affected by the HIV virus, which attacks cells bearing CD4 markers.

Five types of T cells are divided into two groups based on their particular functions, effector cells and regulatory cells. The T cells are known as cytotoxic, helper, suppressor, lymphokine-producing, and memory.

Effector T Cells

Effector T cells directly or indirectly affect immunity. As an indirect effect, they produce **lymphokines,** which are substances that activate inflammatory cells and macrophages. Some effector cells directly attack and destroy antigens. The natural killer T cell (or NK cell), appropriately named, is one effector cell that directly causes cell death of an antigen or tumor cell on contact. Activated cytotoxic cells also attack antigens.

Regulatory T Cells

Regulatory T cells are further divided into two subsets: helper T cells (T4 cells), which enhance the action of B lymphocytes, and suppressor T cells (T8 cells), which suppress or inhibit the action of B lymphocytes.

B Lymphocytes

The B cells are the larger of the lymphocyte cells and have a much shorter life span than the T cells. They mature with exposure to an antigen. Immature B cells are stored in the bone marrow, the lymph nodes, and other lymphatic tissue. They are also found circulating in the bloodstream. It is the B lymphocytes that are primarily responsible for antibody production. Following exposure to an antigen, mature B cells may be transformed into plasma cells, which then secrete antibodies called immunoglobulins. Each plasma cell is specialized to produce only one type of antibody. Several types of antibodies have been identified, and each is active within a given course of events in the immune response. Immunoglobulins are identified as IgA, IgD, IgE, IgG, or IgM. They are discussed in Section Five.

Macrophages

The **macrophage** participates in the immune response by processing the antigen and presenting it in such a way as to increase its recognition and reaction by the B cells and T cells. By means of phagocytosis, the macrophage ingests and digests the antigen, but in the process, the altered antigen is released through the macrophage cell membrane, where it attaches to receptor sites on the surface of the macrophage (Fig. 24–4).

It is at these receptor sites that the interaction takes place with the invading antigen and T cells. Macrophages, as antigen-presenting cells (APCs), are primarily responsible for carrying antigens to the lymph tissue, where the B cells and T cells reside. The macrophage is a critical factor in the immune response to both the T cells and the B cells and is considered to be the link between the inflammatory response and the specific resistance of antibody production and cell mediation by its production of interleukins. In fact, it is also thought that a lymphokine produced by effector T cells (those capable of attacking and destroying antigens) causes migration and activation of the macrophages.

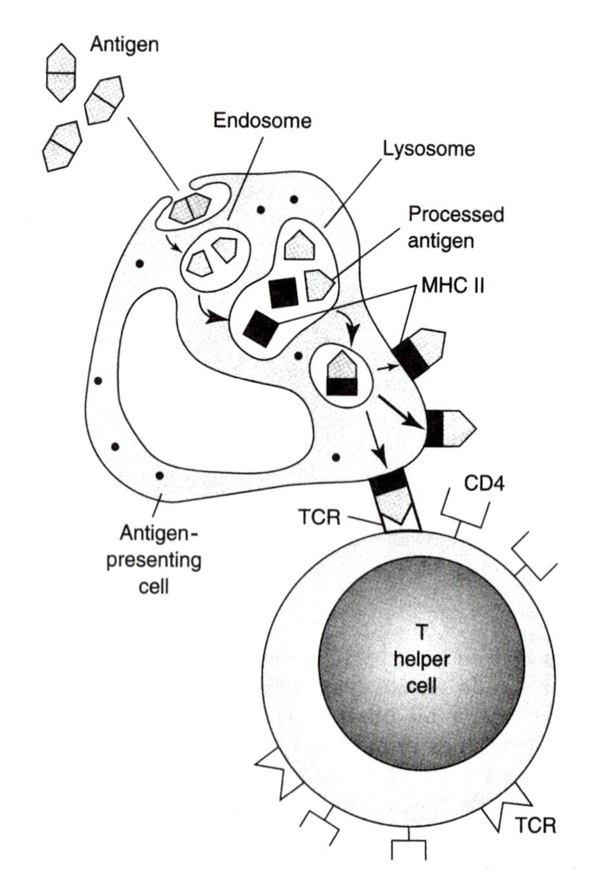

Figure 24–4. Presentation of antigen to T helper cell by an antigen-presenting cell (APC). *(From Porth, C.M. [1998].* Pathophysiology: Concepts of altered health states, *5th ed. [p. 195]. Philadelphia: J.B. Lippincott.)*

Immune Mediators: Cytokines

Cells of the immune system are regulated by chemical messengers, collectively known as **cytokines** or immune mediators, which serve to activate components of the immune system. B cells and T cells produce lymphokines (a type of cytokine). Of particular interest are interleukin (IL), tumor necrosis factor (TNF), and interferons (INF). Because of their ability to activate T4 helper cells (CD4), interleukin-1 (IL-1) and TNF can promote virtually all types of immune responses from T cells and B cells (Oppenheim et al., 1994). Interferons function to activate macrophages, cytotoxic (killer) T cells, and, with IL-2, natural killer (NK) cells.

In summary, all three cell types work together to maintain the integrity of the body against invading antigens. It is the macrophage, however, that plays the important role of preparing the antigen for the T lymphocytes and B lymphocytes. Without adequate macrophage support, the remaining cellular components of the immune system would be severely impaired.

SECTION FOUR REVIEW

1. Which of the following is responsible for direct antigen attack and destruction?
   A. helper T cell
   B. killer T cell
   C. suppressor B cell
   D. memory B cell
2. A major responsibility of the B lymphocytes is
   A. phagocytosis
   B. direct attack on antigens
   C. helper T cell function
   D. antibody production
3. Macrophages are primarily responsible for
   A. interfering with the immune response
   B. protecting against local mucosal invasion of bacteria
   C. triggering the complement system
   D. carrying the antigen to B cells and T cells

Answers: 1. B, 2. D, 3. D

SECTION FIVE: Mechanisms of Immunity

At the completion of this section, the learner will be able to describe mechanisms of specific immunity (humoral and cell-mediated) and mechanisms of nonspecific immunity.

The immune system can be described as providing two types of specific immunity. **Humoral immunity** is based on the activity and characteristics of the B lymphocyte. **Cell-mediated immunity** is based on the role of the T lymphocyte. Figure 24–5 depicts the differential development of cellular and humoral immunity and memory. In contrast, the nonspecific immune response is initiated solely on the recognition of foreign material being nonself antigens and not on their particular identity.

Specific Immunity

Humoral Immunity

Humoral immunity consists of the activity of the B lymphocytes. These lymphocytes mature with exposure to an antigen, develop into **plasma cells,** and produce specific antibodies, or **immunoglobulins.** Each plasma cell is capable of producing only one type of antibody and thus becomes committed to produce antibody only to a specific antigen. Each plasma cell then produces identical cells capable of continuing production of antibody in response to a particular antigen. Some of the offspring of a particular plasma cell continue to produce antibody, while other cells of that set become memory cells for the particular antigen.

The immunoglobulins are in the globulin fraction of the plasma protein. Each has a distinct amino acid chain that creates its specificity to react with a particular antigen. Because of this basic protein matrix of antibodies, the nutritional status of the individual in general and the protein status in particular are critical to an actively functioning immune system. Five classes of immunoglobulins (Ig) have been identified (Table 24–1). The plasma cell becomes the producer of immunoglobulin. Each of the five types plays a particular role in the immune response.

The most common immunoglobulin is IgG. It comprises approximately 75 percent of the immunoglobulins and is found circulating in body fluids. It is the only immunoglobulin that is known to cross the placental barrier, and is responsible for protecting the newborn during the first few months of life. IgG contains several types of antibodies, including antiviral, antibacterial, and antitoxin. It also activates the complement system. IgG can be administered as passive immunity via inoculation.

IgA comprises approximately 15 percent of the total

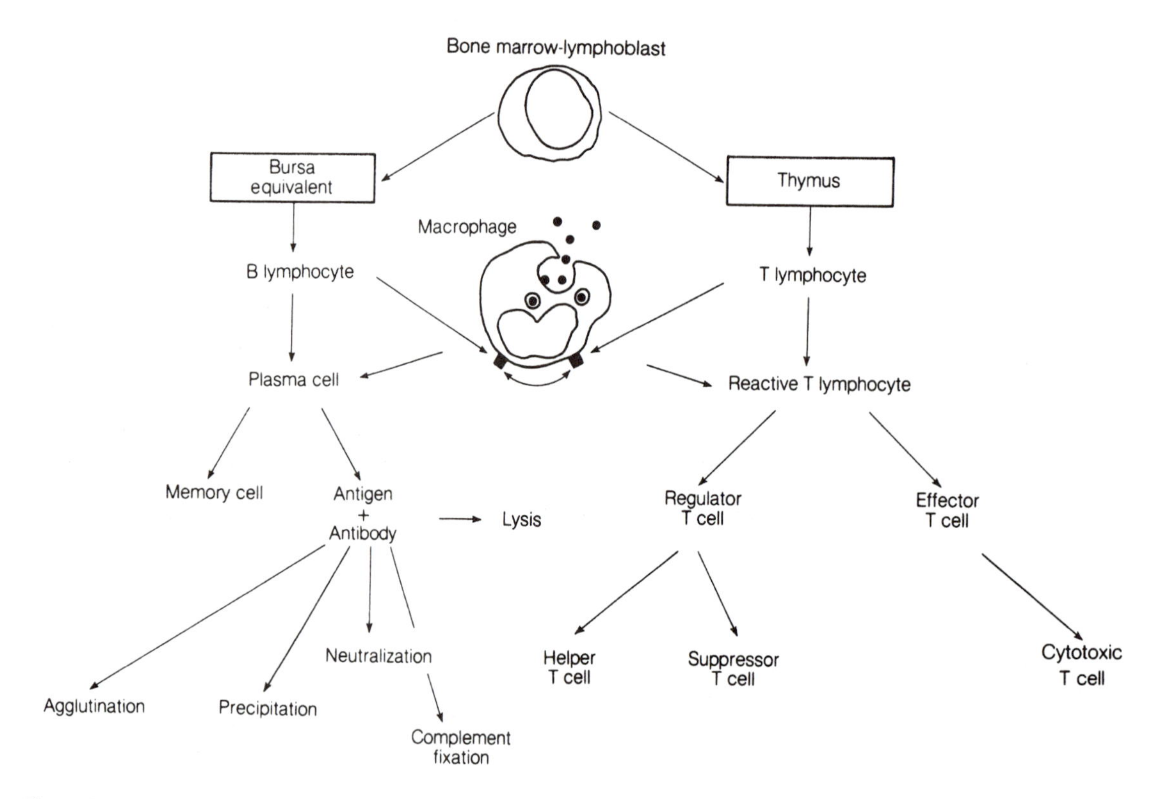

Figure 24–5. Development of cellular and humoral immunity. *(From Porth, C.M. [1994].* Pathophysiology: Concepts of altered health states, *4th ed. [p. 253]. London: J.B. Lippincott.)*

immunoglobulins. It is found in large quantities in secretory body fluids, such as tears, saliva, breast milk, and vaginal, bronchial, and intestinal secretions. IgA is produced by B cells in Peyer's patches, tonsils, and other lymph tissue. IgA affords the body a more local protection against invading organisms. The foreign material might well encounter the IgA antibody long before it encounters the IgG antibody. IgA provides protection at the mucosal level of invasion, whereas IgG provides protection more systemically from the position of circulating body fluids.

TABLE 24–1. CLASSES OF IMMUNOGLOBULINS

CLASS	PERCENTAGE OF TOTAL	CHARACTERISTICS
IgG	75.0	Present in majority of B cells; contains antiviral, antitoxin, and antibacterial antibodies; only immunoglobulin that crosses the placenta; responsible for protection of newborn; activates complement and binds to macrophages
IgA	15.0	Predominant immunoglobulin in body secretions, such as saliva, nasal and respiratory secretions, breast milk; protects mucous membranes
IgM	10.0	Forms the natural antibodies, such as those for ABO blood antigens; prominent in early immune responses; activates complement
IgD	0.2	Action is not known; may affect B cell maturation
IgE	0.004	Binds to mast cells and basophils; involved in allergic and hypersensitivity reactions

Adapted from Porth, C.M. (1998). Pathophysiology: Concepts of altered health states, *5th ed. (p. 197). Philadelphia: J.B. Lippincott.*

Smaller amounts of other immunoglobulins play roles in the immunity processes. IgM is instrumental in forming natural antibodies (e.g., for ABO blood antigens). It occurs early in the immune response to most antigens and is also important in activating the complement system. Comprising only 0.004 percent of the total immunoglobulins, the function of IgE seems to be most prevalent in allergic and hypersensitivity reactions involving the mast cells. The function of IgD is uncertain at the present time, although it may be involved in B cell maturation.

HUMORAL RESPONSE PATTERNS. Humoral immunity—the recognition of antigen and the production of specific antibody—occurs with a primary and secondary response pattern (Fig. 24–6). During the **primary response,** there is a latency period before the antibody can be detected in the serum. This delay may be 48 to 72 hours after exposure. It represents the time needed for the antigen to be recognized as nonself and identified specifically and for antibodies to be formed in response to the antigen's particular molecular makeup. After this latency period, a blood/serum test should reflect the level of antibody to a

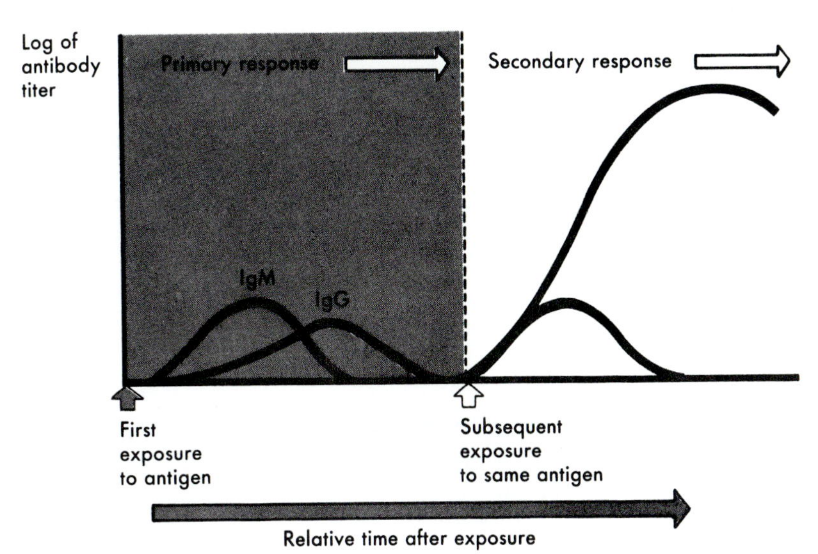

Figure 24–6. Primary and secondary responses of humoral immunity to same antigen. The introduction of antigen induces a response dominated by two classes of immunoglobulins, IgM and IgG. IgM predominates in the primary response, with some IgG appearing later. After the host's immune system is primed, another challenge with the same antigen induces the secondary response, in which some IgM and large amounts of IgG are produced. *(From McCance, K., & Huether, S. [1998].* Pathophysiology: The biologic basis for disease in adults and children, *3rd ed. [p. 177]. St. Louis: C.V. Mosby.)*

particular antigen and the degree of immune response. This level of antibody is called the antibody titer. The antibody titer normally continues to rise for about 10 days to 2 weeks. The peak of the titer generally occurs during recovery from most infectious diseases.

The **secondary response** occurs with subsequent exposures to the same antigen. It is during this time that the memory cells of the plasma clones recognize the antigen almost immediately and initiate the immune response with heightened antibody formation. If a titer were to be drawn at this exposure, one would find the antibody titer to be higher than that of the primary exposure. The follow-up booster regimen of many vaccines, such as tetanus, takes advantage of this secondary response and boosts the titer of specific antibodies to a level that will prevent the disease from occurring. This is the rationale for administering a tetanus booster within 24 hours of a new puncture wound.

Cell-Mediated Immunity

Cell-mediated immunity is based on the activity and characteristics of the T cell. During this portion of the immune response, the T cell and macrophage predominate, creating a direct attack on invading antigens. T cell immunity provides protection from intracellular organisms (such as viruses, fungi, and parasites), cancer cells, and foreign tissue. It is the T cell that is also responsible for much of the **rejection phenomenon** of transplanted organs and grafts. It is, however, one of the body's primary surveillance and attack mechanisms for protection from growth of malignant cells.

Unfortunately, T cell protection is not readily transferred from one individual to another, as humoral protection is. Cell-mediated immunity depends heavily on thymus and lymph node integrity as well as a nutritionally healthy body.

Complement System

The **complement system** is an immune mechanism that resembles the blood coagulation cascade, in that, once initiated, it progresses through several sequential stages, each contributing to the immune response and resulting in cellular destruction or cytolysis. The precursors to the complement pathways are normally circulating in the bloodstream. They are activated only by specific agents, such as IgG and IgM. The complement system is instrumental in facilitating phagocytosis by making antigens more susceptible to digestion, lysis of antigen cell membranes, and attraction of phagocytes to the invading antigen.

Nonspecific Immunity

Phagocytosis

Phagocytosis is a nonspecific immune response whereby invading foreign materials or injured cells are ingested and destroyed by phagocytic cells. Both neutrophils and macrophages are instrumental cellular components to this immune mechanism. Phagocytosis involves **chemotaxis,** the chemical attraction of phagocytic cells to antigens, as well as the engulfing of antigens for purposes of destruction or neutralization. A process known as *opsonization* modifies the antigen, making it more susceptible to phagocytosis. Two circulating factors enhance the opsonization process. The IgG immunoglobulin and C3b, a fragment of the complement system, are called **opsonins** and provide binding sites for attachment of macrophages or neutrophils to the antigen.

Interferons

The **interferons** also play an important but nonspecific role in the immune response. Interferons serve as the first-line defense in the protection of the body against viruses and other intracellular pathogens. Antiviral interferons inhibit the synthesis of viral protein in their reproduction without inhibiting the host's protein synthesis in normal cell reproduction. Immune interferons are known to be one of the strongest activators of macrophage activity. Interferons are lymphokines originating from CD8 and some CD4 T cells and NK cells. Although they are pathogen-nonspecific, they are species-specific. Thus, animal interferons offer little, if any, protection for human beings as vaccines. However, there is growing interest in the possible role of interferons as cell growth regulators in the study of malignant tumor control.

In summary, to maintain a total surveillance function, the immune system must be diverse enough to provide protection from foreign agents with a variety of immune mechanisms. Specific immune response mechanisms include humoral immunity with the formation of antibodies (immunoglobulins) and cell-mediated immunity with its direct-attacking T cells. Nonspecific protection is provided with phagocytes and interferons, which recognize nonself as being foreign but do not specifically program themselves for each individual antigen.

SECTION FIVE REVIEW

1. Humoral immunity is best characterized by
   A. development of antibodies from B cells
   B. recognition of self and nonself
   C. specific recognition and memory of antigens
   D. differentiation of cellular function known as killer, helper, and suppressor cells
2. The immunoglobulin that comprises about 75 percent of the total immunoglobulin in the healthy human body is
   A. IgA
   B. IgE
   C. IgG
   D. IgM
3. The immunoglobulin that locally protects the body at the mucosal level from invading organisms is
   A. IgA
   B. IgE
   C. IgG
   D. IgM
4. Which of the following statements is correct regarding cell-mediated immunity?
   A. it depends on B cell and macrophage activity
   B. it is part of the surveillance mechanism for malignant cells
   C. it is very easily transferred to an individual
   D. it does not protect against invading viruses
5. Antiviral interferons act by inhibiting the synthesis of _____, thus limiting abnormal cell growth.
   A. complement
   B. immunoglobulins
   C. lymphokines
   D. viral proteins

Answers: 1. A, 2. C, 3. A, 4. B, 5. D

SECTION SIX: Pathogenesis of Hypersensitivity and Autoimmunity

At the completion of this section, the learner will be able to explain the theoretical concepts of the occurrence of types I, II, III, and IV immunoglobulin hypersensitivity and autoimmune disorders.

Although several types of **hypersensitivity** reactions are recognized as immune responses, only those particularly associated with the acutely ill adult are discussed here. Historically, hypersensitivity disorders have been described as immediate or delayed reactions based on time from exposure to symptom appearance. Since 1962, hypersensitivity disorders have been commonly described as type I, II, III, and IV, based on descriptions developed by Gell and Coombs (Fig. 24–7). Of the four recognized categories of hypersensitivity reactions, types I, II, and III involve humoral immunity and specific immunoglobulins. Type IV is a cell-mediated response. Whereas some hypersensitivity responses manifest themselves with uncomfortable symptoms of watery eyes, sneezing, and nasal congestion, other more serious manifestations include the anaphylactic shock response, transfusion reactions with decreased oxygenation to major organs, and allergic asthma responses.

Immunoglobulin Hypersensitivity

Type I Response

One type of hypersensitivity is the **allergic response.** The true type I allergic response to an antigen results from IgE activity with mast cells found in the tissues (Fig. 24–8). Mast cells, part of the inflammatory process, are known to release histamine and other vasoactive substances when stimulated by immunoglobulin. In addition to histamine, which increases vascular permeability, an eosinophil chemotactic factor is released that attracts eosinophils, an anaphylactic substance causes constriction of smooth muscle (such as in the bronchiole), and a platelet-activating factor causes platelet aggregation or

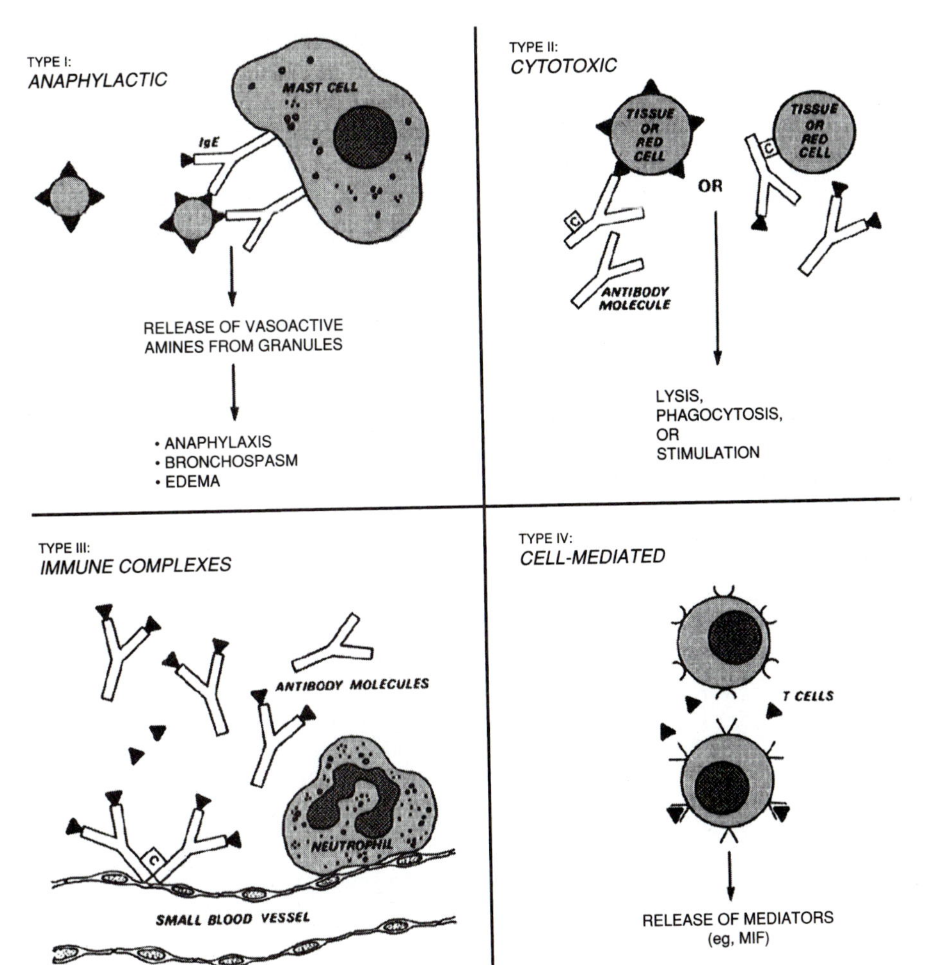

Figure 24–7. Diagrams of four types of immunologic mechanisms that may produce tissue damage. C = complement; ▲ = antigen; U and V = specific receptors for antigens. *(From Stites, D.P., et al. [1984].* Basic and clinical immunology, *5th ed. [p. 133]. Norwalk, CT: Appleton & Lange.)*

clumping and lysis. In sensitized individuals, subsequent exposure to an irritating allergen/antigen initiates the antigen–IgE–mast cell interaction, and the immune response and inflammatory response cause symptoms to develop.

Allergic asthma and allergic rhinitis (hay fever) are especially noteworthy examples of a type I response. In allergic asthma, the anaphylactic substance causing smooth muscle constriction in the bronchioles as well as the histamine release causing edema of the bronchial tissues warrant close monitoring and often emergency treatment to prevent death by asphyxiation. Antihistamines may block the effect of histamine release, but corticosteroids often are used to suppress the entire immune response. Such an allergic response is typically an immediate reaction and may be fatal if not interrupted. There is little if any involvement of T lymphocytes in this process.

ALTERED IMMUNOCOMPETENCE: ANAPHYLAXIS. Although IgE antibodies are primarily responsible for type I hypersensitivity reactions, causing the atopic disorders of allergic rhinitis, latex allergies, and asthma, they are also responsible for the occurrence of anaphylaxis. Systemic anaphylaxis occurs immediately—within minutes—and simultaneously in multiple organs in response to an allergen capable of stimulating the immune system. Most commonly, the causative allergens are food, drugs, or insect venom. Of significance is that the reaction lacks a genetic predisposition and may be fatal in response to prior sensitization to a minute amount of allergen.

Anaphylaxis typically involves the cardiovascular, respiratory, cutaneous, and gastrointestinal systems. Smooth muscle and vascular beds are affected, causing widespread edema and vascular congestion as a result of IgE antibodies interacting with mast cells which contain histamine. Histamine, a potent vasodilator, causes capillary permeability and leaking, smooth muscle contraction, and bronchial constriction. Complement is also a causative factor and further stimulates histamine release as well as a widespread inflammatory response. Anaphylactic shock is the extreme result of this histamine-related generalized vasodilation and vascular permeability causing rapid loss of plasma into interstitial spaces. This shift of fluid causes hypovolemic shock with profound hypotension, decreased cardiac output, myocardial ischemia, and widespread organ death.

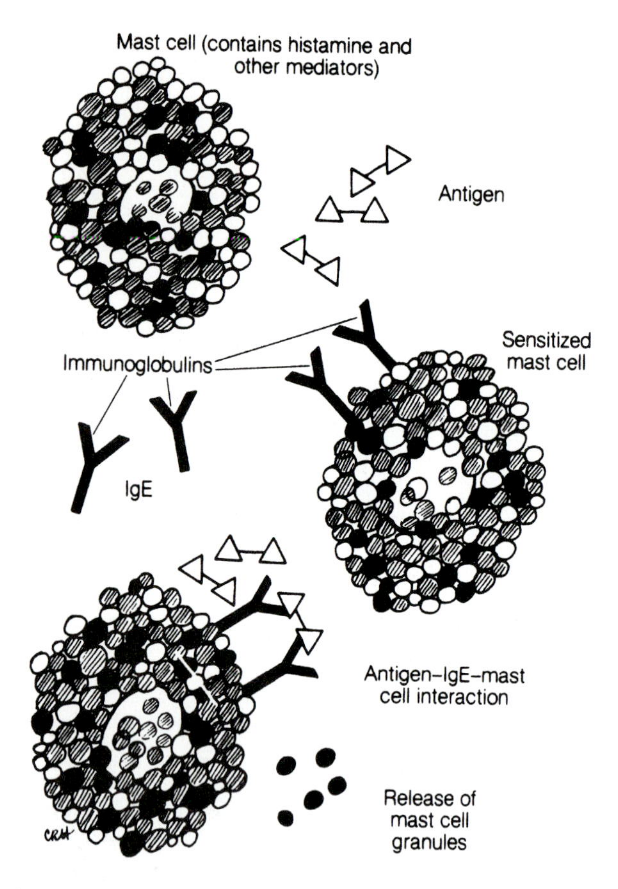

Figure 24-8. Allergen, immunoglobulin, and mast cell interaction, type I. Exposure to the allergen causes sensitization of the mast cell with subsequent binding of the allergen, which causes release of mast cell granules containing inflammatory mediators, such as histamine and SRS-A. *(From Porth, C.M. [1994].* Pathophysiology: Concepts of altered health states, *4th ed. [p. 273]. London: J.B. Lippincott.)*

Urticaria or hives are the result of histamine release from the IgE–mast cell interaction in which receptors in cutaneous blood vessels cause the characteristic redness and swelling. Urticaria alone is not life threatening but heralds the presence of an anaphylactic response. Assessment should include examining the patient for the potential risk of upper airway edema with asphyxiation and the risk of irreversible shock. Gastrointestinal involvement is related to smooth muscle contraction and edema of the mucosa resulting in crampy pain, nausea, and diarrhea. Similar responses can occur within the uterus, causing crampy pelvic pain and a risk of spontaneous abortion.

Treatment must be instituted immediately and includes epinephrine (IV, IM, or SC depending on the intensity). Laryngeal edema may require tracheostomy when edema precludes endotracheal airway placement. Bronchial airway obstruction and/or spasm is often treated with intravenous aminophylline. Other symptoms such as gastrointestinal cramping and urticaria respond well to antihistamine. Diagnostic testing may occur after the patient is stabilized to identify, via careful skin testing, the offending allergen.

Type II Response

A type II hypersensitivity response is referred to as a cytotoxic reaction. The immunoglobulins or antibodies known as IgM and IgG react directly with cell surface antigens, activate the complement system, and produce direct injury to the cell surface. Cellular membranes are disrupted, and target cells such as erythrocytes (RBCs), thrombocytes (platelets), and leukocytes (WBCs) are destroyed. Transfusion reactions are one example of this type of hypersensitivity. Other examples include Rh incompatibility in the neonate, drug reactions causing anemias, and hyperthyroidism caused by Graves' disease.

ALTERED IMMUNOCOMPETENCE: TRANSFUSION REACTION. Type II hypersensitivity reactions are characterized by transfusion reactions. The presence of an antibody in the recipient's serum typically attaches to the donor's erythrocyte (RBC), identifying to the body that the transfused RBC is a target cell. As the immune system becomes active, the RBC is destroyed by alerted macrophages as a hemolytic reaction. Following this destruction, hemoglobin from the red cell is released and is filtered through the glomeruli of the kidneys. This event creates a high risk of oliguria and renal shutdown because obstruction by hemoglobin fragments reduces renal tubular blood flow. Symptoms of a hemolytic transfusion reaction are caused by ABO surface antigen incompatibility and are likely to occur in the first 2 to 5 minutes of the transfusion. Evidence of the reaction includes the sensation of heat and redness at the infusion site, nausea, headache, back pain, chills, fever, and a sense of chest heaviness with difficulty breathing. Tachycardia, hypotension, and death can follow if the transfusion is not interrupted and treatment begun to reestablish cardiovascular stability.

Type III Response

The type III reaction is an example of an immune complex reaction involving antigen–antibody complexes with IgG and IgM. Type III reactions are characterized by deposits of antigen–antibody complexes in the epithelial lining of blood vessels, the kidneys, joints, skin, and other organs, rather than direct cell surface damage as in type II reactions. An acute inflammatory reaction begins as the complement system is initiated by the immune complex, and vessels become occluded with edema, hemorrhage, clotting, and accumulation of neutrophils, causing localized tissue necrosis. Type III reactions may be associated with infections such as hepatitis B and bacterial endocarditis; malignancies; drug therapy; and autoimmune disease.

ALTERED IMMUNOCOMPETENCE: VASCULITIS AND ORGAN DAMAGE. One example of the type III reaction is the **Arthus vasculitis reaction.** Although it may be considered transient and treatable in some body systems, in the case of a graft tissue rejection, the graft may become necrotic from the vasculitis and fail to recover. The Arthus reaction also may occur in other parts of the body unrelated to graft rejection, such as the alveoli, gastrointestinal tract, and skin from fungal antigens, gluten intolerance, and drug therapy. Type III responses are also responsible for lung, joint, and skin damage in autoimmune disorders such as systemic lupus erythematosus (SLE) and kidney damage in glomerulonephritis.

Type IV Response

Cell-mediated type IV hypersensitivity is a delayed-type response involving primarily the T lymphocytes, with no antibody activity. Tissue destruction is its hallmark, most notably through direct cellular killing by T cell toxins, lysosomal enzymes, or phagocytosis by macrophage recruiting following activation by the release of cytokines and lymphokines.

Altered Immunocompetence: Graft and Organ Transplant Rejection. Local reaction to a type IV response can also be demonstrated in the induration of a positive tuberculin test or contact dermatitis such as poison ivy and perhaps latex allergies. Clinical examples include graft or organ transplant rejection in which the HLA antigen is the principal target (graft-versus-host and host-versus-graft diseases). Immunosuppressive drugs, such as azathioprine (Imuran) and cyclosporin (Sandimmune) are given to delay or lessen this acute rejection phenomenon. (Refer to Module 4 for a more in-depth discussion of transplant complications.)

Autoimmune Disorders

For reasons yet unknown, the immune system occasionally begins to recognize self as foreign. With the usual physiologic actions, the immune system can set out to destroy self. Just as it cannot distinguish beneficial foreign material from destructive foreign material in the transplant phenomenon, the system recognizes self as foreign and initiates a destructive response in autoimmune diseases. **Autoimmunity** is intolerance to one's own body tissue and can involve abnormal activity of B cells, T cells, or the complement system. Characteristic of most autoimmune disorders is B cell hyperactivity. Viruses can contribute to autoimmunity by causing proliferation or destruction of lymphocytes. Many diseases are now attributed to such an autoimmune response, and many others are suspected. Table 24–2 provides a list of common autoimmune diseases. Immunodeficiency or immunosuppression may be a therapeutic goal in treating autoimmune disorders. Immune-mediated tissue damage may be suppressed through drug-induced, radiation-induced, or surgically induced immunodeficiency.

Several theories have been postulated to explain the autoimmune phenomenon. Among them are the possibility of alterations of body antigens by chemical or physical means; similarities in exogenous antigens and self-antigens creating a similar immune response to both; mutations of self-antigens to the point where they begin to appear foreign; or an abnormal response to HLA antigens on tissue surfaces. One theory proposes that certain self-antigens in the body were hidden from the immune system over a period of years and on their eventual appearance are recognized as foreign. Another theory suggests that cells reactive to self are always present, but few in number and controlled by regulating factors (Weigle, 1997). Section Seven presents an overview of one autoimmune disease, systemic lupus erythematosus.

TABLE 24–2. COMMON AUTOIMMUNE DISEASES

Respiratory
Goodpasture's disease
Gastrointestinal
Ulcerative colitis
Crohn's disease
Pernicious anemia
Endocrine
Graves' disease (hyperthyroidism)
Insulin-dependent diabetes mellitus
Addison's disease
Partial pituitary deficiency
Neuromuscular
Multiple sclerosis
Cardiomyopathy
Myasthenia gravis
Rheumatic fever
Connective tissue
Systemic lupus erythematosus
Scleroderma (progressive systemic sclerosis)
Rheumatoid arthritis
Ankylosing spondylitis
Hematologic
Autoimmune hemolytic anemia
Autoimmune thrombocytopenic purpura
Renal
Immune-complex glomerulonephritis

In summary, hypersensitivity is an exaggerated or inappropriate immune response to an antigen that results in harm to the body. The allergic response is one type of hypersensitivity reaction and commonly involves an antigen from the environment otherwise considered to be nonpathogenic and not intrinsically harmful to most persons. This section described the four types of hypersensitivity responses, type I, II, III, and IV, and gave examples of each. Finally, the concept of autoimmunity was explored as an altered immunity mechanism, in which the immune system becomes self destructive. To date, no mechanism is known to prevent the abnormal responses of autoimmunity.

SECTION SIX REVIEW

1. The results of a true type I hypersensitivity response are due to
   A. a histamine precursor causing anaphylaxis
   B. antigen–IgE–mast cell interaction
   C. antigen–antibody complexes deposited in vessel walls
   D. massive numbers of destroyed red blood cells
2. Type III hypersensitivity reactions are often characterized by
   A. specific target cells
   B. widespread multiorgan involvement
   C. rapidly progressing symptoms
   D. relatively low-risk patterns
3. Theories of the etiology of the autoimmune phenomenon include all of the following EXCEPT
   A. similarities between self-antigens and nonself antigens
   B. abnormal responses to HLA antigens on tissues
   C. chemical alterations of body antigens
   D. altered mast cell composition
4. Which of the following is correct regarding type IV cell-mediated hypersensitivity responses?
   A. it involves primarily antibody activity
   B. it does not harm body tissues
   C. T cell activity is responsible
   D. it directly interacts with cell surface antigens
5. Disorders thought to be autoimmune in etiology include all of the following EXCEPT
   A. chronic bronchitis
   B. ulcerative colitis
   C. pernicious anemia
   D. diabetes mellitus (insulin-dependent)

Answers: 1. B, 2. B, 3. D, 4. C, 5. A

SECTION SEVEN: Systemic Lupus Erythematosus: A Manifestation of Autoimmunity

Acutely ill patients often present with compounding complicating factors, making assessment, diagnosis, treatment, and recovery difficult. Autoimmune diseases can create a situation in which a chronic disease state causes a state of heightened vulnerability to exist for the patient, or the critical illness allows an otherwise suppressed chronic disease to become quite visible. Either situation can create an exacerbated high-acuity level and an escalated risk to survival.

Systemic lupus erythematosus (SLE) can manifest itself symptomatically from a mild to a fatal form. However, its potential for systemic damage to cardiorespiratory, hematologic, and renal function makes it one of the most complex chronic illnesses to occur simultaneously with other critical illnesses. For example, as many as 40 percent to 50 percent of SLE patients present with pleural effusion or pleuritis; 20 percent to 40 percent present with pericarditis, myocarditis, or hypertension; and 30 percent to 75 percent present with central nervous system involvement such as strokes, seizures, or psychotic symptoms such as dementia, altered consciousness, depression, or euphoria. Approximately 50 percent of SLE patients demonstrate symptoms of renal involvement such as glomerulonephritis, nephrotic syndrome, or renal failure (Porth, 1998).

SLE is thought to be representative of type III hypersensitivity responses. As with other type III responses, SLE is characterized by antigen–antibody complex deposits in the epithelial lining of blood vessels and in tissue surfaces. These create occlusions and inflammation, both of which can cause local damage with edema, hemorrhage, or clotting and an accumulation of neutrophils. Occlusion ultimately leads to tissue death and scar tissue formation, which then impairs organ function.

Why SLE suddenly becomes visible in selected individuals can only be hypothesized. Popular belief holds that the disease is brought about by a combination of genetic, hormonal, and environmental factors. Populations at risk seem to be those who have had repeated exposure to ultraviolet light and various chemicals (drugs such as hydralazine and procainamide, and hair dyes). A familial tendency strongly suggests a genetic link, presumably linked to the HLA genes. The incidence of lupus is statistically higher in African Americans and Asians. The disease is nine times more common in women than in men, and up to 30 times more common in women of childbearing age (Porth, 1998). Studies suggest that estrogens seem to foster the development of SLE, perhaps by enhancing helper T cell function and weakening suppressor T cell function. The net result of helper T cells is the increased production of antibodies; in the case of SLE, it is autoantibodies that develop.

Several theories exist as to the circumstances under which SLE might develop. Tolerance to self-antigens develops normally during the embryonic period. One theory explains autoimmunity as a disease state that occurs when previously sequestered antigens are released from damaged sites following, for example, trauma, infection, or chemical exposure. These self-antigens, hidden immunologically for years, are suddenly recognized by the immune system as foreign, precipitating the immune response and development of autoantibodies against the body's own tissues.

Another theory proposes that during infectious disease, as immune complexes made of pathogenic antigens and antibodies are deposited in tissue sites, a similar production of autoantibodies occurs because of a close resemblance of the self-antigen and the pathologic antigen. The development of autoantibodies then occurs against the body's own tissues, and autodestruction begins. Yet another theory posits that the aging process, with a decrease in T4 cells and increasing hyperactivity of B cells, allows an unchecked increase in antibody formation to occur. Some of these antibodies develop erratically into cells that attack HLA antigens or self-antigens. Several types of immune complexes may be present, thereby increasing the variety of symptoms depending on the tissue and organs to which they have affinity.

Symptoms

Regardless of how or why the disease begins, its symptom presentation and management are highly individualized. Unlike many other autoimmune diseases, SLE is not organ-specific, but its autoantibodies have affinity for DNA. Complex deposits are commonly found in the basement membrane of the glomeruli and renal tubules, as well as in the brain, heart, lung, connective tissues, and spleen. Major clinical findings are illustrated in Figure 24–9.

One of the distinguishing markers of SLE is that affected individuals manifest symptoms of the disease differently depending on the body system affected. Although the majority of patients present symptomatically with cardiopulmonary or renal symptoms at one time or another, nearly all SLE patients experience constitutional symptoms of malaise, fatigue, fever, skin manifestations (rashes and patches), and joint pain.

Chest x-ray reveals cardiomegaly, pleural effusion, and atelectasis. Shortness of breath results from restrictive pulmonary fibrosis, atelectasis, anemia, and the occurrence of congestive heart failure. Cardiac arrhythmias are relatively rare, but chest pain is common owing to pericarditis, myocarditis, or pleurisy. In addition to the cardiopulmonary, renal, and CNS involvement, serious functional symptoms include hemolytic disorders of all three cellular pathways: risk of infection with decreased white blood cells (leukopenia), fatal hemolytic anemia, and bleeding and clotting disorders (thrombocytopenia). Although it is the constitutional symptoms that prompt many patients to seek medical care, for the acutely ill patient, it is the primary organ dysfunction that causes the complex morbidity during times of critical illness.

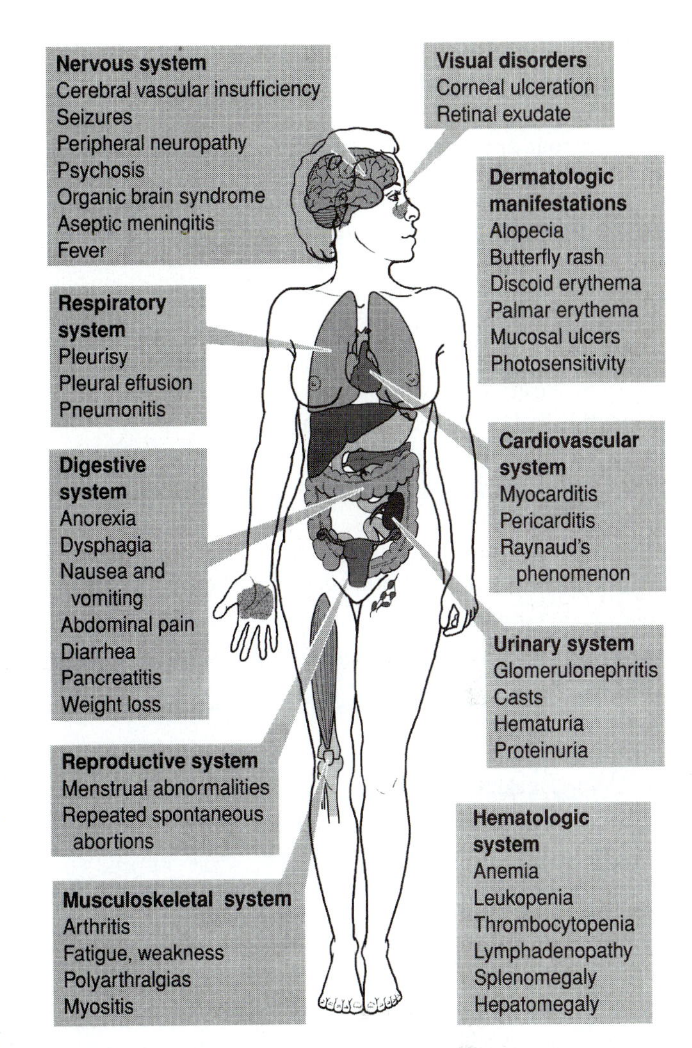

Figure 24–9. Diagram illustrating major clinical findings of systemic lupus erythematosus. *(From Burrell, L.O., et al. [1997].* Adult nursing: Acute and community care *[p. 176]. Stamford, CT: Appleton & Lange.)*

Diagnosis

Diagnosis can be quite difficult and frustrating. Various laboratory tests are available, but no single test is ultimately diagnostic for SLE. Historically, the LE cell test was used in diagnosis, but this test is not specific and several others have replaced it. The most common laboratory test performed is the antinuclear antibody (ANA), which is used for screening; over 95 percent of lupus patients exhibit high ANA levels. However, ANA is not specific for SLE and can be elevated with other diseases such as scleroderma, myositis, and rheumatoid arthritis, and occasionally in various chronic diseases, the aged, and even healthy individuals. A positive ANA is only considered one piece of data toward determining the presence of SLE; other criteria must be present, including a constellation of symptoms and significant history. Although the presence of a positive ANA without other supporting data signifies nothing, the absence of ANA is considered strong evidence that SLE is not present. Anti-DNA and anti-Sm (Smith) antibodies are considered quite specific for SLE and frequently parallel the activity of the disease. Low levels of serum complement (CH50, C4, C3) are also suggestive of SLE.

Data suggesting positive diagnosis includes the presence of four or more of the following criteria as outlined by the American Rheumatism Association:

1. Malar rash (facial butterfly erythema)
2. Discoid rash
3. Photosensitivity
4. Hemolytic anemia, leukopenia, or thrombocytopenia
5. Positive LE prep
6. Oral or nasopharyngeal ulcers
7. Deforming arthritis
8. Anti-DNA
9. Profuse proteinuria
10. Pleuritis or pericarditis; and
11. Seizure or psychotic neurological disorder

Treatment

Treatment of SLE depends on the severity of the illness and the systems involved. Although lupus arthritic-type symptoms and dermatologic symptoms are typically nonfatal and are treated with a regimen of nonsteroidal anti-inflammatory drugs (NSAIDs) and antimalarial drugs, respectively, the more severe symptoms related to cardiac, pulmonary, and renal function are often treated aggressively with high-dose corticosteroids. Uncontrolled lupus "flares" are treated with immunosuppressive agents such as azathioprine (Imuran), cyclophosphamide (Cytoxan), or methotrexate (Fye & Sack, 1994). The risks of aggressive treatment and immunosuppression for severe flares are weighed against the anticipated benefits. Certainly, the complication of systemic lupus erythematosus carries a greater threat of morbidity and mortality in the high-acuity patient.

SECTION SEVEN REVIEW

1. How would you explain the threat of SLE to the immune system in the high-acuity patient?
   A. the T cells are likely to disintegrate
   B. the risk of severe complications is generally low
   C. for some patients renal involvement is a high risk
   D. immature B cells are formed without antibody DNA
2. The course of SLE can be characterized by
   A. a steady increase in intensity of symptoms
   B. a peak of symptoms followed by a slow decline to remission
   C. symptom remission at the onset of old age
   D. individual variation of symptom presentation and intensity
3. What percentage of patients with SLE experience pulmonary involvement?
   A. 20 to 30 percent
   B. 40 to 50 percent
   C. 90 to 99 percent
   D. 75 to 80 percent
4. Which of the following pathologic mechanisms describes lupus involvement with the kidneys?
   A. glomeruli become atrophied
   B. immune complexes deposited in epithelial lining
   C. vascular bed is dramatically dilated
   D. renal artery is obstructed with edema
5. A patient with an uncontrolled "flare" of systemic lupus is likely to be treated with
   A. prednisone
   B. azathioprine (Imuran)
   C. NSAID
   D. hydroxychloroquine (Plaquenil)
6. Describe the physiologic premise on which gender incidence is thought to occur for SLE.
   A. estrogen "protects" the body from autoantibodies
   B. testosterone enhances B cell differentiation to IgA
   C. progesterone stimulates HLA antigen formation
   D. estrogen inhibits T cell function

Answers: 1. C, 2. D, 3. B, 4. B, 5. B, 6. D

SECTION EIGHT: HIV Disease: A Manifestation of Immunodeficiency

At the completion of this section, the learner will be able to characterize the immunodeficiency pattern of human immunodeficiency virus (HIV) disease, including the mechanisms of transmission and intracellular extension of the disease.

Assuming that the immune system and its component parts are intact and functioning normally, one might expect reasonable protection against invading microorganisms, pathogens, and foreign material. Even in such a case, the body often cannot overcome a pathogenic process. The immune system can be subject to inadequate development, disease, and injury from illness or treatments that can result in deficient immune activity. Such a situation is called an **immunodeficiency** state.

Primary Immunodeficiency

Characteristics of **primary immunodeficiency** may vary widely depending on the basic etiology. For example, T cells may fail to develop because of some embryonic anomaly or genetic code. DiGeorge syndrome is an example of a congenital thymic aplasia or hypoplasia in which there are greatly decreased levels of T cells because of partial lack of a thymus. B cell deficiency also may develop from embryonic dysfunction or developmental delay of an infant's immune system and results in lowered levels of immunoglobulins. A condition in which immunoglobulins are almost totally absent from the circulation is known as agammaglobulinemia.

In some instances, both B cells and T cells are affected, as in severe combined immune deficiencies (SCID). In SCID, the bone marrow stem cells for lymphocyte development may be absent. Affected children spend a good portion of their short lives in an environment of total protection from any antigen. The child who lived much of his life in a sterile environment is an example of SCID. Most primary states of immunodeficiency are the result of either embryonic anomaly, genetic predisposition, or congenital failure of the system to develop, thus occurring almost exclusively in infants and toddlers.

Secondary Immunodeficiency

Secondary immunodeficiency states can occur in adults but usually are the result of other primary diseases, drug therapy, or irradiation therapy. For example, the patient with Hodgkin's disease, a malignancy of the lymphatic tissue, might well suffer from subsequent immunodeficiency following malignant invasion of that lymph tissue. Prolonged corticosteroid therapy is known to suppress the adrenal glands through the negative feedback loop (immunosuppression). Eventually, such a suppression creates a situation of immunodeficiency caused by atrophy of lymphoid tissue, decreased antibody formation, decreased development of cell-mediated immunity, and impaired phagocytosis. Finally, immunosuppressive drugs, such as azathioprine (Imuran) and cyclosporine, are administered for the purpose of suppressing the immune response to transplanted organs and grafts (refer to Module 4 for further discussion of immunosuppression).

Human beings can become immune deficient from a direct attack on the immune system by pathogens. When such a situation exists, it is known as acquired immunodeficiency. Acquired immunodeficiency is not primary in that it is not genetically transmitted, nor is it embryonic in the sense of lymphoid tissue failing to develop adequately. It is secondary in the sense that another disease or therapy caused the deficiency.

Cellular Manifestations Characterizing HIV Disease

The immune deficiency characterizing HIV disease is manifested by markedly depressed T lymphocyte functioning, with a reduction of helper T4 cells (CD4), impaired killer T cell activities, and increased suppressor T cells (T8). By selectively invading and infecting T cells, the virus damages the very cell whose function it is to orchestrate the identification and destruction of the virus as antigen. Other cells with the same molecular makeup and surface markers might also become infected. Eventually, the individual's supply of functional T cells becomes depleted. In a person with a competent immune system, the number of T4 lymphocytes ranges from 600 to 1,200/μL, whereas the patient with HIV might have 0 to 500/μL T4 cells. The humoral response in producing antibodies is less directly affected by the HIV virus. B cell production does not seem to be decreased, but the induction and regulation of the humoral response may be affected by the lack of T cell regulators (e.g., T4 cell helpers and T8 cell suppressors).

Epidemiology and Transmission of the HIV Virus

The first populations generally thought to be the major contributors to the current HIV epidemic in the United States were homosexuals and persons using IV drugs while sharing used needles. However, studies now show that the disease has become widely disseminated to include heterosexual groups and all races and ethnic groups represented in the United States. This pattern of homosexual/bisexual men and IV drug users is particular to advanced or industrialized nations. Heterosexual men and women seem to contract the disease at about an equal rate, however, in African and Caribbean countries (CDC, 1997).

The mode of transmission is predominantly by infected blood and body secretions, generally excluding saliva and tears. The most common modes of transmission are sexual contact, administration of contaminated blood and blood products, contaminated needles, and mother to fetus; although blood transfusions of whole blood, packed cells, and fresh frozen plasma are most unlikely to be the cause of transmission with the sophisticated crossmatching and antibody screening measures in use today. However, individuals needing specific blood components (such as factor VIII and frequent plasma replacement) may be at more risk because of the large numbers of donors needed to produce adequate quantities of these components. The risk of acquiring the virus increases with the number of potential carriers involved, just as multiple sexual contacts create higher risk.

Viral Invasion

HIV, or human immunodeficiency virus, formerly known as the human T cell lymphotropic virus (HTLV-III), is known to be a lentivirus of the retrovirus family, carrying genetic information in RNA rather than in DNA. The virus infects the T lymphocyte by binding to it at the CD4 receptor site and penetrating the T cell membrane. Through an enzyme called reverse transcriptase, the HIV RNA is copied as a double-stranded DNA and inserted into the host cell chromosome where non-infectious, immature viral proteins are formed (Fig. 24–10). When the T cell is activated to reproduce, such as during other viral infections, stress, and other causes, its genetic information is programmed to produce more of the infectious HIV virus, and the number of functional T cells diminishes rapidly. Viral load and CD4 T cell counts are reflective of viral activity and disease progression. Unfortunately, reverse transcriptase is highly error-prone and may produce multiple mutations during each replication of the HIV virus. The AIDS patient could have hundreds of viral mutations to transmit. Most antiviral drugs now being tested or used in treatment regimens work by inhibiting the action of reverse transcriptase or by inhibiting an enzyme (protease) needed at a later stage of the HIV's life when maturation of new infectious viruses takes place (Porche, 1999). To date, there are two forms of HIV: HIV-1 and HIV-2. HIV-1 is thought to be the primary pathogenic basis of most AIDS cases. HIV-2 has also been found to cause AIDS, but seems less virulent, less transmissible, and creates lower proportions of infected cells (Stephens, 1997).

HIV Screening

The antibody to this virus has been identified and can be used for screening purposes. However, the latency period—the time the body takes to recognize nonself and program antibodies to the virus, called *seroconversion*—is longer than with many other infectious organisms. The latency period for blood-transmitted HIV infection is thought to be 2 weeks to 3 to 6 months (Bartlett, 1998; Stephens, 1997), and rarely up to 10 months; most people seroconvert by 6 months. The prolonged latency period thus effectively reduces the accuracy and immediacy of host identification. One of the theories concerning this prolonged latency period is that HIV invades T cells and, in effect, sequesters itself from view of the body's surveillance system, meanwhile multiplying anomalous T cells that are ineffective for purposes of immunity. Another theory is that HIV mutates rapidly and B cells may not recognize variations effectively to produce antibodies efficiently.

Screening for the antibody is helpful to the extent that individuals can be identified who have been exposed to HIV. However, not all of these individuals actually carry the virus, nor will all of them show signs of illness. Therefore, several situations are possible.

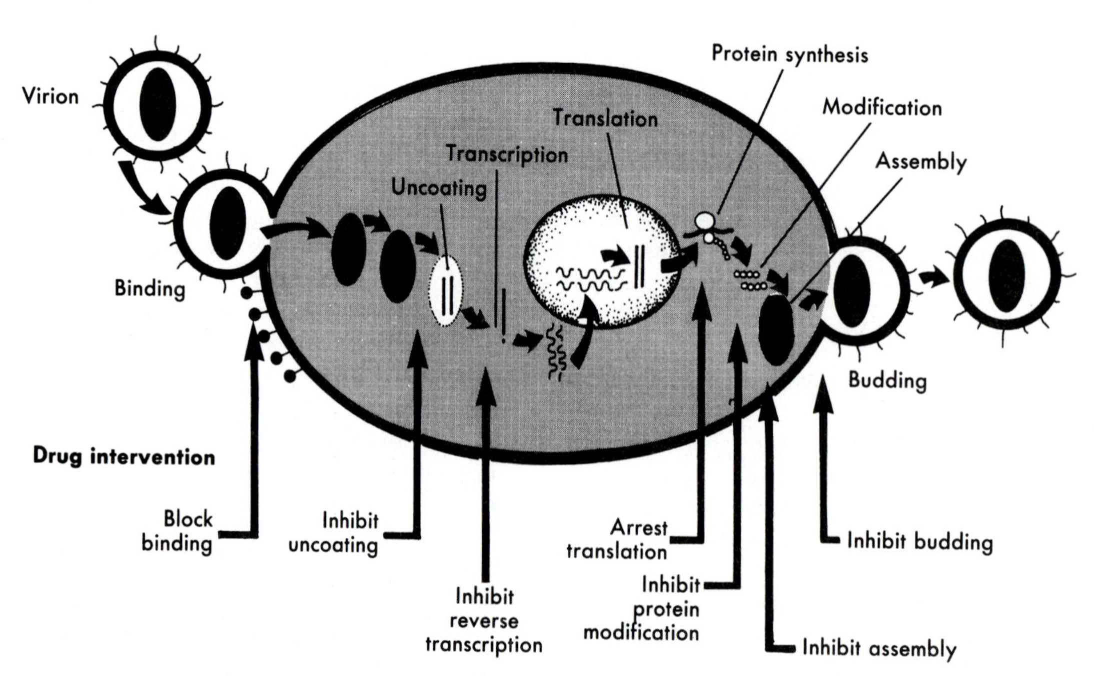

Figure 24–10. HIV life cycle. *(From McCance, K., & Huether, S. [1998].* Pathophysiology: The biologic basis for disease in adults and children, *3rd ed. [p. 273]. St. Louis: C.V. Mosby. [Original but adapted from Yarchoan, Metsurya, and Broder, 1989.])*

- *Exposure*. An individual may be exposed to the virus but neither carry it nor contract the disease.
- *Carrier*. The individual may carry the virus with the capability of infecting others but without accompanying signs and symptoms.
- *Terminal disease*. The individual may be infectious, symptomatic, and terminal. It is only after signs of opportunistic infections begin to develop that an individual is actually determined to have the disease.

Laboratory testing to diagnose HIV infection relies predominantly on the presence of antibody to HIV. Although the virus itself can be detected using p24 antigen capture or polymerase chain reaction (PCR), both of these tests are prohibitively expensive as primary screening tools for adults. They can, however, be useful in detecting the virus prior to antibody formation, called the *window period*, or in cases in which antibody tests are not conclusive. PCR is generally used only as a first-line diagnostic tool in infants.

The enzyme-linked immunosorbent assay (ELISA) is 95 to 99 percent accurate at identifying the presence of antibody. A false-positive ELISA result could occur as a result of cross-reactive antibodies to HLA antigens, hepatic disease, gamma globulin injections, and some malignancies. A positive ELISA must be confirmed with another antibody-reliant test known as the Western blot test. Two positive ELISAs and a positive Western blot test confirm the diagnosis of HIV infection. Indeterminate tests are usually repeated at 3- and 6-month intervals. If tests continue to be negative, the result is seronegative; if the tests are questionable at this time, p24 or PCR tests may be conducted. A newer, noninvasive HIV antibody test uses the Western Blot, but is collected through oral mucosa transudate. This oral test is thought to be as reliable as blood tests using the regular Western blot (Ferri, 1998).

Some authors suggest that the average incubation period for HIV, that is, from infection to clinical symptoms, is estimated to be from 3 months to 10 years. It is also thought that carriers of the virus who test positive for the antibody can remain as carriers for years with the virus in a dormant state. Although approximately one-third of those who now test positive for the disease eventually will begin to show clinical manifestations, some investigators believe that the percentage of those who go on to develop the disease will eventually approach 95 percent. It is estimated that 5 percent of HIV-infected individuals will never develop AIDS. The reason is still unknown, but may be related to an HIV genetic mutation (Stephens, 1997). However, due largely to combination retroviral therapy, there appears to be a decrease in occurrence of AIDS opportunistic infections and in deaths among persons reported with AIDS (Centers for Disease Control and Prevention [CDC], 1997).

Clinical Manifestations

Defining characteristics of AIDS were established in 1981 by the CDC. Based on continued research, the AIDS case definition was revised in 1985, 1989, and 1993 for adolescents and adults and includes 26 or more associated diseases. The 1993 revision defines AIDS as HIV infection (seropositive) with any of the following (CDC, 1992):

1. CD4 count < 200/mL
2. Tuberculosis
3. Recurrent bacterial pneumonia (typically *Pneumocystis carinii* or lymphoid interstitial pneumonia)
4. Invasive cervical cancer

Classification of phases of HIV disease in adults is based either on grouping of disease manifestations or on CD4 levels, both of which reflect disease progression. Classifications are generally referred to as *asymptomatic*, during which there is an intact immune system but active viral replication; *symptomatic*, during which CD4 cells decline and early symptoms develop; and *clinical AIDS*, during which symptoms become severe, CD4 levels drop to < 200/mL, and viral levels (viral load) increases. Further detail of disease progression is evaluated by percentage of CD4 cells and CD4/CD8 ratio (Kirton, Ferri, & Eleftherakis, 1999). Early symptoms include fever, sore throat, fatigue, weight loss, and muscle pain (Stephens, 1997).

Clinical manifestations of HIV infection generally are related to opportunistic infections preying on an impaired immune system. Common diseases include Kaposi's sarcoma, *P. carinii* pneumonia, tuberculosis, and others. The HIV patient commonly succumbs to uncontrollable infection, becoming increasingly debilitated, feverishly ill, malnourished, fatigued, and often in pain (Holzemer, Henry, & Reilly, 1998; Van Servellen, Sarna, & Jablonski, 1998). Lymphadenopathy, pharyngitis, rash, pulmonary infiltrates, wasting syndrome, and neurologic abnormalities, such as dementia, tremors, and encephalitis, contribute to the debilitated state. Because HIV travels from cell to cell rather than through the bloodstream, and because it readily mutates, it is usually not susceptible to circulating antibodies of the body's remaining immune system of B cells. To date, there is no predictable course of curative treatment, and the mortality rate continues to be approximately 95 percent for symptomatic individuals. Two variables to predict outcomes (i.e., time to AIDS, or time to death) include viral load and CD4 count. Average viral burden or load without therapy is 30,000 to 50,000 viral copies/mL (Bartlett, 1998). Individuals with viral levels ≥ 10,000/mL are the most likely to progress to AIDS within 4 years. Viral production and clearance by the immune system daily can reach 1 billion (Stephens, 1997).

AIDS in Children

Pediatric patients with AIDS differ significantly from adult patients in several ways, including transmission, onset, trajectory, and symptom manifestation. HIV/AIDS is transmitted to infants and preschool children either through infected blood, such as during blood transfusions; through a vertical transmission from mother to fetus; through breast-feeding; or more rarely through sexual practices such as incest and sexual abuse.

Although infected blood has been responsible for transmission of the HIV virus in many children over the past decade, blood supply screening has significantly reduced this mode of transmission. The more common transmission is now maternal–fetal, or vertical transmission. Current estimates are that 93 percent of new AIDS cases in children are due to perinatal (vertical) transmission from the mother (Wiznia, Lambert, & Pavlakis, 1996). Preliminary estimates of the risk of maternal vertical transmission were 25 percent to 40 percent, the variability of potential risk resting with the infectious state and viral load of the mother. For example, the mother is most likely to transmit the virus when she is newly infected either with an initial infection or a current reinfection or when she is symptomatic of full-blown AIDS. It is thought that the virus is more actively reproducing and less constrained by the mother's immune system during these times. In 1994, however, experimental studies of HIV-positive pregnant women revealed that the risk of vertical transmission dropped significantly to 8 percent, when taking AZT. Preliminary studies suggest that infants infected in utero tend to have high viral loads at birth, more virulent HIV type, more rapid CD4 decline, and rapid disease progression than infected infants who tested negative at birth who were likely infected during the birth process or from breast feeding. Therefore, recommendations for seropositive HIV pregnant women now include antiretroviral therapy (CDC, 1998).

The infant who tests seropositive at birth presents a complicated and confusing picture. Infants born to HIV-infected mothers will often test positive for HIV antibodies because of the passive transport of maternal antibodies across the placenta at about 32 weeks' gestation. This antibody reflects only maternal infection and may persist up to 15 to 18 months. Only after that time will subsequent antibody titers begin to reflect the infant's actual immune status. Due to recent advances, however, the virus can be cultured from these infants, permitting HIV diagnosis during the first few weeks of life. Other tests can be performed that reflect the presence of the HIV antigen (e.g., p24, PCR assay), but these tests are expensive. PCR assay is the test of choice for HIV diagnosis in children under the age of 15 months (Stephens, 1997). Decreased CD4 counts indicate HIV disease in children as in adults, but the level at which immunocompromise is suspected is much higher than in the adult patient.

Significant distinctions between adults and children are evident. Children tend to exhibit more rapid disease progression; *Pneumocystis carinii* pneumonia (PCP) and encephalopathy occur often, whereas cryptococcus, toxoplasmosis, cytomegalovirus (CMV), and Kaposi's sarcoma are infrequent; and there are age-related changes in CD4 counts and percentages. Pediatric classification of HIV/AIDS status is somewhat different from the adult classification, which is based either on CD4 levels or on the presence of AIDS-defining diseases. Absolute CD4 count and percentages based on age categories of < 12 months, 1 to 5 years, and 6 to 12 years determine evidence and degree of immunosuppression. Table 24–3 out-

TABLE 24–3. CDC 1994 CD4+ T LYMPHOCYTE CATEGORIES FOR HIV-INFECTED CHILDREN < 13 YEARS OF AGE

	Age of Infected Child		
ABSOLUTE CD+ count and percentages	< 12 MONTHS	1–5 YEARS	6–12 YEARS
No evidence of immunosuppression	≥ 1,500 ≥ 25%	≥ 1,000 ≥ 25%	≥ 500 ≥ 25%
Evidence of moderate immunosuppression	750–1,499 15–24%	500–999 15–24%	200–500 15–24%
Severe immunosuppression	< 750 < 15%	< 500 < 15%	< 200 < 15%

CDC 1994 REVISED CLASSIFICATION GRID FOR ASSESSING SEVERITY OF HIV INFECTION IN CHILDREN < 13 YEARS OF AGE

	CLINICAL CATEGORIES (SYMPTOMS)			
IMMUNOLOGIC CLASSIFICATION	NONE (A)	MILD (A)	MODERATE (B)	SEVERE (C)
No evidence of suppression	N1	A1	B1	C1
Moderate suppression	N2	A2	B2	C2
Severe suppression	N3	A3	B3	C3

From Centers for Disease Control and Prevention. (1994). 1994 Revised classification system of human immune deficiency virus infection in children less than 13 years of age. MMWR 43:*1–10.*

lines the classification code recommended for pediatric patients.

While the adult HIV/AIDS patient may be seropositive for up to 15 years without being acutely ill, it is estimated that 50 percent of infants who demonstrate perinatally acquired HIV will be symptomatic by 12 months. Rapid progression is a pattern of illness most common to children < 12 months old who acquired the disease through perinatal transmission. These children are known as *rapid progressors*. *Slow progressors* are children who have acquired HIV perinatally, but do not become symptomatic until > 12 months of age, or who acquire HIV through contaminated blood. Mean survival rates overall appear to be 8 years (Riddel & Moon, 1996).

Symptoms of AIDS in children manifest themselves primarily in the lungs, gastrointestinal tract, and brain. These children are typically recognized for their failure to thrive, with diarrhea, persistent fever, growth below the standard curve, gastric pain and bloody stools, poor muscle development, and decreased ability to eat owing to thrush-related oral pain. Many health care facilities routinely test their pediatric patients exhibiting symptoms of failure to thrive for HIV/AIDS.

Pediatric AIDS patients are commonly developmentally disabled, having experienced incidences of meningitis and encephalitis. (CNS cells carry the CD4 marker to which the HIV virus is attracted.) Finally, HIV/AIDS children frequently present with fever, dry cough, respiratory distress with retractions, and wheezing, indicative of PCP and lymphoid interstitial pneumonia. Because PCP has its highest incidence in HIV-infected infants 3 to 6 months old, the CDC now recommends that all infants born to women with HIV infection receive prophylaxis against PCP beginning at 4 to 6 weeks of age, even before the infant's HIV diagnosis is confirmed.

A variety of opportunistic infections, including potentially fatal rubella, chickenpox, flu, *Streptococcus*, and *Staphylococcus*, make scrupulous infection control critical. All HIV children should be immunized against measles (MMR), pneumococcus, and influenza since the risk of developing the diseases outweighs possible risks of the vaccines. The child's immune system may need support with monthly IV gamma globulin. HIV in children beyond infancy is characterized by periods of sickness and relative wellness. To make the situation more complex, often the parent or parents are also ill, the family may be stigmatized and isolated from interpersonal support systems, or the family may be separated due to the parents' inability to care for the child.

Adolescents and school-age children are most likely to acquire HIV through contaminated blood, either through transfusion (although this mode is becoming more rare) or contaminated drug-related needles. Sexual transmission also occurs in this age group. However, the number of seropositive (HIV-1) adolescents is a better indicator for this age group than the actual number of AIDS cases because of the long latency period. Less than 1 percent of AIDS patients are adolescents age 13 to 19 years, but the subclinical HIV-1 incidence is rising and produces a large population of young adults age 20 to 29 with manifestations of defining symptoms of AIDS.

Treatment Approaches

Various approaches to treatment have been theorized and tested. Restoration of immune function has been attempted by bone marrow transplant, transfusions of white blood cells, and interferon treatments. Unfortunately, the newest healthy cells are quickly infected by the virus. The HIV is so variable (much like the variations of flu virus) that a medication formulated against one genetic mutation of the virus may not provide protection against other strains. Pharmacological approaches using combination antiretroviral therapy rather than monotherapy (one drug) using some of the newer protease inhibitors has been successful in maintaining viral load suppression and in treating AIDS as a long-term chronic disease in adults (Williams, 1999). Antiretroviral combination therapy with reverse transcriptase inhibitors, such as zidovudine (ZBV, AZT) and lamivudine (3TC), and protease inhibitors, such as indinavir (Crixivan), has been most successful to date. Such therapy is known as *highly active antiretroviral therapy*. Antiretroviral therapy for children, however, has differed in that some agree that monotherapy with reverse transcriptase inhibitors is the treatment of choice. Research continues toward the most effective antiretroviral therapy for infants and children.

CD4 cell counts are evaluated to determine degree of immune deficiency. Viral load testing reflects viral activity and disease progression. Effective viral suppression is considered as < 400 to 500 copies/mL. Rising viral load indicates disease progression (5,000 to 10,000 copies/mL) as does falling CD4 levels (< 500 cells/mL) (Porche, 1999).

Antiretroviral drug resistance is one of the most difficult challenges in HIV management. Incomplete HIV suppression can result in HIV resistance and while antiretroviral drugs can have significant unpleasant side effects, patient compliance is a must because sustained, uninterrupted therapy is required for HIV inhibition. To date there are relatively few effective drugs available; drug resistance puts the patient at risk for rapid decline (Williams, 1999). Because of the prolonged latency period of HIV, anti-HIV agents may be required for an individual's protection for up to 10 years or longer to eradicate the virus.

Drug prophylaxis protocols for opportunistic infections of HIV/AIDS have shown some promising results in delaying or avoiding symptomatic infections. The goal of primary prophylaxis is to avoid or delay the onset of disease symptoms; secondary prophylaxis seeks to prevent or delay recurrent symptomatic infection. Other treatment approaches are symptomatic, and still others continue to be under experimental investigation. By and large, the most common infectious manifestation of the immunosuppressed HIV patient is PCP and its recurrence. This disease was one of the first opportunistic infections to be identified as an AIDS case-defining phenomenon. Since its prevalence in the AIDS population has been followed, it continues to be the most life-threatening opportunistic infection to both adult and pediatric AIDS patients. Although the PCP organism is not considered particularly pathogenic in the immunocompetent individual, its virulence increases as the T4 cell count falls below 200/μL in the adult and 1,500/μL in the child. The infected patient presents with fever, fatigue, and weight loss months before actual respiratory symptoms occur. Coughing, shortness of breath, hypoxemia, and abnormal pulmonary function studies contribute to the clinical picture of progressive illness. Prophylaxis therapy is indicated when the T4 cell count falls below 200 to 300 μL in the adult HIV-1 patient. Typical preventive and treatment therapy for PCP includes trimethoprim-sulfamethoxazole (TMP-SMX, Bactrim, Septra) or an aerosol of pentamidine.

Prevention of other opportunistic infections such as toxoplasmosis, tuberculosis, *Mycobacterium avium* complex (MAC), cytomegalovirus (CMV), and fungi is crucial. High-priority vaccine recommendations include pneumonia and influenza. Other vaccines may be contraindicated because of their imposed risk as live viruses such as measles, mumps, and rubella (MMR) and chickenpox (varicella zoster). Immune globulins can be given before or after exposures to measles, chickenpox, or hepatitis A (Bartlett, 1998). Neupogen, a granulocyte stimulant, may be given to counteract the neutropenia related to antiretroviral therapy or to the HIV itself.

Finally, although relatively few health care professionals are at risk for HIV, treatment approaches for occupational exposure to needle sticks, blood and body fluids, or contaminated instruments have been developed. Postexposure prophylaxis protocols include determining the source and severity of the exposure, determining HIV status of the source, and recommendations for treatment. According to the Public Health Service guidelines (1998), a basic postexposure prophylactic regimen begins within 2 hours of exposure and includes four weeks of zidovudine (ZDV, AZT) and lamiduvine (3TC). Other protocols recommend triple combination therapy for needlestick exposure, which includes protease inhibitors (Rich, Ramratnam, & Flanigan, 1997).

In summary, the basic concepts of HIV transmission, cellular transformation, epidemiology, treatment, and outcome have been discussed. Great strides have been made in the past few years in an attempt to understand this disease and to begin to research its detection, treatment, and cure. It is impossible to cover all aspects of this immune deficiency disease adequately in such a brief space and to approach currency in information. The learner is encouraged to seek out current information as it becomes available while building on the basic concepts presented in this section.

SECTION EIGHT REVIEW

1. Immunodeficiency originating from embryonic anomaly, genetic predisposition, or congenital failure is categorized as
   A. primary
   B. secondary
   C. acute
   D. chronic
2. Which of the following best characterizes HIV disease?
   A. symptoms result from opportunistic pathology
   B. HIV invades cells primarily through the bloodstream
   C. clinical manifestation is a characteristic and predictable sequence
   D. people testing positive for HIV are carriers and contagious
3. Fluids known to be modes of transmission for HIV include
   A. tears
   B. perspiration
   C. plasma
   D. saliva
4. Opportunistic diseases associated with AIDS are all of the following EXCEPT
   A. PCP
   B. Kaposi's sarcoma
   C. tuberculosis
   D. acute tubular necrosis

Answers: 1. A, 2. A, 3. C, 4. D

SECTION NINE: Aging, Malnutrition, Stress, Trauma, and the Immune System

At the completion of this section, the learner will be able to describe the pathogenesis of aging, malnutrition, trauma, and stress related to the function of the adult immune system.

Aging

The function of the immune system diminishes with increasing age. T lymphocyte function and specific antibody responses are particularly depressed, but in contrast there is an increasing number of autoantibodies. In the older population, the thymus is quite minimal in size and function. T cells, although continuing to be produced and circulated, are deteriorating in function and proliferation, thus impairing cell-mediated immunity (Tortorella et al., 1997). The very purpose of the immune system as a surveillance system is compromised, as manifested in more frequent infections, diminished capability to overcome infection, and increased evidence of cancer. Whereas helper T cells are less functional, it also seems that suppressor T cells are more active, a major factor in impaired humoral immunity in the elderly. In effect, as the body becomes older, it is less capable of responding to invading antigens and instead turns its immune response more toward self. It is not uncommon to see sharply elevated incidences of diseases thought to be autoimmune in the elderly (see Table 24–2).

Malnutrition

Nutritional deficiencies, always a possibility in the acutely ill adult and which should always be a concern to caregivers, can have a profound impact on the immune system. Basic components of calorie and protein intake play key roles in the formation and integrity of T cells and immunoglobulins (antibodies). Malnutrition contributes to immunocompromise by causing impaired response of lymphocyte to pathogens, to vaccines, and to components of defense such as complement and macrophage function (Shronts, 1993). Severe deficits affect both the number and function of these cells. The humoral response seems to be less affected by malnutrition, although the activity of macrophages and the complement system is depressed, and more frequent infections occur. Zinc plays a major role in the structure and function of both B cells and T cells and in collagen synthesis for wound healing. As a cofactor, zinc is required for normal function of lymphocytes in their production of enzymes. Although zinc deficiencies do not normally occur with regular eating habits, it can be lost from the body in dangerous amounts through the gastrointestinal tract by malabsorption syndrome or inflammatory bowel disease, characterized by severe diarrhea. It also can be lost through the skin in burn victims. Several vitamins also serve as cofactors in enzyme production and, during deficient states, affect the function of both T cells and B cells. These vitamins include A, E, pyridoxine, folic acid, and pantothenic acid.

Malnutrition is also believed to contribute to sepsis as the malnourished gut becomes atrophied and more permeable to bacteria following trauma. When bacteria seep out of the gut, immune system mediators are released and trigger systemic lymphocyte activity. TNF, a major immune mediator, is primarily responsible for precipitating multiple system organ dysfunction. Early enteral feedings, which prevent gut atrophy in the acutely ill patient, are also instrumental in preventing sepsis, excess circulating immune mediators, and subsequent multiple organ dysfunction in the critically ill patient (Secor, 1994). Multiple organ dysfunction syndrome is presented in more depth in Module 11.

Stress

Stress affects the immune system primarily through the effects of cortisol. During periods of stress, either physical or psychologic, the adrenal glands produce more cortisol in response to needs based on increased metabolism, but cortisol has a direct suppressing effect on the immune system. Normally, when an antigen enters the body, a series of reactions takes place. The antigen is recognized as nonself, and it is presented to T cells by macrophages. The macrophages secret interleukin-1, which activates helper T cells, and these helper T cells produce interleukin-2, which stimulates more T cell production. Finally, B cells may be stimulated to program antibodies to the antigen. Cortisol inhibits the production of IL-1 and IL-2, thus decreasing the T cell response and the subsequent B cell response.

Trauma

Trauma, both intentional (such as surgery) and accidental (such as burns, motor vehicle crashes, and falls) suppresses both T cell and B cell function. Research shows that trauma can cause cellular dysfunction, characterized by decreased chemotactic and phagocytic activities and decreased antibody and lymphocyte levels (Chaudry and Ayala, 1993; Gann and Amaral, 1985). Impaired T-cell activity and depressed lymphokines have been linked to multiple organ dysfunction and poor clinical outcomes in the trauma patient (Puyana et al., 1998). Although the degree of immunosuppression directly correlates with the severity of the injury, the cause for such changes is not fully understood. Additionally, several medications can suppress the immune response. Among these are glucocorticoids, general anesthetic agents, and cytoxic drugs.

The immune system is complex and is highly sensitive to changes in the body. Trauma, hemorrhage, blood transfusions, and surgery/anesthesia all contribute to immunosuppression (Secor, 1994). Immune consequences of trauma most likely are related to neurohormonal stress responses and altered cytokine/immune mediator activity. Hypovolemic shock has been found to decrease antigen-specific antibody production, cellular immunity, and macrophage function for approximately 2 weeks following hemorrhage (Chaudry and Ayala, 1993; Zellweger et al., 1995). The critically ill trauma patient enters the intensive care unit immunosuppressed from the outset owing to a stress response to the injury and as a result of hemorrhage and shock. Subsequent malnutrition, organ dysfunction, hypoxia, and multiple invasive procedures all create a potential scenario of vulnerability to virulent nosocomial pathogens.

The serum of a burn patient contains substances that suppress all immune responses regardless of the origin of the antigen. For patients with extensive burns, T cell impairment leaves them vulnerable to massive infectious episodes, often leading to multiple organ failure (Puyana et al., 1998). Most aspects of cell-mediated immunity are depressed following a major thermal injury. Complement component concentrations are reduced by massive activation at the burn site, limiting macrophage activity in preparing antigens for T cell and B cell immune activity (Robins, 1989). Concentrations of lymphokines, derived from T cells, also are decreased, including IL-2, which promotes antibody formation by the humoral immune response. Humoral immunity is depressed as IgG is markedly reduced, as are IgA and IgM levels. These immunoglobulins return to normal levels in approximately 2 weeks postburn (Robins, 1989). It is also the burn patient who is likely to become malnourished over time due to pain, immobility, and depression and who might also experience immune suppression related to increased cortisol in response to stress.

In summary, the stressors of illness, age, and trauma play a significant role in immunosuppression, seemingly just when the body is in acute need of protection against invading antigens. The maintenance of one's nutritional status is a common problem in most instances of trauma and illness, as is the excess production of cortisol during periods of psychological or physical stress. Nutritional deficits of protein, zinc, and calories, along with atrophic changes with aging and the added circulating cortisol during stress, can prove to be devastating to the body's immune system.

SECTION NINE REVIEW

1. What is the function of zinc in the competent immune system?
   A. it is required for normal lymphocyte function
   B. it protects B cells from being destroyed by macrophages
   C. T cells require zinc for production of gamma globulin
   D. macrophages are composed primarily of zinc
2. What effect does the normal aging process have on the immune system?
   A. B cell function in general is particularly depressed
   B. T cells begin to deteriorate in functioning
   C. autoantibodies begin to diminish with increasing age
   D. immune system becomes hypervigilant to invading organisms
3. In the acutely ill adult, which of the following nutritional losses is a critical factor in immune system integrity?
   A. iron
   B. vitamin C
   C. complex carbohydrate chains
   D. protein
4. Stress primarily affects the immune system through the effects of
   A. lymphokines
   B. interleukin
   C. cortisol
   D. epinephrine

Answers: 1. A, 2. B, 3. D, 4. C

SECTION TEN: Care of the Immunocompromised Patient

Focused Assessment

The physical examination for level of immunocompetence primarily reflects the patient's nutritional status since the proper functioning of the immune system is dependent on nutritional status. Consequently, if the patient is malnourished, immune status will be negatively affected. Physical assessment techniques and critical thinking must be focused on seeking evidence of infection, either acute or chronic. This includes assessing for skin lesions, open wounds, the presence of adventitious breath sounds and abnormal sputum, enlarged liver or spleen, or palpable lymph nodes or masses.

Nursing History

The patient history gives important clues to possible altered immunocompetence. Ferri (1998) suggests obtaining the following historical data:

- Complaints of fever, fatigue, weakness, swollen glands, lightheadedness, visual disturbances
- Slow wound healing history
- Unexplained rashes, mouth sores, or oral patches
- Presence of increased levels of stress, infection, malignancy, or autoimmune disease
- Changes in menstrual patterns, unusual bleeding or bruising (reflective of platelet dysfunction)
- Recent use of immunosuppressant drugs
- Allergy history
- Exposure to work environment chemicals
- At-risk factors for development of AIDS:
  - Homosexual orientation or sexual partner of homosexual
  - Transfusion of blood or blood products
  - IV illegal drug users or sexual partner of drug user
  - Child born of mother with AIDS
- Family history of autoimmune disorders or cancer

Immunocompetence in the High-Acuity Patient

The high-acuity patient is at high risk for development of immunocompetence problems secondary to prolonged stress, severe infections, malnutrition, diabetes, and other problems. The nurse must monitor the patient for critical cues of an underlying immunocompetence problem. Some of these major critical cues include the presence of:

- Fever
- Poor wound healing
- Joint pain
- White oral patches
- Level of consciousness and mental status changes
- Abnormal CBC with differential
- Abnormal coagulation studies
- Recurrent, prolonged, or severe infections
- Secondary infections
- Immunosuppressive drug therapy, such as corticosteroids or cytotoxic drugs
- Other at-risk factors, such as splenectomy, diabetes mellitus, chronic alcohol abuse, malnutrition, or renal failure

Laboratory Findings

Laboratory testing is the major diagnostic tool for establishing immune status. Tests may include common ones, such as the WBC with differential and total lymphocyte count (TLC), as well as tests establishing nutritional status, such as serum albumin. These tests are relatively inexpensive and easy to perform and are used as screening tests for general immune status. The nurse should be able to monitor these levels for abnormal trends.

A variety of cell-specific and disorder-specific laboratory tests are available if further evaluation of immunocompetence is necessary. Many of these tests, however, are both time consuming and expensive. Immunoglobulins, T cells, and B cells can be measured both quantitatively and functionally. Skin testing may be ordered to evaluate cellular immunocompetence. Protein and immunoglobulin levels through electrophoresis can help detect diseases associated with excess or deficient immune function. The ELISA can show exposure to HIV, to rheumatoid factor, and to lupus cells (Ferri, 1998).

WBC with Differential

The WBC with differential cell count indicates whether a person has abnormally high numbers of leukocytes (leukocytosis) or abnormally low numbers of leukocytes (leukocytopenia). The normal white blood cell count is 4,500 to 10,000 mL. In general, leukocytosis is associated with inflammation, infection, and leukemia, and leukocytopenia is associated with malnutrition, severe infection, autoimmune diseases, malignancies, and bone marrow depression. Leukocytes can be differentiated further into specific cell types including neutrophils, lymphocytes, monocytes, eosinophils, and basophils. Each of these cell types provides a unique service that is essential in maintaining protection against invading organisms or substances.

NEUTROPHILS. One-half to three-fourths of the circulating WBCs consist of neutrophils. They are the "rapid response team" of the immune system, rushing to a site of tissue injury in massive quantities; thus providing the first line of defense. Normally, an adult has approximately 50 billion neutrophils circulating in the bloodstream. Neutrophils are short-lived phagocytes, however, with a life span of only 1 to 2 days (Parslow, 1994). This requires the bone marrow to dedicate more than half of its activity to producing an adequate supply. Neutrophils consist of mature cells, called segmented neutrophils or "segs" (also known as *polymorphonuclear leukocytes, PMNs*, or *polys*), and immature cells, called *bands*.

LYMPHOCYTES. Lymphocytes are the second most numerous leukocyte cell type. Lymphocytes (T cells and B cells) respond to viral and chronic infections, providing longer-term protection than neutrophils. Lymphocytes are discussed in Section Four.

MONOCYTES. Monocytes (macrophages) are mononuclear phagocytes that normally comprise about 5 percent of the total WBC count. They are slower to respond but more powerful than neutrophils, providing the immune system's second line of defense. Monocytes ingest and destroy large substances (e.g., foreign particles) as well as bacteria. They are resident in many of the body's tissues (e.g., Kupffer cells in the liver, alveolar macrophages in the lungs) rather than primarily circulating in the blood stream. Macrophage activity increases as an acute infection progresses and remains active during a chronic infection. Macrophages are discussed further in Section Four.

EOSINOPHILS AND BASOPHILS. Eosinophils and basophils normally exist in very small quantities. Increased eosinophil levels are most commonly associated with parasitic infections and allergic conditions, and basophil levels increase during tissue healing.

Table 24–4 provides a summary of the WBC differential cell count, including normal ranges (in percent of total WBC) and some of the more common disease conditions that cause increased and decreased levels.

Nursing Management

General Goals

The goals for care of the immunocompromised patient include the goals appropriate to the malnourished patient. Additional goals include reestablishing immunocompetence and preventing/treating complications.

Collaborative Interventions

1. *Laboratory testing*. Various tests may be ordered to evaluate immune status, as discussed previously. Since many of the cell-specific blood tests are not commonly performed and are both expensive and time consuming to obtain or measure, the nurse must clarify nursing responsibilities and expectations regarding the tests before drawing samples or having them drawn, to prevent nursing error.
2. *Drug therapy*. Two types of drugs have a direct impact on the immune system: immunosuppressive therapy agents and agents that enhance immunity. Immunosuppressants decrease immune function. Uses include control of chronic inflammatory problems, prevention of organ transplant rejection, and others. Examples of immunosuppressant drugs are steroids and cyclosporin A. Drugs that enhance immune function in some way include immunotherapy agents, primarily used in cancer therapy; monoclonal antibodies, antibodies that act against specific antigens; and interleukin, a lymphokine used to enhance immune responses. Drug therapy is presented in more detail in Module 4.
3. *Environmental protection*. Severe leukopenia places the patient at high risk for infection. The severely immunocompromised patient is placed in a controlled environment. Hospitals have protocols establishing the exact nature of the environmental protection. A private room is ordered. Some hospitals have special positive airflow rooms that diminish airflow of possibly contaminated air into the protected patient's room.

Independent Nursing Interventions

In caring for the immunocompromised patient, the nurse's role centers around monitoring and prevention of

TABLE 24–4. WBC DIFFERENTIAL CELL SUMMARY

CELL TYPE NORMALS (% OF TOTAL WBC COUNT)[a]	ASSOCIATED DISORDERS	
	INCREASED LEVELS	DECREASED LEVELS
Neutrophils (50–70%) Segmented (50–65%) Bands (0–5%)	Acute infections, inflammatory diseases, tissue damage, Hodgkin's disease, leukemia (myelocytic), acute cholecystitis, acute appendicitis, acute pancreatitis.	Viral diseases, leukemias (monocytic, lymphocytic), agranulocytosis, anemias (aplastic, iron deficiency); drug related: antibiotic therapy, immunosuppressive agents
Lymphocytes (25–35%)	Leukemia (lymphocytic), viral infections, chronic infections, Hodgkin's disease, multiple myeloma.	Cancer, leukemia, adrenocortical hyperfunction, agranulocytosis, aplastic anemia, multiple sclerosis, renal failure, nephrotic syndrome, systemic lupus erythematosus
Monocytes (4–6%)	Viral diseases, parasitic diseases, leukemia (monocytic), cancer, anemias (hemolytic, sickle cell), systemic lupus erythematosus, rheumatoid arthritis, ulcerative colitis.	Leukemia (lymphocytic), aplastic anemia
Eosinophils (1–3%)	Allergies, parasitic disease, cancer, phlebitis thrombophlebitis, asthma, emphysema, renal disease.	Stress (e.g., shock, burn)
Basophils (0.4–1.0%)	Inflammatory process, leukemia, infection (healing stage), inflammation, acquired hemolytic anemia.	None

[a]Normal WBC count: 4,500–10,000 µL (mm^3)

Data from Kee, J.L. (1999). Laboratory & diagnostic tests with nursing implications, *5th ed. Stamford, CT: Appleton & Lange.*

infection, regaining or maintaining adequate nutrition, and meeting the psychosocial needs of the patient and family. Patient and family teaching to prevent and recognize infection is essential. Monitoring for infection should focus on the mucous membranes, skin, and lungs, which are the most common sites of infection in this patient population.

There are two nursing diagnoses appropriate in meeting the first two goals.

- *High risk for infection* related to deficient immune protection
- *Nutrition, alteration in* less than body requirements

HIGH RISK FOR INFECTION RELATED TO DEFICIENT IMMUNE PROTECTION, NEUTROPENIA. Desired patient outcome: the patient will show no evidence of infection.

I. Monitor patient every 2 to 4 hours for signs and symptoms of infection
   A. Temperature increases. A persistent fever of 100.5°F or higher for more than 12 hours may be the only sign of infection
   B. Signs and symptoms of inflammation, such as pain, redness, heat, swelling (some or all of these may be absent if neutrophils are too low)
   C. Skin or mucous membrane lesions
      1. Check all skin folds, mouth, and perianal area
      2. Check wounds and areas noted in 1. for yeast invasion (white patches)
   D. Gastrointestinal lesions
      1. Check all stools for occult blood
      2. Monitor for diarrhea or constipation
   E. Genitourinary problems
      1. Check urine for color, odor
      2. Monitor patient for pain or fever
   F. Respiratory
      1. Monitor for adventitious breath sounds, cough, dyspnea, pain. Early in the course of a pulmonary infection, the patient may only develop dyspnea, tachypnea, and fever.
   G. Invasive line/tube sites
      1. Observe all sites closely for signs or symptoms of actual or potential infection

The severely neutropenic patient will not be able to muster a normal immune response, which significantly alters the clinical findings. The inability to form pus (a byproduct of normal neutrophil activity) can significantly reduce common infection findings; such as:

- Cloudy urine
- Purulent sputum, including adventitious breath sounds
- Purulent wound drainage

II. Institute measures to protect patient environmentally
   A. Place in private room; keep door closed
   B. Screen all persons coming into contact with patient for signs and symptoms of infection
      1. Apply mask if respiratory infection is suspected or confirmed
   C. Excellent handwashing before contact (gloves recommended)
   D. Maintain strict aseptic technique for all sterile procedures
   E. Minimize foods and objects brought into the room from outside environment. Fresh fruits and vegetables may need to be peeled before being taken into the room. Flowers and vases with standing water may be restricted
   F. Special daily room cleaning with disinfectants is recommended

III. Provide ongoing protection against development of infection
   A. Monitor hydration status every shift
   B. Turn every 1 to 2 hours
   C. Skin care
      1. Thorough bathing every day
      2. Keep skin clean and lubricated at all times
   D. Keep linens clean and wrinkle free
   E. Pulmonary exercises every 4 hours
      1. Incentive spirometry, deep breathing
      2. As ordered: percussion, postural drainage, vibration (percussion is contraindicated if coagulopathy exists)
   F. Minimize invasive procedures: no rectal temperatures or enemas and no injections
   G. Protect patient against injury
      1. Instruct patient
         a. No straining
         b. Use no sharp objects: use electric razor
         c. Report any infection signs and symptoms
         d. Brush teeth with very soft bristle brush or toothette

IV. Institute measures that foster drug regimen compliance
   A. Clarify critical importance of regimen to prevent development of drug resistance to antiretrovirals
   B. Tailor medication regimen to patient lifestyle
   C. Direct observation, as needed
   D. Help patient and family plan ahead for changes in routine

ALTERATION IN NUTRITION: LESS THAN BODY REQUIREMENTS. The nutritional needs of the high-acuity patient are presented in detail in Module 22. Immunocompromised patients often develop stomatitis, which can interfere with consumption of food.

I. Perform actions to minimize stomatitis problems
   A. Mouth care before mealtime
   B. Offer lidocaine viscous immediately before mealtime
   C. Provide a soft food diet with frequent small meals

Many other nursing diagnoses might apply to the immunosuppressed patient based on individual physiologic and psychosocial needs. Some of the more common ones include:

- High risk for injury
- Anxiety
- Coping, ineffective individual
- Pain
- Knowledge deficit
- Powerlessness
- Activity intolerance
- Social isolation
- Self-care deficit

SECTION TEN REVIEW

1. Common patient complaints associated with altered immunocompetence include all of the following EXCEPT
   A. abnormal bleeding
   B. pain
   C. swollen glands
   D. fatigue
2. The nurse is assessing a patient for possible underlying immunocompetence problems. Which of the following assessments might indicate reduced immunocompetence?
   A. leukocytosis
   B. high-grade fever
   C. poor wound healing
   D. inflammation at fresh wound site
3. A severely immunocompromised hospitalized patient should receive environmental protection, including
   A. screening visitors for infection
   B. using bedding brought from home
   C. wearing clean gloves for dressing changes
   D. placing in semiprivate room with door closed
4. Which of the following clinical findings is most suggestive of a gastrointestinal complication associated with an immunocompromised state?
   A. diminished bowel sounds
   B. distended abdomen
   C. increased flatulence
   D. occult blood in stool
5. Nursing actions that provide ongoing protection against development of infection in a patient with neutropenia, include
   A. restrict patient's fluid intake
   B. turn patient every 1 to 2 hours
   C. bathe the patient every third day
   D. encourage patient's use of incentive spirometer once per shift

Answers: 1. B, 2. C, 3. A, 4. D, 5. B

POSTTEST

1. In defending the body, the immune system is activated after which of the following defenses is unsuccessful?
   A. inflammatory response
   B. skin integrity
   C. phagocytosis
   D. interferons
2. Which of the following is primarily responsible for production of B cells?
   A. bursa equivalent
   B. thymus
   C. stem cells
   D. spleen
3. By which of the following ways is passive immunity acquired?
   A. exposure to live antigen through inoculation
   B. vaccination with antiserum, such as tetanus toxoid
   C. genetic determination
   D. exposure to IgA antibodies
4. The best definition of antibody titer is the
   A. amount of a specific antibody in a serum
   B. presentation of processed T lymphocytes
   C. synthesis of circulating immunoglobulins
   D. molecular weight of an antigenic determinant
5. Specific immunity is best described as
   A. antigen–antibody response
   B. foreign material filtration
   C. phagocytosis
   D. interferon antiviral activity
6. Matching of HLA antigens is particularly critical before
   A. blood transfusions
   B. factor VIII replacement
   C. organ transplantation
   D. in vitro fertilization
7. Which of the following cells is responsible for the synthesis of circulating immunoglobulins?
   A. suppressor T cells
   B. B cells

C. macrophages
D. memory cells

8. The macrophage is primarily responsible for antigen destruction by
A. lysis
B. neutralization
C. differentiation
D. phagocytosis

9. Cell-mediated immunity is best characterized by
A. specific recognition and memory of antigen
B. primary and secondary response patterns
C. subsets of IgG, IgA, IgE, IgM, IgD
D. direct attack on invading antigens

10. Which of the following immunoglobulins is found in large quantities in secretory body fluids?
A. IgA
B. IgE
C. IgG
D. IgM

11. IgG comprises several types of antibodies and
A. provides local antibody protection in the mucosa
B. crosses the placental barrier
C. can be administered as active acquired immunity
D. functions with mast cells in hypersensitivity responses

12. The best definition of the complement system is
A. a nonspecific immune response of engulfing and ingesting foreign antigens by neutrophils
B. the body's first line of defense against viruses
C. the body's surveillance system for malignant cells
D. a progressive, sequential immune response activated by IgG and IgM

13. Which of the following is an example of a type IV hypersensitivity reaction?
A. blood transfusion reaction
B. host transplant rejection
C. allergic asthma
D. Arthus reaction

14. Which of the following is commonly thought of as being an autoimmune phenomenon?
A. transplant rejection
B. polio
C. *Pneumocystis carinii*
D. ulcerative colitis

15. Of the following laboratory tests, which is most specific for the differential diagnosis of SLE?
A. LE cell
B. B and T cell levels
C. antinuclear antibodies (ANA)
D. anti-DNA

16. For which of the following reasons has HIV treatment been largely disappointing?
A. treatment against one genetic strain may not provide protection against other evolving strains
B. the virus does not attach to immunoglobulin antigenic sites as other antigens do
C. the HIV blocks the complement system
D. HIV invades B cells and sequesters itself from view of the body's immune system

17. Why are individuals who receive specific blood components more at risk for acquiring HIV than the average person who receives whole blood or packed cell transfusion?
A. the screening procedures lack the sophistication of whole blood testing
B. the risk increases with the large numbers of donors required to produce therapeutic amounts
C. HIV is more difficult to detect in blood components than in whole blood or packed cells
D. the virus attaches to large amounts of factor VIII and platelets

18. How do increased levels of cortisol released during stress affect the immune system?
A. increases the production of glycogen
B. cortisol inhibits the production of interleukin-1 and -2
C. stimulation of T cell production is enhanced by cortisol
D. higher levels of cortisol cause accelerated production of immunoglobulins by B cells

19. Zinc plays a major role in B cell and T cell production. For what reasons might an acutely ill adult have a zinc deficiency?
A. prolonged periods of IV potassium replacement
B. malabsorption syndromes accompanied by severe diarrhea
C. third-space fluid deficit
D. hyperosmolar dehydration

20. In what ways is the immune system thought to be compromised in the patient with extensive burns?
A. their serum contains substances that suppress all immune responses
B. zinc levels may become dangerously high, with extensive epidermal loss
C. T cells are suppressed, but B cell activity and antibody production generally are unaffected
D. dehydration creates an imbalance between humoral and cell-mediated immunity

21. When assessing a patient with neutropenia for infection, the nurse should focus on which three body areas?
A. gastrointestinal tract, skin, lungs
B. lungs, mucous membranes, urine
C. urine, skin, gastrointestinal tract
D. mucous membrane, skin, lungs

22. The most important indicator of the presence of infection in a neutropenic patient is
A. rubor
B. edema
C. fever
D. pus

Posttest Answers

Question	Answer	Section	Question	Answer	Section
1	B	Introduction	12	D	Five
2	A	One	13	B	Six
3	B	Two	14	D	Six
4	A	Two	15	D	Seven
5	A	Three	16	A	Eight
6	C	Three	17	B	Eight
7	B	Four	18	B	Nine
8	D	Four	19	B	Nine
9	D	Five	20	A	Nine
10	A	Five	21	D	Ten
11	B	Five	22	C	Ten

REFERENCES

Appelbaum, J. (1992). The role of the immune system in the pathogenesis of cancer. *Semin Oncol Nurs* 8(1):51–62.

Bartlett, J. (1998). *Medical management of HIV infection*. Baltimore, MD: Johns Hopkins University.

Centers for Disease Control and Prevention. (1998). Public Health Service Task Force recommendations for the use of antiretroviral drugs in pregnant women infected with HIV-1 for maternal health and for reducing perinatal HIV-1 transmission in the United States. *MMWR 47*, RR-2:1–30.

Centers for Disease Control and Prevention. (1992). Revised classification system for HIV infection and expanded surveillance case definitions for AIDS among adolescents and adults. *MMWR 41*, RR-17:19.

Centers for Disease Control and Prevention. (1997). *HIV/AIDS Surveillance Report* 4(2):1–6.

Chaudry, I., & Ayala, A. (1993). Immune consequences of hypovolemic shock and resuscitation. *Curr Opin Anaesthesiol* 6:385–392.

Ferri, R. (1998). Oral mucosal transudate testing for HIV-1 antibodies: A clinical update. *J Assoc Nurses AIDS Care* 9(2):68–72.

Fye, K., & Sack, K. (1994). Rheumatic diseases. In D.P. Stites, A.I. Terr, & T.G. Parslow (eds.), *Basic and clinical immunology* (8th ed.) (pp. 387–392). Norwalk, CT: Appleton & Lange.

Gann, D., & Amaral, J. (1985). Pathophysiology of trauma and shock. In G. Zuidema, R. Rutherfore, & W. Ballinger (eds.), *The management of trauma* (4th ed.) (pp. 37–103). Philadelphia: W.B. Saunders.

Goodman, J. (1994a). Immunogens and antigens. In D.P. Stites, A. I. Terr, & T.G. Parslow (eds.), *Basic and clinical immunology* (pp. 50–57). Norwalk, CT: Appleton & Lange.

Goodman, J. (1994b). The immune response. In D.P. Stites, A.I. Terr, & T.G. Parslow (eds.), *Basic and clinical immunology* (pp. 40–49). Norwalk, CT: Appleton & Lange.

Greenberg, P. (1994). Mechanisms of tumor immunology. In D.P. Stites, A.I. Terr, & T.G. Parslow (eds.), *Basic and clinical immunology* (pp. 569–577). Norwalk, CT: Appleton & Lange.

Holzemer, W., Henry, S., & Reilly, C. (1998). Assessing and managing pain in AIDS care: The patient perspective. *J Assoc Nurses AIDS Care* 9(1):22–30.

Imboden, J. (1994). T lymphocytes and natural killer cells. In D.P. Stites, A.I. Terr, & T.G. Parslow (eds.), *Basic and clinical immunology* (pp. 94–104). Norwalk, CT: Appleton & Lange.

Kirton, C., Ferri, F., & Eleftherakis, V. (1999). Primary care and case management of persons with HIV/AIDS. *Nurs Clin North Am 34*(1):71–93.

McCance, K., & Huether, S. (1998). *Pathophysiology: The biologic basis for disease in adults and children* (3rd ed.). St. Louis: C.V. Mosby.

Oppenheim, J., Ruscetti, F., & Faltynek, C. (1994). Cytokines. In D.P. Stites, A.I. Terr, and T.G. Parslow (eds)., *Basic and clinical immunology* (pp. 105–123). Norwalk, CT: Appleton & Lange.

Parslow, T.G. (1994). The phagocytes: Neutrophils and macrophages. In D.P. Stites, A.I. Terr, & T.G. Parslow (eds.), *Basic and clinical immunology* (pp. 9–39). Norwalk, CT: Appleton & Lange.

Porche, D. (1999). State of the art: Antiretroviral and prophylactic treatments in HIV/AIDS. *Nurs Clin North Am* 34(1):95–111.

Porth, C. (1998). *Pathophysiology: Concepts of altered health states* (5th ed.). Philadelphia: J.B. Lippincott.

Puyana, J., Pellegrini, J., De, A., et al. (1998). Both T-helper-1 and T-helper-2 type lymphokines are depressed in posttrauma anergy. *J Trauma: Injury, Infection, and Critical Care* 44(6):1037–1045.

Rich, J., Ramratnam, B., & Flanigan, T. (1997). Triple combination antiretroviral prophylaxis for needlestick exposure to HIV. *Infection Control Hosp Epidemiol 18*(3):161.

Riddel, J., & Moon, M. (1996). Children with HIV becoming adolescents: Caring for long term survivors. *Pediatr Nurs 22*(3):220–227.

Robins, E. (1989). Immunosuppression of the burned patient. *Crit Care Nurs Clin North Am 1*(4):767–774.

Secor, V. (1994, September). Sepsis in the trauma patient. Paper presented at the workshop for Advanced Trauma Management, Georgia Baptist College of Nursing, Atlanta, GA.

Shronts, E. (1993). Basic concepts of immunology and its application to clinical nutrition. *Nutr Clin Pract* 8:177–183.

Stephens, P. (1997). HIV infection and AIDS: A review and update. *Curr Rev Nurse Anesth 20*(11):97–108.

Tortorella, C., Loria, M., Piazolla, G., et al. (1997). Age-related impairment of T cell proliferative responses related to the decline of CD28+ T cell subsets. *Arch Gerontol Geriatr 26*:55–70.

Van Servellen, G., Sarna, L., & Jablonski, K. (1998). Women with HIV: Living with symptoms. *West J Nurs Res 20*(4): 448–464.

Weigle, W. (1997). Advances in basic concepts of autoimmune disease. *Clin Laboratory Med 17*(3):329–340.

Williams, A. (1999). Adherence to highly active antiretroviral therapy. *Nurs Clin of North Am 34*(1):113–129.

Wiznia, A., Lambert, G., & Pavlakis, S. (1996). Pediatric HIV infection. *Med Clin North Am 80*(6):1309–1335.

Zellweger, R., Ayala, A., DeMaso, C., & Chaudry, I. (1995). Trauma hemorrhage causes prolonged depression in cellular immunity. *Shock* 4:149–153.

ADDITIONAL READINGS

Flaskerud, J., & Ungvarski, P. (1992). *HIV/AIDS: A guide to nursing care* (2nd ed.). Philadelphia: W.B. Saunders.

Secor, V. (1994). The inflammatory/immune response in critical illness: Role of the systemic inflammatory response syndrome. *Crit Care Nurs Clin North Am* 6:251–264.

Stites, D., Terr, A., & Parslow, T. (1994). *Basic and clinical immunology* (8th ed.). Norwalk, CT: Appleton & Lange.

Zurlinden, J., & Verheggen, R. (1994, January). HIV vaccines: A report from the front. *RN*. pp. 36–40.

Module 25

Altered Glucose Metabolism

Diane Orr Chlebowy, Kathleen Dorman Wagner

This self-study module focuses on physiologic processes involved in normal glucose metabolism, as well as the pathophysiologic basis of altered glucose metabolism. The three major diabetic crises are presented. Each is described in terms of pathophysiology, clinical presentation, and management. The module is composed of nine sections. Sections One and Two discuss normal glucose metabolism and the effects of insulin on metabolism. The focus then shifts to abnormal glucose metabolism. Section Three describes the impact of insulin deficit on metabolism. Section Four defines and then differentiates the two major types of diabetes mellitus (type 1 and type 2). Sections Five through Seven discuss the three acute life-threatening consequences of diabetes: therapy-induced hypoglycemia, diabetic ketoacidosis, and hyperglycemic hyperosmolar nonketotic syndrome. Section Eight reviews exogenous insulin therapy, focusing on types of insulin therapy used during acute illness. Finally, Section Nine presents an overview of chronic diabetic complications, and their effects on the nursing management of the acutely ill client. Each section includes a set of review questions to help the learner evaluate his or her understanding of the section's content before moving on to the next section. All Section Reviews and the module Pretest and Posttest include answers. It is suggested that the learner review those concepts answered incorrectly in the review questions before proceeding to the next section.

OBJECTIVES

Following completion of this module, the learner will be able to

1. Discuss normal glucose metabolism.
2. Describe the effects of insulin on metabolism.
3. Explain the effects of insulin deficit.
4. Differentiate the two major types of diabetes mellitus.
5. Discuss the pathophysiology, clinical manifestations, and nursing care management of therapy-induced hypoglycemia.
6. Discuss the pathophysiology, clinical manifestations, and nursing care management of diabetic ketoacidosis.
7. Discuss the pathophysiology, clinical manifestations, and nursing care management of hyperosmolar hyperglycemic nonketotic syndrome.
8. Explain the use of exogenous insulin in the management of the client with diabetes mellitus.
9. Discuss the acute care nursing implications of chronic diabetic complications.

PRETEST

1. Insulin promotes use of glucose by
   A. breaking down glucose
   B. assisting glucose into the cells
   C. converting glucose to glycogen
   D. transporting glucose in the blood

2. Which of the following is true regarding the effect of insulin on fat metabolism? It inhibits
   A. synthesis of fatty acids
   B. glucose use by tissues
   C. release of fatty acids
   D. transport of glucose into fat cells
3. When an insulin deficiency exists, the liver responds by converting
   A. fatty acids to glucose
   B. glycogen to glucose
   C. glucagon to glucose
   D. amino acids to glucose
4. Insulin-dependent cells use which of the following nutritional substances FIRST when insulin is not available?
   A. fatty acids
   B. glycogen
   C. glucagon
   D. amino acids
5. The etiology of type 1 diabetes is believed to be
   A. obesity
   B. an autoimmune reaction
   C. a bacterial infection
   D. general pancreatic dysfunction
6. A client experiencing rapid onset hypoglycemia is most likely to have predominantly __________ symptoms.
   A. cell dysfunction
   B. gastrointestinal
   C. stimulated sympathetic nervous system
   D. stimulated parasympathetic nervous system
7. Central nervous system symptoms associated with hypoglycemia are caused by lack of _____ rather than insulin deficit.
   A. glucose
   B. amino acids
   C. fatty acids
   D. glucagon
8. Clinical manifestations of severe hypoglycemia include
   A. bradycardia
   B. fruity odor of the breath
   C. mental confusion
   D. ketonuria
9. Clinical manifestations of diabetic ketoacidosis include
   A. weight gain
   B. fluid overload
   C. electrolyte depletion
   D. hypoventilation
10. Which of the following statements is correct regarding hyperglycemic hyperosmolar nonketotic syndrome?
    A. it has a higher mortality rate than DKA
    B. it is most common in young clients with type 1 diabetes
    C. it causes severe fluid volume overload
    D. significant ketosis is present
11. Exogenous insulin is
    A. used only in the treatment of type 1 diabetes
    B. often used in management of type 2 diabetes during periods of stress
    C. most often derived from animal sources
    D. seldom used in the treatment of HHNS
12. Diabetic retinopathy causes blindness by
    A. glucose deposits on the retina
    B. thickening of the retina
    C. destruction of the optic nerve
    D. infarction of retinal tissue
13. Diabetic nephropathy damages the nephrons by causing
    A. glomerulosclerosis
    B. glomerulonephritis
    C. chronic nephritis
    D. renal hypertension

Pretest answers: 1. B, 2. C, 3. B, 4. A, 5. B, 6. C, 7. A, 8. C, 9. C, 10. A, 11. B, 12. D, 13. A

GLOSSARY

Acetoacetic acid. Produced by fat catabolism, it is one component of ketone bodies

Acetone (dimethyl ketone). Produced by fat catabolism, it is a component of ketone bodies

Acetyl-coA (acetylcoenzyme A). A product of the reaction between acetic acid and coenzyme A

Aminoacidemia. Amino acids in the blood

Anion gap. A measurement of excessive unmeasurable anions

Atherosclerosis. A form of arteriosclerosis characterized by plaque deposits

β-Hydroxybutyric acid. One component of ketone bodies

Carbohydrates. Nutritional substances composed of complex and simple sugars

Catabolism. Breakdown of a substance

Diabetes mellitus. A complex metabolic disorder in which the person has either an absolute or a relative insulin deficiency; this insulin deficiency results in disordered carbohydrate, protein, and fat metabolism

Diabetic ketoacidosis (DKA). A potentially devastating form of metabolic acidosis, characterized by a clinical syndrome of symptoms associated with elevated serum blood glucose and serum ketones and metabolic acidosis

Glucagon. A hormone produced by the alpha cells of the islets of Langerhans of the pancreas

Gluconeogenesis. Formation of glycogen in the liver from a noncarbohydrate substance

Glycogen. The stored form of carbohydrate for conversion into glucose

Glycogenolysis. Conversion of glycogen to glucose

Glycosuria. Excretion of glucose in the urine

Glycosylated hemoglobin (HbA, c). Hemoglobin with glucose attached to it

Hormone-sensitive lipase. A fat-splitting enzyme

Hyalinization. A degenerative cell process affecting the basement membrane of arteries and arterioles; hyalinized cells take on a glassy appearance

Hyperglycemia. Abnormally high level of glucose in the blood

Hyperglycemic hyperosmolar nonketotic syndrome (HHNS). A hyperglycemic complication of diabetes mellitus that results from insulin deficiency

Hypoglycemia. Abnormally low level of glucose in the blood

Infarction. Death of tissue

Insulin. An anabolic hormone produced by the beta cells of the islets of Langerhans of the pancreas

Insulin-dependent cells. Cells that require insulin to facilitate diffusion of glucose through the cell membrane

Ketonuria. The presence of ketones in the urine

Ketosis. The presence of ketones in the blood

Lipogenesis. Formation of fat

Lipolysis. Breakdown or splitting of fat

Lipoprotein. A protein that is conjugated (joined) with lipid molecules, such as triglycerides, cholesterol, and phospholipids; lipids exist in the plasma primarily as lipoproteins

Macroangiopathy. Disease of the large and medium-sized blood vessels; essentially atherosclerosis

Microangiopathy. Small blood vessel disease

Microvascular disease. Disease of the capillaries

Metabolic acidosis. An alteration in acid-base balance characterized by an arterial blood gas pH of < 7.35 (normal is 7.35 to 7.45) with a bicarbonate level of < 22 mEq/L (normal is 22 to 28 mEq/L)

Osmotic diuresis. Excessive urinary excretion caused by osmotic shifting of fluids

Polydipsia. Excessive thirst

Polyuria. Excessive urination

Somogyi effect. A nocturnal hypoglycemia rebound phenomenon characterized by wide swings in serum glucose levels

Synthesis. Formation of a substance

Uptake. To take a substance into a cell

ABBREVIATIONS

CO. Cardiac output

DKA. Diabetic ketoacidosis

FFA. Free fatty acid

Hb A. Hemoglobin A

HbA, c. Glycosylated hemoglobin

HHNS. Hyperglycemic hyperosmolar nonketotic syndrome

ICA. Islet cell antibodies

SECTION ONE: Normal Glucose Metabolism

At the completion of this section, the learner will be able to discuss normal glucose metabolism.

Glucose is used by most body cells as an energy source. Some cells (e.g., brain cells) can use only glucose for energy. Glucose, however, does not cross muscle and fat cell membranes using the same mechanisms, as do most other molecules. It requires a protein carrier, facilitated by insulin, to transport it into these cells. Fat and muscle cells are, therefore, sometimes referred to as **insulin-dependent cells.** After combining with the protein carrier in the cell membrane, glucose is able to diffuse across the membrane into the cell, where the carrier releases it. Supplying the cells with glucose is a complex physiologic task based on important feedback mechanisms for regulating blood glucose levels. This mechanism is primarily controlled by two hormones, insulin and glucagon, with important support by three other hormones, epinephrine, growth hormone, and cortisol. The normal serum glucose level is 70 to 110 mg/dL (fasting) (Kee, 1999).

Insulin

Insulin is a polypeptide (small protein) produced by the beta cells of the islets of Langerhans in the pancreas. Its underlying role is to lower the blood glucose level, and it sometimes is referred to as the hypoglycemic factor. Insulin plays a crucial part in regulating carbohydrate, fat, and protein metabolism.

Insulin must bind to special insulin receptor proteins in the cell membrane to carry out its functions. Once it is attached to a receptor site, insulin combines with the carrier protein in the cell membrane. The carrier protein, with help from insulin, promotes glucose diffusion across the cell membrane. Insulin's exact role is to enhance the function of the carrier protein.

Glucagon

Glucagon, a small protein, is secreted by alpha cells in the islets of Langerhans in the pancreas. It is the major hormone responsible for raising serum glucose levels and sometimes is referred to as the hyperglycemic factor. Its effects are in opposition to those of insulin. The stimulus for glucagon release is a blood glucose level < 70 mg/dL (Guyton & Hall, 1997). Glucagon counterbalances the effects of insulin by converting hepatic **glycogen** (via **glycogenolysis**) into glucose. Once converted, hepatic glucose rapidly moves into the circulation, increasing blood glucose levels. The reciprocal relationship between insulin and glucagon assists in maintaining homeostatic blood glucose levels.

Epinephrine, Growth Hormone, and Cortisol

When serum glucose drops below normal ranges, the sympathetic nervous system is stimulated. Consequently, the adrenal glands secrete epinephrine. Epinephrine increases serum glucose levels in a manner similar to glucagon but to a lesser extent.

Pituitary growth hormone and cortisol both respond to prolonged periods of hypoglycemia. They help reestablish a more normal glucose level by decreasing the rate of glucose use by the cells. Growth hormone decreases the body's ability to use carbohydrates, which spares them as an energy source. It facilitates the transport of amino acids into the cells. Growth hormone also has a synergistic relationship with insulin in the promotion of growth (Guyton & Hall, 1997).

In summary, glucose is the body's main source of fuel. Its control and use are dependent primarily on two hormones, insulin and glucagon. Three other hormones also contribute to regulating serum glucose levels. Epinephrine elevates glucose in response to a hypoglycemic state in a similar manner to glucagon. Growth hormone and cortisol decrease cellular use of glucose, promoting hyperglycemia.

SECTION ONE REVIEW

1. Insulin is produced in the
   - **A.** kidneys
   - **B.** pituitary gland
   - **C.** liver
   - **D.** pancreas
2. Insulin promotes use of glucose by
   - **A.** breaking down glucose
   - **B.** assisting glucose into the cells
   - **C.** converting glucose to glycogen
   - **D.** transporting glucose in the blood
3. Glucagon promotes
   - **A.** decreased use of glucose
   - **B.** conversion of hepatic glycogen
   - **C.** protein synthesis and transport
   - **D.** transport of glucose into the cells
4. Which of the following is true regarding growth hormone?
   - **A.** it decreases cellular use of glucose
   - **B.** it promotes storage of fat
   - **C.** it decreases blood glucose levels
   - **D.** it increases breakdown of glycogen
5. Release of cortisol
   - **A.** increases mobilization of fats
   - **B.** decreases use of glucose
   - **C.** decreases secretion of insulin
   - **D.** increases breakdown of muscle glycogen

Answers: 1. D, 2. B, 3. B, 4. A, 5. B

SECTION TWO: The Effects of Insulin on Metabolism

At the completion of this section, the learner will be able to describe the effects of insulin on metabolism.

Carbohydrate Metabolism

The body is dependent on adequate levels of glucose to provide energy for normal functioning. **Carbohydrates,** nutritional substances composed of complex and simple sugars, normally provide most of the body's glucose needs. Directly after consumption of carbohydrates, the serum glucose level increases, triggering a rapid increase in insulin secretion. Under the influence of insulin, glucose is moved into cells (cellular **uptake**) for immediate use or stored for later use. The liver plays a major role in glucose storage and to a lesser extent fat and muscle tissues also provide glucose storage.

Insulin and the Liver in Glucose Metabolism

Directly after a meal, glucose that is not used immediately by the cells is stored rapidly in the liver as glycogen. With the help of insulin, glucose is converted into glycogen, diffusing into the liver cells where it becomes trapped until the serum glucose level becomes low. Insulin levels alter in direct response to glucose levels. Consequently, as serum glucose levels drop (such as between meals) insulin is no longer needed and thus its level rapidly declines. The lack of insulin triggers a reversal of the process, breaking down the liver glycogen into glucose phosphate and releasing it from the liver cells to move back into the circulation. Approximately 60 percent of glucose is stored in the liver in this manner (Guyton & Hall, 1997).

Insulin and Muscle Tissue in Glucose Metabolism

During normal daily activity, muscle tissue uses fatty acids, not glucose, as its major source of energy. This is because the resting membrane of the muscle does not allow glucose into the cell without the presence of insulin. Insulin levels, however, are very low between meals, thereby requiring use of energy sources other than glucose.

Muscle cells use glucose under two circumstances. First, during heavy exercise, muscle cell membranes become highly permeable to glucose. Second, for several hours after meals, the high level of insulin in the serum enhances transport of glucose into the muscle cells. Muscle cells store available glucose as muscle glycogen for their own use. They are, however, unable to convert it back into glucose or transport it back out of the muscle tissue into the general circulation. Muscle tissue, therefore, does not contribute to counteracting the effects of insulin because it does not increase serum glucose levels (Guyton & Hall, 1997).

Insulin and Fat Metabolism

Insulin also has important effects on fat metabolism. Normal levels of insulin help regulate fat metabolism by:

- Facilitating glucose use by most tissues, thereby sparing fat as the major energy source
- Promoting synthesis of fatty acids primarily in the liver; fatty acids are then transported to adipose tissue for storage
- Inhibiting fatty acid release into the circulation
- Facilitating transport of glucose into fat cells for fatty acid synthesis

The blood glucose level is the major determining factor as to whether the cells will use carbohydrates or fats for energy. Once the decision is made, the switch from one energy source to the other is done rapidly. When there is a lack of insulin (such as between meals), cells must rely on fat as the primary energy source in insulin-dependent tissues. When insulin is again made available in sufficient quantities, glucose resumes its function as the major energy source. Insulin, then, is a crucial factor in determining which energy source is used (Guyton & Hall, 1997).

Insulin and Protein Metabolism

Insulin plays an important part in the storage of protein following ingestion of nutrients. Insulin helps regulate protein metabolism by:

- Facilitating transport of amino acids across the cell membrane
- Promoting protein **synthesis**
- Decreasing protein **catabolism**

In addition to glucose, amino acids also act as a trigger for insulin secretion. Thus, when amino acid levels increase after ingestion of nutrients, insulin is secreted to facilitate cellular uptake, synthesis, and storage of proteins.

In summary, the effects of normal levels of insulin on carbohydrate, fat, and protein metabolism are profound. Insulin helps regulate glucose metabolism in fat and muscle (insulin-dependent) tissues. It plays an important part in the cellular uptake, synthesis, and storage of both amino acids and fatty acids. Blood glucose and amino acid levels are the major triggers of insulin secretion. Blood glucose levels are the decisive factor in the type of food (carbohydrate or fat) used as the energy source for the insulin-dependent cells.

SECTION TWO REVIEW

1. Which of the following substance supplies the primary source of cell energy?

   A. fat
   B. protein
   C. carbohydrate
   D. glucagon

2. Cells requiring insulin to facilitate diffusion of glucose into them are called
   A. insulin-dependent
   B. glucose-dependent
   C. glycogen-dependent
   D. carbohydrate-dependent
3. Excess glucose is stored in the
   A. pancreas
   B. muscle tissues
   C. adipose tissues
   D. liver
4. During normal daily activities, muscle cells use which of the following as their major energy source?
   A. glucose
   B. fatty acids
   C. amino acids
   D. glucagon
5. Which of the following is true regarding the effect of insulin on fat metabolism? It inhibits
   A. synthesis of fatty acids
   B. glucose use by tissues
   C. release of fatty acids
   D. transport of glucose into fat cells

Answers: 1. C, 2. A, 3. D, 4. B, 5. C

SECTION THREE: The Effects of Insulin Deficit

At the completion of this section, the learner will be able to explain the impact of insulin deficit on metabolism.

Insulin deficiency results in disordered carbohydrate, protein, and fat metabolism. If carbohydrates are unable to be the major glucose energy source, the liver initiates conversion of glycogen to glucose. The principal metabolic alterations associated with insulin deficiency include: (1) impaired cellular uptake and use of glucose; (2) increased extracellular (serum) glucose; (3) increased mobilization of fats; and (4) tissue depletion of protein (Fig. 25–1).

Movement of glucose into insulin-dependent cells occurs in direct proportion to the amount of insulin available. When insulin-dependent tissues are deprived of glucose as a result of either insulin deficiency or insulin resistance their functional capacities become restricted. Table 25–1 summarizes the effects of insulin deficiency on insulin-dependent tissues.

Insulin Deficit and Carbohydrate Metabolism

Insulin deficit dramatically alters carbohydrate metabolism. Carbohydrates are the major supplier of simple and complex sugars, producing glucose as the primary energy source. Insulin deficit causes cessation in glucose uptake by insulin-dependent cells and a decrease in glucose use by the cells. The combination of decreased glucose uptake and decreased glucose use causes a rapid buildup of serum glucose, hyperglycemia.

In an insulin-poor environment, insulin-dependent cells are actually starving. Though abundant potential energy is available in the form of glucose, it is of no use to the cells. Other sources of energy are used, including fatty acids (the primary backup energy source) and amino acids once fat reserves are depleted. Clinically, dysfunctional carbohydrate metabolism is evidenced as hyperglycemia, and if not controlled, ketosis and aminoacidemia may result, each with its own set of complications.

Insulin Deficit and Fat Metabolism

Insulin deficit alters fat metabolism by increasing **lipolysis** (fat breakdown) and decreasing **lipogenesis** (fat formation). The decreased availability of intracellular glucose results in increased breakdown of stored triglycerides by **hormone-sensitive lipase,** causing lipolysis. Free fatty acids become the major energy source for the tissues, with the major exception of the brain. Clinically, this is evidenced as increased blood levels of free fatty acids and glycerol. The liver also converts some of the excess fatty acids into cholesterol and phospholipids. Excess fatty acid breakdown causes increased levels of **acetyl-coA,** which either is used by the liver for energy or the excess is converted into **acetoacetic acid.** Some of the acetoacetic acid is further converted into **β-hydroxybutyric acid** and **acetone.** These three substances (acetoacetic acid, β-hydroxybutyric acid, and acetone) move into the circulation as ketone bodies (see Fig. 25–1).

Clinically, this sequence of events has both acute and chronic consequences. Acutely, the increased levels of ketone bodies result in **ketosis** and **ketonuria.** When ketosis is extreme, severe acidosis and coma result (e.g., diabetic ketoacidosis). The use of fat as energy is evidenced as a significant increase in plasma lipoproteins (as much as three times normal). In the long term, high levels of lipoproteins are associated with the rapid onset of atherosclerosis, especially when high cholesterol levels are present. Many of the complications of diabetes mellitus are secondary to atherosclerotic changes.

Insulin Deficit and Protein Metabolism

Without insulin, the body is unable to store protein. There is an increase in protein catabolism and cessation

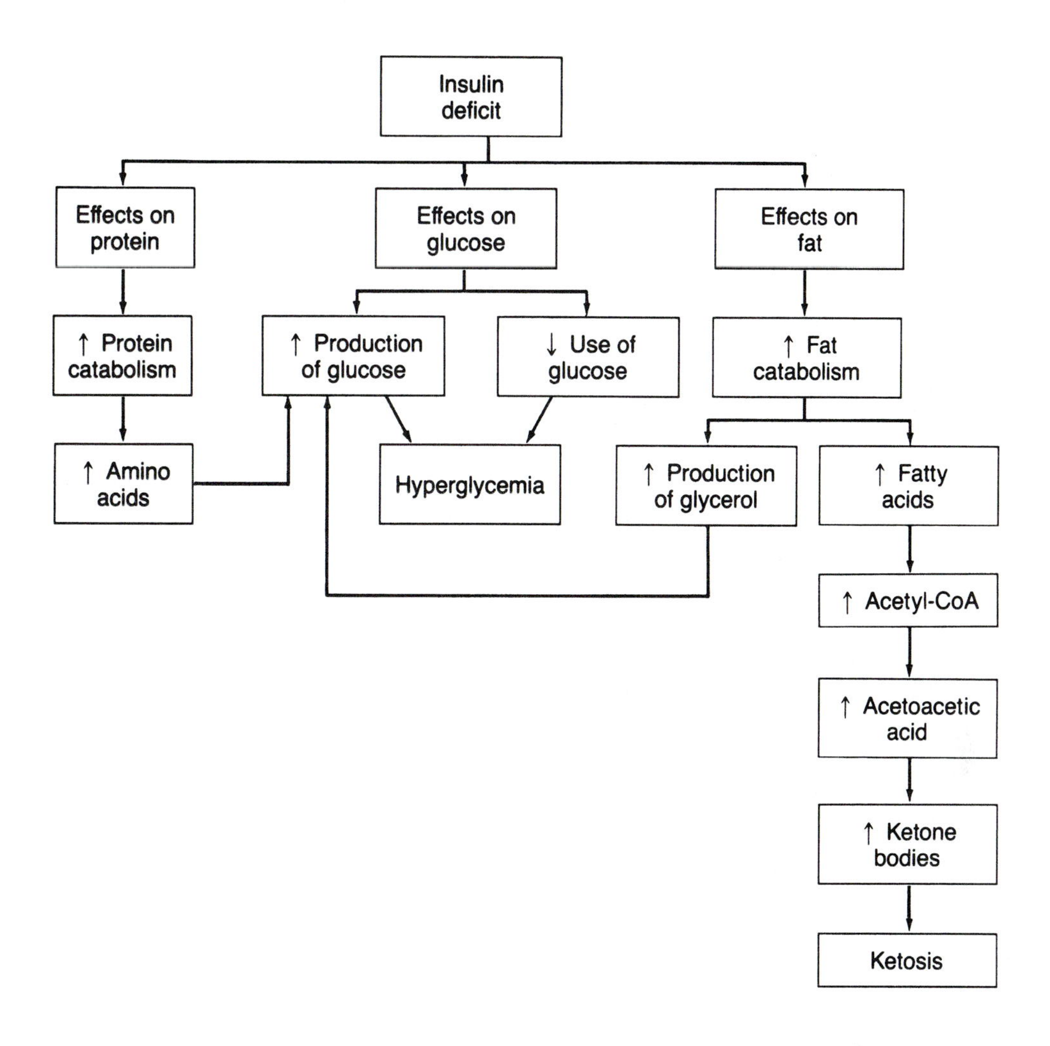

Figure 25–1. Consequences of insulin deficit.

of protein synthesis. Protein catabolism causes large quantities of amino acids to move into the circulation. The amino acids are then used either directly as an energy source or as part of the **gluconeogenesis** process.

TABLE 25–1. EFFECTS OF INSULIN DEFICIT ON INSULIN-DEPENDENT TISSUES

TISSUES	EFFECTS
Glucose Transport Problems	
Skeletal muscle	Fatigue; decreased strength
Cardiac muscle	Weaker contractions; decreased cardiac output; decreased peripheral circulation
Smooth muscle	Poor bowel tone; decreased vascular tone
Leukocytes	Depressed leukocyte function; impaired inflammatory response
Crystalline lens of eye	Opacity/cataracts
Fibroblasts	Impaired healing
Pituitary gland	Retarded growth; impaired regeneration of tissue; other endocrine problems
Insulin Resistance Problem	
Adipose tissue	Lipolysis; lipidemia; elevated serum ketone levels

Clinically, protein catabolism is evidenced by muscle wasting, multiple organ dysfunction, aminoacidemia, and increased urine nitrogen. If nitrogenous wastes accumulate in the body faster than they can be excreted in the urine, the client exhibits an altered level of consciousness and mentation. In addition, as gluconeogenesis is initiated, hyperglycemia is further aggravated.

Insulin Deficit and Fluid and Electrolyte Balance

When an insulin deficit exists, the serum glucose level increases, which causes plasma osmotic pressure to increase. The resulting change in pressure produces a shifting of body fluids from the tissues into the intravascular compartment. This shifting of fluids leads to intracellular dehydration.

As the level of hyperglycemia increases beyond the kidney's ability to reabsorb the extra glucose, **glycosuria** (excretion of glucose in the urine) develops. Urinary excretion of glucose produces an **osmotic diuresis** evidenced as

polyuria (excessive urination). Osmotic diuresis results in excessive loss of water, potassium, sodium, chloride, and phosphate ions. Loss of these ions further increases both extracellular and intracellular dehydration. Deficits in potassium and sodium are manifested by weakness, fatigue, and other signs and symptoms associated with the specific electrolyte imbalances. As fluid is lost, serum osmolality increases. Dehydration stimulates the hypothalamic thirst center, causing excessive thirst **(polydipsia).** Dehydration also produces hemoconcentration as fluid from the vascular space is lost, which causes decreased cardiac output (CO). If the dehydration is allowed to progress, the CO may become critically low, ultimately leading to circulatory failure.

Circulatory failure has two major consequences. First, it causes poor tissue perfusion and tissue hypoxia. Decreased perfusion to the brain results in cerebral hypoxia and symptoms related to altered cerebral tissue perfusion. Second, it causes severe hypotension, which is responsible for decreased renal perfusion and may eventually result in acute renal failure. Circulatory failure is fatal if an adequate CO is not reestablished in a timely manner.

In summary, insulin deficiency severely alters metabolism of carbohydrates, proteins, and fats. When glucose is unable to move into insulin-dependent cells, cell function becomes rapidly impaired. Fluid and electrolyte balance becomes impaired as plasma osmotic pressure changes due to glycosuria. As fluids shift, the cells become dehydrated, and electrolytes become deranged. Osmotic diuresis, if prolonged, causes hypovolemia and decreased CO, eventually leading to circulatory failure.

SECTION THREE REVIEW

1. When an insulin deficiency exists, the liver responds by converting
   A. fatty acids to glucose
   B. glycogen to glucose
   C. glucagon to glucose
   D. amino acids to glucose
2. Insulin-dependent cells use which of the following nutritional substances FIRST when insulin is not available?
   A. fatty acids
   B. glycogen
   C. glucagon
   D. amino acids
3. Insulin deficit alters fat metabolism by
   A. increasing lipogenesis
   B. synthesizing triglycerides
   C. increasing lipolysis
   D. synthesizing glycerol
4. When acetoacetic acid converts to acetone and β-hydroxybutyric acid, _____ is/are formed.
   A. amino acids
   B. acetyl-coA
   C. glycerol
   D. ketone bodies
5. Protein catabolism is evidenced by
   A. muscle wasting
   B. hyperexcitability
   C. decreased urine urea nitrogen
   D. increased triglyceride levels

Answers: 1. B, 2. A, 3. C, 4. D, 5. A

SECTION FOUR: Types of Diabetes Mellitus

At the completion of this section, the learner will be able to differentiate the two major types of diabetes mellitus.

Diabetes mellitus (diabetes) is a complex metabolic disorder in which the person has either an absolute or relative insulin deficit. It is divided into two major types: type 1 and type 2 diabetes mellitus.

Type 1 Diabetes Mellitus

Type 1 diabetes occurs when there is an absolute lack of endogenous insulin caused by autoimmune beta cell destruction. It can develop at any age but most commonly occurs before the age of 30. The HLA genotype, HLA DR-3 and/or DR-4, is strongly associated with the occurrence of type 1 diabetes among certain racial groups. Viral and chemical agents are also proposed to be triggers for the development of type 1 diabetes (Funnell, Hunt, & Kulkarni, 1998). Regardless of the triggering event, it is believed that an autoimmune reaction destroys the beta cells.

Type 2 Diabetes Mellitus

Approximately 90 percent of individuals in the United States with diabetes have type 2 diabetes. Type 2 diabetes is usually diagnosed after the age of 30 years but may also occur in children and adolescents. It is associated with a relative insulin deficiency (less insulin secretion) and/or insulin resistance rather than a total deficit. The major etiology of type 2 diabetes is progressive pancreatic dysfunction secondary to **hyalinization** of the islets of Langerhans. Over the course of the disease, both the pancreas and the liver develop fatty deposits due to high serum lipid levels. They also undergo tissue atrophy, associated with a decrease in size and number of functioning pancreatic and liver cells. Obesity in the presence of hereditary tendencies is considered a major risk factor for development of type 2 diabetes. It has many different characteristics than does type 1 diabetes. Table 25–2 presents a comparison of type 1 and type 2 diabetes.

Diabetic Crises

Diabetes mellitus is associated with many clinical manifestations that are multisystemic in nature. Prolonged hyperglycemia may result in three acute complications: diabetic ketoacidosis (DKA), hyperosmolar hyperglycemic nonketotic syndrome (HHNS), and hypoglycemic coma. DKA and HHNS are produced by an abnormally high blood glucose level, hyperglycemia. In contrast, hypoglycemic coma is produced by an abnormally low blood glucose level, hypoglycemia. Many clients with diabetes are admitted to the hospital for a diagnosis other than their chronic diabetic state. However, the physiologic stress caused by the acute problem may precipitate a diabetic crisis, which further complicates the client's prognosis.

The Focused History

When a diabetic crisis is suspected, specific parts of the nursing history should be obtained rapidly.

- Preexisting history of type 1 or type 2 diabetes
- Self-maintenance activities
- Special diet, including compliance with diet
- Insulin or oral hypoglycemics (type, dosage, compliance to regimen)
- Glucose testing history (blood glucose monitoring, urine testing)
- Exercise and weight loss
- Usual pattern of glucose control (stable vs. occasional-to-frequent loss of glucose control)
- Possible precipitating factors (e.g., infection, presence of other physiologic or psychologic stressors, failure to follow diet or drug therapy)
- Preexisting neurologic or vascular complications of diabetes (e.g., decreased kidney function, peripheral or cardiovascular disease)
- Unexplained weight loss of $\geq$ 10 percent.

Sections Five, Six, and Seven present the three acute complications, including assessment and management.

In summary, diabetes mellitus is a complex metabolic disorder associated with an absolute or relative insulin deficit or insulin resistance. There are two major types of diabetes mellitus: type 1 and type 2. Type 1 is associated with autoimmune destruction of the beta cells in the pancreas. Type 2 is associated with heredity, obesity, insulin resistance, or general dysfunction of the pancreas and the liver. There are many differences between these two types of diabetes. However, both cause progressive deterioration of multiple body systems.

TABLE 25–2. COMPARISON OF THE TWO TYPES OF DIABETES MELLITUS

CHARACTERISTIC	TYPE 1	TYPE 2
Usual age of onset	< 30 years of age	> 40 years of age
Rate of onset	Rapid	Slow
Weight status	Not associated with obesity	Commonly associated with obesity
Insulin secretion (beta cell status)	Total loss of beta cells within 1 year of diagnosis; no insulin secretion	Decrease in size and number of beta cells; decreased insulin secretion
Glucagon secretion (alpha cell status)	Abnormal alpha cell function, but relative excess of glucagon in relation to insulin	Decrease in size and number of alpha cells; glucagon and insulin secretion decreased but often balanced
Ketone status	Ketone prone; high risk for ketoacidosis	Not ketone prone unless under stress; low risk for ketoacidosis
Insulin resistance	Usually only present with elevated glucose levels	Usually present
Insulin supplement status	Insulin-dependent	Usually not insulin-dependent
Diabetic crises associated with disorder(s)	Diabetic ketoacidosis (DKA); hypoglycemic coma	Hyperosmolar hypoglycemic nonketotic syndrome (HHNS); hypoglycemic coma

SECTION FOUR REVIEW

1. The etiology of type 1 diabetes is believed to be
   A. obesity
   B. an autoimmune reaction
   C. a bacterial infection
   D. general pancreatic dysfunction
2. By 1 year after diagnosis of type 1 diabetes, there is _____ percent of functioning beta cells remaining in the pancreas.
   A. 0
   B. 10
   C. 30
   D. 50
3. Type 2 diabetes is associated with which of the following major risk factors?
   A. smoking
   B. viral infection
   C. obesity
   D. autoimmune reaction
4. In what way is pancreatic function altered in the client with type 2 diabetes?
   A. beta cells become hyalinized
   B. beta cells become overactive
   C. alpha cell activity predominates
   D. alpha cells break down insulin
5. Which of the following statements is true regarding type 2 diabetes? Type 2 diabetes __________ than type 1 diabetes.
   A. is less common
   B. has a slower rate of onset
   C. usually occurs at a younger age
   D. is more commonly associated with ketones

Answers: 1. B, 2. A, 3. C, 4. A, 5. B

SECTION FIVE: Hypoglycemic Coma

At the completion of this section, the learner will be able to discuss the diabetic complication, hypoglycemic coma.

Hypoglycemia—an abnormally low blood glucose level—is the most common diabetic complication. It may occur with any type of diabetes. Hypoglycemia is triggered by an imbalance between exercise, diet, and medication. Onset of symptoms is usually rapid, and if prolonged, coma may result.

Clinical Presentation

Hypoglycemia can be defined clinically as a blood glucose level of < 70 mg/dL or 3.9 mMol/L (Funnell et al., 1998). Some clients, however, develop symptoms of hypoglycemia even with a serum glucose of > 70 mg/dL, or if the drop in glucose is very rapid. Hypoglycemia becomes symptomatic when there is insufficient glucose available to meet the energy needs of the central nervous system. Common precipitating conditions for development of hypoglycemia include:

- Excessive administration of insulin or oral antidiabetes agents
- Consumption of too little food
- High activity levels
- Certain medications (e.g., propranolol) and alcohol, which potentiate the effects of the pharmacologic regimen
- Hormonal changes

Clients receiving oral hypoglycemic therapy are at risk for severe and prolonged symptoms of hypoglycemia due to the extended half-life of these agents.

A client's clinical presentation is primarily related to central nervous system (CNS) effects and catecholamine effects.

Central Nervous System Effects

The CNS depends on available glucose for its energy source and is sensitive to insufficient levels of glucose. CNS effects reflect the inability of brain cells to function normally without an adequate energy source. Progressive symptoms include:

- Decreased ability to reason and remember (slow thinking)
- Changing mental status
- Emotional lability
- Headache, dizziness
- Thickened, slurred speech
- Loss of coordination
- Loss of proprioception
- Numbness
- Drowsiness
- Convulsions
- Coma

Catecholamine Effects

The lack of circulating glucose triggers the secretion of stress hormones, subsequently causing production of glucose from alternate body sources, such as hepatic gluconeogenesis. The presence of increased levels of the hormone epinephrine, a catecholamine, triggers a sympathetic response. This stress response accounts for many of the symptoms of hypoglycemia such as:

- Anxiety
- Tremors, nervousness
- Cold, clammy skin
- Tachycardia, palpitations
- Hyperventilation
- Tingling in extremities
- Nausea and vomiting
- Hunger
- Diaphoresis

The rate of onset and the client's age influence the type of symptoms that predominate.

Rapid Onset

When the onset of hypoglycemia is rapid, sympathetic nervous system symptoms often predominate. A significant, rapid drop of blood glucose level stimulates the sympathetic nervous system, which initiates secretion of epinephrine. Epinephrine causes gluconeogenesis in the liver, thereby increasing the serum glucose level. Concurrently, growth hormone and cortisol also are secreted to assist in increasing glucose levels by decreasing glucose use by the cells.

Slow Onset

When the onset of hypoglycemia is slow, the symptoms of CNS dysfunction may predominate. Over a period of time, the body is able to adapt to a slow decline in blood glucose. Brain cells are not insulin dependent and take in glucose directly. Central nervous system symptoms, therefore, are caused by lack of available glucose rather than an insulin deficit. The brain is a high-energy tissue, requiring large amounts of glucose to maintain normal functioning. Without glucose, particularly over a prolonged period, the brain can sustain permanent damage that may be either minor or severe (irreversible coma).

The Influence of Age

The age of the client has an impact on the clinical presentation of hypoglycemia. The elderly tend to have more severe symptoms and may become symptomatic at higher serum glucose levels. CNS symptoms, particularly those relating to altered levels of consciousness, may be misdiagnosed in chronically ill elderly if the onset is very slow. In the elderly, the hypoglycemic symptoms may be masked as worsening dementia.

Medical Interventions

The major goal of interventions is rapid restoration of normal serum glucose levels. The specific type of intervention is based partially on the client's level of consciousness.

The Conscious Hypoglycemic Client

Reversal of hypoglycemia in the conscious client is relatively simple to accomplish. Clients with blood glucose levels less than 70 mg/dL should eat or drink 10 to 15 g of carbohydrate. If blood glucose levels are less than 50 mg/dL, 20 to 30 g of carbohydrate may be needed. If after treatment blood glucose levels remain low, the treatment should be repeated. Immediate treatment should be followed with high-protein foods (e.g., cheese with crackers).

The Unconscious Hypoglycemic Client

If a hospitalized client with diabetes becomes hypoglycemic, the following regimen is suggested (Johnson, 1998):

1. Administer glucagon 1 mg (IM).
2. Reevaluate blood glucose every 30 minutes until stabilized.
3. If no response within 10 to 15 minutes, administer 50 mL of 50 percent glucose (IV).
4. If hypoglycemia episode is long lasting, Andreoli et al. (1997) suggest following up the 50 percent glucose with an intravenous feeding of 10 percent glucose at a rate that is sufficient to maintain the serum glucose at > 100 mg/dL.

In summary, hypoglycemia is a condition in which there is insufficient glucose to meet cellular energy needs. It may be due to excessive administration of insulin or antidiabetes agents, too little food, high activity levels, certain medications and foods, or hormones. Hypoglycemia triggers the sympathetic response, causing secretion of epinephrine, which initiates the conversion of glycogen to glucose. The clinical presentation of hypoglycemia is due to sympathetic nervous system stimulation and starvation of neural cells. The primary goal of treatment is restoration of blood glucose levels to as close to normal as possible.

Section Five Review

1. Which of the following statements is TRUE regarding hypoglycemia?
   A. it is defined only in terms of blood glucose levels
   B. it is defined only in terms of clinical presentation
   C. it becomes symptomatic only when excessive insulin is present
   D. it becomes symptomatic at different blood glucose levels
2. Conditions that increase the risk of hypoglycemia include
   A. dietary fasting
   B. high-fat diet
   C. little exercise
   D. too little insulin

3. Of the following, the clinical presentation of hypoglycemia partially reflects
   A. lack of glucose within the cells
   B. excessive glucose within the cells
   C. stimulation of parasympathetic nervous system
   D. excessive circulating insulin
4. A client experiencing rapid onset hypoglycemia is most likely to have predominantly __________ symptoms.
   A. cell dysfunction
   B. gastrointestinal
   C. stimulated sympathetic nervous system
   D. stimulated parasympathetic nervous system
5. Central nervous system symptoms associated with hypoglycemia are caused by lack of _____ rather than insulin deficit
   A. glucose
   B. amino acids
   C. fatty acids
   D. glucagon
6. In the unconscious hypoglycemic client with a venous access, the treatment of choice is
   A. 50 percent glucose (IV)
   B. 0.5 to 2 mg glucagon (IM)
   C. 10 percent dextrose and water (IV)
   D. 8 ounces of orange juice (orally)

Answers: 1. D, 2. A, 3. A, 4. C, 5. A, 6. A

SECTION SIX: Diabetic Ketoacidosis

At the completion of this section, the learner will be able to describe the diabetic complication, diabetic ketoacidosis.

Diabetic ketoacidosis (DKA) results from an absolute or relative deficiency in insulin. It is a potentially severe, sometimes deadly complication characterized by ketosis, acidosis, hyperglycemia, and dehydration (Funnell et al., 1998).

Focused Assessment

A rapid assessment of the severity and state of compensation of DKA helps establish management priorities. The signs and symptoms of DKA are multisystemic in nature. Thus, a systematic assessment is necessary. Not every client exhibits all the clinical manifestations of DKA, and confirmation is made by evaluation of appropriate laboratory tests. Table 25–3 summarizes the major cardinal signs and their specific associated signs and symptoms. A brief description of the pathophysiologic basis of the cardinal signs of diabetic ketoacidosis follows.

TABLE 25–3. CARDINAL SIGNS AND SPECIFIC SIGNS AND SYMPTOMS OF DIABETIC KETOACIDOSIS

CARDINAL SIGNS	SPECIFIC SIGNS AND SYMPTOMS
Hyperglycemia	Elevated serum glucose (usually > 300 mg/dL, may increase to 700 mg/dL)
	Elevated urine glucose
Metabolic acidosis	Elevated serum and urine ketones
	Acidotic serum pH (< 7.30)
	Acidotic serum HCO_3 (< 15 mEq/L)
	Positive high anion gap (> 17 mEq/L)
	Alkalotic serum Pco_2 (< 35 mm Hg)
	Elevated respiratory rate and depth (Kussmaul breathing)
	Fruity odor to breath
Osmotic diuresis	Polyuria
	Polydipsia
	Dehydration
	Hypotension
	Hemoconcentration
	Electrolyte abnormalities
	Azotemia (elevated BUN and creatinine)
	Elevated serum osmolarity (but < 350 mg/dL)
Compensation	Decreased urine output
	Increased serum sodium levels
	Increased blood pressure, pulse, respirations
	Peripheral vasoconstriction

Pathophysiologic Basis of DKA Symptomatology

HYPERGLYCEMIA. The origin of **hyperglycemia** is an absolute or relative deficit in insulin, which causes the inability of glucose to move into cells, thus increasing serum glucose levels. Fat from adipose tissue is converted into free fatty acids (FFAs). The FFAs, in turn, are converted to glucose by gluconeogenesis in the liver. The liver also causes glycogenolysis, which converts glycogen to glucose. All these factors contribute to worsening hyperglycemia (see Fig. 25–1)

METABOLIC ACIDOSIS. Free fatty acids are broken down by the CNS into ketone bodies for energy faster than they can be converted to glucose. Due to the lack of insulin, muscle cells cannot oxidize the ketone bodies sufficiently, causing a buildup of ketone bodies. Increased levels of circulating ketone bodies decreases the pH, and as the pH falls below 7.20, the respiratory center is stimulated to excrete carbonic acid via the lungs in the form of carbon dioxide and water. Acetone, which is contained in ketone bodies, is excreted through the lungs (ketone breath) and the kidneys (ketonuria). Bicarbonate reserves become overwhelmed and then exhausted by the severity and prolonged state of the acidosis, which causes a drop in serum bicarbonate levels.

Osmotic Diuresis. Elevated serum glucose levels increase intravascular osmotic pressure. The increased pressure draws extravascular fluids into the intravascular compartment. As the levels of glucose and intravascular volume increase, the kidneys respond by dramatically increasing excretion of glucose and urine. This is associated with increased loss of electrolytes, hemoconcentration, and increasing dehydration. Gastrointestinal symptoms associated with DKA may be related to abnormally low electrolyte levels.

Compensatory Mechanisms. The renin–angiotensin–aldosterone system is activated to increase sodium and water reabsorption. Antidiuretic hormone (ADH) is secreted by the posterior pituitary to cause retention of water and sodium. Urine output also is controlled by compensatory vasoconstriction, which limits renal blood flow. The autonomic nervous system is stimulated to secrete catecholamines and glucocorticoids, which results in vasoconstriction; thus increasing the blood pressure and decreasing urine output. Blood pressure, pulse, and respirations are all increased as a result.

Decompensation. The client with severe DKA can eventually develop failure of compensatory mechanisms. Decompensation represents exhaustion of compensatory mechanisms, which rapidly leads to cardiovascular collapse. The level of consciousness deteriorates and blood pressure and pulse can no longer maintain adequate organ perfusion. The supply of catecholamines becomes exhausted, causing loss of the body's ability to maintain peripheral vasoconstriction. Urine output decreases and ceases as hypoperfusion to the kidneys causes them to fail.

Anion Gap

DKA is only one cause of metabolic acidosis. Measuring **anion gap** is one way to help isolate DKA from some other acidotic conditions. Gaining a basic understanding of the concept of anion gap may facilitate early diagnosis and treatment of DKA.

Metabolic acidosis exists either as normal anion gap acidosis (from loss of bicarbonate ions) or as high anion gap acidosis (from an accumulation of fixed acids in the serum).

Anions are negatively charged particles (e.g., CO_2^-, HCO_3^-, and Cl^-). They are the opposite of cations, or positively charged particles (e.g., Na^+ and K^+). Normally, cations and anions are in balance with each other. Anion gap represents the level of unmeasurable anion excess that exists in the body. Measurement of the anion gap is helpful in differentiating the type of metabolic acidosis present. It is expressed as:

$$\text{Anion gap} = (Na^+ + K^+) - (CL^- + HCO_3^-)$$

Anion gap has a normal range of 10 to 17 mEq/L (Kee, 1999). This normal range is a function of such unmeasured serum anions as phosphates, sulfates, ketones, and lactic acid.

High Anion Gap Acidosis

An anion gap of > 17 mEq/L indicates an accumulation of these unmeasured anions and warrants immediate attention. When metabolic acidosis is caused by elevations in organic acids, the anion gap increases. Such states as starvation, lactic acidosis, and DKA cause a high anion gap.

Normal Anion Gap Acidosis

When metabolic acidosis is caused by a loss of bicarbonate (buffer) anions, the anion gap remains normal. This occurs in such states as high chloride intake, renal failure, and diarrhea.

A person admitted with a potential or actual DKA may have an anion gap determination performed. Although anion gap alone is inconclusive for DKA, it is used as adjunctive data in clustering critical cues for differential diagnosis.

Causes of Diabetic Ketoacidosis

DKA is caused by extreme insulin deficiency. Illness and infection are the primary causes in approximately 25 to 30 percent of the DKA cases (Funnell et al., 1998). Illness and infection increase the production of glucocorticoids by the adrenal gland supporting the production of new glucose by the liver (gluconeogenesis). Epinephrine and norepinephrine levels are also increased causing further breakdown of glycogen into glucose (glycogenolysis). Diabetic ketoacidosis is seen most commonly in type 1 diabetics.

Any condition or situation that increases the insulin deficit can precipitate DKA; for example: infection, pregnancy, emotional or physical stress, and extreme anxiety (Guven & Kuenzi, 1998). In about 20 percent of cases, no specific precipitating event is found (Johnson, 1998).

Stress as a Major Precipitating Factor

An increased level of stress causes further production of stress hormones (e.g., epinephrine, growth hormone, and cortisol). As discussed in Section One, when secreted, these hormones increase blood glucose levels by either increasing conversion of glycogen to glucose or decreasing cellular use of glucose. When the stress is severe, as in a severe acute infection, the increase in glucose can be substantial, thus precipitating an imbalance in the glucose/insulin relationship.

Severe infection with systemic involvement also is typically accompanied by hyperthermia (fever). Hyperthermia increases the metabolic rate; thus greatly increasing cellular need for insulin. Therefore, in the presence of infection, there is both an increased supply and an increased demand for glucose. In such a situation, it would seem that a balance in glucose would exist. This is not the case, however, with type 1 diabetes. A balance can be maintained or regained only when sufficient insulin is present to meet the increased glucose needs of the cells. DKA is precipitated by a relative insulin deficiency in this situation. If insulin dosage is not increased in response, there is insufficient insulin to meet the increased glucose supply as well as the increased metabolic demand.

A similar situation can occur with a client with type 2 diabetes, whose condition normally is controlled by diet, antidiabetes agents, or both. In situations of high stress (infection, trauma, surgery), the level of insulin secretion in the pancreas often is insufficient to meet the increased supply of and demand for glucose. Thus, this type of client clinically exhibits hyperglycemia, which often requires temporary exogenous insulin therapy. Insulin is then administered until the level of physiologic stress is sufficiently reduced and balance is regained between the glucose level and the endogenous insulin supply.

Management of Diabetic Ketoacidosis

The DKA-related treatment goals include:

- Correcting fluid and electrolyte imbalances
- Decreasing serum glucose
- Preventing further complications
- Clearing urine and serum ketones
- Providing client education (Halloran, 1998; Funnel et al., 1998)

Nursing interventions are based on activities that help the client meet expected outcomes. They consist of collaborative interventions: (1) activities ordered by the physician but requiring some actions by the nurse; and (2) activities that are within the nursing scope of practice (independent nursing orders).

Collaborative Interventions

The physician's orders may include the following (see Fig. 25–2 for an example of a DKA treatment plan):

1. *IV therapy*. The client's initial management requires rapid rehydration. Osmotic diuresis precipitated by elevated glucose levels severely depletes body fluids. Initial fluid replacement will be with one-half normal (0.45 percent) or normal (0.9 percent) saline. As soon as the serum glucose level is decreased to approximately 300 mg/dL, IV fluids should contain glucose (usually 5 percent dextrose with 0.45 percent saline) (Funnell et al., 1998). The client will receive nothing by mouth until the crisis state is resolved.
2. *Insulin therapy*. Correction of the hyperglycemic state is dependent on careful use of insulin. During the crisis state, only short-acting or rapid-acting insulins are used because of their fast results in reducing glucose levels, which facilitate better control. Insulin management generally is via continuous, low-dose intravenous infusion.
3. *Sodium bicarbonate therapy*. Sodium bicarbonate is the drug of choice for rapid correction of most metabolic acidosis problems. However, with DKA treatment with sodium bicarbonate ($NaHCO_3$) is controversial and not recommended by the majority of endocrinologists. Sodium bicarbonate may be recommended with severe cases of metabolic acidosis if the arterial pH is 7.0 or less or if the serum bicarbonate level is less than 5 mEq/L. If used, serum potassium levels may drop rapidly and must be monitored closely (Funnell et al., 1998). Also, when the ketoacidosis is corrected too rapidly, it can precipitate cerebrospinal fluid (CSF) acidosis, causing potentially severe neurologic complications. Cerebrospinal fluid acidosis is difficult to correct because sodium bicarbonate does not cross the blood–brain barrier. Diabetic ketoacidosis often corrects itself with the use of insulin, electrolyte therapy, and IV fluid replacement.
4. *Electrolyte replacement*. Potassium, sodium, and phosphate are three of the major electrolytes requiring replacement during a DKA episode. Sodium is replaced primarily during the initial rehydration phase of treatment in the 0.9 percent and 0.45 percent normal saline IV solutions. Particular care is taken in managing potassium replacement since serum levels decrease as the acidotic state is corrected and normal urine output is regained. Unless the serum potassium is low at the time of admission, potassium replacement is contraindicated for the first 3 to 4 hours of management. However, if T wave changes occur, potassium may be added in the second to fourth hour of treatment or sooner. Once potassium shifts have stabilized, insulin therapy has been instituted and the urine output has been stabilized, potassium replacement is instituted. Phosphate, a buffer, may become depleted during periods of acidosis, particularly if the acidosis is prolonged. Adequate levels of phosphate are important in managing the acidosis. When replacement is warranted, it is generally administered IV in the form of potassium phosphate.
5. *Correction of underlying problems*. A key to successful management of a hyperglycemic crisis is finding and aggressively treating the underlying cause. If an infection is the underlying problem, antibiotic therapy is initiated, and if a wound is present (such as an open ulcer), it may be debrided. The pathophysiologic effects of diabetes prevent the client from healing well, increasing the risk of further infectious complications.

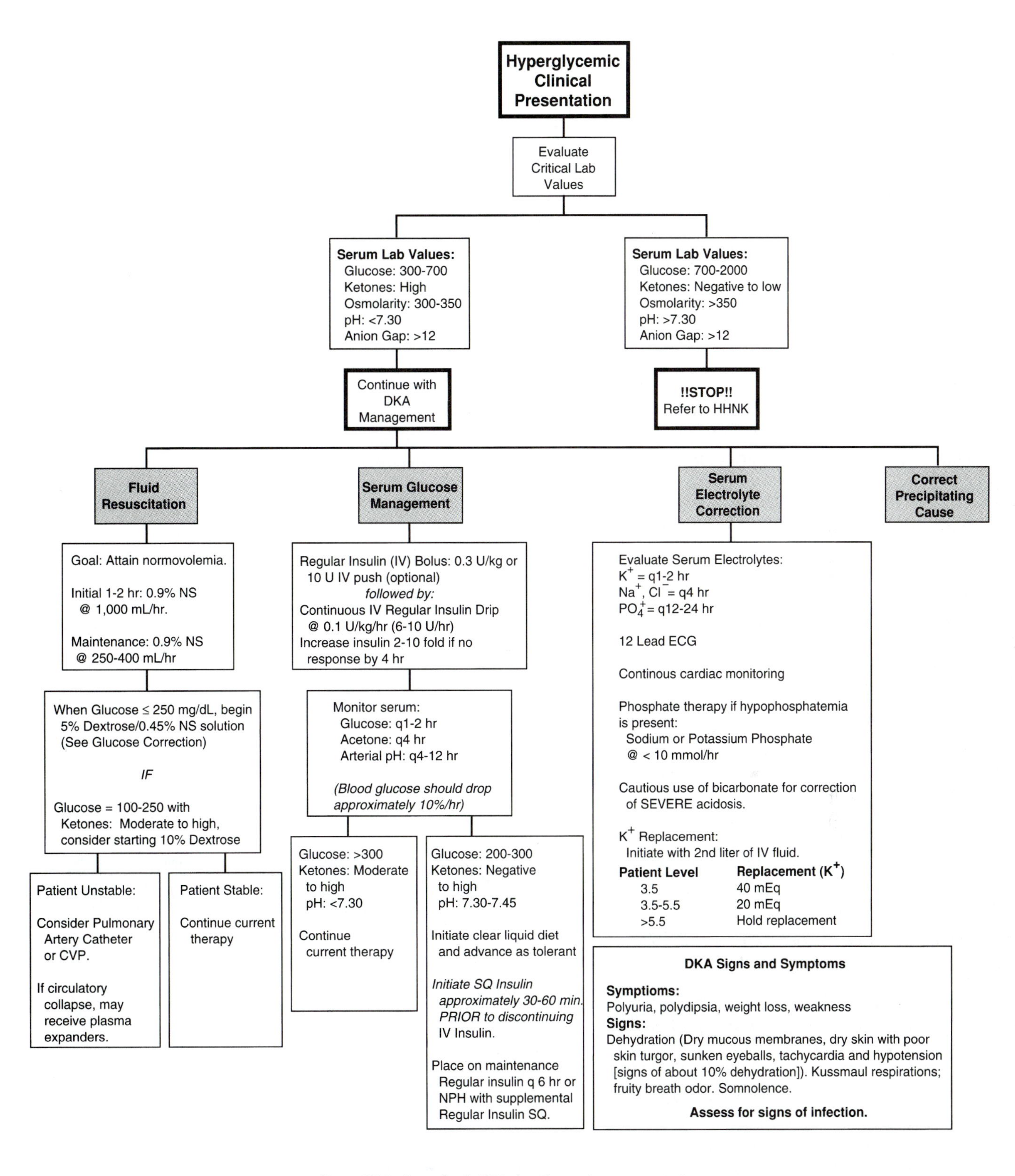

Figure 25–2. Example of a DKA algorithm and management plan.

6. *Laboratory and other tests*. The client's status will be closely monitored throughout the DKA period. Initially, close monitoring of serum pH, glucose, ketones, osmolality, and electrolytes is necessary. The client may have an electrocardiogram (ECG) ordered to monitor serum potassium effects on the heart. A culture and Gram stain of potentially infected secretions or fluids confirm the type of organism so that IV antibiotic therapy can be most effective.

Independent Nursing Interventions

Fluid Volume Deficit

1. Assess for signs and symptoms of fluid volume deficit; report abnormals.
2. Monitor hemodynamics as available; report worsening trends: pulmonary artery pressure, pulmonary artery wedge pressure, and central venous pressure.
3. Monitor laboratory and other test results; report abnormals: blood urea nigrogen (BUN) and creatinine, electrolytes, hemoglobin, and hematocrit.
4. Monitor for therapeutic and nontherapeutic effects of fluid replacement therapy; report abnormals.
5. When taking oral fluids, encourage intake to 2,500 mL/24 hr if underlying problems permit.

Altered Nutrition: Less Than Body Requirements

1. Monitor for therapeutic and nontherapeutic effects of insulin therapy; report abnormals.
2. Monitor laboratory and other test results; report abnormals: serum glucose, ketones, albumin, transferrin, CBC with differential.
3. Monitor and document dietary intake.
4. Encourage intake of prescribed diet.
   a. Avoid painful procedures immediately before meals or feedings.
   b. Administer pain medications before meals, when needed; assess effectiveness of PRN medications.
5. Implement measures to reduce energy requirements.

PC: Electrolyte Imbalances
PC: Metabolic Acidosis

1. Assess for signs and symptoms of electrolyte imbalances; report abnormals (specify imbalances based on specific disorder).
2. Assess for signs and symptoms of metabolic acidosis; report abnormals.
3. Monitor laboratory (e.g., serum electrolytes) and other test results; report abnormals
4. Monitor for therapeutic and nontherapeutic effects of electrolyte and acidosis drug therapy; report abnormals.
5. Monitor ECG for changes consistent with electrolyte imbalance, such as dysrhythmias, T wave changes, ST segment changes.
6. Encourage intake of appropriate nutrients.
7. Restrict intake of undesirable nutrients based on electrolyte levels.
8. Encourage intake of fluids if fluid volume deficit exists.

In summary, DKA is an acute life-threatening consequence of diabetes mellitus, which can be prevented by thorough rapid intervention, client education, and medical management. It is a type of high anion gap metabolic acidosis caused by accumulation of ketone bodies. Anion gap is one method of differentiating DKA from several other types of acidosis. DKA may be precipitated by any event that increases the insulin deficit. Physiologic stress and acute infection are two major precipitating conditions.

SECTION SIX REVIEW

1. Which of the following set of laboratory results best reflects diabetic ketoacidosis?
   A. pH 7.28, HCO_3 34 mEq/L, blood glucose 260 mg/dL
   B. pH 7.18, HCO_3 13 mEq/L, blood glucose 120 mg/dL
   C. pH 7.26, HCO_3 14 mEq/L, blood glucose 450 mg/dL
   D. pH 7.38, HCO_3 24 mEq/L, blood glucose 620 mg/dL
2. Typical clinical manifestations of diabetic ketoacidosis include
   A. absence of ketonuria
   B. fluid overload
   C. electrolytes within normal range
   D. progressive dehydration
3. Ketosis results from mobilization of
   A. amino acids
   B. glucagon
   C. glucose
   D. fatty acids
4. A high anion gap acidosis is consistent with which of the following problems?
   A. diarrhea
   B. high intake of chloride
   C. starvation
   D. high intake of sodium
5. A common precipitating factor for development of diabetic ketoacidosis is
   A. stress-free lifestyle
   B. decreased exercise
   C. infection
   D. food/insulin balance

Answers: 1. C, 2. D, 3. D, 4. C, 5. C

SECTION SEVEN: Hyperglycemic Hyperosmolar Nonketotic Syndrome

At the completion of this section, the learner will be able to discuss the diabetic complication, hyperglycemic hyperosmolar nonketotic syndrome.

Hyperglycemic hyperosmolar nonketotic syndrome (HHNS) is a hyperglycemic complication of diabetes mellitus that results from insulin deficiency and/or insulin resistance. It is sometimes overlooked and primarily occurs in elderly clients, particularly sick elderly, with type 2 diabetes. HHNS has a higher mortality rate than DKA because of its severe metabolic changes and the delay in diagnosis. The major precipitating factor for development of HHNS is infection, particularly pneumonia and urinary tract infections (Johnson, 1998). See Table 25–4 for a summary of other precipitating factors.

Pathophysiologic Basis of HHNS

The client with type 2 diabetes produces moderate levels of insulin. In the presence of a precipitating event, the type 2 diabetic's relative lack of insulin can trigger hyperglycemia by way of acceleration of hepatic gluconeogenesis and decreased peripheral glucose utilization. The result of these events is extreme hyperglycemia (may be in excess of 2,000 mg/dL) while avoiding significant ketoacidosis. Failure to develop significant ketoacidosis is attributed to the type 2 diabetic's ability to produce sufficient insulin to prevent or minimize lipolysis and ketogenesis.

The excess glucose accumulates in the extracellular spaces because it cannot be transported into the cells or metabolized normally, resulting in a progressive increase in osmolality. As extracellular osmolality increases, water is pulled from the intracellular spaces into the extracellular spaces. As the level of hyperglycemia increases and exceeds the renal threshold, osmotic diuresis significantly increases, precipitating progressive dehydration of intracellular and extracellular spaces. Severe dehydration of the intracellular and extracellular spaces results in hyperosmolar coma if the serum osmolality increases to 350 mOsm/L or higher (Johnson, 1998).

TABLE 25–4. PRECIPITATING FACTORS OF HHNS

Inadequate fluid intake
Infection
Severe stress
Severe burns
Peritoneal dialysis
Thiazide and diuretic usage
Chronic illness
Infirmity, institutionalization (elderly)
Hypertonic feeding
Mental impairment

Sources: Siperstein, M.D. (1992). Diabetic ketoacidosis and hyperosmolar coma. Endocrinol Metab Clin North Am *21(2):415–432; and Funnell, M.M., Hunt, C., Kulkarni, K., et al. (1998).* A core curriculum for diabetes education, *3rd ed. Chicago: American Association of Diabetes Educators.*

Clinical Presentation

DKA and HHNS have many similarities, as both are associated with

- An absolute or relative insulin deficit
- Hyperosmolality secondary to hyperglycemia and water loss
- Depletion of volume secondary to osmotic diuresis
- Electrolyte abnormalities secondary to the osmotic diuresis
- Altered mental status

There are also many major differences between DKA and HHNS that assist the clinician in differentiating the two disorders. Some of the major differences include:

- DKA is associated with rapid onset, whereas HHNS develops more slowly and insidiously.
- Hyperglycemia is more severe with HHNS.
- Hyperosmolality is more severe in HHNS, causing profound dehydration.
- Water loss associated with HHNS is significantly greater than with DKA.
- HHNS is associated with severe neurologic signs (e.g., coma, seizures); in addition, mental status changes may occur over a period of days with HHNS.

The clinical manifestations as well as a comparison of HHNS with DKA are presented in Table 25–5.

Medical Interventions

Medical goals for management of the client with HHNS are essentially the same as for the client with DKA. In management of HHNS, the first priority is rehydration and restoration of normal electrolyte levels. Other goals include correction of the precipitating event (if possible) and prevention of complications. Fluid replacement needs in the HHNS client are greater than in the DKA client due to the more profound state of dehydration. Careful monitoring is necessary to prevent complications associated with too rapid rehydration, though complications associated with fluid volume overload during fluid resuscitation of the HHNS client is rare. Because the individual with type 2 diabetes may be sensitive to exogenous insulin, insulin generally is administered in lower doses in treatment of the HHNS client than in the DKA client. Table 25–6 provides a brief overview of a medical protocol for fluid replacement and insulin therapy for treatment of pure HHNS.

TABLE 25–5. DIFFERENTIATING DKA FROM HHNC

FACTOR	DKA	HHNS
Population affected	< 40 years of age	> 60 years of age
Diabetic type	Type 1	Type 2
Previous history of diabetes	Almost always	In about 50 percent
Predisposing factors	Noncompliance to type 1 treatment plan; surgery, stress	Elderly; presence of acute illness or other physiologic stress
Rate of onset	Sudden (hours)	Slow, insidious (days–weeks)
Usual duration	< 5 days	> 5 days
Complications	Rare	Frequent
Symptomatology	Ketoacidosis; fruity breath odor; respirations rapid and deep (Kussmaul type); mental disorientation	Absent to mild ketosis; no acetone breath odor; respirations non-Kussmaul type; profound coma; convulsions
Laboratory data		
Anion gap	Positive high (> 17 mEq/L)	Negative (< 17 mEq/L)
Serum glucose	300–800 mg/dL	> 700 mg/dL; often > 1,000 mg/dL
Serum ketones	Positive ketoacids	Absence of significant ketones
Serum osmolality	< 350 mOsm/L	> 350 mOsm/L
Free fatty acids	Significantly elevated	Not significantly elevated
Acid–base status	pH low; bicarbonate low	pH normal; bicarbonate normal
Urine glucose	Elevated	Elevated
Urine ketones	Positive	Absence or not significant

Sources: Andreoli, T.E., Carpenter, C.C., Bennett, J.C., & Plum, F. (1997). Cecil's essentials of medicine, *4th ed. Philadelphia: W.B. Saunders; and Thelan, L.A., Urden, L.D., Lough, M.E., & Stacy, K.M. (1998). Endocrine disorders and therapeutic management. In L.A. Thelan et al. (eds.),* Critical care nursing: Diagnosis and management, *3rd ed. St. Louis: C.V. Mosby.*

DKA–Hyperosmolar Coma (or Mixed) Syndrome

Siperstein (1992) and Andreoli et al. (1997) suggested that DKA and HHNS can be viewed as existing on a continuum, with pure DKA being at one end and pure hyperosmolar coma at the other end (Fig. 25–3). The common factors between these two disorders are hypoinsulinemia and hyperglycemia. Some clients develop an intermediate combination of these two disorders, a syndrome of signs and symptoms that exhibit aspects of both. The syndrome is primarily found in clients who develop an acute bacterial infection or experience a significant physiologic stress during the time that they are developing type 2 diabetes. Other contributing factors that can precipitate the syndrome are the same as those listed for both of the individual metabolic disorders. DKA–hyperosmolar coma (mixed) syndrome should be suspected when a client is admitted in a comatose state with severe hyperglycemia that is accompanied by mild to moderate ketoacidosis. Pure DKA is rarely associated with coma, whereas severe hyperosmolality (> 350 mOsm/L) is strongly associated with it.

TABLE 25–6. A MEDICAL INTERVENTION PROTOCOL FOR HHNS

TREATMENT	PROTOCOL
Fluid replacement	Initial hour: 2 L of 0.9% NS (especially with circulatory collapse) Maintenance: 6–10 L of 0.45% NS as needed for fluid replacement for first 10 hours (requires close monitoring of sodium and water balance) When serum glucose is 250–300 mg/dL, begin 5% dextrose in 0.9% or 0.45% NS
Insulin (regular)	Initial IV bolus of 10 to 15 U Alternative choices for maintenance doses: 0.1 U/kg/hr IV until serum glucose is 250–300 mg/dL Maintenance doses are discontinued when glucose level is 250 mg/dL

Sources: Thelan, L.A., Urden, L.D., Lough, M.E., & Stacy, K.M. (1998). Endocrine disorders and therapeutic management. In L.A. Thelan et al. (eds.), Critical care nursing: Diagnosis and management, *3rd ed. St. Louis: C.V. Mosby.*

In summary, HHNS is a type of hyperglycemic diabetic crisis associated with type 2 diabetes mellitus. The hallmark of HHNS is a hyperosmolar hyperglycemic state without significant ketosis. The degree of hyperglycemia and dehydration is more severe in HHNS than in DKA. Treatment of DKA and HHNS is similar, although HHNS requires higher volumes of fluids and lower doses of insulin. The diabetic client may also develop an intermediate hyperglycemic crisis called DKA–hyperosmolar (or mixed) syndrome. This syndrome is characterized by a clinical presentation that includes signs and symptoms of both DKA and HHNS.

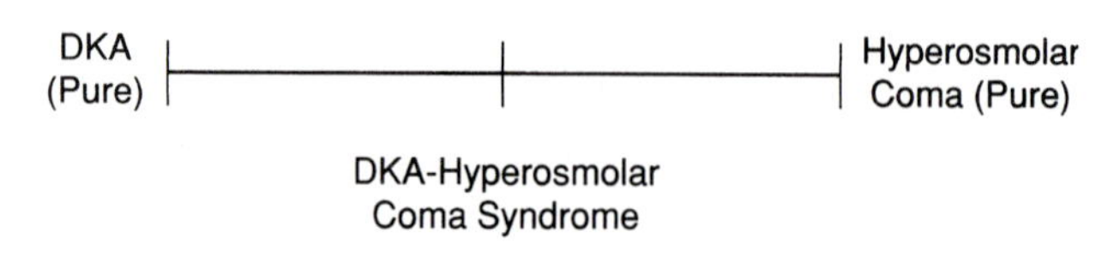

Figure 25–3. DKA–hyperosmolar coma (or mixed) syndrome. Pure diabetic ketoacidosis (DKA) is characterized by a predominance of signs and symptoms owing to metabolic acidosis. Pure hyperosmolar coma is characterized by a predominance of signs and symptoms owing to profound hyperglycemia. DKA–hyperosmolar coma exists between the two pure disorders and is characterized by signs and symptoms related to both DKA and hyperosmolar coma.

Section Seven Review

1. Which of the following statements is correct regarding HHNS?
   A. it has a high mortality rate
   B. it is most common in type 1 diabetes
   C. it causes severe fluid volume overload
   D. death occurs from severe metabolic acidosis
2. Common precipitating events causing HHNS include which of the following?
   A. hemodialysis
   B. hyperalimentation
   C. chronic infection
   D. high-fat diet
3. HHNS does not cause ketosis because
   A. lipolysis does not occur
   B. protein catabolism is occurring
   C. high glucagon levels prevent it
   D. hyperglycemia is not sufficiently severe
4. Which of the following statements regarding the differences between DKA and HHNS is correct?
   A. the onset of HHNS is faster
   B. dehydration is less severe in HHNS
   C. hyperosmolality is more severe in HHNS
   D. mental status changes more rapidly in HHNS
5. Which of the following statements is correct regarding insulin management of the client with HHNS?
   A. insulin management is contraindicated
   B. usually requires low-dose insulin management
   C. the type 2 diabetic is resistant to exogenous insulin
   D. the type 1 diabetic is resistant to exogenous insulin

Answers: 1. A, 2. B, 3. A, 4. C, 5. B

SECTION EIGHT: Exogenous Insulin Therapy

At the completion of this section, the learner will be able to explain the use of exogenous insulin in the management of the client with diabetes mellitus.

Individuals with type 1 diabetes require exogenous insulin replacement. Type 2 diabetics do not always require exogenous insulin. However, during a period of stress (e.g., illness or surgery), the type 2 diabetic may experience hyperglycemia, requiring temporary insulin therapy until the condition is resolved and glucose levels return to normal.

Sources of Exogenous Insulin

Insulin is derived from the pancreases of animals or synthesized in a laboratory. Insulin produced from animal pancreases is further divided into three types: beef (bovine), pork (porcine), and bovine–porcine combination. Of all types of exogenous insulin, bovine insulin differs most from human insulin and, therefore, generally is not used as commonly as other forms. Porcine insulin is structurally similar to human insulin and usually is well accepted by the body. Bovine–porcine combination insulin also is available as a less expensive insulin alternative.

Synthetic insulin is rapidly replacing animal-based insulins and is used almost exclusively in the United States. Synthetic insulin is developed in a laboratory setting and involves structural conversion of a substance into the amino acid chains identical to human insulin. Various substances such as porcine insulin and *Escherichia coli* are used to manufacture human insulin using recombinant DNA technology.

Certain factors dictate which type of insulin is best suited to a specific person. Some of these factors include the presence of the following:

- Insulin allergy
- Insulin resistance
- Adipose tissue atrophy at injection sites
- Religious restriction against pork
- Cost of insulin

The final choice of insulin often is based on trial and error in finding which product best meets the individual needs of the person. Insulins are not interchangeable, since they have differing efficacy levels and possible allergy implications. For this reason, it is important for the nurse to be aware of the type of insulin ordered and to take precautions that the same type of insulin is being administered. For example, the client who normally receives synthetic insulin should not be given porcine or bovine insulin without specific orders to do so.

Factors That Influence Insulin

Many factors have an impact on insulin dosage or effectiveness. Table 25–7 lists some of the major factors and how they influence insulin dosages.

Types of Insulin

Insulin is divided into four major categories according to its duration of action. The four categories include ultrashort-acting, short-acting, intermediate-acting, and long-acting. There are also several insulins that are categorized as premixed. These insulins combine neutral protamine

TABLE 25–7. FACTORS AFFECTING INSULIN DOSAGE

FACTOR	EFFECT
Drug interactions	
Beta-adrenergic blocking agents	May mask hypoglycemic symptoms; propranolol is associated with causing hyperglycemia when given concurrently with insulin
Steroids	Use of steroids is associated with increased glucose levels; may require increased dosage of insulin
Oral antidiabetic agents	Enhance hypoglycemic effects; may require reduction in insulin dosage
Other	
Exercise	An unusually high level of exercise may reduce glucose levels, producing hypoglycemia; may require reduction in insulin dosage
Acute illness	Increases blood glucose levels and insulin needs; often requires sliding scale insulin administration
Nutritional support	Elevates blood glucose, increasing insulin need; often requires sliding insulin administration

Source: McHenry, L.M., & Salerno, E. (eds.). (1992). Mosby's pharmacology in nursing, *18th ed. St. Louis: C.V. Mosby.*

Hagedorn (NPH) with regular insulins. Lispro insulin (Humalog), a new synthetic insulin, has a change in structure that results in a shortened action time. This ultra-rapid-acting insulin has a peak of 30 to 90 minutes and duration of 4 hours or less. It has become the preferred meal coverage insulin for many diabetics (Lewis, Heitkemper, & Dirksen, 2000). Table 25–8 differentiates the various insulins according to these categories. Figure 25–4 differentiates between the categories based on the extent and duration of action.

Side Effects of Insulin

Administration of too much insulin causes **hypoglycemia.** The client is at greatest risk for hypoglycemia during peak action time. It is crucial to be aware of the type of insulin administered (e.g., rapid acting), when the dose was administered, and what type of nutrition has been consumed after administration. A person receiving a rapid-acting insulin, such as regular insulin, at 8:00 A.M. would have peak within 2 to 4 hours after subcutaneous administration. This would mean that the risk for hypoglycemia is greatest between the hours of 10:00 A.M. and 12:00 noon.

A client receiving an intermediate-acting insulin (such as NPH) at 8:00 A.M. would peak about 6 to 12 hours later, placing him at greatest risk for hypoglycemia between the hours of 2:00 P.M. and 8:00 P.M. Many acutely ill clients require supplemental rapid-acting insulin (regular insulin) as well as their usual intermediate- or long-acting insulin. Mixing types of insulin gives the client multi-

TABLE 25–8. EXAMPLES OF INSULIN PREPARATIONS AVAILABLE IN THE UNITED STATES[a]

PREPARATION	SPECIES SOURCE
Ultra-short-acting insulin	
Insulin lispro, Humalog (Lilly)	Human analog (recombinant)
Short-acting insulins	
Standard	
Regular Iletin (Lilly)	Beef and pork
"Purified"	
Regular (Novo Nordisk)[b]	Pork or human
Regular Humulin (Lilly)[c]	Human
Regular Iletin II (Lilly)[c]	Pork
Velosulin (Novo Nordisk)[d]	Human
Intermediate-acting insulins	
Standard	
Lente Iletin I (Lilly)	Beef and pork
NPH Iletin I (Lilly)	Beef and pork
"Purified"	
Lente Humulin (Lilly)	Human
Lente Iletin II (Lilly)	Pork
Lente (Novo Nordisk)	Pork or human
NPH Humulin (Lilly)	Pork or human
NPH Iletin II (Lilly)	Pork
NPH (Novo Nordisk)	Human
Premixed insulins (% NPH, % regular)	
Novolin 70/30 (Novo Nordisk)	Human
Humulin 70/30 (Lilly)	Human
Long-acting insulins	
"Purified"	
Ultralente Humulin (Lilly)	Human

[a]All are available in U100 concentration.
[c]Also available in U500 concentration.
[b]Novo Nordisk human insulins are termed Novolin R, L, and N.
[d]Velosulin contains phosphate buffer, which favors its use to prevent insulin aggregation in pump tubing but precludes its being mixed with lente insulin.
Modified and reproduced, with permission, from Katzung, BG (ed.). (1998). Basic & clinical pharmacology, *7th ed. Stamford, CT: Appleton & Lange.*

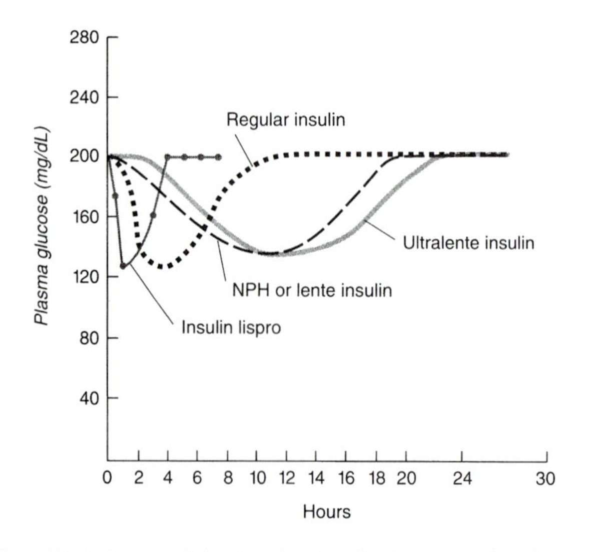

Figure 25–4. Extent and duration of action of various types of insulin (in a fasting diabetic). *(From Katzung, B.G. [1998].* Basic and clinical pharmacology, *7th ed. (p. 689). Stamford, CT: Appleton & Lange.)*

ple insulin peak periods throughout a 24-hour period. Other factors commonly seen in acutely ill clients, such as prolonged NPO status and nutritional support, all have an impact on glucose levels and insulin needs.

Continuous Low-Dose Intravenous Insulin Infusion

Fleckman (1993) stated that historically, treatment of DKA in its early stages consisted of large doses of insulin (hundreds of units). Over time, clinicians found that continuous low-dose IV insulin made regulation easier and provided better control of glucose levels. Other advantages include fewer complications associated with hypokalemia and hypoglycemia and rapid rate of insulin dissipation.

During a hyperglycemic crisis, a continuous infusion of regular insulin may be ordered to provide better control of serum insulin levels. When preparing to administer IV insulin, it is important to remember that:

- Only regular insulin is administered IV.
- Insulin binds to polyvinylchloride in IV bags and tubing, lowering the insulin concentration in the fluid. One form of insulin, Velosulin, has been buffered with phosphate, which prevents the insulin from binding to plastic tubing.
- Blood glucose levels must be monitored frequently to avoid hypoglycemia.

Sliding-Scale Insulin Administration

During periods of physiologic stress, glucose levels may be very unstable, requiring supplemental insulin in addition to the client's usual insulin coverage. Consequently, insulin dosage must reflect current blood glucose levels. Orders may be written to titrate the insulin dose to specific glucose levels. This type of insulin regimen is called *sliding-scale insulin* coverage. Table 25–9 gives an example of a sliding-scale insulin order.

It is recommended that sliding-scale insulin administration be carried out based on blood glucose rather than urine glucose measurements. Urine glucose does not reflect hour-by-hour changes in glucose levels. Thus, its value for tight glucose control is diminished.

TABLE 25–9. EXAMPLE OF SLIDING-SCALE INSULIN REGIMEN

BLOOD GLUCOSE LEVEL (MG/DL)	REGULAR INSULIN DOSE (SUBCUTANEOUSLY)
200–250	5 units
251–300	10 units
301–350	15 units
351–400	Call physician

The Somogyi Effect: An Insulin Dosage Problem

Some clients, particularly those who are acutely ill, have wide swings in serum glucose levels from early morning to postprandial testings caused by an excessive insulin dosage. One explanation of this phenomenon is the **Somogyi effect.** The effect is triggered by nocturnal hypoglycemia. Hypoglycemia causes release of stress hormones, ultimately increasing serum glucose, which, in turn, creates a state of hyperglycemia. Morning urine ketones may be noted as well as an elevated serum glucose caused by catabolic processes. The resulting hyperglycemia, if accompanied by increased insulin dosage, precipitates another episode of hypoglycemia that may be worse than the preceding episode (Fig. 25–5).

Recognition of the presence of the Somogyi effect has important treatment implications. The administration of more insulin worsens the level of nocturnal hypoglycemia, further aggravating the problem. When the Somogyi effect is suspected, the insulin dosage may actually need to be decreased, or a bedtime snack of protein may be added to the diet to slow down the rebound cycle.

In summary, exogenous insulin therapy is a necessity for the client with type 1 diabetes. The type 2 diabetic may require it, particularly during periods of physiologic stress. Exogenous insulin is available from either animal or synthetic sources. Animal sources of insulin are similar but not identical to human insulin, making them potentially less acceptable to the body. Synthetic insulin is a laboratory duplication of human insulin. Choice of type of insulin based on source usually is decided by trial and error.

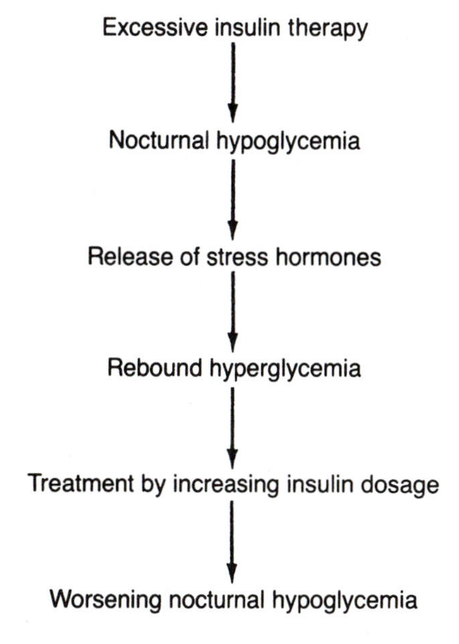

Figure 25–5. The Somogyi effect.

SECTION EIGHT REVIEW

1. Which of the following situations would be most likely to necessitate exogenous insulin use in the type 2 diabetic client?
   A. a localized toe infection
   B. a mild common cold
   C. a high carbohydrate meal
   D. an abdominal hysterectomy
2. All of the following are sources of insulin EXCEPT
   A. pork
   B. beef
   C. *Staphylococcus aureus*
   D. *Escherichia coli*
3. Exogenous insulin is
   A. seldom used in the treatment of HHNS
   B. most often derived from animal sources
   C. used only in the treatment of type 1 diabetes
   D. often required in management of type 2 diabetes during stress periods
4. All of the following are factors that dictate the type of insulin that is best suited for a specific person EXCEPT
   A. client's weight
   B. insulin resistance
   C. client's allergies
   D. adipose tissue condition
5. Which of the following factors would most likely decrease insulin need?
   A. acute illness
   B. steroid therapy
   C. nutritional support
   D. oral antidiabetic agents

Answers: 1. A, 2. C, 3. D, 4. A, 5. D

SECTION NINE: Acute Care Implications of Chronic Complications

At the completion of this section, the learner will be able to discuss the acute care implications of chronic diabetic complications.

Glucose Control and Complications

The acutely ill client has many factors that influence client outcomes, such as preexisting chronic diseases. Diabetes is a chronic disease that profoundly affects client outcomes because of the many acute and chronic complications that can result from it. Though diabetes mellitus is caused by dysfunction of one organ—the pancreas—it causes dysfunction of virtually all organs. Maintaining long-term glucose control is essential in the prevention or reduction of diabetes-related complications.

Overall glucose control can be monitored using the **glycosylated hemoglobin** (Hb A_1c) test. According to Kee (1999) the predominant type of hemoglobin is hemoglobin A (Hb A). Normally, about 4 percent to 8 percent of hemoglobin A has glucose attached to it and is referred to as glycosylated hemoglobin (Hb A_1). Hb A_1 forms slowly throughout the 120-day life span of hemoglobin. Hb A_1 is made up of three different molecules, one of which is Hb A_1c. This particular molecule is about 70 percent glycosylated. The amount of glycosylated hemoglobin is dependent on the amount of glucose in the blood and is a good indicator of the average serum glucose level over a 120-day period. The normal range of glycosylated hemoglobin (Hb A_1c) is 4.5 percent to 7.5 percent of the total hemoglobin (Kee, 1999). Uncontrolled diabetes mellitus is present if a glycosylated hemoglobin level is more than 15 percent of the total hemoglobin.

Chronic Complications

Chronic complications can be divided into three types: peripheral neuropathy, microvascular, and macrovascular. The remainder of this section presents an overview of major long-term complications associated with diabetes mellitus.

Diabetic Peripheral Neuropathies

Peripheral neuropathies are the most common complications of diabetes mellitus. They begin early in the course of the disease, affecting both type 1 and type 2 diabetics. Peripheral neuropathies primarily alter sensory perception. The underlying cause of neuropathies is poorly understood. They may result from thickening of vessel walls that supply peripheral nerves, thus impairing nutrition to the nerves. They may result from a segmental demyelinization that results in slowed or disrupted conduction. There is also some evidence that sorbitol may accumulate in the nerve cells, impairing conduction. Whatever the cause, the result is an alteration in sensory perception.

Neuropathies initially may cause pain or abnormal sensations or both. As nerve degeneration progresses, the client may experience loss of the ability to discriminate fine touch, a decrease in proprioception, and local anesthesia.

The autonomic nervous system also may be affected. As the myelin sheath undergoes degenerative changes, functions governed by the autonomic nerves are affected adversely. The client may experience an increase in gut motility and diarrhea, postural hypotension, or other autonomic nervous system–related complications.

The neuropathies experienced by diabetics vary in type, severity, and clinical manifestations. Because of this diversity, it is not possible to predict which neuropathy any individual will develop.

Acute Care Implications. When feasible, clients with diabetes should be assessed for the presence and degree of peripheral neuropathy. The presence of a diminished sense of touch and pain may mask injury or infection. The client must be protected from injury at all times to prevent damage to affected tissues. The diabetic client must also be protected from hyperthermic burns. Excessive heat may not be sensed, which increases the risk of burns by heating pads, hyperthermia blankets, and bathing. Some neuropathies are associated with progressive, permanent damage to the neurons. However, others are reversible when good glucose control is maintained.

Microvascular Disease

Microvascular disease is associated with capillary membrane thickening, which causes **microangiopathy** (small blood vessel disease). As the capillary membrane thickens, the tissues become increasingly hypoperfused, and organs become hypoxic and ischemic. Prolonged ischemia eventually causes **infarction** (death of tissue). The degree of microvascular disease may be influenced most by the duration of diabetes rather than the level of glucose control. Two organs are at particular risk for microvascular disease secondary to diabetes mellitus: the retina of the eyes and the kidneys.

Retinopathy

Diabetic retinopathy is responsible for a significant portion of newly diagnosed blindness in the United States. It is caused by an underlying microangiopathy of the retina, leading to retina microvascular occlusion. Once occlusion exists, the retina undergoes increasing areas of ischemia and infarction, eventually leading to blindness. Damage occurs in two complex stages. Stage I is associated with increased capillary permeability, aneurysm formation, and hemorrhage. Stage II is associated with increasing retinal ischemia and eventual infarction, causing blindness. Diabetic retinopathy is associated with both type 1 and type 2 diabetes.

Acute Care Implications. The acutely ill diabetic client may have moderate to severe visual impairment. Early assessment of visual status is important, either by questioning of the client directly or by interviewing the family. Medical and nursing management and teaching must be altered to meet the needs of a visually impaired client. In the high-acuity client, blindness affects pupillary changes and must be taken into consideration when performing a neurologic assessment. A visually impaired client in a critical care environment may have more difficulty making sense of distracting noises and equipment surrounding the bedside. Frequent explanation and reorientation may be necessary.

Nephropathy

Diabetic nephropathy is a disease of the glomeruli. The glomerular basement membrane becomes thickened, resulting in intracapillary glomerulosclerosis (hardening and thickening of the glomeruli). Glomeruli become enlarged and eventually are destroyed, ultimately resulting in renal failure. As the degree of renal failure increases, the client may require a decreased insulin dosage to prevent hypoglycemia. Reduced renal function decreases the ability of the kidneys to metabolize insulin. Insulin not metabolized remains available to facilitate glucose metabolism.

Acute Care Implications. The acutely ill client with some degree of preexisting renal impairment is at risk for further impairment from hypotensive episodes, nephrotoxic drug therapy, or the multisystemic complications associated with many acute illnesses. Kidney function must be carefully monitored at regular intervals. Drug therapy may need to be altered based on kidney function. Kidney failure, as a disease entity, has its own set of actual and potential complications.

Macrovascular Disease

Macrovascular disease (**macroangiopathy**) refers to atherosclerosis. **Atherosclerosis** is a form of arteriosclerosis (thickening and hardening of arterial walls), characterized by plaque deposits of lipids, fibrous connective tissue, calcium deposits, and other blood substances. Atherosclerosis, by definition, affects only large arteries (excluding arterioles). The cause of rapid development of atherosclerosis in the diabetic client is described in Section Three.

Macrovascular disease is associated with the development of coronary artery disease, peripheral vascular disease, brain attack (stroke), and increased risk of infection. Type 2 diabetes is more closely associated with macrovascular diseases than type 1 diabetes. Peripheral vascular disease and increased risk of infection have important implications in the care of the acutely ill client.

Peripheral Vascular Disease

Progressive atherosclerotic changes in peripheral arterial circulation lead to decreasing arterial blood flow to peripheral tissues. As the disease progresses, small arteries become occluded, precipitating a tissue ischemia/infarction sequence of events. In the type 2 diabetic, this is typically noted as small isolated patches of gangrene, particularly on the feet and toes. As circulation becomes increasingly compromised, areas of gangrene become larger, and amputation may be required.

ACUTE CARE IMPLICATIONS. The client with peripheral vascular disease is at increased risk for complications secondary to poor tissue perfusion and loss of skin integrity. Of particular concern in the acutely ill client is the development of decubitus ulcers and infection. Development of either of these two problems could potentially lead to gangrene and possible amputation. Careful limb positioning, excellent skin hygiene, and close monitoring of skin integrity are extremely important.

Increased Risk of Infection

The diabetic client is at high risk for development of infection for a variety of reasons (Ludwig-Beymer, Huether, & Zekauskus, 1996).

1. *Diminished early warning system*. Impaired vision and peripheral neuropathy contribute to the decreased ability of the diabetic client to perform self-monitoring. Breaks in skin integrity may not be seen or felt due to the underlying disease process.
2. *Tissue hypoxia*. Vascular disease causes tissue hypoxia. When skin integrity is broken, there is a decreased ability to heal, secondary to lack of oxygen. Glycosylated hemoglobin in RBCs decreases release of oxygen to the tissues, thus contributing to hypoxia.
3. *Rapid proliferation of pathogens*. Once inside the body, pathogens rapidly multiply because of increased glucose in body fluids, which acts as an energy source for the pathogens.
4. *Impaired white blood cells*. Diabetes is associated with the development of abnormal white blood cells, particularly phagocytes, and also alters with chemotaxis (movement of WBCs to the site of infection).
5. *Impaired circulation*. A diminished blood supply decreases the ability of WBCs to move into the infected area.

ACUTE CARE IMPLICATIONS. The acutely ill diabetic client is at increased risk for development of severe, difficult-to-treat infections. Any infection, no matter how minor it begins, may become life threatening in this client population. Close monitoring for infection and rapid, aggressive intervention are needed. Decreased kidney function may be a complicating factor in aggressive antibiotic therapy.

Wound healing also is impaired in the diabetic for several reasons. Impaired tissue perfusion, especially in the peripheral body area, interferes with healing in those areas due to lack of circulation and tissue hypoxia. Hyperglycemic states adversely affect wound healing by interfering with collagen concentrations in a wound. Good control of blood glucose significantly facilitates wound healing.

In summary, the multisystemic nature of the chronic complications of diabetes strongly influences client outcome in acute illness. There are three major categories of complications: (1) peripheral neuropathies, (2) microvascular complications, including retinopathy and nephropathy, and (3) macrovascular complications, including coronary artery disease, brain attack (stroke), peripheral vascular disease, and increased risk of infection.

SECTION NINE REVIEW

1. Peripheral neuropathies primarily affect
   A. motor functions
   B. sensory functions
   C. optic functions
   D. vascular functions
2. Microvascular diseases are associated with
   A. deposits of lipoproteins
   B. deposits of calcium products
   C. large blood vessel disease
   D. small blood vessel disease
3. Diabetic retinopathy causes blindness by
   A. glucose deposits on the retina
   B. thickening of the retina
   C. destruction of the optic nerve
   D. infarction of retinal tissue
4. Diabetic nephropathy damages the nephrons by causing
   A. glomerulosclerosis
   B. glomerulonephritis
   C. chronic nephritis
   D. renal hypertension
5. Diabetes-induced atherosclerosis is associated with all of the following complications EXCEPT
   A. peripheral vascular disease
   B. cerebrovascular accidents
   C. gastrointestinal ulcers
   D. coronary artery disease
6. Diabetes increases a client's chance of infection for which of the following reasons?
   A. abnormal white blood cells
   B. abnormal platelet function
   C. slow proliferation of pathogens
   D. decreased body fluid glucose levels

Answers: 1. B, 2. D, 3. D, 4. A, 5. C, 6. A

POSTTEST

The following Posttest is constructed in a case study format. A client is presented. Questions are asked based on available data. New data are presented as the case study progresses.

Connie D is a 44-year-old housewife with a history of diabetes mellitus. She has been admitted to the hospital for reevaluation of insulin dosage. She has been having periods of drowsiness and confusion at home.

1. Connie's brain cells
   A. do not require glucose for energy
   B. require fatty acids as their major energy source
   C. do not require insulin for cellular uptake of glucose
   D. require high levels of insulin for cellular uptake of glucose
2. When Connie's blood glucose drops below normal, the sympathetic nervous system stimulates secretion of
   A. epinephrine
   B. cortisol
   C. glucagon
   D. growth hormone
3. Which of the following statements best reflects the effect of insulin on glucose metabolism in Connie's liver? Insulin facilitates conversion of ______.
   A. excess amino acids into glucose
   B. excess fatty acids into glycogen
   C. excess glycogen into glucose
   D. excess glucose into glycogen
4. When Connie's blood amino acid levels increase, insulin
   A. facilitates storage of proteins
   B. inhibits synthesis of protein
   C. facilitates protein catabolism
   D. inhibits transport of amino acids into cell

Connie has an absolute insulin deficit.

5. An absolute insulin deficit would affect her carbohydrate metabolism in which of the following ways?
   A. brain cells rapidly become glucose starved
   B. insulin-dependent cells become glucose starved
   C. brain cells convert glycogen to glucose directly
   D. insulin-dependent cells take in glucose directly
6. In which of the following ways does insulin deficit affect Connie's protein metabolism?
   A. protein synthesis is increased
   B. protein catabolism is halted
   C. protein cannot be stored without insulin
   D. protein cannot be used as energy without insulin

Connie's diabetes is characterized by the following. Her mother also had diabetes. Connie was diagnosed with diabetes at the age of 32. She is 5 feet 5 inches tall and weighs 173 pounds. She requires insulin on a daily basis.

7. Which of the preceding data is most diagnostic of type 1 diabetes?
   A. her mother also had diabetes
   B. she was diagnosed at the age of 32
   C. she is 5 feet 5 inches tall and weighs 173 pounds
   D. she requires insulin on a daily basis
8. If Connie had type 2 diabetes, the most common etiologic factors include
   A. viral infection and obesity
   B. obesity and genetic predisposition
   C. immune reaction and viral infection
   D. obesity and autoimmune reaction

During her hospitalization, Connie was kept NPO for 8 hours for a particular set of blood tests. She, however, did receive her usual morning insulin dosage. Consequently, Connie experiences symptoms typical of a hypoglycemic episode.

9. Typical clinical manifestations of Connie's hypoglycemia would include all of the following EXCEPT
   A. bradycardia
   B. tremor
   C. diaphoresis
   D. vomiting
10. Common causes of hypoglycemic episodes include
    A. lack of dietary intake
    B. heavy carbohydrate meal
    C. insufficient insulin dose
    D. decreased exercise level

Connie has developed an infection from an ingrown toenail. She currently has a temperature of 100°F (oral). A rapid assessment showed the following: opens eyes and groans to mild shaking but closes them immediately after stimulation.

11. What other clinical manifestations would help confirm a diagnosis of diabetic ketoacidosis at this time?
    A. polydipsia
    B. hand tremors
    C. fruity breath odor
    D. shallow respirations
12. Which of the following laboratory results would be most diagnostic of diabetic ketoacidosis?
    A. pH 7.34
    B. anion gap 18 mEq/L
    C. HCO_3 17 mEq/L
    D. $PaCO_2$ 28 mmHg

It has been decided that Connie's diabetic ketoacidosis was precipitated by her foot infection.

13. Infection can precipitate a diabetic ketoacidosis episode due to
    - A. stress response
    - B. increased insulin resistance
    - C. increased glucagon levels
    - D. diminished cortisol activity
14. Connie's diabetic ketoacidosis can be differentiated best from hyperosmolar hyperglycemic nonketotic coma by measuring
    - A. pH
    - B. ketones
    - C. bicarbonate
    - D. blood glucose

Connie is experiencing large swings in her glucose levels throughout the day. The physician orders a larger insulin dose to better control the hyperglycemia. The next day, her hyperglycemia is worse. It is decided that she may be experiencing the Somogyi effect. Connie is confused but conscious.

15. The Somogyi effect is characterized by a rebound phenomenon caused by release of
    - A. glucagon
    - B. amino acids
    - C. fatty acids
    - D. stress hormones
16. Considering her status, which of the following interventions would be most appropriate?
    - A. 5 units of regular insulin
    - B. glucagon 1.5 mg (IM)
    - C. 8 ounces of orange juice
    - D. 50 percent dextrose (IV)

During her diabetic ketoacidosis, Connie receives a continuous drip of IV insulin.

17. Important rules to remember in infusing IV insulin include all of the following EXCEPT
    - A. only regular insulin is used IV
    - B. insulin binds to plastic bags and tubing
    - C. obtain urine glucose every hour
    - D. IV doses usually are small

On Connie's history, you note that she has a long history of peripheral neuropathy, poor vision, and peripheral vascular disease.

18. Connie's peripheral neuropathy is best controlled by
    - A. steroid therapy
    - B. good glucose control
    - C. vitamin supplementation
    - D. nothing; there is no slowing the process
19. Connie's vision has become progressively impaired over the duration of her diabetes. Diabetic retinopathy is due to
    - A. glucose deposits on retina
    - B. macrovascular occlusion
    - C. fatty deposits on retina
    - D. microvascular occlusion
20. Connie's peripheral vascular disease may lead to further complications because it causes
    - A. tissue ischemia
    - B. acute infection
    - C. peripheral edema
    - D. coronary artery disease

POSTTEST ANSWERS

Number	Answer	Section	Number	Answer	Section
1	C	One	11	C	Six
2	A	One	12	B	Six
3	D	Two	13	A	Six
4	A	Two	14	B	Seven
5	B	Three	15	D	Eight
6	C	Three	16	C	Eight
7	D	Four	17	C	Eight
8	B	Four	18	B	Nine
9	A	Five	19	D	Nine
10	A	Five	20	A	Nine

REFERENCES

Andreoli, T.E., Carpenter, C.C., Bennett, J.C., & Plum, F. (1997). *Cecil's essentials of medicine* (4th ed.). Philadelphia: W.B. Saunders.

Fleckman, A.M. (1993). Diabetic ketoacidosis. *Endocrinol Metab Clin North Am 22*(2):181–206.

Funnell, M.M., Hunt, C., Kulkarni, K., et al. (1998). *A core curriculum for diabetes education* (3rd ed.). Chicago: American Association of Diabetes Educators.

Guven, S., & Kuenzi, J. (1998). Diabetes mellitus. In C.M. Porth (ed.). *Pathophysiology: Concepts of altered health states* (5th ed.) (pp. 805–830). Philadelphia: J.B. Lippincott.

Guyton, A.C., & Hall, J.E. (1997). *Human physiology and mechanisms of disease* (6th ed.). Philadelphia: W.B. Saunders.

Halloran, T. (1998). Common endocrine disorders. In C.M. Hudak, B.M. Gallo, & P.G. Morton (eds.). *Critical care nursing: A holistic approach* (7th ed.) (pp. 829–849). Philadelphia: J.B. Lippincott.

Johnson, D. (1998). Endocrine disorders. In M.R. Kinney et al. (eds.). *AACN's clinical reference for critical-care nursing* (4th ed.) (pp. 849–872). St. Louis: C.V. Mosby.

Kee, J.L. (1999). *Laboratory and diagnostic tests with nursing implications* (5th ed.). Stamford, CT: Appleton & Lange.

Lewis, S.M., Heitkemper, M.M., & Dirksen, S.R. (2000). *Medical–surgical nursing: Assessment and management of clinical problems* (5th ed.). St. Louis: C.V. Mosby.

Ludwig-Beymer, P., Huether, S.E., & Zekauskus, S.B. (1996). Alterations of hormonal regulation. In S.E. Huether & K.L. McCance (eds.). *Understanding pathophysiology* (pp. 471 506). St. Louis: C.V. Mosby.

Siperstein, M.D. (1992). Diabetic ketoacidosis and hyperosmolar coma. *Endocrinol Metab Clin North Am 21*(2):415–432.

Module 26

Acute Renal Dysfunction

Kathleen Dorman Wagner

This self-study module focuses on the physiologic as well as pathophysiologic processes involved in acute renal failure. It is composed of eight sections. Sections One and Two discuss normal renal function. The module then shifts its focus to abnormal kidney function, specifically acute renal dysfunction. Sections Three and Four present causes, types, and stages of acute renal failure. Section Five presents assessment of renal dysfunction, including the nursing assessment, and laboratory tests and procedures used for diagnosing acute renal failure. Section Six describes the effects of acute renal failure on fluid and electrolyte balance. Section Seven gives an overview of collaborative and independent nursing management. Section Eight completes the module, with an overview of dialysis concepts. Each section includes a set of review questions to help the learner evaluate his or her understanding of the section's content before moving on to the next section. All Section Reviews and the module Pretest and Posttest include answers. It is suggested that the learner review those concepts answered incorrectly in the review questions before proceeding to the next section.

OBJECTIVES

Following completion of this module, the learner will be able to

1. Briefly explain normal kidney function.
2. Discuss the influences of selected body systems on renal function.
3. Identify the causes of acute renal failure as prerenal, intrarenal, or postrenal.
4. Describe the stages of acute renal failure.
5. Discuss assessment of renal dysfunction.
6. Describe the effects of acute renal dysfunction on fluid and electrolyte balance.
7. Provide a brief overview of the management of the patient with acute renal dysfunction.
8. Discuss dialysis as a treatment modality for acute renal failure.

PRETEST

1. The functional unit of the kidney is the
   A. nephron
   B. glomerulus
   C. renal tubule
   D. Bowman's capsule

2. Fluid and solutes are moved from the vascular system into the tubular system of the nephron by
   A. tubular reabsorption
   B. glomerular filtration
   C. vascular resistance
   D. tubular secretion

3. A receptor that increases the blood pressure by increasing production of antidiuretic hormone (ADH) is
   A. baroreceptor
   B. chemoreceptor
   C. osmoreceptor
   D. stretch receptor
4. Aldosterone's influence on the maintenance of body fluid levels is based on which of the following principles?
   A. sodium follows water
   B. potassium follows sodium
   C. water follows sodium
   D. sodium follows potassium
5. Approximately _____ percent of patients treated early in the course of acute renal failure have little to no residual loss of renal function.
   A. 10
   B. 25
   C. 50
   D. 75
6. Acute tubular necrosis (ATN) is caused primarily by which of the following two factors?
   A. myoglobin and nephrotoxic drugs
   B. hypoperfusion and myoglobin
   C. myoglobin and hemoglobin
   D. nephrotoxic drugs and hypoperfusion
7. Renal ischemia has which of the following effects on renal blood flow?
   A. vasospasm
   B. vasodilation
   C. vasoconstriction
   D. decreased vascular resistance
8. The early diuretic stage ends when the blood urea nitrogen (BUN) and creatinine
   A. cease increasing
   B. begin to drop
   C. slow their increase
   D. return to normal
9. Which of the following laboratory values can be used to differentiate acute tubular necrosis from prerenal hypoperfusion?
   A. BUN and chloride
   B. calcium and chloride
   C. sodium and potassium
   D. specific gravity and urine osmolality
10. Renal biopsy would most likely be used to further investigate
    A. prerenal failure
    B. intrarenal failure
    C. renal thrombosis
    D. renal calculi obstruction
11. Which of the following imbalances most commonly occur secondary to acute renal failure?
    A. hyperkalemia, hyperphosphatemia, metabolic acidosis
    B. hypokalemia, hyponatremia, hypercalcemia
    C. hyperkalemia, hypocalcemia, metabolic alkalosis
    D. hypernatremia, hypermagnesemia, hypercalcemia
12. Potassium imbalance secondary to acute renal dysfunction is associated with all of the following factors EXCEPT
    A. increased excretion
    B. metabolic acidosis
    C. decreased excretion
    D. increased tissue breakdown
13. Which of the following statements is true regarding the cardiovascular effects of acute renal failure?
    A. it causes hypotension
    B. it causes congestive heart failure
    C. it causes atherosclerosis
    D. it causes increased renal blood flow
14. Acute renal failure can precipitate gastrointestinal bleeding due to increased levels of
    A. uric acid
    B. creatinine
    C. urea
    D. ammonia
15. Common rapid access sites for short-term hemodialysis are
    A. subclavian and femoral veins
    B. femoral and brachial arteries
    C. radial and femoral arteries
    D. internal jugular and subclavian veins
16. Which of the following statements is correct regarding diffusion?
    A. it occurs up a concentration gradient
    B. it moves particles (solute) across a membrane
    C. it occurs down a concentration gradient
    D. it disperses solute within a solution with no membrane
17. Catabolic processes that are present in patients with acute renal failure make restriction of __________ necessary.
    A. carbohydrates
    B. fats
    C. protein
    D. essential amino acids
18. The major cause of death from acute renal failure is
    A. hyperkalemia
    B. metabolic acidosis
    C. fluid excess
    D. infection

Pretest answers: 1. A, 2. B, 3. A, 4. C, 5. C, 6. D, 7. C, 8. A, 9. D, 10. B, 11. A, 12. A, 13. B, 14. D, 15. A, 16. C, 17. C, 18. D

Glossary

Acid–base balance. A stable concentration of hydrogen ions in body fluids

Acidosis. An increased hydrogen ion concentration in the blood or a pH less than 7.35

Active transport. Movement of substances across a membrane without a pressure gradient, using energy

Acute renal failure. The rapid onset of impaired renal function associated with oliguria/anuria and azotemia

Acute tubular necrosis (ATN). A destructive process of the renal tubules

Aldosterone. A hormone produced by the adrenal cortex, responsible for excretion of potassium and absorption of sodium in the renal tubules, leading to reabsorption of water into the blood volume

Anions. Electrons with a negative charge

Antidiuretic hormone (ADH). A hormone produced by the hypothalamus and secreted by the posterior pituitary

Anuria. Cessation of urine production

Autoregulation. A compensatory mechanism that maintains renal blood flow even when there is a great variance in perfusion pressure

Azotemia. The accumulation of uremic toxins (urea, uric acid, and creatinine) in the blood

Bowman's capsule. The initial structure of the tubular system of the nephron

Cardiac output. The amount of blood the heart pumps in 1 minute

Cations. Electrons with a positive charge

Dialysis. A process of diffusion by which dissolved particles can be transported across a semipermeable membrane from one fluid compartment to another

Diuretic. Medication that reduces the reabsorption of sodium and water in the kidneys, resulting in an increase in urine excretion

Electrolytes. Elements or compounds that when dissolved in a fluid dissociate into ions and can carry an electrical current

Glomerular filtration. The process by which fluid and solutes are moved from the vascular system into the tubular system of the nephron

Glomerular filtration rate (GFR). Measurement of the plasma volume that can be cleared of any given substance within a certain time frame

Glomerulus. A cluster of capillaries located in the nephron; its primary function is to filter solutes

Homeostasis. The normal state of chemical balance within the body

Hyperkalemia. A greater than normal amount of potassium in the blood

Hypertension. Abnormally elevated blood pressure persistently exceeding 150/90 mm Hg

Hypervolemia. Increase in the amount of fluid in the circulating blood volume

Hypotension. Abnormally low blood pressure, inadequate for normal tissue perfusion and oxygenation

Intrarenal acute renal failure. Kidney dysfunction caused by direct damage to the renal parenchyma

Nephron. The functional unit of the kidney

Oliguria. Excretion or formation of an abnormally small amount of urine

Passive transport (diffusion). Movement of molecules from an area of high concentration to an area of lower concentration; does not require the expenditure of energy

Permeability. The capability of spreading or flowing through small holes or gaps

Postrenal acute renal failure. Kidney dysfunction caused by bilateral obstruction of urine flow distal to the kidney parenchyma

Prerenal acute renal failure. Kidney dysfunction caused by inadequate renal blood flow

Tubular secretion. The process by which substances are secreted into the tubules to be excreted in the final stage of urine formation

Uremia. Clinical symptoms of azotemia

Uremic syndrome. A general term used to describe the clinical manifestations associated with renal failure

Abbreviations

ADH. Antidiuretic hormone

ATN. Acute tubular necrosis

BUN. Blood urea nitrogen

CAVH. Continuous arteriovenous hemofiltration

CAVH-D. Continuous arteriovenous hemofiltration–dialysis

CRRT. Continuous renal replacement therapy

CVP. Central venous pressure

CVVH. Continuous venovenous hemofiltration

CVVH-D. Continuous venovenous hemofiltration–dialysis

GFR. Glomerular filtration rate

SECTION ONE: Normal Kidney Function

At the completion of this section, the learner will be able to explain briefly normal kidney function.

The Urinary System

The urinary system, with all of its structures intact, includes two kidneys, two ureters, a urinary bladder, and a urethra (Fig. 26–1). This system maintains **homeostasis** by removing waste products and by either conserving or excreting fluid and electrolytes. An individual requires only one functioning kidney to maintain normal regulatory mechanisms. The kidneys are the only means by which urine is transported and excreted.

The Kidney

A cross-section view of the kidney reveals the cortex, medulla, and pelvis (Fig. 26–2). The cortex and medulla are called the *renal parenchyma*. The medulla contains the renal pyramids, or collecting ducts. The cortex and medulla house all of the nephrons, which are composed primarily of tubular structures and blood vessels surrounding the nephrons. The nephrons produce urine, which then drains to the papilla, located at the base of the pyramid. The papilla acts as a collecting area, funneling urine to the renal pelvis, where it flows out of the kidney via the ureter. Renal blood supply to the kidney is from the renal artery, a direct branch of the abdominal aorta. The renal artery subdivides further, with some branches nourishing the kidney and others taking part in the filtration process. Almost all of the blood being filtered returns to the normal circulation via the renal vein.

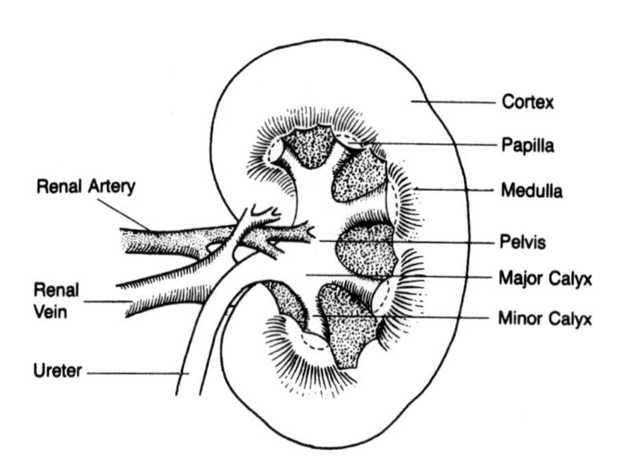

Figure 26–2. Gross anatomy of the kidney. *(From Ulrich, B.T. [1989]. Nephrology nursing: Concepts and strategies [p. 3]. Norwalk, CT: Appleton & Lange.)*

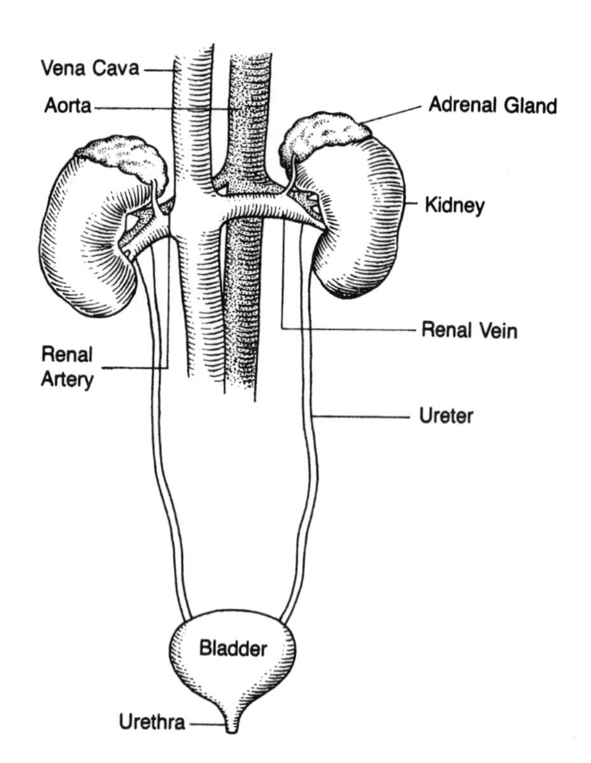

Figure 26–1. Gross anatomy of the renal system. *(From Ulrich, B.T. [1989]. Nephrology nursing: Concepts and strategies [p. 2]. Norwalk, CT: Appleton & Lange.)*

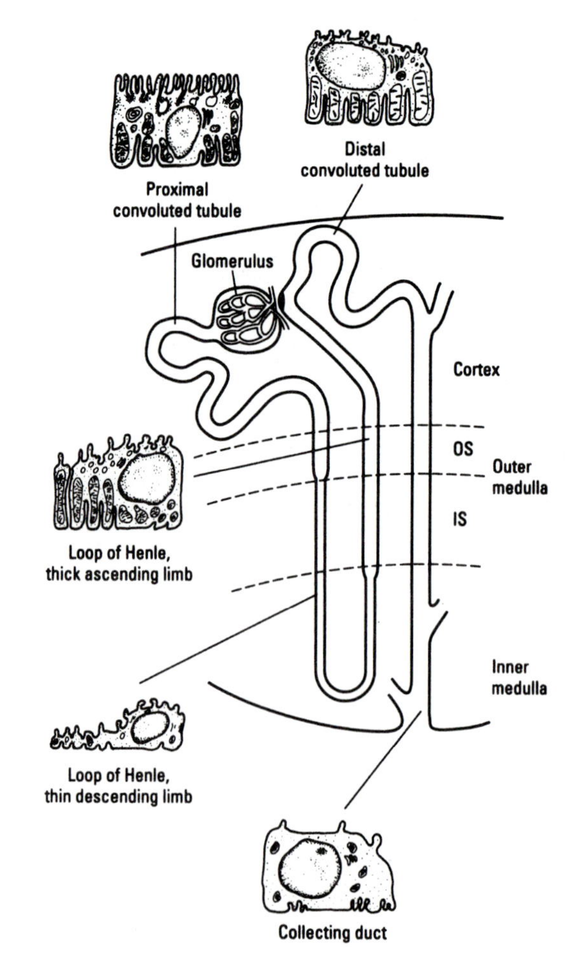

Figure 26–3. The nephron. *(From Ganong, W.F. [1985]. Review of medical physiology, 13th ed. [p. 581]. East Norwalk, CT: Appleton & Lange.)*

Nephron

The **nephron** is the functional unit of the kidney. Each nephron is composed of three major structures: a glomerulus, tubular apparatus, and collecting duct (Fig. 26–3). There are approximately 1.25 million nephrons in each kidney composed of vascular (blood flow) and tubular (urine flow) systems that promote the formation of urine. The vascular system of a nephron includes the glomerulus and vasa recta. The **glomerulus** is composed of a tight cluster of capillaries, and the afferent and efferent loops. The afferent loop becomes the glomerulus, and the efferent loop continues distal to the glomerulus to become the vasa recta, encircling the convoluted tubules and the loops of Henle.

Surrounding each glomerulus is a **Bowman's capsule,** the initial structure of the tubular system. Connected to the Bowman's capsule is the proximal convoluted tubule, which then becomes the loop of Henle. The loop of Henle is a hairpin-shaped section of the tubule. At the distal end of the loop of Henle is the distal convoluted tubule. This section is continuous with a system of collecting ducts that becomes progressively larger, eventually dumping urine into the renal pelvis.

The primary function of the nephron unit is to filter waste products from the blood as it flows through the kidneys. Approximately 1,200 mL of blood (around 21 percent of the resting cardiac output) passes through the kidneys every minute (Guyton & Hall, 1997). This large amount of blood is needed to produce the volume of filtrate necessary for glomerular filtration to occur. Urine formation is made possible by glomerular filtration and tubular reabsorption and secretion. Figure 26–4 shows nephron transport of substances, as well as their fate in the filtration process.

GLOMERULAR FILTRATION. **Glomerular filtration** is the process by which fluid and solutes are moved from the vascular system into the tubular system of the nephron, from an area of relatively high pressure to an area of low pressure. The glomerulus is a high-pressure, semipermeable capillary bed. For filtration to occur, there must be adequate blood volume in the intravascular space and adequate hydrostatic pressure from the cardiac output and vascular resistance. Glomerular filtrate is composed of:

- Water (H_2O), hydrogen ions (H^+)
- Electrolytes: sodium (Na^+), potassium (K^+), calcium (Ca^{++}), magnesium (Mg^{++}), chloride (Cl^-), bicarbonate (HCO_3^-), phosphate (PO_4^-).
- Waste products: urea, creatinine, uric acid
- Metabolic substrates: glucose and amino acids

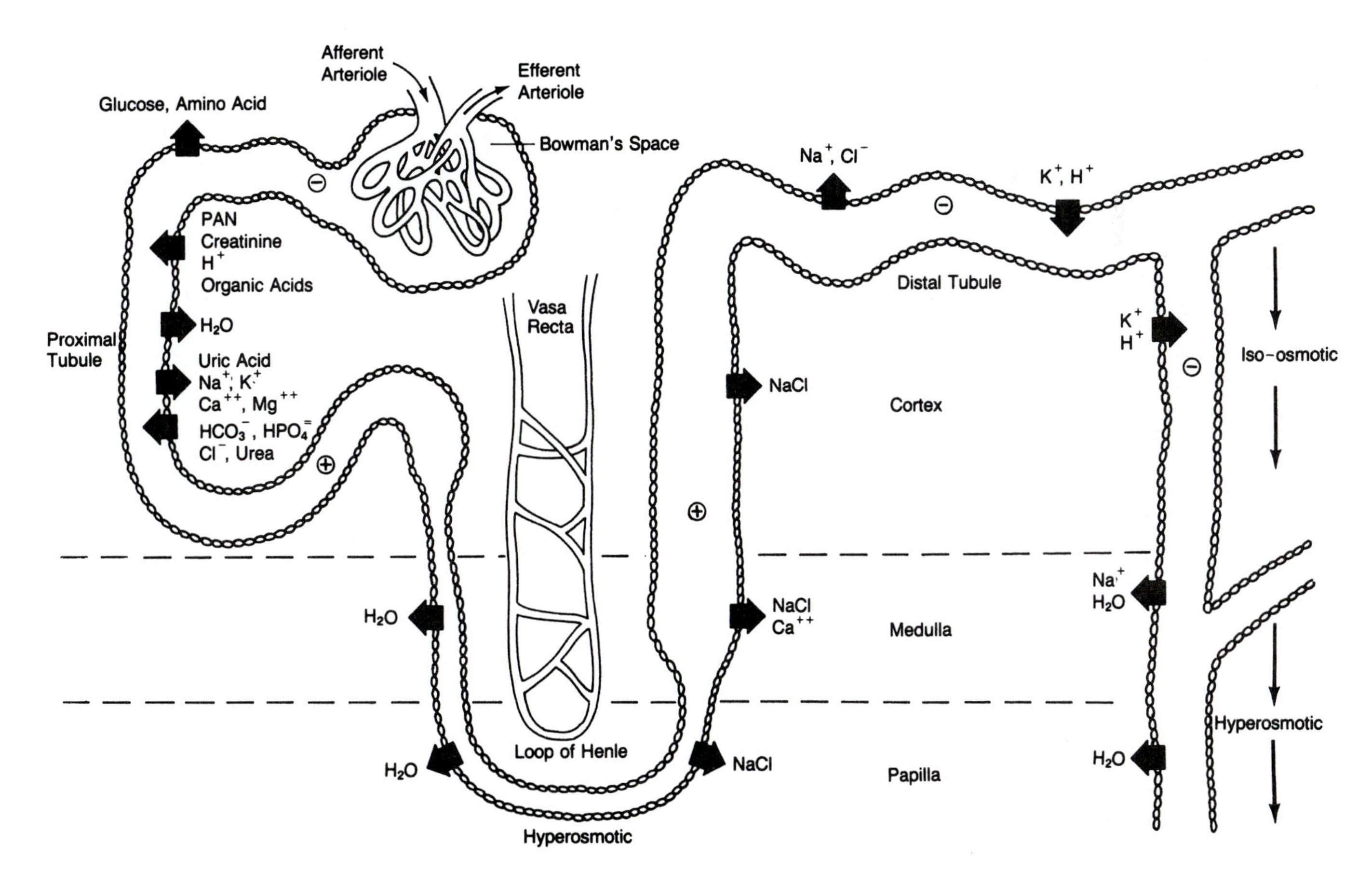

Figure 26–4. Nephron transport. *(From Ulrich, B.T. [1989].* Nephrology nursing: Concepts and strategies *[p. 15]. Norwalk, CT: Appleton & Lange.)*

The **glomerular filtration rate (GFR)** measures the plasma volume that can be cleared of any given substance within a certain time frame. In a person with normal renal function, the GFR is about 180 L/day. The GFR can be used as an indicator of the adequacy of renal function. The rate of glomerular filtration is altered by any disease condition that alters plasma flow through the glomeruli or the **permeability** of the cell membrane.

TUBULAR REABSORPTION. Not all filtrate is excreted. Some is reabsorbed and returned to the blood through tubular reabsorption. Tubular reabsorption is accomplished in the proximal convoluted tubules of the kidneys. Reabsorption occurs due to two transport systems:

1. **Active transport.** Movement of substances across a membrane without a pressure gradient, using the expenditure of energy. Potassium, sodium, calcium, phosphates, glucose, and amino acids all require active transport.
2. **Passive transport (diffusion).** Movement of molecules from an area of higher concentration to an area of lower concentration. Passive transport does not require an expenditure of energy. Water, chloride, urea, and some phosphate and bicarbonate are reabsorbed by passive transport.

TUBULAR SECRETION. Tubular secretion is the process by which substances, such as potassium, hydrogen, and antibiotics, are secreted into the tubules to be excreted in the final stage of urine formation. The final concentration or dilution of urine occurs in the distal tubules and collecting ducts that lead to the bladder. The volume of urine excreted is about 1,500 mL/day.

In summary, the kidneys are the primary organs responsible for excretion of body wastes and excess fluid, electrolytes, and metabolites. The nephron is the functioning unit of the kidneys and is composed of a glomerulus, Bowman's capsule, and tubular system. Glomerular filtration is the process by which fluid and substances are moved across the nephron vascular cell membrane into the tubular system for either reabsorption or eventual excretion. Glomerular filtration occurs by either an active or a passive transport system.

SECTION ONE REVIEW

1. The functional unit of the kidney is the
   A. nephron
   B. ureter
   C. medulla
   D. glomerulus
2. The term *renal parenchyma* refers to
   A. renal pelvis
   B. renal tubules
   C. renal cortex and medulla
   D. renal blood supply
3. Fluid and solutes are moved from the vascular system into the tubular system of the nephron by
   A. tubular reabsorption
   B. glomerular filtration
   C. vascular resistance
   D. tubular secretion
4. The movement of substances across a membrane without a pressure gradient using energy is called
   A. active transport
   B. tubular secretion
   C. passive transport
   D. tubular reabsorption
5. The urinary system controls the level of waste products by
   A. excreting hydrogen ions
   B. conserving body water
   C. conserving or excreting excess nutrients
   D. excreting or conserving fluid and electrolytes

Answers: 1. A, 2. C, 3. B, 4. A, 5. D

SECTION TWO: Influences of Body Systems on Renal Function

At the completion of this section, the learner will be able to discuss the influences of selected body systems on renal function.

Renal function depends on the interrelated functioning of the cardiovascular, nervous, and endocrine systems.

Cardiovascular System

The heart and blood vessels provide the kidneys with sufficient plasma to permit regulation of water and electrolytes in the body fluids. The cardiovascular system delivers blood to be filtered, sustains the blood pressure necessary for filtration to occur, and provides the nephron vascular system. The average GFR is about 180 L/day, which means that about 20 percent of the plasma is filtered as it flows through the kidney (Guyton & Hall, 1997).

Nervous System

The nervous system helps regulate blood pressure through the sympathetic nervous system. Several types of receptors located in large arteries of the neck and chest help maintain normal arterial blood pressure. Baroreceptors are sensitive to blood pressure changes, activating the hypothalamus when stimulated to alter antidiuretic hormone (ADH) production appropriately.

Chemoreceptors in the carotid and aortic bodies send messages to the vasomotor center to increase blood flow when hydrogen and carbon dioxide content is high and oxygen levels are low. In addition, hypothalamic osmoreceptors are sensitive to changes in water osmolality. As water osmolality changes, the osmoreceptors communicate these changes to the hypothalamus, which results in altered ADH production.

The nervous system influences fluid balance by regulating the thirst mechanism. The thirst center is located in the brain's hypothalamus and is highly sensitive to fluid osmolality. In circumstances such as cellular dehydration, the hypothalamus sends impulses to stimulate thirst. Conversely, the drive to drink is diminished when overhydration is present.

Endocrine System

The endocrine system affects renal function directly through secretion of two hormones, ADH and aldosterone. **Antidiuretic hormone (ADH)** is produced by the hypothalamus and secreted by the posterior pituitary. It is responsible for the ability of water to follow sodium as it is excreted or reabsorbed. ADH secretion is stimulated by baroreceptors, which are sensitive to changes in arterial blood pressure, and by osmoreceptors, which are sensitive to changes in serum osmolarity. It increased the permeability of the nephron cell membranes to water, allowing more water to be reabsorbed. Urinary output declines in response to the action of ADH.

Aldosterone, produced by the adrenal cortex, is influenced by serum levels of sodium and potassium. Aldosterone causes the kidney tubules to excrete potassium and absorb sodium, leading to a reabsorption of water into the blood volume. Fluid deficit stimulates production of this hormone. Angiotensin is a major controller of aldosterone secretion and thus is crucial in control of sodium levels. It also is an important part of the renin–angiotensin system, which strongly influences arterial blood pressure, as well as water and sodium regulation.

Compensatory Mechanisms

Compensatory mechanisms for maintaining renal perfusion and prevention of ischemic damage are the renin–angiotensin mechanism and autoregulation.

RENIN–ANGIOTENSIN SYSTEM. The renin–angiotensin system is important in control of blood pressure. Renin is an enzyme secreted by the juxtaglomerular apparatus of the kidneys. It is theorized that a decreased blood pressure **(hypotension),** low intratubular sodium, or possibly catecholamines may stimulate renin production. Once produced, renin combines with angiotensin I. Angiotensin I, which originates in the liver, is converted to angiotensin II in the lungs. Angiotensin II causes peripheral vasoconstriction and stimulates aldosterone release. Aldosterone stimulates the expansion of the circulatory volume through the reabsorption of sodium and water in the distal tubules. Figure 26–5 shows the sequence of events involved in the renin–angiotensin system.

AUTOREGULATION. Autoregulation maintains a constant renal blood flow by regulating resistance of flow of blood even when there are great variances in perfusion pressure. Through autoregulatory feedback mechanisms, the GFR and renal blood flow remain normal as long as the perfusion pressure remains between 75 mm Hg and 160 mm Hg, a wide variance (Guyton & Hall, 1997).

Even with compensatory mechanisms, the GFR is decreased when blood flow in the glomerulus diminishes, passing less water into the filtrate. Thus, with less water being filtered and sodium and water being conserved through compensatory measures, an increase in overall body fluid and hypervolemia can occur.

In summary, renal function is dependent on multiple body systems. The cardiovascular system provides blood to the kidneys for filtering and sufficient blood pressure for perfusion. The nervous system provides special receptors to help control blood pressure and fluid balance. Receptors stimulate the hypothalamus to alter production of ADH to either stimulate or inhibit production. The hypothalamus is also responsible for regulation of thirst in response to the level of hydration. The endocrine system in conjunction with the nervous system is responsible for secretion of ADH and aldosterone. ADH alters water reabsorption, and aldosterone alters sodium and potassium serum levels, influencing water balance and arterial blood pressure.

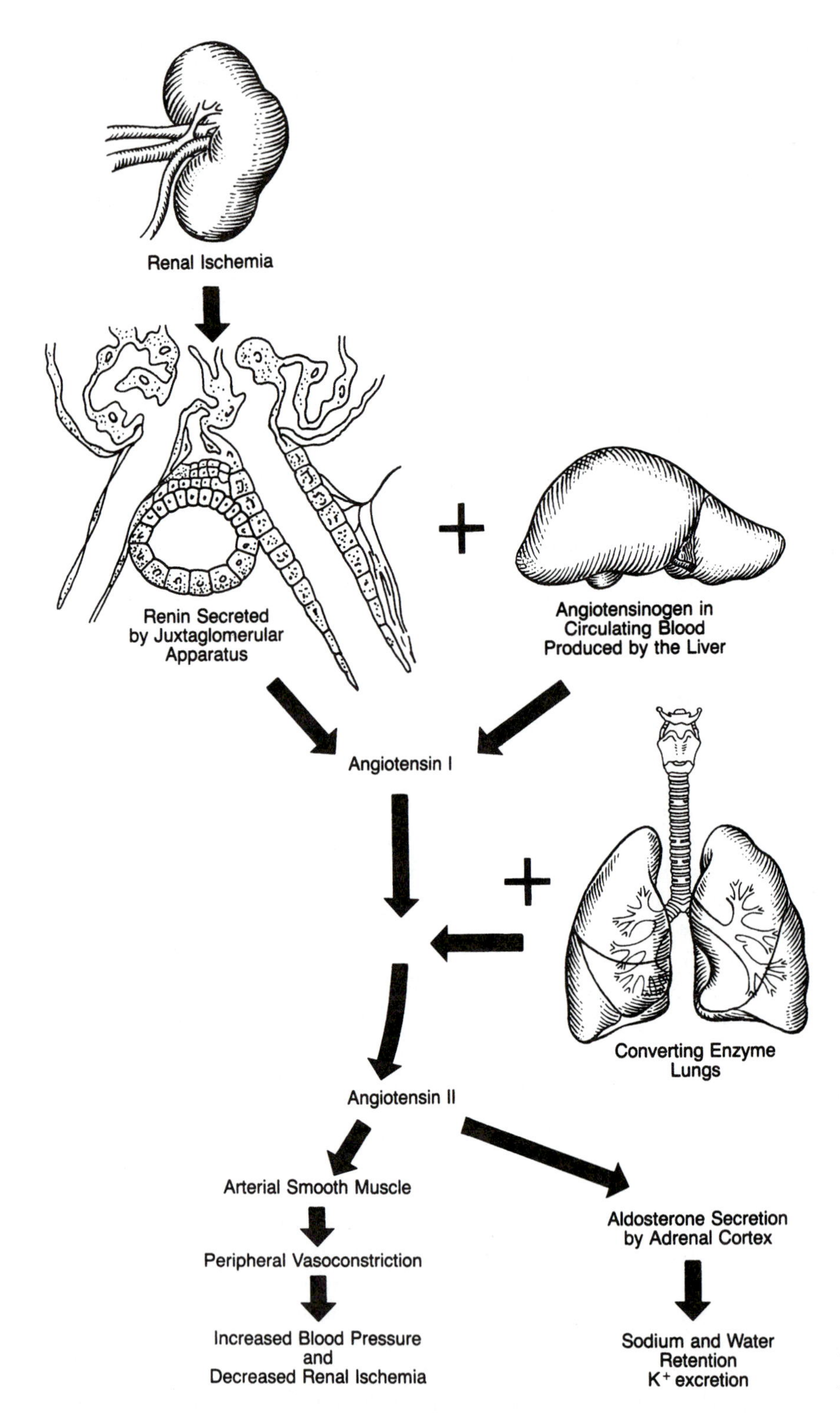

Figure 26–5. The renin–angiotensin system. *(From Ulrich, B.T. [1989].* Nephrology nursing: Concepts and strategies *[p. 22]. Norwalk, CT: Appleton & Lange.)*

SECTION TWO REVIEW

1. About _____ percent of the cardiac output comprises the total renal blood flow.
   A. 10
   B. 20
   C. 30
   D. 40
2. A receptor that increases the blood pressure by increasing production of ADH is

A. baroreceptor
B. chemoreceptor
C. osmoreceptor
D. ADH receptor

3. Aldosterone's influence on the maintenance of body fluid levels is based on which of the following principles?
   A. sodium follows water
   B. potassium follows sodium
   C. water follows sodium
   D. sodium follows potassium
4. The renin–angiotensin system is important in control of
   A. autoregulation
   B. blood pressure
   C. potassium excretion
   D. ADH production

Answers: 1. B, 2. A, 3. C, 4. B

SECTION THREE: Causes of Acute Renal Failure

At the completion of this section, the learner will be able to identify the causes of acute renal failure as prerenal, intrarenal, or postrenal.

Acute renal failure is the rapid onset of impaired renal function associated with **oliguria/anuria** and **azotemia** (the accumulation of uremic toxins). It is associated with loss of renal ability to excrete waste products and loss of the ability to regulate fluid, **electrolytes,** and **acid–base balance.** Acute renal failure may occur suddenly, within hours, or over a period of days. It is often reversible if diagnosed and treated early. Acute renal failure develops in 10 to 20 percent of patients in critical care units (Price, 1994). If left unrecognized or if inadequately treated, acute renal failure can progress, causing permanent damage of the renal parenchyma.

Acute renal failure is categorized based on the location of the insult, being designated as prerenal, intrarenal, or postrenal.

Prerenal Acute Renal Failure

Prerenal acute renal failure stems from problems that interfere with renal perfusion, causing renal hypoperfusion. Underlying conditions that can precipitate prerenal failure include decreased cardiac output and vascular obstruction.

Decreased Cardiac Output

Any problem that significantly diminishes **cardiac output** can cause prerenal failure (e.g., congestive heart failure, burns, sepsis, myocardial infarction, shock, and hemorrhage). When cardiac output drops, one of the first compensatory mechanisms to increase it is vasoconstriction of the kidney capillary beds, to provide more blood to the more critical core organs. Although this serves the immediate needs of the heart and brain, if it is prolonged, renal tissue ischemia results.

Vascular Obstruction

Whereas decreased cardiac output is a systemic cause of acute renal failure, vascular obstruction is a localized cause. When the vessels serving the kidneys suddenly lose their patency, perfusion distal to the obstruction becomes compromised and can precipitate acute renal failure. Examples of obstructions include tumor, embolus, or dissecting aortic aneurysm.

Intrarenal Acute Renal Failure

Intrarenal acute renal failure is caused by problems involving the renal parenchyma (renal tissue). The most common type of intrarenal failure is acute tubular necrosis, which accounts for about 75 percent of cases of acute renal failure.

Other causes of intrarenal failure include renal vascular disease (e.g., renal artery stenosis, diabetic sclerosis, renal vein thrombosis), glomerulonephritis, and interstitial nephritis (e.g., pyelonephritis, hypercalcemia).

Acute Tubular Necrosis

Acute tubular necrosis (ATN) refers to necrosis (death) of renal tubule tissue. It is caused by renal tissue ischemia caused by inadequate treatment of prerenal failure or by nephrotoxic agents. Because ATN is associated with tissue destruction, the incidence of permanent renal damage is high. According to Parker (1998), tissue ischemia occurs when the mean arterial blood pressure falls below 50 mm Hg to 70 mm Hg for > 25 minutes. Damage may be mild and reversible if the duration of the ischemia is < 25 minutes. Prolonged ischemia (> 60 to 90 minutes) usually causes severe, permanent renal damage.

Andreoli et al. (1997) explains that nephrotoxicity can develop from exogenous or endogenous agents. Common exogenous agents include radiographic contrast agents, aminoglycosides, nonsteroidal anti-inflammatory drugs (NSAIDs), and others. Risk for nephrotoxicity caused by many of these agents can be reduced by keeping the patient well hydrated and maintaining an adequate hemodynamic status. Two major problems associated with endogenous nephrotoxicity include rhabdomyolysis and hepatorenal syndrome. Rhabdomyolysis is a disorder that is characterized by excessive skeletal muscle breakdown, which causes release of muscle cell contents (such as myoglobin) in large quantities (Hansen, 1998). It is commonly caused by alcohol abuse, compression of muscle, multiple injuries or burns, and seizure activity.

Postrenal Acute Renal Failure

Postrenal acute renal failure refers to renal dysfunction caused by an obstruction to the outflow of urine from the kidneys. To precipitate renal failure, the obstruction must block urine outflow bilaterally, or unilaterally when there is only one functioning kidney. Renal failure is caused by a buildup of pressure caused by the increasing volume of urine proximal to the obstruction. Postrenal failure can be caused by obstruction of the bladder, ureters, or urethra, which may be of mechanical or functional origin. Mechanical causes include blood clots, calculi, tumors, prostatic hypertrophy, and urethral strictures. Functional causes include diabetic neuropathy, neurogenic bladder, and certain drugs (e.g., ganglionic blockers).

In summary, there are three causes of acute renal failure: prerenal, which stems from decreased renal perfusion; intrarenal (usually ATN), caused by problems involving the renal tissue; and postrenal, which results from obstruction of urine flow. Should acute renal failure be left unrecognized or inadequately treated, increased kidney tissue damage will result and lead to permanent damage, regardless of the cause.

SECTION THREE REVIEW

1. Congestive heart failure, hemorrhage, and shock are examples of possible etiologic factors for development of which type(s) of renal failure?
   A. prerenal
   B. intrarenal
   C. postrenal
   D. prerenal and postrenal
2. Approximately _____ percent of patients treated early in the course of acute renal failure have little to no residual loss of renal function.
   A. 10
   B. 25
   C. 50
   D. 75
3. ATN is caused primarily by which of the following two factors?
   A. myoglobin and nephrotoxic agents
   B. hypoperfusion and myoglobin
   C. myoglobin and hemoglobin
   D. nephrotoxic agents and hypoperfusion
4. Renal tissue ischemia occurs when the mean arterial blood pressure drops to below _____ mm Hg.
   A. 5 to 60
   B. 6 to 70
   C. 7 to 80
   D. 8 to 90
5. Drugs that are considered highly nephrotoxic include all of the following EXCEPT
   A. cephalosporins
   B. aminoglycosides
   C. cardiac glycosides
   D. NSAIDs

Answers: 1. A, 2. C, 3. D, 4. B, 5. C

SECTION FOUR: The Stages of Acute Renal Failure

At the completion of this section, the learner will be able to explain the stages of acute renal failure.

Changes in renal function can be considered on a continuum that ranges from mild renal impairment to complete renal failure. Renal impairment begins when the kidneys are not able to meet the demands of dietary or metabolic stress. Renal impairment may not be discovered until as much as 80 percent of the nephrons have lost normal functioning. Hypertrophy and hyperplasia of the remaining nephrons permit an increase in their workload and in their ability to maintain function. The progressive course of acute renal failure can be divided into four stages: onset, oliguric/anuric, diuretic (early and late), and convalescent.

Onset Stage

The onset stage begins at the time of injury. During this stage, the patient is acutely ill due to the underlying disorder, as well as the rapid onset of acute renal failure. There is a noticeable drop in urine output to approximately 20 percent of normal. The onset stage lasts about 2 days and ends either when the oliguric/anuric stage begins or when azotemia develops in the absence of an oliguric/anuric stage.

Oliguric/Anuric Stage

The oliguric/anuric stage begins when the patient's urine output falls to less than 400 mL/24 hr, which usually occurs by about 48 hours postinjury. It lasts 1 to 2 weeks, until the early diuresis stage begins. The term anuria is used when the urine output falls to less than 50 mL/24 hr. The longer the patient remains in the oliguric/anuric stage, the higher the risk of irreversible renal damage and chronic renal failure.

During this stage, the GFR significantly decreases and metabolites (e.g., creatinine, urea, and potassium) rapidly accumulate since they are normally excreted through the kidneys. Fluid excess develops in the extracellular and intracellular compartments, which can result in edema, congestive heart failure, and water intoxication (Gallagher-Lepak, 1998). Not all patients with acute renal failure go through the oliguric/anuric stage. This is at least partially due to significant improvements in the treatment regimen for improving heart performance and circulatory failure (Gallagher-Lepak, 1998).

Diuretic Stage

The diuretic stage is divided into two divisions based on time: the early diuretic stage and the late (recovery) diuretic stage.

Early Diuretic Stage

The onset of the early diuretic stage begins when the patient's urine output increases to over 400 mL/24 hr. It continues until the BUN and creatinine stabilize (stop increasing), and it lasts approximately 1 to 2 weeks. During the early diuretic stage, the renal tubules are beginning to heal, regaining their integrity. As this stage progresses, the urine output may be 1 to 2 L/24 hr due to the inability of the kidneys to concentrate urine and the diuretic effect of an elevated BUN. Fluid and electrolyte levels become difficult to manage.

Late (Recovery) Diuretic Stage

The late diuretic stage begins when the patient's BUN and creatinine begin to decrease. It continues until the BUN and creatinine levels return to normal, which takes approximately 10 days. During the late stage, renal function continues to improve as the nephrons heal. A high urine output continues, which requires careful monitoring and control of fluid and electrolyte balance.

Convalescent Stage

The convalescent stage begins when the patient's laboratory values have returned to normal. It ends with the return of normal renal function, lasting 6 months to a year. During this stage, the patient's urine output returns to normal with return of the patient's ability to concentrate urine. The kidneys are extremely vulnerable during this stage; thus, it is important to avoid use of nephrotoxic agents. The patient requires close monitoring and management of fluid and electrolyte levels and evaluation of the degree of permanent renal damage.

In summary, there are four stages of acute renal failure, including onset, oliguric/anuric, diuretic (early and late), and convalescent. These stages occur in the same progressive order, though some patients do not experience a distinct oliguric/anuric stage. Fluids and electrolytes must be monitored carefully and controlled during each stage. Early diagnosis and treatment are crucial to prevent or minimize permanent renal damage.

Section Four Review

1. As many as _____ percent of the nephrons may be lost before significant renal dysfunction is noted.
   A. 40
   B. 60
   C. 80
   D. 100
2. The oliguric/anuric stage of acute renal failure begins when urine output falls to below _____ mL/24 hr.
   A. 50
   B. 100
   C. 200
   D. 400
3. Renal ischemia has which of the following effects on renal blood flow?
   A. vasospasm
   B. vasodilation
   C. vasoconstriction
   D. decreased vascular resistance
4. The early diuretic stage ends when the BUN and creatinine
   A. cease increasing
   B. begin to drop
   C. slow their increase
   D. return to normal
5. During the diuretic stage, urine output remains high due to
   A. lack of secretion of antidiuretic hormone
   B. loss of ability to concentrate urine
   C. lack of secretion of aldosterone
   D. loss of ability to reabsorb sodium

Answers: 1. C, 2. D, 3. C, 4. A, 5. B

SECTION FIVE: Assessment of Acute Renal Dysfunction

At the completion of this section, the learner will be able to discuss assessment of renal dysfunction.

The Focused Renal Dysfunction Assessment

In the acutely ill patient, renal dysfunction often has an insidious onset. It may be suspected first when urine output stays below normal despite attempts to increase it. It also may be detected first when electrolyte or BUN values develop abnormal trends.

Nursing History

Important recent history data to be aware of include:

- Recent use of nephrotoxic substances (e.g., nephrotoxic antibiotics, particularly aminoglycosides)
- Recent exposure to heavy metals or organic solvents
- Recent hypotensive episode of > 30 minutes
- Presence of tumor or multiple clots that might cause renovascular or urine outflow obstruction bilaterally

Physical Assessment

Acute renal failure affects multiple body functions and systems. The collective term used to describe the clinical manifestations of renal failure is **uremia.** The following sections provide a brief description of the effects of renal failure on body systems and related clinical manifestations.

Neurologic Effects

Accumulation of nitrogenous waste products from impaired renal excretion and metabolic acidosis contributes to a decrease in mental functioning. As uremic toxins build up in the brain tissue, uremic encephalopathy develops. Peripherally, accumulation of uremic toxins can slow peripheral nerve conduction, which causes peripheral neuropathy. In addition, fluid volume excess, caused by renal failure, can precipitate cerebral edema, which may increase intracranial pressure and alter level of consciousness.

NEUROLOGIC CLINICAL MANIFESTATIONS

- Decreased alertness, energy, and thought processing
- Decreased level of consciousness that progresses from drowsiness to coma
- Seizures
- Itching, tingling, numbness, twitching of extremities

Cardiovascular and Pulmonary Effects

Hypertension is a common manifestation of acute renal failure. It is caused by (1) systemic and central fluid volume excess and (2) increased renin production. When renal ischemia is present, the renin–angiotensin system is triggered, which results in increased blood pressure and increased renal blood flow (see Section Two). Fluid volume excess and electrolyte imbalances are the basis of most cardiovascular symptoms. The presence of fluid volume excess may cause congestive heart failure accompanied by peripheral and pulmonary edema. Electrolyte imbalances can precipitate cardiac arrhythmias. The inability of the kidneys to excrete hydrogen ions and electrolytes adequately causes them to accumulate in the body.

The patient with acute renal failure needs to be monitored closely for the signs and symptoms of pneumonia. He or she is at high risk for developing this complication owing to decreased level of consciousness, weakness, thick secretions, decreased cough reflex, and decreased pulmonary macrophage activity.

CARDIOVASCULAR AND PULMONARY CLINICAL MANIFESTATIONS

- **Cardiovascular**
  Hypertension
  Cardiac arrhythmias
  Peripheral edema
  Signs and symptoms of congestive heart failure
- **Pulmonary**
  Adventitious breath sounds
  Decreased cough reflex
  Thick secretions
  Kussmaul-type breathing pattern
  Infiltrates on x-ray
  Signs and symptoms of pneumonia

Gastrointestinal Effects

Electrolyte imbalances and increasing levels of uremic toxins are the primary contributors to gastrointestinal (GI) manifestations. As urea decomposes in the GI tract, it releases ammonia. Ammonia in the GI tract is associated with capillary fragility and GI mucosal irritation. As the ammonia levels increase, small mucosal ulcerations may develop, causing GI bleeding. Acute renal failure alters GI motility largely due to electrolyte imbalances. The patient may develop constipation or diarrhea, depending on the GI motility status.

GASTROINTESTINAL CLINICAL MANIFESTATIONS

- Weight loss
- Positive guaiac stools
- Anorexia
- Nausea and vomiting
- Constipation or diarrhea

Hematopoietic Effects

The kidneys produce erythropoietin, which is necessary for normal red blood cell (RBC) production. When kidney function fails, red blood cell production becomes compromised and the life span of existing RBCs may decrease. Platelet function is also impaired by the presence of uremic toxins, which increases the risk of bleeding problems. The combination of hematopoietic factors, GI irritation, and blood loss from hemodialysis all contribute to development of anemia.

Hematopoietic Clinical Manifestations

- Anemia
- Pale mucous membranes
- Fatigue, weakness

Integumentary Effects

Because the uremic toxins cannot be excreted via the kidneys, they may accumulate on the skin surface causing pruritus and dry skin. The patient's skin appears pale and may develop a yellow cast. The yellow skin coloring is different from the jaundice associated with liver disease. The color is duller and does not affect the sclera of the eyes. Bruising is frequently noted due to dysfunctional platelets. The development of uremic frost, a late-stage phenomenon of renal failure, has become less common in the acute care setting because of earlier, more effective management. The term *uremic frost* refers to a fine, white layer of urate crystals that develops on the skin. In addition, protein wasting may cause thin hair and brittle, thin nails.

Integumentary Clinical Manifestations

- Pale, dry, dull, yellow skin
- Bruising
- Pruritus
- Thin hair and brittle, thin nails

Skeletal Effects

Under normal circumstances, about seven-eighths of ingested calcium is excreted in the feces without being absorbed. The remaining eighth is absorbed by the intestines and is eventually excreted by the kidneys (Guyton & Hall, 1997). Because of the limited ability of the kidneys to metabolize vitamin D in acute renal failure, absorption of calcium in the intestines is further impaired. In long-term renal failure, skeletal disorders occur related to decreased calcium absorption.

Laboratory Tests

BUN and Creatinine

The diagnosis and management of renal failure are largely dependent on laboratory tests, measuring uremic toxins and renal excretion. BUN and creatinine are the two most important laboratory measurements of renal status. BUN is the end product of protein metabolism. Creatinine is the end product of muscle metabolism. Under normal circumstances, BUN and creatinine maintain a 20:1 ratio to each other. When the kidneys go into failure, the nephrons are unable to cleanse the waste products (e.g., BUN and creatinine) from the blood. This results in increasing levels of serum BUN and creatinine. Creatinine is a more stable indicator of kidney function than BUN because protein metabolism is less stable than muscle metabolism. Table 26–1 summarizes major laboratory values measuring kidney function. Note that serum and urine values have an inverse relationship.

Glomerular Filtration Rate

The onset of symptoms brought about by a decrease in the GFR varies with differences in etiology, course of the disease, and secondary contributing factors. When the GFR falls to 5 to 10 percent of normal and continues to decline, the catchall term **uremic syndrome** can be used to symptomatically describe the clinical manifestations.

Osmolality

The relationship of urine and blood osmolality is monitored as an indicator of adequate renal function. When renal function is normal, the urine and blood (plasma) osmolality maintain a direct relationship (i.e., as one rises, the other also will increase). If renal perfusion becomes diminished, the urine osmolality becomes more elevated than the blood osmolality, and urine specific gravity increases. If there is damage to the renal tubules (e.g., ATN), the urine osmolality will be ≤ 50 mOsm/kg of the blood osmolality. This symptom is accompanied by a low specific gravity due to the lost ability to concentrate urine secondary to nephron damage.

Assessment of Electrolyte Imbalances

Electrolyte imbalances are the result of some type of body system dysfunction or lack of proper nutrition. Electrolyte imbalances cause a wide range of functional problems,

TABLE 26–1. MAJOR LABORATORY VALUES MEASURING KIDNEY FUNCTION

LABORATORY TEST	NORMAL VALUES	ABNORMAL TREND
Serum		
Blood urea nitrogen	5–25 mg/dL	Increased
Creatinine	0.5–1.5 mg/dL	Increased
Uric acid		
Male	3.5–8.0 mg/dL	Increased
Female	2.8–6.8 mg/dL	Increased
Potassium	3.5–5.3 mEq/L	Increased
Calcium	9–11 mg/dL	Decreased
Chloride	95–105 mEq/L	Increased
Phosphorus	2.5–4.5 mg/dL	Increased
Albumin	3.5–5.0 g/dL	Decreased
Urine		
Protein	0–5 mg/dL/24 hr	Increased
Creatinine clearance	85–135 mL/min	Decreased
Urea clearance	64–100 mL/min	Decreased

Normal serum values are from Kee, J.L. (1999). Laboratory and diagnostic tests with nursing implications *(5th ed.). Stamford, CT: Appleton & Lange.*

particularly in the neurologic, musculoskeletal, cardiovascular, and gastrointestinal systems. The signs and symptoms of imbalances often reflect either hyperactive or hypoactive system function, depending on the nature of the imbalance.

Special Procedures

Occasionally, the acutely ill patient requires radiographic testing or invasive procedures to help verify the exact etiology of acute renal failure. The following is a brief description of some of the more common tests performed to help make a differential diagnosis.

Renal Biopsy

Renal biopsy is an invasive procedure performed by needle aspiration of renal tissue. Once obtained, the tissue is examined microscopically. Renal biopsy may be used when the exact nature of intrarenal acute renal failure is unknown.

Intravenous Pyelogram

Intravenous pyelogram (IVP) uses a flat plate film of the abdomen before and after injection of a contrast medium into the kidneys via the bloodstream. The IVP is able to outline the kidneys, showing size, shape, and the ability to concentrate and excrete the dye.

Renal Ultrasound

Renal ultrasound uses high frequency sound waves directed at the kidneys to measure various densities. Ultrasound can distinguish tumors, fluid masses, and obstruction. Major advantages of renal ultrasound are that it is noninvasive, and it can be performed at the bedside with minimal discomfort to the acutely ill patient.

Computed Tomographic Scan

The computed tomographic (CT) scan uses a three-dimensional concept of radiography by taking x-ray slices of an organ. The CT scan provides information regarding the size and shape of the kidneys and the presence of lesions, cysts, calculi, and congenital anomalies. Masses are detected more easily with this method.

Renal Arteriogram

The renal arteriogram requires injection of a contrast dye into the renal artery via the femoral artery. The arteriogram visualizes blood flow through the renal vessels. Prerenal obstruction can be diagnosed using this method.

In summary, early diagnosis of acute renal failure generally is made based on urine and blood chemistry alterations. Certain tests help differentiate the exact nature of the acute renal failure. The acutely ill patient may require a combination of blood, urine, radiographic, or other tests to help differentiate the etiology.

SECTION FIVE REVIEW

1. When a patient experiences diminished renal perfusion, how will the urine/plasma osmolality relationship change?
   - **A.** plasma osmolality decreases more than urine osmolality
   - **B.** urine osmolality decreases more than plasma osmolality
   - **C.** plasma osmolality increases more than urine osmolality
   - **D.** urine osmolality increases more than plasma osmolality
2. Which of the following laboratory values can be used to differentiate acute tubular necrosis from prerenal hypoperfusion?
   - **A.** BUN and chloride
   - **B.** calcium and chloride
   - **C.** sodium and potassium
   - **D.** specific gravity and osmolality
3. Renal biopsy would most likely be used to further investigate which of the following?
   - **A.** prerenal failure
   - **B.** intrarenal failure
   - **C.** renal thrombosis
   - **D.** renal calculi obstruction
4. Which of the following tests would most likely be performed to diagnose a prerenal vascular obstruction?
   - **A.** CT scan
   - **B.** IVP
   - **C.** renal biopsy
   - **D.** renal arteriogram
5. A renal diagnostic procedure requiring contrast dye is
   - **A.** arteriogram
   - **B.** biopsy
   - **C.** ultrasound
   - **D.** CT scan
6. Alterations in mental function secondary to acute renal failure are caused primarily by
   - **A.** uremic toxins
   - **B.** magnesium imbalance
   - **C.** hypoglycemia
   - **D.** fluid overload

7. Peripheral neuropathy can manifest itself in all of the following ways EXCEPT
   A. tingling
   B. numbness
   C. itching
   D. seizures
8. Which of the following statements is true regarding the cardiovascular effects of acute renal failure?
   A. it causes hypotension
   B. it causes congestive heart failure
   C. it causes atherosclerosis
   D. it causes increased renal blood flow
9. Acute renal failure can precipitate gastrointestinal bleeding due to increased levels of
   A. uric acid
   B. creatinine
   C. urea
   D. ammonia
10. Which of the following statements best reflects the effects of acute renal failure on the integumentary system?
   A. thickened hair follicles
   B. excessively oily skin
   C. excessive bruising
   D. thickened nailbeds

Answers: 1. D, 2. D, 3. B, 4. D, 5. A, 6. A, 7. D, 8. B, 9. D, 10. C

SECTION SIX: The Effect of Acute Renal Dysfunction on Fluid and Electrolyte Balance

At the completion of this section, the learner will be able to describe the effects of acute renal failure on fluid and electrolyte balance.

When a patient develops acute renal failure, the kidneys are no longer able to function normally, ceasing to regulate reabsorption and excretion of fluids and electrolytes. The body's fluids (primarily composed of water and electrolytes) are found in essentially every organ system. Therefore, because acute renal failure profoundly alters fluid and electrolyte balance, it also has negative influences on all body systems.

Fluid Balance

The importance of fluid regulation is apparent, considering that 60 percent to 70 percent of the body's composition consists of water. Body water is divided into two compartments, intracellular (fluid within the cells) and extracellular (fluid outside the cells). Extracellular fluid can be further subclassified into intravascular fluid within the blood vessels (plasma) and interstitial water in the tissue spaces.

Failure of the kidneys to excrete water unbalances the normal homeostasis of the body, causing serious consequences. Fluid imbalance triggers one of two problems: hypervolemia, an increase in circulatory and body water, or hypovolemia, an inadequate amount of circulating fluid volume. Acute renal failure (during the oliguric/anuric stage) is associated with development of an accumulation of fluids **(hypervolemia)** produced by failure of the kidneys to perfuse and filter fluids properly. Hypervolemia is associated with many complications, including congestive heart failure, pulmonary edema, and hypertension.

Electrolyte Balance

In addition to the regulatory mechanisms of the endocrine system, the kidneys control the balance of electrolytes within the body fluid. These electrolytes help maintain fluid osmolality. The major **cations** regulated by the kidneys are potassium, sodium, calcium, and magnesium. Major **anions** under renal regulation include chloride and bicarbonate.

Electrolyte imbalance caused by acute renal failure is associated with the following major conditions: hyperkalemia, hypernatremia, hyponatremia, hypocalcemia, hypermagnesemia, and metabolic acidosis.

Potassium Imbalance

Acute renal failure is associated most commonly with hyperkalemia. **Hyperkalemia** is caused by decreased excretion of potassium by the kidneys and increased cellular release of potassium through tissue breakdown and acidosis. Hyperkalemic changes manifest most frequently in cardiac and neuromuscular changes. Occasionally, hypokalemia is associated with acute renal failure as a possible causative factor. Hypokalemia can alter the interstitium of the renal medulla, impairing renal function and precipitating acute renal failure.

Sodium Imbalance

Acute renal failure generally causes increased serum sodium; however, this is not always true. Hypernatremia occurs when the GFR is decreased and sodium is unable to be excreted in sufficient amounts. Because sodium conservation occurs mainly in the renal medulla, any deterioration of this area of the kidney may cause excessive sodium loss (hyponatremia). For these reasons, sodium levels are variable in acute renal failure.

Calcium and Phosphate Imbalances

Calcium follows a similar reabsorption pathway as sodium. Serum calcium is reduced in acute renal failure due to decreased absorption from the gastrointestinal tract caused by an inability of the kidneys to produce the active component of vitamin D, 1,25–dihydroxycholecalciferol. Lack of active vitamin D results in diminished use of calcium, causing hypocalcemia. Calcium maintains an inverse relationship with phosphate (PO_4^{2-}). Therefore, as calcium levels decrease, phosphate levels increase, causing hyperphosphatemia.

Magnesium Imbalance

Acute renal failure is a major cause of hypermagnesemia. Hypermagnesemia occurs because, like potassium, magnesium is excreted primarily by the kidneys. When the kidneys lose their ability to excrete magnesium, serum levels increase. Hypermagnesemia may also result from use of magnesium-containing drugs, such as antacids.

Metabolic Acidosis

The kidneys play an important role in maintaining normal pH by urinary excretion of excess hydrogen ions. Metabolic **acidosis** arises as the result of the kidneys' inability to excrete hydrogen ions. As hydrogen ions build up in the body, the pH falls, becoming increasingly acid. Acute renal failure also can cause metabolic acidosis by loss of bicarbonate buffering capabilities.

Fluid and electrolyte problems are presented in detail in Module 3.

In summary, acute renal failure has a profound impact on fluid and electrolyte balance. Hypervolemia is caused by an inability of the kidneys to excrete adequate volumes of body fluids, which leads to fluid volume excess. Acute renal failure causes electrolyte imbalances primarily through loss of the ability to excrete adequate amounts of electrolytes, such as potassium and sodium. This, in turn, interferes with vitamin D production, precipitating hypocalcemia and hyperphosphatemia. The loss of the kidneys' ability to excrete sufficient amounts of hydrogen ions results in metabolic acidosis.

SECTION SIX REVIEW

1. Interstitial fluid is located
   A. inside the cells
   B. inside the blood vessels
   C. within the tissue spaces
   D. within the intracellular compartment
2. Which of the following sets of imbalances most commonly occur secondary to acute renal failure?
   A. hyperkalemia, hyperphosphatemia, metabolic acidosis
   B. hypokalemia, hyponatremia, hypercalcemia
   C. hyperkalemia, hypocalcemia, metabolic alkalosis
   D. hypernatremia, hypermagnesemia, hypercalcemia
3. Potassium imbalance secondary to acute renal failure is associated with all of the following factors EXCEPT
   A. increased excretion
   B. metabolic acidosis
   C. decreased excretion
   D. increased tissue breakdown
4. An inability of the kidneys to produce 1,25-dihydroxycholecalciferol, the active component of vitamin D, lowers the serum levels of which electrolyte?
   A. sodium
   B. magnesium
   C. phosphate
   D. calcium
5. Metabolic acidosis is closely associated with acute renal failure because of the kidneys' inability to
   A. retain sodium ions
   B. excrete hydrogen ions
   C. retain bicarbonate ions
   D. excrete potassium ions

Answers: 1. C, 2. A, 3. A, 4. D, 5. B

SECTION SEVEN: Management of the Patient in Acute Renal Failure

At the completion of this section, the learner will be able to provide a brief overview of the management of the patient with acute renal failure.

Management of the patient in acute renal failure is composed primarily of collaborative interventions. The interventions focus on correction of the precipitating event (e.g., hypotensive episode, obstruction), support of the body systems until kidney function stabilizes, and prevention or treatment of complications. Nursing care is complex, as these patients are extremely sick and unstable during the early stages of the disorder.

Acute renal failure is a physiologic complication that has the capacity to cause dysfunction of multiple other body systems. A major part of management of acute renal failure is prevention and treatment of complications. Four major potential complications are routinely addressed:

- Fluid overload
- Catabolic processes
- Electrolyte/acid–base imbalance
- Infection

Fluid Overload

Fluid overload is the result of two mechanisms; retention of sodium and water, and the renin–angiotensin–aldosterone system. Fluid overload can result in development of congestive heart failure (CHF) and pulmonary edema. Interventions focus on preventing fluid excess or, if it is present, regaining fluid balance. There are a variety of ways that these goals are accomplished, including fluid restriction, diuretic therapy, and dialysis.

Fluid Restriction

Collins (1998) suggests that fluid replacement should be restricted to urine output plus insensible water loss (about 800 mL to 1 L/day). Accurate measurement of output (urine, nasogastric, tube or fistula drainage, diarrhea, etc.) is crucial to be able to replace fluid on a one-to-one basis. The free water can be distributed evenly over the 2-hour day or it can be divided up by shifts, to provide the patient with fluid to drink with meals or to take with oral medications. The free water also can be used for tube feeding flushes. Uremic patients may experience extreme thirst; thus, oral fluids in small quantities often increase patient comfort.

Diuretic Therapy and Dialysis

If the kidneys have maintained some level of function, **diuretic** therapy may decrease fluid excess to varying degrees. Dialysis is an invasive but effective means of controlling fluid excess. Because it is an invasive procedure, it places the patient at increased risk for multiple complications. Dialysis is presented in Section Eight.

NURSING DIAGNOSES. Nursing diagnoses that readily apply to fluid overload include:

- *Fluid volume excess*
- *Decreased cardiac output*

Nursing interventions focus on monitoring the patient for fluid volume excess and heart failure, following through on physician's orders related to fluid overload, and evaluating patient outcomes.

Catabolic Processes

The high-acuity patient in acute renal failure generally is undergoing accelerated catabolic processes due to hypermetabolism that is triggered by high stress levels, infection, trauma, or other acute problems. Hypermetabolism significantly increases nutritional requirements, particularly protein; thus, it increases formation of nitrogen waste products. The injured kidneys, however, cannot rid the body of nitrogen waste and the uremic toxins. They accumulate rapidly and produce azotemia. Elevated concentrations of nitrogenous waste products impair function of multiple body systems (refer to Section Five). At particular risk for serious complications are the brain (renal encephalopathy) and the gastrointestinal tract (GI bleeding).

To combat the accelerated catabolic processes, the patient requires nutritional support. The diet should be restricted in protein, sodium, potassium, and fluids; and high in carbohydrates, fats, and essential amino acids. Nutrition given orally or via tube feeding routes is preferable to the IV route to minimize the risk of infection. If dietary restrictions are insufficient in maintaining acceptable nitrogenous waste levels (e.g., BUN and creatinine) dialysis may be initiated.

NURSING DIAGNOSES. Nursing diagnoses that frequently occur during catabolic processes include:

- *Altered nutrition: Less than body requirements*
- *Potential complication: GI bleeding*
- *Altered thought processes*
- *Altered bowel elimination: Diarrhea*
- *Altered bowel elimination: Constipation*

Electrolyte/Acid–Base Imbalance

Electrolyte imbalances are a frequent complication associated with acute renal failure. Two major electrolytes that require close monitoring and management are potassium and sodium.

Potassium

Hyperkalemia is an ongoing, potentially lethal complication of acute renal failure. Treatment may include drug therapy or dialysis. Drug therapy may consist of several options. Cation exchange resins may be used either rectally or orally to physically remove the potassium from the body. Sodium, bicarbonate, insulin, or hypertonic glucose may be ordered to attempt to drive potassium back into the cells. Dialysis may be ordered to control potassium, particularly when the hyperkalemia is accompanied by excess fluid volume.

Sodium

Sodium levels vary in the acute renal failure patient and management depends on whether levels are normal, high, or low. The close relationship between sodium and water make it important to control; therefore, values are monitored closely. Sodium is restricted in the diet and in IV fluids to control fluid excess and prevent dilutional hyponatremia. Maintaining a balance of intake and output helps prevent or control hypernatremia. If renal function is sufficient, diuretic therapy may be ordered to lower sodium levels.

Metabolic Acidosis

Metabolic acidosis can become severe in acute renal failure, creating disruption of normal cellular functions. Sodium bicarbonate may be used sparingly, to minimize the hypernatremic effects. Dialysis may also be initiated to help control acidosis.

NURSING DIAGNOSES. Nursing diagnoses that apply to electrolyte and acid–base balance include:

- *Potential complication: Metabolic acidosis*
- *Potential complication: Electrolyte imbalance*
- *Fluid volume excess*

The nurse monitors the patient for the clinical manifestations of electrolyte imbalances, particularly potassium, sodium, calcium, phosphate, and magnesium.

Infection

Infection is the major cause of death from acute renal failure, due to an immunocompromised status. Minimal use of invasive lines and tubes is crucial. If the patient becomes symptomatic of infection, potential sources should be cultured and antibiotic therapy initiated. Antibiotic therapy requires dose adjustments based on the severity of renal impairment.

NURSING DIAGNOSES. The nursing diagnosis that applies to the patient with a potential infection is:

- *High risk for infection*

The nurse focuses care on monitoring the patient for signs and symptoms of infection. Scrupulous hygienic maintenance is necessary to minimize the risk of infection. Major sources of infection in the acute renal failure patient include urinary tract infection, pneumonia, septicemia, and skin/wound infections.

Related Nursing Diagnoses

In addition to the nursing diagnoses previously listed, the patient in acute renal failure frequently meets the critical criteria for the following:

- *Activity intolerance*
- *High risk for injury*
- *High risk for altered mucous membranes*
- *High risk for altered skin integrity*
- *Altered renal tissue perfusion*
- *Pain*
- *Anxiety*
- *Knowledge deficit*

In summary, a general overview of management of the high-acuity patient in acute renal failure has been presented. Since acute renal failure is a complication that results in further complications, it requires a strong collaborative effort between physicians and nurses. The nurse performs frequent assessments to evaluate the function of multiple body systems, implements and evaluates actions based on physician's orders, and performs independent nursing actions based on the individual needs of the patient. Four major potential complications are routinely addressed: fluid overload, catabolic processes, electrolyte/acid–base imbalance, and infection.

SECTION SEVEN REVIEW

1. Major complications that are routinely addressed in the patient with acute renal failure include all of the following EXCEPT
   - **A.** fluid overload
   - **B.** acid–base imbalance
   - **C.** anabolic processes
   - **D.** infection
2. To restrict fluid intake of the patient with acute renal failure, a common method is to
   - **A.** maintain strict NPO status
   - **B.** match the intake to the output
   - **C.** restrict intake to less than 50 mL/hr
   - **D.** infuse IV fluid at 400 mL/24 hr
3. Catabolic processes that are present in patients with acute renal failure make restriction of ________ necessary.
   - **A.** carbohydrates
   - **B.** fats
   - **C.** proteins
   - **D.** essential amino acids
4. Hyperkalemia is frequently treated with which of the following drugs?
   - **A.** cation exchange resin
   - **B.** sodium bicarbonate
   - **C.** calcium chloride
   - **D.** phosphate
5. The major cause of death from acute renal failure is
   - **A.** hyperkalemia
   - **B.** metabolic acidosis
   - **C.** fluid excess
   - **D.** infection

Answers: 1. C, 2. B, 3. C, 4. A, 5. D

SECTION EIGHT: Dialysis—An Acute Renal Failure Treatment Modality

At the completion of this section, the learner will be able to discuss dialysis as a treatment modality for acute renal failure.

A major portion of the management of acute renal failure focuses on maintaining fluid and electrolytes within acceptable limits. During the oliguric/anuric stage, severe kidney dysfunction can cause life-threatening abnormalities in fluid, electrolyte, and uremic toxin levels. Medical management of acute renal failure varies with the type of failure (prerenal, intrarenal, or postrenal). This section focuses on dialysis as one distinct feature in the management of acute renal failure.

Early in the course of the disorder, tests may be performed to define the type of renal failure (e.g., diminished renal function secondary to a postshock state [prerenal] versus parenchymal tubular damage [intrarenal]). To differentiate between these two etiologies, a diuretic challenge may be given, using either mannitol (an osmotic diuretic) or furosemide (a loop diuretic). If the kidneys are able to respond to the diuretic by increasing urinary output, fluid replacement and additional diuretics are given to treat a prerenal type of problem. If, however, there is no response from the diuretic challenge, ATN is considered seriously, and dialysis may be a viable treatment option. Patients who experience the oliguric/anuric stage for more than 4 to 5 days generally require dialysis. Dialysis has significantly improved the prognosis of patients experiencing ATN.

Dialysis

Dialysis is a process of diffusion by which dissolved particles are transported across a semipermeable membrane from one fluid compartment to another. Dialysis does not correct renal dysfunction. It only corrects fluid, electrolyte, and acid-base imbalances. Return of normal renal function is dependent on treatment of the underlying problem and the ability of the body to heal the damaged tubules. Hemodialysis, continuous renal replacement therapy (CRRT), and peritoneal dialysis are three types of treatment for acute renal failure. Table 26–2 provides a comparison of the three treatment modalities.

Hemodialysis

Hemodialysis requires a direct access into the vascular compartment. For short-term use, as is seen frequently in the high-acuity patient, temporary access sites may be used. The two most common sites are the subclavian and femoral veins, using a relatively simple percutaneous venous access, which is effective for hemodialysis on a temporary basis. For long-term use, an internal arteriovenous fistula, shunt, or graft may be formed surgically, usually in the lower arm. Figure 26–6 illustrates three types of venous access.

Hemodialysis cleans the blood by pumping it out of the patient via the venous access. The blood then passes through a dialyzer, which removes fluid and solutes, returning the filtered blood back to the patient. The semipermeable membrane necessary for diffusion in hemodial-

TABLE 26–2. COMPARISON OF ACUTE RENAL FAILURE TREATMENT MODALITIES

FACTORS	HEMODIALYSIS	CONTINUOUS RENAL REPLACEMENT THERAPY	PERITONEAL DIALYSIS
Indications for use	Acute poisoning Acute/chronic renal failure Transfusion reaction Hepatic coma	Multiple organ dysfunction syndrome Sepsis Acute renal failure Inability to tolerate hemo- or peritoneal dialysis	Hemodynamic instability Severe cardiovascular disease Hemodialysis not available Less rapid treatment is appropriate Inadequate vascular access
Disadvantages	Requires vascular access and heparin Restricts activity level	Requires vascular access Slow process Restricts activity level Risk of contamination	Slower than hemodialysis Abdominal discomfort Decreased mobility Risk of peritonitis
Contraindications	Coagulopathy Age extremes Hemodynamic instability	Acute poisoning Hematocrit > 45% Inability to anticoagulate Low mean arterial pressure Congestive heart failure	Adhesions of peritoneum or abdomen Peritonitis Recent abdominal surgery
Complications	Infection Decreased cardiac output Cardiac arrhythmias Disequilibrium syndrome[a] Air embolism Disconnection hemorrhage	Infection Bleeding Infiltration Air embolus	Infection Decreased cardiac output Fluid overload Hyperglycemia Metabolic alkalosis Respiratory insufficiency Abdominal pain

[a]Symptoms of disequilibrium syndrome include disorientation, seizures, headache, agitation, and nausea and vomiting.

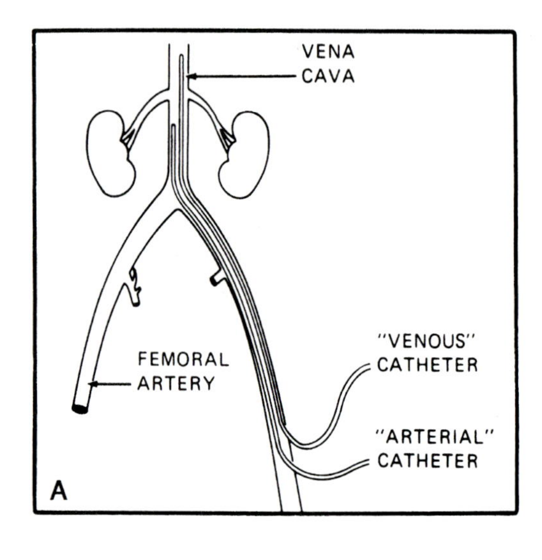

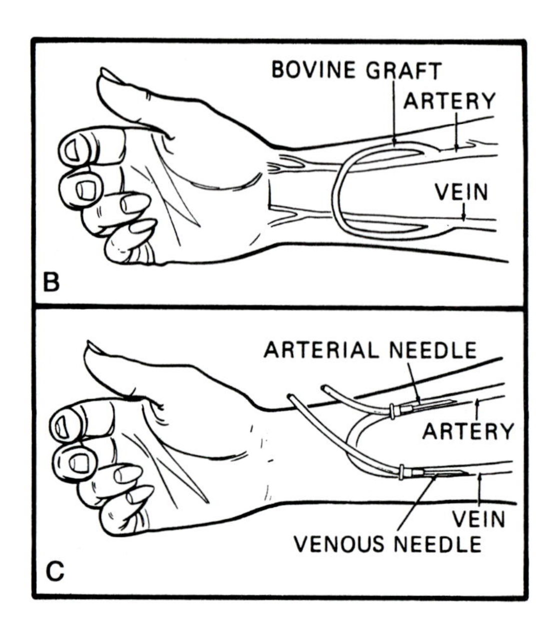

Figure 26–6. Three types of venous access. **A.** Shunt using Shaldon catheters, provide short-term access. **B.** A graft in place. **C.** Anastomosis to form an arteriovenous fistula. A graft is a type of fistula that anastomoses some type of graft material (e.g., bovine carotid). A fistula anastomoses an artery directly to a vein. Grafts and fistulas provide long-term access and require a period of healing prior to use. *(From Ahrens, T., and Prentice, D. [1993].* Critical care certification preparation and review, *3rd ed. Norwalk, CT: Appleton & Lange.)*

ysis is penetrable, thin cellophane. The blood comprises the first fluid compartment, and the dialysate is the second one. The semipermeable membrane pores are large enough to allow small substances to pass across (e.g., creatinine, urea and uric acid, and water molecules) but too small to allow larger particles to diffuse (e.g., proteins, blood cells, and bacteria).

Diffusion occurs down a concentration gradient because the blood has a higher solute concentration than the dialysate has. This causes the flow of urea, creatinine, and other relatively concentrated solutes to move across the semipermeable membrane (the cellophane) into the dialysate solution.

Continuous Renal Replacement Therapy

Continuous renal replacement therapy (CRRT) is a relatively new type of dialysis that is used when hemodialysis is not feasible (e.g., hemodynamic instability or intolerance to peritoneal dialysis). At this time, CRRT is being used in the critical care setting because frequent assessments and ongoing monitoring are essential.

CRRT, a continuous form of therapy (8 hours or more), is used primarily to remove fluid and, if necessary, waste products and excess electrolytes. The two most commonly used forms of CRRT are continuous arteriovenous hemofiltration (CAVH) and continuous venovenous hemofiltration (CVVH). When continuous dialysis is added to CAVH or CVVH, it is referred to as CAVH-D and CVVH-D, respectively.

CONTINUOUS ARTERIOVENOUS HEMOFILTRATION (CAVH). Blood enters the CAVH circuit using the patient's own arterial blood pressure. Therefore, both an arterial and a venous access are necessary. The most common access site is the femoral artery and vein because of easy access and large vessel size. The volume within the extracorporeal circuit at any one time is small, making it less hemodynamically traumatic than conventional hemodialysis.

Blood in the circuit flows past a hemofilter, which maintains a lower pressure than the blood. This pressure difference facilitates movement of solutes and water across its semipermeable membrane. The resulting ultrafiltrate drains into a collection apparatus. The level at which the collection device is hung determines the ultrafiltration rate. The ultrafiltration rate can also be adjusted by several other means such as clamping the ultrafiltrate line or using an infusion control device. Once the blood passes the hemofilter, it is rediluted with a predetermined bath of electrolytes, water, and nutrients, based on the patient's fluid, electrolyte, and nutritional status.

CONTINUOUS ARTERIOVENOUS HEMOFILTRATION–DIALYSIS (CAVH-D). CAVH-D is the addition of continuous dialysis to CAVH. CAVH-D uses a dialysate solution that infuses into the hemofilter at the venous end. The dialysate solution flows in the opposite direction of the blood, which creates a continual diffusion gradient throughout the hemofilter; thus, the removal of waste products and excess electrolytes is facilitated. Figure 26–7 provides an illustration of the CAVH-D circuit.

CONTINUOUS VENOVENOUS HEMOFILTRATION (CVVH). CVVH uses only a double-lumen catheter placed in a vein, which eliminates the need for an arterial catheter with its potential complications. CVVH uses a small pump to propel the blood from one side of the catheter

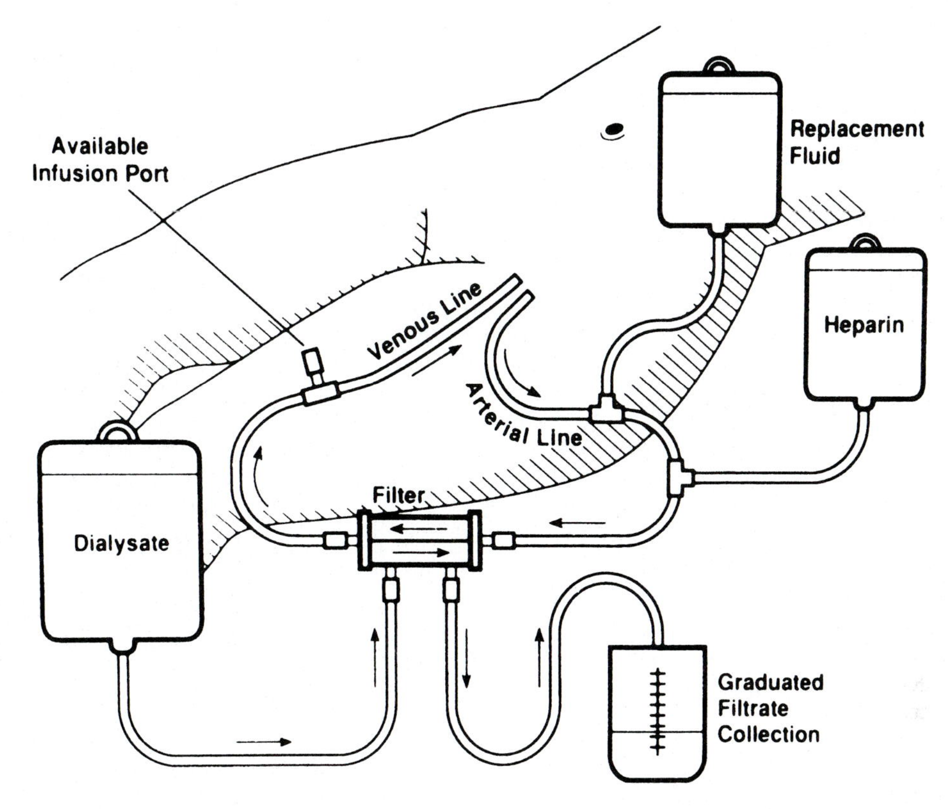

Figure 26–7. Configuration of continuous arteriovenous hemodiafiltration (CAVH-D) circuit used. Arrows denote direction of flow. Arterial blood leaves the circulation via the femoral arterial catheter and flows across the hemofilter. Dialysate is run countercurrent within the filter, and dialysate with ultrafiltrate is collected in a separate chamber. Blood is returned to the circulation via the femoral venous catheter. *(From Tominaga, G. [1993]. Continuous arteriovenous hemodiafiltration in postoperative and traumatic renal failure. Reprinted from* Am J Sur *166:6:612–616.)*

through the hemofilter and back into the vein through the second lumen of the catheter. The pump serves to control the blood flow and fluid removal rate.

CONTINUOUS VENOVENOUS HEMOFILTRATION–DIALYSIS (CVVH-D). CVVH-D is the addition of continuous dialysis to the process of CVVH. The dialysate solution is infused through the hemofilter in the same manner as in CAVH-D.

Peritoneal Dialysis

Peritoneal dialysis uses the patient's own peritoneal lining to serve as the semipermeable membrane through which diffusion, osmosis, and filtration occur. The desired outcome of peritoneal dialysis is the same as other forms of dialysis—to remove metabolic wastes and correct fluid and electrolyte imbalances. It can be performed either manually or by use of automatic cycling machines. Dialyzing fluid is introduced into the peritoneal cavity via a peritoneal catheter, which is secured in place. Once in the abdominal cavity, it is held there for a specified period of time, allowing adequate time for the transfer of fluid and solutes across the peritoneal lining. Once the dialyzing pass time is completed, the dialyzing fluid, with its additional fluid and solutes, is drained out of the abdomen.

Nursing management of the patient undergoing dialysis or hemofiltration focuses on activities that maintain catheter or venous access patency and prevention of complications. Many nursing interventions apply to all treatment modalities. Table 26–3 summarizes nursing activities based on type of treatment modality.

Dialysate Solutions

The exact nature of the dialysate is based on the fluid and electrolyte status of the patient. It consists of a combination of water and variable concentrations of electrolytes. Electrolytes common to dialysate solutions include potassium, sodium, chloride, magnesium, and calcium. Electrolyte concentrations are manipulated carefully depending on whether the serum level of each electrolyte is high, low, or within normal range. Acute renal failure usually is associated with higher than normal levels of potassium, sodium, magnesium, and phosphate. For this reason, the electrolyte levels in the dialysate solution will be either within normal range or below normal to pull excess electrolytes out of the blood and into the dialysate solution (down the concentration gradient).

Glucose may be added to the solution to increase filtration of fluid. A buffer is included, either bicarbonate or acetate. Buffers help stabilize any existing metabolic aci-

TABLE 26–3. NURSING MANAGEMENT OF ACUTE RENAL FAILURE TREATMENT MODALITIES

	HEMODIALYSIS	CRRT	PERITONEAL DIALYSIS
Goals	Maintain shunt, fistula, or catheter patency	Maintain catheter patency Prevent complications	Maintain catheter patency Prevent complications Maintain balanced intake and output
Nursing care	Monitor vital signs and hemodynamic status Monitor for signs and symptoms of complications Daily sterile shunt site care Daily fistula care until site is healed No blood pressure cuff, injection, IV insertions, or tourniquets on limb with shunt or fistula Keep clamps at bedside at all times Monitor laboratory values Weigh before and after dialysis	Monitor vital signs and hemodynamic status Monitor daily for signs and symptoms of complications Assess for patency (presence of palpable thrill and warmth on both tubings) Monitor hourly intake and output Monitor laboratory values for therapeutic effects Weights daily Daily catheter care Observe color if ultrafiltrate is used	Monitor vital signs and hemodynamic status Weigh daily Monitor laboratory values for therapeutic effects Obtain intermittent cultures of drainage dialysate and catheter tip (if removed) Precise documentation of intake and output with every exchange Turn side to side to facilitate drainage Daily catheter care Observe color of drainage dialysate

dosis and keep electrolytes in solution form. Table 26–4 shows a typical example of the composition of hemodialysis dialysate, including normal serum levels of each component.

Drug Therapy and Dialysis

Administration of drugs requires special consideration when the patient is receiving dialysis. First, between intermittent dialysis treatments, drugs that do not break down fully in the body continue to circulate in active form, since they cannot be excreted via the kidneys. Continuing to deliver the usual normal doses in such a patient can lead to severe toxic effects. Second, during dialysis, many drugs are able to cross the semipermeable membrane to be cleansed from the blood, thereby rendering those drug levels as nontherapeutic. This capability makes dialysis a useful option for rapid removal of intentional or accidental overdoses of dialyzable drugs.

The nurse caring for the patient receiving dialysis should be aware of which drugs are dialyzable. Many hospitals have a listing of drugs that will be dialyzed out. These drugs should be scheduled appropriately to avoid undesired dialysis. Table 26–5 is a partial listing of the dialyzability of some common drugs.

TABLE 26–4. COMPOSITION OF DIALYSATE

COMPONENT	DIALYSATE LEVEL	NORMAL SERUM LEVELS
Sodium	133–142 mEq/L	135–145 mEq/L
Potassium	0.0–4.0 mEq/L	3.5–5.3 mEq/L
Chloride	103–105 mEq/L	95–105 mEq/L
Calcium	2.5–3.5 mEq/L	2.2–2.5 mEq/L
Magnesium	1.0–1.5 mEq/L	1.5–2.5 mEq/L
Glucose	0.0–200 mg/100 mL	70–110 mg/dL
Acetate	33–38 mEq/L	—
Bicarbonate	As ordered	24–28 mEq/L

Adapted from Ulrich, G.T. (1989). Nephrology nursing: Concepts and strategies, *p. 130. Norwalk, CT: Appleton & Lange. Normal serum levels from Kee, J.L. (1999).* Laboratory and diagnostic tests with nursing implications *(5th ed.) Stamford, CT: Appleton & Lange.*

In summary, when the kidneys are no longer able to adequately cleanse the blood of excess waste products, fluid, and electrolytes, artificial means often are required to correct the imbalances. Three methods were described: hemodialysis, peritoneal dialysis, and continuous renal replacement therapy (CRRT). Each modality carries with it indications, contraindications, and disadvantages. The nurse must be aware of the effect of hemodialysis on drug therapy. Problems of either toxic or subtherapeutic drug levels are associated with acute renal failure and dialysis.

TABLE 26–5. DIALYZABILITY OF COMMON DRUGS

DRUGS DIALYZED OUT OF BLOOD	DRUGS NOT SIGNIFICANTLY DIALYZED OUT OF BLOOD
Acetaminophen	Albumin (large protein molecule)
Aspirin	Diazepam (protein bound, low distribution volume)
Captopril	Digoxin (middle molecular weight, stored in tissues)
Mannitol 25%	Furosemide (protein bound)
Methyldopa	Heparin (protein bound)
Metoclopramide (partially)	Hydralazine (protein bound, low distribution volume)
Protamine sulfate	Iron products (protein bound)
Pyridoxine	Levothyroxine (protein bound)
Theophylline	Nifedipine (protein bound) Prazosin HCl (protein bound) Prochlorperazine (protein bound) Propranolol HCl (protein bound) Quinidine (protein bound) Verapamil (protein bound)

Section Eight Review

1. If the patient responds to a diuretic challenge by increasing urine output, the nurse would anticipate which type of follow-up intervention?
   A. hemodialysis
   B. peritoneal dialysis
   C. large doses of diuretics
   D. fluid replacement and diuretics
2. The major purpose of using dialysis is to
   A. remove proteins from the blood
   B. correct imbalances of fluid and electrolytes
   C. remove drugs from the blood
   D. correct renal dysfunction
3. Common rapid access sites for short-term hemodialysis are
   A. subclavian and femoral veins
   B. femoral and brachial arteries
   C. radial and femoral arteries
   D. internal jugular and subclavian veins
4. Which of the following statements is correct regarding diffusion?
   A. it occurs up a concentration gradient
   B. it moves particles (solute) across a membrane
   C. it occurs down a concentration gradient
   D. it disperses out within a solution with no membrane
5. CRRT would most likely be used on which of the following patients?
   A. 6-year-old patient diagnosed with prerenal failure
   B. hemodynamically stable, 7-year-old cardiac patient
   C. 2-year-old patient diagnosed with postrenal failure
   D. hemodynamically unstable 4-year-old trauma patient
6. When peritoneal dialysis is performed, the semipermeable membrane is the
   A. peritoneal lining
   B. hemofilter
   C. cellophane membrane
   D. renal lining
7. Assuming that a patient's electrolytes have undergone the typical imbalances associated with acute renal failure, the dialysate solution will contain low levels of which of the following electrolytes?
   A. calcium
   B. chloride
   C. potassium
   D. bicarbonate

Answers: 1. D, 2. B, 3. A, 4. C, 5. D, 6. A, 7. C

Posttest

The following Posttest is constructed in a case study format. A patient is presented. Questions are posed based on available data. New data are presented as the case study progresses.

Maria G, a 3-year-old teacher, has been admitted through the emergency department after sustaining multiple injuries in a motor vehicle crash (MVC). The emergency medical team relates that when found at the scene of the event, she was noted to have an arterial blood pressure of 76/42. It was believed that the ambulance had arrived 35 to 45 minutes after the crash. In the emergency department, she was found to have a ruptured spleen. She was prepared immediately for surgery. She has no known history.

It has been almost 48 hours since the event. You note that Maria's urine output has been approximately 25 mL for 2 successive hours.

1. For glomerular filtration to take place, it is important that Maria maintain
   A. a low hydrostatic pressure
   B. an adequate cardiac output
   C. a low renal blood volume
   D. a high renal vascular resistance
2. Certain substances, such as potassium and hydrogen, undergo renal tubular secretion. This term refers to the process by which substances are moved
   A. into the tubules for excretion
   B. back into the vascular system
   C. into the interstitial compartment
   D. back into the glomerulus from Bowman's capsule
3. Assuming Maria's nervous system is intact, it would respond to her low blood pressure in which of the following ways?
   A. osmoreceptors inhibit antidiuretic hormone production
   B. stretch receptors vasoconstrict peripheral arterioles
   C. chemoreceptors stimulate production of aldosterone
   D. baroreceptors stimulate antidiuretic hormone production

4. The renin–angiotensin system assists in increasing Maria's arterial blood pressure by
   A. causing vasoconstriction
   B. decreasing circulatory volume
   C. increasing hydrogen ion concentration
   D. inhibiting reabsorption of sodium

The following data are now available. It is believed that Maria's blood pressure remained low for at least 1 hour directly after the crash. The emergency team had difficulty obtaining a vascular access with which to administer fluids. Her daughter has informed you that Maria has no known chronic conditions except for mild arthritis, which she controls with aspirin on a daily basis.

5. Considering Maria's recent history, which type of acute renal failure is she initially at most risk of developing?
   A. acute tubular necrosis
   B. postrenal
   C. prerenal
   D. intrarenal

Five days have passed since the accident. Maria's urine output has fallen to 350 mL over the past 24 hours. She has just received a diuretic challenge, to which she had no response. Her blood pressure is now 165/94.

6. Considering the latest changes, what specifically is Maria most likely developing?
   A. prerenal failure
   B. acute tubular necrosis
   C. postrenal failure
   D. intrarenal failure
7. Maria is at high risk for developing renal failure because ischemia occurs when the mean arterial blood pressure drops to below _____ mm Hg for more than 30 minutes.
   A. 50 to 60
   B. 60 to 70
   C. 70 to 80
   D. 80 to 90

Maria is now in acute renal failure secondary to acute tubular necrosis. Her urine output has been approximately 350 mL/24 hr and her BUN is now 100 mg/dL. She is confused and drowsy.

8. According to the latest data, Maria is experiencing the _____ stage of acute renal failure.
   A. oliguric/anuric
   B. onset
   C. early diuresis
   D. late diuresis

It has been approximately 12 days since the onset of Maria's acute renal failure. Her urine output is now 450 mL over the past 24 hours, and her BUN and creatinine have both leveled off.

9. According to the latest available data, Maria is in which of the following stages of acute renal failure?
   A. oliguric/anuric
   B. late diuresis
   C. onset
   D. early diuresis

Maria's laboratory values are as follows:

48 Hours Postinjury:	**5 Days Postinjury:**
BUN/creatinine ratio 24:1	BUN/creatinine ratio 13:1
Urine sodium 38 mEq/L	Urine sodium 52 mEq/L
Specific gravity 1.028	Specific gravity 1.008
Serum osmolality 650 mOsm/L	Serum osmolality 285 mOsm/L

10. Maria's pattern of renal laboratory findings are consistent with an initial __________ failure which became a(n) __________ failure.
    A. postrenal, intrarenal
    B. prerenal, postrenal
    C. prerenal, intrarenal
    D. intrarenal, acute tubular necrosis
11. A renal ultrasound is ordered. Which of the following statements is correct regarding ultrasound?
    A. it is an invasive procedure
    B. it requires use of a contrast dye
    C. it can be performed at the bedside
    D. it requires a local anesthetic

Maria is experiencing some of the clinical manifestations of uremic syndrome. She is complaining of tingling and numbness of her hands and feet. She also has developed skin bruising associated with minimal trauma.

12. Maria's new symptoms of tingling and numbness are most likely caused by
    A. hyperkalemia
    B. hypocalcemia
    C. stimulated stretch receptors
    D. peripheral neuropathy
13. Skin bruising in acute renal failure is secondary to the effects of
    A. increased erythropoietin
    B. decreased ammonia levels
    C. severe hypocalcemia
    D. excessive uremic toxins
14. Maria's serum phosphate is elevated. Which of the following reasons is most likely the cause?
    A. hypermagnesemia
    B. hypocalcemia
    C. hypomagnesemia
    D. hypercalcemia
15. She is at risk for developing metabolic acidosis primarily due to
    A. decreased excretion of potassium
    B. increased excretion of hydrogen ions
    C. increased excretion of potassium
    D. decreased excretion of hydrogen ions

Maria had the following hourly urine outputs recorded:

3:00: 32 mL
4:00: 41 mL
5:00: 43 mL

16. Based on common fluid restriction practice, and assuming that she has no other output during this period, you would anticipate giving Maria _________ mL of fluid between 5:00 and 6:00.
    A. 41
    B. 43
    C. 84
    D. 116
17. Maria is to begin receiving nutritional support. The nurse would anticipate that the preferred route to be used is
    A. oral
    B. Hickman catheter
    C. peripheral parenteral nutrition
    D. central venous IV line

It has been decided that Maria needs dialysis. Her present status is as follows. She is hemodynamically stable, and she is 8 days postabdominal surgery. She has generalized edema and severe electrolyte abnormalities.

18. Based only on the available data, which type of dialysis is most likely to be ordered for Maria?
    A. hemodialysis
    B. peritoneal dialysis
    C. continuous ultrafiltration
    D. combination of hemodialysis and peritoneal dialysis
19. She is receiving a drug that is highly protein bound while in circulation. What would be the significance of drug protein binding and hemodialysis if this treatment were ordered?
    A. protein-bound drugs will be released during dialysis
    B. protein-bound drugs break down rapidly in the blood
    C. protein-bound molecules are too large to dialyze out
    D. protein-bound drugs in tissues move into circulation during dialysis

POSTTEST ANSWERS

Question	Answer	Section	Question	Answer	Section
1	B	One	11	C	Five
2	A	One	12	D	Five
3	D	Two	13	D	Five
4	A	Two	14	B	Six
5	C	Three	15	D	Six
6	B	Three	16	B	Seven
7	B	Three	17	A	Seven
8	A	Four	18	A	Eight
9	D	Four	19	C	Eight
10	C	Five			

REFERENCES

Andreoli, T.E., Bennett, J.C., Carpenter, C.C.J., & Plum, F. (eds.). (1997). Acute renal failure. In author, *Cecil's essentials of medicine* (4th ed.) (pp. 235–251). Philadelphia: W.B. Saunders.

Collins, S.T. (1998). Common renal disorders. In C.M. Hudak, B.M Gallo, & P.G. Morton, *Critical care nursing: A holistic approach* (7th ed.) (pp. 569–590). Philadelphia: J.B. Lippincott.

Gallagher-Lepak, S. (1998). In C.M. Porth (ed.), *Pathophysiology: Concepts of altered health states* (5th ed.) (pp. 667–683). Philadelphia: J.B. Lippincott.

Guyton, A.C., & Hall, J.E. (1997). *Human physiology and mechanisms of disease* (6th ed.). Philadelphia: W.B. Saunders

Hansen, M. (1998). Pathophysiology: Foundations of Disease and Clinical Interventions. Philadelphia: Saunders.

Parker, K.P. (1998). Acute renal failure. In M.R. Kinney, S.B. Dunbar, J.A. Brooks-Brunn, N. Molter, & J.M Vitello-Cicciu (eds.). *AACN clinical reference for critical care nursing* (4th ed.) (pp. 797–820). St. Louis: C.V. Mosby.

Price, C.A. (1994). Acute renal failure. A sequelae of sepsis. *Crit Care Nurs Clin of North Am* 6(2):359–372.

Module 27

Nursing Care of the Patient with Altered Metabolic Function

Kathleen Dorman Wagner

This module is designed to integrate the major points discussed in Modules 22 through 26. This module summarizes relationships between key concepts and assists the learner in clustering information to facilitate clinical application. The module applies content in an interactive learning style using a case study format. The learner is encouraged to cluster data and derive as well as prioritize nursing diagnoses. The module ends with a brief summary of major points.

All normal ranges for laboratory values are taken from Kee (1999).

Objectives

At the completion of this module, given a specific clinical situation, the learner will be able to

1. Interpret the significance of laboratory data.
2. Interpret the significance of assessment data.
3. Develop appropriate expected patient outcomes.
4. Apply knowledge of the patient with altered nutrition/metabolism to develop a plan of nursing interventions.
5. Describe the nursing management of the patient with altered nutrition/metabolism status.

DEVELOPING A PLAN OF CARE

Assessment

Each module in Part VI: Metabolic-presented material on assessment appropriate to the module's specific topic. Once data collection is complete, the nurse clusters the critical cues based on the presence of abnormal data or missing normal data, collects any necessary additional data, and develops a list of nursing diagnoses.

Nursing Diagnoses

Nursing diagnoses are based on frequently recurring functional problems rather than body systems, which is characteristic of medical diagnoses. Therefore, the disorders presented in the modules in Part VI have many nursing diagnoses in common even though they may disturb different body systems. Although the etiologic factors associated with each nursing diagnosis may differ based on the underlying pathophysiologic problem, the desired patient outcomes and nursing management remain essentially the same. This nursing care-oriented module presents some of the major nursing diagnoses and desired patient outcomes (evaluative criteria) commonly associated with problems of nutrition and metabolism.

Problems of Nutrition

Three North American Nursing Diagnosis Association (NANDA)-approved nursing diagnoses directly reflect nutrition:

- *Altered nutrition: Less than body requirements*
- *Altered nutrition: More than body requirements*
- *Potential for altered nutrition: More than body requirements.*

The disorders presented in Part VI are associated primarily with nutritional deficits rather than excesses.

Problems of Metabolism

Many metabolic alterations, such as starvation, renal failure, and diabetes, are associated with shifts in body fluid and electrolytes, placing the high-acuity patient at risk for developing problems in these areas.

Fluid Imbalance

Problems of metabolism often affect fluid balance, though in different ways. Three NANDA-approved nursing diagnoses focus on fluid balance:

- *Fluid volume deficit*
- *Fluid volume excess*
- *High risk for fluid volume deficit*

Fluid volume excess is presented in Part I: Special Topics and Part IV: Perfusion, and will not be discussed here.

Electrolyte Imbalances

Electrolyte imbalances are not addressed directly in any NANDA-approved nursing diagnosis. They are physiologic complications that are collaborative problems. Collaborative problems are based on physiologic complications. The nurse focuses on monitoring the patient for clinical manifestations that indicate onset of the complication, as well as monitoring the patient for changes in clinical status. Collaborative problems require a combination of physician-ordered and nurse-ordered interventions to treat the complication effectively. Using a collaborative problem model, electrolyte imbalance can be addressed in a plan of care as follows:

- *Potential complication: Electrolyte imbalances*

Ulrich and associates (1998) suggest an alternative nursing/collaborative diagnosis that combines fluid and electrolyte problems. They recommend the following:

- *Altered fluid and electrolyte balance*

Altered Immunocompetence

Metabolic problems frequently alter immune function. Infection, therefore, is a relatively common complication. The following NANDA-approved nursing diagnosis addresses infection:

- *Risk for infection*

Carpenito (1999) and Ulrich et al. (1998) suggest the following additional collaborative problems related to immunocompetence (PC = potential complication):

- PC: Opportunistic infections
- PC: Sepsis
- PC: Allergic reaction
- PC: Donor tissue rejection
- PC: Immunodeficiency

An additional nursing diagnosis, *Hyperthermia*, may be included in the plan of care if the nurse views fever as a distinctly separate problem.

Additional Nursing Diagnoses

Many other nursing diagnoses potentially could be included in the plan of care for the patient with a disorder affecting nutrition and metabolism. Some of these include:

- *Activity intolerance (high risk for or actual)*
- *Altered cardiac output: decreased*
- *Altered comfort (specify)*
- *Altered oral mucous membrane*
- *Altered respiratory function*
- *Altered thought processes*
- *Altered tissue perfusion (specify)*
- *Anxiety*
- *Fatigue*
- *Impaired skin integrity (high risk for or actual)*
- *Impaired tissue integrity*
- *Knowledge deficit*
- *Pain*
- *Self-care deficit*

Desired Patient Outcomes

The desired outcomes (evaluative criteria) presented here are standard ones as suggested by Ulrich and colleagues (1998). On an actual plan of care, each outcome would need to be written more specifically, reflecting outcomes that are realistic for the individual needs and capabilities of the patient.

Altered Nutrition: Less than Body Requirements

Desired outcomes: The patient will maintain adequate nutrition, as evidenced by:

1. Serum glucose, albumin, transferrin, hemoglobin and hematocrit, lymphocyte, BUN, and creatinine within acceptable ranges
2. Weight trends moving toward normal for patient
3. Mucous membranes healthy
4. Strength and activity tolerance usual or improved

Fluid Volume Deficit Related to (Applicable Etiologies)

Desired outcomes: The patient will regain fluid and electrolyte balance as evidenced by:

1. Stable weight
2. Normal skin turgor
3. Normal mental status for patient
4. Blood pressure and pulse within normal range for patient
5. Serum osmolality within normal range
6. Serum BUN, creatinine, glucose, hemoglobin, and hematocrit within acceptable ranges
7. Urine output ≥ 30 mL/hr
8. Moist mucous membranes
9. Intake = output
10. Capillary refill < 3 to 5 seconds
11. Urine specific gravity within normal range

PC: *Electrolyte Imbalances*

Desired outcomes: The patient will maintain/regain electrolyte balance, as evidenced by:

1. Electrolyte levels within normal ranges
2. Absence of cardiac dysrhythmias
3. Normal neurologic status for patient
4. Normal muscle strength and tone for patient
5. Normal neuromuscular status for patient
6. Normal blood pressure, pulse, and respirations for patient
7. Absence of abdominal pain, nausea, or vomiting

The desired outcomes presented here are generic. If the patient is experiencing several specific significant electrolyte abnormalities, the plan can separate each abnormality. When split up, each specific abnormality would include its own listings of desired patient outcomes and interventions.

Infection, Risk For

Desired outcomes: The patient will be free of infection as evidenced by:

1. Pulse and temperature within normal range
2. Absence of lesions with redness, swelling, heat, or drainage
3. Absence of chills
4. Negative cultures
5. Skin integrity intact
6. Absence of adventitious breath sounds
7. WBC/differential counts within acceptable range
8. Urine clear
9. Voiding asymptomatic

Interventions

Collaborative and independent nursing interventions are presented in each module. In addition, interventions are applied in the upcoming case study.

CASE STUDY

BEATRICE J, A PATIENT WITH COMPLEX METABOLIC DYSFUNCTION

Beatrice J, a 53-year-old woman, was brought into the emergency department by her husband, who simply stated that his wife "just looks real bad."

The Initial Appraisal

On approaching Beatrice's stretcher, you make the following rapid assessment.

GENERAL APPEARANCE. Beatrice is a moderately obese Caucasian female. Her hair is gray and unkempt, and she is wearing a soiled nightgown.

SIGNS OF DISTRESS. Beatrice's breathing is even but deep. No facial grimacing is noted, and her limbs are outstretched in a relaxed fashion. She is mumbling in a confused manner. She appears drowsy.

OTHER. You note a foul odor emanating from Beatrice, suggesting infection. She does not have any tubes or IV lines attached at this time. A man who states that he is Beatrice's husband, George, is standing beside the stretcher.

Recent History

George gives you the following brief history. Beatrice has a 15-year history of type 1 (insulin-dependent) diabetes. About 3 weeks ago, she had a left heel spur removed in an outpatient surgery. Four days before this admission, Beatrice began experiencing abdominal pain and nausea, with intermittent vomiting. Her husband relates that for the past 2 days, his wife had omitted her insulin because "she didn't need it since she hadn't been able to eat anything." Although she was complaining of her foot hurting, she adamantly refused to have her husband call the doctor. Over the past week, her foot had become increasingly swollen and red, with a bad odor. For the past 3 days, she required frequent assistance into the bathroom to urinate, but she had not urinated in the last 8 hours. George adds that Beatrice has become increasingly confused and disoriented. Because of these developments, he felt the need to bring her into the hospital.

QUESTION

Based on these preliminary data, you would focus your assessment first on her __________ status.

A. renal
B. diabetes
C. nutrition
D. immunocompetence

ANSWER

The correct answer is B. During the initial appraisal, a critical cue was noted: no insulin in 2 days. Based on this single cue, the nurse can quickly cluster other similar critical cues, including history of type 1 diabetes, recent and acute physiologic stressors (surgery, probable wound infection), abdominal pain, nausea and vomiting, change in level of consciousness, failure to take insulin, no food consumption for several days, and a pattern of polyuria changing to diminished urine output. The exact nature of the diabetic crisis remains uncertain until laboratory results are evaluated. While waiting for laboratory results, if available, the nurse can obtain a capillary glucose specimen or urine sample for sugar and acetone.

The Focused Diabetic Assessment

Beatrice's initial appraisal, brief recent history, and data clustering are suggestive of a diabetic crisis. Immediate attention should be focused on obtaining more data to test this hypothesis. The results are as follows. Beatrice is drowsy and responds rapidly to light shaking. Her respirations are deep and even at 28/min (Kussmaul type). When bending down to examine her eyes, a fruity odor is noted on her breath. Her blood pressure is now 88/64, pulse 115/min, and temperature 102°F. Her skin is flushed, hot, and dry. Her mucous membranes also are dry. You note that her jugular veins are collapsed when she is lying in a flat position.

Stat laboratory samples are drawn, and the results come back as follows:

Arterial Blood Gas (ABG)
pH = 7.20
P_{CO_2} = 28 mm Hg
P_{O_2} = 88 mm Hg
HCO_3 = 14 mEq/L

Serum Glucose	
400 mg/dL	(Normal, 70 to 110 mg/dL)
Serum Ketones	
Positive	(Normal, negative)
Serum Electrolytes	
Na = 110 mEq/L	(Normal, 135 to 145 mEq/L)
Cl = 95 mEq/L	(Normal, 95 to 105 mEq/L)
K = 5.8 mEq/L	(Normal, 3.5 to 5.3 mEq/L)
Ca = 8.3 mg/dL	(Normal, 9 to 11 mg/dL)
Anion Gap	
19 mEq/L	(Normal, 10 to 17 mEq/L)
Hemoglobin	
15.4 g/dL	(Normal for females, 12 to 15 g/dL)
Hematocrit	
48.2%	(Normal for females, 36 to 46%)

QUESTION

Based on the data collected thus far, you hypothesize that Beatrice's clinical presentation is most consistent with which type of crisis?

A. hypoglycemia
B. Somogyi effect
C. diabetic ketoacidosis
D. hyperosmolar hyperglycemic nonketotic syndrome (HHNS)

ANSWER

The correct answer is C. Beatrice's laboratory data are consistent with DKA. The positive high anion gap metabolic acidosis, the positive serum ketones, the level of glucose elevation, as well as her presenting history, suggest DKA rather than HHNS.

The Systematic Bedside Assessment

Beatrice has a No. 18 IV catheter inserted, and appropriate medical interventions for DKA are initiated based on her laboratory results. Interventions include an IV insulin drip and fluid and electrolyte replacement. She is then moved from the emergency department to an intermediate care unit.

On arrival in the intermediate care unit, Beatrice is transferred to a bed. An updated report from the emergency department nurse is given, and a systematic bedside assessment is performed.

HEAD AND NECK. Beatrice's face appears flushed, and her lips are dry and cracked. She now moans and opens her eyes when moderately shaken. Her pupils are equal and react briskly to light. Her neck veins are flat. No abnormalities are noted.

CHEST

Pulmonary Status. Breath sounds are present and equal bilaterally. No adventitious breath sounds are auscultated. Rate and quality are the same as previously noted.

Cardiac Status. S_1 and S_2 with no murmur is auscultated. Tachycardia is present at 120/min. Rhythm is regular.

ABDOMEN. The abdomen is slightly distended. Hypoactive bowel sounds are auscultated in all quadrants. The abdomen is soft to palpation.

PELVIS. A urinary catheter is in place. The urine output over the past 2 hours is 25 mL. The urine is clear, dark amber, with a specific gravity of 1.045.

EXTREMITIES. There is poor skin turgor. The skin is hot and dry. No peripheral edema is noted. The nailbeds are pale. Peripheral pulses are present in all four extremities but weak. The left foot is hot and edematous. You note a 15-cm open wound on the left heel, with a moderate amount of green purulent drainage. Touching the foot causes Beatrice to moan and grimace.

POSTERIOR. No skin breakdown is noted and no sacral edema. Posterior breath sounds are clear.

Developing the Plan of Care: Diabetic Ketoacidosis

Beatrice's DKA is brought under control through appropriate medial management.

The nurse writes the following initial list of nursing diagnoses based on Beatrice's current status.

- *Altered nutrition: less than body requirements*
- *Altered cardiac output: decreased*
- *Pain*
- *Altered tissue perfusion: peripheral*
- *Fluid volume deficit*
- *Risk for infection*
- *Self-care deficit*

QUESTION

Which of the preceding nursing diagnoses would be considered as top priority during the first 4 hours after admission?

A. infection
B. fluid volume deficit
C. altered tissue perfusion: peripheral
D. altered nutrition: less than body requirements

ANSWER

The correct answer is B. A second cluster of critical cues is as follows: blood pressure 88/64 mm Hg, pulse 115/min. Lips and mucous membranes are dry. There is poor skin turgor. Neck veins are collapsed when lying flat. A history is given of an elimination pattern change from polyuria to oliguria over the past few days. These critical cues are very suggestive of fluid volume deficit. Correction of the fluid volume deficit is a priority if complications of hypovolemic shock are to be avoided. Correcting the fluid volume deficit also should increase Beatrice's cardiac output, assuming her cardiovascular system remains intact.

The presence of a large-bore IV catheter is necessary to allow rapid IV infusion rates. Central venous pressure line placement early in the course of treatment will facilitate appropriate management of fluid rates to meet her needs. If closer monitoring of fluid and cardiac status is considered desirable, a flow-directed pulmonary artery catheter may be inserted.

QUESTION

Fluid resuscitation has been initiated on Beatrice. The nurse can anticipate that the second set of priority interventions will focus on initiating

A. electrolyte replacement
B. sodium bicarbonate
C. antibiotic therapy
D. insulin therapy

ANSWER

The correct answer is D. Beatrice's hyperglycemia must be addressed as soon as there is IV access and fluid replacement has been initiated. These two collaborative interventions will be performed in rapid succession. Electrolyte levels will be monitored carefully until her condition has stabilized. She will probably receive sodium chloride in her IV fluid replacement solution. Her serum potassium is currently high; however, it will drop rapidly when her insulin therapy begins to drive potassium back into the cells. Potassium therapy is often held initially unless it is low at admission. In addition, her phosphate level should be obtained and monitored carefully. Since phosphate is a buffer, the acidotic state may have depleted. If replacement therapy is needed, it may be administered in the form of potassium phosphate (K-Phos).

EXERCISE

The nurse is developing a list of desired patient outcomes that are appropriate for the nursing diagnosis: *Fluid volume deficit*. List at least six evaluative criteria that would be appropriate for this nursing diagnosis.

1.
2.
3.
4.
5.
6.

ANSWER

1. Weight stable
2. Normal skin turgor
3. Blood pressure and pulse within normal range for patient
4. Serum osmolality within normal range
5. Serum BUN, creatinine, glucose, hemoglobin, and hematocrit within acceptable ranges
6. Urine output ≥ 30 mL/hr
7. Normal mental status for patient
8. Capillary refill < 3 to 5 seconds
9. Urine specific gravity within normal range
10. Moist mucous membranes

Case Study Update: 7 Days Postadmission

Beatrice remains in the intermediate care unit. Although her DKA was resolved within the first 48 hours, her glucose levels remain elevated. An updated systematic assessment shows the following.

HEAD AND NECK. Neurologically, Beatrice is confused and drowsy, oriented to name only. A Salem sump tube is in place in her right nostril, and correct placement is confirmed. Mucous membranes are pink and moist. Positive jugular vein distention (JVD) is noted at a 45-degree angle.

CHEST

Cardiovascular status. S_1, S_2, and S_3 are present, with no murmurs. Rhythm is regular with a sinus tachycardia at 110 to 115/min. T waves are peaked on ECG. Blood pressure is 174/92.

Respiratory status. Breath sounds are heard in all lung fields. Bases are diminished, with crackles to midfields bilaterally. Occasional nonproductive cough is noted.

ABDOMEN. A nasogastric tube is connected to intermittent low wall suction. Nasogastric drainage is dark green and negative for blood. Bowel sounds are hypoactive in all four quadrants. The abdomen is moderately distended and tight.

PELVIS AND GENITOURINARY TRACT. Urinary catheter remains in place. Urine output for the last 24 hours has been a total of 425 mL.

EXTREMITIES. Edema (4+) is noted in all extremities. The skin is dry and flaky. Pulses are difficult to palpate secondary to edema.

Left foot wound status: The wound remains open and draining. It appears pale, with large areas of blackened tissue and patches of white. No healthy tissue is evident.

POSTERIOR. The coccyx is reddened, although the skin is still intact. With Beatrice positioned on her right side, crackles are auscultated over the posterior fields (right more than left).

OTHER. Temperature is 100°F to 102°F. A 5-pound weight gain is noted over the past 48 hours. Beatrice continues to receive 5 percent dextrose in normal saline at 125 mL/hr. No type of diet or supplement has yet been ordered.

Current Drug Therapy

Current drug therapy includes regular and NPH Humulin insulin (SQ), gentamicin (IV), heparin (SQ), and ranitidine (IV).

QUESTION

Of the following, which assessment is most suggestive of the presence of an underlying nutritional problem?

A. edema
B. flaky, dry skin
C. hypoactive bowel sounds
D. absence of wound healing

ANSWER

The correct answer is D. Following Beatrice's wound debridement and antibiotic therapy, some degree of wound healing would be expected. However, her wound is again deteriorating according to the latest assessment data. Beatrice's ability to heal is further complicated by her long-standing diabetes as well as possible renal failure, since both of these conditions suppress healing.

QUESTION

Besides Beatrice's prolonged hypotensive episode as a major risk factor for development of acute renal failure, which of the following drugs is particularly associated with nephrotoxicity?

A. gentamicin
B. insulin
C. heparin
D. ranitidine

ANSWER

The correct answer is A. Aminoglycosides, such as gentamicin, are highly nephrotoxic. Gentamicin peak and trough levels should be drawn routinely to monitor for toxic blood levels. To monitor renal function for development of nephrotoxicity, serum BUN and creatinine also are measured routinely.

Current Serum Laboratory Results (Abnormal Values Only)

Glucose	
320 mg/dL	
Albumin	
2.2 g/dL	(Normal, 3.5 to 5.0 g/dL)
Transferrin	
112 mg/dL	(Normal, 200 to 430 mg/dL)
White Blood Cell Count	
4,300/mL	(Normal, 4,500 to 10,000/mL)
WBC Differential	
Neutrophils = 75%	(Normal, 50 to 70%)
Bands = 15%	(Normal, 0 to 5%)
Lymphocytes = 20%	(Normal, 25 to 35%)
BUN	
54 mg/dL	(Normal, 5 to 25 mg/dL)
Creatinine	
2.7 mg/dL	(Normal, 0.5 to 1.5 mg/dL)
Electrolytes	
Na = 162 mEq/L	
Cl = 115 mEq/L	
K = 6.0 mEq/L	
Ca = 11.2 mEq/L	

QUESTION

Which of the following statements best reflects the reason that Beatrice's serum creatinine is elevated?

A. controlled diabetes causes increased breakdown of protein
B. malnutrition causes increased excretion of creatinine
C. gluconeogenesis increases the amount of serum creatinine
D. nephrons are unable to cleanse the waste products from the blood

ANSWER

The correct answer is D. Creatinine is a waste product of muscle metabolism. When the kidneys go into failure, they can no longer perform their normal functions, and creatinine remains in the blood rather than being excreted. While Beatrice is in acute renal failure, you would anticipate that while her serum creatinine and BUN increase, creatinine and urea nitrogen clearance in the urine will decrease.

QUESTION

Beatrice's leukopenia is most likely caused by which combination of physiologic insults?

A. hyperglycemic crisis and hypotension
B. malnutrition and overwhelming infection
C. acute renal failure and hyperglycemia
D. hypotension and malnutrition

ANSWER

The correct answer is B. Beatrice's malnutrition is a major factor in failure of the immune system. This has been complicated by a severe infection of prolonged duration that may well have exhausted available neutrophils and lymphocytes.

QUESTION

A disadvantage of using serum albumin as an indicator of malnutrition is that it

A. reflects muscle protein
B. has a short half-life
C. reflects plasma protein
D. has a long half-life

ANSWER

The correct answer is D. Although considered to be a good indicator of nutritional status, the long half-life of serum albumin can make the laboratory values misleading as to current status. Serum prealbumin, another indicator, is better at reflecting current status because of its short half-life.

Beatrice's malnourished state is severely hindering her recovery. Goals for managing this problem include:

1. Halt the state of catabolism
2. Regain positive nitrogen balance
3. Prevent/treat complications

Collaborative Interventions

1. *Laboratory testing*. High-acuity patients need to have blood drawn for intermittent laboratory tests that measure various aspects of nutritional status. These tests include CBC with differential, serum albumin (and/or transferrin), BUN, and creatinine. Urine clearance testing of urea and creatinine may be ordered. Clearance testing helps determine the extent of damage to the nephrons, the effectiveness of renal disease treatment, and the baseline function of the kidneys before initiating treatment.
2. *Dietary orders*. Nutritional support is needed. The decision of route of intake (oral, gastric tube, IV) and type of support (diet, tube feeding, TPN) may be made on the basis of an educated guess of nutritional need, or it may result from a more complex and thorough assessment of nutritional needs via the various nutrition-related tests. Generally speaking, the more physiologically compromised the patient is, the more complex the nutritional needs are. It is essential that Beatrice's nutritional needs be met to facilitate healing and to build up her immune system, which is dangerously compromised. For 7 days, she has had no nutritional supplementation except for fluid and electrolytes. If Beatrice did not have acute renal failure, she would be placed on a high-protein diet to facilitate regaining immunocompetence and the healing process.
3. *Nutritional supplementation*. Various supplements consisting of vitamins and minerals may be ordered to meet Beatrice's current nutritional needs, which are important in healing and blood cell formation. These supplements may include vitamins, iron, zinc, and folic acid.

Nutritional support is presented in depth in Module 22.

Independent Nursing Interventions

Altered nutrition: Less than body requirements is the primary nursing diagnosis that is included on Beatrice's plan of care to address her state of malnutrition. Other significant nursing diagnoses pertinent to care of the malnourished patient include the following.

- *High risk for infection*
- *Activity intolerance*
- *Self-care deficit*
- *Pain*
- PC: *Electrolyte imbalance* or *Altered fluid and electrolyte balance*

QUESTION

Based on available data, which type of acute renal failure is Beatrice most likely experiencing?

A. prerenal
B. postrenal
C. intrarenal
D. insufficient data to decide

ANSWER

The correct answer is C. Beatrice's clinical picture and laboratory data are most consistent with intrarenal acute renal failure.

Case Update

Though her DKA has been resolved, Beatrice's general condition has not significantly improved over the past week. Her renal function has stabilized over the past 24 hours, however, with her last BUN being 69 mg/dL and a creatinine of 3.3 mg/dL. Today, the nurse has noted progressive mental changes in Beatrice. The latest neurologic assessment resulted in the following data:

> Over the past 24 hours, her Glasgow Coma Scale has dropped from 15 to 11. She is disoriented to place and time, and her speech pattern has become slurred and confused. She is drowsy and lethargic, requiring mild shaking before she opens her eyes. She has been vomiting. Her temperature is 100°F, blood pressure is 164/95 mm Hg, pulse is 106/min, and respirations are rapid at 30 breaths/min; light crackles are auscultated in her bilateral lung bases. Her skin is diaphoretic and hand tremors are noted.

EXERCISE

Based on the available data, what problems could Beatrice be developing? List at least three potential medical problems.

1.
2.
3.

ANSWER

Beatrice's current assessment could have several possible sources. Based on her history of diabetes, vital signs, changes in clinical presentation, and recent development of acute renal failure, potential sources of her new signs and symptoms include hypoglycemia, a gas exchange problem, electrolyte imbalances, worsening of her acute renal failure with developing renal encephalopathy, or she possibly could be developing hepatic encephalopathy. To make matters more difficult, her recent changes may be a combination of problems due to multiple organ dysfunction.

QUESTION

Is there sufficient data to develop nursing diagnoses? If YES, list the diagnoses. If NO, what further data do you need to obtain to write a nursing diagnosis (or diagnoses)?

ANSWER

Through clustering existing data, it has been hypothesized that Beatrice may be having a problem with hypoglycemia, gas exchange, electrolyte imbalances, renal encephalopathy, or hepatic encephalopathy (all physiologic complications). Currently, however, there is insufficient data to write a complete diagnostic statement since the potential origins of the problem have not been investigated. Since physiologic complications are collaborative problems that require laboratory or other tests to diagnose, it is most expedient for the nurse to contact the physician to discuss the status change and receive orders. Prior to contacting the physician, however, the nurse may want to obtain additional critical data that will help differentiate the diagnosis, including a finger-stick glucose level, S_{pO_2} by pulse oximetry, and rapid focused assessment of nailbeds and mucous membranes—the finger-stick glucose level and S_{pO_2} can be obtained rapidly, cheaply, and often as independent nursing functions.

The change in Beatrice's status is communicated to the physician, who orders diagnostic laboratory tests, including arterial blood gas, serum glucose, BUN and creatinine, serum electrolytes, and liver function profile (LFP). The laboratory test results are as follows:

ABGs
- pH = 7.48
- P_{CO_2} = 32 mm Hg
- P_{O_2} = 88 mm Hg
- HCO_3 = 31 mEq/L
- Sa_{O_2} = 97%

Serum Glucose
- 65 mg/dL

Serum Electrolytes
- Na = 130 mEq/L
- K = 5.2 mEq/L

Renal Function Profile
- BUN = 68 mg/dL
- Creatinine = 3.2 mg/dL

Liver Function Profile
- ALT = 1,200 U/mL (Normal, 5 to 35 U/mL)
- AST = 1,500 U/L (Normal, 0 to 35 U/L)
- ALP = 120 U/L (Normal, 20 to 90 U/L)

QUESTION

Based on the laboratory results, which hypotheses can be discarded? Circle your decision.

Hypoglycemia	Discard / Do not discard
Gas exchange problem	Discard / Do not discard
Electrolyte imbalances	Discard / Do not discard
Renal encephalopathy	Discard / Do not discard
Hepatic encephalopathy	Discard / Do not discard

ANSWER

Based on the available data, the ABGs are not sufficiently abnormal to cause Beatrice's new clinical signs and symptoms—discard gas exchange. Her renal function labs, while abnormal, continue to be stable and would probably not account for the acute status change—discard renal encephalopathy as the most probable source of the change in status. Her electrolyte imbalances are not consistent with her acute status changes—discard. Her serum glucose as well as some of her acute changes are consistent with hypoglycemia—do not discard. Her clinical presentation is suspicious of hepatic encephalopathy and her LFP is consistent with liver dysfunction—do not discard. Her hypoglycemia problem may be due to the hepatic dysfunction.

Based on Beatrice's clinical manifestations and current laboratory data, the physician makes a tentative diagnosis of acute hepatic failure. Acute hepatic dysfunction is presented in Module 29.

Since Beatrice has had a series of nutrition/metabolic problems, her care plan already contains most of the nursing diagnoses associated with hepatic dysfunction. The nurse can anticipate adding the following nursing diagnoses to Beatrice's plan of care:

- *Altered respiratory function*
- *Altered comfort: Nausea and vomiting*
- *Pain: Upper abdominal*
- *PC: Bleeding*

EXERCISE

List three desired outcomes that would be appropriate for the following collaborative problem:

PC: Bleeding

1.
2.
3.

ANSWER

PC: Bleeding

1. Blood pressure and pulse within normal range
2. No blood in urine, stool, or vomitus

3. No purpura, petechiae, ecchymoses of skin or mucous membranes
4. Improved or stable hemoglobin and hematocrit
5. Stable abdominal girth

The nurse is developing nursing interventions that will help protect Beatrice from developing bleeding problems. Ulrich et al. (1998) suggest the following interventions:

1. Injection and venous access sites: use small-gauge needles; apply prolonged, gentle pressure to site after removal of needle/catheter
2. Blood pressures: avoid overinflation of cuff and inflate cuff only as needed
3. Place pads on side rails if restless or confused
4. Avoid trauma to gums: no stiff toothbrush or floss
5. Avoid rectal trauma (no rectal temps, no rectal tubes, no straining during bowel movement)
6. As ordered, administer and monitor for therapeutic effects of
   a. vitamin K
   b. fresh plasma (or blood)
   c. platelets
7. If bleeding occurs, take immediate steps to control it:
   a. apply firm pressure over site, when appropriate
   b. for epistaxis:
      1. position in high-Fowler's position
      2. apply pressure, apply ice pack
   c. for gastric or esophageal bleeding:
      1. position on side
      2. administer vasopressin, as ordered
      3. assist with esophageal-gastric balloon insertion, as ordered
      4. administer vitamin K and blood products, as ordered
   d. monitor for signs and symptoms of hypovolemic shock
   e. provide patient and family with emotional support

Evaluation and Revision of the Plan of Care

Evaluation of the effectiveness of Beatrice's plan of care is based on how well she meets the desired outcomes within each nursing diagnosis. The care plan is a working document subject to frequent changes. Interventions that have not been effective must be scrutinized to pinpoint why they are ineffective. Revision of the plan is then made, removing ineffective actions and adding alternative ones.

Beatrice's problems are complex and require aggressive interventions, both collaborative and independent, if she is to regain her prehospitalization state of health.

Ultimately, following failure of her left heel wound to heal and subsequent development of sepsis, Beatrice required amputation of her left leg to below the knee. On removal of this major physiologic stressor, she rapidly recovered and was able to be discharged home.

In summary, this module has provided the learner with the opportunity to apply the concepts learned in Part VI, Metabolic, to a complex patient situation. In addition, the case study has attempted to show how one type of metabolic disorder can precipitate an imbalance in another body function. This case study presented a sequence of events that in reality do occur, profoundly affecting the patient's prognosis. Although each disorder had a different etiology, they shared many of the same nursing diagnoses.

REFERENCES

Carpenito, L.J. (1999). *Handbook of nursing diagnosis* (8th ed.). Philadelphia: Lippincott-Williams & Wilkins.

Kee, J.L. (1999). *Laboratory and diagnostic tests with nursing implications* (5th ed.). Stamford, CT: Appleton & Lange.

Ulrich, S.P., Canale, S.W., & Wendell, S.A. (1998). *Medical–surgical nursing care planning guides* (4th ed.). Philadelphia: W.B. Saunders.

PART VII

Gastrointestinal

MODULE 28

Acute Gastrointestinal Dysfunction

Melanie Hardin–Pierce

This self-study module presents the physiologic and pathophysiologic processes involved in acute gastrointestinal (GI) dysfunction and management of the patient with acute GI bleeding, problems in motility, and intestinal ischemia. The module is composed of 10 sections. Section One presents an overview of the anatomy and physiology of the GI system, including organs, and functions. Section Two explains the GI blood supply and nervous system innervation. Section Three explains the defense mechanisms of the GI tract, including lymphatic and immune function. Section Four describes the various laboratory and diagnostic tests utilized to evaluate GI function. Section Five describes the incidence and clinical manifestations of acute GI bleeding. Section Six describes the etiology and pathophysiology of acute upper GI bleeding. Section Seven describes the etiology and pathophysiology of acute lower GI bleeding. Section Eight provides an overview of the collaborative management of acute GI bleeding including pharmacotherapy and therapeutic and surgical interventions. Section Nine explains the etiology, pathophysiology, and management of acute intestinal obstruction and paralytic ileus. Finally, Section Ten describes the nursing diagnosis and management of acute GI bleeding and paralytic ileus.

OBJECTIVES

Following completion of this module, the learner will be able to

1. Identify the anatomic structures of the GI tract.
2. Discuss the functions of the GI tract.
3. Discuss factors influencing circulation to the GI tract.
4. Describe the neurologic control of the GI tract.
5. Describe the mechanisms that exist to protect the integrity of the GI tract.
6. Describe the evaluation of GI function utilizing laboratory and diagnostic tests.
7. Describe the incidence and clinical manifestations associated with acute GI bleeding.
8. Describe the etiology and pathophysiology of acute upper GI bleeding.
9. Describe the etiology and pathophysiology of acute lower GI bleeding.
10. Describe an overview of the management of acute GI bleeding.
11. Describe the etiology, pathophysiology, and management of acute intestinal obstruction and paralytic ileus.
12. Describe the nursing diagnosis and management of acute GI bleeding and bowel obstruction.

PRETEST

1. The primary function of the GI tract is to
   A. metabolize toxic agents
   B. produce clotting factors
   C. provide nutrients needed for metabolism
   D. eliminate carbon dioxide
2. The outermost layer of the GI tract is the
   A. peritoneum
   B. submucosa
   C. mucosa
   D. serosa
3. Blood flow through the gut, spleen, pancreas, and liver comprise the
   A. portal circulation
   B. mesenteric circulation
   C. splanchnic circulation
   D. extrinsic circulation
4. The arterial blood supply to the mesentery and intestines is known as the _______ circulation.
   A. mesenteric
   B. portocaval
   C. visceral
   D. aortic
5. Gut-associated lymphoid tissue (GALT) includes
   A. thyroid, duodenum, gastric mucosa
   B. tonsils, appendix, Peyer's patches
   C. adrenal glands, cecum, stomach
   D. goblet cells, salivary glands, parietal cells
6. The main aerobic bacteria within the GI tract is
   A. *Escherichia coli*
   B. *Bacteroides fragilis*
   C. *Staphylococcus aureus*
   D. beta-hemolytic streptococcus
7. Which laboratory measures are important in evaluating the need for clotting factor replacement?
   A. hemoglobin and hematocrit
   B. platelet count and hematocrit
   C. thrombin time and mean corpuscular volume
   D. prothrombin time and partial thromboplastin time
8. Elevations in the white blood cell count (WBC) suggests a(n)
   A. inflammatory or infectious process
   B. immunocompromised host
   C. normal nonimmunologic gut defense response
   D. hemoconcentration due to fluid volume deficit
9. The appearance of melena is described as
   A. bright red in color from a lower GI tract source
   B. black and tarry in color from an upper GI source
   C. light brown in color from an upper GI source
   D. "coffee ground" in appearance from the colon
10. A client passes a large amount of loose, maroon-colored stool. After notifying the medical practitioner, the nurse documents the stool as being
    A. melena
    B. diarrhea
    C. hematochezia
    D. hematemesis
11. Infections associated with peptic ulcer disease include
    A. *Escherichia coli* infection
    B. *Helicobacter pylori*
    C. beta-hemolytic streptococcus
    D. *Staphylococcus aureus*
12. Drugs known to disrupt the mucosal barrier are
    A. nonsteroidal anti-inflammatory drugs (NSAIDs)
    B. angiotensin-converting enzyme (ACE) inhibitors
    C. cephalosporins
    D. histamine receptor antagonists
13. The elderly are at increased risk of developing ischemic bowel complications. What is another risk factor for the development of bowel ischemia in this population?
    A. atrial fibrillation
    B. hypertension
    C. immobility
    D. obesity
14. Twenty-five percent of all bleeding from ischemic bowel disease is associated with
    A. recreational drug use
    B. severe malnutrition
    C. anticoagulant use
    D. traumatic injury
15. A good measure of perfusion for the nurse to monitor is
    A. arterial blood gas (ABG)
    B. complete blood count (CBC)
    C. urine output
    D. skin temperature
16. Complications of vasopressin include
    A. hypoglycemia
    B. hypernatremia
    C. decreased coronary blood flow
    D. increased portal pressures
17. Acute paralytic ileus (adynamic ileus) is associated with
    A. adhesions following abdominal surgery
    B. a loss of intestinal peristalsis
    C. volvulus of the intestines
    D. hyperperistalsis of the intestines
18. Medications which are known to contribute to the development of acute paralytic ileus include
    A. ACE inhibitors
    B. aminoglycosides
    C. opioids
    D. beta blockers
19. The _______ system inhibits GI motility.

A. sympathetic
B. parasympathetic
C. intrinsic
D. enteric

20. Colonoscopy allows inspection of the
A. duodenal bulb
B. large intestine
C. gastric mucosa
D. small intestine

21. Prophylactic measures to prevent the development of peptic ulcers in acutely ill patients include
A. early enteral feeding, and histamine receptor antagonists
B. surgical resection of all affected mucosa, and antacids
C. total parenteral nutrition, and proton pump inhibitors
D. sclerotherapy and sucralfate

Pretest answers: 1. C, 2. D, 3. C, 4. A, 5. B, 6. A, 7. D, 8. A, 9. B, 10. C, 11. B, 12. A, 13. A, 14. C, 15. C, 16. C, 17. B, 18. C, 19. A, 20. B, 21. A

Glossary

Cholecystokinin. Hormone that stimulates pancreatic enzymes, increases contractility of the gallbladder; inhibits gastric motility

Chyme. A mixture of partly digested food and digestive secretions within the stomach and small intestine

Gastric inhibitory peptide. Hormone that helps to digest carbohydrates and fats

Gut. Refers to the bowel or intestine

Hematemesis. Vomiting of bright red blood or blood that resembles "coffee grounds"

Hematochezia. Bright red or maroon stool secondary to bleeding

Intestinal strangulation. Intestine twists to such an extent that circulation to the twisted area is impaired

Melena. Black, tarry, foul-smelling stools containing blood

Mesenteric circulation. Blood flow to the intestines

Mesentery. Part of the peritoneum that suspends the small intestine to the abdominal wall

Mucosa. Innermost layer of the GI wall

Muscularis. Muscular layer of the GI wall

Peritoneum. Serous membrane that lines the abdominal cavity and abdominal organs

Peyer's patches. Lymph tissue on the outer wall of the intestine

Secretin. Hormone that stimulates release of pancreatic bicarbonate water

Serosa. Outermost layer of the GI wall

Splanchnic circulation. Blood flow through the gut, spleen, pancreas, and liver

Submucosa. Layer of the GI wall that contains blood and lymphatic vessels

Villi. Fingerlike projections covering intestinal folds

Abbreviations

AVM. Arteriovenous malformation

BUN. Blood urea nitrogen

CNS. Central nervous system

EGD. Esophagogastroduodenoscopy

GALT. Gut-associated lymphoid tissue

GI. Gastrointestinal

ICU. Intensive care unit

IV. Intravenous

mEq/L. Milliequivalents per liter

mm Hg. Millimeters of mercury

NSAIDs. Nonsteroidal anti-inflammatory drugs

PUD. Peptic ulcer disease

SECTION ONE: Anatomy and Physiology of the Gastrointestinal Tract

At the completion of this section, the learner will be able to identify the anatomic structures and functions of the gastrointestinal (GI) tract.

The primary function of the GI system is to provide the necessary nutrients needed by cells to sustain function and growth. The GI tract provides the mechanisms for the digestion and absorption of those nutrients through the processes of ingestion, digestion, and absorption. The anatomic structures of the GI tract are the mouth, pharynx, esophagus, stomach, and the small and large intestines (see Fig. 28–1).

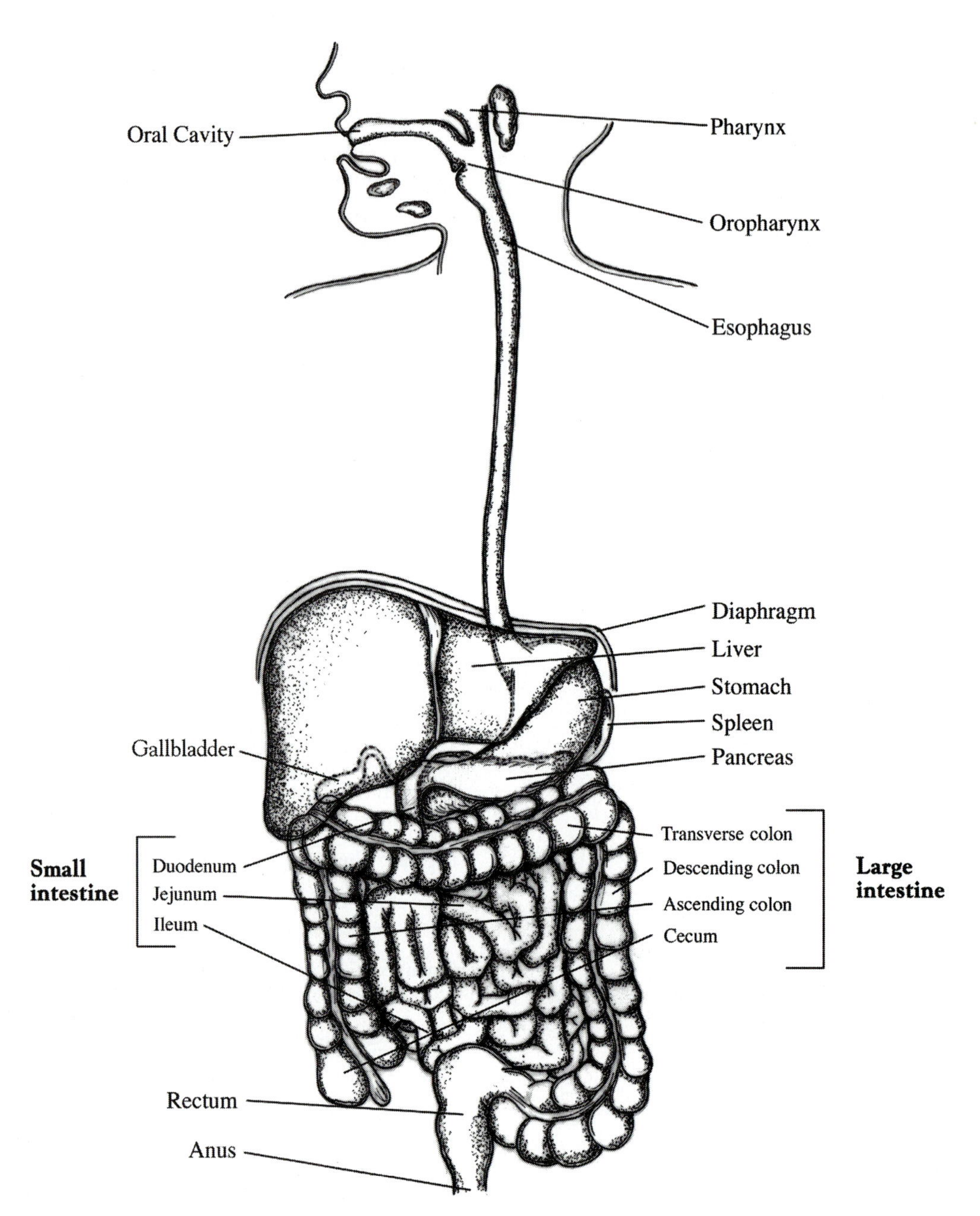

Figure 28–1. The gastrointestinal tract.

Gastrointestinal Wall

The gastrointestinal wall is comprised of four major layers. These layers, from the inside out, are the mucosa, submucosa, muscularis, and serosa (Fig. 28–2). The outermost layer is called the **serosa.** The serosa is derived from the visceral peritoneum, as it adheres to the visceral organs of the abdomen. The serosa secretes mucus, which prevents friction between the abdominal organs. The **muscularis** is a muscular layer, providing the rhythmic contraction needed to mechanically break down food, mix it with enzymes, and propel it through the GI tract. The next layer, the **submucosa,** contains loose, connective tissue and elastic fibers, blood vessels, and lymphatic vessels. The submucosa also contains one plexus of the enteric nervous system (Meissner's nerve plexus), a part of the autonomic nervous system (Andreoli et al., 1997; Wilson & Lindseth, 1996).

The **mucosa,** the innermost layer, absorbs both nutrients and fluids and receives the majority of the blood supply. The mucosa contains specialized cells throughout the GI tract whose function varies depending on the anatomic location. These cells mostly secrete mucus or digestive enzymes to aid in the passage or digestion of food (Gray, 1995; Guyton, 1996). In critical illness, the integrity of the mucosa can break down as a result of

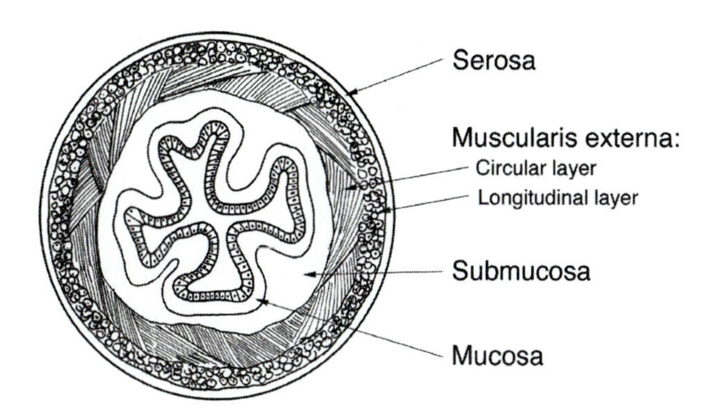

Figure 28–2. Cross-section of the gut wall.

trauma, hypoperfusion, stress, medications, or surgery. The result of the impaired mucosal integrity can be bleeding, inflammation, and infection.

The **peritoneum,** the largest serous membrane in the body, consists of a visceral and a parietal layer. The parietal peritoneum lines the wall of the abdominal cavity. The visceral peritoneum covers most of the abdominal organs and constitutes their serosa. The peritoneum contains large folds that weave in and out between the organs. These folds function to bind the organs to each other and contain the blood vessels, lymph tissue, and the nerves that supply the abdominal organs. The potential space between the visceral and parietal layers of the peritoneum is called the *peritoneal space*. Inflammation of the peritoneum is called *peritonitis*. One of the most important functions of the peritoneum is to prevent friction between contiguous organs.

The **mesentery** is the large outward fold of peritoneum that suspends the small intestine to the abdominal wall. It functions to bind the small intestine to the abdominal wall and facilitates intestinal motility while supporting blood vessels, nerves, and lymphatics. Impaired blood flow through the mesentery can result in intestinal ischemia. This can occur due to shock in critically ill patients (Bucher & Melander, 1999).

Gastric Enzymes

The primary function of the GI tract is digestion of food and absorption of nutrients. The cardiac (proximal) and pyloric (distal) sphincters of the stomach control the rate of food passage through the GI tract. Secretion of gastric enzymes is necessary for digestion. Enzymes are secreted by the cardiac and fundic glands, which are located in the stomach. The cardiac glands secrete mucus, a lubricant and a mucosal barrier from acids. The fundic glands consist of the chief cells and the parietal cells. The chief cells secrete pepsinogen, which converts to its active form (pepsin) in an acid environment. Pepsin is necessary for protein digestion. Parietal cells secrete (1) hydrochloric acid, which lowers pH and kills bacteria, and (2) intrinsic factor, which is necessary for vitamin B_{12} absorption. Gastrin, a hormonal regulator produced by cells located in the pyloric region of the stomach, stimulates the gastric glands to produce the hydrochloric acid and pepsinogen (Wilson & Lindseth, 1996; Guyton & Hall, 1997).

Small Intestine

The small intestine extends from the pylorus to the ileocecal valve and consists of the duodenum, the jejunum, and the ileum (see Fig. 28–1). Its primary function is absorption of nutrients and water. The mucosa and submucosal layers of the small intestine are arranged in folds, which actually project out into the lumen of the intestine. These folds function to slow the passage of **chyme** through the small intestine in order to allow more time for digestion and absorption to occur. Fingerlike projections covering the intestinal folds are called **villi.** Each individual villus is covered with tiny absorptive fingerlike projections called microvilli. The villi and the microvilli collectively make up the brush border of the small intestine. The folds, villi, and microvilli greatly increase the absorptive surface of the small intestine. The villi contain two cell types: (1) goblet cells, which produce mucus, and (2) absorptive cells (microvilli), which are responsible for absorption of nutrients. The villi also produce digestive enzymes along the brush border which complete the process of digestion as absorption takes place (see Fig. 28–3). Diseases of the small intestine that cause atrophy and flattening of the brush border greatly reduce the surface area for absorption, resulting in malabsorption (Wilson & Lindseth, 1996; Markey, 1999).

The small intestine secretes hormones that have both stimulatory and inhibitory effects necessary in the regulation of intestinal digestion. Remember, the gastric pH is acidic. When acidic chyme comes into contact with the duodenal mucosa, hormones are secreted that regulate the digestive process. These hormones include cholecystokinin, secretin, and gastric inhibitory peptide. **Cholecystokinin (CCK)** is secreted in response to the presence of fat, protein, and an acidic pH. The role of cholecystokinin is to (1) stimulate the release of pancreatic digestive enzymes necessary for the digestion of protein and fat, (2) increase the contractility of the gallbladder so that bile is released into the duodenum to aid in the absorption of fats, and (3) inhibit gastric motility in order to slow things down a little so that digestion and absorption can take place. Gastric acid in contact with the intestinal mucosa causes the release of another hormone, **secretin.** Secretin stimulates the release of pancreatic bicarbonate and water ("pancreatic juice"). Pancreatic juice is alkaline and therefore functions to increase the pH of the chyme within the duodenum. Pancreatic digestive enzymes are active only in an alkaline environment. **Gastric inhibitory peptide (GIP)** is another hor-

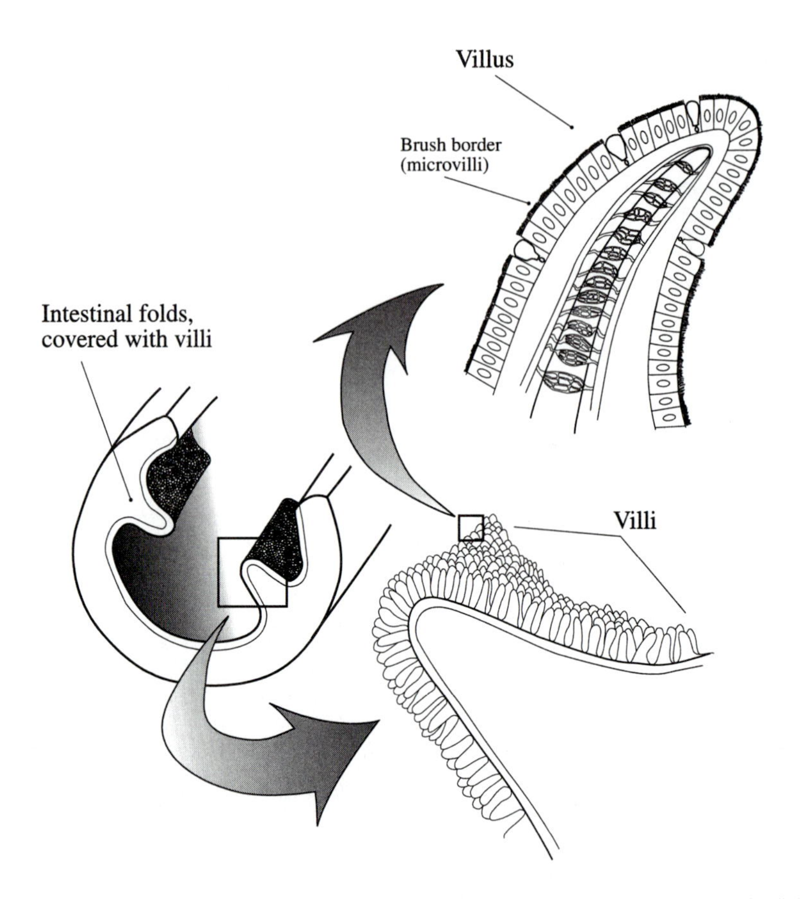

Figure 28–3. Cross-section of small intestine. This cross-section of the intestinal wall shows an intestinal fold covered with villi from three different magnifications.

mone secreted by the small intestine to facilitate the digestion of carbohydrates and fats. GIP is secreted in response to the presence of carbohydrates and fats within the small intestine. GIP inhibits motility, and the secretion of gastric acid. Furthermore, GIP stimulates insulin secretion. The inhibition of gastric acid is to maintain a basic pH environment, necessary for the pancreatic proteolytic enzymes to metabolize proteins and fats. The inhibition of gastric motility aids absorption by decreasing transit time. See Table 28–1 for a summary of the hormones.

Large Intestine

The large intestine is a hollow, muscular tube, extending from the terminal ileum at the ileocecal valve to the anus (approximately 5 feet in length). The main functions of the large intestine are the completion of water and nutrient absorption, the manufacture of certain vitamins, the formation of feces, and the expulsion of feces from the body. The large intestine is divided into the cecum, colon, and rectum (see Fig. 28–1). The cecum lies below the ileocecal valve, which controls the flow of chyme from the ileum of the small intestine into the cecum. This valve also prevents backflow of fecal material from the large intestine into the small intestine. The opposite end of the cecum joins with the colon. The colon is divided into four portions: ascending, transverse, descending, and sigmoid. The absorption of water and electrolytes is largely

TABLE 28–1. INTESTINAL HORMONES

HORMONE	ACTION
Secretin—secreted in response to acidic chyme and alcohol entering the duodenum	Stimulates release of pancreatic bicarbonate and water Stimulates release of bile Potentiates the action of CCK
Cholecystokinin (CCK)—secreted in response to the presence of fat, protein, and acidic chyme	Stimulates release of pancreatic digestive enzymes Increases contractility of gallbladder Inhibits gastric motility
Gastric inhibitory peptide (GIP)—secreted in response to carbohydrates and fat	Inhibits gastric acid secretion and motility Stimulates insulin secretion

Sources: Wilson, L.M., & Lindseth, G.N. (1997). Disorders of the small intestine. In S.A. Price & L.M. Wilson (eds), Pathophysiology: Clinical concepts of disease processes, *5th ed. St. Louis: C.V. Mosby; and Guyton, A.C., & Hall, J.E. (1997).* Human physiology and mechanisms of disease, *6th ed. (pp. 530–531). Philadelphia: W.B. Saunders.*

completed in the ascending colon. In fact, the colon absorbs approximately 1,000 mL/day of water and electrolytes (Smith, 1998). The last portion of the large intestine is the rectum. The rectum extends from the sigmoid colon to the anus, which is the opening to the outside of the body. The anus is regulated by internal and external sphincter muscles (Guyton & Hall, 1997).

The wall of the large intestine differs from the wall of the small intestines. The mucosal layer of the large intestine is thicker and contains no villi or folds. The mucosa of the large intestine contains more mucus-producing goblet cells than does the mucosa of the small intestine. The mucus facilitates the passage of fecal contents through the colon by lubricating and protecting the mucosa (Guyton & Hall, 1997).

The digestion that does occur in the large intestine results from bacterial rather than enzymatic action. The normal flora bacteria that reside within the large intestine break down dietary cellulose and synthesize folic acid, vitamin K, riboflavin, and nicotinic acid.

The movements of the large intestine are called haustral churning. These movements are slow and cause the intestinal contents to move back and forth in a kneading action, thus allowing time for absorption to occur. As the rectal wall becomes full of stool and distends, the defecation reflex is initiated.

SECTION ONE REVIEW

1. The innermost layer of the GI tract which is responsible for secretion of mucus and enzymes is the
   A. submucosa
   B. muscularis
   C. mucosa
   D. mesentery
2. The _______ line(s) the wall of the abdominal cavity.
   A. peritoneum
   B. mucosa
   C. microvilli
   D. brush border
3. Parietal cells secrete
   A. gastrin
   B. pepsinogen
   C. hydrochloric acid
   D. mucus
4. CCK is secreted in response to
   A. fats, acidic pH, protein
   B. alkaline pH, secretin, protein
   C. fats, carbohydrates, alkaline pH
   D. acidic pH, secretin, carbohydrates
5. Absorption of water and electrolytes takes place in the
   A. transverse colon
   B. descending colon
   C. sigmoid colon
   D. ascending colon

Answers: 1. C, 2. A, 3. C, 4. A, 5. D

SECTION TWO: Blood Supply and Nervous System Innervation of the GI Tract

At the completion of this section, the learner will be able to discuss factors influencing circulation to the GI tract and describe the neurologic control of the GI tract.

The GI system receives about one-fourth of the resting cardiac output, more than any other organ system (Hudak, Gallo, & Morton, 1998). The organs of the abdomen are known as *viscera.* The term *splanchnic* refers to the viscera. The combination of the portal and mesenteric circulatory systems is called the **splanchnic circulation.** The splanchnic circulatory system includes blood flow through the **gut,** spleen, pancreas, and liver (Guyton & Hall, 1997) (see Fig. 28–4).

Arterial Blood Supply to the Intestines

The arterial blood supply to the mesentery and the intestines is called the **mesenteric circulation,** a part of the extensive splanchnic circulation. The mesenteric circulation begins its flow at the aorta, flowing through the aortic arch to the celiac artery and the superior and inferior mesenteric arteries. Arteries that branch off of the larger celiac artery supply blood to the stomach, esophagus, duodenum, gallbladder, pancreas, and spleen. The superior mesenteric artery supplies arterial blood to the small intestine, the ascending colon, and part of the transverse colon. The inferior mesenteric artery supplies the remainder of the transverse colon, the descending colon, sigmoid colon, and the rectum (Krumberger, 1998; Guyton & Hall, 1997). Table 28–2 summarizes the arterial blood supply to the gut via the branches of the celiac artery and the superior and inferior mesenterics.

Venous Drainage

Venous drainage from the GI tract and the liver passes through the portal vein system (see Module 29, Fig. 29–3). Venous drainage passes through the inferior vena cava and

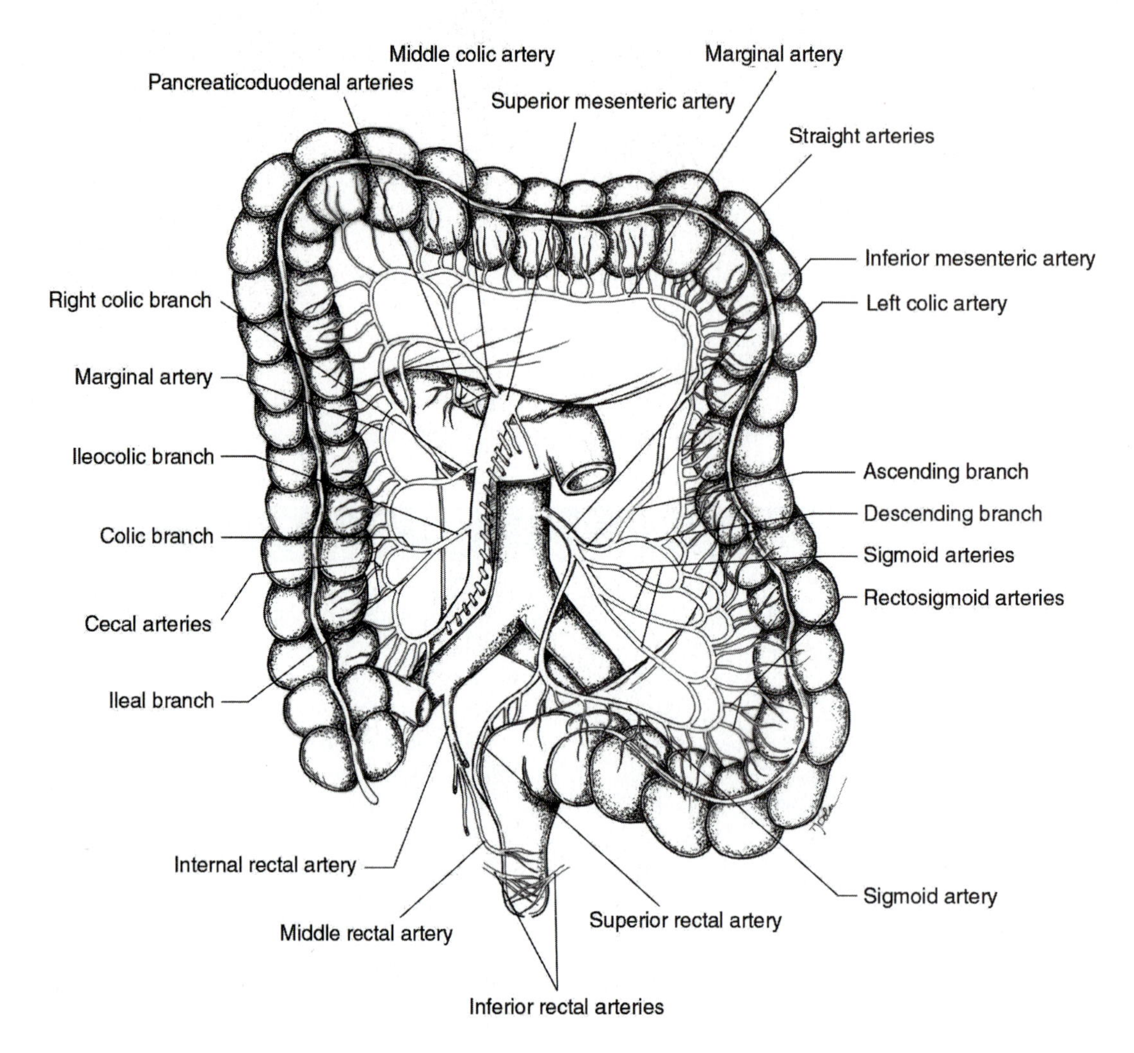

Figure 28–4. Blood supply to the gut. Arterial and venous blood supplies to the primary and accessory organs of the GI system.

the external iliac vein. Table 28–3 summarizes the veins that branch off from the portal vein and the specific sites from which they drain (Guyton & Hall, 1997; Hudak, Gallo, & Morton, 1998; Krumberger, 1998; Markey, 1999).

TABLE 28–2. ARTERIAL BLOOD SUPPLY

ARTERY (BRANCH OF CELIAC)	AREA SUPPLIED WITH BLOOD
Left gastric	Stomach and esophagus
Hepatic to right gastric	Stomach
Gastroduodenal	Duodenum, gallbladder, stomach
Cystic	Gallbladder
Splenic	Stomach, spleen, pancreas
Superior mesenteric	Ascending colon, cecum, ileum, jejunum, transverse colon
Inferior mesenteric	Rectum, sigmoid colon, transverse colon

Adapted from Krumberger, J.M. (1998). Gastrointestinal clinical physiology. In M.R. Kinney et al. (eds.), AACN's clinical reference for critical care nursing, *4th ed. (p. 985). St. Louis: C.V. Mosby.*

Sympathetic stimulation directly affects the splanchnic circulation by causing vasoconstriction of the arterioles within the gut wall, resulting in a decrease in blood flow. Prolonged vasoconstriction, as occurs in shock states or with high doses of vasopressor drugs, can lead to ischemia and ulceration of the gut mucosal lining. The breakdown in the integrity of the intestinal walls results

TABLE 28–3. PORTAL VEIN BRANCHES AND THEIR DRAINAGE SITES

PORTAL VEIN BRANCH	DRAINAGE SITE
Gastric	Esophagus, stomach
Splenic	Duodenum, esophagus, gallbladder, stomach, pancreas
Superior mesenteric	Ascending and transverse colon, small intestine
Inferior mesenteric	Descending and sigmoid colon, rectum

Source: Krumberger, J.M. (1998). Gastrointestinal clinical physiology. In M.R. Kinney et al. (eds.) AACN's clinical reference for critical care nursing, *4th ed. St. Louis: C.V. Mosby.*

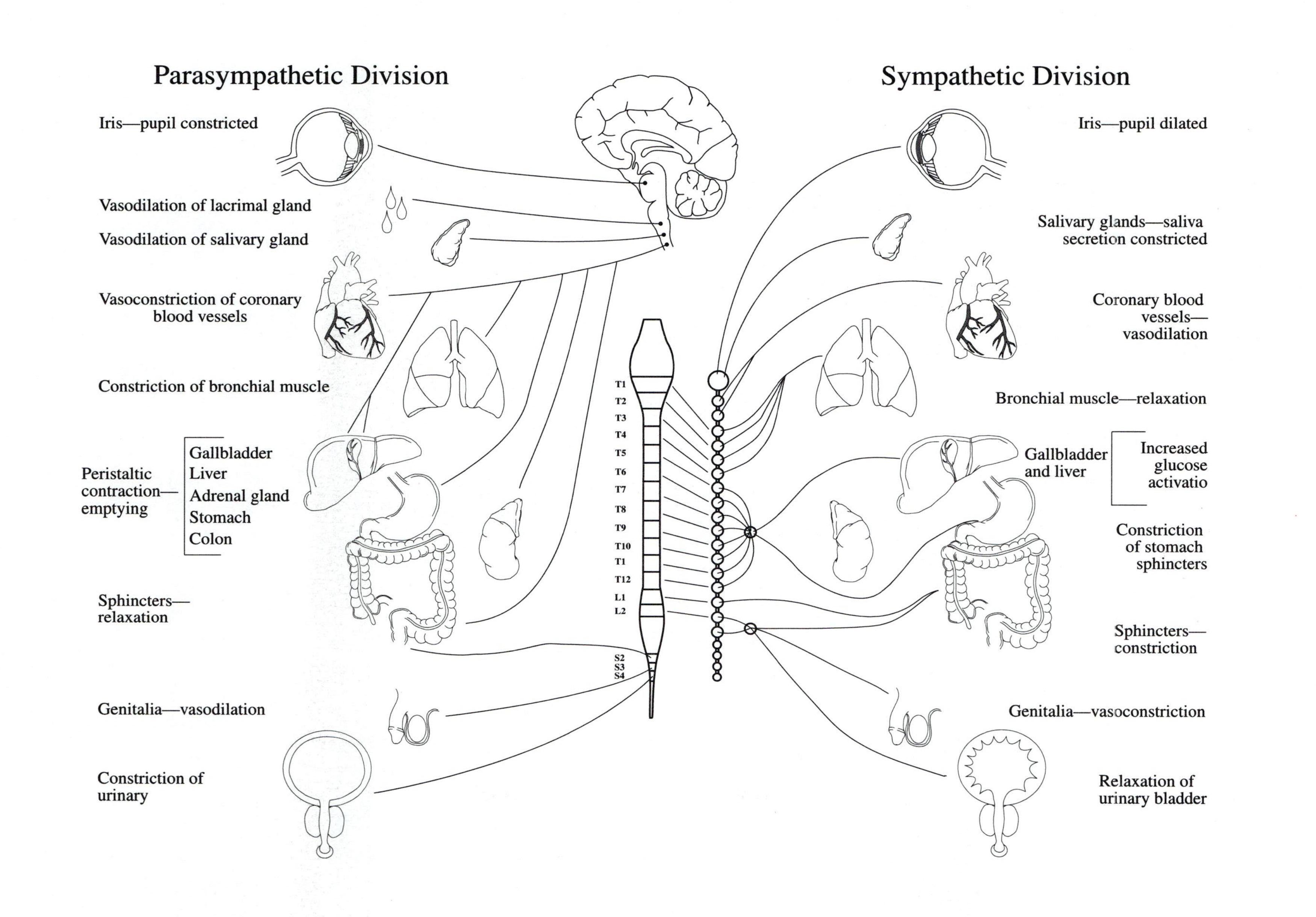

Figure 28–5. Parasympathetic and sympathetic divisions of the autonomic nervous system.

in an inability to serve as a barrier against bacteria and foreign toxins. Gram-negative bacteria from within the intestines can translocate through the damaged mucosal lining to the general circulation, resulting in sepsis. Ulceration of the mucosal barrier can lead to ulcers and GI bleeding (Guyton & Hall, 1995; Heitkemper & Westfall, 1993; Hudak, Gallo, & Morton, 1998; Markey, 1999).

Innervation of the GI Tract

The stomach receives its nerve supply from the autonomic nervous system, which can be further divided into the extrinsic and intrinsic nervous systems.

Extrinsic Nervous System

The extrinsic nervous system consists of the parasympathetic and sympathetic systems. Parasympathetic fibers arise from the medulla and spinal segments (vagus nerves). This parasympathetic system (1) enhances GI functions by secretion of the neurotransmitter acetylcholine, (2) increases glandular secretion and muscle tone, and (3) decreases sphincter tone. The net result of parasympathetic stimulation is increased propulsion of contents through the GI tract. The sympathetic motor and sensory fibers arise from the thoracic and lumbar segments of the spinal cord with distribution via the sympathetic ganglia (celiac plexus). Sympathetic fibers run alongside the blood vessels secreting the neurotransmitter norepinephrine. Stimulation of the sympathetic nervous system inhibits activity in the GI tract, causing effects essentially opposite to those of the parasympathetic stimulation (inhibits peristalsis and increases sphincter tone). The net result of sympathetic stimulation is greatly slowed propulsion of contents through the GI tract (Hudak, Gallo, & Morton, 1998; Smith, 1998). Figure 28–5 compares the sympathetic and parasympathetic nervous systems.

Intrinsic Nervous System

The GI tract also has an intrinsic nervous system, known as the enteric nervous system, which coordinates GI motility and secretion. The enteric nervous system is considered the third component of the autonomic nervous system. It consists of two networks located within the wall of the GI tract: the myenteric (Auerbach's) plexus and the submucosal (Meissner's) plexus (Fig. 28–6). The myenteric plexus influences muscle tone, contractions, velocity, and excitation of the stomach. The submucosal plexus influences secretions of the stomach (Guyton & Hall, 1997; Smith, 1998).

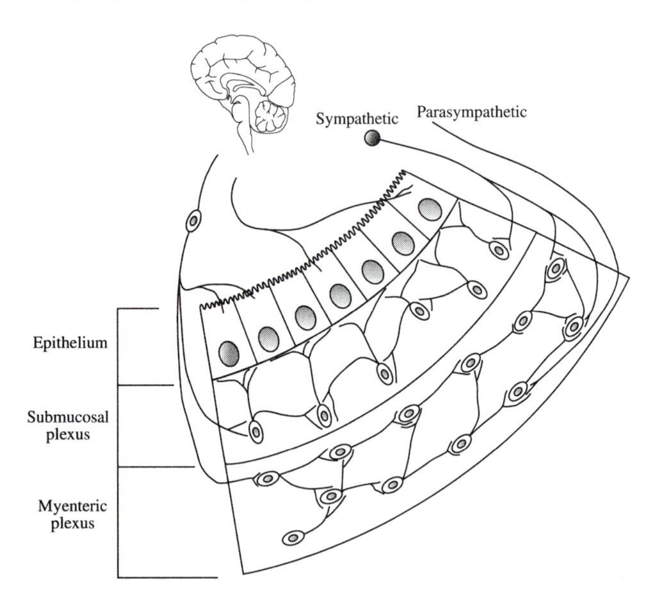

Figure 28–6. Neural control of the gut wall.

SECTION TWO REVIEW

1. The mesenteric circulation begins its flow at the
   A. celiac artery
   B. hepatic artery
   C. aorta
   D. superior vena cava
2. The portal venous system drains the GI tract and the
   A. spleen
   B. liver
   C. pancreas
   D. kidneys
3. Sympathetic stimulation of the splanchnic circulation results in
   A. vasoconstriction of the arterioles within the gut wall
   B. vasodilation of the arterioles within the gut wall
   C. translocation of bacteria across the gut wall
   D. ulceration of the gut wall mucosa
4. The portal venous system includes the
   A. superior vena cava and the external iliac vein
   B. inferior vena cava and the external portal vein
   C. superior vena cava and the inferior celiac vein
   D. inferior vena cava and the external iliac vein
5. The Meissner's (submucosal) plexus influences
   A. muscle tone
   B. stomach secretions
   C. muscle contractions
   D. stomach excitation

Answers: 1. C, 2. B, 3. A, 4. D, 5. B

SECTION THREE: Gut Defenses

At the completion of this section, the learner will be able to describe the mechanisms that exist within the GI tract to protect the integrity of the gut.

When food is ingested, so are foreign antigens and microorganisms. Simply licking the lips or placing the fingers into the mouth allows multitudes of bacteria to gain entry into the GI tract. Because of its easy accessibility to potentially pathologic organisms, the GI system must play a major role in the body's defense against bacteria, parasites, and other toxic pathogens. The GI system has two major mechanisms of defense: nonimmunologic and immunologic.

Nonimmunologic Defense Mechanisms

Nonimmunologic defense mechanisms are those provided by salivary secretions, gastric acid, peristalsis, mucous coat, and commensal bacteria. Food enters the mouth, where it comes into contact with saliva. Saliva contains substances that are active against foreign antigens and bacteria ingested with the food. Pathogenic microorganisms surviving the mouth pass along to the stomach, where the effects of the gastric acidity ($pH < 4.0$) create an environment that is unfavorable to pathogen growth. The acid environment inhibits bacteria from entering the small intestine, where the pH must remain basic (pH of ≥ 7.0) in order for the pancreatic proteolytic enzymes to become active and participate in the digestive process. Offending organisms that survive the gastric acidic environment have difficulty adhering to the epithelial surface of the GI tract in order to colonize and invade the gut wall. This difficulty in attachment to the epithelial surface is partly due to the tight junctions that exist between the epithelial mucosal cells, preventing colonization and invasion. Peristaltic motility further inhibits pathogen attachment to the gut mucosa by pushing contents along, decreasing contact time needed by the pathogens to colonize. Continuous peristalsis movement prevents stagnation of chyme and reflux of duodenal contents back up into the stomach (Guyton & Hall, 1997; Markey, 1999; Smith, 1998).

Further mechanical resistance to offending pathogenic invaders is provided by the overlying mucous coat covering the epithelial surface. Goblet cells within the submucosa of the GI tract secrete mucus which covers the intestinal surface, providing a physical barrier to the passage of potential pathogens. The mucous coat may actually facilitate the removal of these microorganisms by allowing them to "slide through" the GI tract.

Commensal or indigenous bacteria are the normal flora existing within the ileum and large intestine that limit proliferation and adherence of potentially pathologic bacteria. *Bacteroides fragilis* is the main anaerobic bacteria, and *Escherichia coli* is the main aerobic bacteria that prevent overgrowth of other gram-negative and gram-positive bacteria. These normal flora are stable and protective in healthy persons. They break down cellulose and synthesize vitamin K, folic acid, riboflavin, and nicotinic acid. They limit pathologic infections by competing with nutrients, adhesion sites, and producing inhibitory fatty acids within the epithelium (Markey, 1999). The stomach, duodenum, and jejunum are sterile.

Immunologic Defense Mechanisms

The immunologic defenses are provided by the gut-associated lymphoid tissue (GALT). "Approximately 25% of the intestinal mucosa is lymphoid tissue and 70 to 80% of all immunologic secreting cells are within the intestinal wall, making the GI tract a major immune organ within the body" (Markey, 1999). GALT includes the tonsils, lymph tissue within the intestinal wall, and the appendix. The tonsils are strategically located to intercept airborne and ingested pathogens. **Peyer's patches** are nodules of lymph tissue located on the outer wall of the intestines. The appendix is a blind tube about the size of the little finger located in the ileocecal region of the small intestine. These tissues include T-helper cells (of the CD4 type), B cells, plasma cells, mucosal mast cells (goblet cells), and macrophages that respond to gastrointestinal pathogens. Immunoglobulins produced by GALT migrate to the GI tract, tear ducts, and salivary glands to defend against pathogen penetration of epithelial surfaces (Guyton & Hall, 1997; Sommers, 1997).

Mechanisms That Maintain Mucosal Integrity

Superficial epithelial cells secrete mucus and bicarbonate, which aid in maintaining a pH gradient between the lumen and the mucosa to protect the underlying epithelial tissues from damage by gastric acid and pepsin. Mucosal blood flow is also believed to be an important mechanism to maintain mucosal integrity (Andreoli et al., 1997; Guyton & Hall, 1997) (see Fig. 28–7).

Trauma, shock, intestinal obstruction, protein malnutrition, and parenteral nutritional therapy can all cause disruption of the intestinal mucosal integrity. When patients are treated with total parenteral nutrition (TPN), it has been observed that the lack of enteral stimulation results in mucosal atrophy and bacterial overgrowth. Impaired gut barrier function facilitates bacterial translocation of bacteria across the mucosal barrier and into the lymphatic vessels and portal circulation. This potentially pathologic bacterium may enter the systemic circulation and cause sepsis. Intestinal bacteria have been observed to cause systemic disease in immunodeficient patients, such as the critically ill (Andreoli et al., 1997; Hudak, Gallo, & Morton, 1998; Smith, 1998).

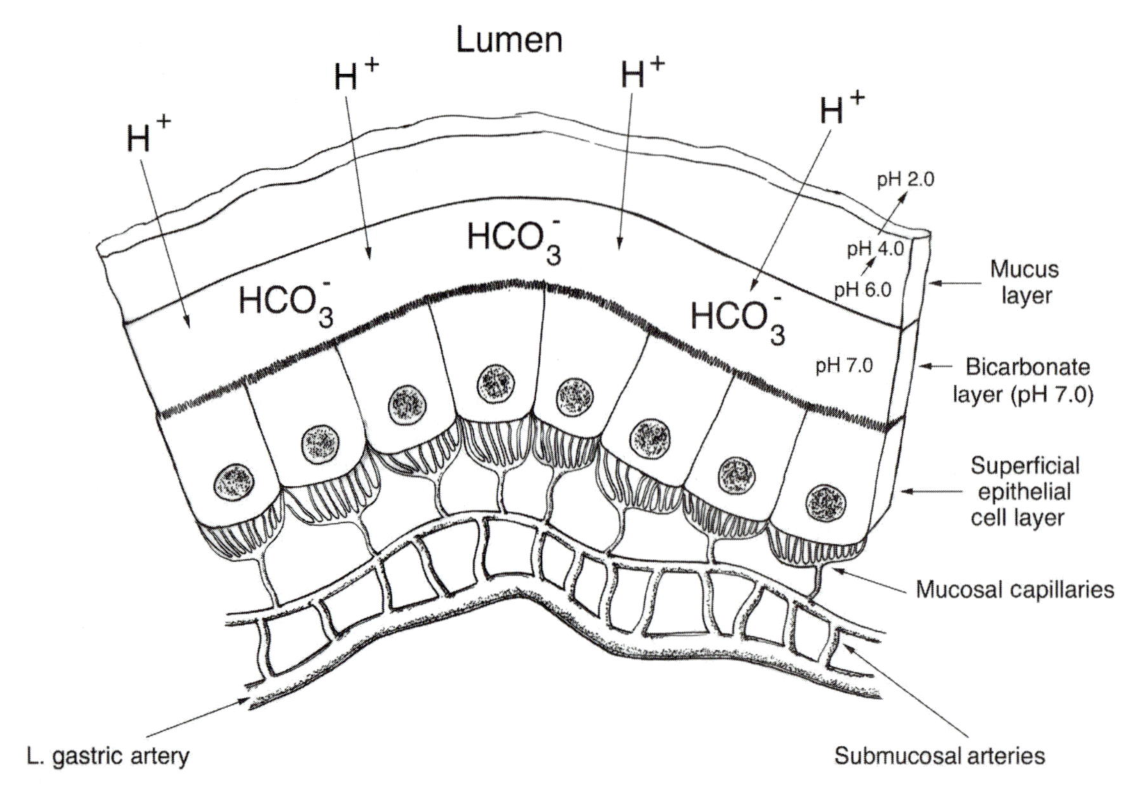

Figure 28–7. Mechanisms maintaining mucosal integrity. Superficial epithelial cells secrete mucus and bicarbonate, which aid in maintaining a pH gradient between lumen and mucosa, and protect the underlying epithelial cells from damage by acid and pepsin. Mucosal blood flow is also believed to be a mechanism important in maintaining mucosal integrity.

SECTION THREE REVIEW

1. Commensal bacteria are a part of the gut's
   A. enteric defense mechanism
   B. nonimmunologic defense mechanism
   C. gut-associated lymphatic tissue
   D. immunologic defense mechanism
2. Peristalsis promotes gastrointestinal health by
   A. pushing intestinal contents along the GI tract and preventing reflux
   B. creating an acid environment that is unfavorable to pathogen growth
   C. secreting substances active against foreign antigens
   D. covering the epithelial surface with mucus
3. The mucous coat
   A. maintains an acid environment
   B. activates protective digestive enzymes
   C. provides a physical barrier against invasion by pathogens
   D. interferes with bacterial replication
4. Goblet cells secrete
   A. gastrin
   B. hydrochloric acid
   C. secretin
   D. mucus
5. The initial nonimmunologic defense mechanism that is active against antigens is provided by
   A. salivary secretions
   B. intestinal peristalsis
   C. *Escherichia coli* bacteria
   D. Peyer's patches

Answers: 1. B, 2. A, 3. C, 4. D, 5. A

SECTION FOUR: Laboratory and Diagnostic Studies

At the completion of this section, the learner will be able to describe the laboratory and diagnostic tests utilized in the management of acute GI problems.

Laboratory Findings

Laboratory tests used to make a differential diagnosis in GI bleeding and acute abdominal pain include electrolytes, end products of metabolism, enzymes, hematology, and arterial blood gases (ABGs). They are summarized in Table 28–4.

Electrolyte levels that should be monitored with GI dysfunction include calcium, chloride, magnesium, potassium, and sodium. These electrolytes are primarily absorbed by the small intestine and may be depleted, or increased with gastrointestinal disorders (e.g., potassium loss occurs with diarrhea and vomiting). Blood urea nitrogen (BUN) elevation (> 40 mg/dL) in the absence of underlying renal disease, as evidenced by a normal serum creatinine, may indicate significant blood loss (loss of two or more units of blood). Furthermore, an elevated BUN/creatinine ratio may occur in upper GI bleeding and volume depletion due to hemoconcentration from a fluid volume deficit. Bowel obstruction can cause azotemia because stasis of intestinal contents within the intestines allows more digestion to take place, which produces more by-products of protein metabolism. Following a GI bleed, old blood may be within the intestines. When there is blood present, digestion of the blood cells takes place and results in the production of by-products of metabolism, thus raising the BUN (Andreoli et al., 1997; Haist, Robbins, & Gorwella, 1997; Hudak, Gallo, & Morton, 1998; Kee, 1999; McQuaid, 1999).

Aspartate aminotransferase (AST) and lactic dehydrogenase (LDH) may be elevated in liver disease. Elevated AST and LDH levels may be significant in the

TABLE 28–4. LABORATORY TESTS

TEST	NORMAL VALUES	COMMENTS
Electrolytes		
Calcium	Total, 4.5–5.5 mEq/L Ionized, 4.4–5.0 mg/dL	Absorbed by the small intestine and may be lost, depleted, or increased with GI disorders
Chloride	95–105 mEq/L	
Magnesium	1.5–2.5 mEq/L	
Potassium	3.5–5.3 mEq/L	
Sodium	135–145 mEq/L	
Chemistry		
Blood urea nitrogen	5–25 mg/dL	Bowel obstruction can cause azotemia; lactic acid is elevated in bowel infarction and metabolic acidosis
Lactic acid	Arterial: 0.5–2.0 mEq/L Venous: 0.5–2.0 mEq/L	
Enzymes		
Alkaline phosphatase	20–90 U/L	Found in bone, intestine, and liver, and released with destruction of those tissues
Amylase	25–125 U/L	Elevated in peptic ulcer disease, intestinal obstruction, mesenteric thrombosis, and after abdominal surgery
Hematologic		
Complete blood count with differential		Hct, Hgb are decreased with GI bleeding and with malabsorption; with acute blood loss, Hct may not decrease for several hours
Hemoglobin	M: 14–18 g/dL F: 12–16 g/dL	
Hematocrit	M: 40–54% F: 37–47%	
White blood cells	4,500–10,000/mm^3	White blood cell count elevated with infection, and inflammation
Arterial blood gases	pH 7.35–7.45 $Paco_2$ 35–45 mm Hg Pao_2 80–100 mm Hg Sao_2 > 95% HCO_3 22–26 mEq/L BE +2 to −2 mEq/L	Metabolic acidosis may result from ischemic bowel
***Helicobacter* antibodies**	Negative	Used to detect *Helicobacter pylori* infection in peptic ulcer disease

Sources: Hudak, C.M., Gallo, B.M., Morton, P.G. (1998). Critical care nursing: A holistic approach, *7th ed. Philadelphia: J.B. Lippincott; Kee, J. (1999).* Laboratory diagnostic tests with nursing implications, *5th ed. Stamford, CT: Appleton & Lange; McQuaid, K.R. (1999). Alimentary tract. In L.M. Tierney, S.J. McPhee, & M.A. Papadakis (eds.),* Current medical diagnosis and treatment, *3rd ed. Stamford, CT: Appleton & Lange; and Westfall, U.E. (1999). Gastrointestinal laboratory and diagnostic tests. In L. Buchee & S. Melander (eds.),* Critical care nursing. *Philadelphia: W.B. Saunders.*

presence of GI bleeding since liver dysfunction may contribute to GI bleeding (see Module 29). Alkaline phosphatase elevations occur with intestinal, liver, and bone tissue injury. Serum amylase elevations occur with pancreatitis, peptic ulcer disease (PUD), small bowel obstruction, and ischemic bowel.

Hematologic levels, which may be abnormal in gastrointestinal bleeding, include serum hematocrit (Hct) and hemoglobin (Hgb). Serial measures are most helpful. However, in acute hemorrhage, the Hct may not reflect the amount of blood loss. Prior to fluid resuscitation, the Hct may be higher than one would expect secondary to hemoconcentration from volume loss. The Hct may fall precipitously after aggressive fluid resuscitation due to hemodilution effects. It takes 24 to 72 hours for the Hct to equilibrate with the extravascular fluid following administration of large amounts of fluids or blood products (Haist, Robbins, & Gorwella, 1997). Platelets may be increased or decreased with GI bleeding. A prolonged prothrombin time (PT) and partial thromboplastin time (PTT) can make stabilization of the patient with a GI bleed very challenging. Platelets and clotting factors are also lost with rapid bleeding. It is important to evaluate PT and PTT levels in order to determine requirements for replacement of clotting factors. A decreased mean corpuscular volume (MCV) suggests the possibility of iron-deficiency anemia secondary to chronic GI blood loss.

Elevations in the WBC suggests an inflammatory or infectious process. This can occur with peptic ulcer with perforation, and with ischemic bowel.

ABG measures are useful to evaluate respiratory status and pH deviations. Hypoxemia is an early sign of sepsis. Metabolic acidosis may result from sepsis, ischemic bowel, or peptic ulcer perforation. Decreased oxygen-carrying capacity, secondary to acute blood loss, is a common complication from severe upper GI hemorrhage.

Helicobacter antibodies may be detected in the serum of persons with *H. pylori* infection. *H. pylori* infection is associated with PUD and will be discussed further in another section of this module.

Diagnostic Studies

Both noninvasive and invasive tests are used to diagnose GI disorders. X-ray exam or flat plate of the abdomen is helpful in diagnosing intra-abdominal problems such as intestinal obstruction, rupture, masses, abnormal fluid/air levels, and foreign bodies. Upper GI series with contrast medium is another type of x-ray exam, which allows visualization of the GI tract in order to diagnose tumors, masses, hernias, obstructions, ulcers, fistulas, or diverticular disease. The patient must ingest a contrast material, usually barium, prior to the actual x-ray. The contrast medium allows visualization of any abnormalities. It is important to ask about the client's allergy history prior to administration of the contrast medium in order to prevent serious allergic reactions. Furthermore, it is important to assist the patient in expelling the contrast (barium).

Computed tomographic (CT) scan is another test allowing visualization of the abdomen, retroperitoneal structures, masses, abscesses, and abnormal fluid/air levels, which might be visible if perforation has occurred. This exam requires the person to ingest a barium contrast solution prior to the exam.

Ultrasound sonography allows visualization of abdominal and retroperitoneal soft tissue structures to diagnose fluid/air pockets, abscesses, masses, and to observe movement. This procedure may be done at the bedside. Transducing gel is applied to the skin, and mild pressure is applied with a transducer. Adipose tissue, air, and barium may diminish ultrasound wave transmission.

Magnetic resonance imaging (MRI) is useful to assess abdominal and retroperitoneal structures for masses, abscesses, and fluid/air pockets. All external metal objects and dental appliances must be removed. Internal metal objects or foreign bodies are a contraindication to MRI. It is very important that the patient lie still for this test and therefore he or she must be able to cooperate.

Nuclear scan allows visualization of organs, gastrointestinal motility, and bleeding. An intravenous contrast medium is administered, making allergic reactions a risk with this test; therefore, an allergy history should be obtained. Nuclear scan is contraindicated in pregnancy, breast-feeding, or recent nuclear exposure. All metal must be removed from these patients also. Nonuniform radioactive uptake in tissues often indicates disease.

Angiography allows visualization of blood flow in selected vascular beds. Bleeding vessels can be identified with this test. A contrast medium is administered intravenously; therefore, allergy history is important (Westfall, 1999).

A series of diagnostic tests for the GI system called endoscopies use fiber-optic light and a lens system. This light allows inspection of internal surfaces of organs. Removal of tissue for testing (biopsy), as well as some treatments such as sclerotherapy, suction, and cauterization of bleeding vessels, may be performed during endoscopy of the upper or lower GI tract. Endoscopic exam of the upper GI tract, known as esophagogastroduodenoscopy (EGD) can include inspection of structures from the mouth to the ligament of Treitz (the junction of the duodenum and jejunum) to diagnose source of bleeding, or ulceration of the GI tract mucosa. Colonoscopy allows inspection of the large intestine to identify a lower GI bleeding source or other disease (McQuaid, 1999; Westfall, 1999). Common endoscopic tests are summarized in Table 28–5.

TABLE 28–5. ENDOSCOPIES OF THE GASTROINTESTINAL SYSTEM

TEST	INDICATIONS	CONTRAINDICATIONS
Esophagogastroduodenoscopy (EGD)	Visualization of upper GI tract for diagnosis or treatment; locate upper GI bleeding source	Cardiovascular and/or respiratory instability
Colonoscopy	Visualization of the large intestine for diagnosis or treatment; locate lower GI bleeding source	Perforation, peritonitis, recent bowel surgery, cardiovascular and/or respiratory compromise, inability of the patient to tolerate bowel prep
Proctoscopy, sigmoidoscopy, proctosigmoidoscopy, anoscopy	Visualization of sigmoid colon and rectal/anal mucosa for diagnosis or treatment; locate source of sigmoid, rectal, or anal bleeding	Perforation, infection, peritonitis, surgery, cardiovascular and/or respiratory compromise

Sources: McQuaid, K.R. (1999). Alimentary tract. In L.M. Tierney, S.J. McPhee, & M.A. Papadakis (eds.), Current medical diagnosis and treatment, *38th ed. Stamford, CT: Appleton & Lange; and Westfall, U.E. (1999). Gastrointestinal laboratory and diagnostic tests. In L. Buchee & S. Melander (eds.)* Critical care nursing. *Philadelphia: W.B. Saunders.*

Section Four Review

1. BUN is commonly elevated following a GI bleeding event. Which of the following best explains why this abnormal laboratory measure occurs?
   A. acute renal failure
   B. fluid volume overload
   C. metabolic acidosis
   D. hemoconcentration of the blood
2. BUN elevation (> 40 mg/dL), in the absence of underlying renal disease, may suggest
   A. loss of two or more units of blood
   B. impaired circulation to renal tissues
   C. significant fluid volume overload
   D. onset of acute renal failure
3. Bowel obstruction can cause a(n)
   A. elevated AST
   B. elevated BUN
   C. decreased LDH
   D. decreased MCV
4. *H. pylori* infection is associated with
   A. upper GI bleeding
   B. chronic lower GI bleeding
   C. liver disease
   D. PUD
5. _______ may contribute to GI bleeding.
   A. Pulmonary disease
   B. Hepatic dysfunction
   C. Autoimmune complications
   D. Connective tissue disease

Answers: 1. D, 2. A, 3. B, 4. D, 5. B

SECTION FIVE: Incidence and Clinical Manifestations of Acute GI Bleeding

Following the completion of this section, the learner will be able to describe the incidence of and clinical manifestations of acute GI bleeding.

Incidence

GI bleeding is a common clinical problem. The incidence per year of upper GI bleeding is 150 per 100,000 people (Huether, McCance, & Tarmina, 1994), with a mortality of 5 to 10 percent (Longstreth, 1995). GI bleeding can range in severity from a very slow occult blood loss to a sudden, massive hemorrhage. About 80 percent of acute GI bleeding stops without intervention, but some recurrent bleeding can become a life-threatening emergency (Andreoli et al., 1997; McQuaid, 1999). Upper GI bleeding, from vessels proximal to the ligament of Treitz, is more likely to produce arterial hemorrhage because of the large arterial blood supply needed for digestion, whereas lower GI bleeding is more commonly of venous origin. In persons with acute upper GI hemorrhage, comorbid or concurrent disease is the cause of death approximately 70 percent of the time. Patients with acute lower GI bleeding tend to be older than those with upper GI bleeding, have more concomitant medical problems, and experience increased morbidity. The mortality rate for acute lower GI bleeding is the same as for acute upper GI bleeding (Bono, 1996).

Clinical Manifestations

Gastrointestinal blood loss may be (1) acute (sudden or massive with hypovolemia) or (2) chronic (slow and often unnoticed by the patient). Blood that is present in the GI tract but not really visible is called *occult blood.* Occult bleeding is often detected by chemical testing of a stool or nasogastric specimen. This process is known as *hemoccult* or *guaiac testing.* Acute GI bleeding may present in one of several ways:

1. **Hematemesis**—vomiting of bright red blood or blood that looks like coffee grounds. This bleeding is often brisk, and is usually from an upper GI arterial source.
2. **Melena**—black, tarry, foul-smelling stools passed after a bleed of 100 to 500 mL of blood, usually from an upper GI source. However, a small intestine or right colon bleeding source may also be the cause.
3. **Hematochezia**—bright red blood or maroon stool from the rectum, usually due to lower GI bleeding or massive upper GI bleeding.

Clients with chronic GI bleeding often present with fatigue, dyspnea, syncope, angina, a positive fecal occult blood test, or iron-deficiency anemia (Andreoli et al., 1997; Haist, Robbins, & Gorwella, 1997; Krumberger, 1998).

SECTION FIVE REVIEW

1. The section of the GI tract that is involved in an upper GI hemorrhage is
   A. proximal to the ligament of Treitz
   B. proximal to the ileocecal valve
   C. distal to the pyloric sphincter
   D. distal to the duodenal bulb
2. The mortality rate for acute lower GI bleeding is
   A. twice as high as the mortality rate for acute upper GI bleeding
   B. less than the mortality rate for acute upper GI bleeding
   C. the same as the mortality rate for acute upper GI bleeding
   D. slightly higher than the mortality rate for acute upper GI bleeding
3. Characteristics of acute lower GI bleeding include
   A. bleeding is commonly arterial in origin
   B. bleeding is commonly of venous origin
   C. bleeding is massive 80 percent of the time
   D. bleeding is always occult
4. A client presents to the emergency department after vomiting bright red blood. The client becomes hypotensive soon after and is admitted into the hospital with GI bleeding. The presentation of this episode of bleeding is
   A. occult
   B. chronic
   C. subacute
   D. acute
5. Clients with occult GI bleeding often present with
   A. nausea and vomiting
   B. mental status changes
   C. headache and abdominal pain
   D. fatigue and syncope

Answers: 1. A, 2. C, 3. B, 4. D, 5. D

SECTION SIX: Acute Upper GI Bleeding

At the completion of this section, the learner will be able to describe the etiology and pathophysiology of acute upper GI bleeding.

Etiology

Greater than 90 percent of upper GI bleeding cases are caused by peptic ulcer, erosive gastritis, Mallory–Weiss tears, or esophagogastric varices (Andreoli et al., 1997). Other etiologies of upper GI bleeding include tumors, arteriovenous malformations, and stress ulcers. Table 28–6 summarizes the causes of upper GI bleeding.

The amount and degree of upper GI bleeding is variable. When an ulcer erodes through an artery, the bleeding is profuse. Therefore, the manifestations of GI bleeding depend on the source, the rate of bleeding, and comorbid disease. Severe GI bleeding may seriously aggravate coronary artery disease, hypertension, diabetes mellitus, pulmonary disease, and renal failure, and it often presents as shock. Lesser degrees of bleeding may present as orthostatic changes in pulse (a change of > 10

TABLE 28–6. CAUSES OF UPPER GI BLEEDING

ETIOLOGY	OCCURRENCE (PERCENTAGE OF TOTAL UPPER GI BLEED CASES)
Peptic ulcers	45%
Gastric	23%
Duodenal	22%
Gastritis	20–30%
Varices	15–20%
Esophagitis	13%
Mallory–Weiss tear	5–10%
Arteriovenous malformation	< 5%

Source: Beers, M.H., & Berkhow, R. (eds.). (1999). The Merck manual of diagnosis and therapy, *17th ed. Whitehouse Station, NJ: Merck Research Laboratories.*

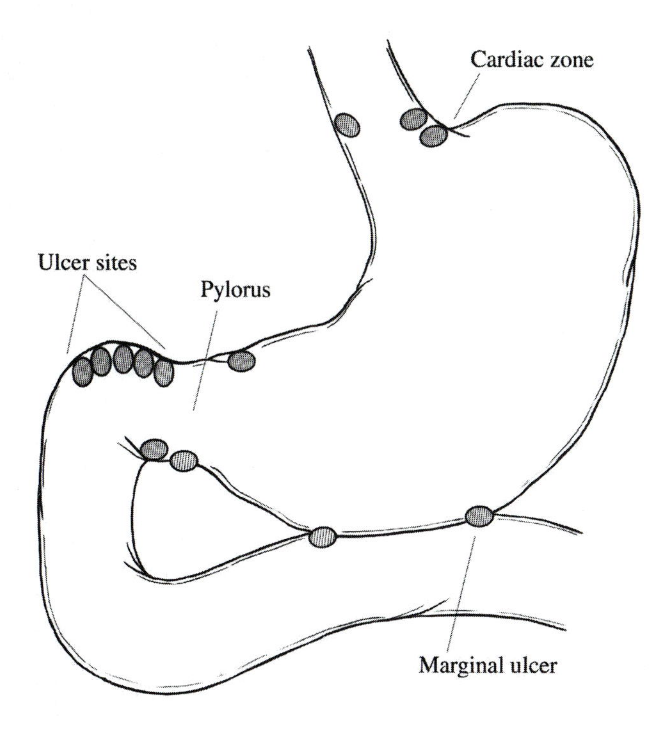

Figure 28–8. Common sites of peptic ulcers. Causes of peptic ulcers: 1. high acid and pepsin content; 2. irritation; 3. poor blood supply; 4. poor secretion of mucus; and 5. infection.

beats/min) or blood pressure (a drop of ≥ 10 mm Hg) secondary to compensatory mechanisms (Beers & Berkhow, 1999). Studies have found that the most common cause of death in GI hemorrhage is the result of exacerbation of the underlying disease rather than intractable hypovolemic shock (Andreoli et al., 1997; Chojkler, 1986; McQuaid, 1999). However, GI hemorrhage, if unrecognized or treated too late, can lead to hypovolemic shock and ultimately death.

Peptic Ulcer Disease

PUD is the most common cause of upper GI bleeding. Ulcers range in size from several millimeters to several centimeters and are characterized by a break in the mucosa extending through the muscularis mucosae. Peptic ulcers occur in the portion of the GI tract exposed to acid–pepsin secretion, which includes the stomach and the duodenum (see Figs. 28–8 and 28–9).

Traditional theories on the cause of PUD have been focused on acid hypersecretion and/or the inability of the mucosa to secrete mucus for protection. It is now known that hypersecretion is not the primary mechanism by which ulceration occurs. It appears that certain associated factors, namely, infection with *H. pylori* bacteria and the use of NSAIDs, disrupt the mucosal defense barrier, making it susceptible to the damaging effects of acid. Cigarette smoking has been linked to an increased incidence of ulcer disease, slower healing rates, and higher rates of ulcer recurrence (Isenkery et al., 1995). Other risk factors include a family history of ulcer disease and the use of aspirin (Hudak, Gallo, & Morton, 1998). Mortality, as a result of PUD is quite low; however, patients suffer substantial pain as a result of the chronic nature of this disease. Interestingly, PUD is the most common cause of upper GI bleeding in critically ill patients. PUD accounts for approximately 40

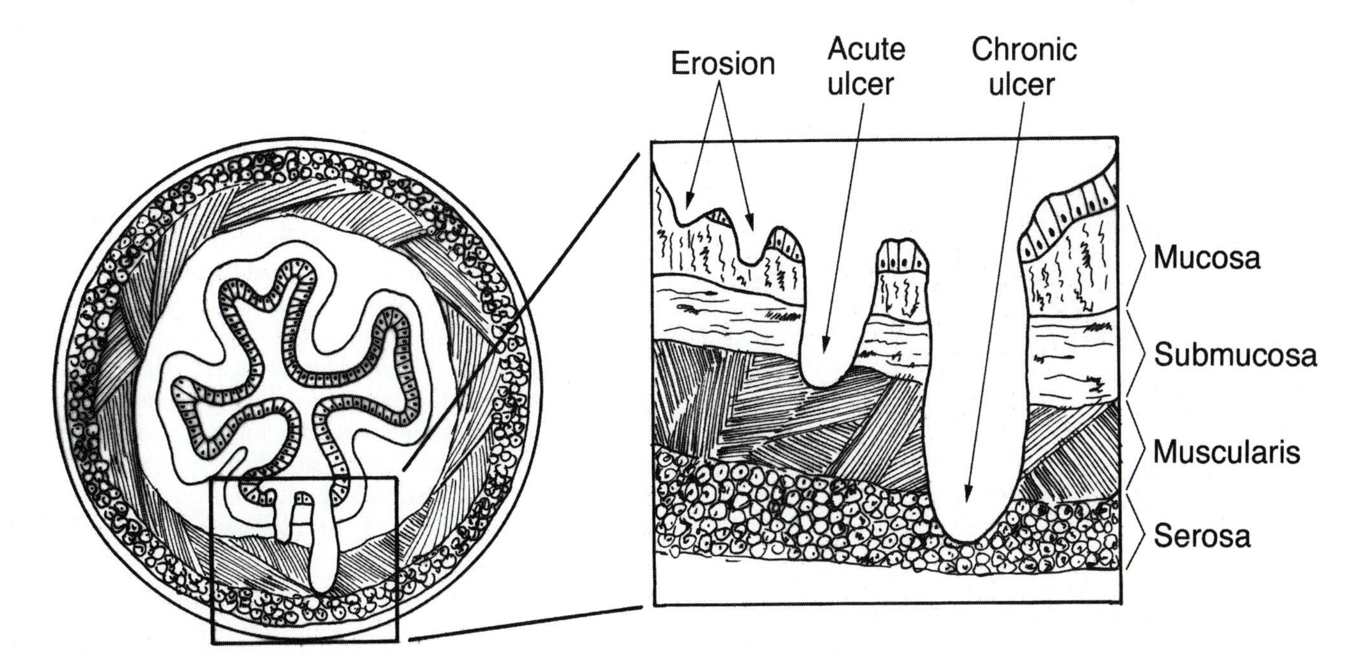

Figure 28–9. Degrees of ulceration in peptic ulcer disease. This cross-section of the gut wall shows degrees of ulceration, including erosion, acute ulcer, and chronic ulcer. Acute and chronic ulcers may penetrate the entire wall of the stomach.

percent of patients admitted to an intensive care unit (ICU) specifically for bleeding and 50 percent of patients admitted for some other reason who develop upper GI hem- orrhage during their stay (Passaro, 1994).

H. pylori can be cultured from the stomachs of approximately 70 to 90 percent of patients with gastric ulcers, and 90 to 100 percent of patients with duodenal ulcers (Passaro, 1994). *H. pylori* is able to secrete its own protective covering that protects it from gastric acid, allowing it to thrive in a high-acid environment. The mechanism by which *H. pylori* impairs mucosal integrity is poorly understood. The organism is responsible for the production of ammonia, cytotoxins, and mucolytic enzymes that erode the mucous barrier, making the mucosa more susceptible to acid damage. NSAIDs inhibit prostaglandin production and action. Inhibition of prostaglandins is believed to be the most important causative factor to the development of ulcers. Prostaglandins function to increase mucous secretion, bicarbonate secretion, and mucosal blood flow as well as inhibit gastric acid secretion. Because NSAIDs interfere with the normal prostaglandin actions, they contribute to the formation of peptic ulcers (see Fig. 28–10).

PUD can be subdivided into duodenal ulcers and gastric ulcers. Duodenal ulcers constitute approximately 80 percent of peptic ulcers (Smith, 1998). The most frequent sites for duodenal ulcers are the gastric pylorus and the first portion of the duodenum. Duodenal ulcers can occur at any age, but are most common among young adults, especially in persons with type A blood, who smoke, abuse alcohol, and who report a positive family history of peptic ulcers. Duodenal ulcer pain tends to be consistent. The pain is absent upon awakening, but returns around midmorning. It is relieved by food but recurs 2 to 3 hours after eating. Antacids will provide some temporary relief. Intense pain that awakens the patient from sleep at night is common to duodenal ulcer.

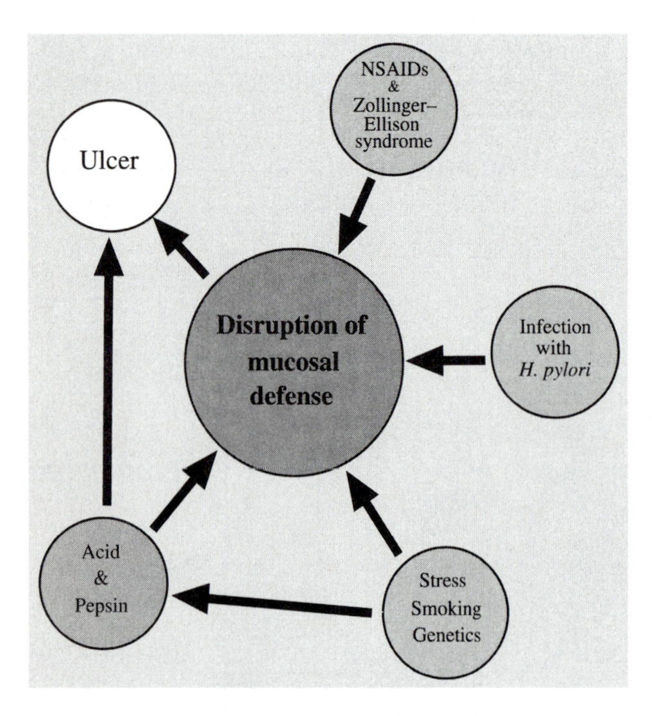

Figure 28–10. Etiological factors in ulcer development. Acid and pepsin activity overpowers mucosal defense to produce ulcers most commonly when mucosal defense is impaired. Two factors, nonsteroidal anti-inflammatory drugs and *H. pylori* infection, appear to be linked to the impairment of mucosal defense.

Gastric ulcer symptoms usually do not follow a consistent pattern. For example, eating often causes pain. Gastric ulcers affect older adults and are associated with malignancy. Gastric ulcers tend to be chronic, usually involving branches of the left gastric artery, and can produce severe hemorrhage if erosion into the arterial wall occurs. If the gastric ulcer is located in the pyloric canal (the narrow region of the stomach that opens through the pylorus into the duodenum), the symptoms are often associated with obstruction (e.g., bloating, nausea, vomiting) (Andreoli et al., 1997; Beers & Berkhow, 1999; Passaro, 1994).

Diagnosis and Treatment

Diagnosis of PUD is largely suggested by history and is confirmed by visualization with fiber-optic endoscopy, the diagnostic tool of choice. Conversely, approximately 10 percent (Beers & Berkhow, 1999) of duodenal ulcers may be missed using endoscopy. For this reason, a follow up barium x-ray exam may be ordered if clinical suspicion for peptic ulcer is high. Determination of a duodenal or gastric ulcer by upper endoscopy or radiographic study should be followed by confirmation of *H. pylori* infection. *H. pylori* infection can be definitively diagnosed using endoscopy. Diagnostic tests for the presence of *H. pylori* vary and include serologic testing, carbon-labeled urea breath tests, rapid urease assay (Clotest), and culture or histologic analysis of endoscopic biopsies (Carey, Lee, & Woeltze, 1998).

Treatment of PUD involves antibiotics (eradication of *H. pylori*), histamine receptor antagonist agents (antisecretory), proton pump inhibitors (acid secretion inhibition), prostaglandins (inhibits acid secretion and enhances mucosal barrier), sucralfate (promotes mucosal barrier), and antacids (gives symptomatic relief, raises gastric pH). Many high-acuity patients have nasogastric as well as small-bore enteric feeding tubes. The appropriate route of administration for sucralfate and antacids is through the nasogastric tube to allow for direct contact with the gastric mucosa. If the nasogastric tube is attached to suction, it must be interrupted for 30 to 60 minutes. Eliminating foods that cause distress is helpful. Surgery is indicated only to manage severe bleeding and perforation complications of peptic ulcers. The pharmacologic interventions will be discussed further in upcoming sections of this module.

Acute Erosive or Hemorrhagic Gastritis

Acute erosive or hemorrhagic gastritis involves severe inflammation of the gastric mucosa. The most common clinical manifestation of erosive gastritis is upper GI bleeding, which presents as hematemesis, "coffee ground" emesis, or bloody aspirate in a patient receiving nasogastric suction, or as melena. Because erosive gastritis involves superficial lesions, bleeding is not as rapid as with a lesion that extends deeper into the mucosa and may erode into a blood vessel. The slow loss of blood can be noted in a continuously decreasing hemoglobin and hematocrit level. Causes of erosive gastritis include NSAIDs, alcohol, and acute stress. Uncommon causes of gastric mucosal erosion include radiation, viral infections, caustic ingestion, and direct trauma (e.g., nasogastric tubes). Gastritis is often asymptomatic, but may cause epigastric pain, nausea, vomiting, and bleeding. GI bleeding due to gastritis is usually not severe, except in the critically ill. Diagnosis of gastritis is accomplished by direct visualization with endoscopy (McQuaid, 1999).

NSAID Gastritis

Thirty percent of patients receiving long-term NSAID therapy have gastritis at one time or another. NSAID-induced ulcers are more common in persons 55 years of age or older (Smith, 1997). Other factors that may increase the risk of NSAID-induced ulcers include a previous history of PUD, corticosteroid use, high doses of NSAIDs, and recent use of NSAIDs. Also, the incidence is slightly higher in females (Smith, 1997). NSAIDs compete with prostaglandin receptor sites in the gastric mucosa. Prostaglandins, particularly prostaglandin E, have been linked to mucosal repair and maintenance of mucosal integrity (Wilson & Lindseth, 1996). When these prostaglandin defense mechanisms are inhibited by the action of NSAIDs, severe inflammation and erosive injury can occur to the gastric mucosa. The incidence of NSAID gastritis may decrease with greater use of Cox 2 inhibitors. These new NSAIDs do not produce GI side effects since they do not inhibit prostaglandin E.

Alcoholic Gastritis

Chronic alcohol ingestion can result in inflammation of the gastric mucosa. The inflammation can progress to erosions and hemorrhage. Episodes of upper GI bleeding due to gastritis are usually mild and respond to withdrawal of alcohol and to pharmacologic therapy (2 to 3 weeks of H_2 receptor antagonists or sucralfate therapy) (McQuaid, 1999).

Stress Gastritis

Bleeding associated with stress-related gastritis comes from diffuse, superficial lesions or erosions in the gastric mucosa. Decreased blood flow to the gut during times of severe stress may contribute to the breakdown in normal mucosal defenses (McGuirk & Coyle, 1994). Risk factors for stress gastritis include severe burns, sepsis, central nervous system trauma, shock, respiratory failure with mechanical ventilation, hepatic and renal failure, multiorgan dysfunction, and high doses of vasopressor agents (dopamine, Levophed). Increased length of stay in an ICU and increased length of time the patient has gone without enteral nutrition are associated with higher risk of developing stress-related gastritis. Endoscopic studies have shown that stress-related mucosal damage occurs in 52 to 100 percent of patients within 18 to 24 hours of admission to an ICU (Chamberlain, 1993). Diagnosis of gastritis is confirmed by direct endoscopic visualization.

Prevention and Treatment

Once significant GI bleeding from gastritis occurs (in about 2 percent of ICU patients), the mortality rate is > 60 percent (Beers & Berkhow, 1999). Severe bleeding from a localized lesion may be treated with endoscopic sclerotherapy to cauterize the bleeding lesion. Diffusely bleeding lesions may respond to vasopressin, administered intravenously or intra-arterially into a bleeding vessel. Vasopressin (also known as antidiuretic hormone) is a potent stimulator of smooth muscle, particularly those of capillaries and arterioles. It exerts its therapeutic effect in the management of GI bleeding by vasoconstriction of the splanchnic vessels, which reduces blood flow through the bleeding vessel. Vasopressin exerts its vasoconstricting effects systemically; therefore, untoward side effects of abdominal cramping, angina, hypertension, arrhythmias, and headache may occur. Concomitant use of nitroglycerin may reduce vasopressin's effects on the coronary arteries, especially in persons with coronary artery disease (Carey, Lee, & Woeltze, 1998). Surgical resection of the involved portions of the stomach is indicated if bleeding does not respond to more conservative treatment.

The incidence of stress-related gastritis can usually be decreased or prevented if the gastric pH is maintained above 4.0. This can be accomplished with the prophylactic administration of histamine receptor antagonists or oral antacids to all at-risk patients to raise the gastric pH above 4.0 (Beers & Berkhow, 1999; McQuaid, 1999). Sucralfate, a mucosal binding agent that forms a protective barrier over the erosion, given orally is also effective in reducing stress-related bleeding. Early enteral feeding has been advocated as a means of lowering the incidence of bleeding in acutely ill persons.

Conservative treatment for NSAID-induced gastritis includes discontinuation of the drug, reduction to the lowest effective dose, or administration with meals. Patients with persistent gastritis or who are at increased risk of developing gastric mucosal injury should be treated with sucralfate, histamine receptor antagonists, or with a proton pump inhibitor (omeprazole). Misoprostol can be administered along with NSAID therapy to prevent ulcer formation. Misoprostol is a synthetic prostaglandin E analog that replaces the protective prostaglandins consumed with prostaglandin-inhibiting therapies (e.g., NSAIDs). Misoprostol is reserved for use with long-term NSAID therapy in high-risk persons (Lacy et al., 1998). If the patient has adequate renal function, switching the patient to a Cox 2 inhibitor NSAID (Rofecoxib/Vioxx, Celecoxib/Celebrex) may prevent NSAID-induced gastritis.

Esophageal and Gastric Varices

Upper GI bleeding from esophageal or gastric varices is associated with cirrhosis, portal hypertension, and portal and/or splenic vein thrombosis. Bleeding from esophagogastric varices is usually massive and occurs without warning. Portal hypertension causes the development of collateral venous pathways, called *varices*, which are located in the esophagus and stomach. Hepatic cirrhosis due to alcohol abuse is the most common cause of variceal bleeding in the United States. (See Module 29 for an overview of the etiology, pathophysiology, and treatment of bleeding esophageal or gastric varices.)

Mallory–Weiss Tears

A Mallory–Weiss tear is a small laceration in the mucosa at the gastroesophageal junction. Fifty percent of these patients give a history of vomiting that precedes the hematemesis (Andreoli et al., 1997). High-risk patients are those with a history of alcohol abuse. Bleeding due to a Mallory–Weiss tear often presents with mild to massive hematemesis. Most tears stop bleeding spontaneously, and rebleeding is infrequent. Diagnosis is confirmed by upper GI endoscopy, and treatment consists of histamine receptor antagonists, antacids, and embolization or selective infusion of vasopressin into the bleeding vessel (Passaro, 1994).

Arteriovenous Malformation

An arteriovenous malformation (AVM), sometimes referred to as an *angiodysplasia*, is a small, abnormal mucosal or submucosal blood vessel that has a tendency to bleed. AVMs can occur in both the upper GI and the lower GI tracts, but they are most commonly located in the cecal region of the lower GI tract. The cause of AVMs is unknown but appears to be genetic. Once GI bleeding from an AVM occurs, recurrent GI bleeding, chronic anemia, or severe acute GI bleeding is the usual clinical course (Beers & Berkhow, 1999). Gastrointestinal AVMs are common in the elderly with other comorbid illness such as valvular heart disease, chronic renal failure, liver disease, and collagen vascular disease and those undergoing radiotherapy. Upper GI bleeding due to an AVM is most commonly diagnosed by upper GI endoscopy. Definitive treatment of the underlying or concomitant conditions (e.g., valvuloplasty, kidney transplantation) can cure bleeding AVMs. Endoscopic sclerotherapy is used palliatively because new AVMs can continue to develop in high-risk patients (Graham, 1996).

SECTION SIX REVIEW

1. Which of the following is a cause of acute upper GI bleeding?
   A. Mallory–Weiss tear
   B. diverticula
   C. ischemic bowel disease
   D. ulcerative colitis
2. _______ is the most common cause of upper GI bleeding.
   A. Esophageal varices
   B. PUD
   C. AVM
   D. Stress gastritis
3. Peptic ulcers occur in the
   A. stomach and ileum
   B. duodenum and colon
   C. stomach and peritoneum
   D. stomach and duodenum
4. A 35-year-old male is diagnosed with PUD. His father had a gastric ulcer. He smokes one pack of cigarettes per day, takes a diuretic to treat his hypertension, and is obese (310 pounds at 6 feet tall). He takes aspirin every day for his "arthritis." How many risk factors for PUD does this person have?
   A. two
   B. three
   C. four
   D. five
5. Peptic ulcers are caused by
   A. colonization of bacteria within the GI tract
   B. hypersecretion of pancreatic enzymes
   C. underproduction of bicarbonate
   D. disruption of the mucosal barrier
6. Gastric ulcer symptoms
   A. are relieved by eating
   B. are aggravated by eating
   C. are not affected by eating
   D. follow a consistent pattern
7. Stress-related mucosal damage occurs in 52 to 100% of patients within _______ hours of admission to an ICU.
   A. 24 to 48
   B. 8 to 16
   C. 18 to 24
   D. 48 to 72

8. Which drug is often prescribed along with long-term NSAID therapy in high risk patients to prevent the development of ulcers?
   A. neomycin
   B. misoprostol
   C. sucralfate
   D. antacids

9. GI bleeding due to a Mallory–Weiss tear often presents with
   A. hematemesis
   B. hematochezia
   C. melena
   D. pain

Answers: 1. A, 2. B, 3. D, 4. B, 5. D, 6. B, 7. C, 8. B, 9. A

SECTION SEVEN: Acute Lower GI Bleeding

At the completion of this section, the learner will be able to describe the etiology and pathophysiology of acute lower GI bleeding.

The two most common causes of acute lower GI bleeding are diverticulosis and AVM. Other common causes of chronic lower GI bleeding are internal hemorrhoids and malignant tumor. Table 28–7 summarizes the causes and characteristics of lower GI bleeding. Bleeding stops spontaneously in 80 to 90 percent of patients, with a risk of recurrence in 25 percent of the patients (Passaro, 1994). Most lower GI bleeding, unlike upper GI bleeding, is slow and intermittent and does not require hospitalization (Driscoll, 1999). Less frequent causes of lower GI bleeding include ischemic bowel disease and inflammatory bowel disease. Because 10 to 20 percent of the acute lower GI bleeding cases do not resolve spontaneously and therefore require high-acuity nursing lower GI bleeding is included in this module (Driscoll, 1999).

TABLE 28–7. CAUSES AND CHARACTERISTICS OF LOWER GI BLEEDING

CAUSE	CHARACTERISTICS
Diverticula	Sustained, dark, occasionally massive bleeding throughout the colon
Arteriovenous malformation	Intermittent, both dark and bright red bleeding, clots, coming from cecal area
Internal hemorrhoids	Bright red blood per rectum, intermittent with bowel movements
Ischemic bowel disease	Intermittent, mostly dark blood; abdominal tenderness, fever, leukocytosis
Carcinoma	Occult bleeding with intermittent melena, right colon tumors
Inflammatory bowel disease	Intermittent bleeding, mixed with frequent bowel movement

Sources: Krumberger, J.M., & Hammer, B. (1998). Gastrointestinal disorders. In M.R. Kinney et al. (eds.), AACN's clinical reference for critical care nursing, *4th ed. St. Louis: C.V. Mosby; Passaro, E. (1994). Gastrointestinal bleeding. In F.S. Bongard & D.Y. Sue (eds.),* Current critical care diagnosis and treatment. *Norwalk, CT: Appleton & Lange; and Driscoll, C.J. (1999). Acute gastrointestinal bleed. In L. Bucher & S. Melander (eds.).* Critical care nursing. *Philadelphia: W.B. Saunders.*

Diverticular Bleeding

Diverticular bleeding can be massive and life threatening but occurs in only 3 percent of patients with diverticulosis. It is the most common etiology of major lower GI bleeding. Bleeding from a diverticulum occurs when an artery penetrates and ruptures into the sac of the diverticulum, a result of pressure erosion (Driscoll, 1999). Bleeding stops spontaneously in 80 percent of patients, with no further intervention necessary. However, 25 percent of these cases rebleed requiring surgical intervention or angiography with intra-arterial infusion of vasopressin (Beers & Berkhow, 1999; Spencer, 1994).

Arteriovenous Malformations

Bleeding from an AVM is usually slow, chronic, and can be occult. Patients usually present with weakness, fatigue, dyspnea on exertion, and guaiac-positive stools. Bleeding from an AVM is rarely massive. A typical bleeding episode requires less than two to four units of blood and is not associated with hypotension. The elderly have increased risk of severe blood loss from this type of GI bleed. AVMs are angiodysplastic lesions that are usually small, superficial, multiple, and located in the colon and cecum. The cause of AVMs is not clear, but they appear to be associated with cardiac disease, low flow states, and the aging process. Bleeding occurs from weakened, friable vessel wall lesions caused from chronic tension and dilation of blood vessels most commonly located in the cecal area of the intestine. In cases in which the bleeding does not stop spontaneously, arterial embolization and surgery may be necessary.

Ischemic Bowel Disease

Ischemic bowel disease can be defined as inflammation of the colon resulting from an interruption of the colonic blood supply (Beers & Berkhow, 1999). It may result from occlusion of a major artery, small-vessel disease, venous obstruction, low flow states (e.g., cardiogenic shock), or intestinal obstruction. Intestinal ischemia can occur postoperatively following vascular bypass or colon resection with anastomosis. In the elderly, risk factors for developing ischemic bowel disease include atherosclerosis, atrial fibrillation, and hypotension. Older patients are most commonly affected, although younger patients with diabetes, pancreatitis, heart disease, sickle cell disease, or systemic lupus erythematosus are also at risk.

Bleeding from ischemic bowel disease is often associated with anticoagulant use (25 percent of all bleeding cases) (Beers & Berkhow, 1999). The bleeding is usually intermittent, with mixed dark and bright red blood and clots visible from the rectum. Fever and abdominal pain are usually present. Lower GI endoscopy reveals purple discoloration of the bowel, often in the presence of erosion and ulceration. Radiographic x-rays are nonspecific, but may reveal abnormal air pockets if perforation is present. Barium contrast studies reveal characteristic "thumbprints," suggesting a necrotic process. Arterial or venous occlusion of the mesenteric vasculature should be suspected and ruled out when ischemia of the bowel is included in the differential diagnosis. Treatment of ischemic bowel disease involves restoration of blood circulation to the intestines and might include fluid resuscitation, optimization of cardiac output, and treatment of any underlying disease. Antibiotics may be required for infections. Resection of affected bowel may be necessary for fulminant disease and/or severe bleeding. Patients with ischemic bowel disease often have other medical problems including multiple organ failure, and therefore have a mortality of 50 percent (Crittormson & Burbick, 1989).

Inflammatory Bowel Disease

Bloody diarrhea is the most common symptom of inflammatory bowel disease. The degree of bleeding is usually small to moderate but it can be massive. In very rare instances, life-threatening bleeding can result when the underlying inflammation ulcerates into adjacent arteries (Bono, 1996). The treatment of bleeding associated with inflammatory bowel disease is management of the underlying disorder with corticosteroids (Elta, 1995). If the bleeding is uncontrollable by medical means, then surgical resection of the affected portion of the bowel is necessary.

Neoplasms

Benign and malignant tumors and polyps are common among the elderly, with 10 to 20 percent of these patients developing bleeding lesions (Bono, 1996). Bleeding from neoplasms is usually slow, chronic, and self-limiting. Only rarely is there acute blood loss of significant proportions from a neoplasm. In these cases, bowel resection and tumor excision are indicated.

SECTION SEVEN REVIEW

1. Diverticula are found throughout the
   A. stomach
   B. small intestine
   C. colon
   D. GI tract
2. Sustained, dark red lower GI bleeding from the large intestine is a characteristic of a bleeding
   A. diverticula
   B. hemorrhoid
   C. tumor
   D. angiodysplasia
3. Angiodysplasia (AVM) of the lower GI tract is associated with
   A. renal disease
   B. cardiac disease
   C. a high-fat diet
   D. an inflammatory process
4. Ischemic bowel disease is defined as a(n)
   A. malignant process
   B. infectious process
   C. chronic stress process
   D. inflammatory process
5. Treatment of ischemic bowel disease involves
   A. steroid administration
   B. high-dose narcotics
   C. fluid resuscitation
   D. enemas until clear

Answers: 1. C, 2. A, 3. B, 4. D, 5. C

SECTION EIGHT: Management of Acute Gastrointestinal Bleeding

At the completion of this section, the learner will be able to describe the management of acute GI bleeding.

Patients who are experiencing acute GI bleeding must be approached in a systematic manner (see Fig. 28–11). This approach should be collaborative and include (1) initial assessment, (2) resuscitation, (3) definitive diagnosis, and (4) treatment.

Caring for the patient with acute GI bleeding is a collaborative endeavor. The nurse's role includes the following (in collaboration with the physician):

- Assess the severity of blood loss.
- Replace a sufficient amount of fluids and blood products to counteract shock.
- Assist in the diagnosis of the cause of the bleeding.
- Plan and implement treatment.
- Manage the ongoing plan of care and monitor progress.

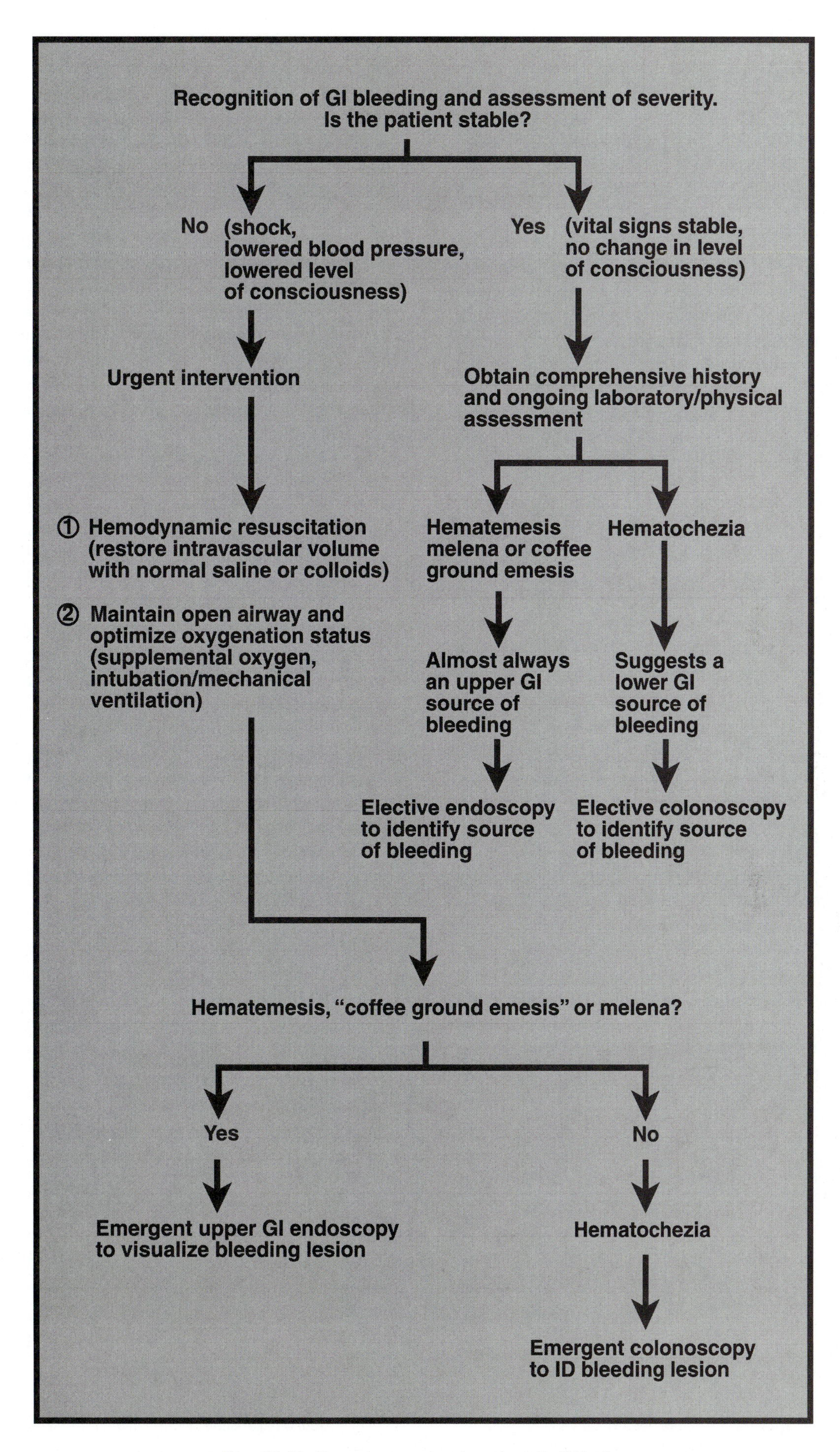

Figure 28–11. Diagnostic approach to the patient with GI bleeding.

- Provide supportive care and education to the patient and significant others, since any bleeding experience is potentially life threatening.

Initial Assessment

To assess severity of blood loss, the nurse must determine hemodynamic stability. Evidence of instability includes decreased blood pressure and/or orthostatic hypotension, decreased or altered level of consciousness, and decreased urine output (which is suggestive of fluid volume deficit). Evidence of hemodynamic instability in the presence of hematemesis, hematochezia, or melena should be considered an emergency until proven otherwise, and admission to an ICU is recommended. The following are guidelines for admission to an ICU:

1. Clearly documented frank hematemesis
2. Coffee-ground emesis and either melena or hematochezia
3. Hemodynamic instability (hypotension, tachycardia, or orthostatic hypotension)
4. A drop in hematocrit of five points after fluid resuscitation
5. A significant unexplained increase in the BUN when GI bleeding is suspected (increased BUN suggests fluid volume deficit and/or metabolism of blood within the GI tract)

Resuscitation

Resuscitation is the primary goal of early management in the hemodynamically unstable patient, and mandates the maintenance of intravascular volume and tissue oxygenation. Blood specimens for type and crossmatching, CBC, PT/PTT, and chemistries should be obtained. Nasal oxygen and pulse oximetry are useful, especially in the elderly or in patients with a history of cardiac or pulmonary disease. Close nursing assessment of the patient's level of consciousness and oxygenation status is important in the acute phase. Endotracheal intubation should be considered for decreased level of consciousness, shock, or massive bleeding, and the nurse should have emergency intubation and oxygen equipment ready if needed. Vital signs, orthostatic blood pressure changes, and urine output are valuable clinical indicators of perfusion and blood volume. An indwelling catheter should be placed to monitor urine output, since this is a good measure of perfusion. Central venous pressures or pulmonary capillary wedge pressures are also helpful to monitor volume status. Volume resuscitation is accomplished with crystalloid (normal saline or lactated Ringer's) at a rate to maintain a systolic blood pressure of > 90 mm Hg through at least two large-bore IV lines. If after 2 to 3 L of crystalloid infusion, the patient remains unstable, an infusion of blood products (packed red cells, whole blood) should be considered. Vasoconstricting drugs (vasopressors) are generally not indicated because hypovolemia is usually the cause of the hypotension. Packed red cells are transfused for massive bleeding to keep the hematocrit > 28 to 30 percent. Patients with cardiac or pulmonary disease may require transfusion to a higher hematocrit (> 30 percent). Transfusions of whole blood may be considered in massively bleeding patients because they provide increased colloid osmotic pressure, thus decreasing the patient's total fluid requirements. O-negative blood can be used until the patient's blood has been crossmatched. A blood warmer should be considered for rapid fluid or blood administration to prevent hypothermia. Each unit of blood should elevate the hematocrit by three points. Fresh frozen plasma is considered for patients who have a coagulopathy (increased PT or PTT) or who have been on Coumadin therapy. If the patient has thrombocytopenia, platelet transfusion should be considered to maintain the platelet count above 50,000/mm^3 (Andreoli et al., 1997; Beers & Berkhow, 1999; Carey, Lee, & Woeltze, 1998). An early surgical consult is essential and should be obtained within the first few hours of the onset of bleeding.

For patients with persistent bleeding, some type of therapeutic intervention is necessary. This intervention can be pharmacotherapy, mechanical (balloon) tamponade

TABLE 28–8. THERAPEUTIC PHARMACOLOGIC INTERVENTIONS IN ACUTE GI BLEEDING

INTERVENTION	EFFECTS	COMMENTS
Antacids	Neutralize gastric acidity	Therapy for peptic ulcer disease and gastritis Must act in the stomach, in direct contact with the gastric mucosa
Histamine receptor antagonists (H_2 blockers)	Block histamine stimulation of acid-secreting cells; reduce acid secretion	Therapy for peptic ulcer disease and gastritis
Sucralfate	Forms a protective barrier, allowing ulcer healing	Therapy for peptic ulcer disease and gastritis Must act in the stomach, in direct contact with the gastric mucosa
Proton pump inhibitors	Inhibits acid secretory pump (H^+, K^+-ATPase)	Therapy for peptic ulcer disease and gastritis
Prostaglandins (misoprostol)	Inhibits gastric secretion, and stimulates mucosal defense mechanisms	Adjunct prophylactic therapy to prevent development of ulcers with chronic nonsteroidal anti-inflammatory drug use

Source: McQuaid, K.R. (1999). Alimentary tract. In L.M. Tierney, S.J. McPhee, & M.A. Papadakis (eds.), Current medical diagnosis and treatment, *38th ed. Stamford, CT: Appleton & Lange.*

TABLE 28–9. INTERVENTIONS FOR SEVERE GI HEMORRHAGE (EVIDENCE OF HEMODYNAMIC INSTABILITY AND/OR PERSISTENT BLEEDING)

INTERVENTION	EFFECTS	COMMENTS
Vasopressin	Decreases portal pressure by vasoconstricting splanchnic arteries Untoward effects include decreased coronary blood flow, increased blood pressure	Treatment of severe hemorrhage due to upper GI variceal bleeding, erosive gastritis, arteriovenous malformations, and Mallory–Weiss tears
Somatostatin	Decreases portal pressure by vasoconstriction of splanchnic circulation	See above
Octreotide	A synthetic analog of somatostatin; has same action as somatostatin	See above
Mechanical tamponade	Provides tamponade to actively bleeding gastric/esophageal varices	Treatment of bleeding esophageal and gastric varices

Source: McQuaid, K.R. (1999). Alimentary tract. In L.M. Tierney, S.J. McPhee, & M.A. Papadakis (eds.), Current medical diagnosis and treatment, *38th ed. Stamford, CT: Appleton & Lange.*

(Sengstaken–Blakemore tube), endoscopic therapy (sclerotherapy), or surgery. Once blood volume is restored, the patient is monitored for evidence of further bleeding (e.g., tachycardia, decreased blood pressure, hematemesis, bloody or tarry stools). Specific therapy depends on the bleeding site (refer to previously discussed etiologies of GI bleeding for specific treatments). Tables 28–8, 28–9, and 28–10 summarize therapeutic pharmacologic and interventional therapies in the setting of acute GI bleeding. Definitive diagnosis of the source of the GI bleeding should be undertaken as soon as the patient is stable. Table 28–5 summarizes the various endoscopies of the GI system.

Arterial Angiotherapy Interventions in Persistent GI Hemorrhage

Selective arterial infusion of vasopressin is used to control massive bleeding in patients who have PUD, stress ulcers, erosive gastritis, Mallory–Weiss tear, and AVM. Selective catheterization of the bleeding artery is required for infusion of vasopressin. Arterial embolization is an alternative to arterial vasopressin where the bleeding vessel is selectively catheterized, and a coagulant is placed in the vessel (Andreoli et al., 1997; Beers & Berkhow, 1999; Carey, Lee, & Woeltze, 1998).

Therapy for Specific Lesions

Bleeding peptic ulcers can often be diagnosed and treated with endoscopy. Surgery is considered for severe hemorrhage or recurrent bleeding. Arterial angiography can be used to control massive bleeding from peptic ulcers in patients who are considered to be poor surgical risks.

Bleeding from esophageal or gastric varices requires ICU admission. These patients will need endotracheal intubation and early endoscopy. Sclerotherapy should be performed as soon as a diagnosis of variceal bleeding is confirmed. Rebleeding occurs in 50 percent of cases following sclerotherapy (Carey, Lee, & Woeltze, 1998). Intravenous vasopressin or octreotide (somatostatin analog) may be used as an alternative to sclerotherapy or concomitantly to reduce portal pressures (see Module 29). Balloon tamponade therapy is an effective, temporary method to stop variceal bleeding while awaiting more definitive therapy. Shunt surgery or transjugular intrahepatic portosystemic shunt (TIPS) should be considered if the risk is high for recurrent variceal bleeding (see Module 29).

Bleeding Mallory–Weiss tears that do not stop spontaneously require therapeutic endoscopy or selective arterial angiotherapy, whereas bleeding AVMs of the colon can be treated with arterial angiotherapy or therapeutic endoscopic procedures. In diverticular bleeding, selective arterial vasopressin is often effective in stopping the bleeding. Selective arterial therapy requires catheterization of the bleeding vessel for infusion of vasopressin. Surgery is needed when the bleeding is severe (Andreoli et al., 1997; Beers & Berkow, 1999; McQuaid, 1999).

TABLE 28–10. ENDOSCOPIC INTERVENTIONS IN GI HEMORRHAGE

INTERVENTION	DESCRIPTION	COMMENTS
Endoscopic injection sclerotherapy	Sclerosing agent is injected into bleeding vessel	Treatment bleeding from varices, Mallory–Weiss tears, arteriovenous malformations, ulcers
Endoscopic electrocoagulation	Direct electric current is applied to bleeding lesion = fibrosis	See above
Endoscopic laser therapy	Direct application of heat to coagulate bleeding lesion	See above
Endoscopic heater probe	Direct electric current is applied to coagulate bleeding lesion	See above

Sources: McQuaid, K.R. (1999). Alimentary tract. In L.M. Tierney, S.J. McPhee, & M.A. Papadakis (eds.), Current medical diagnosis and treatment, *38th ed. Stamford, CT: Appleton & Lange; and Graham, D. (1996). Management of upper gastrointestinal hemorrhage. In J.C. Bennett et al. (eds.),* Cecil's textbook of medicine, *20th ed. Philadelphia: W.B. Saunders.*

SECTION EIGHT REVIEW

1. The first step in the collaborative treatment of a patient who is experiencing an acute GI bleed is
   A. assessment
   B. resuscitation
   C. diagnosis
   D. treatment
2. To assess the severity of blood loss, the nurse should determine
   A. respiratory status
   B. hemodynamic status
   C. level of consciousness
   D. the degree of impairment
3. Signs and symptoms that provide supporting evidence of a fluid volume deficit are
   A. abdominal distention
   B. unchanged level of consciousness
   C. orthostatic hypotension
   D. increased urine output
4. In a patient who has had a GI bleed, an increased BUN suggests fluid volume deficit and/or
   A. onset of acute renal failure
   B. development of systemic inflammatory response
   C. an acute infectious process
   D. metabolism of blood in the gut
5. Laboratory tests needed in the management of a patient with an acute GI hemorrhage include
   A. hourly ABG measurements
   B. blood and urine cultures
   C. type and crossmatch blood for possible transfusion
   D. stool culture for occult blood
6. Volume resuscitation is usually accomplished with
   A. intravenous crystalloid infusion
   B. vasoconstricting drugs
   C. blood transfusion
   D. normal saline via a nasogastric tube

Answers: 1. A, 2. B, 3. C, 4. D, 5. C, 6. A

SECTION NINE: Acute Intestinal Obstruction and Paralytic Ileus

At the completion of this section, the learner will be able to describe the etiology, pathophysiology, and management of acute intestinal obstruction and paralytic ileus.

Acute Small-Bowel Obstruction

Obstruction of the small intestine is a common surgical complication often due to the development of adhesions following abdominal surgery. Other causes of obstruction are hernias, volvulus, Crohn's disease, and tumors. Most obstructions result from actual occlusion of the intestinal lumen (mechanical or physical), resulting in distention and gas and fluid accumulation above the obstruction. When the small bowel is obstructed, distention with gas and fluid occurs proximal to the obstruction. Swallowed air is the major cause of the distention. Bacterial fermentation within the lumen of the intestine produces other gases (methane). Inflammation leads to transudation of fluid from the extracellular space into the intestinal lumen and peritoneal cavity. Fluid and electrolytes become trapped within the obstructed bowel and may leak out into the peritoneum, further disturbing electrolyte and fluid balance. The inflammatory process causes large amounts of fluid and sodium to accumulate within the intestine (mass effect). Fluid losses may be so severe that hypotension results, which can result in cardiovascular collapse unless the condition is recognized and treated. In severe cases, perforation of the intestinal wall can occur, with spillage of the bowel contents into the peritoneal cavity (Alle, Stewart, & Maselly, 1994; Krumberger, 1998).

In severe cases of bowel obstruction, the intestine can become strangulated. **Intestinal strangulation** occurs when the intestine "twists" itself to such an extent that circulation is interrupted. Strangulation can result in necrosis, perforation, and sepsis. Corrective surgery is generally the treatment of choice to prevent ischemic bowel problems. Appropriately treated simple obstruction has a low mortality rate (< 2 percent), whereas strangulation is associated with a high mortality rate (up to 25 percent if surgery is delayed). When the obstruction is located in the colon, it usually stems from a malignant tumor (McQuaid, 1999).

Acute Paralytic Ileus

Paralytic ileus (adynamic ileus) involves bowel obstruction due to a loss of intestinal peristalsis in the absence of any mechanical (physical) obstruction commonly seen in hospitalized patients. It can occur anywhere along the GI tract as a complication from trauma, handling of the bowel during surgery, electrolyte disturbances (hypokalemia, hypocalcemia, and hypomagnesemia), intestinal ischemia, peritonitis, and sepsis. In addition, there are multiple medications that reduce gastric motility (e.g., opioids, anticholinergics, and phenothiazines), thus contributing to the development of paralytic ileus (Alle, Stewart, & Maselly, 1994).

Ogilvie's syndrome involves paralytic ileus of the colon. This is a severe form of ileus that often arises in bedridden patients who have serious systemic illnesses. The abdomen is usually silent, and abdominal cramping is not present, but tenderness may be noted. Abdominal x-rays show a dilated colon. Dehydration is usually present as a consequence of fluid translocation into distended loops of intestine (Alle, Stewart, & Maselly, 1994).

Clinical Manifestations

Laboratory and radiologic examinations, along with history and physical findings, aid in diagnosing intestinal obstruction. The hallmark clinical manifestation of intestinal obstruction is abdominal distention. Small-bowel obstruction is characterized by cramping, periumbilical pain that occurs in waves, with periods of relative comfort in between the waves of pain. Vomiting, possibly profuse, soon follows the onset of pain and is usually bilious with a large quantity of mucus. Electrolyte imbalances and intraluminal loss of fluids occur, with dehydration soon following. Visible peristaltic waves may be observed on the abdomen, and high-pitched tinkles are auscultated during the painful spasms. The abdomen may be tender to palpation. If rebound tenderness develops, the nurse should observe for signs and symptoms of shock due to perforation. Symptoms of colonic paralytic ileus (Ogilvie's syndrome) include abdominal distention and diminished bowel sounds without pain (Alle, Stewart, & Maselly, 1994).

Laboratory Findings

Hematology, electrolyte, and chemistry studies will reflect inflammation, fluid, and electrolyte imbalances. Mild leukocytosis ($< 15,000$) is common, whereas WBC elevations from 15,000 to 25,000 may occur with strangulation and perforation (Hudak, Gallo, & Morton, 1998). Serum BUN, creatinine, sodium, and osmolality levels become elevated as fluid and electrolytes leak out of the obstructed bowel and third spacing (translocation of electrolytes and fluid into the intestinal lumen) occurs. Increases in serum amylase levels are common.

Radiologic Findings

Radiology films are taken with the patient in upright, flat, and side-lying positions. Distended bowel loops will reveal air–fluid levels in a "ladderlike" pattern. Distention is more pronounced within the colon in patients with paralytic ileus. Direct visualization and barium studies may help to confirm the diagnosis (Andreoli et al., 1997; McQuaid, 1999).

Treatment

It is imperative to identify those patients at risk of developing a bowel obstruction or motility problem. Patients at risk of developing bowel obstruction are the elderly, postoperative, bedridden, and those with dysfunction of multiple body systems. Initial therapy is directed toward fluid resuscitation and stabilization of the patient. Oral food and fluids are withheld, and a nasogastric tube (Salem-sump) is inserted and attached to low, intermittent suction to relieve vomiting and to decompress abdominal distention. Colonoscopy with decompression is sometimes useful in Ogilvie's syndrome. Isotonic intravenous fluid administration should be used to treat dehydration. Electrolyte losses should be replaced and continually monitored by the nurse. The extent of fluid resuscitation is best guided by the urine output, though in the elderly or those with cardiopulmonary disease, a pulmonary artery catheter (Swan–Ganz) is the best means of determining fluid volume needs. The nurse should closely monitor the patient's urine output, utilizing an indwelling urinary drainage catheter. (Refer to Module 14 for explanation of pulmonary artery catheters.) If the patient demonstrates peritoneal signs (boardlike abdominal distention with severe pain) and strangulation is suspected, broad-spectrum antibiotics should be considered to provide anaerobic and gram-negative coverage. Early surgical consult is advised in high-risk patients. All cases of complete obstruction require surgical resection of the affected bowel (Beers & Berkow, 1999; Hudak, Gallo, & Morton, 1997; McQuaid, 1999).

SECTION NINE REVIEW

1. Common mechanical causes of small-bowel obstruction are
   A. adhesions
   B. myocardial infarction
   C. closed head injury
   D. inflammatory bowel disease
2. A patient with a small-bowel obstruction develops rebound tenderness with "boardlike" distention. The nurse should suspect
   A. constipation
   B. perforation
   C. Ogilvie's syndrome
   D. retroperitoneal bleeding
3. _______ accumulates in the bowel proximal to the actual bowel obstruction, resulting in distention.
   A. Fluid
   B. Blood
   C. Stool
   D. Pus
4. Bowel that "twists" itself to such an extent that circulation is interrupted is known as
   A. peritonitis
   B. perforation
   C. strangulation
   D. peristalsis
5. Strangulation is associated with a mortality rate of
   A. < 2 percent
   B. ≤ 50 percent
   C. ≤ 80 percent
   D. ≤ 25 percent

Answers: 1. A, 2. B, 3. A, 4. C, 5. D

SECTION TEN: Gastrointestinal Nursing Diagnosis and Management

At the completion of this section, the learner will be able to describe the nursing diagnosis and management of acute GI bleeding and paralytic ileus.

The care of patients with acute GI bleeding is complex and requires close assessment and monitoring of the patient's condition and progress. Collaborative management of physiologic problems as well as concern for the patient's psychosocial response to the acute illness are priorities for the nurse. Because fear and anxiety often accompany acute GI bleeding, patients and their significant others need information and support during this time. Nurses coordinate plans for the patient's ongoing care based on accurate and ongoing nursing assessment. Nursing diagnoses that are appropriate for patients diagnosed with GI bleeding, paralytic ileus, and acute intestinal ischemia are listed in Table 28–11.

A life-threatening complication of acute GI bleeding and bowel infarction is shock (hypovolemic and/or septic shock). Key nursing goals for the patient with hypovolemic or septic shock include maintenance of adequate tissue perfusion/oxygenation, prevention of fluid volume deficit related to blood loss and third spacing of fluids, and optimization of hemodynamic status. Regardless of what has caused the shock (GI hemorrhage, sepsis), the nurse must first see that venous access is achieved so that fluid and blood resuscitation therapy can begin. Table 28–12 lists common interventions used to stop the hem-

TABLE 28–11. NURSING DIAGNOSES

PROBLEM STATEMENT	ETIOLOGIC FACTOR
GASTROINTESTINAL BLEEDING	
Fluid volume deficit, risk for	Hypovolemia secondary to blood loss; NPO; vomiting; diarrhea
Tissue perfusion, altered: cerebral, cardiac, respiratory, renal, peripheral, mesenteric	Hypovolemia and decreased oxygenation secondary to anemia, hypotension, shock
Gas exchange, impaired	Hypovolemia, anemia
Anxiety	Fear of bleeding, threat of death
Aspiration, risk for	Hematemesis and potential changes in level of consciousness
Nutrition, less than body requirements, altered	Decreased appetite secondary to bowel irritability; NPO
Pain	Bleeding and discomfort
Diarrhea	Decrease in intestinal transit time secondary to cathartic effects of blood in GI tract
Thought processes, altered	Hypoxia secondary to anemia
Infection, risk for	Immune suppression; intestinal ischemia/infarction secondary to hypotension and shock
Fatigue	Anemia, decreased oxygenation
Knowledge deficit	Precipitating factors; therapeutic procedures/interventions; discharge information
PARALYTIC ILEUS	
Ineffective breathing pattern	Abdominal distention
Fluid volume deficit, actual	Vomiting, distention, electrolyte imbalance, hypovolemia (loss of fluid/electrolytes due to stasis of bowel contents)
Tissue perfusion, risk for, bowel	Decreased oxygenation to tissues secondary to bowel strangulation, perforation, and/or shock
Infection, risk for	Perforation, strangulation, bowel ischemia → infarction → necrosis → sepsis
Bowel elimination, altered	Absent bowel sounds; NPO; electrolyte loss; constipation
Pain/discomfort, actual	Distention; intestinal angina; perforation
Knowledge deficit, actual	Illness, treatments, procedures, and outcome
INTESTINAL ISCHEMIA	
Pain/comfort, actual	Intestinal angina; distention; infarction; peritonitis
Infection, risk for	Infarction → necrosis → sepsis
Fluid volume deficit, risk for	Electrolyte imbalance; NPO; vomiting; diarrhea; third spacing; shock if perforation occurs
Knowledge deficit, actual	Illness, treatments, procedures, and outcome

Sources: Carpenito, L.J. (1999). Nursing care plans and documentation, *3rd ed. Philadelphia: J.B. Lippincott; and Krumberger, J.M., & Hammer, B. (1998). Gastrointestinal disorders. In M.R. Kinney et al. (eds.).* AACN's clinical reference for critical care nursing, *4th ed. St. Louis: C.V. Mosby.*

TABLE 28–12. ARTERIAL ANGIOTHERAPY INTERVENTIONS IN GI HEMORRHAGE

INTERVENTION	DESCRIPTION	COMMENTS
Selective arterial infusion of vasopressin	Requires selective catheterization of the bleeding artery for infusion of vasopressin.	Used to control massive bleeding in those patients who have peptic ulcer disease, stress ulcers, erosive gastritis, and Mallory–Weiss tear
Arterial embolization	An alternative to arterial vasopressin where the bleeding vessel is selectively catheterized, and a coagulant is placed in the vessel	

Sources: Andreoli, T.E., Bennett, J.C., Carpenter, C., & Blum, F. (eds.). (1997). Cecil's essentials of medicine, *4th ed. Philadelphia: W.B. Saunders; Beers, M.H., & Berkhow, R. (eds.). (1999).* The Merck manual of diagnosis and therapy, *17th ed. Whitehouse Station, NJ: Merck Research Laboratories; and Carey, C.F., Lee, H.H., & Woeltze, K.F. (eds.). (1998).* Washington Manual *Philadelphia: Lippincott-Raven.*

morhage. Ensuring adequacy of intravenous infusions remains a nursing priority for the duration of the treatment of shock. In order to maintain adequate gas exchange and tissue perfusion, the nurse should:

1. Ensure an open airway and administer supplementary oxygen.
2. Initiate continuous monitoring for cardiac dysrhythmias.
3. Prepare for insertion of a pulmonary artery catheter and record and monitor cardiac filling pressures once placement has been achieved.
4. Prepare the patient for emergent surgical intervention to control bleeding and/or resect necrotic bowel (Andreoli et al., 1997; Driscoll, 1999; Krumberger, 1998).

Table 28–13 summarizes some nursing interventions specific to the care of the patient at risk for hypovolemia due to GI bleeding. These interventions also apply to the patient who is in shock secondary to sepsis.

TABLE 28–13. CLINICAL APPLICATION: NURSING INTERVENTIONS FOR PATIENTS AT RISK FOR HYPOVOLEMIA DUE TO GI BLEEDING

- Assess for signs and symptoms of shock; vital signs, urine output, hemodynamic measures (PAP, PCWP, CI, CO, SVR, CVP), Sao_2 (oxygen saturation), diminished peripheral pulses, restlessness, agitation, cool, pale, or moist skin
- Assess fluid status; intake and output (urine output, gastric drainage)
- Assess electrolyte levels (may become altered from fluid loss or fluid shifts)
- Assess hemoglobin, hematocrit, RBC, coagulation studies (PT, PTT), renal function (BUN, serum creatinine)
- Test gastric drainage, emesis, or stools for occult blood
- Assess gastric pH; consult with physician/practitioner about specific pH range and antacid administration
- Consult with physician/practitioner about replacing fluid losses based on assessment findings
- Administer replacement fluids and blood products as directed
- Assess for adverse reaction to blood products

PAP, pulmonary artery pressure; PCWP, pulmonary capillary wedge pressure; CI, cardiac index; CO, cardiac output; SVR, systemic vascular resistance; CVP, central venous pressure; RBC, red blood count; PT, prothrombin time; PTT, partial thromboplastin time; BUN, blood urea nitrogen.

Source: Krumberger, J.M., & Hammer, B. (1998). Gastrointestinal disorders. In M.R. Kinney et al. (eds.). AACN clinical reference for critical care nursing, *4th ed. (pp. 1105–1152). St. Louis: C.V. Mosby.*

SECTION TEN REVIEW

1. A life-threatening complication of acute GI bleeding and bowel infarction is
   A. renal failure
   B. abdominal aorta aneurysm
   C. shock
   D. pancreatitis

2. When providing nursing care for a patient experiencing GI bleeding or paralytic ileus/necrotic bowel, the nurse should prepare the patient for
   A. surgery
   B. placement of a urinary catheter
   C. endotracheal intubation
   D. obtaining blood cultures

Answers: 1. C, 2. A

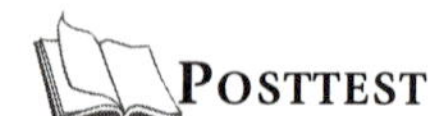

POSTTEST

1. The normal flora that reside within the large intestine break down cellulose and synthesize
   A. hydrochloric acid, vitamin C, calcium, carbolic acid
   B. vitamin E, phosphorous, creatine, folic acid
   C. vitamin K, carbon dioxide, methane, riboflavin
   D. vitamin K, folic acid, riboflavin, nicotinic acid

2. The ileocecal valve
   A. prevents backflow of feces from large to small intestine
   B. prevents backflow of chyme from the duodenum to the stomach

C. allows stomach contents to move into the small intestine
D. allows passage of feces through the rectum

3. The stomach receives its nerve supply from the
A. autonomic nervous system
B. gastrointestinal nervous system
C. mesenteric nervous system
D. splanchnic nervous system

4. The enteric nervous system coordinates
A. sphincter tone and glandular secretion
B. splanchnic blood supply and sensation
C. GI motility and secretion activities
D. absorption of fluid and electrolytes

5. Chronic total parenteral nutritional therapy without enteral stimulation may result in
A. regeneration of intestinal mucosa cells
B. enhanced immunologic defense mechanisms
C. mucosal atrophy and bacterial overgrowth
D. enhanced production of mucus by goblet cells

6. Intact gut barrier function inhibits
A. bacterial translocation across mucosal barriers
B. GALT defense mechanisms
C. rapid response of macrophages to pathogens
D. immunoglobulin production by GALT

7. _______ may contribute to gastrointestinal bleeding.
A. Pulmonary disease
B. Hepatic dysfunction
C. Autoimmune complications
D. Cardiac disease

8. In the case of GI bleeding, angiography allows visualization of
A. vascular beds and flow
B. GI motility
C. abscesses
D. masses

9. All external metal objects must be removed in order for a(n) _______ to be performed.
A. ultrasound sonography
B. angiography
C. CT scan
D. MRI

10. Occult bleeding is usually
A. unnoticed by the patient
B. massive in its presentation
C. acute in its presentation
D. bright red in appearance

11. NSAIDs interrupt mucosal integrity by
A. inhibiting gastric acid production
B. increasing mucus production
C. inhibiting prostaglandin function
D. decreasing bicarbonate secretion

12. Upper GI bleeding from esophageal or gastric varices is associated with
A. acute renal failure
B. gastric acid hypersecretion
C. chronic renal failure
D. portal hypertension

13. Gastrointestinal AVMs are most common in
A. the young, healthy adult population
B. the elderly with chronic disease
C. females with diabetes mellitus
D. males with human immunodeficiency virus (HIV)

14. Duodenal ulcer pain is characteristically
A. consistent
B. sporadic
C. worse upon awakening
D. aggravated by food

15. The mortality rate for patients with ischemic bowel disease is
A. 20 percent
B. 30 percent
C. 40 percent
D. 50 percent

16. _______ is the most common symptom of inflammatory bowel disease.
A. Nausea and vomiting
B. Bloody diarrhea
C. Constipation
D. Abdominal distention

17. A patient requires a blood transfusion. The blood bank has not typed and crossmatched the patient's blood; therefore, packed red cells cannot be transfused due to the risk of allergic reaction. The patient needs blood now, and the decision is made to transfuse whole blood that does not require type and crossmatch. Which type of whole blood can be used in this situation?
A. type A
B. type AB
C. type B
D. type O

18. The nurse notes that the patient's heart rate is 125 beats/min (increased from 85). The patient's blood pressure is decreased to 88/40 from 126/62, and the patient is suddenly anxious. These assessment findings can indicate
A. rebleeding
B. pain
C. hypervolemia
D. hyperglycemia

19. Ogilvie's syndrome involves paralytic ileus of the
A. colon
B. ileum
C. jejunum
D. duodenum

20. Complete bowel obstruction requires
A. rapid initiation of enteral feeding
B. stat soapsuds enema
C. surgical resection of bowel
D. evacuation by colonoscopy

POSTTEST ANSWERS

Question	Answer	Section	Question	Answer	Section
1	D	one	11	C	six
2	A	one	12	D	six
3	A	two	13	B	six
4	C	two	14	A	six
5	C	three	15	D	seven
6	A	three	16	B	seven
7	B	four	17	D	eight
8	A	four	18	A	eight
9	D	four	19	A	nine
10	A	five	20	C	nine

REFERENCES

Alle, K., Stewart, D.E., & Maselly, M.J. (1994). Gastrointestinal failure in the ICU. In F.S. Bongard & D.Y. Sue (eds.), *Current critical care diagnosis and treatment* (pp. 117–130). Norwalk, CT: Appleton & Lange.

Andreoli, T.E., Bennett, J.C., Carpenter, C., Blum, F. (eds.). (1997). *Cecil's essentials of medicine* (4th ed.). Philadelphia: W.B. Saunders.

Beers, M.H., & Berkhow, R. (eds.). (1999). *The Merck manual of diagnosis and therapy* (17th ed.). Whitehouse Station, NJ: Merck Research Laboratories.

Bono, M.J. (1996). Lower gastrointestinal tract bleeding, Part 1. *Emerg Med Clin North Am Gastrointest Emerg 14*:547–556.

Carey, C.F., Lee, H.H., & Woeltze, K.F. (eds.). (1998). *Washington manual* (pp. 302–309). Philadelphia: Lippincott-Raven.

Chamberlain, C.E. (1993). Acute hemorrhagic gastritis. *Gastroenterol Clin North Am 22*:843–873.

Chojkler, M. (1986). Predictors of outcome in massive upper GI hemorrhage. *J Clin Gastroenterol* 8:16–22.

Crittormson, W.L., & Burbick, M.P. (1989). Mortality from ischemic colitis. *Dis Colon Rectum 32*:469–472.

Driscoll, C.J. (1999). Acute gastrointestinal bleed. In L. Bucher & S. Melander (eds.). *Critical care nursing*. Philadelphia: W.B. Saunders.

Elta, G.H. (1995). Approach to the patient with gross gastrointestinal bleeding. In T. Yamada et al. (eds.), *Textbook of gastroenterology* (pp. 671–698). Philadelphia: J.B. Lippincott.

Graham, D. (1996). Management of upper gastrointestinal hemorrhage. In J.C. Bennett et al. (eds.). *Cecil's textbook of medicine* (20th ed.). Philadelphia: W.B. Saunders.

Gray, H. (1995). *Gray's anatomy: The anatomical basis of medicine and surgery* (38th ed.). New York: Churchill.

Guyton, A.C. (1996). *Textbook of medical physiology* (8th ed.) (pp. 736–742). Philadelphia: W.B. Saunders.

Guyton, A., & Hall, J.E. (1996). *Textbook of medical physiology* (9th ed.). Philadelphia: W.B. Saunders.

Guyton, A.C., & Hall, J.E. (1997). *Human physiology and mechanics of disease* (6th ed.). Philadelphia: W.B. Saunders.

Haist, S.A., Robbins, J.B., & Gorwella, L.G. (1997). *Internal medicine on call* (2nd ed.). Stamford, CT: Appleton & Lange.

Heitkemper, M., & Westfall, U. (1993). Gastrointestinal physiology. In J. Clochesy, C. Breu, S. Cardin, & A. Whittaker (eds.), *Critical care nursing* (pp. 929–944). Philadelphia: W.B. Saunders.

Hudak, C.M., Gallo, B.M., & Morton, P.G. (1998). *Critical care nursing: A holistic approach* (7th ed.) (pp. 743–804). Philadelphia: J.B. Lippincott.

Huether, S.E., McCance, K.L., & Tarmina, M.S. (1994). Alterations of digestive function. In K.L. McCance & S.E. Heuther (eds.), *Pathophysiology: The biologic basis for disease in adults and children* (pp. 1212–1266). St. Louis: C.V. Mosby.

Isenkery, J.I., McQuaid, K.R., Laine, I., et al. (1995). Acid peptic disorders. In T. Yamada et al. (eds.), *Textbook of gastroenterology*. Philadelphia: J.B. Lippincott.

Kee, J. (1999). *Laboratory diagnostic tests with nursing implications* (5th ed.). Stamford, CT: Appleton & Lange.

Krumberger, J.M., & Hammer, B. (1998). Gastrointestinal disorders. In M.R. Kinney, S.B. Dunbar, J.A. Brooks-Brunn, N. Molter, & J.M. Vitello-Cicciu (eds.). *AACN's clinical reference for critical care nursing* (4th ed.) (pp. 1033–1037). St. Louis: C.V. Mosby.

Krumberger, J.M. (1998). Gastrointestinal clinical physiology. In M.R. Kinney, S.B. Dunbar, J.A. Brooks-Brunn, N. Molter, & J.M. Vitello-Cicciu (eds.). *AACN's clinical reference for critical care nursing* (4th ed.). St. Louis: C.V. Mosby.

Lacy, C., Armstrong, L.L., Ingrim, N.B., & Lance, L.L. (1998). *Drug information handbook*. Cleveland, OH: American Pharmaceutical Association.

Longstreth, G.F. (1995). Epidemiology of hospitalization for acute upper gastrointestinal hemorrhage: A population-based study. *Am J Gastroenterol 90*:206–210.

Markey, D.W. (1999). Gastrointestinal anatomy and physiology. In L. Bucher & S. Melander (eds.), *Critical care nursing* (pp. 675–691). Philadelphia: W.B. Saunders.

McGuirk, T.D., & Coyle, W.J. (1994). Upper gastrointestinal tract bleeding in emergency medicine, Part 1. *Emerg Med Clin North Am 14*:523–543.

McQuaid, K.R. (1999). Alimentary tract. In L.M. Tierney, S.J. McPhee, & M.A. Papadakis (eds.), *Current medical diagnosis and treatment* (38th ed.). Stamford, CT: Appleton & Lange.

Passaro, E. (1994). Gastrointestinal bleeding. In F.S. Bongard & D.Y. Sue (eds.), *Current critical care diagnosis and treatment*. Norwalk, CT: Appleton & Lange.

Smith, S.L. (1998). The gastrointestinal system. In J.G. Alspach (ed.), *AACN's core curriculum for critical care nursing* (5th ed.). Philadelphia: W.B. Saunders.

Smith, C. (1997). Upper gastrointestinal disorders. In L.Y. Young & M.A. Koda-Kimble (eds.), *Applied therapeutics: The clinical use of drugs* (6th ed.). Vancouver, WA: Applied Therapeutics Inc.

Sommers, M.S. (1997). Response of the body to immunologic challenge. In S.A. Price & L.M. Wilson, *Pathophysiology: Clinical concepts of disease processes* (5th ed.) (p. 68). St. Louis: C.V. Mosby.

Spencer, J. (1994). Lower gastrointestinal bleeding. In I. Bouchier, R. Allan, H. Hodgson, & M. Keighley (eds.), *Gastroenterology: Clinical science and practice* (pp. 975–988). London: W.B. Saunders.

Westfall, U.E. (1999). Gastrointestinal laboratory and diagnostic tests. In L. Buchee & S. Melander (eds.), *Critical care nursing*. Philadelphia: W.B. Saunders.

Wilson, L.M., & Lindseth, G.N. (1996). Disorders of the stomach and duodenum. In S.A. Price & L.M. Wilson, *Pathophysiology: Clinical concepts of disease processes* (5th ed.). St. Louis: C.V. Mosby.

Module 29

Acute Hepatic Dysfunction

Kathleen D. Wagner, Melanie Hardin-Pierce

This self-study module presents the physiologic and pathophysiologic processes involved in acute hepatic dysfunction and management of the patient with acute hepatic failure. The module is composed of eight sections. Sections One through Three present a review of the anatomy and physiology of the liver, including liver functions and evaluation of liver function through laboratory testing. Section Four provides an overview of acute hepatitis. Section Five describes acute hepatic failure based on causative factors. It then describes the clinical manifestations of acute hepatic failure. Section Six explains the multisystem complications of hepatic dysfunction. Sections Seven and Eight complete the module, with an overview of medical management, therapeutic goals, nursing assessment, and frequently occurring nursing diagnoses. Each section includes a set of review questions to help the learner evaluate his or her understanding of the section's content before moving on to the next section. All Section Reviews and the module Pretest and Posttest include answers. It is suggested that the learner review those concepts answered incorrectly in the review questions before proceeding to the next section.

Objectives

Following completion of this module, the learner will be able to

1. Identify the anatomic structures of the liver.
2. Discuss the functions of the liver.
3. Discuss liver function through evaluation of laboratory tests results.
4. Describe the etiology and clinical manifestations associated with acute hepatitis.
5. Describe the etiology and clinical manifestations associated with acute hepatic dysfunction and failure.
6. Describe the complications of acute hepatic dysfunction.
7. Describe an overview of medical management of the patient with acute hepatic dysfunction.
8. Describe the nursing implications appropriate to management of the patient experiencing acute hepatic dysfunction.

Pretest

1. The functional unit of the liver is called the
   A. hepatocyte
   B. lobule
   C. canaliculi
   D. capsule

2. Bile is secreted by the
   A. terminal bile ducts
   B. quadrate lobe
   C. canaliculi
   D. hepatocytes

3. The primary substance in bile is
   A. bile salts
   B. bilirubin
   C. cholesterol
   D. electrolytes
4. The major function of bile salts is to assist with
   A. absorption of fat products
   B. blood clotting
   C. conversion of vitamin D
   D. protein synthesis
5. The majority of iron is located in
   A. the liver
   B. bone
   C. fat
   D. hemoglobin
6. The major by-product of amino acid deamination is
   A. bilirubin
   B. ammonia
   C. fatty acids
   D. glucose
7. Serum enzyme levels are obtained to measure
   A. clotting factors
   B. organ function
   C. cellular injury
   D. tissue oxygenation
8. Serum isoenzyme levels often provide better data than parent enzyme levels because they are
   A. faster to obtain
   B. more tissue specific
   C. more plentiful
   D. easier to measure
9. Which combination of lactic dehydrogenase (LDH) isoenzymes best reflects hepatic injury?
   A. LDH1 and LDH2
   B. LDH2 and LDH3
   C. LDH3 and LDH4
   D. LDH4 and LDH5
10. Acute hepatitis is most commonly caused by
    A. bacterial invasion
    B. viral invasion
    C. yeast invasion
    D. an autoimmune reaction
11. The major cause of acute and chronic hepatitis and cirrhosis is
    A. cytomegalovirus
    B. hepatitis C virus
    C. Epstein–Barr virus
    D. hepatitis B virus
12. Classic hepatitis is characterized by
    A. localized necrosis
    B. a greatly enlarged liver
    C. the development of fibrosis
    D. the development of fulminant hepatic failure
13. Which of the following statements is true regarding fulminant hepatic failure?
    A. it causes necrosis of liver tissue
    B. it has a mortality of less than 50 percent
    C. it is characterized by stage I to II encephalopathy
    D. it has a slow, insidious onset
14. A major hepatotoxin that is known to cause fulminant hepatic failure is
    A. acetaminophen
    B. gentamicin
    C. aspirin
    D. cephalosporin
15. In the United States cirrhosis of the liver is most commonly caused by
    A. hepatitis A virus
    B. alcohol abuse
    C. hepatitis B virus
    D. Epstein–Barr virus
16. A major cause of ascites is
    A. hyperalbuminemia
    B. low colloid osmotic pressure
    C. hepatorenal syndrome
    D. fluid volume overload
17. A major factor contributing to the onset of acute renal failure as a complication of hepatic failure is
    A. hepatotoxins
    B. a hypotensive episode
    C. high ammonia levels
    D. portal vein shunting
18. The onset of type II hepatorenal syndrome usually occurs in the presence of
    A. hepatotoxins
    B. a hypotensive episode
    C. high ammonia levels
    D. severe ascites
19. Dietary management of the patient with acute viral hepatitis would include
    A. high protein, low fat
    B. low fat, high carbohydrate
    C. low carbohydrate, low fat
    D. low protein, high fat
20. A patient with acute viral hepatitis will most likely be admitted to the hospital if he or she is experiencing
    A. severe fatigue
    B. occasional nausea
    C. elevated bilirubin
    D. hepatic encephalopathy
21. The patient with fulminant hepatic failure will require strict nutritional control of
    A. protein
    B. fat
    C. carbohydrate
    D. fiber

Pretest answers: 1. B, 2. D, 3. A, 4. A, 5. D, 6. B, 7. C, 8. B, 9. D, 10. B, 11. D, 12. A, 13. A, 14. A, 15. B, 16. B, 17. B, 18. D, 19. B, 20. D, 21. A

GLOSSARY

Acute hepatitis. An inflammatory liver disease, usually of viral origin, that results in liver injury and necrosis

Alanine aminotransferase (ALT, SGPT). An enzyme primarily found in the cells of the liver, kidneys, heart, and skeletal muscles

Alkaline phosphatase (ALP). An enzyme primarily found in the cells of the liver and kidneys

Ascites. A collection of fluid (hepatic lymph) in the abdominal cavity

Aspartate aminotransferase (AST, SGOT). An enzyme primarily found in the cells of the liver, kidneys, heart, pancreas, and brain

Bile. A substance produced by the hepatocytes that is essential to normal digestion, particularly fats

Bilirubin. The end product of hemoglobin degradation

Conjugated bilirubin. Bilirubin that has been joined with glucuronic acid to make it water soluble

Enzymes. Catalyst substances found in cells that assist in cellular activities

Fulminant hepatic failure (FHF). A rapidly developing (< 8 weeks) acute failure of the liver, characterized by severe encephalopathy (stage III or IV), that develops in a person with no preexisting liver dysfunction

Hepatic encephalopathy. An altered neurologic status that is caused by a buildup of circulating toxins of hepatic origin

Hepatic failure. The inability of the liver to perform its normal functions

Hepatorenal syndrome (HRS). Acute renal failure associated with advanced liver dysfunction

Isoenzymes. A subgrouping of parent enzymes that are more specific to a particular cell type

Jaundice. A yellow cast of the skin, sclera, and mucous membranes caused by elevated bilirubin, a yellow pigment

Kupffer's cells. Fixed tissue macrophages found in the liver

Lobule. The functional unit of the liver

Portal hypertension. Elevated portal vein pressure that is sustained at above-normal levels

Prothrombin time (PT). Measures the coagulation extrinsic pathway

Splanchnic circulation. The combination of the portal venous and arterial circulatory systems of the viscera

Unconjugated bilirubin. Fat-soluble bilirubin that has not yet joined with glucuronic acid

Urobilinogen. Bilirubin in the urine

Urea. A nitrogen substance produced by the liver from ammonia

Varices. Dilated veins

ABBREVIATIONS

AHF. Acute hepatic failure

ALP. Alkaline phosphatase

ALT. Alanine aminotransferase (SGPT)

AST. Aspartate aminotransferase (SGOT)

BUN. Blood urea nitrogen

FHF. Fulminant hepatic failure

GI. Gastrointestinal

GFR. Glomerular filtration rate

GGT. Gamma glutamyl transpeptidase

HAV. Hepatitis A virus

HBsAg. Hepatitis B surface antigen

HBV. Hepatitis B virus

HCV. Hepatitis C virus

HDV. Hepatitis D virus

HEV. Hepatitis E virus

HIV. Human immunodeficiency virus

HRS. Hepatorenal syndrome

LDH. Lactic dehydrogenase

OCT. Ornithinecarbamoyl transferase

PT. Prothrombin time

SIRS. Systemic inflammatory response syndrome

STD. Sexually transmitted disease

5′-N. 5′-Nucleotidase

SECTION ONE: Anatomy of the Liver

At the completion of this section, the learner will be able to identify the anatomic structures of the liver.

Located in the right upper quadrant of the abdominal cavity, the liver lies directly underneath the diaphragm. The liver has two major lobes, the right and the left. The right lobe can be further differentiated into the caudate and quadrate lobes, located on the posterior and inferior liver surfaces, respectively (Fig. 29–1). It is enclosed in visceral peritoneum and covered with Glisson's capsule, a connective tissue structure that provides support to the liver. The capsule subdivides into branches, called septa that extend into the liver parenchyma to form individual liver lobules.

The **lobule** is the functional unit of the liver (Fig. 29–2). It is a cylindrically shaped unit that surrounds a central vein in a spokelike fashion. Each lobule is composed of hepatic cellular plates that radiate out from the central vein. The hepatic cells (hepatocytes) secrete bile, which flows into the bile canaliculi, a small space separating the hepatic cellular plates. From the canaliculi, bile flows into terminal bile ducts located in the septa, or spaces, lying between adjoining lobules. The septa contain the portal venules, which provide blood flow from the portal veins. The portal venules supply the blood that flows by the hepatic cellular plates, and ultimately flows into the central vein of the lobule. The physiologic structure of the lobule allows continuous exposure of blood to the hepatic cells.

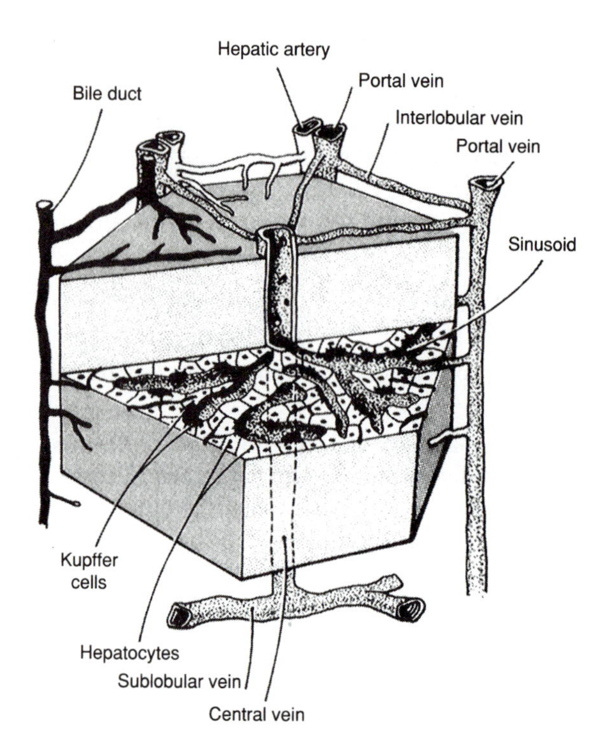

Figure 29–2. Microscopic structure of hepatic function unit (liver lobule). *(From Wilson, L.M., & Lester, L.B. [1992]. Liver, biliary tract, and pancreas. In S.A. Price & L.M. Wilson [eds].* Pathophysiology: Clinical concepts of disease processes, *4th ed. [p. 338]. St. Louis: Mosby-Year Book.)*

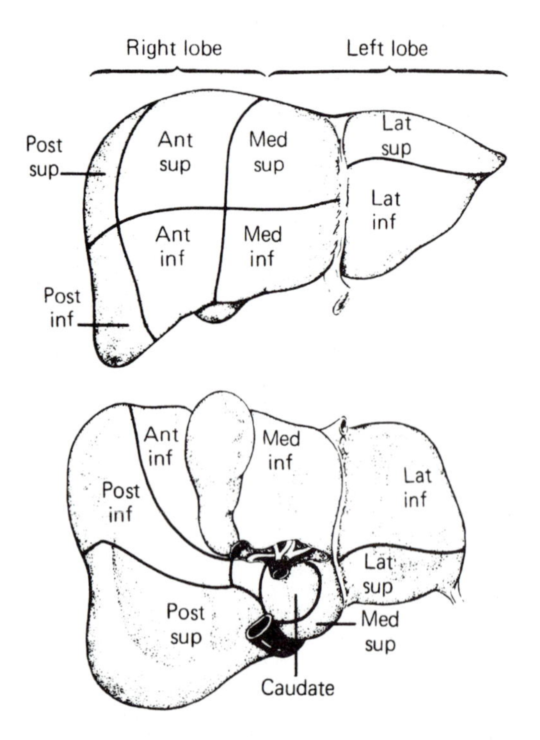

Figure 29–1. Segmental anatomy of the liver. The major lobar fissure, separating the right and left lobes, passes from the inferior vena cava through the gallbladder bed. *(Reproduced with permission from Way, L.W. [1985].* Current surgical diagnosis and treatment, *7th ed. [p. 398]. Norwalk, CT: Appleton & Lange.)*

Bile is composed primarily of bile salts. It also contains bilirubin, cholesterol, electrolytes, and other substances. Bile flows through the bile duct system, which ultimately dumps bile into either the gallbladder or the duodenum. Approximately 0.5 to 1.0 L of bile is formed each day; the capacity of the gallbladder is only about 50 mL. Once in the gallbladder, the bile's water and inorganic salt content is absorbed by blood vessels and lymphatics, increasing the bile concentration by about 10 times. Bile is intermittently emptied from the gallbladder via contraction, which is stimulated by the presence of chyme in the duodenum. Foods with high fat content provide the strongest contraction stimulus (Wilson & Lester, 1992).

Splanchnic Circulation

The term *splanchnic* refers to the viscera (the abdominal organs). The combination of the portal venous and arterial circulatory systems of the viscera is called the **splanchnic circulation** (Fig. 29–3). Approximately 30 percent of the cardiac output (about 1.5 L/min) flows through the liver. The volume of blood flowing into the liver is pri-

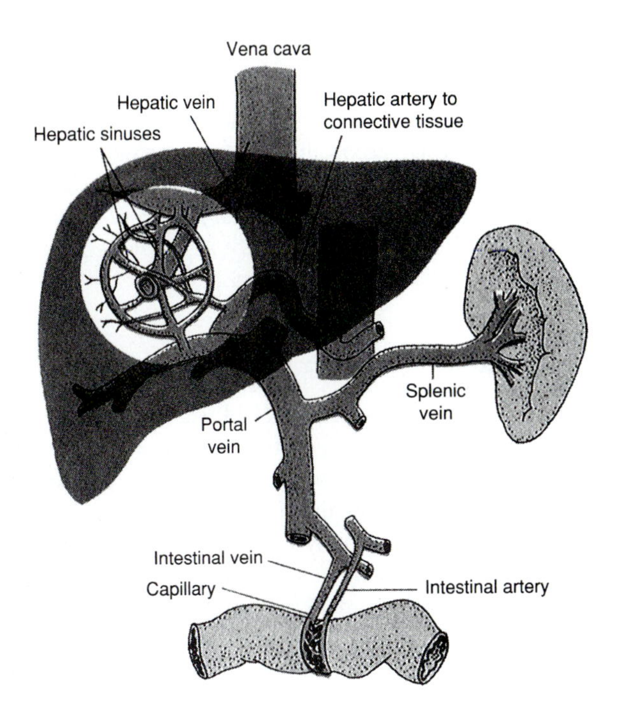

Figure 29–3. The splanchnic circulation. *(Reproduced with permission from Guyton, A.C. [1992].* Human physiology and mechanisms of disease. *5th ed. [p. 485]. Philadelphia: W.B. Saunders.)*

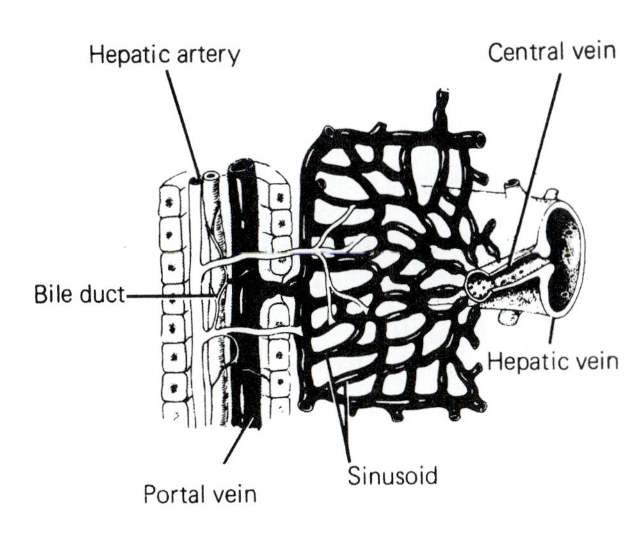

Figure 29–4. Vascular anatomy of the liver lobule. *(Reproduced with permission from Way, L.W. [1985].* Current surgical diagnosis and treatment, *7th ed. [p. 404]. Norwalk, CT: Appleton & Lange.)*

marily determined by the volume of blood flow through the spleen and gastrointestinal (GI) tract, both of which are parts of the splanchnic circulation. The liver is richly supplied with both arterial and venous blood (Fig. 29–4). The arterial blood supply is the hepatic artery, a branch of the aorta. The portal vein brings in blood from the spleen, intestines, pancreas, and stomach. The hepatic veins drain blood away from the liver to the inferior vena cava.

In summary, the liver is located in the right upper quadrant of the abdominal cavity. The lobule is the functional unit and consists of hepatic cellular plates. Hepatocytes secrete bile, which is stored in the gallbladder in a highly concentrated state until it is needed. Splanchnic circulation accounts for a significant portion of the cardiac output. Both the spleen and GI tract are important in determining the volume of hepatic blood flow.

Section One Review

1. The functional unit of the liver is called the
   - **A.** hepatocyte
   - **B.** lobule
   - **C.** canaliculi
   - **D.** capsule
2. Bile is secreted by
   - **A.** terminal bile ducts
   - **B.** the quadrate lobe
   - **C.** canaliculi
   - **D.** hepatocytes
3. The primary substance in bile is
   - **A.** bile salts
   - **B.** bilirubin
   - **C.** cholesterol
   - **D.** electrolytes
4. The blood volume flowing through the liver represents what percentage of cardiac output?
   - **A.** 10 percent
   - **B.** 20 percent
   - **C.** 30 percent
   - **D.** 40 percent
5. The portal vein brings in blood from all of the following organs EXCEPT the
   - **A.** kidneys
   - **B.** spleen
   - **C.** intestines
   - **D.** pancreas

Answers: 1. B, 2. D, 3. A, 4. C, 5. A

SECTION TWO: The Functions of the Liver

At the completion of this section, the learner will be able to discuss the functions of the liver.

The liver provides multiple functions that are essential to life, including metabolism, blood filtration, blood clotting, and acting as a blood volume reservoir.

Metabolic Functions

Fat Metabolism

The liver is responsible for the synthesis of phospholipids and cholesterol. Through oxidation of fatty acids, the liver can supply the body with massive amounts of energy. A major function of the liver is the production and excretion of bile. The major component of bile—bile salts—are necessary for normal digestion. In the intestines, bile salts assist in absorption of fat products such as fatty acids, cholesterol, and fat-soluble vitamins. Bile salts also assist in the breakdown of fat molecules through a detergentlike action. The second major component of bile is bilirubin, a bile pigment (discussed in Section Three).

Vitamin- and Mineral-Related Functions

Adequate levels of bile are needed for absorption of the fat-soluble vitamins A, D, E, and K. Should the production of bile be deficient, fat absorption will decrease and the levels of these vitamins will be significantly reduced. The liver requires vitamin K for production of clotting factors. If the level of vitamin K is low, clotting factor production will be reduced, possibly causing coagulation deficit complications. The liver also plays a crucial role in the early steps of the conversion of vitamin D into its active product 1,25-dihydroxycholecalciferol, which helps control the concentration of calcium.

The liver is the major storage center for iron, which is stored as ferritin and is released into the body as iron levels become depleted. Iron is an important part of hemoglobin synthesis; more than half the body's iron is located in hemoglobin. Liver damage (e.g., cirrhosis) can decrease levels of serum iron (Kee, 1999). If iron stores become depleted, iron-deficiency anemia develops.

Carbohydrate Metabolism

The liver plays a major role in maintaining normal blood glucose levels. Glucose is stored in the liver as glycogen, which is converted back into glucose as needed by the body through the process of glycogenolysis. The liver is also able to convert amino acids to glucose through the process of gluconeogenesis.

Protein Metabolism

Protein metabolism is essential to life. The liver is responsible not just for synthesis of the majority of the body's proteins; it also degrades amino acids for energy use through the process of deamination. The major byproduct of deamination is ammonia, which is toxic to tissues. The liver is responsible for converting ammonia into **urea,** a nontoxic substance. Urea diffuses from the liver into the circulation for urinary excretion. When liver failure occurs, ammonia cannot be converted to urea and levels rapidly build in the blood.

Blood Volume Reservoir

The liver serves as a reservoir for blood. Its massive vascular bed and its ability to expand and compress provide a large potential overflow receptacle. During periods of high fluid volume states in the right heart, the liver is able to accept approximately 1 L of the excess volume by distending, which decreases circulating fluid volume. In periods of fluid volume deficit, the liver is able to compress, shift blood into the intravascular space, and thereby increase circulating fluid volume.

Blood Filter

Blood flowing through the intestines becomes contaminated with bacteria. Special tissue macrophages in the liver called **Kupffer's cells** efficiently and rapidly engulf and destroy bacteria before the blood moves back into general circulation. The Kupffer's cells are part of the tissue macrophage system (also called the reticuloendothelial system). The tissue macrophage system consists of mobile macrophages that are able to move freely through the tissues, and fixed macrophages that are attached to tissues. Fixed macrophages, such as the Kupffer's cells, are

TABLE 29–1. MAJOR FUNCTIONS OF THE LIVER

GENERAL FUNCTION	COMMENTS
Metabolic	Fat metabolism—massive energy source; produces bile Carbohydrate metabolism—maintains normal blood glucose Protein metabolism—synthesis of proteins and deamination of amino acids; converts ammonia to urea Vitamin and minerals—major role in absorption of fat-soluble vitamins (A, D, E, and K); major storage area for iron
Blood volume reservoir	Able to distend and compress to alter circulating blood volume
Blood filter	Tissue macrophages, Kupffer's cells, purify the blood of bacteria
Blood clotting factors	Produces clotting factors including prothrombin and fibrinogen
Drug metabolism and detoxification	Responsible for metabolism of drugs; is able to deactivate potentially harmful substances and ready them for excretion in a harmless form

able to detach from their tissue when stimulated in order to carry out their phagocytic activities.

Blood Clotting Factors

The liver is responsible for the formation of most blood clotting factors. Normal formation of clotting factors requires synthesis of vitamin K by the intestines. When vitamin K synthesis is hindered, the formation of clotting factors is inhibited, leading to bleeding tendencies. The liver also produces fibrinogen, a protein that forms fibrin threads and blood clots when acted on by thrombin.

Drug Metabolism and Detoxification

The liver plays a major role in the metabolism of fat-soluble drugs. Through biotransformation, it changes potentially harmful drugs into harmless substances that are then excreted by the kidneys. The liver also has the ability to detoxify harmful endogenous substances such as phenol, which is formed by bacterial action on amino acids in the large intestines (Wilson et al., 1997).

In summary, the liver lobule is the functional unit of the liver. It plays a crucial role in many body functions. Table 29–1 lists the major functions of the liver.

SECTION TWO REVIEW

1. The major function of bile salts is to assist with
   A. absorption of fat products
   B. blood clotting
   C. conversion of vitamin D
   D. protein synthesis
2. The majority of iron is located in
   A. the liver
   B. bone
   C. fat
   D. hemoglobin
3. The major by-product of amino acid deamination is
   A. bilirubin
   B. ammonia
   C. fatty acids
   D. glucose
4. The blood filtering capabilities of the liver are primarily due to the presence of
   A. Kupffer's cells
   B. immunoglobulins
   C. ammonia
   D. bile

Answers: 1. A, 2. D, 3. B, 4. A

SECTION THREE: Evaluation of Liver Function through Laboratory Tests

At the completion of this section, the learner will be able to discuss liver function through evaluation of laboratory tests results.

A variety of common laboratory tests are required to evaluate the liver's ability to carry out its major metabolic and blood clotting activities.

Serum Enzyme Studies

Many cell activities require **enzymes** acting as catalysts to carry out their normal functions. Under normal circumstances, intracellular enzymes remain within their cell confines. When cell walls are damaged, however, these enzymes are able to escape their usual environment and can be found in surrounding tissues and in the serum. Most enzymes are found in two or more types of cells. For example, alanine aminotransferase is most highly concentrated in the liver, but is also found in the kidneys, heart, and skeletal muscles. For this reason, a diagnosis of hepatic dysfunction is made based on clinical presentation and serum tests.

Hepatic Enzymes

The liver's multiple metabolic functions require the assistance of a variety of enzymes. Three of the most common are:

- **Alanine aminotransferase (ALT, SGPT)**
- **Aspartate aminotransferase (AST, SGOT)**
- **Alkaline phosphatase (ALP)**

Table 29–2 summarizes information on the three major liver enzymes.

While of great value, enzyme levels cannot be used as a definitive test for hepatic dysfunction because they are nonspecific to the liver. If the patient's clinical presentation and initial enzyme levels do not give a clear diagnostic picture, the physician may order isoenzyme levels.

Isoenzymes

Isoenzymes are a subgrouping of the parent enzymes and are more specific to a particular type of cell. Several ALP

TABLE 29–2. ENZYME STUDIES MEASURING LIVER FUNCTION

ENZYME	NORMAL RANGE	TREND IN LIVER DISEASE	COMMENTS
Alanine aminotransferase (ALT, SGPT)	5–35 U/mL	Increased up to 20 times normal	False elevations noted with various drugs and alcohol; more specific to liver than to other organs. The ratio of AST/ALT usually is > 1 in alcoholic cirrhosis and liver congestion and < 1 in acute hepatitis.
Aspartate aminotransferase (AST, SGOT)	0–35 U/L (female values slightly lower)	Increased	False elevations noted with various drugs; rises with damage to kidneys, heart, pancreas, and brain as well as liver
Alkaline phosphatase (ALP)	20–90 U/L	Increased; levels will elevate two to three times normal when bile duct obstruction is present	False high or low values occur with a variety of drugs; rises with damage/disease of kidneys and bone as well as liver; a sensitive measure of biliary tract obstruction

Normal ranges from Kee, J. (1999). Laboratory and diagnostic tests with nursing implications, *5th ed. Stamford, CT: Appleton & Lange. Comments from Kee, J. (1999) and Krumberger, J.M. (1998). Gastrointestinal patient assessment. In M.R. Kinney et al. (eds.),* AACN's clinical reference for critical care nurses, *4th ed. (pp. 1011–1012). St. Louis: C.V. Mosby.*

isoenzymes found in the liver include 5′-nucleotidase (5′-N), gamma glutamyl transpeptidase (GGT), and ornithinecarbamoyl transferase (OCT). Two isoenzymes of lactic dehydrogenase (LDH) also predominate in the liver. These are LDH isoenzymes 4 and 5 (LDH4 and LDH5). Table 29–3 summarizes information concerning these isoenzymes.

Bilirubin

Bilirubin is the end product of hemoglobin degradation, which occurs in the liver. It is the pigmented portion of heme. Through the oxidation process, heme is turned into bilirubin and then is released into the bloodstream. There are two types of bilirubin: fat soluble and water soluble. Fat-soluble bilirubin has not yet passed through the liver (prehepatic). Prior to undergoing a conversion in the liver, it is called unconjugated. Once in the liver, bilirubin is first split from albumin molecules by the hepatocytes and then is conjugated (joined) with glucuronic acid. In this conjugated state, it becomes water-soluble bilirubin.

Water-soluble bilirubin is also called **conjugated,** or posthepatic, **bilirubin.** In this state, it is transported as bile from the liver into the intestines. From the intestines, most of the bilirubin is excreted through the feces. A small amount is excreted through the urine (urobilinogen). Very little conjugated bilirubin remains in the circulation to return to the liver; therefore, when bilirubin is measured, it is primarily the unconjugated (prehepatic) level that is being measured.

Testing for Bilirubin

Conjugated (or "direct") bilirubin (posthepatic, water soluble) is measured using a direct method since it requires no modifications before being measured. **Unconjugated** (or "indirect") **bilirubin** (prehepatic, fat soluble) is measured using an indirect method since it must be altered to a water-soluble state using a solvent before it can be measured. **Urobilinogen** is a sensitive test for hepatic damage.

TABLE 29–3. ISOENZYMES FOR EVALUATION OF LIVER FUNCTION

ISOENZYME	NORMAL RANGE	TREND IN DYSFUNCTION	COMMENTS
LDH isoenzymes (LDH4 and LDH5)	LDH4: 8–16% LDH5: 6–16%	Increased	This combination of LDH isoenzymes is common only to the liver and skeletal muscle injury; many drugs result in false elevations of LDH
ALP isoenzymes (5′-nucleotidase [5′-N])	< 17 U/L	Increased	5′-N is the most hepatobiliary tissue-specific ALP isoenzyme; elevated levels suggest a hepatobiliary problem
Gamma glutamyl transpeptidase (GGT)	0–45 U/L	Increased	GGT is fairly specific to hepatobiliary tissues; it is, however, also present in pancreatic and renal cells; elevated GGT is present in serum of alcohol abusers
Ornithinecarbamoyl transferase (OCT)	8–20 U/L	Increased	Helps the liver convert ammonia to urea; an increase is associated with hepatic cell damage and hepatotoxic chemicals or drugs

All normal ranges except OCT are from Kee, J. (1999). Laboratory and diagnostic tests with nursing implications, *5th ed. Stamford, CT: Appleton & Lange. Other data from Cavenaugh, B.M. (1999).* Nurse's manual of diagnostic and laboratory tests, *3rd ed. Philadelphia: F.A. Davis.*

It may increase before serum bilirubin levels increase. In early hepatitis or mild liver cell damage, the urine urobilinogen level will increase despite an unchanged serum bilirubin level. However, with severe liver failure, the urine urobilinogen level may decrease, since less bile will be produced. This test might be ordered along with a urinalysis. Table 29–4 summarizes the different types of bilirubin testing. Note the very small normal serum levels.

Bilirubin is a yellow pigment that provides a yellow cast to its surroundings. For example, bilirubin provides the brown color of stool. When normal elimination of bilirubin is obstructed, the characteristic yellow color becomes noticeably absent from stool and becomes evident in body fluids, as well as on the skin, sclera, and mucous membranes. This condition is called **jaundice.**

Prothrombin and Partial Thromboplastin Time

The **prothrombin time (PT)** measures the extrinsic coagulation pathway. Prothrombin is known as factor II of the coagulation cascade and is dependent on vitamin K, which is produced by the liver. Measuring the PT does not evaluate liver function, but it may be useful as supportive data when making a diagnosis of liver dysfunction. Increased levels may be seen with chronic liver disease (i.e., cirrhosis) or vitamin K deficiency. Normal prothrombin time is 11 to 15 seconds. Partial thromboplastin time (PTT) is a more sensitive test than PT in detecting clotting deficiencies in all factors except VII and XIII. Elevations of PTT are seen with severe liver disease or heparin therapy. Normal PTT is 60 to 70 seconds (Kee, 1999; Krumberger, 1998b).

Serum Ammonia

Elevated levels of serum ammonia indicate that the liver is not adequately converting ammonia to urea for proper elimination in the urine. Serum ammonia levels may be drawn intermittently to evaluate trends. As levels increase, the patient will present with increasing signs of hepatic encephalopathy. Arterial ammonia levels are recommended over venous specimens because they more accurately reflect the stage of encephalopathy. The normal range for serum ammonia is 15 to 45 μg/dL (Kee, 1999). Ammonia will be discussed in more detail in Section Five.

Serum Albumin

Elevated levels of serum ammonia may be seen with liver dysfunction, hepatic failure, and congestive heart failure (Krumberger, 1998b). As liver function decreases, protein levels will also decrease, since the liver cells synthesize albumin and other proteins. Serum albumin is a good indicator of general protein levels. Serum level trends are evaluated in conjunction with other nutritional and liver function data. Reduced levels are associated with several severe illnesses. The normal range for serum albumin is 3.5 to 5.0 g/dL (Kee, 1999). Refer to Module 22 for a detailed discussion of other nutritional measurement data that reflect liver function.

In summary, laboratory tests are a major source of diagnostic data. While enzyme studies can give general information regarding tissue injury, isoenzymes often provide data that is more specific to liver tissue injury. Other laboratory tests that provide important data include serum bilirubin, prothrombin time, and ammonia and albumin levels. Data from these tests are used in conjunction with clinical presentation to diagnose a particular liver dysfunction and differentiate it from other disease processes. These tests are generally obtained intermittently to evaluate trends.

TABLE 29–4. BILIRUBIN TESTING

TYPE	NORMAL VALUES	COMMENTS
Total bilirubin	0.1–1.2 mg/dL	Measures both conjugated and unconjugated bilirubin Elevations seen with biliary obstruction
Indirect bilirubin	0.1–1.0 mg/dL	Measures prehepatic, unconjugated bilirubin; elevations associated with viral hepatitis and other disease processes where lysis of red blood cells occur
Direct bilirubin	0.1–0.3 mg/dL	Measures posthepatic conjugated bilirubin; elevations associated with multiple intrahepatic and bile duct dysfunctions
Urobilinogen	Negative in freshly voided urine	Measures posthepatic urobilinogen in the urine; elevations associated with early or recovery phase liver cell damage Antibiotics may decrease levels

Normal ranges from Kee, J. (1999). Laboratory and diagnostic tests with nursing implications, *5th ed. Stamford, CT: Appleton & Lange. Comments from Kee (1999) and Krumberger, J. M. (1998). Gastrointestinal patient assessment. In M.R. Kinney et al. (eds.),* AACN's clinical reference for critical care nurses, *4th ed. (pp. 1011–1012). St. Louis: C. V. Mosby.*

SECTION THREE REVIEW

1. Serum enzyme laboratory levels are obtained to measure
   A. clotting factors
   B. organ function
   C. cellular injury
   D. tissue oxygenation
2. Serum isoenzyme levels often provide better data than parent enzyme levels because they are
   A. faster to obtain
   B. more tissue specific
   C. more plentiful
   D. easier to measure
3. Which combination of LDH isoenzymes best reflects hepatic injury?
   A. LDH1 and LDH2
   B. LDH2 and LDH3
   C. LDH3 and LDH4
   D. LDH4 and LDH5
4. Bilirubin is
   A. secreted by hepatocytes
   B. broken down into bile salts
   C. produced primarily in the pancreas
   D. the end product of hemoglobin degradation
5. When a serum bilirubin is obtained, it primarily measures _______ bilirubin.
   A. unconjugated
   B. posthepatic
   C. conjugated
   D. water-soluble

Answers: 1. C, 2. B, 3. D, 4. D, 5. A

SECTION FOUR: Acute Hepatitis

At the completion of this section, the learner will be able to describe the etiology and clinical manifestations associated with acute hepatitis.

Acute hepatitis is defined as an inflammatory liver disease, usually of viral origin, that results in liver injury and necrosis. The term "acute" implies that the condition lasts less than 6 months and ends either in complete resolution of the injured hepatic tissue or in rapid deterioration to liver failure and death (Andreoli et al., 1997). Acute hepatitis affects multiple body systems.

Etiology and Epidemiology

It is estimated that 200,000 to 300,000 new hepatitis B cases occur each year in the United States, with about 10,000 requiring hospitalization. Approximately 250 people die each year with fulminant liver failure, the most severe form of acute failure (Doughty & Jackson, 1993; Wilson et al., 1997).

Three common viruses are associated with acute hepatitis—hepatitis A, hepatitis B, and non-A, non-B hepatitis. Other viral sources include hepatitis D, cytomegalovirus, and Epstein–Barr virus. Less common causes of acute hepatitis include drug toxicity (e.g., acetaminophen, erythromycin, and isoniazid) and alcohol abuse.

Hepatitis A (infectious hepatitis, HAV) is transmitted through the fecal–oral route only during acute infection, and is most commonly found in young adults. It is transmitted primarily through contaminated food or water and often occurs as an epidemic. There is a high incidence of HAV in underdeveloped countries. Eating contaminated raw shellfish is sometimes responsible for HAV. Immunity occurs following acute illness. HAV is not associated with development of chronic hepatitis. A vaccine against HAV has recently been approved in the United States. It is recommended for high-risk populations (e.g., health care and child care workers, travelers to endemic areas of the world, and persons who are immunosuppressed). Immune globulin should be administered to close contacts with HAV as prophylaxis therapy (Jacobs, 1999; Carey et al., 1998).

Hepatitis B (serum hepatitis, HBV) is transmitted through contaminated blood serum or body fluids. Thus, people who come into contact with contaminated needles or body fluids are at risk for contracting hepatitis B. The at-risk population for HBV is similar to the HIV (human immunodeficiency virus) at-risk group (Table 29–5); it is considered a significant sexually transmitted disease (STD). Hepatitis B is seen in all age groups. It occurs throughout the world and is endemic in many parts of the world, though not in the United States. It is a major cause of acute and chronic hepatitis and cirrhosis. A vaccine is available to protect the at-risk population from HBV.

Non-A, non-B hepatitis was discovered in the mid 1970s. Since that time, research in finding the causative agent has shown that there are actually two causes of non-

TABLE 29–5. AT-RISK POPULATION FOR HEPATITIS B VIRUS (HBV)

- Illicit drug users
- Health care workers
- Male homosexuals
- People who require frequent transfusions (i.e., hemophiliacs)
- People with decreased immunocompetence
- Sexual partners of people infected with HBV
- Newborns of mothers infected with HBV

A, non-B hepatitis. These are now designated as hepatitis C (HCV), which is believed to be transmitted primarily through blood serum, and hepatitis E (HEV), which is believed to be transmitted through the fecal–oral route. The development of hepatitis C places a person at high risk (approximately 50 percent) for development of chronic liver disease (Doughty & Jackson, 1993). Like HBV, HCV is also considered a sexually transmitted disease. No vaccine is yet available for protection against either HCV or HEV.

Hepatitis D (HDV), also known as delta virus, is not a complete virus and requires the surface antigen of the hepatitis B virus (HBsAg) to act as its outer shell in order to be a viable virus. Patients who do not test positive for HBV need not be tested for HDV. HDV is primarily transmitted through the blood serum and in the United States is primarily found in hemophiliacs and drug addicts.

Pathophysiologic Basis of Acute Hepatitis

The pathologic effects of acute hepatitis are the same regardless of the causative agent. Acute hepatitis can be divided into three categories based on the severity of the disease—classic hepatitis, submassive hepatic necrosis, and massive hepatic necrosis. Acute hepatitis is generally considered a reversible disease unless complications develop.

Classic hepatitis is characterized by a liver that is normal in size and color, or by one that has mild enlargement and edema with bile staining present. Necrosis is localized but inflammation is generalized. The liver tissue structures remain intact throughout the disease process.

Submassive hepatic necrosis is characterized by more generalized necrosis, with a large number of necrotic hepatocytes. Inflammation is severe and injury leads to the collapse of hepatic tissues with subsequent loss of lobule structure. Fibrosis of hepatic tissue may develop during the healing stage.

Massive hepatic necrosis is characterized by extensive necrosis with loss of entire lobules. This type of acute hepatitis is associated with the development of fulminant hepatic failure, which is discussed further in Section Five of this module.

Clinical Manifestations of Acute Hepatitis

Viral hepatitis is generally associated with a prodromal period in which the person develops flulike symptoms.

TABLE 29–6. CLINICAL MANIFESTATIONS OF ACUTE VIRAL HEPATITIS

Prodromal period

"Flulike" symptoms: malaise, headache, anorexia, hyperpyrexia, nausea and vomiting, arthritis, myalgia, abdominal pain

Jaundice

Anicteric hepatitis—no jaundice is present

Cholestatic hepatitis—jaundice that may be severe; dark urine is present several days before jaundice appears; stool is clay colored; serum bilirubin = 20–30 mg/dL

The urine may become dark several days before bilirubinemia causes jaundice to be present. Jaundice usually peaks by week 2 of the disease and is gone by week 4 to 6 (Andreoli et al., 1997; Doughty & Jackson, 1993).

Only about 25 percent of people with acute hepatitis develop jaundice. Based on this manifestation, hepatitis can be divided into anicteric and cholestatic hepatitis. Anicteric hepatitis refers to hepatitis with no jaundice. Patients with anicteric hepatitis may have severely compromised liver function that is overlooked due to lack of jaundice. Cholestatic hepatitis refers to hepatitis with retention of bile due to a biliary obstruction (usually secondary to the inflammatory process). Persons with cholestatic hepatitis usually are severely jaundiced. Urine is dark and feces is clay colored. Serum bilirubin is greatly increased (20 to 30 mg/dL) with obstructive disease (Doughty & Jackson, 1993). The clinical manifestations of acute viral hepatitis are summarized in Table 29–6.

In summary, acute hepatitis is primarily of viral origin. Multiple viruses can cause acute hepatitis, including hepatitis A, B, C, D, and E; cytomegalovirus; and Epstein–Barr virus. Hepatitis B is a major health concern. It is transmitted via body fluids and is a major cause of chronic hepatitis and cirrhosis. Acute hepatitis causes hepatic injury and necrosis that is generalized throughout the organ. The severity of acute hepatitis can be divided into three categories: classic, submassive, and massive. Acute hepatitis is usually reversible. The clinical manifestations of acute hepatitis typically include a prodromal period in which the patient experiences flulike symptoms. If the patient has cholestatic hepatitis, jaundice will develop and serum bilirubin levels will significantly increase.

SECTION FOUR REVIEW

1. Acute hepatitis is most commonly caused by
   - **A.** bacterial invasion
   - **B.** viral invasion
   - **C.** yeast invasion
   - **D.** an autoimmune reaction

2. The major cause of acute and chronic hepatitis and cirrhosis is
   A. cytomegalovirus
   B. hepatitis C virus
   C. Epstein–Barr virus
   D. hepatitis B virus
3. Classic hepatitis is characterized by
   A. localized necrosis
   B. a greatly enlarged liver
   C. development of fibrosis
   D. development of fulminant hepatic failure
4. If a patient has anicteric hepatitis the nurse would expect to see
   A. dark urine
   B. clay-colored stool
   C. normal-colored urine
   D. black stool
5. If a patient has cholestatic hepatitis the nurse would anticipate serum bilirubin levels to
   A. fall below normal range
   B. remain within normal range
   C. elevate slightly above normal
   D. rise significantly above normal

Answers: 1. B, 2. D, 3. A, 4. C, 5. D

SECTION FIVE: Acute Hepatic Failure

At the completion of this section, the learner will be able to describe the etiology and clinical manifestations associated with acute hepatic failure.

The term **hepatic failure** refers to the inability of the liver to perform its normal functions. Acute hepatic failure (AHF) results from one of the three following situations:

1. A primary disease process in the absence of preexisting hepatic disease
2. A complication of chronic liver disease
3. A part of multiple organ failure in the critically ill

Regardless of the cause of AHF, many of the clinical manifestations are the same.

Acute Hepatic Failure as a Primary Disease

Though uncommon, AHF can occur without preexisting liver disease. Four possible etiologies include shock, virulent viral infection, hepatotoxins, and systemic inflammatory response (see multiple organ failure, below).

Shock

The liver is extremely vulnerable to ischemic injury, as are the other splanchnic organs. A sustained hypotensive episode (shock) can result in insufficient oxygenation of liver tissue, which can precipitate ischemic hepatitis. In response to hypoxia, the delicate endothelial lining of the hepatic capillaries becomes damaged and more permeable. Increased permeability allows fluid to leak from the capillaries into the hepatic tissue. As fluid shifts out of the vasculature, microthrombi develop, partly due to the high concentration of particulate matter remaining in the vessels. Microthrombi can cause a blockage of blood flow with subsequent tissue ischemia and necrosis distal to the blockages. Though the liver has a large reserve, if tissue destruction exceeds this reserve, acute liver failure will result. Ischemic hepatitis may spontaneously resolve or it may degenerate into AHF. The longer the initial hypotensive episode continues, the more severe the liver destruction will be.

Viral Infection and Hepatotoxins

A particularly severe form of acute hepatic failure is called **fulminant hepatic failure (FHF).** Fulminant hepatic failure can result from multiple causes. Two major causes are acute viral infections and hepatotoxins. Hepatitis viruses A, B, C, and D account for approximately 75 percent of cases of FHF in the United States. The most common hepatotoxin precipitating FHF is acetaminophen. In some cases no cause is found, although an undetected viral etiology is generally suspected. A more extensive listing of known causes of FHF is presented in Table 29–7 (Andreoli et al., 1997).

Definitions of FHF vary widely, from being synonymous with AHF to being an extreme form of AHF. For the purposes of this module, the definition of FHF is based on the following criteria: the level of encephalopathy, the preexisting liver status, and the rate of onset. Fulminant hepatic failure is defined as a form of AHF in a

TABLE 29–7. CAUSES OF FULMINANT HEPATIC FAILURE (FHF)

- Viral infections
  Hepatitis A, B, C, and D (hepatitis B and D are implicated in > 50% of FHF cases); cytomegalovirus; Epstein–Barr virus
- Hepatotoxins
  Acetaminophen, mushroom poisoning, isoniazid (INH), hydrocarbons
- Traumatic vascular injury
  May be part of multiple organ failure

Data from Wilson, L.M., & Lester, L.B. (1997). Liver, biliary tract, and pancreas. In S.A. Price & L.M. Wilson (eds). Pathophysiology: Clinical concepts of disease processes, *4th ed. (pp. 372–408). St. Louis: C.V. Mosby.*

patient with no preexisting history of liver disease that develops rapidly (in less than 8 weeks) in the presence of stage III or IV encephalopathy (Andreoli et al., 1997). FHF has a high mortality rate (over 80 percent).

FHF causes rapid, massive deterioration and destruction of liver tissue with widespread hepatocellular necrosis. The end result is severe hepatic dysfunction with subsequent development of encephalopathy.

Acute Hepatic Failure as a Complication of Chronic Liver Disease

Cirrhosis of the liver is the third leading cause of death in males between 35 and 54 years of age in the United States (Krumberger, 1998a). Andreoli and colleagues define cirrhosis as "the irreversible end result of fibrous scarring and hepatocellular regeneration that constitute the major responses of the liver to a variety of longstanding inflammatory, toxic, metabolic, and congestive insults" (p. 339). The onset of cirrhosis is insidious and progressive. In the United States, the two most common causes of cirrhosis are alcohol abuse and hepatitis C (non-A, non-B hepatitis). Over time, the progressive deterioration of hepatic function becomes sufficient to compromise the normal functioning of the liver.

Acute Hepatic Failure as Part of Multiple Organ Failure

A major body insult, such as sepsis, can set off a systemic inflammatory response that, in turn, leads to a series of physiologic events. This response is called the *systemic inflammatory response syndrome (SIRS)*. When SIRS develops, the normally localized inflammatory response becomes a systemic, malignant process. SIRS results in a single or multiple organ inflammatory insult. In the liver, the inflammatory response sets off a massive release and assault by the liver macrophages (Kupffer's cells), causing destruction of liver tissue. The inflammatory response also causes the endothelial lining of the vessels to become more permeable, allowing fluids to leak into the liver parenchyma and resulting in organ edema and microthrombi. The microthrombi and inflammation eventually lead to the damage of hepatocytes and the blockage of bile flow. When damage becomes severe, hepatic failure ensues (Harvey, 1998). Acute hepatic failure as part of the multiple organ dysfunction syndrome is discussed in Module 11.

Clinical Manifestations of Acute Hepatic Failure

The massive tissue destruction caused by AHF produces essentially the same manifestations regardless of its etiology. The clinical manifestations of AHF reflect severe hepatic encephalopathy and multiple metabolic dysfunctions.

Hepatic Encephalopathy

Encephalopathy is the hallmark of AHF. Hepatic encephalopathy, also called hepatic coma or "portosystemic encephalopathy," is defined as an altered neurologic status caused by a buildup of circulating toxins of hepatic origin (e.g., ammonia). Hepatic encephalopathy has been staged (graded) according to clinical manifestations for clarity (Table 29–8). Hepatic encephalopathy is also considered a complication of AHF and is further discussed in Section Six.

Metabolic Dysfunction

Liver failure develops when more than 60 percent of hepatocytes are injured, reflected in the organ's inability to perform its multiple metabolic functions. Liver failure results in the following metabolically related clinical manifestations:

- *Protein metabolic dysfunction:* ascites, hypoalbuminemia, hepatic encephalopathy, evidence of impaired clotting factors (hemorrhage, epistaxis, purpura)
- *Carbohydrate metabolism dysfunction:* hypoglycemia
- *Fat metabolism dysfunction:* nausea and vomiting, anorexia, constipation or diarrhea, prolonged PT

These metabolic dysfunctions are expressed in alterations in body systems, as noted in Table 29–9.

TABLE 29–8. STAGES OF HEPATIC ENCEPHALOPATHY

STAGE[a]	CLINICAL MANIFESTATIONS
I	Awake, apathetic, restless, sleep pattern changes, mental clouding, impaired computational ability, impaired handwriting, subtle intellectual function changes, diminished muscle coordination; electroencephalogram (EEG) shows mild-to-moderate abnormalities
II	Decreased level of consciousness, lethargy, drowsiness, disorientation to time and place, confusion, asterixis, diminished reflexes, slurring of speech; EEG shows moderate-to-severe abnormalities
III	Stupor (arousable), no spontaneous eye opening, hyperactive reflexes, seizures, rigidity, abnormal posturing: decorticate, decerebrate, extensor plantar responses; EEG shows severe abnormalities
IV	Coma (may or may not respond to painful stimuli), seizures, pupillary dilation, flaccidity; EEG shows severe abnormalities

[a] Stage 0 encephalopathy may be used to describe subclinical intellectual impairment.

Data from Andreoli, T.E., Bennett, J.C., Carpenter, C.C., & Plum, F. (eds.). (1997). Cecil's essentials of medicine, *4th ed. Philadelphia: W.B. Saunders; and Clochesy, J., et al. (eds.). (1992). The patient with liver dysfunction. In* Critical care nursing. *Philadelphia: W.B. Saunders.*

TABLE 29–9. EFFECTS OF HEPATIC FAILURE ON BODY SYSTEMS

SYSTEM	CLINICAL MANIFESTATIONS
Neurologic	Stage I to IV encephalopathy
Cardiovascular	Pulmonary edema, hypotension
Gastrointestinal	Nausea and vomiting, constipation or diarrhea, anorexia, ascites
Hematopoietic	Impaired coagulation, prolonged PT
Pulmonary	Tachypnea, crackles (rales)

In summary, acute hepatic failure can develop as a primary disease process or as a complication of either chronic liver disease or multiple organ failure. The clinical manifestations of acute hepatic failure reflect encephalopathy and the loss of many liver functions. Fulminant hepatic failure is a critical illness with a high mortality, characterized by massive hepatic necrosis and severe encephalopathy. The presence of hepatic encephalopathy, primarily from high ammonia levels, is considered the hallmark of hepatic failure.

SECTION FIVE REVIEW

1. Which of the following statements is true regarding fulminant hepatic failure?
   A. it causes necrosis of liver tissue
   B. it has a mortality of less than 50 percent
   C. it is characterized by stage I and II encephalopathy
   D. it has a slow, insidious onset
2. A major hepatotoxin that is known to cause fulminant hepatic failure is
   A. acetaminophen
   B. gentamicin
   C. aspirin
   D. cephalosporin
3. In the United States, cirrhosis of the liver is most commonly caused by
   A. hepatitis A virus
   B. alcohol abuse
   C. hepatitis B virus
   D. Epstein–Barr virus
4. Stage III and IV hepatic encephalopathy are characterized by
   A. stupor, coma
   B. lethargy, asterixis
   C. restlessness, slurred speech
   D. sleep pattern changes, drowsiness
5. Hepatic encephalopathy is primarily caused by high levels of
   A. bilirubin
   B. bile
   C. ammonia
   D. blood urea nitrogen (BUN)

Answers: 1. A, 2. A, 3. B, 4. A, 5. C

SECTION SIX: Complications of Hepatic Dysfunction

At the completion of this section, the learner will be able to describe complications of hepatic dysfunction.

The inability of the liver to meet all of the demands placed on it by other systems places the patient at risk for many multisystem complications. The severity of the complications is related to the level of liver dysfunction. Table 29–10 lists the major complications of hepatic dysfunction.

Hepatic Encephalopathy

As previously discussed, **hepatic encephalopathy** is caused by toxic levels of circulating ammonia, which readily crosses the blood–brain barrier. Normally, the level rapidly converts ammonia into urea, which is then excreted in the urine. When the liver is unable to convert ammonia to urea, toxicity rapidly develops.

Contributing Factors

A variety of factors contribute to increased nitrogenous waste, thus contributing to increased ammonia levels (Thompson et al., 1997), including:

- *Constipation*—nitrogenous wastes remain in the GI tract longer, providing more opportunity for conversion to ammonia
- *Blood in the GI tract*—as blood in the tract is broken down, ammonia is released

TABLE 29–10. COMMON COMPLICATIONS OF HEPATIC FAILURE

- Hepatic encephalopathy
- Portal hypertension
- Ascites
- Esophageal varices
- Infection: sepsis and spontaneous bacterial peritonitis
- Acute renal failure

- *Azotemia*—decreases the ability of the kidneys to excrete nitrogenous wastes
- *Dietary protein consumption*—provides amino acids, thus more ammonia buildup
- *Certain drugs*—tranquilizers, sedatives, and analgesics, for example

Portal Hypertension

Normal hepatic venous flow is through a moderate resistance system (8 to 10 mm Hg) when compared with the very low resistance level (2 to 8 mm Hg) of the connecting vena cava. When hepatic tissue is injured or destroyed, blood flowing through the damaged areas requires more pressure to maintain organ blood flow. Consequently, increased hepatic capillary resistance occurs in a fashion similar to that which is created in the lungs when they sustain parenchymal damage.

Portal hypertension refers to sustained portal vein pressure elevation. Portal hypertension results from increased vascular resistance of the portal vein, an increase in blood flow, or both (Raper, 1994). The pressure can increase to ≥ 30 mm Hg. Over time, as in chronic hepatic dysfunction, the liver develops a system of collateral circulation that helps to relieve the increase in pressure. These collateral veins are called **varices** and are characterized by their dilated, tortuous appearance. In AHF, however, collateral circulation does not have sufficient time to develop, and back flow leads to congestion of other organs in the splanchnic circulation. Figure 29–5 illustrates how circulation is affected by portal hypertension.

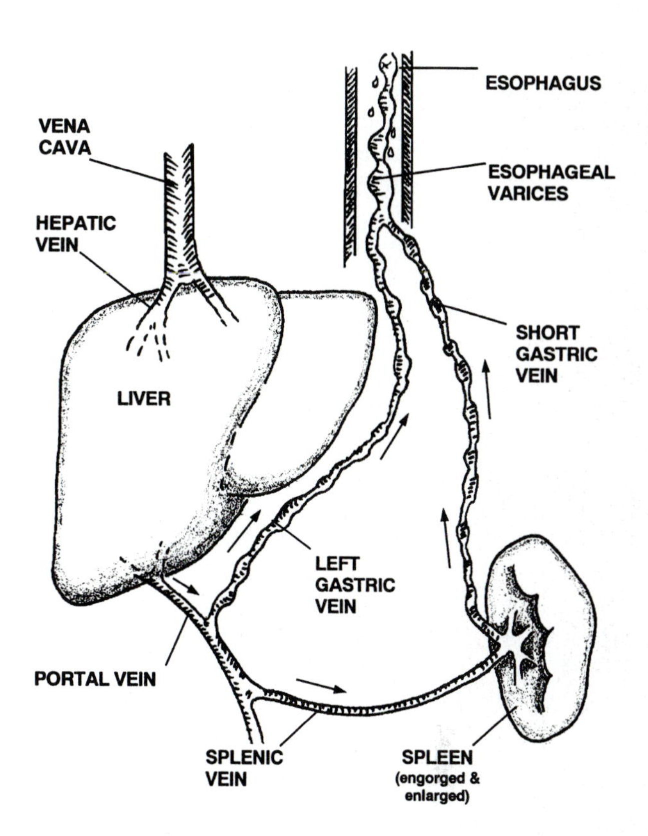

Figure 29–5. Portal hypertension. Damage to liver tissue increases vascular resistance. Venous flow becomes blocked in the liver, causing portal vein pressure to increase. Blood backs up through the splenic vein into the spleen and collateral venous circulation (such as the short and left gastric veins).

Esophageal Varices

Esophageal varices are a major complication of portal hypertension. Blood naturally flows through the vessels with the least resistance; thus, blood naturally seeks an easier path to take. This diversion of flow is called shunting. The esophageal veins (varices) in the lower portion of the esophagus provide a common collateral flow diversion. Esophageal varices dilate to accept shunted blood. A rapid increase in pressure (e.g., coughing, vomiting, straining) can cause the dilated varices to rupture, precipitating hemorrhage. Bleeding esophageal varices are considered a medical emergency. Esophageal varices occur in approximately 70 percent of patients with advanced cirrhosis (Wilson et al., 1997).

Ascites

Ascites is defined as a collection of fluid in the abdominal cavity. Ascites develops during advanced-stage hepatic dysfunction. Two major causes of ascites are decreased colloid osmotic pressure and portal hypertension. Colloid osmotic pressure decreases owing to a reduction in albumin. Hypoalbuminemia is caused by the inability of the liver to carry out its usual protein metabolism functions. When colloid osmotic pressure becomes too low, fluid shifts (third spaces) out of the intravascular compartment and into other body compartments, such as the intra-abdominal cavity. In addition, cirrhosis patients can develop extreme sodium retention by the kidneys, which leads to ascites. This phenomenon is caused by an alteration in renal sodium and water excretion related to hypoalbuminemia, hyperaldosteronism, and increased antidiuretic hormone levels (Andreoli et al., 1997; Raper, 1994).

Hepatorenal Syndrome

Hepatorenal syndrome (HRS) refers to acute renal failure that occurs as a complication of hepatic failure. A diagnosis of HRS should not be made until other types of acute renal failure are ruled out. Hepatorenal syndrome can be divided into two subgroups: type I and type II.

Type I Hepatorenal Syndrome

Acute renal insufficiency and failure are fairly common complications of hepatic failure. Type I HRS is a prerenal type of renal failure that is precipitated by inadequate renal arterial blood volume. The third-spacing of fluids associated with advanced hepatic disease places the patient at risk for a significant drop in mean arterial blood pressure. When the mean arterial pressure of blood flowing through the kidneys drops below 60 mm Hg, the kidneys no longer receive sufficient blood to meet oxygenation needs; thus, ischemia and renal injury occur. This type of renal failure may be reversed with appropriate fluid resuscitation to increase circulating blood volume.

Type II Hepatorenal Syndrome

Type II HRS develops in patients with advanced liver disease and FHF. While the exact cause of this functional renal failure is unknown, it is believed that it may be a complication of impaired renal perfusion caused by increased renal vascular resistance. Hepatorenal syndrome typically occurs in the presence of severe ascites. More specifically, it often follows vigorous therapies to significantly reduce ascites (diuretics, paracentesis), and sepsis (Andreoli et al., 1997). Type II HRS is progressive in nature and is usually fatal. With a liver transplant, Type II HRS patients have a 90 percent chance for full renal recovery and a 10 percent chance of developing end-stage renal disease. Without a liver transplant, it carries a 90 percent mortality rate.

The clinical characteristics of hepatorenal syndrome are presented in Table 29–11.

TABLE 29–11. CLINICAL CHARACTERISTICS OF HEPATORENAL SYNDROME

- Presence of liver failure
- Decreasing glomerular filtration rate (GFR)
- Reduced urine sodium (< 10 mEq/24 hours)
- Presence of azotemia (elevated creatinine and blood urea nitrogen [BUN])
- Oliguria or anuria
- High BUN/creatinine ratio

Data from Andreoli, T.E., Bennett, J.C., Carpenter, C.C., & Plum, F. (eds.). (1997). Cecil's essentials of medicine, *4th ed. Philadelphia: W.B. Saunders; and Raper, S.E. (1994). Hepatobiliary disease. In F.S. Bongard & D.Y. Sue (eds.).* Current critical care diagnosis and treatment *(pp. 576–591). Norwalk, CT: Appleton & Lange.*

Infections: Sepsis and Spontaneous Bacterial Peritonitis

The Kupffer's cells play a crucial part in controlling the inflammatory response and in cleansing gram-negative intestinal bacteria from the blood. Their ability to detoxify bacteria and vasoactive substances inhibits development of a systemic inflammatory response and hemodynamic instability. In addition, the liver produces special proteins and enzymes that assist in controlling the inflammatory response (Thelan et al., 1998). The loss of the liver's Kupffer's cells to cleanse the blood and loss of protein synthesis places the hepatic failure patient at risk for development of sepsis and SIRS.

The patient with acute hepatic failure is also at risk for development of spontaneous bacterial peritonitis. This form of peritonitis occurs when ascites becomes infected. Bacteria are able to translocate (migrate) into the ascites when the bowel wall loses its integrity due to endothelial damage secondary to tissue ischemia and/or infarct. Intestinal bacteria move across injured intestinal wall and seed themselves in the ascites fluid. A hypotensive episode is the most common cause of intestinal wall injury in this patient population. The bowel is the primary source of bacteria in both sepsis and spontaneous bacterial peritonitis.

In summary, there are multiple serious complications associated with hepatic failure, significantly reducing the patient's prognosis. Complications of acute hepatic failure include hepatic encephalopathy, hypoglycemia, metabolic abnormalities, gastrointestinal (GI) hemorrhage, cerebral edema, hepatorenal syndrome, spontaneous bacterial peritonitis, and sepsis. Portal hypertension can result in esophageal varices.

SECTION SIX REVIEW

1. Portal hypertension is caused by
   A. increased vascular resistance
   B. decreased portal vein blood flow
   C. increased hepatic artery volume
   D. decreased hepatic blood flow
2. Esophageal varices dilate in response to
   A. decreased hepatic blood flow
   B. hepatic vasoconstriction
   C. shunted splanchnic blood
   D. increased cardiac output
3. A major cause of ascites is
   A. hyperalbuminemia
   B. low colloid osmotic pressure
   C. hepatorenal syndrome
   D. fluid volume overload
4. A major factor contributing to onset of acute renal failure as a complication of hepatic failure is
   A. hepatotoxins
   B. a hypotensive episode
   C. high ammonia levels
   D. portal vein shunting

5. The onset of type II HRS usually occurs in the presence of
   A. hepatotoxins
   B. a hypotensive episode
   C. high ammonia levels
   D. severe ascites

6. The hepatic failure patient is at risk for spontaneous bacterial peritonitis due to
   A. translocation of intestinal bacteria
   B. increased bacterial growth in intestines
   C. secondary hepatic bacterial infection
   D. unknown causes

Answers: 1. A, 2. C, 3. B, 4. B, 5. D, 6. A

SECTION SEVEN: Medical Management

At the completion of this section, the learner will be able to describe an overview of the medical management of the patient with hepatic dysfunction.

Management of the patient with acute hepatic dysfunction is primarily supportive regardless of the causative agent.

Management of Acute Viral Hepatitis

There is no specific therapy for treatment of viral hepatitis. Table 29–12 summarizes the general focuses for medical management of acute viral hepatitis. Patients with this diagnosis do not necessarily require hospitalization.

TABLE 29–12. SUPPORTIVE MEDICAL MANAGEMENT OF ACUTE VIRAL HEPATITIS

FOCUS	GENERAL MANAGEMENT
Activity/rest	Limit activities based on level of fatigue Require rest based on severity of symptoms
Hydration/nutritional needs	Maintain balanced hydration status Diet: high carbohydrate, low fat; no alcohol intake Nausea management: metoclopramide and hydroxyzine in small doses Vitamin K, if needed
Hospitalization criteria	Hospitalization is indicated if severe nausea and vomiting develops, deteriorating liver function is noted (e.g., hepatic encephalopathy and/or prolonged prothrombin time)

Data from Andreoli, T.E., Bennett, J.C., Carpenter, C.C., & Plum, F. (eds.). (1997). Cecil's essentials of medicine, *4th ed. Philadelphia: W.B. Saunders.*

Management of Acute Hepatic Failure Complications

Hepatic Encephalopathy

Management of hepatic encephalopathy centers around four general principles (Andreoli et al., 1997):

- Identify and treat the precipitating factors when possible
- Eliminate or reduce generation of ammonia toxins
- Reduce the amount of bacteria in the bowel
- Prevent movement of ammonia toxins from the bowel

Identify and Treat the Precipitating Factors. Hepatic encephalopathy is known to be triggered or worsened by certain precipitating factors (Table 29–13). It is important to rapidly identify and aggressively treat precipitating factors to reduce the severity of the encephalopathy.

Eliminate or Reduce Ammonia Toxins. Protein intake must be either eliminated or tightly controlled. There is evidence that controlling protein intake rather than totally eliminating it may be useful in decreasing hepatic encephalopathy. Raper (1994) suggests that intake of branched-chain amino acids (e.g., leucine and valine) be increased while eliminating the intake of aromatic amino acids (e.g., tyrosine and phenylalanine). Branched-chain amino acids do not cross the blood–brain barrier and act as an excellent source of energy, which serves to reduce muscle wasting as an energy source. Aromatic amino acids, however, cross the blood–brain barrier and worsen the encephalopathy.

Reduce Bacteria in the Bowel. The aminoglycoside neomycin is frequently ordered to suppress ammonia-producing intestinal bacteria. One gram of neomycin administered orally every 6 to 8 hours can maintain long-term suppression for the treatment of hepatic

TABLE 29–13. PRECIPITATING FACTORS ASSOCIATED WITH HEPATIC ENCEPHALOPATHY

- Infection
- Elevated protein intake
- Worsening hepatic function
- Constipation
- Azotemia (elevated blood urea nitrogen and creatinine)
- Gastrointestinal bleeding
- Hypovolemia

encephalopathy. Neomycin does not absorb well through the gastrointestinal tract; thus, its effects are primarily local. As with all aminoglycosides, the patient must be monitored for the potential side effects of ototoxicity and nephrotoxicity (Andreoli et al., 1997; Deglin & Vallerand, 1997; Jawetz, 1995).

Gastrointestinal bleeding and constipation can precipitate hepatic encephalopathy. In the event of gastrointestinal bleeding or constipation, the bowels should be cleansed of all residual blood and stool by administration of enemas. This will prevent further buildup of nitrogenous waste (Andreoli et al., 1997).

Prevent Movement of Ammonia Toxins. The synthetic disaccharide lactulose may be ordered to help prevent absorption of ammonia from the bowel. Lactulose may be administered for its laxative effect. When stool is excreted more rapidly, it has less opportunity to form ammonia. It is also believed that lactulose facilitates trapping of ammonia ions in the intestines, for unknown reasons. Lactulose breaks down into lactic acid and other organic acids that may facilitate the ammonia-trapping action. It is also theorized that lactulose may modify the intestinal flora in some manner, thereby causing a reduction in absorption of bacteria through the bowel. Typically, 15 to 30 mL of lactulose is administered qid (oral or enema) or adjusted as necessary to attain three to five soft stools per 24 hours (Altman, 1995).

Hypoglycemia

Liver failure interferes with normal carbohydrate metabolism. Thus, the patient develops hypoglycemia secondary to decreased gluconeogenesis. Management consists of frequent monitoring of serum glucose levels and close observation for the development of hypoglycemic symptoms. Treatment of hypoglycemia may consist of a continuous IV infusion of 10 percent dextrose solution. If the hypoglycemia is severe, 50 percent dextrose may be ordered as immediate treatment.

Metabolic Abnormalities

Electrolyte abnormalities such as hyponatremia and hypokalemia are common in patients with liver failure. Hyponatremia results from sodium loss due to diuretic therapy, the hemodilution effect, and sodium restriction. Hypokalemia is caused by diuretic therapy and elevated aldosterone levels, which result from the loss of the liver's ability to metabolize aldosterone. In addition, the renin–angiotensin–aldosterone system is activated by diminished renal blood flow.

Acid–base imbalances are also common occurrences. The AHF patient is at risk of developing metabolic acidosis for two major reasons. First, hepatic cellular damage releases lactic acid, which results in lactic acidosis. Second, metabolic acidosis is a complication of acute renal failure, a common sequela of hepatic failure. Respiratory alkalosis may develop from hyperventilation associated with compensatory mechanisms. Treatment of acid–base imbalances consists of correcting the underlying problems and administering bicarbonate if necessary.

Gastrointestinal Hemorrhage

The AHF patient is at risk for development of GI hemorrhage for several reasons. One is the stress associated with severe illness, which can precipitate development of stress ulcers. Another is the presence of abnormal clotting factors, which increases the risk for abnormal bleeding. The mortality rate is high for the first episode of GI bleeding and, should the patient survive the first episode, repeated bleeds are common. Therapy generally consists of prevention of stress ulcers using histamine antagonists or antacids, and controlling the coagulopathy through use of vitamin K and blood products.

Cerebral Edema

Cerebral edema is an ominous complication of AHF. Its etiology is unknown yet its presence significantly reduces the patient's chances of survival. If edema cannot be adequately controlled, intracerebral herniation may result and is generally fatal.

Table 29–14 summarizes the supportive medical management of AHF based on common complications.

Fulminant Hepatic Failure

As soon as fulminant hepatic failure is suspected, the patient is transferred to a critical care unit. When feasible, it is also recommended that FHF patients be transferred to medical centers that specialize in FHF management since the patient's survival may often depend on rapid identification and management of multisystem complications. The causative problem of FHF is not usually treatable; therefore, the primary focus of medical management is supportive. Liver transplantation is usually required in patients who do not spontaneously recover from FHF. This requires transfer of the patient to a liver transplant center as soon as the decision is made. The survival rate of patients with FHF restricted to medical management is < 20 percent, while the survival rate associated with liver transplantation is > 55 percent (Chapman, 1997; Smith & Ciferni, 1990). Transplantation is discussed in detail in Module 4.

Esophageal Varices

Portal hypertension leads to formation of venous collateral vessels between the portal and systemic circulations. These collateral vessels become dilated, tortuous veins (varices) within the submucosa of the esophagus and stomach. Esophageal varices are unpredictable—they can

TABLE 29–14. SUPPORTIVE MEDICAL MANAGEMENT OF ACUTE HEPATIC FAILURE COMPLICATIONS

COMPLICATION	MANAGEMENT
Hepatic encephalopathy	Correct the precipitating cause, if possible No protein intake, or consider control of protein intake: Increase intake of branched-chain amino acids Eliminate intake of aromatic amino acids present Enema if constipation and/or GI bleeding Lactulose (PO, NG, rectal), 15–30 mL administered qid or as necessary to attain three to five soft stools/24 hr Intubate and mechanically ventilate Neomycin, 1–4 g (PO or enema) q6–8h
Hypoglycemia	10% dextrose continuous IV infusion 50% dextrose IV, as required Monitor for low serum glucose and clinical manifestations of hypoglycemia
Metabolic abnormalities	Frequent monitoring of serum electrolytes and pH Correct electrolyte abnormalities Administer bicarbonate, as necessary
Gastrointestinal hemorrhage	Vitamin K Oral antacids or H_2 receptor antagonists (IV) to keep gastric pH > 5 Fresh frozen plasma, possibly platelets
Cerebral edema	Intracranial pressure monitoring IV mannitol Consider barbiturate-induced coma, if indicated
Hepatorenal syndrome	Type I Fluid resuscitation May consider shunt Type II Dopamine, 5–10 mg/kg/min (to increase renal blood flow) Liver transplantation
Spontaneous bacterial peritonitis	Antibiotic therapy Third-generation cephalosporin, usually administered for 5 to 7 days (until ascitic fluid cell count is normal)

Data from Andreoli, T.E., Bennett, J.C., Carpenter, C.C., & Plum, F. (eds.). (1993). Cecil's essentials of medicine, *4th ed. Philadelphia: W.B. Saunders; Marini, J.J., & Wheeler, A.P. (1989).* Critical care medicine—the essentials. *Baltimore: Williams & Wilkins; and Raper, S.E. (1994). Hepatobiliary disease. In F.S. Bongard & D.Y. Sue (eds).* Current critical care diagnosis and treatment *(pp. 576–591). Norwalk, CT: Appleton & Lange.*

TABLE 29–15. MANAGEMENT OF THE PATIENT WITH ESOPHAGEAL VARICES

FOCUS OF TREATMENT	INTERVENTIONS
Control bleeding	**IV vasopressin** Reduces splanchnic blood flow Initial dose of 20 units followed by continuous IV infusion of 0.4–0.6 u/min **Somatostatin** (or synthetic analog octreotide) Reduces splanchnic blood flow & portal pressure Less systemic vasoconstrictive effects than vasopressin Initial dose of 50 μg/hour continuous IV infusion **Nitroglycerin** Given with vasopressin to decrease systemic vasoconstrictive effects (i.e., cardiac or mesenteric ischemia) **Fresh frozen plasma** A replacement of clotting factors; Platelets may be ordered, although their efficacy is controversial
Aggressive correction of bleeding varices	**Sengstaken-Blakemore** or Minnesota tube placement An inflated balloon that tamponades bleeding varices (see Fig. 29–6) **Portal systemic shunt surgery** Portocaval anastomosis Transjugular intrahepatic shunt (TIPS) Distal splenorenal shunt (see Fig. 29–7)
Preventive therapy	Therapy to reduce portal pressure: Nonselective beta blockers, i.e., propanolol, nadolol Mononitrates, i.e., isosorbide mononitrate Elective shunt surgery Endoscopic sclerotherapy Endoscopic variceal banding The varix is isolated and banded, which results in oblation

Data from Andreoli, T.E., Bennett, J.C., Carpenter, C.C., & Plum, F. (eds.). (1997). Cecil's essentials of medicine, *4th ed. Philadelphia: W.B. Saunders; and Passaro, E. (1994).* Gastrointestinal bleeding. *In F.S. Bongard & D.Y. Sue (eds.).* Current critical care diagnosis and treatment *(pp. 562–575). Norwalk, CT: Appleton & Lange*

rupture at any time. Their close association with cirrhosis, and its specific pathologic features, places the patient at high risk for hemorrhage. Management of the patient with bleeding esophageal varices is summarized in Table 29–15.

In summary, medical management of the patient with hepatic dysfunction is primarily supportive. The person with acute viral hepatitis may be managed at home unless complications develop. Rest, control of activities,

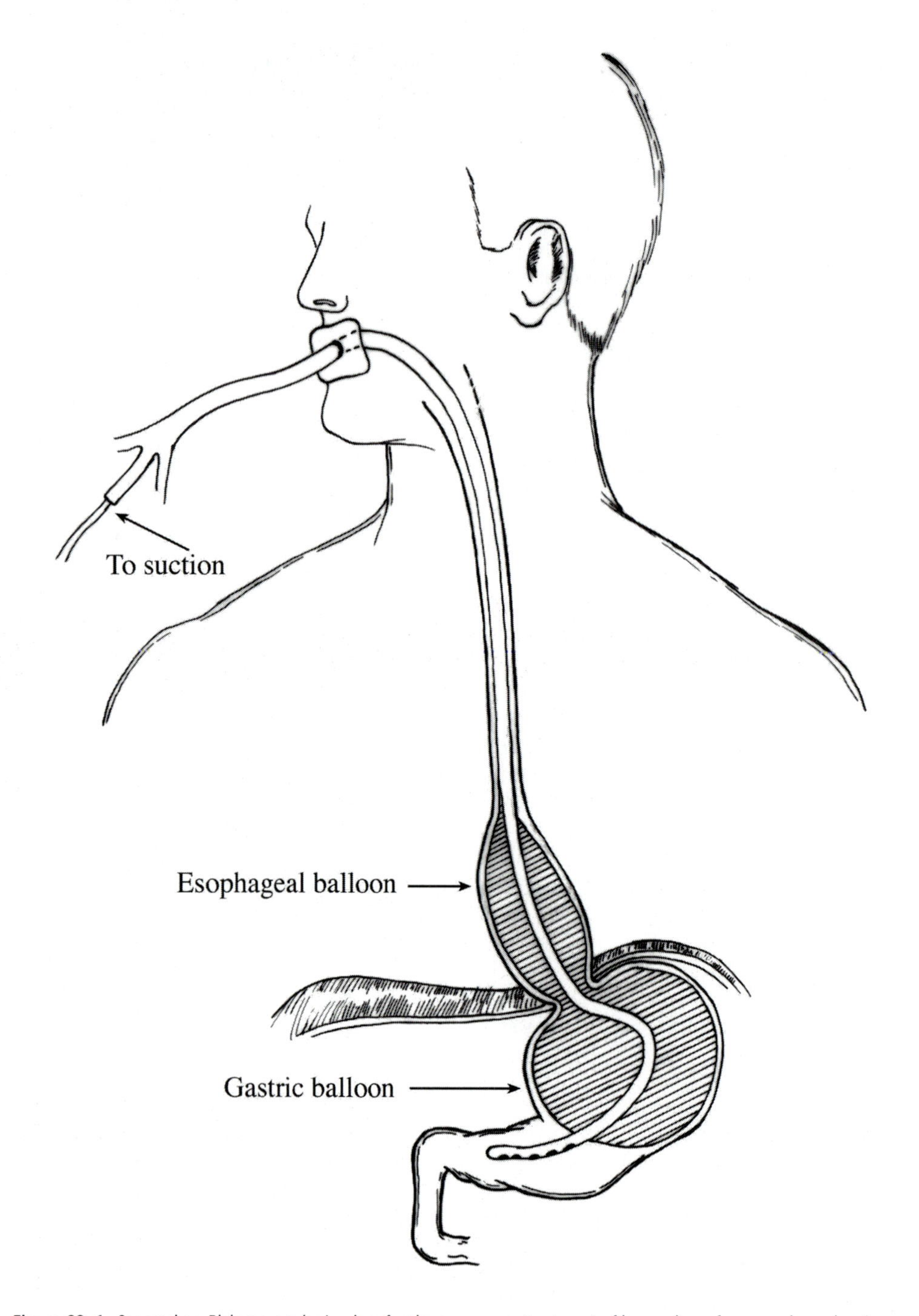

Figure 29–6. Sengstaken–Blakemore tube in place for the emergency treatment of hemorrhage from esophageal varices.

hydration, and special diet are baseline interventions. Management of the complications associated with AHF and FHF requires specialized multisystem treatment in a critical care unit. Management is primarily supportive and based on complications that develop. Esophageal varices are best treated prior to rupture. If variceal hemorrhage occurs, a medical emergency exists that demands rapid treatment to control bleeding and prevent further bleeding. Fulminant hepatic failure usually requires organ transplantation if the patient is to survive.

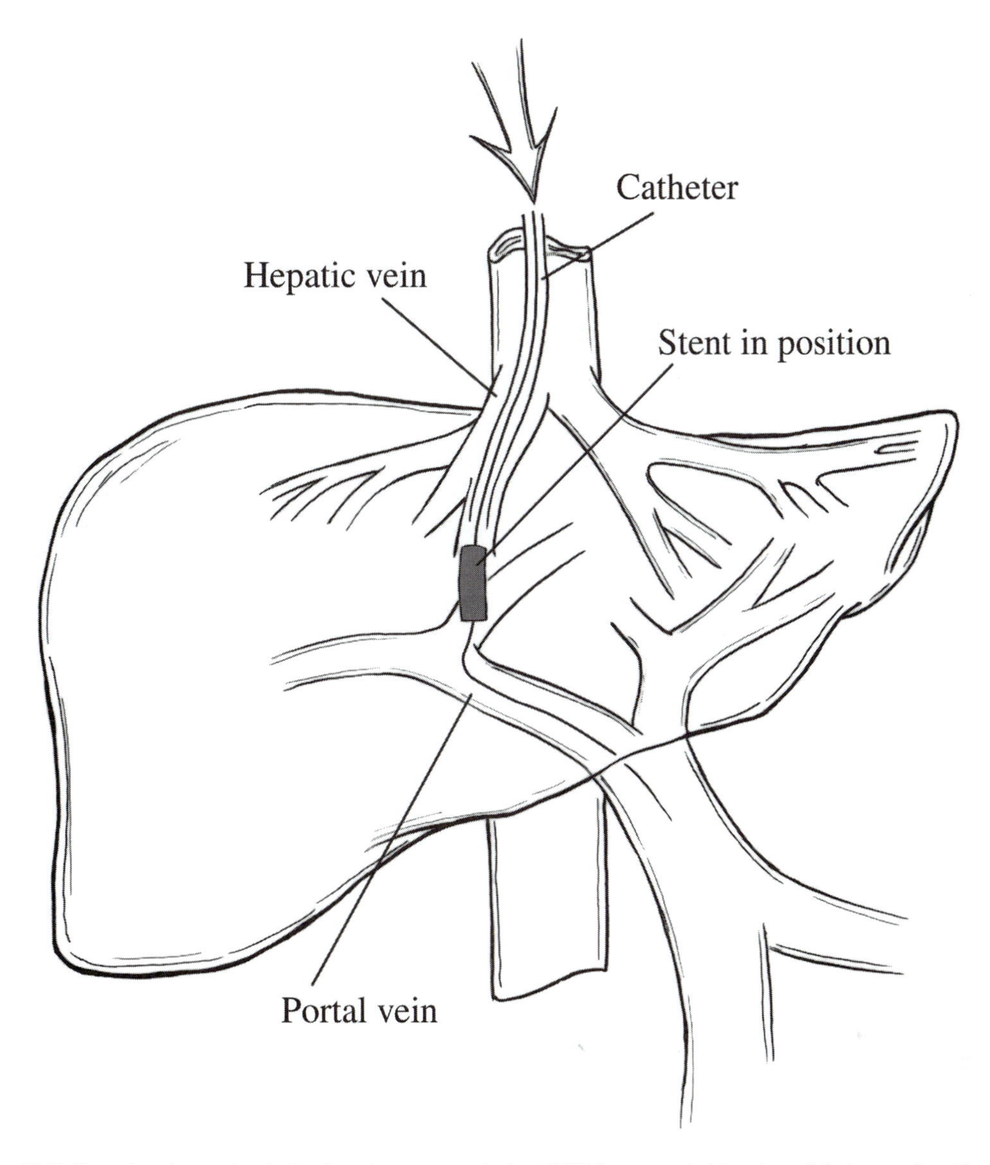

Figure 29–7. Illustration of a transjugular intrahepatic portosystemic shunt "TIPS," a nonsurgical, invasive radiologic procedure. The goal of this procedure is to decrease the portal to hepatic vein gradient to 10 mm Hg or less.

SECTION SEVEN REVIEW

1. Dietary management of the patient with acute viral hepatitis should include
   A. high protein, low fat
   B. low fat, high carbohydrate
   C. low carbohydrate, low fat
   D. low protein, high fat
2. A patient with acute viral hepatitis will most likely be admitted to the hospital if he or she experiences
   A. severe fatigue
   B. occasional nausea
   C. elevated bilirubin
   D. hepatic encephalopathy
3. The patient with acute hepatic failure will require strict nutritional control of
   A. protein
   B. fat
   C. carbohydrate
   D. fiber

4. The patient with acute hepatic failure would most likely receive which of the following continuous IV infusions based on altered glucose metabolism?
   A. lactated Ringer's
   B. 5 percent dextrose
   C. 10 percent dextrose
   D. normal saline
5. To correct bleeding in the patient with bleeding esophageal varices, the treatment of choice is
   A. sclerotherapy
   B. portosystemic shunt
   C. packed red blood cells
   D. Hespan
6. As a treatment for hepatic encephalopathy, intestinal bacteria levels are suppressed by
   A. lactulose
   B. neomycin
   C. tyrosine
   D. H_2 antagonists
7. Acute hepatic failure is associated with development of hyponatremia, which is precipitated by all of the following EXCEPT
   A. hemodilution
   B. diuretic therapy
   C. sodium restriction
   D. hepatic cell damage

Answers: 1. B, 2. D, 3. A, 4. C, 5. A, 6. B, 7. D

SECTION EIGHT: Nursing Implications

At the completion of this section, the learner will be able to describe the nursing implications appropriate to managing care of the patient experiencing acute hepatic dysfunction.

General Goals

Medical management of acute hepatic dysfunction, particularly during the most active disease stages, is collaborative. Evaluation of hepatic function is performed through laboratory testing and other diagnostic procedures (noninvasive and invasive), which typically require a physician's orders and diagnostic expertise. The two goals that drive the majority of management activities are:

1. Determine and correct underlying cause.
2. Support the patient until liver function returns.

Activities to support the patient center around two goals: (1) promote stable hemodynamic and ventilatory status; and (2) prevent or minimize secondary complications.

The nurse plays a crucial role in improving patient outcomes by being responsible for bedside assessment and analysis of the patient's status on a continual basis. A major focus of the nursing assessment is monitoring the patient for the signs and symptoms of multisystem complications. The nurse facilitates the medical diagnostic process by preparing the patient and family for procedures, assisting with procedures, and monitoring the patient's status during and after procedures. The nurse also develops nursing hypotheses and subsequent independent nursing diagnoses based on the patient's response to the illness, rather than the illness itself. This section provides a description of that part of a comprehensive nursing history and physical assessment, which focuses specifically on hepatic function.

The Focused Nursing Database

On admission, it is crucial that the nurse obtain a comprehensive nursing database. The nurse particularly focuses on data that may have a positive or negative impact on patient outcomes.

The Focused Nursing History

General historical data to collect include preexisting medical conditions, surgeries, and recent history information, such as the events leading up to the patient's admission and a description of the patient's symptoms.

Focused Health Maintenance History

When obtaining the health maintenance portion of the history, the nurse should focus on obtaining information regarding:

- Diet and eating pattern
- Usual appetite prior to admission
- Weight fluctuations
- History of skin or wound healing problems

Focused Cognitive–Perceptual History

Information regarding the patient's usual mental status, ability to communicate, and presence of discomfort or pain provides important baseline data.

Focused Value–Belief History

Acute hepatic dysfunction may place the patient at significant risk. Information regarding the value–belief patterns of the patient and family can assist the nurse with planning appropriate supportive interventions.

The Focused Nursing Assessment

Assessment of the patient with acute hepatic dysfunction has two major focuses: (1) monitoring for potential complications, a collaborative effort; and (2) monitoring the progress of the independent nursing diagnoses. The following sections present some of the major assessments that may be obtained on an ongoing basis during an acute hepatic dysfunction episode to monitor the patient for potential complications.

Respiratory/Circulatory Assessment

Hepatic failure can significantly alter cardiopulmonary function, primarily through severe third spacing of fluids with subsequent intravascular fluid volume deficit. The nurse must monitor the patient for:

- Signs and symptoms of fluid volume deficit
- Edema, which may be peripheral or generalized, and/or may be present in the form of pulmonary edema
- Diminished and/or adventitious breath sounds (crackles, in particular)
- Abnormal trends in blood pressure and pulse

Elimination Assessment

The adequacy of renal function is closely monitored because of the risk for development of hepatorenal syndrome. This is accomplished through observation of ordered renal function laboratory tests (e.g., BUN, creatinine, urine sodium), and evaluation of renal function through measuring intake and output balance and urinary output volume.

Neurologic Assessment

The patient's neurologic status requires close monitoring throughout the duration of the acute illness since hepatic failure can lead to hepatic encephalopathy and is also known to cause cerebral edema. The clinical manifestations of hepatic encephalopathy are described in Section Five and contributing factors are presented in Section Six. The neurologic assessment should minimally include the following.

FOCUSED COGNITIVE-PERCEPTUAL ASSESSMENT

- *Glasgow Coma Scale* (GCS). The GCS is a useful trending tool that assesses the arousal component of consciousness. An altered level of consciousness is an early finding in hepatic encephalopathy. The GCS specifically addresses eye opening, verbal response, and motor response.

FOCUSED MUSCULAR–SKELETAL ASSESSMENT

- *Coordination*. Coordination becomes increasingly impaired in the early stages of encephalopathy.
- *Reflexes*. Reflexes become hypoactive in the early stages of hepatic encephalopathy and hyperactive in the later stages.
- *Movement*. Asterixis (also called *liver flap* when associated with liver failure) refers to an involuntary tremor that is particularly noted in the hands but may also be seen in the feet and tongue. It becomes evident at the stage II level of hepatic encephalopathy.

FOCUSED NEURO/SENSORY ASSESSMENT

- *Seizures*. Seizures may develop in the later stages of hepatic encephalopathy.

Metabolic and Integumentary Assessment

FOCUSED METABOLIC ASSESSMENT. Hepatic dysfunction is associated with a variety of GI signs and symptoms. The nurse should assess for:

- *Nausea and vomiting, anorexia*
- *Presence of diarrhea or constipation*
- *Ascites*. Enlarging abdominal girth; shifting dullness on percussion of the abdomen; abdominal fluid wave; protruding umbilicus. In addition, the patient may develop dyspnea, diminished breath sounds, and/or the clinical manifestations of fluid volume deficit.
- *Bleeding esophageal varices*. The nurse does not independently evaluate the patient for the existence of varices. Instead, the nurse monitors the patient for active variceal bleeding. This is most directly accomplished through assessing nasogastric fluids for blood. If blood is present, the assessment should also include the volume and characteristics of the blood; as well as close assessment for development of the signs and symptoms of hypovolemic shock.
- *Hepatic tenderness and enlargement on palpation*

FOCUSED INTEGUMENTARY ASSESSMENT. The increasing levels of hepatotoxins and the fluid shifts are two major causes of dermatologic findings, which include:

- Jaundice
- Pruritus
- Edema
- Dry, flaky skin
- Poor skin turgor
- Caput medusa (visible veins over the umbilical area caused by congestion and dilation of superficial abdominal wall veins associated with portal vein obstruction)

In addition, the skin can be assessed for several clinical manifestations of problems with coagulation, bleeding, and diminished proteins that usually occur with severe hepatic dysfunction, including:

- Evidence of poor wound healing
- Ecchymosis or petechiae
- Bleeding gums
- Pale mucous membranes and nailbeds

The Nursing Care Plan

The nursing care plan of the patient experiencing an acute hepatic dysfunction episode usually includes both collaborative problems and independent nursing diagnoses.

Frequently Occurring Collaborative Problems
According to Carpenito (1999) and Ulrich and colleagues (1998), the following potential complications (PCs) are commonly associated with hepatic dysfunction:

- PC: Hemorrhage (bleeding)
- PC: Metabolic disorders
- PC: Drug toxicity
- PC: Renal insufficiency
- PC: Progressive liver degeneration
- PC: Portal systemic encephalopathy

Frequently Occurring Nursing Diagnoses
On completion of the nursing database, the nurse clusters data and develops a set of nursing hypotheses based on the available data. Additional critical data that may either support or eliminate each hypothesis should also be identified and obtained. Once the hypotheses have been established, the nurse is ready to develop a list of nursing diagnoses.

In the patient with acute hepatic dysfunction, a variety of nursing diagnoses frequently occur during the crisis period. The following is a partial list of some of these frequently occurring nursing diagnoses, as suggested by Carpenito (1999), Ulrich and colleagues (1999), and Krumberger (1998a):

- *Ineffective breathing pattern* related to pressure on diaphragm from ascites, weakness, pleural effusion, thought processes impairment from ammonia toxins
- *Fluid volume deficit* related to reduced intravascular volume, variceal bleeding, coagulopathy
- *Activity intolerance* related to decreased energy secondary to impaired liver metabolism, tissue hypoxia, decreased nutritional intake
- *Altered nutrition: Less than body requirements* related to impairment of nutrient absorption and metabolism, decreased nutritional intake, fat-soluble vitamin malabsorption
- *Altered comfort* related to pruritus secondary to buildup of bile salts and bilirubin pigment
- *Pain: Upper abdominal* related to ascites and enlarged liver
- *Altered thought processes* related to impaired clearance of drugs and ammonia, bleeding, dehydration
- *High risk for infection* related to leukopenia secondary to hypoproteinemia; and splenic hyperactivity

Many of these nursing diagnoses and their interventions are addressed in other modules. Nursing care of the patient with coagulopathy, a collaborative problem (PC: bleeding) that is frequently caused by hepatic dysfunction, is addressed in Module 27.

In summary, care of the patient with acute hepatic dysfunction requires both collaborative and independent nursing activities. Collaborative interventions center around the medical management goals of supporting the patient and preventing secondary complications until the liver tissue heals and function returns. Monitoring the patient for potential complications during the acute phase of illness requires ongoing, frequent multiple body system assessments. Independent nursing activities are based on the patient's responses to his or her illness rather than the disease process itself. A listing of some of the more frequently occurring nursing diagnoses is provided.

SECTION EIGHT REVIEW

1. A major underlying management goal that drives the majority of medical management activities is to
   A. promote stable hemodynamic status
   B. prevent secondary complications
   C. promote stable ventilatory status
   D. support the patient until liver function returns
2. In the later stages of hepatic encephalopathy, the reflexes typically become
   A. nonactive
   B. hypoactive
   C. normoactive
   D. hyperactive
3. The presence of asterixis indicates that _______ is/are present.
   A. involuntary tremor
   B. loss of coordination
   C. focal seizures
   D. skeletal muscle rigidity
4. The nurse notes the presence of ascites. All of the following are assessments for the presence of ascites EXCEPT
   A. abdominal fluid waves
   B. retracting umbilicus
   C. shifting abdominal dullness
   D. enlarging abdominal girth
5. Dermatologic findings commonly noted in the patient with acute hepatic dysfunction include
   A. oily skin
   B. generalized rash
   C. pruritus
   D. shiny skin

Answers: 1. D, 2. D, 3. A, 4. B, 5. C

POSTTEST

The following Posttest is constructed in a case study format. Questions are asked based on available data. New data are presented as the case study progresses.

Jerome J, 32 years old, was admitted 7 days ago with a severe drug overdose of acetaminophen. He has been in the medical intensive care unit since admission. Jerome's Glasgow Coma Scale peaked at 15 and over the past 24 hours has steadily decreased. The nurse notifies the physician of the change in neurologic status. Following an assessment, the medical team suspects liver dysfunction.

1. Jerome's liver is extremely important. Blood flowing through the liver accounts for what percentage of his total cardiac output?
   A. 20 percent
   B. 30 percent
   C. 40 percent
   D. 50 percent
2. If Jerome's splanchnic blood flow is altered, it would directly affect all of the following organs EXCEPT the
   A. intestines
   B. spleen
   C. liver
   D. kidneys
3. If Jerome is experiencing liver dysfunction, his altered fat metabolism will cause
   A. a decrease in his energy availability
   B. an inability to convert glycogen
   C. an increase in serum ammonia
   D. a decrease in stored iron
4. If he is experiencing congestive heart failure, the liver will respond by
   A. vasoconstricting
   B. expanding in size
   C. secreting more bile
   D. secreting antidiuretic hormone

Jerome has serum enzymes ordered. The results are as follows:

ALT = 1500 U/L
AST = 1500 U/L
ALP = 140 U/L

5. Jerome's serum enzyme levels indicate that _______ is present.
   A. hepatorenal syndrome
   B. encephalopathy
   C. severe hepatocellular injury
   D. severe cellular injury
6. The physician orders alkaline phosphatase (ALP) isoenzymes on Jerome. Which ALP isoenzyme is considered to be most hepatobiliary specific?
   A. 5′-nucleotidase
   B. gamma glutamyl transpeptidase (GGT)
   C. OCT
   D. LDH isoenzymes 4 and 5

The nurse notes that Jerome's urine has become dark amber. The quantity was 150 mL in the past hour.

7. Based on the early diagnosis of an acute hepatic dysfunction, the color of Jerome's urine suggests that the nurse can expect
   A. ammonia to decrease
   B. low serum proteins
   C. acute renal failure
   D. jaundice to develop
8. If Jerome is diagnosed as having acute hepatitis, he will most likely receive _______ therapy.
   A. antibiotic
   B. antiviral
   C. antifungal
   D. no specific
9. Which of the following types of hepatitis do health care workers most commonly develop?
   A. hepatitis A
   B. hepatitis B
   C. hepatitis C
   D. hepatitis D
10. If Jerome develops mild hepatic enlargement and edema, with generalized inflammation but localized necrosis, it would be classified as _______ hepatitis.
    A. classic
    B. submassive
    C. massive
    D. anicteric
11. If he has developed cholestatic hepatitis, you would anticipate assessing for
    A. the absence of jaundice
    B. the presence of gallstones
    C. severe jaundice
    D. an inflamed gallbladder
12. Typical prodromal symptoms of the patient developing acute hepatitis includes all of the following EXCEPT
    A. hyperpyrexia
    B. increased intracranial pressure
    C. nausea and vomiting
    D. arthritis and myalgia
13. If Jerome had developed stage III encephalopathy, you would anticipate a neurologic presentation to include
    A. restlessness, reversal of sleep rhythm
    B. lethargy, drowsiness
    C. disorientation, asterixis
    D. stupor, hyperactive reflexes

14. Based on Jerome's history, he is at risk for developing fulminant hepatic failure based on which cause?
    A. hepatotoxin ingestion
    B. hepatitis virus
    C. multiple organ failure
    D. complication of chronic failure
15. Jerome has no preexisting history of hepatic dysfunction. It is unlikely that he will develop
    A. acute renal failure
    B. esophageal varices
    C. sepsis
    D. acid–base disorders
16. If he develops spontaneous bacterial peritonitis, it is probably caused by
    A. septicemia
    B. translocation of intestinal bacteria
    C. spread of hepatic infective agent
    D. autoimmune reaction
17. Jerome's encephalopathy is worsening. The nurse notes that he has not had a bowel movement in 3 days. What physician order can the nurse anticipate?
    A. increase dietary protein
    B. neomycin 1 to 2 times per day
    C. daily milk of magnesia
    D. lactulose qh until desired effect
18. The majority of patients experiencing fulminant hepatic failure ultimately require which of the following interventions?
    A. liver transplantation
    B. portosystemic shunt
    C. sclerotherapy
    D. Sengstaken–Blakemore tube
19. The majority of Jerome's plan of care will focus on which of the following as the underlying goal?
    A. evaluate renal function
    B. promote stable hemodynamic status
    C. support the patient until liver function resumes
    D. prevent secondary complications
20. While assessing his integumentary status, the nurse notes visible veins over the umbilical area. In a patient with hepatic dysfunction, this finding is called
    A. asterixis
    B. ecchymosis
    C. ascites
    D. caput medusa
21. Based on the typical fluid status of the patient with acute hepatic dysfunction, the most appropriate nursing diagnosis to be added to Jerome's plan of care would be
    A. *Fluid volume deficit*
    B. *Fluid volume excess*
    C. *Cardiac output: Decreased*
    D. *Nutrition: More than body requirements*

POSTTEST ANSWERS

Question	Answer	Section	Question	Answer	Section
1	B	One	12	B	Four
2	D	One	13	D	Five
3	A	Two	14	A	Five
4	B	Two	15	B	Six
5	D	Three	16	B	Six
6	A	Three	17	D	Seven
7	D	Three	18	A	Seven
8	D	Four	19	C	Eight
9	B	Four	20	D	Eight
10	A	Four	21	A	Eight
11	C	Four			

REFERENCES

Altman, D.F. (1995). Drugs used in gastrointestinal diseases. In B.G. Katzung (ed). *Basic and clinical pharmacology* (6th ed.) (pp. 949–961). Norwalk, CT: Appleton & Lange.

Andreoli, T.E., Bennett, J.C., Carpenter, C.C., & Plum, F. (eds.). (1997). *Cecil's essentials of medicine* (4th ed.). Philadelphia: W.B. Saunders.

Carey, C.F., Lee, H.H., & Woeltze, K.F. (eds.) (1998). *Washington manual* (29th ed.) pp. 329–342. Philadelphia: Lippincott-Raven.

Carpenito, L.J. (1999). *Nursing care plans and documentation* (3rd ed.) (p. 130). Philadelphia: J.B. Lippincott.

Chapman, J.R. (ed.). (1997). *Organ and tissue donation for transplantation*. New York: Oxford University Press.

Deglin, J.H., & Vallerand, A.H. (1997). *Davis's drug guide for nurses* (6th ed.). Philadelphia: F.A. Davis.

Doughty, D.B., & Jackson, D.B. (1993). Gastrointestinal disorders. In *Mosby's clinical nursing series*. St. Louis: C.V. Mosby.

Harvey, M.A. (1998). Multisystem organ failure. In M.R. Kinney, S.B. Dunbar, J.A. Brooks-Brunn, N. Molter, & J.M. Vitello-Cicciu (eds.). *AACN's clinical reference for critical care nurses* (4th ed.) (pp. 1125–1149). St. Louis: C.V. Mosby.

Jacobs, R.A. (1999). General problems in infectious disease. In L.M. Tierney, S.J. McPhee, & M.A. Papadakis (eds.). *Current medical diagnosis and treatment* (38th ed.) (p. 1174). Stamford, CT: Appleton & Lange.

Jawetz, E. (1995). Aminoglycosides and polymyxins. In B.G. Katzung (ed.). *Basic and clinical pharmacology* (6th ed.) (pp. 699–703). Norwalk, CT: Appleton & Lange.

Kee, J. (1999). *Laboratory and diagnostic tests with nursing implications* (5th ed.). Stamford, CT: Appleton & Lange.

Krumberger, J.M. (1998a). Gastrointestinal disorders. In M.R. Kinney, S.B. Dunbar, J.A. Brooks-Brunn, N. Molter, & J.M. Vitello-Cicciu (eds.). *AACN's clinical reference for critical care nurses* (4th ed.) (pp. 1033–1037). St. Louis: C.V. Mosby.

Krumberger, J.M. (1998b). Gastrointestinal patient assessment. In M.R. Kinney, J.A. Brooks-Brunn, N. Molter, & J.M. Vitello-Cicciu (eds.). *AACN's clinical reference for critical care nurses* (4th ed.) (pp. 1003–1014). St. Louis: C.V. Mosby.

Raper, S.E. (1994). Hepatobiliary disease. In F.S. Bongard and D.Y. Sue (eds.). *Current critical care diagnosis and treatment* (pp. 576–591). Norwalk, CT: Appleton & Lange.

Smith, S.L., & Ciferni, M. (1990). Liver transplantation. In S.L. Smith (ed.), *Tissue and organ transplantation* (pp. 273–300). St. Louis: Mosby-Year Book.

Thelan, L.A., Urden, L.D., Lough, M.E., & Stacy, K.M. (1998). *Critical care nursing: Diagnosis and management* (3rd ed.) (pp. 917–973). St. Louis: C.V. Mosby.

Thompson, J.M., McFarano, G.K., Hirsch, J.E., Tucker, S.M., & Bowers, A.C. (1997). *Mosby's manual of clinical nursing* (4th ed.). St. Louis: C.V. Mosby.

Ulrich, S.P., Canale, S.W., & Wendell, S.A. (1998). *Medical–surgical nursing care planning guides* (4th ed.) (pp. 682–704). Philadelphia: W.B. Saunders.

Wilson, L.M., & Lester, L.B. (1992). Liver, biliary tract, and pancreas. In S.A. Price & L.M. Wilson (eds.). *Pathophysiology: Clinical concepts of disease processes* (4th ed.) (pp. 337–367). St. Louis: Mosby-Year Book.

Wilson, L.M., et al. (1997). Liver, biliary tract, and pancreas. In S.A. Price & L.M. Wilson (eds.), *Pathophysiology: Clinical concepts of disease processes* (5th ed.) (pp. 372–408). St. Louis: Mosby.

Module 30

Acute Pancreatic Dysfunction

Kathleen D. Wagner, Melanie Hardin-Pierce

This self-study module focuses on assessment and management concepts related to the patient with a disruption of normal pancreatic function. Sections One and Two provide a brief review of basic anatomy and physiology of the pancreas, including pancreatic exocrine functions. Section Three describes the pathophysiologic basis of pancreatic dysfunction, including etiologic factors. Section Four describes laboratory tests and diagnostic procedures used to diagnose acute pancreatitis. Section Five discusses the nursing assessment of a patient with acute pancreatitis. Section Six offers a brief overview of the major complications associated with acute pancreatitis, and Section Seven describes the medical management. The module closes with Section Eight, which provides the reader with a list of independent nursing diagnoses and collaborative problems. The nursing diagnosis *Altered comfort: nausea and vomiting*, is developed, including expected patient outcomes and interventions. With the exception of Section Eight, each section includes a set of review questions to help the learner evaluate his or her understanding of the section's content before moving on to the next section. All Section Reviews and the module Pretest and Posttest include answers. It is suggested that the learner review those concepts that have been missed in the review questions before proceeding to the next section.

Objectives

Following completion of this module, the learner will be able to

1. Describe the anatomy of the pancreas.
2. Explain the exocrine functions of the pancreas.
3. Describe the pathophysiologic basis of acute pancreatic dysfunction.
4. Describe medical data used in the diagnosis of acute pancreatic dysfunction.
5. Discuss assessment of the patient with acute pancreatic dysfunction.
6. Explain the complications of acute pancreatitis.
7. Describe the medical management of a patient with acute pancreatitis.
8. Discuss the nursing plan of care for a patient with acute pancreatic dysfunction.

Pretest

1. The functional unit of the pancreas is called the
   A. ampulla of Vater
   B. pancreatic acinus
   C. alpha cell
   D. islets of Langerhans

2. The duct of Wirsung shares the opening into the duodenum with the
   A. acinar cells
   B. common bile duct
   C. gallbladder
   D. duct of Santorini

3. The pH of pancreatic juice is
   A. highly acidic
   B. moderately acidic
   C. neutral
   D. highly alkaline
4. The pancreas is protected from autodigestion by
   A. bicarbonate and water
   B. the presence of the hormone secretin
   C. protective pancreatic cell wall coverings
   D. the production of enzymes in their inactive states
5. A common cause of acute pancreatitis is
   A. chronic alcohol abuse
   B. steroid therapy
   C. duodenal ulcers
   D. viral infections
6. Regardless of the etiology of acute pancreatitis, the primary physiologic event is
   A. hemorrhage
   B. edema
   C. autodigestion
   D. pain
7. Alcohol has which of the following affects on the pancreas?
   A. decreases enzyme secretion
   B. depresses secretion of secretin
   C. inhibits the inflammatory response
   D. causes spasm of the sphincter of Oddi
8. The primary laboratory test used to help make a diagnosis of pancreatitis is serum
   A. amylase
   B. calcium
   C. lactic dehydrogenase (LDH)
   D. elastase
9. The typical pain of acute pancreatitis is characterized as all of the following EXCEPT
   A. severe
   B. relieved by vomiting
   C. radiating to the flank
   D. continuous
10. Shock associated with acute pancreatitis can be caused by all of the following EXCEPT
    A. dehydration
    B. vasodilation
    C. hemorrhage
    D. third spacing
11. Pulmonary complications are attributed to which of the following pancreatic enzymes?
    A. trypsin
    B. elastase
    C. amylase
    D. phospholipase A
12. If a pancreatic pseudocyst were to rupture into the peritoneal cavity, the patient would most likely develop
    A. peritonitis
    B. acute renal failure
    C. paralytic ileus
    D. septicemia
13. The release of myocardial depressant factor by injured pancreatic tissue is believed to have what effect on the heart?
    A. decreases heart rate
    B. decreases cardiac output
    C. increases blood pressure
    D. increases cardiac output
14. Peritoneal signs include all of the following EXCEPT
    A. rebound tenderness
    B. rigid abdomen
    C. hyperactive bowel sounds
    D. leukocytosis
15. Cullen's sign may be noted under which of the following circumstances?
    A. acute tubular necrosis (ATN)
    B. hemorrhage
    C. hypovolemic shock
    D. respiratory failure
16. The highest priority in management of the patient with severe acute pancreatitis is
    A. control of pain
    B. correct the underlying problem
    C. minimize pancreatic stimulation
    D. stabilize hemodynamic status
17. The drug of choice in pain management of the patient with acute pancreatitis is
    A. morphine sulfate
    B. codeine
    C. meperidine (Demerol)
    D. ibuprofen

Pretest answers: 1. B, 2. B, 3. D, 4. D, 5. A, 6. C, 7. D, 8. A, 9. B, 10. A, 11. D, 12. A, 13. B, 14. C, 15. B, 16. D, 17. C

GLOSSARY

Acinus. The exocrine functional unit of the pancreas; composed of acinar cells that secrete digestive enzymes (pleural, acini)

Ampulla of Vater. A dilated area of the main pancreatic duct, formed by the junction at the duodenum of the main pancreatic duct and the common bile duct

Amylolytic. Facilitating the breakdown of carbohydrates

Autodigestion. Breakdown of pancreatic tissues by its own enzymes

Chyme. The partially digested mixture of food and secretions of digestion found in the stomach and small bowel

Chymotrypsin. A proteolytic pancreatic enzyme

Duct of Santorini. An accessory duct of the pancreas that exists in approximately 70 percent of the population

Duct of Wirsung. The main pancreatic duct

Elastase. A proteolytic pancreatic enzyme; its proenzyme, proelastase, requires trypsin to become activated; responsible for erosion of blood vessels contributing to hemorrhage in severe acute pancreatitis

Kallikrein. An enzyme found in plasma, body tissues, and urine that forms kinin. It normally circulates in the plasma in its inactive state, as the proenzyme kallikreinogen. When activated by trypsin, it is an extremely potent vasodilator

Lipase. A lipolytic pancreatic enzyme; its action contributes to necrosis of fatty tissue surrounding the pancreas in the presence of pancreatitis

Lipolytic. Facilitating the breakdown of fats

Pancreatitis. Inflammation of the pancreas; it may occur as an acute or chronic condition

Phospholipase A. A lipolytic pancreatic enzyme, activated by either bile salts or trypsin; contributes to the development of pulmonary complications (ARDS) by decreasing surfactant in the lungs

Proteolytic. Facilitating the breakdown of proteins

Secretin. A hormone present in the small bowel mucosa that stimulates sodium bicarbonate secretion by the pancreas and bile secretion by the liver. It decreases gastrointestinal peristalsis and motility

Sphincter of Oddi. A circular muscle that surrounds the ampulla of Vater; it helps control the rate of pancreatic enzyme and bile flow into the duodenum

Trypsin. A proteolytic pancreatic enzyme. It exists in the pancreas in its proenzyme (inactive) state as trypsinogen. Most of the other pancreatic enzymes require trypsin for activation

Abbreviations

CCK. Cholecystokinin

ERCP. Endoscopic retrograde cholangiopancreatogram

GCS. Glasgow Coma Scale

LDH. Lactic dehydrogenase

MDF. Myocardial depressant factor

SECTION ONE: Anatomy of the Pancreas

At the completion of this section, the learner will be able to describe the anatomy of the pancreas.

The pancreas is a multifunctional organ, having both endocrine and exocrine functions. It is located in the upper abdominal cavity, lying in a horizontal position (Fig. 30–1). It has three divisions: the head, the body, and the tail. The head lies adjacent to the duodenum, within its curve. The pancreatic body lies directly behind the stomach, and the tail is adjacent to the spleen.

Exocrine Anatomic Structure

The majority of the pancreatic tissue consists of exocrine tissues. The functional exocrine unit is called the **acinus** (Fig. 30–2). Acini are composed of digestive enzyme–secreting acinar cells that are necessary for digestion. Acini are clustered into larger units called pancreatic lobules. The lobules are separated from each other by septa.

The digestive enzymes flow through a ductal system (Fig. 30–3) into the duodenum. Once enzymes have been released from the acinar lumina, they flow into small duct lumina and on into a connecting network of ducts, eventually terminating at the main pancreatic duct (the **duct of Wirsung**). The main pancreatic duct runs through the center of the organ from head to tail. It joins with the common bile duct, sharing the same opening into the duodenum at the **ampulla of Vater,** which is surrounded by the **sphincter of Oddi** (Fig. 30–4). Located at the junction of the common bile duct and the duodenum, the sphincter of Oddi helps control the rate of pancreatic enzyme and bile flow into the duodenum. A second duct, the accessory pancreatic duct (**duct of Santorini**) exists in approximately 70 percent of people (Andreoli et al., 1997). When present, it joins the duodenum at the minor duodenal papilla, which is located proximal to the main pancreatic duct.

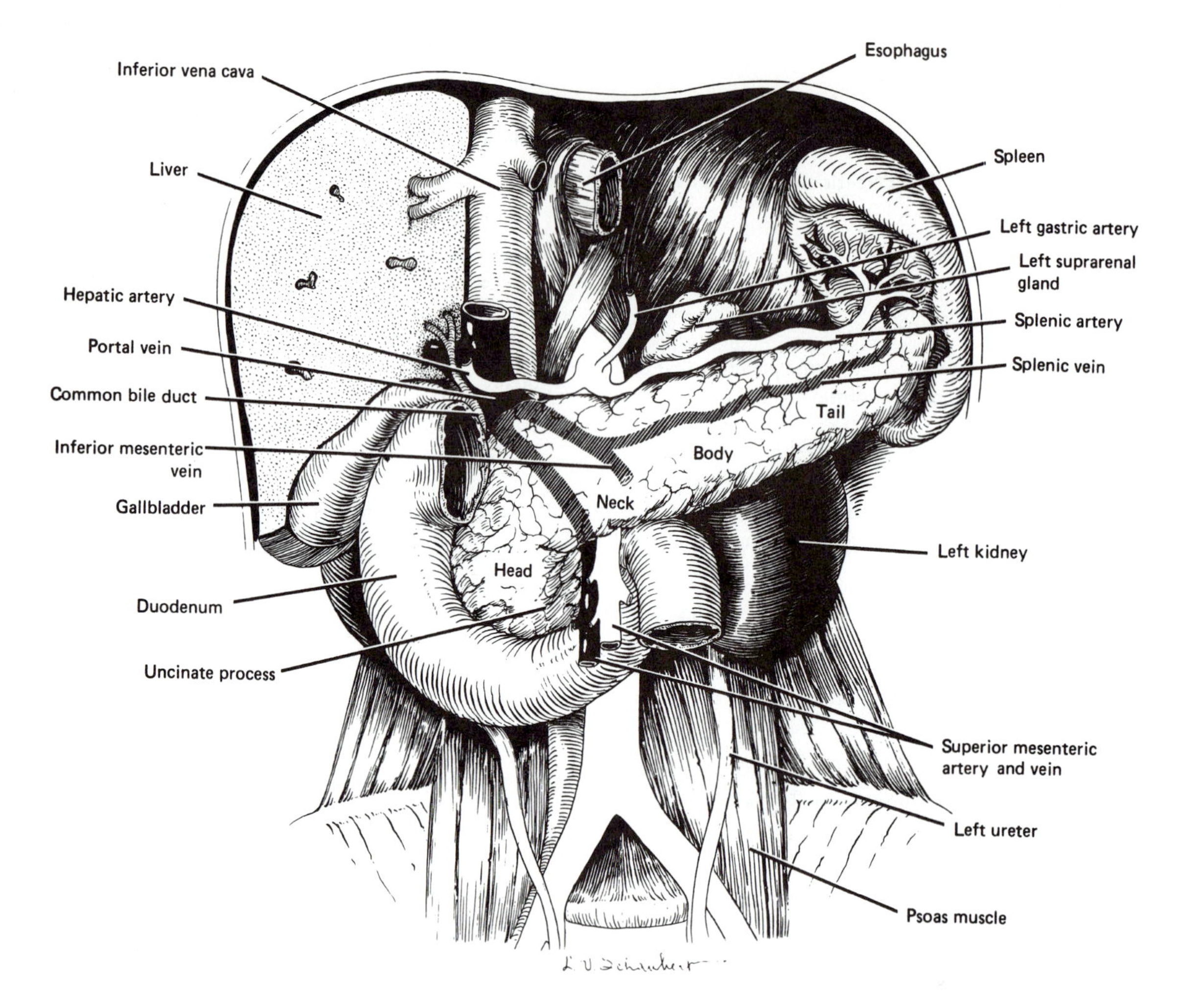

Figure 30–1. The pancreas, showing relations of the major vessels, venous drainage, and adjoining structures. *(From Lindner, H.H. [1989].* Human anatomy *[p. 426]. Norwalk, CT: Appleton & Lange.)*

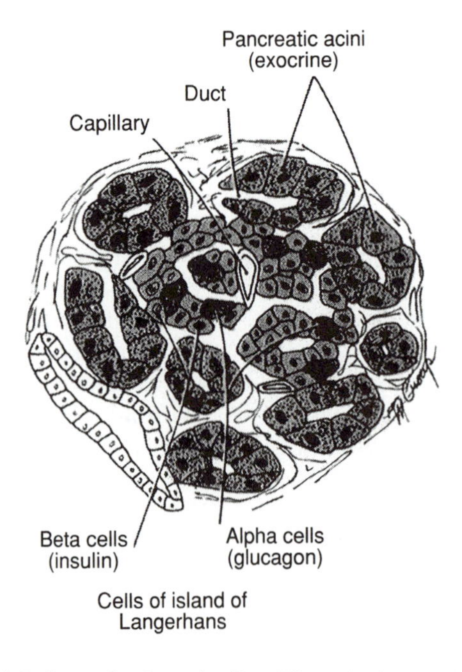

Figure 30–2. Pancreatic acinar units. *(From Wilson, L.M., & Lester, L.B. [1992]. Liver, biliary tract, and pancreas. In S.A. Price & L.M. Wilson [eds].* Pathophysiology: Clinical concepts of disease processes, *4th ed. [p. 338]. St. Louis: Mosby-Year Book.)*

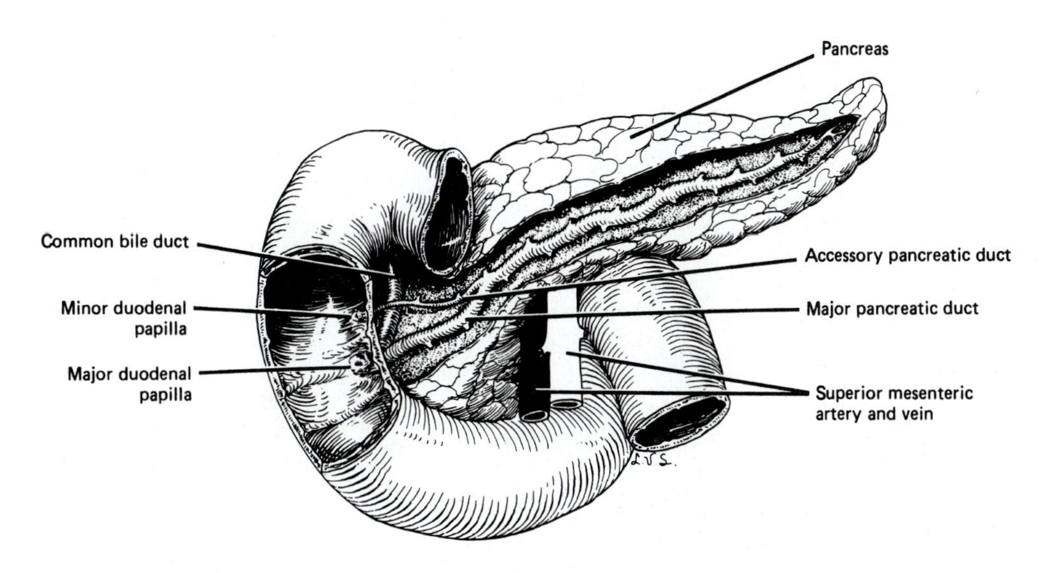

Figure 30–3. The ductal system of the pancreas. *(From Lindner, H.H. [1989].* Human anatomy *[p. 430]. Norwalk, CT: Appleton & Lange.)*

In summary, the pancreas has both exocrine and endocrine functions. It is located in the upper abdominal cavity. The pancreatic acinus is the functional unit of the pancreas. It secretes digestive enzymes capable of breaking down carbohydrates, proteins, and fats. Once secreted, the pancreatic juice flows through a network of duct systems and eventually passes through the ampulla of Vater and flows into the small intestines (Marieb, 1998).

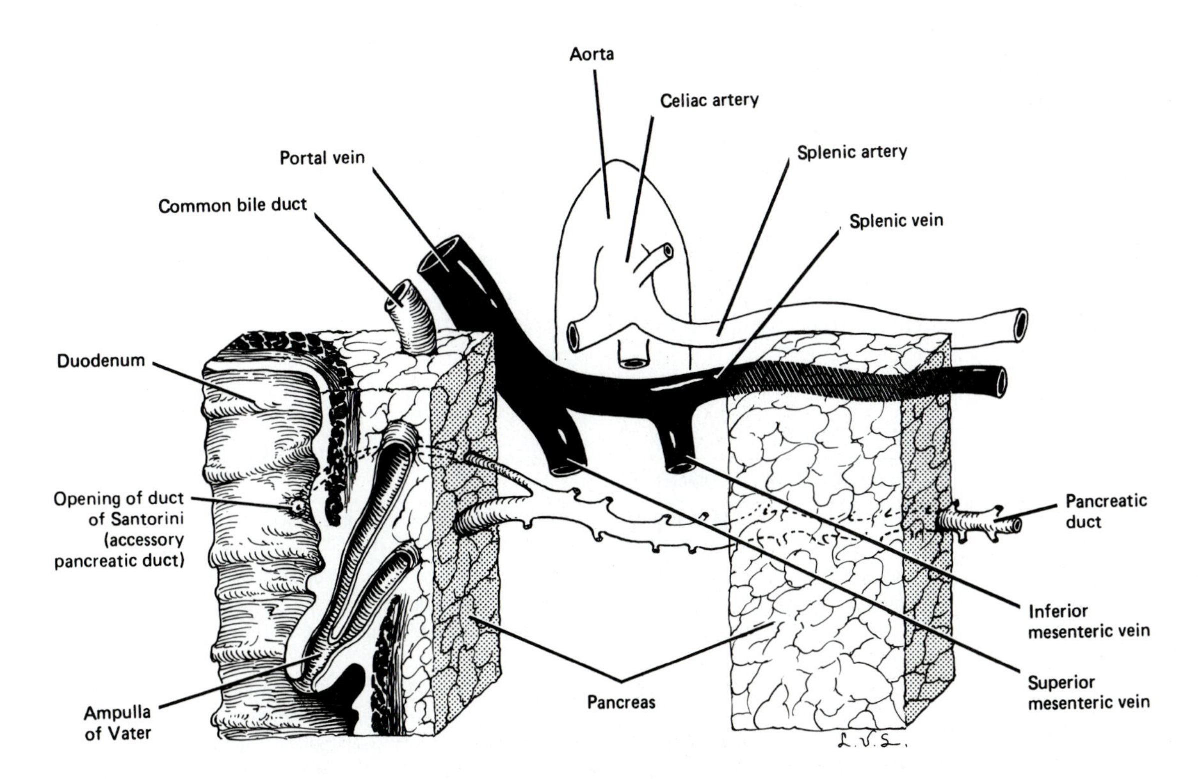

Figure 30–4. Diagram of blocks of the pancreas and the descending duodenum to illustrate the common bile and pancreatic ducts, the splenic vein, the portal vein, and the course of the splenic artery. *(From Lindner, H.H. [1989].* Human anatomy *[p. 431]. Norwalk, CT: Appleton & Lange.)*

SECTION ONE REVIEW

1. The functional unit of the pancreas is called the
   A. ampulla of Vater
   B. acinus
   C. alpha cell
   D. islets of Langerhans
2. All of the following are part of the pancreatic anatomic structure EXCEPT the
   A. body
   B. tail
   C. arm
   D. head
3. The sphincter of Oddi primarily serves which of the following purposes?
   A. control of rate of pancreatic enzyme flow into intestines
   B. control of the activation of the pancreatic enzymes
   C. regulation of the level of intestinal secretin
   D. regulation of the rate of bicarbonate secretion
4. The duct of Wirsung shares the opening into the duodenum with the
   A. acinar cells
   B. duct of Santorini
   C. gallbladder
   D. common bile duct

Answers: 1. B, 2. C, 3. A, 4. D

SECTION TWO: The Exocrine Functions of the Pancreas

At the completion of this section, the learner will be able to explain the exocrine functions of the pancreas.

Exocrine Functions

The pancreas normally secretes up to 4 L of pancreatic juice per day, with a pH of approximately 8.3. Pancreatic juice is composed of water, bicarbonate, electrolytes (particularly potassium and sodium), and digestive enzymes (American Association of Critical Care Nurses [AACN], 1998). The pancreas is important in neutralizing the acids in the small intestines and in providing digestive enzymes.

Control of pH

Chyme is the mixture of partially digested food and intestinal secretions as it exists in the stomach and small bowel. The acidic pH of the chyme that enters the duodenum from the stomach stimulates mucosal secretion of the hormone **secretin** by the proximal end of the small intestines. Secretin is essential in the regulation of intestinal pH. Release of secretin is stimulated by a drop in pH to < 4.5. This serves several functions. First, when intestinal pH becomes too acidic, secretin stimulates the pancreas to secrete large quantities of bicarbonate and water. Bicarbonate raises the intestinal pH, which protects the mucosa. Second, pancreatic enzymes work best within a pH level that is neutral to slightly alkaline. The alkaline pH of the small bowel is important in the formation of pepsin, which protects the delicate intestinal mucosa and facilitates normal digestive enzyme processes.

Pancreatic Enzymes

Normal digestion is dependent on the digestive enzymatic activities of the pancreatic enzymes. Pancreatic digestive enzymes are responsible for the breakdown of proteins (proteolytics), fat (lipolytics), and carbohydrates **(amylolytics).** Table 30–1 summarizes the major pancreatic enzymes.

TABLE 30–1. MAJOR PANCREATIC ENZYMES

ENZYME	TARGET	PRECURSOR NAME	COMMENTS
Trypsin	Proteins	Trypsinogen	Most abundant proteolytic enzyme; activated in intestinal mucosa by enterokinase or by preexisting trypsin
Elastase	Proteins	Proelastase	Activated by trypsin; breaks down elastic tissue; can break down blood vessel walls
Chymotrypsin	Proteins	Chymotrypsinogen	Activated by trypsin; splits (via hydrolyzing) proteins into peptones
Pancreatic amylase	Carbohydrates	—	Splits glycogen, starches, and other carbohydrates, with the exception of cellulose, into disaccharides (primarily)
Lipase	Fats	—	Requires bile salts; splits fats into monoglycerides and fatty acids
Phospholipase A	Fats	—	Activated by trypsin or bile salts; splits phospholipids into fatty acids; breaks down cell membranes and is capable of causing pancreatic and fat tissue necrosis

Data from Guyton, A.C., & Hall, J.E. (1997). Human physiology and mechanisms of disease, *6th ed. (pp. 530–531). Philadelphia: W.B. Saunders; and Wilson, L.M., & Lester, L.B. (1997). Liver, biliary tract, and pancreas. In S.A. Price & L.M. Wilson (eds).* Pathophysiology: Clinical concepts of disease processes, *5th ed. (pp. 372–408). St. Louis: Mosby-Year Book.*

Pancreatic Secretion Regulation

Secretion of pancreatic enzymes is regulated by both hormonal and neural factors, though hormonal influences are more important. There are four major stimuli of pancreatic secretion: gastrin, cholecystokinin (CCK), secretin, and acetylcholine. Large quantities of gastrin are secreted by the stomach in response to neural stimulation. The intestinal hormones, secretin, and CCK, are stimulated by stomach acids, and amino acids and fats, respectively. Gastrin, secretin, and CCK stimulate the pancreatic acinar cells and are responsible for the release of large quantities of pancreatic enzymes. Acetylcholine is secreted by parasympathetic vagal and other cholinergic nerve endings throughout the gut. Vagal influence stimulates secretion of pancreatic enzymes, which are then placed in temporary storage in the acini, awaiting a transport mechanism to move them into the intestines (Marieb, 1998).

Pancreatic Self-Protective Properties

The **proteolytic** pancreatic enzymes (e.g., **trypsin, chymotrypsin,** and elastase) are responsible for the breakdown of proteins. Proteolytic enzymes make up about 90 percent of pancreatic digestive enzymes. The **lipolytic** pancreatic enzyme, phospholipase A, is responsible for breaking down phospholipids into fatty acids. Without some protective mechanism, these enzymes are capable of digesting the pancreatic tissues, a process called **autodigestion.** Under normal circumstances, several mechanisms exist to prevent autodigestion. First, pancreatic proteolytic enzymes (refer to Table 30–1) are produced in an inactive, precursor form, remaining inactive while in the pancreas. Second, a trypsin inhibitor is secreted by the acinar cells that maintains trypsin in its inactive (inhibited) state while it is present in the pancreatic ducts and cells (Doughty & Jackson, 1993).

In summary, pancreatic juice, composed of water, electrolytes, pancreatic enzymes, and bicarbonate, maintains a highly alkaline pH and is used to increase the pH of chyme. Two major pancreatic exocrine functions are control of intestinal pH and secretion of digestive enzymes. Regulation of pancreatic enzyme secretion is influenced by hormonal and neural factors. Secretin plays an important role in intestinal pH regulation. Normally, the pancreas is protected from digesting itself by several protective mechanisms (Marieb, 1998).

SECTION TWO REVIEW

1. The pH of pancreatic juice is
   A. highly acidic
   B. moderately acidic
   C. neutral
   D. highly alkaline
2. The function of secretin is to
   A. lower the pancreatic pH
   B. stimulate secretion of pancreatic enzymes
   C. directly activate pepsin production
   D. inhibit secretion of pancreatic enzymes
3. The most abundant pancreatic enzyme is
   A. chymotrypsin
   B. lipase
   C. trypsin
   D. elastase
4. The pancreas is protected from autodigestion by
   A. bicarbonate and water
   B. the presence of the hormone secretin
   C. protective pancreatic cell wall coverings
   D. the production of enzymes in their inactive states

Answers: 1. D, 2. B, 3. C, 4. D

SECTION THREE: Pathophysiologic Basis of Acute Pancreatitis

At the completion of this section, the learner will be able to describe the pathophysiologic basis of acute pancreatitis.

Pancreatitis is defined as inflammation of the pancreas. It can occur either as an acute or chronic condition. Acute pancreatitis is the sudden onset of pancreatic inflammation. It is characterized by varying degrees of abdominal pain, pancreatic tissue edema, necrosis of pancreatic tissue and, possibly, hemorrhage. It can be further subdivided into two more specific categories based on pathologic findings: acute hemorrhagic and acute nonhemorrhagic pancreatitis.

Acute nonhemorrhagic pancreatitis (also known as interstitial or mild edematous pancreatitis) is the most common form of pancreatitis (approximately 95 percent) and is associated with a low mortality rate (5 to 15 percent) (Brown, 1991; Reece-Smith, 1997; Smith & Butler, 1993). Acute hemorrhagic pancreatitis (also known as necrotizing pancreatitis) is associated with a high mortality of up to 50 percent due to systemic complications (Brown, 1991; Oleynikov et al., 1998). Table 30–2 summarizes the characteristics of these two types of acute pancreatitis.

TABLE 30–3. MAJOR ETIOLOGIES OF ACUTE PANCREATITIS

Common
Alcohol abuse
Gallstone obstruction
Blunt trauma to abdomen
Scorpion bite
Less Common
Epstein–Barr virus
Mycoplasma infection
Autoimmune disorders (e.g., thrombotic thrombocytopenic purpura, necrotizing angiitis)
Drug side effect
Shock (associated with multiple organ dysfunction syndrome [MODS])

Etiologies

Pancreatitis most commonly develops in men with a history of alcohol abuse and women with biliary tract disease associated with gallstones. It occurs less commonly as the result of adverse effects of certain drugs, duodenal ulcers, trauma, and viral infections. Sometimes, no specific cause can be found. Table 30–3 lists some of the major etiologies of acute pancreatitis.

Pathophysiology

The exact mechanisms of injury associated with acute pancreatitis are unclear at this time. Regardless of the cause, the primary pathophysiologic event is autodigestion, or breakdown of pancreatic tissues by its own enzymes. Autodigestion is caused by premature activation of pancreatic digestive enzymes while they are still within the pancreas. Multiple theories have been proposed to explain the mechanisms that trigger autodigestion, including (1) pancreatic duct obstruction, (2) alcohol-induced pancreatic irritation, and (3) reflux of bile or duodenal contents into the pancreatic ducts at the sphincter of Oddi.

Pancreatic Duct Obstruction

Obstruction of the pancreatic duct is a common cause of acute pancreatitis. It is associated with the following risk factors: obesity; female gender; age over 60 years. Since the common bile duct and duct of Wirsung share a common exit at the ampulla of Vater, obstruction by a gallstone can readily occur, causing blockage of the main pancreatic duct. The stone may lodge in either duct. Inflammation and edema of the terminal end of the common bile duct or main pancreatic duct from any cause can also precipitate obstruction to flow of pancreatic juices into the duodenum (Alle, Stewart, & Maselly, 1994; Smith & Butler, 1993). Obstruction of the main pancreatic duct for any reason causes a backup of pancreatic flow, which increases ductal pressures. When pressures become too great, the enzymes begin leaking out of the duct into the pancreatic tissues, which in turn triggers premature activation of digestive enzymes.

TABLE 30–2. CHARACTERISTICS OF NONHEMORRHAGIC AND HEMORRHAGIC ACUTE PANCREATITIS

NONHEMORRHAGIC (INTERSTITIAL)	SEVERE HEMORRHAGIC (NECROTIZING)
• Short term	• Longer duration
• Pancreatic edema and swelling	• Pancreatic hemorrhage
• Little to no necrosis	• Extensive fat and tissue necrosis
• Localized inflammation	• Extrapancreatic invasion of pancreatic enzymes
• Reversible	• Irreversible damage to pancreas and surrounding tissues
• Good prognosis	• Poor prognosis—associated with sepsis and multiple organ dysfunction

Alcoholic Pancreatitis

Long-term alcohol consumption accounts for about 40 percent of acute pancreatitis cases in the United States. Alcoholic pancreatitis is associated with recurrent acute attacks that are destructive to pancreatic tissues. The pancreas becomes increasingly scarred with each attack. The resulting destruction replaces functional acinar cells with nonfunctioning fibrous tissue (Alle, Stewart, & Maselly, 1994). Alcoholic pancreatitis is most commonly found in men 30 to 40 years of age (Smith & Butler, 1993). The effects of alcohol on the pancreatic tissue are not clearly understood. Alcohol stimulates secretion of secretin and hydrochloric acid which, in turn, are known to stimulate the secretion of pancreatic enzymes. Alcohol can also cause the sphincter of Oddi to spasm, which can obstruct normal enzyme flow out of the main pancreatic duct, initiating the pancreatic obstruction sequence of events. It is also theorized that chronic use of alcohol may precipitate inflammation of the duodenal wall, which could interfere with normal pancreatic enzyme flow out of the pancreas (Guyton & Hall, 1997; Smith & Butler, 1993).

Reflux of Bile or Duodenal Contents

The following is one possible sequence of events that helps explain reflux of bile or duodenal contents as an initiating event.

Duodenal contents, including digestive juices, reflux through the sphincter of Oddi. The acidic digestive juices damage the delicate epithelium of the pancreatic duct.

The damaged epithelial layer loses its integrity and becomes more permeable and leaky, thereby allowing digestive juices to leak through the duct walls into the pancreatic tissues. The presence of the acidic digestive juices triggers activation of the pancreatic enzymes, primarily trypsin, which then activate other pancreatic enzymes.

Activation of two pancreatic enzymes is thought to cause the most damage. These enzymes are phospholipase A and elastase. **Phospholipase A** digests the phospholipids on the cell membranes, and **elastase** digests elastic tissue of vessel walls. As vessel walls sustain increasing damage, both capillary and lymphatic vessels become injured, which results in hemorrhage and edema, respectively. As the damage progresses, more acini are triggered to activate and secrete their digestive enzymes, which further increases autodigestive activities.

As a part of the inflammatory process, kallikrein is activated by the trypsin. **Kallikrein** is a basophil mediator of inflammation. It is responsible for causing bradykinin formation. Kallikrein is thought to increase local damage and precipitate systemic hypotension. It causes vasodilation and increases permeability of blood vessels, pain, and leukocyte invasion. Once kallikrein has been activated, systemic hypotension may lead to shock and multisystem dysfunction or failure (such as acute respiratory distress syndrome and acute renal failure). Thus, the initial local insult of acute pancreatitis may become a complex multisystemic dysfunction disease process (Andreoli et al., 1997; Wilson & Lester, 1997).

Drug-Induced Pancreatitis

In addition to the more common causes of acute pancreatitis, certain drugs, at toxic levels, have also been implicated (Krumberger, 1998). Some of these drugs are:

- Tetracycline
- Sulfonamides
- Furosemide (thiazide diuretics)
- Estrogen
- Azathioprine
- Methyldopa

In summary, pancreatitis is an inflammation of the pancreas. Acute pancreatitis can be divided into hemorrhagic and nonhemorrhagic types. The mortality rate is significantly higher with the hemorrhagic type. The majority of pancreatitis cases are precipitated by either alcohol abuse or biliary tract disease. Other possible causes include reflux of bile or duodenal contents and drug toxicity. The exact pathophysiologic mechanisms of injury are not yet clearly understood. The major pathophysiologic event is autodigestion of the organ, which activates an inflammatory cascade resulting in local, and in severe cases, systemic complications.

SECTION THREE REVIEW

1. Acute hemorrhagic pancreatitis is characterized by all of the following EXCEPT
   A. severe bleeding
   B. vasoconstriction
   C. tissue necrosis
   D. extrapancreatic invasion
2. A common cause of acute pancreatitis is
   A. chronic alcohol abuse
   B. steroid therapy
   C. duodenal ulcers
   D. viral infections
3. Regardless of the etiology of acute pancreatitis, the primary physiologic event is
   A. hemorrhage
   B. edema
   C. autodigestion
   D. pain
4. It is theorized that acute pancreatitis can be triggered by reflux of
   A. digestive juices through the sphincter of Oddi
   B. pancreatic enzymes into the common bile duct
   C. digestive juices through the common bile duct
   D. pancreatic enzymes into the duodenum
5. Premature activation of the pancreatic enzymes _______ and _______ is thought to cause the most pancreatic damage.
   A. trypsin, amylase
   B. lipase, chymotrypsin
   C. phospholipase A, elastase
   D. elastase, amylase
6. Obstruction by gallstones is most commonly seen in all of the following EXCEPT
   A. obesity
   B. alcoholics
   C. persons older than 60 years
   D. women
7. Alcohol has which of the following affects on the pancreas?
   A. decreases enzyme secretion
   B. depresses secretion of secretin
   C. inhibits the inflammatory response
   D. causes spasm of sphincter of Oddi

Answers: 1. B, 2. A, 3. C, 4. A, 5. C, 6. B, 7. D

SECTION FOUR: Diagnosing Acute Pancreatitis

At the completion of this section, the learner will be able to describe medical data used in the diagnosis of acute pancreatitis.

The initial clinical presentation of the patient with acute pancreatitis is similar to that of a variety of other acute abdominal disorders. Diagnosing acute pancreatitis requires data from multiple sources, including laboratory tests and other diagnostic procedures. In addition, the patient history and physical assessment provide valuable information that will support or help rule out a diagnosis of acute pancreatitis. The nursing history and assessment are presented in Section Five.

Laboratory Assessment of Acute Pancreatitis

Pancreatic Enzyme Levels

Measurement of pancreatic enzyme levels is usually obtained from the serum and urine. Cellular enzymes leak into the blood when pancreatic tissue is injured, thereby increasing serum enzyme levels. The most commonly measured pancreatic enzymes include serum amylase and **lipase.**

Serum amylase levels rise early in the course of acute pancreatitis and return to normal within 2 to 3 days after disease onset. Serum amylase can increase for a variety of reasons, since the enzyme is nonspecific to the pancreas. Altered serum amylase levels, therefore, are examined in the context of other supportive clinical data. Amylase is secreted from both the salivary glands and pancreas, each with a distinct isoenzyme. Measurement of amylase isoenzyme P (P = pancreatic) is useful in ruling out nonpancreatic elevations in serum amylase. An amylase/creatinine clearance ratio may also be ordered. A ratio of > 5 percent may indicate the presence of acute pancreatitis. This test is not specific for pancreatitis, however, as other conditions may also cause elevation (e.g., severe burns, diabetic ketoacidosis) (Dolan, 1996).

Serum lipase levels rise later than amylase and remain elevated for approximately 1 to 2 weeks post onset. Measuring lipase levels provides a longer period for trending values than that provided by serum amylase levels. Serum lipase levels can be elevated by use of opioids or consumption of food within 8 hours before the serum level is drawn (Kee, 1999).

Other Laboratory Tests

A variety of laboratory tests may be helpful in evaluating acute pancreatitis and multisystem involvement, particularly the liver and gallbladder. Table 30–4 summarizes some of the major laboratory tests used in making a differential diagnosis of acute pancreatitis.

TABLE 30–4. DIFFERENTIAL LABORATORY DIAGNOSIS OF ACUTE PANCREATITIS

LABORATORY TEST	NORMAL VALUES[a]	TRENDS	TREND VALUES	COMMENTS
Serum				
Amylase	30–170 U/L	↑↑	> 500 U/dL	Peaks 2–12 hr post-onset; may remain elevated 3–5 days; ≥ times normal; level does not correlate well with severity
Isoamylase P (pancreatic)	30–55%	↑	> 55%	
Amylase/creatinine ratio	< 5%	↑	> 5%	Useful as supportive data; it is nondiagnostic for acute pancreatitis since it also occurs in other disorders
Lipase	14–280 U/L	Rapid ↑	> 280 U/L	May remain elevated after amylase returns to normal
Glucose	70–110 mg/dL	Transient ↑	> 180 mg/dL	Secondary to islet cell malfunction; criteria used in absence of preexisting history of hyperglycemia
Calcium	9–11 mg/dL	↓	< 7.5 mg/dL	Secondary to necrosis of fat causing calcium soap formation; also attributed to hypoalbuminemia (decreased availability of protein for calcium binding)
White blood cell count	4,500–10,000/mL	↑	> 15,000/mL	Secondary to inflammatory process
Blood urea nitrogen	5–25 mg/dL	↑	> 45 mg/dL	Level remains elevated following correction of fluid volume deficit
Direct bilirubin (posthepatic)	0.1–0.3 mg/dL	↑	> 0.3 mg/dL	Associated with biliary obstruction
LDH	70–250 U/L	↑	> 350 IU/L	Associated with biliary obstruction and pancreatitis; LDH3 isoenzyme is found in pancreas and other organs
AST (SGOT)	5–40 U/L	↑↑	> 250 IU/mL	
Serum albumin	3.5–5.0 g/dL	↓	< 3.2 g/dL	Associated with protein deficiency
Pao_2	80–100 mm Hg	↓	< 60 mm Hg	Associated with pulmonary involvement
Stool				
Fat	< 6 g/24 hr	—	> 6 g/24 hr	Steatorrhea; stool is pale or gray, smells foul; caused by deficiency in pancreatic enzymes in bowel

[a] Values may vary slightly according to the laboratory performing the test

Source: All normal values (except amylase/creatine ratio) are from Kee, J.L. (1999). Laboratory and diagnostic tests with nursing implications, *5th ed. Stamford, CT: Appleton & Lange. Other data from AACN. (1998).* Core curriculum for critical care nursing, *5th ed. Philadelphia: W.B. Saunders; Andreoli, T.E., Bennett, J.C., Carpenter, C.C., & Plum, F. (1997).* Cecil's essentials of medicine, *4th ed. Philadelphia: W.B. Saunders; and Cavenaugh, B.M. (1999).* Nurses' manual of laboratory and diagnostic tests, *3rd ed. Philadelphia: F.A. Davis.*

Diagnostic Tests

Diagnosis of acute pancreatitis requires data from a variety of sources. Frequently ordered major diagnostic tests include abdominal x-rays, ultrasound, computed tomographic (CT) scan, endoscopic retrograde cholangiopancreatogram (ERCP), and aspiration biopsy.

Abdominal and Chest X-Rays

The abdominal x-ray may be used initially as a quick means of revealing abdominal distention as well as gross abdominal abnormalities, such as an ileus. It is limited in its usefulness as a tool for diagnosing organ disorders. Chest films are valuable in revealing pulmonary complications associated with acute pancreatitis, such as atelectasis and pleural effusion.

CT Scan and Ultrasound

The CT scan provides a noninvasive means of viewing the structure of the pancreas, the bile ducts, and the gallbladder. Damaged pancreatic tissue and lesions can be visualized. CT scan is currently considered one of the best tests for assessing pancreatic necrosis (Alle, Stewart, & Maselly, 1994). Ultrasound uses high-frequency sound waves rather than radiation. It provides a "real-time" view of the structure being tested. In diagnostic testing for acute pancreatitis, ultrasound is particularly valuable in viewing the bile ducts and can identify gallstones more readily than the CT scan (Andreoli et al., 1997). Ultrasound is also useful in revealing pseudocysts and edema.

Endoscopic Retrograde Cholangiopancreatogram

The ERCP is an invasive endoscopic test that provides direct viewing of the ampulla of Vater, and the pancreatic and bile ducts. It requires injection of a radiographic contrast medium followed by a series of x-rays. ERCP is particularly useful in diagnosing obstructions. In addition, the ERCP provides the opportunity for direct removal of mechanical obstructions such as a gallstone or pancreatic stone, or allows a stent to be placed to provide drainage through a stricture (Andreoli et al., 1997).

Aspiration Biopsy

Aspiration biopsy involves the removal of a small plug of tissue using a syringe and needle technique. It is useful in diagnosing the severity of pancreatic tissue damage, diagnosing types of lesions, and draining pseudocysts. Aspiration biopsy can be performed during ultrasound or CT scan, to enable visualization of correct needle placement.

Predicting the Severity of an Acute Pancreatitis Episode

The Ranson criteria (Table 30–5) are commonly used to predict patient outcome, having been shown to be highly accurate (96 percent accuracy). Using these criteria, the following assumptions can be made:

- A person who has less than three criteria at the time of admission has a mortality risk < 1 to 2 percent
- A person who is admitted with three or four criteria has a mortality risk of 15 percent
- A person who is admitted with five or six criteria present has a mortality risk of 40 percent
- A person who is admitted with seven or more criteria present has a 100 percent risk of mortality (Alle, Stewart, & Maselly, 1994; Andreoli et al., 1997)
- A person who is admitted with more than three criteria should be managed in a critical care unit (Alle, Stewart, & Maselly, 1994; Carey, Lee, & Woeltze, 1998)

TABLE 30–5. RANSON CRITERIA FOR PREDICTING SEVERITY OF ACUTE PANCREATITIS

RISK FACTOR	PRESENT AT TIME OF ADMISSION	RISK FACTOR	PRESENT AT TIME INITIAL 48 HOURS
Age	> 55	Hct	Decrease of > 10%
WBC	> 16,000 mm^3	BUN	Rise of > 5 mg/dL
Serum glucose	> 200 mg/dL	Serum calcium	< 8 mg/dL
Serum LDH	> 350 IU/L	PaO_2	< 60 mg/dL
Serum SGOT	> 250 U/dL	Base deficit	> 4 mEq/L
		Estimated fluid sequestration	> 6 L

Associated Mortality Based on Number of Risk Factors:[a]

# Risk Factors	Mortality (%)
< 3	0.9
3–4	15
5–6	40
≥ 7	Near 100

[a] Additional risk factors: Respiratory failure with intubation, shock, hypocalcemia, and massive colloid administration (if ≥ 3 of these factors are present, mortality increases to near 65%)

Adapted from Ranson, J.C. (1985). Risk factors in acute pancreatitis. Hosp Pract *20(4):69–73.*

In summary, the diagnosis of acute pancreatitis primarily is made on the basis of laboratory findings and presenting symptoms. The hallmark of the disease is a rapid, significant increase in serum amylase and lipase levels in the presence of risk factors and complaints of severe abdominal pain. A variety of diagnostic tests can be used in differentiating the diagnosis, such as ultrasound, CT scan, ERCP, and aspiration biopsy. Ranson's criteria provide an accurate method of predicting patient mortality associated with acute pancreatitis. A differential diagnosis cannot be made on the basis of the patient history and physical assessment alone.

SECTION FOUR REVIEW

1. The primary laboratory test obtained to help make a diagnosis of pancreatitis is serum
   A. amylase
   B. calcium
   C. LDH
   D. elastase
2. What effect will severe acute pancreatitis most likely have on serum glucose?
   A. severe hypoglycemia
   B. transient hypoglycemia
   C. no effect
   D. transient hyperglycemia
3. According to Ranson's criteria for predicting the risk of mortality in acute pancreatitis patients, a patient who is admitted with five criteria would have a mortality risk of _______ percent.
   A. < 1
   B. 40
   C. 60
   D. 100

Answers: 1. A, 2. D, 3. B

SECTION FIVE: Nursing Assessment of the Patient with Acute Pancreatitis

At the completion of this section, the learner will be able to discuss nursing assessment of the patient with acute pancreatitis.

Pain History and Assessment

Pain is the most consistent complaint associated with acute pancreatitis and is a high-priority assessment. The classic pattern of pain is described as a sudden onset of sharp, knifelike, twisting and deep, upper abdominal (epigastric) pain that frequently radiates to the flank, chest, or other parts of the abdomen. The pain may be further described as severe and relentless (Krumberger, 1998). The patient may report some degree of relief by assuming a leaning forward or fetal position (Andreoli et al., 1997; Krumberger, 1998), and may report an increase in pain when doing activities that increase abdominal pressure (e.g., coughing). The pain intensity varies greatly from patient to patient. The pain may be described as vague and mild, or it may be excruciating and refractory to analgesic therapy. The intensity often reflects the degree to which the disease process has extended beyond the confines of the pancreas. If localized, the pain is usually more vague and mild; however, once pancreatic functions infiltrate extrapancreatic tissues (into the peritoneum), the pain becomes well defined and sharp, and the intensity increases significantly. The pain is believed to be a result of edema and distention of the pancreatic capsule, chemical burn of the peritoneum by pancreatic enzymes, and the release of kinin peptides or biliary obstruction (Krumberger, 1998). Initially, the patient's complaints of pain intensity may seem out of proportion to other clinical manifestations (Smith & Butler, 1993). The pain intensity does not always correlate with the degree of pancreatic inflammation (Alle, Stewart, & Maselly, 1994).

The Focused History and Assessment

The majority of the clinical manifestations of acute pancreatic dysfunction are of gastrointestinal (GI) origin; thus, while taking the nursing history, the nurse should particularly focus on gaining information related to this system. The remainder of this section presents the major signs and symptoms associated with acute pancreatitis.

Gastrointestinal Assessment

The presence of abdominal pain is a major finding in acute pancreatitis. Additional GI clinical manifestations include:

- Anorexia
- Upper abdominal tenderness without rigidity
- Abdominal distention
- Nausea and vomiting
- Steatorrhea

- Diarrhea
- Peritoneal signs (noted in severe cases):
  Diminished or absent bowel sounds (ileus may develop)
  Increased pain
  Abdominal rigidity, guarding, rebound tenderness
  Other: leukocytosis, tachycardia, and fever

Additional Assessments

In addition to the major GI clinical manifestations, a variety of other common or classic signs and symptoms are commonly associated with the disease process.

Integumentary
If the patient has hemorrhagic pancreatitis, two uncommon but classic signs may be observed:

1. *Cullen's sign*—a bluish discoloration around the umbilicus
2. *Grey Turner's sign*—a bluish discoloration of the flank region

Other observations that may be noted by skin inspection are jaundice and edema. If the patient develops shock, the skin will become pale, cold, and moist.

Cardiopulmonary
Cardiac signs and symptoms usually present themselves in conjunction with the complication of shock or the release of myocardial depressant factor (MDF), which is discussed in Section Six. The nurse should observe the patient for the signs and symptoms of hypovolemic shock: decreased cardiac output (tachycardia, hypotension with decreased systemic vascular resistance); and MDF (decreased cardiac output with increased systemic vascular resistance).

Respiratory signs and symptoms include those typical of:

- Pleural effusion—adventitious breath sounds, particularly crackles
- Respiratory insufficiency or failure (refer to Module 5)
- Pulmonary edema (noncardiogenic)
- Pneumonia

Neurologic
The patient with acute pancreatitis frequently develops an alteration in level of consciousness. The nurse can rapidly trend the state of arousal using the Glasgow Coma Scale (GCS). Common neurologic manifestations include confusion, restlessness, and agitation.

Renal
The patient must be closely monitored for the development of acute tubular necrosis (refer to Module 26). The urine can also be observed. As increased levels of bile are excreted through the urine, it develops a brownish color and may become foamy.

Hematologic
The nurse should monitor the patient for clinical manifestations of disseminated intravascular coagulation (refer to Module 11).

Electrolyte Imbalances
Hypocalcemia may develop owing to fat necrosis because serum calcium migrates to the extravascular space surrounding the pancreas where the fat necrosis is taking place. Two classic signs of hypocalcemia are:

1. *Chvostek's sign*—the facial nerve is tapped directly in front of the ear. A positive sign is present when the facial muscles contract on the same side of the face as the tapping.
2. *Trousseau's sign*—a blood pressure cuff is inflated on the upper arm to a level directly above the patient's systolic blood pressure for 2 minutes. A positive sign is present when the hand flexes (carpopedal spasm) in response to the test.

In addition to hypocalcemia, the patient should be monitored for the hypokalemia and hypomagnesemia that may result from GI loss and insufficient intake (Carey, Lee, & Woeltze, 1998; Hudak, Gallo, & Morton, 1998; Noone, 1995). (Refer to Module 3 for a listing of the clinical manifestations of hypocalcemia, hypokalemia, and hypomagnesemia.)

In summary, assessment of the patient with acute pancreatitis focuses primarily on pain and the gastrointestinal system. The severity of the signs and symptoms varies greatly and is largely dependent on whether the disease process is localized or has extended beyond the confines of the pancreas. Extrapancreatic invasion into the peritoneal spaces can cause chemical peritonitis, which carries with it multiple additional signs and symptoms.

SECTION FIVE REVIEW

1. The classic pattern of pain typically described by the patient with acute pancreatitis is

   A. dull, diffuse, and poorly defined
   B. sharp and confined to the epigastric area
   C. well defined, dull, localized in the flank area
   D. sharp, knifelike, often radiating to the flank

2. The intensity and description of pain associated with acute pancreatitis varies, often based on the
   A. pH of the pancreatic enzymes
   B. degree to which extrapancreatic invasion has occurred
   C. pain threshold of the individual patient
   D. degree of release of myocardial depressant factor (MDF)
3. Peritoneal signs include all of the following EXCEPT
   A. rebound tenderness
   B. rigid abdomen
   C. hyperactive bowel sounds
   D. leukocytosis
4. Cullen's sign may be noted under which of the following circumstances?
   A. acute tubular necrosis
   B. hemorrhage
   C. hypovolemic shock
   D. respiratory failure
5. The cardiopulmonary assessment of the patient with acute pancreatitis focuses on monitoring for the development of
   A. hypercapnia
   B. hypertension
   C. cardiac arrhythmias
   D. decreased cardiac output
6. If the pancreatitis is localized, assessment of the abdomen would show all of the following EXCEPT
   A. tenderness
   B. rigidity
   C. distention
   D. diminished bowel sounds

Answers: 1. D, 2. B, 3. C, 4. B, 5. D, 6. B

SECTION SIX: Complications of Acute Pancreatitis

At the completion of this section, the learner will be able to explain the complications of acute pancreatitis.

Acute pancreatitis is considered a multisystemic disease process. Complications are common and can be divided into two types: local and systemic.

Local Complications

Pancreatic abscess and pseudocyst are two local complications. Pancreatic abscess results from a localized infectious process. It generally occurs late in the course of a severe episode and may be fatal if not aggressively treated, usually with surgery and antibiotics. A pancreatic pseudocyst is composed of pancreatic enzymes, necrotic tissue, and possibly blood. While not truly encapsulated, the pseudocyst is enclosed either by some type of adjacent tissue or by pancreatic tissues. Some pseudocysts resolve on their own; however, while present, they run the risk of becoming infected or of rupturing into the peritoneal cavity, which can precipitate chemical peritonitis.

Systemic Complications

The complications of acute pancreatitis have the potential to interfere with virtually all of the body's functions.

Neurologic

A decreased level of consciousness is a common problem in severe pancreatitis and is related to several potential etiologies; including analgesia and pancreatic encephalopathy. The alleviation of pain associated with acute pancreatitis requires large doses of opioids and possibly sedation. Cerebral function is altered by either of these therapies. The pathophysiologic basis of pancreatic encephalopathy is unclear but may be attributed to pancreatic lipase activity (AACN, 1998; Alle, Stewart, & Maselly, 1994).

Pulmonary

Hypoxemia is present in the majority of severe acute pancreatitis patients within the first 2 days of onset. Respiratory insufficiency and failure are common complications of acute pancreatitis. They are attributed to the release of pancreatic enzyme phospholipase A, which destroys the phospholipid surfactant. Loss of surfactant decreases vital capacity and lung compliance and damages the pulmonary capillary endothelium (Horne, Heitz, & Swearingen, 1991; Wilson & Lester, 1998). The patient is at risk of developing pneumonia and/or pleural effusion and, in severe cases, acute respiratory distress syndrome (ARDS).

Cardiovascular

Pancreatic enzyme released into the bloodstream can have devastating effects on the cardiovascular system through two mechanisms: release of myocardial depressant factor (MDF) and hypovolemic shock.

MYOCARDIAL DEPRESSANT FACTOR. MDF is a chemical mediator that is believed to originate from ischemic pancreatic tissue (Rauen & Munro, 1998). When MDF is released, it depresses myocardial function, resulting in decreased cardiac output with increased systemic vascular resistance (compensatory) (Hudak, Gallo, & Morton, 1998; Smith & Butler, 1993). MDF is one of the chemical mediators implicated in the sequence of events leading to shock.

Hypovolemic Shock. Vasoactive substances are released from damaged pancreatic tissue. Trypsin activates the powerful vasodilating circulating enzyme, kallikrein, which forms two plasma kinins (kallidin and bradykinin). These two substances are responsible for vasodilation, decreased systemic vascular resistance, and increased permeability of endothelial linings of vessels. As vessels become more porous, intravascular fluids are able to shift into other compartments and into the retroperitoneal cavity, causing hypovolemia and third spacing. Fluid shifts can account for up to 12 L of fluid, which can produce hypovolemic shock (Krumberger, 1998; Wilson & Lester, 1997).

Hemorrhage is also a major cause of hypovolemic shock in hemorrhagic pancreatitis. When prematurely activated, the pancreatic enzyme elastase is able to break down duct and blood vessel elastic fibers, causing hemorrhage (Thelan et al., 1998). Hemorrhage can also occur due to other complications such as a bleeding ulcer or tissue necrosis.

Renal

Acute tubular necrosis (ATN), a type of renal failure, is a fairly common sequela in severe acute pancreatitis. It results from renal ischemia secondary to hypotension. If fluid resuscitation is timely and adequate, the kidney damage may be temporary.

Hematologic

Disseminated intravascular coagulation (DIC) is associated with severe acute pancreatitis. It may be due to activation of the coagulation cascade by trypsin (Krumberger, 1998; Smith & Butler, 1993).

TABLE 30–6. MAJOR SYSTEMIC COMPLICATIONS OF ACUTE PANCREATITIS

BODY SYSTEM/FUNCTION	COMPLICATIONS
Neurologic	Encephalopathy
Pulmonary	Hypoxia, respiratory failure, pneumonia, pleural effusion, atelectasis, acute respiratory distress syndrome (ARDS)
Cardiovascular	Hemorrhage, hypotension, shock, pericardial effusion, pericardial tamponade
Gastrointestinal	Bleeding
Renal	Acute renal failure
Metabolic	Metabolic acidosis, hypocalcemia, hyperglycemia
Hematologic	Vascular thrombosis, disseminated intravascular coagulation (DIC)

In summary, acute pancreatitis is capable of precipitating both local and systemic complications. Locally, the pancreas can develop abscesses and pseudocysts. The presence of a pancreatic abscess is a critical complication that may cause death if not treated rapidly. Systemically, most body systems can become involved. Many of the complications are multisystemic in nature and are due to hypotension and tissue hypoxia. Table 30–6 summarizes the major systemic complications.

Section Six Review

1. Pancreatic pseudocyst is composed of all the following EXCEPT
   - **A.** necrotic tissue
   - **B.** air
   - **C.** blood
   - **D.** pancreatic enzymes
2. If a pseudocyst were to rupture into the peritoneal cavity the patient would most likely develop
   - **A.** septicemia
   - **B.** acute renal failure
   - **C.** paralytic ileus
   - **D.** peritonitis
3. In the acute pancreatitis patient, hypovolemic shock usually results from all of the following EXCEPT
   - **A.** hemorrhage
   - **B.** third spacing
   - **C.** renal failure
   - **D.** kallikrein release
4. Pulmonary complications are attributed to which of the following pancreatic enzymes?
   - **A.** trypsin
   - **B.** elastase
   - **C.** amylase
   - **D.** phospholipase A
5. The release of myocardial depressant factor by injured pancreatic tissue is believed to have what effect on the heart?
   - **A.** decreases cardiac output
   - **B.** decreases heart rate
   - **C.** increases blood pressure
   - **D.** increases cardiac output

Answers: 1. B, 2. D, 3. C, 4. D, 5. A

SECTION SEVEN: Medical Management

At the completion of this section, the learner will be able to describe the medical management of the patient with acute pancreatitis.

The medical management of the patient with acute pancreatitis may be either supportive or curative; it is often a combination of both. Supporting the patient's hemodynamic and oxygenation status is essential while either correcting the underlying problem (mechanical obstruction) or allowing the underlying problem to resolve itself (alcohol induced).

Supportive Therapy

Medical management is based on prioritized goals, including stabilizing hemodynamic status, controlling pain, minimizing pancreatic stimulation, correcting the underlying problem, and preventing or treating complications. A summary of general physician orders related to supportive management of the acute pancreatitis patient is listed in Table 30–7.

TABLE 30–7. SUPPORTIVE THERAPY FOR ACUTE PANCREATITIS

TYPE OF SUPPORT	GENERAL PHYSICIAN ORDERS
Fluid resuscitation	May consist of up to 10–20 L of fluid during the first 24 hours, as required Fluids may be crystalloids or colloids If hypoalbuminemic, consider albumin replacement If hemoglobin ≤ 10 mg/dL, consider blood transfusion As experimental therapy to deactivate systemic proteolases, fresh frozen plasma may be ordered
Inotropic	When hypotension predominates, consider dopamine therapy When poor tissue perfusion predominates, consider dobutamine therapy
Respiratory	If Pao_2 < 60 mm Hg in the presence of high oxygen concentration, and/or respiratory rate is > 30/min, consider early intubation and mechanical ventilation with sedation and analgesia
Renal	In the presence of impaired renal function, consider dopamine at a low "renal" dose to increase renal perfusion; timely and adequate fluid resuscitation is essential to prevent permanent damage
Nutritional	Once hemodynamic stability has been achieved, total parenteral nutrition (TPN) is initiated Monitor serum glucose closely, maintaining levels at approximately 150 mg/dL if possible High doses of insulin may be necessary due to severe insulin resistance

Data from Alle, K.M., Stewart, D.E., & Maselly, M. (1994). Gastrointestinal failure in the ICU. In F.S. Bongard & D.Y. Sue (eds). Current critical care diagnosis and treatment *(pp. 120–121). Norwalk, CT: Appleton & Lange; and Hennessy, K. (1996). Patients with acute pancreatitis. In J. Clochesy et al. (eds.).* Critical care nursing, *2nd ed. (pp. 1091–1103). Philadelphia: W.B. Saunders.*

Goal #1: Stabilize the Patient's Hemodynamic Status

Hypovolemia must be identified and treated aggressively. Hemodynamic stability is accomplished primarily through two types of interventions: fluid resuscitation and inotropic therapy. Fluid resuscitation includes crystalloids and possibly colloids and plasma expanders. As treatment progresses, it is essential to monitor closely the hemodynamic status. Hemodynamic status monitoring might include:

- Blood pressure and pulse
- Pulmonary artery pressure
- Pulmonary artery wedge pressure
- Central venous pressure
- Cardiac output
- Cardiac index
- Intake and output, daily weights
- Hematocrit and serum BUN levels

Goal #2: Control the Patient's Pain

Acute pancreatitis is extremely painful. Controlling the level of pain is essential for comfort and to decrease secretion of pancreatic enzymes. The drug of choice is meperidine (Demerol) rather than morphine sulfate. Dilaudid (hydromorphone) may also be effective in pain management. Opiates, such as morphine, can cause spasms of the sphincter of Oddi, which may further aggravate the disease process.

Goal #3: Minimize Pancreatic Stimulation

It is important to reduce the stimulation of pancreatic secretion as much as possible. Keeping the GI tract at rest facilitates pancreatic rest and reduces the amount of pancreatic juice secreted. Organ rest will need to continue until serum amylase levels have returned to normal and pain has subsided. This may take up to 7 weeks. The physician may order the following:

- Strict NPO status
- Placement of a nasogastric tube to low wall suction
- Drug therapy such as antacids or anticholinergics (anticholinergics reduce GI motility)

Patients who are experiencing acute pancreatitis are especially hypermetabolic. They have extremely high nutritional demands but are unable to consume nutrients orally for a prolonged period. Nutritional support is essential to improving the patient's outcome.

Curative Therapy

Goal #4: Correct the Underlying Problem

Generally, medical interventions are more desirable than surgical ones. Some triggering events, such as binge alcohol abuse, may subside spontaneously if given sufficient rest time using supportive therapy. If the etiology is mechanical, however, the underlying problem can be corrected surgically. For example, if a patient has a biliary obstruction such as a gallstone, a cholecystectomy may be performed to relieve the obstruction. Certain surgical procedures to relieve obstructions can be performed during an ERCP, as explained in Section Four.

Goal #5: Prevent or Treat Complications

It is imperative that complications be recognized early in their early development and then treated aggressively. Close patient monitoring is a crucial part of meeting this goal. Medical interventions are based on correcting or supporting system dysfunctions as they develop. In addition to the various supportive physician orders listed in Table 30–7, the physician may need to order any of the following:

- electrolyte replacement
- insulin therapy
- antibiotic therapy
- arterial blood gases
- oxygen therapy
- pulmonary toilet (e.g., incentive spirometry)
- radiographic studies
- cardiac monitoring
- Swan–Ganz catheter

Peritoneal lavage is an alternative treatment modality that is sometimes used to reduce the risk of sepsis. A typical procedure for peritoneal lavage is continual lavage of the peritoneum with 2 L of fluid at the rate of one exchange per hour (Alle, Stewart, & Maselly, 1994). Research is still inconclusive regarding the effectiveness of this therapy.

If the patient develops an abscess, surgery will be needed for debridement. Surgical incisions of pancreatic tissue may lead to the development of pancreatic fistulas, which may or may not resolve spontaneously. Fistulas can move pancreatic juice into other tissues, causing further damage and new complications. Multiple surgeries are often required to correct continuing problems.

In summary, the medical management of the patient with acute pancreatitis is based on complex multisystem needs. Five major supportive treatment focuses provide the basis for the majority of medical care: fluid resuscitation; inotropes; and respiratory, renal, and nutritional support. There are also major prioritized goals that help organize medical management of acute pancreatitis. These include stabilizing hemodynamic status, controlling pain, minimizing pancreatic stimulation, correcting the underlying cause, and preventing or treating complications. Many physician orders will be written as the patient's status changes.

Section Seven Review

1. The highest priority in management of the patient with severe acute pancreatitis is to
   A. control pain
   B. stabilize hemodynamic status
   C. minimize pancreatic stimulation
   D. correct the underlying problem
2. The drug of choice in pain management of the patient with acute pancreatitis is
   A. morphine sulfate
   B. codeine
   C. meperidine
   D. ibuprofen
3. Anticholinergics may be ordered for the patient with acute pancreatitis for the primary purpose of
   A. reducing GI motility
   B. reducing pain
   C. increasing pancreatic stimulation
   D. increasing gastric pH
4. The effective management of complications is dependent on all of the following EXCEPT
   A. close monitoring
   B. early recognition
   C. aggressive treatment
   D. severity of the pancreatitis

Answers: 1. B, 2. C, 3. A, 4. D

SECTION EIGHT: The Nursing Care Plan

At the completion of this section, the learner will be able to discuss the nursing plan of care for a patient with acute pancreatic dysfunction.

The nursing care plan for the patient experiencing an acute pancreatic dysfunction episode includes both collaborative problems and independent nursing diagnoses.

Frequently Occurring Collaborative Problems

Acute pancreatitis carries the risk of many potential complications. On a nursing plan of care, potential complications are dealt with as collaborative problems (Carpenito, 1999). Collaborative problems require a combination of physician and nursing orders to manage the problem optimally. Potential complications (PCs) that are commonly noted in patients with acute pancreatitis include:

- Hyperglycemia
- Hemorrhage
- Peritonitis
- Sepsis
- Noncardiogenic pulmonary edema
- Fluid and electrolyte imbalances
- Pleural effusion
- Hypovolemic shock
- Acute tubular necrosis
- Disseminated intravascular coagulation
- Pancreatic abscess
- Pancreatic pseudocyst

Frequently Occurring Nursing Diagnoses

Upon completion of the nursing database, the nurse clusters data and develops a set of nursing hypotheses based on the available data. Additional critical data that may either support or eliminate each hypothesis should also be identified and obtained. Once the hypotheses have been established, the nurse is ready to develop a list of nursing diagnoses based on the patient's response to the illness rather than on the illness itself.

In the patient with acute pancreatic dysfunction, a variety of nursing diagnoses frequently occur during the crisis period. The following is a partial list of some of these nursing diagnoses as suggested by Carpenito (1999) and Ulrich and associates (1998):

- *Pain: Epigastric or abdominal* related to localized peritonitis, pancreatic capsule distention and nasogastric suction
- *Altered nutrition: Less than body requirements* related to vomiting, anorexia, impaired digestion secondary to decreased pancreatic enzymes
- *Ineffective breathing pattern* related to abdominal pain, depressant effects of opioid therapy, decreased lung expansion
- *Anxiety* related to unfamiliar environment; discomfort; lack of understanding of diagnosis, diagnostic tests, and interventions; fear of death
- *Altered comfort: Nausea and vomiting* related to stimulation of the vomiting center

Many of the nursing diagnoses listed here are presented in other modules. Two nursing diagnoses—*Alteration in comfort: Nausea and vomiting*, and *Pain*—are of particular interest to this patient population.

Nausea and Vomiting

Nausea and vomiting frequently accompany and further aggravate abdominal pain in the patient with acute pancreatitis. Some patients develop dry heaves rather than actual vomiting. The following is a plan of care for managing nausea and vomiting as suggested by Ulrich and colleagues (1998).

Alteration in comfort: Nausea and vomiting related to vomiting center stimulation

DESIRED PATIENT OUTCOMES. The patient will experience relief of nausea and vomiting as evidenced by:

- No vomiting
- No dry heaves
- Patient states relief of nausea

NURSING INTERVENTIONS

1. Assess patient for nausea, vomiting, and dry heaves.
2. Implement interventions to relieve nausea, vomiting, and dry heaves.
   a. Prevent/relieve gastric distention:
      Potential collaborative action: insertion of nasogastric tube
      Related independent actions: maintain tube patency
   b. Restrict oral intake, as ordered (NPO status is often ordered).
   c. When nauseated:
      Encourage deep, slow breathing.
      Change positions slowly.
   d. Oral hygiene every 2 hours and as necessary postvomiting.
   e. Administer antiemetic therapy as ordered: monitor for therapeutic and nontherapeutic effects of therapy.
3. Consult with physician if current therapy fails to meet desired outcomes.

Pain

The severe pain associated with acute pancreatitis is a major nursing concern. It negatively effects patient outcomes and can be difficult to control. The following presents a partial care plan for addressing this problem, as suggested by Ulrich and colleagues (1998).

Pain: Epigastric or abdominal related to localized peritonitis, pancreatic capsule distention, and nasogastric suction

DESIRED PATIENT OUTCOMES. The patient will experience decreased pain, as evidenced by:

- Verbalizes pain relief
- Relaxed body positioning
- Relaxed facial expression
- Blood pressure, pulse, and respirations

NURSING INTERVENTIONS

1. Assess patient's perception of pain experience through self-report methods.

2. Assess patient for factors that increase and decrease the pain.
3. Implement interventions to decrease pain.
   a. Nothing by mouth during acute phase.
   b. Insert nasogastric tube, as ordered.
   c. Administer medications to reduce gastric acid quantity and neutralize acid.
   d. Administer analgesics as ordered; avoid use of morphine sulfate. Encourage use of patient-controlled analgesia (PCA), if ordered.
   e. Monitor for therapeutic and nontherapeutic effects of analgesic therapy.
   f. Help patient assume body positioning that reduces pain (e.g., sit/lie with knees flexed and trunk slightly flexed).
4. Consult with physician if current interventions are not adequately meeting desired outcomes.

For further information regarding acute pain management, refer to Module 2.

In summary, acute pancreatic dysfunction is a potentially severe health problem that requires complex management. This section has presented collaborative problems based on potential complications and frequently occurring nursing diagnoses that may apply to the care of the patient with acute pancreatitis. Two nursing diagnoses—*Altered comfort: Nausea and vomiting*, and *Pain*—have been presented in more detail.

POSTEST

The following Posttest is constructed in a case study format. A patient is presented. Questions are asked based on available data. New data are presented as the case study progresses.

Joan M, 63 years old, presents in the emergency department with complaints of severe abdominal pain. Due to her past history, she is admitted with a diagnosis of "rule out pancreatitis."

1. Joan's pancreas is located
   A. adjacent to the liver
   B. in front of the stomach
   C. behind the spleen
   D. within the curve of the duodenum
2. Under normal circumstances, Joan's pancreas empties into the small bowel at the
   A. ampulla of Vater
   B. duct of Wirsung
   C. acinus
   D. tail
3. Joan's pancreatic regulation of pH is accomplished by
   A. formation of pepsin
   B. release of secretin
   C. activation of enzymes
   D. secretion of cholecystokinin
4. Under normal circumstances, Joan's pancreas is protected from autodigestion because the pancreatic enzymes
   A. are inhibited by acetylcholine
   B. are activated only by an acid pH
   C. exist in precursor form in the pancreas
   D. are used immediately, with no storage capabilities
5. Joan's pancreas secretes the enzyme trypsin, which
   A. is responsible for breakdown of fats
   B. splits phospholipids into fatty acids
   C. splits carbohydrates into disaccharides
   D. is the most abundant proteolytic enzyme

Joan is 5 feet 4 inches tall and weighs 73 kg. She gives a history of smoking about one pack per day for 40 years. She drinks a glass of wine several days a week with her evening meal. She denies a history of diabetes or heart problems but states that she has had several "gallbladder attacks" over the past several years.

6. Joan is more likely to have which type of pancreatitis?
   A. acute nonhemorrhagic
   B. chronic nonhemorrhagic
   C. acute hemorrhagic
   D. chronic hemorrhagic
7. Which piece of Joan's history represents the strongest etiologic factor for development of pancreatitis?
   A. smoking history
   B. gallbladder disease
   C. alcohol consumption
   D. obesity
8. If Joan is diagnosed with nonhemorrhagic acute pancreatitis, it typically is characterized by
   A. a long duration
   B. fat necrosis
   C. irreversible damage
   D. localized inflammation
9. If Joan's pancreatitis has been caused by pancreatic duct obstruction, the obstruction is most likely caused by
   A. a gallstone
   B. edema
   C. a stricture
   D. severe spasms

The physician orders a battery of diagnostic tests that include, among others, serum amylase, serum lipase, and ERCP.

10. Serial serum lipase levels may be ordered in preference to serum amylase levels since serum lipase
    A. is more accurate
    B. is more specific to pancreatitis
    C. remains elevated for a longer period
    D. requires no special analysis technique
11. A major advantage of performing an ERCP is that
    A. it is a noninvasive procedure
    B. it can be performed at the bedside
    C. it provides access to the gallbladder and pancreas
    D. mechanical obstructions can be directly removed
12. If Joan's description of her pain is typical of the classic pattern associated with acute pancreatitis, it would have all of the following characteristics EXCEPT
    A. piercing
    B. slow onset
    C. epigastric
    D. sharp
13. The nurse should check Joan's stool for characteristic
    A. leukocytes
    B. green coloring
    C. steatorrhea
    D. positive guaiac
14. If Joan develops peritoneal signs due to extrapancreatic invasion of enzymes, the nurse would assess
    A. abdominal rigidity
    B. hyperactive bowel sounds
    C. dulling of abdominal pain
    D. onset of bradycardia
15. The nurse will be able to assess Joan for Grey Turner's sign if Joan is positioned
    A. on her back
    B. on her side
    C. in high-Fowler's position
    D. in semi-Fowler's position
16. If Joan should develop cardiovascular complications associated with her acute pancreatitis, no matter what the mechanism is, the consistent end result is
    A. increased systemic vascular resistance
    B. increased cardiac output
    C. decreased systemic vascular resistance
    D. decreased cardiac output
17. The major pulmonary complications of acute pancreatitis include all of the following EXCEPT
    A. cor pulmonale
    B. pleural effusion
    C. hypoxia
    D. respiratory failure
18. If Joan develops a severe case of acute pancreatitis, the initial medical management will focus on
    A. controlling pain
    B. minimizing pancreatic stimulation
    C. stabilizing hemodynamic status
    D. correcting the underlying problem
19. Joan is complaining of severe abdominal pain. The nurse can anticipate administering which of the following drugs as a first choice?
    A. meperidine
    B. morphine
    C. hydromorphone
    D. codeine

POSTTEST ANSWERS

Question	Answer	Section	Question	Answer	Section
1	D	One	11	D	Four
2	A	One	12	B	Five
3	B	Two	13	C	Five
4	C	Two	14	A	Five
5	D	Two	15	B	Five
6	A	Three	16	D	Six
7	B	Three	17	A	Six
8	D	Three	18	C	Seven
9	A	Three	19	A	Seven
10	C	Four			

REFERENCES

Alle, K.M., Stewart, D.E. and Maselly, M. (1994). Gastrointestinal failure in the ICU. In F.S. Bongard & D.Y. Sue (eds). *Current critical care diagnosis and treatment* (pp. 117–123). Norwalk, CT: Appleton & Lange.

American Association of Critical Care Nurses. (1998). *Core curriculum for critical care nursing* (5th ed.). Philadelphia: W.B. Saunders.

Andreoli, T.E., Bennett, J.C., Carpenter, C.C., & Plum, F. (1997). *Cecil's essentials of medicine* (4th ed.). Philadelphia: W.B. Saunders.

Brown, A. (1991). Acute pancreatitis: Pathophysiology, nursing diagnoses, and collaborative problems. *Focus Crit Care AACN 18*(2):121–130.

Carpenito, L.J. (1999). *Nursing care plans and documentation* (3rd ed.) (pp. 177–184). Philadelphia: J.B. Lippincott.

Carey, C.F., Lee, H.H., & Woeltze, K.F. (eds). (1998). *Washington manual* (29th ed.) (pp. 323–324). Philadelphia: Lippincott-Raven.

Dolan, J.T. (1996). *Critical care nursing: Clinical management through the nursing process* (2nd ed.). Philadelphia: F.A. Davis.

Doughty, D.B., & Jackson, D.B. (1993). *Gastrointestinal disorder: Mosby clinical nursing series*. St. Louis: C.V. Mosby.

Guyton, A.C., & Hall, J.E. (1997). *Human physiology and mechanisms of disease* (6th ed.) (pp. 530–531). Philadelphia: W.B. Saunders.

Horne, M.M., Heitz, U.E., & Swearingen, P.L. (1991). *Fluid, electrolyte, and acid–base balance: A case study approach* (p. 388). St. Louis: C.V. Mosby.

Hudak, C.M., Gallo, B.M., & Morton, P.G. (eds). (1998). *Critical care nursing: A holistic approach* (7th ed.) (pp. 796–803). Philadelphia: Lippincott-Raven Publishers.

Kee, J. (1999). *Laboratory and diagnostic tests with nursing implications* (5th ed.). Stamford, CT: Appleton & Lange.

Krumberger, J.M. (1998). Gastrointestinal disorders. In M.R. Kinney, S.B. Dunbar, J.A. Brooks-Brunn, N. Molter, & J.M. Vitello-Cicciu (eds.), *AACN's clinical reference for critical care nursing* (4th ed.) (pp. 1033–1037). St. Louis: C.V. Mosby.

Marieb, E.N. (1998). *Human anatomy and physiology* (4th ed.). Menlo Park, CA: Benjamin Cummings.

Noone, J. (1995). Acute pancreatitis: An Oram approach to nursing assessment and care. *Crit Care Nurs 15*(4): 27–37.

Oleynikov, D., Cook, C., Sellers, B., Mone, M.C., & Barton, R. (1998). Decreased mortality from necrotizing pancreatitis. *Am J Surg 176*(6):648–653.

Rauen, C.A., & Munro, N. (1998). Shock. In M.R. Kinney, S.B. Dunbar, J.A. Brooks-Brunn, N. Molter, & J.M. Vitello-Cicciu (eds.), *AACN's clinical reference for critical care nursing* (4th ed.) (pp. 1151–1179). St. Louis: C.V. Mosby.

Reece-Smith, H. (1997, July–August). Pancreatitis. *Care Crit Ill 13*(4):135–138.

Smith, S.L., & Butler, R.W. (1993). Acute pancreatitis, Part I: An overview. In S.L. Smith & R.W. Butler, *Critical Care Nurse presents acute pancreatitis* (pp. 1–11). Aliso Viejo, CA: American Association of Critical Care Nurses.

Thelan, L.A., Urden L.D., Lough, M.E., & Stacy, K.M. (1998). *Critical care nursing: Diagnosis and management* (3rd ed.) (pp. 950–957). St. Louis. C.V. Mosby.

Ulrich, S.P., Canale, S.W., & Wendell, S.A. (eds). (1998). *Medical–surgical nursing care planning guides* (4th ed.). Philadelphia: W.B. Saunders.

Wilson, L.M., & Lester, L.B. (1997). Liver, biliary tract, and pancreas. In S.A. Price & L.M. Wilson (eds.). *Pathophysiology: Clinical concepts of disease processes* (5th ed.) (pp. 372–408). St. Louis: Mosby-Year Book.

ADDITIONAL READINGS

Guyton, A.C., & Hall, J.E. (1997). *Human physiology and mechanisms of disease* (6th ed.) (pp. 543–545). Philadelphia: W.B. Saunders.

Toskes, P., & Greenberger, N. (1998). Pancreas. In Fauci et al. (eds). *Harrison's principles of internal medicine*, vol. 2 (14th ed.). New York: McGraw-Hill

Module 31

Nursing Care of the Patient with Altered Gastrointestinal Function

Melanie Hardin-Pierce

This module is designed to integrate major points discussed in Modules 29 through 30. This module summarizes key relationships between concepts and assists the learner in clustering information to facilitate clinical application. Content is presented in an interactive learning style. Using a case study format, the learner is encouraged to identify nursing actions based on the assessment of a patient experiencing gastrointestinal (GI) dysfunction. The consequences of selecting a particular action are discussed. Rationale for all answers is presented.

Objectives

Following completion of this module, the learner will be able to

1. Describe an appropriate database for a patient with GI dysfunction.
2. Explain the assessment of a patient with GI dysfunction.
3. Discuss the development of nursing diagnoses appropriate for a patient with GI dysfunction.
4. Discuss the development of a plan of care for the patient with GI dysfunction.

Abbreviations

ABG. Arterial blood gas

ADH. Antidiuretic hormone

ALT. Alanine aminotransferase

ARDS. Acute respiratory distress syndrome

BP. Blood pressure

BUN. Blood urea nitrogen

GCS. Glasgow Coma Scale

GI. Gastrointestinal

GGT. Glutamyl transpeptidase

HCT. Hematocrit

HR. Heart rate

ICU. Intensive care unit

IV. Intravenous

JVD. Jugular venous distention

LOC. Level of consciousness

NG. Nasogastric

NSAID. Nonsteroidal anti-inflammatory drug

PTT. Partial thromboplastin time

RBC. Red blood cell

SpO_2. Peripheral arterial oxygen saturation

TPN. Total parenteral nutrition

WBC. White blood cell

CASE STUDY 1

Case Study 1: Upper GI Bleed

Mr. Mike Pierce is a 45-year-old white male admitted to your unit with a diagnosis of acute upper GI bleeding. He was brought by car to the emergency department by two of his friends after he vomited blood earlier in the day. He was intoxicated on arrival at the hospital. His friends, who were also intoxicated, left immediately. He was transferred to the medical intensive care unit (ICU). Upon arrival to the ICU, the patient promptly vomited coffee ground emesis. His medical diagnoses are: (1) acute upper GI bleed and (2) hypovolemic shock.

Initial Appraisal

On approaching Mike's bed, you make the following rapid assessment.

GENERAL APPEARANCE. Mike is a thin, Caucasian male with a distended abdomen. His hair is blond and dirty, with typical male pattern baldness. He appears older than his stated age.

SIGNS OF DISTRESS. Mike's respiration rate is approximately 24/minute; shallow and even without apparent distress. No facial grimacing is noted, and his limbs are outstretched in a relaxed manner. He is mumbling and is disoriented. He appears drowsy. His pulse is weak and thready; skin is pale and diaphoretic.

OTHER. You note the odor of alcohol on Mike's breath. He has one 18-gauge intravenous (IV) catheter in each of his arms with 0.9% normal saline solution infusing at 125 cc/hour. There is evidence of dried blood around the patient's mouth. His abdomen is distended, while his face and extremities are thin and emaciated. The nurse notes that his skin has a yellowish cast to it.

Focused Nursing History

Hospital records reveal that the patient was last hospitalized 3 months ago for decreased level of consciousness (LOC) and pneumonia. His pneumonia was treated with antibiotics, and his LOC returned to baseline. He was discharged home, where he resides with his elderly aunt. He did not show up for his scheduled follow-up appointment. His past medical history includes the following: alcohol abuse and hypertension, for which he has been prescribed a diuretic. There is documentation of one previous episode of bleeding esophageal varices 3 years ago for which he was hospitalized. The patient is unable to provide any further history or information.

QUESTION

You note that he is ventilating without apparent distress. Based on the patient's past medical history and his history of present illness (vomiting blood), you would next focus your assessment on his _______ status.

A. renal
B. neurological
C. fluid volume
D. nutritional

ANSWER

C is the correct answer. During initial appraisal, the nurse noted a critical cue, hematemesis (vomiting blood, dried blood around patient's mouth). Based on this single cue, the nurse can quickly cluster other similar critical cues, including a weak pulse and history of alcohol abuse and therefore possible hepatic dysfunction. Additionally, there are some cues that direct the nurse to consider the possibility of hepatic dysfunction such as distended abdomen (possible ascites); thin, emaciated extremities indicative of a poor nutritional status; and jaundice.

You scan his admission orders. An arterial blood gas (ABG); pulse oximetry; oxygen at 2 L per nasal cannula; nasogastric (NG) tube to low, intermittent suction; and urinary catheter have been ordered.

QUESTION

You decide that the NG tube and urinary catheter can wait. Which of the remaining orders would you implement first?

A. pulse oximetry
B. oxygen
C. arterial blood gas (ABG)

ANSWER

B is the correct answer. You should administer the oxygen first because you have noted the critical cues: rapid but shallow respirations, decreased LOC, confusion, and probable upper GI bleeding event signifying blood loss. Reduced oxygen-carrying capacity accompanies active blood loss. In Mike's case, because he is symptomatic of a decreased oxygen-carrying capacity and has obviously experienced acute blood loss, oxygen should be administered first. It is also important to obtain a baseline ABG, and sometimes this should be done initially before applying oxygen in persons who are not symptomatic. In Mike's case, you should notify the laboratory regarding how much oxygen Mike is receiving and for how long he has been receiving it in order to get a true baseline ABG measurement. This intervention should be followed by a measurement of his SpO_2, which will help you to monitor Mike's response to the oxygen therapy. If you delay the oxygen administration, Mike could become hypoxic and go into respiratory failure. An NG tube is placed and Mike is lavaged with room temperature normal saline. The return aspirate consists of "coffee ground" emesis.

Focused Nursing Assessment

Mike's initial appraisal, brief recent and past histories, and data clustering are suggestive of an upper GI bleeding crisis. Immediate action should be focused on obtaining more data to confirm this hypothesis. Focused neurological and respiratory assessments are indicated because Mike has a decreased LOC and there exists the possibility that he may have aspirated some of the vomitus into his lungs.

Focused Neurological Assessment

Mike is drowsy and oriented to his name only. He is mumbling inappropriate word phrases, and his Glasgow Coma Scale (GCS) score is 13 (opens eyes spontaneously, verbalizes inappropriate words; appears confused but able to obey simple commands). He moves all of his extremities to command, and has a weak but equal hand grasp. Pupils are equal in size (4 mm), round, midline, and briskly reactive to light.

Focused Respiratory Assessment

Auscultation of his lungs reveal fine bibasilar crackles. Respiratory rate is 32 breaths/min and shallow. SpO_2 per pulse oximetry is 86 percent on 4 L of oxygen per nasal cannula.

Focused Gastrointestinal and Fluid Volume Assessment

A focused GI and fluid volume assessment reveals two-plus pitting edema in his lower extremities. His skin and sclera are markedly icteric, and spider angiomas are noted over a grossly distended abdomen. He has ascites. Bowel sounds are noted on auscultation of his abdomen. Abdomen is mildly tender over the right upper quadrant. He demonstrates significant orthostatic hypotension of > 10 points difference when lying and sitting (with legs dangling over the side of the bed). He complains of "lightheadedness" when in sitting position.

Focused Cardiovascular Assessment

A focused cardiovascular assessment reveals sinus tachycardia with a heart rate of 135, blood pressure 88/52, and absent jugular venous distention (JVD). Auscultation of his heart reveals an audible S_1S_2, without murmur or gallop.

Focused Integument and Temperature Assessment

Skin is cool and dry to touch with palpable peripheral pulses. The nurse notes a yellowish tinge to the skin, and scleras are also yellow. Rectal temperature is 100°F.

Mike suddenly vomits a large amount of bright red blood. Measurement of his vital signs at this time reveals the following: blood pressure 80/45, heart rate 152, with a respiratory rate of 36 breaths/min. Pulse oximetry reveals an oxygen saturation (SpO_2) of 85 percent. His LOC has further deteriorated.

QUESTION

How would you interpret Mike's blood pressure and pulse?

A. they are directly related to his loss of skeletal muscle mass
B. they are indicative of alcohol withdrawal
C. they are directly related to his hypovolemia
D. they are indicative of severe fluid volume overload

ANSWER

The correct answer is C. Patients with acute blood loss may become hypotensive and tachycardic due to hypovolemic shock. On arrival at the hospital, Mike also demonstrated orthostatic hypotension of > 20 points when going from a supine position to sitting up with his feet dangling. Orthostasis suggests fluid volume deficit.

Significant admission laboratory results were as follows:

Hematocrit: 17 (normal, 40 to 54 percent [males]; 36 to 46 percent [females])
Hemoglobin: 7 (normal, 13.5 to 17g/dL [males]; 12 to 15 g/dL [females])
WBC: 17,000 (normal, 45,000 to 10,000)
Coagulation panel
Prothrombin time (PT): 15.1 seconds (normal, 11 to 15 seconds) with an international normalized ratio (INR) of 1.9 (normal, 1.0)
Partial thromboplastin time (PTT): 62 seconds (normal, 60 to 70 seconds)

Liver function tests
  Alanine aminotransferase (ALT or SGPT): 1,000 (normal, 3 to 35 U/mL)
  Gamma-glutamyl transferase (GGT): 210 (normal, 4 to 23 IU/L)
  Total bilirubin: 5.0 (normal, 0.1 to 1.2 mg/dL)
Blood alcohol level: 252 mg/dL (normal, 00.0 mg/dL; indicative of alcohol intoxication, > 150 mg/dL; severe alcohol intoxication, 250 mg/dL; comatose, 300 mg/dL; fatal > 400 mg/dL)
Blood urea nitrogen (BUN): 67 mg/dL (normal, 5 to 25 mg/dL in adults)
Serum creatinine: 1.0 mg/dL (normal, 0.5 to 1.5 mg/dL)
Sodium: 148 (normal, 135 to 145 mEq/L)
Potassium: 3.1 mEq/L (normal, 3.5 to 5.3 mEq/L)
Glucose: 78 (normal, 70 to 110 mg/dL
ABG
  pH: 7.35 (7.35 to 7.45)
  $Paco_2$: 44 (35 to 45 mm Hg)
  Pao_2: 82 (75 to 100 mm Hg)
  Sao_2: 90% (> 95%)
Chest x-ray: right lower lobe infiltrate

(All normal values from Kee [1999]).

QUESTION

What is the significance of the laboratory and radiographic data?

ANSWER

1. The hematocrit (Hct) is low, perhaps in response to the actual blood loss. This patient's bleeding is probably significant since the hematocrit is so low. Usually, the hema-tocrit value does not change substantially during the first hours after an episode of acute GI bleeding and therefore is not a reliable measure of the amount of blood loss (Kee, 1999). Serial measurements of hematocrit values are useful to evaluate continued blood loss and adequacy of red blood cell (RBC) replacement. Because the hematocrit value represents a percentage of RBC mass to total intravascular volume, the absolute value for the hematocrit must be evaluated in relation to other parameters of fluid status. The hematocrit value may be normal or even elevated during the hypovolemic event. Once rehydration occurs with IV fluids, significant decreases of hematocrit can occur without any significant change in the amount of RBCs.

2. The BUN level is also important to monitor, since elevated levels may be seen with hypovolemia and renal failure. If the BUN is rising and the creatinine level remains relatively unchanged, a decreased intravascular volume is suggested. In fact, BUN elevations of two to five times normal are associated with blood loss of > 1,000 cc. The BUN level also increases because of the intestinal absorption of blood proteins (Krumberger & Hammer, 1998). This patient's BUN is elevated while the creatinine is normal, suggesting hypovolemia.

3. This patient's hemoglobin (Hgb) is low. Decreased Hgb values are seen with severe hemorrhage, cirrhosis of the liver, and with large amounts of IV fluids due to hemodilution. Chronic anemia may also be an underlying problem with this patient.

4. This patient's WBC is decreased, suggesting immunosuppression, possibly secondary to chronic malnutrition.

5. The coagulation panel values consisting of the PT and the PTT are normal. Liver function values (ALT or SGPT, GGT, and total bilirubin) are elevated and suggest underlying liver disease.

6. This patient's blood alcohol level is elevated, suggesting severe alcohol intoxication.

7. The serum sodium value is slightly elevated, suggesting hypo-volemia due to hemoconcentration. This level should decrease following fluid resuscitation. The potassium level is decreased and will need replacement to promote optimal myocardial function.

8. The serum glucose level is normal, but should be monitored closely for decreased levels.

9. This patient's ABG values are adequate on 2 L of oxygen per nasal cannula. The Spo_2 should be monitored continuously per pulse oximetry for decreased levels. Protection of the airway is critical in this patient. Endotracheal intubation should be considered by the medical team since a risk of aspiration exists (vomiting, continued decreased LOC, hypoxia).

10. The patient's chest x-ray reveals a right lower lobe infiltrate. Close surveillance of this patient's oxygenation status is indicated because of the high risk of aspiration pneumonia.

Development of Nursing Diagnoses

You are now ready to develop the nursing diagnoses based on the available subjective and objective data. To cluster your data, look for abnormal values and findings discovered during the assessment. Mike's major symptoms at this time are bleeding, hypotension, and decreased LOC. Thus, these primary symptoms can initiate your first cluster of critical cues.

CLUSTER 1

Subjective data. The patient has a decreased LOC and is unable to give you any information. His friends reported that he had vomited blood prior to arrival.

Objective data. Mike is hypotensive and vomiting bright red blood. His LOC has deteriorated from his initial GCS score of 13. His Hct is markedly decreased, while his BUN value is elevated. His serum creatinine is normal. Cardiac monitoring reveals sinus tachycardia.

QUESTION

Based on the above data, which of the following nursing diagnoses is the priority diagnosis at this time for Mike?

A. *Decreased cardiac output*
B. *Impaired gas exchange*
C. *Fluid volume excess*
D. *Fluid volume deficit*

ANSWER

The correct answer is D. Mike is experiencing hypovolemic shock from active blood loss. The nursing diagnosis of *Fluid volume deficit* related to active blood loss is supported by the data. A Foley catheter is inserted, resulting in only 35 cc of "tea"-colored urine. This finding of a decreased urine output further supports the diagnosis of *Fluid volume deficit*.

Other nursing diagnoses that apply to this patient include:

- *Tissue perfusion, altered: Cerebral, respiratory, renal, peripheral,* as evidenced by the decreased Hct/Hgb with decreased oxygen-carrying capacity, altered LOC, tachycardia, tachypnea, decreased urine output, cool skin, and weakly palpable pulses.
- *Aspiration, risk for* related to decreased level of consciousness, and vomiting.
- *Thought processes, altered* related to alcohol intoxication, risk for alcohol withdrawal symptoms, and anemia.
- *Anxiety* related to fear of bleeding, threat of death, and decreased oxygenation.

Plan of Care

1. Stop the bleeding and achieve hemostasis.
2. Replace lost blood volume.
3. Correct hypovolemic shock.
4. Maintain adequacy of oxygenation status.

To deal with a presumed variceal bleed, Mike is started on intravenous vasopressin at 0.4 U/min. Aggressive fluid resuscitation is begun. He received a total of 8 units of packed red blood cells to replace blood loss, 4 units of fresh frozen plasma to correct clotting factors, and 7 L of crystalloid solution (lactated Ringer's and 0.9 percent normal saline). Because of vomiting and hypotension, Mike was electively intubated to protect his airway. Diagnostic endoscopy is performed and large esophageal varices 2 to 4 cm above the gastroesophageal junction are found. Sclerotherapy is then performed.

QUESTION

What is the purpose of sclerotherapy?

ANSWER

Endoscopic sclerotherapy is now the most common method of treatment in acute variceal hemorrhage. The purpose of this treatment is to sclerose (scar) the bleeding vessel, thus halting or preventing further hemorrhage. A sclerosing agent is injected into or around the bleeding vessel (Krumberger & Hammer, 1998).

QUESTION

What nursing interventions are important in caring for a patient undergoing this procedure?

ANSWER

Nursing interventions during the procedure include providing the patient and family with information concerning the procedure, positioning the patient, and administering sedation if the patient is agitated. The nurse also continuously observes the patient for any signs of distress during the procedure. The focus of care following the procedure includes assessing for further bleeding and monitoring for complications. Complication of sclerotherapy can include dysphagia, aspiration, esophageal perforation, mediastinitis, substernal pain, mucosal ulcerations, esophageal strictures, septicemia, fever, and pulmonary complications (Krumberger & Hammer, 1998).

QUESTION

What is vasopressin? What should the nurse assess for in patients who are receiving intravenous vasopressin?

ANSWER

Vasopressin cause systemic vasoconstriction, especially of the splanchnic arteriolar system. It occurs naturally in the body as antidiuretic hormone (ADH), which is produced by the posterior pituitary. Vasopressin increases mesenteric vascular resistance, causing a reduced portal venous blood flow. These actions result in a concomitant decrease in portal venous pressure and esophageal variceal pressure, thus reducing bleeding. Unfortunately, vasopressin has some undesirable and dangerous systemic effects. These other side effects include decreased cardiac output, myocardial ischemia, and decreased coronary blood flow. In fact, chest pain is not uncommon in patients receiving intravenous vasopressin, particularly in those who have a positive history for coronary artery disease. Nitroglycerin is often used simultaneously with a vasopressin infusion to maximize coronary blood flow and perfusion. Other complications of vasopressin for which the nurse should monitor are abdominal cramping secondary to splanchnic vasoconstriction and mesenteric ischemia, hyponatremia secondary to free water retention and antidiuretic action, hypertension secondary to systemic vasoconstriction, and bradycardia secondary to reflex responses to hypertension. Vasopressin must be weaned off slowly in order to avoid rebound effects such as hypotension. Hypotension may also signal rebleeding. Nitroglycerin is weaned off along with the vasopressin. Diuresis may occur as the circulating ADH returns to a physiologic level, necessitating close monitoring of electrolytes, especially sodium and potassium. Octreotide, a somatostatin analogue, has an action similar to vasopressin (splanchnic vasoconstriction/reduced portal pressure) but with fewer systemic side effects. Octreotide is administered intravenously and may offer efficacy similar to vasopressin with fewer side effects (Cello, 1995; Passaro, 1995).

Therapeutic Goals and Desired Patient Outcomes

The following are critical therapeutic goals and outcomes as outlined by Krumberger and Hammer (1998):

Hemodynamic Stability

Systolic BP > 90 mm Hg
Mean arterial pressure > 70 mm Hg
HR < 110 beats/min
Hematocrit value > 30 percent
Hemoglobin value 12 to 14 g/100 mL

Restored Tissue Perfusion

Urine output > 0.5 cc/kg body weight/hr
Capillary refill ≤ 3 seconds
Warm skin with strongly palpable peripheral pulses
Clear lung sounds
Oxygen saturation > 90 percent or equal to baseline
Mental status returned to baseline
Absence of chest pain, dysrhythmia, or electrocardiographic abnormalities

Achieve Hemostasis/Correct Coagulation Deficits

Bleeding stopped
PT/PTT within normal limits

Respiratory Stability

Respiratory rate returned to baseline (< 20 to 24 breaths/min)
Absence of shortness of breath and crackles
ABG values within normal limits with baseline SpO_2 > 90 percent

Serum Electrolytes within Normal Limits

Sodium, potassium, calcium, glucose, magnesium

Comfort Achieved

Absence of anxiety, pain, fear

Treatment Plan Understood

Patient and family verbalize understanding of and participate in treatment plan

Medical and Nursing Management and Patient Outcome

Fourteen hours after ICU admission, Mike's bleeding was stabilized. No further bleeding ensued. Fluid volume balance was maintained effectively, with urine output 50 to 100 cc/hr and electrolytes within normal limits. BUN and creatinine also were within normal limits. Mike still required sedation while on the ventilator, demonstrating agitation and thrashing about in bed as the sedation wore off. Although vital signs were stable (blood pressure 102/52; heart rate 110; respiratory rate 16), his rectal temperature rose to 100.4°F, and rhonchi were audible in both lung fields. WBC was 15,000 and ABG values were pH 7.51; PCO_2 36 mm Hg; PO_2 68 mm Hg; O_2 saturation 90 percent.

Revised Medical and Nursing Diagnoses

Medical Diagnoses

Acute GI bleeding (resolving)
Pneumonia
Delirium tremens/alcohol withdrawal syndrome

Nursing Diagnoses

Impaired gas exchange related to alveolar hypoventilation secondary to pneumonia
Sensory/perceptual alterations related to alcohol withdrawal

Revised Plan of Care

Culture sputum, blood, and urine
Chest x-ray to evaluate for presence of infiltrates
Replace all invasive lines with new ones
Begin empiric antibiotic therapy
Sedation as needed
Continue respiratory ventilator support as needed
Begin aggressive pulmonary hygiene measures

Independent Nursing Interventions

The onset of acute upper GI bleeding and the resultant crisis-oriented interventions present a terrifying ordeal for the patient and family. Therefore, emotional and spiritual support is needed. Additionally, the nurse should provide comfort measures. The patient needs frequent mouth care. Because of the presence of tubes (endotracheal, nasogastric, and in some cases a Sengstaken–Blakemore tube) in the nasal and oral cavities, the patient becomes a mouth breather. Hematemesis leads to the accumulation of blood in the oral cavity. The presence of tubes causes difficulty in swallowing saliva. To prevent undue discomfort from these invasive tubes, an emesis basin, tissues, and suction catheter should be kept within easy reach of the patient. The patient can be taught to suction out his mouth with a special handheld suction device sometimes called a "Yaunker." To prevent undue irritation of the nares they should be regularly cleansed and lubricated with a water-soluble substance. Epigastric discomfort can occur. Mike was kept NPO (nothing by mouth) until all evidence of bleeding was absent. Occasional ice chips or specially prepared oral lubricants per physician order may be provided to relieve mouth dryness. Humidification of supplemental oxygen is beneficial to prevent drying of delicate tissues as well as thinning pulmonary secretions so that they may be more easily expectorated.

Psychological and Family Implications

GI bleeding episodes create a crisis for the patient and the family. Not only can independent nursing intervention affect the outcome of this crisis, but it can also influence the adaptation that the patient and family continue to make to the situation.

THE PATIENT. The loss of any quantity of blood may evoke panic and fear of death in the patient. The response is more complicated, with additional behavioral problems, if the patient is an alcoholic or drug abuser. Based on the idea that crisis situations have predictable outcomes, timely explanations of ongoing interventions and anticipated results help the patient to cope with the overwhelming anguish and anxiety (Kuenzi & Fenton, 1975). Decisive and supportive nursing care will help Mike to regain control of his own behavior and cooperate with the health team in therapy.

THE FAMILY. The family may display a variety of emotional reactions similar to those experienced by the patient. The need for the nurse to be keenly aware of the family and to assess the family as well as the patient should be self-evident if optimal crisis care is to be given. It is important for the patient and the family to be offered counseling following discharge to home. The family/significant others will play a critical role in the patient's eventual recovery and rehabilitation from alcohol.

Patient Outcome

The remainder of Mike's stay was uneventful. His urine culture was positive for *Escherichia coli;* blood and sputum cultures were positive for *Staphylococcus aureus*. His sputum culture was also positive for *Hemophilus influenzae*. He was started on the appropriate antibiotics and was given aggressive pulmonary toilet by his nurses. Sedation was decreased, and ventilatory support was withdrawn without complications. Mike was effectively coughing up copious pulmonary secretions, his temperature had decreased to 99°F, and he was taken off all supplemental oxygen. His LOC returned to baseline (GCS score of 15). No further evidence of GI bleeding occurred, and he was discharged to home to live with his sister, who agreed to help him make his follow-up clinic appointments. Mike's nurse referred him to a local support group to help him deal with his alcohol abuse.

CASE STUDY 2

BLEEDING PEPTIC ULCER

Mrs. Hardin is an 80-year-old woman with rheumatoid arthritis. She visited her local emergency department with complaints of dizziness, shortness of breath, and chest pain. Her daughter, with whom she resides, drove her to the hospital. She is a poor historian, but her daughter relates that her symptoms have been occurring with increasing frequency over the past 2 weeks.

Initial Appraisal

On approaching Mrs. Hardin, you make the following assessment.

GENERAL APPEARANCE. Mrs. Hardin is a mildly obese, Caucasian female who appears her stated age. Her hair is gray and well kept. Her clothes are clean and appropriate. She is carrying a small handbag, and a paper sack filled with her prescribed medications. Her daughter is appropriately attentive and concerned.

SIGNS OF DISTRESS. Mrs. Hardin's breathing is rapid and even. No facial grimacing is noted, and her posture is relaxed. Her speech is clear and appropriate. She is oriented to her surroundings. Her skin is pale and cool to touch.

OTHER. Initial evaluation reveals a heart rate of 110, respiratory rate of 28, and peripheral oxygen saturation (SpO_2) of 92 percent. Continuous cardiac monitoring and

4 L of oxygen supplementation are initiated. A 12-lead electrocardiogram (ECG) is performed.

Focused Nursing History

Additional questioning reveals that Mrs. Hardin has smoked two packs of cigarettes a day for the past 60 years, has a history of coronary disease, and has been taking corticosteroids and nonsteroidal anti-inflammatory drugs (NSAIDs) for the management of her rheumatoid arthritis. Hospital records reveal that she was last hospitalized 3 months ago for a kidney infection. Her infection was treated with antibiotics, and she was discharged to home without further complications.

Focused Nursing Assessment

On physical examination, Mrs. Hardin's lungs are clear to auscultation. Respirations are unlabored but rapid. No dysrhythmias are noted, and her ECG is normal, although her pulse is weak. Nailbeds are pale and capillary refill is sluggish. Her skin is pale, cool, and dry. Her heart sounds are audible, and no murmurs or gallops are present. She is alert and cooperative. She states that her chest pain has stopped since she has been resting. She also states that her chest pain occurs with exertion, which she describes as brisk walking and climbing stairs. Her abdomen is soft and nontender, bowel sounds are hyperactive, and rectal exam reveals tarry-colored stool that tests positive for blood. During this time, Mrs. Hardin tells you that she has been having black, tarry stools for several weeks, which she thought started after she began taking iron supplements. She also shares with you that she has been having burning abdominal pain precipitated by eating food for the past 2 weeks. Blood work reveals the following:

Complete blood count
- WBC: 4,500 (normal, 5,000 to 10,000)
- Hemoglobin: 8.2 (normal, 13.5 to 17 g/dL [males]; 12 to 15 g/dL [females])
- Hematocrit: 26.6 (normal, 40 to 54 percent [males]; 36 to 46 percent [females])
- Platelets: 276,000 (normal, 150,000 to 400,000)

Coagulation studies are all within normal limits.

Arterial blood gas
- pH: 7.37
- PaO_2: 70
- $PaCO_2$: 43
- O_2 saturation: 96 percent on 4 L of oxygen per nasal cannula

Vital signs:

	Lying	Sitting
Blood pressure	130/70	110/50
Heart rate	110	130
Respiration	24	28
Temperature	98.5°F	

The decision was made to admit Mrs. Hardin to the hospital for further evaluation and management. She was admitted to a "step-down" unit and placed on continuous cardiac monitoring because of her age and complaints of chest pain. An upper endoscopy is performed on Mrs. Hardin, which reveals a large gastric ulcer. The ulcer appears to be oozing blood. This finding is compatible with her reports of pain following eating, her "tarry" stools, and her low hematocrit. She is diagnosed with peptic ulcer disease: gastric ulcer.

QUESTION

How do the clinical features of a gastric peptic ulcer compare to those of a duodenal peptic ulcer?

ANSWER

Characteristics of Duodenal and Gastric Ulcers

INCIDENCE. The incidence ratio of duodenal and gastric ulcers is approximately 4:1. The most common age group affected is 25 to 50 year olds, with men being affected four times more than women.

PATHOGENESIS OF DUODENAL ULCERS. Hyperacidity is the most important factor in the pathogenesis of duodenal ulcers. Diseases associated with hyperacidity include hyperparathyroidism, chronic pulmonary disease, chronic pancreatitis, alcoholism, and cirrhosis. Duodenal ulcers are also associated with tobacco use and high stress levels.

PATHOGENESIS OF GASTRIC ULCERS. Disruption of the GI mucosal barrier is the most important factor in the pathogenesis of duodenal ulcers. However, hydrochloric acid production is normal to low in most patients. Some drugs contribute to the development of gastric ulcers, such as alcohol, tobacco, and NSAIDs. *Helicobacter pylori* infection increases the risk of developing both gastric and duodenal ulcers.

LOCATION. The location of duodenal ulcers is within the duodenal bulb in 90 percent of cases. The location of gastric ulcers is in the antrum and lesser curvature of the stomach in 90 percent of cases.

CLINICAL FEATURES OF DUODENAL ULCERS. Duodenal ulcers exhibit a pain–food relief pattern. When food is eaten, the pain from a duodenal ulcer is relieved. Night pain is common. Weight loss seldom affects the occurrence of a duodenal ulcer.

CLINICAL FEATURES OF GASTRIC ULCERS. Eating may relieve or exacerbate the pain from a gastric ulcer. Night pain is less common than with a duodenal ulcer. Anorexia and weight loss are common with a gastric ulcer (Hursch & Caswell, 1999).

QUESTION

What presenting symptoms influenced the decision to admit Mrs. Hardin to the hospital?

ANSWER

The symptoms that hastened her hospital admission were her complaints of dizziness, shortness of breath, and chest pain, and the fact that these symptoms have recently been occurring with increased frequency. These presenting symptoms combined with her advanced age indicate a potentially life-threatening situation. Furthermore, she demonstrated orthostatic hypotension when her blood pressure measurements was compared between lying (supine) and sitting (erect) positions. Significant orthostatic hypotension exists if the patient becomes dizzy, has a pulse increase of ≥ 20 beats/min, or has a systolic blood pressure decrease of ≥ 20 mm Hg (Thomas, 1997). Because Mrs. Hardin's systolic blood pressure decreased from 130 to 110 and her heart rate increased from 110 to 130 when going from a sitting to a lying position, it can be concluded that she demonstrates orthostasis. This significant change in her vital signs signifies hypovolemia or dehydration. Furthermore, her hematocrit is low, and her stool is positive for blood. Her report of "tarry" stools lends support to a diagnosis of GI bleeding.

Based on the available data, you make the following nursing diagnoses and goals:

- *Fluid volume deficit* related to gastric ulcer bleeding and fluid loss

  Goal—Patient's circulating blood and fluid volume will be maintained.

  Supporting data—Melena (tarry stools); abdominal pain (especially after eating); hyperactive bowel sounds; orthostasis; low Hct and Hgb; dizziness; weak pulse; bleeding gastric ulcer per endoscopic evaluation.
- *Alteration in tissue perfusion* related to bleeding and fluid loss

  Goal—Patient's circulating blood volume will be restored and maintained.

  Supporting data—Low Hct and Hgb; chest pain; shortness of breath; increased heart rate.
- *Alteration in comfort: Pain* related to peptic ulcer disease and GI bleeding

  Goal—Patient will verbalize minimal discomfort or absence of pain.

  Supporting data—Abdominal and chest discomfort.
- *Alteration in nutrition: Less than body requirements* related to GI bleeding, abdominal pain, and NPO status (nothing by mouth)

  Goal—Patient's body weight will be maintained.
- *Anxiety/fear* related to emergent situation and hospitalization

  Goal—Patient will verbalize anxieties and fears and demonstrate progress toward positive coping behaviors.
- *Knowledge deficit* regarding treatments, interventions, and home care needs

  Goal—Patient and/or significant other will demonstrate understanding of all interventions, treatments, medications, home care, and follow-up instructions.

QUESTION

From the history, what factors increase Mrs. Hardin's risk for the development of peptic ulcer disease (PUD)?

ANSWER

Mrs. Hardin takes NSAIDs for her rheumatoid arthritis. Chronic use of NSAIDs can increase the risk for the development of ulcer disease by causing damage to the gastric mucosa. Overwhelming evidence associates chronic NSAID use with PUD, particularly gastric ulcers. NSAIDs and aspirin impair ulcer healing and induce ulcer formation through prostaglandin inhibition and directly irritate the gastric and duodenal mucosa. Prostaglandins, which are produced by the cells in the GI tract, play an important role in preventing injury to the gastroduodenal mucosa by inhibiting gastric acid secretion, maintaining blood flow, and stimulating mucus and bicarbonate production. Mrs. Hardin has smoked two packs of cigarettes a day for the past 60 years. Cigarette smoking causes decreased biliary bicarbonate secretion, thus causing duodenal gastric reflux, which contributes to ulcer formation. Furthermore, her advanced age is in itself a risk factor for ulcer development. Other risk factors that may contribute to the development of PUD include chronic aspirin use and alcohol use, both of which cause damage to the gastric mucosa, and heredity, which may be responsible for an increased number of parietal cells, resulting in hypersecretion of gastric acid. *Helicobacter pylori* infection also has been implicated in the pathogenesis of peptic ulcers. The inflammatory response associated with *H. pylori* infection is thought to disrupt the mucosal resistance to injury from gastric acid. This disruption in the mucosal defense mechanism allows the gastric acid to contribute to ulcer formation.

QUESTION

What was the cause of Mrs. Hardin's chest pain?

ANSWER

This patient has a history of coronary artery disease, which, when combined with an impaired tissue perfusion secondary to blood loss from a gastric ulcer, could contribute to myocardial ischemia and chest pain. The blood loss and decreased Hct could be causing a decreased perfusion to the myocardium, resulting in ischemic chest pain. On the other hand, since her ECG was normal (without evidence of ischemia/infarct), her chest pain could be a referred pain symptom of her gastric ulcer.

QUESTION

What is the rationale for performing the upper endoscopy?

ANSWER

Because GI bleeding was suspected, the endoscopic procedure was needed to directly observe the GI tract mucosa for the source of the bleeding. After the bleeding ulcer was confirmed, a sclerosing agent was injected directly into the bleeding vessel to stop the bleeding. The sclerosing agent actually traumatizes the endothelium, causing necrosis and eventually sclerosis of the bleeding vessel. Her bleeding is stopped, and she is started on a clear liquid diet.

QUESTION

What possible complications should the nurse assess for in a patient who has undergone sclerotherapy of a bleeding gastric ulcer?

ANSWER

Several complications can result from endoscopic sclerotherapy, including ulcer perforation, strictures, bacteremia, increased bleeding (especially if coagulation abnormalities exist), aspiration, dysphagia, fever, venous thrombosis involving the mesentery, and systemic effects of sclerosis such as acute respiratory distress syndrome (ARDS).

QUESTION

What pharmaceutical options exist for the control of gastric pH?

ANSWER

Pharmaceutical options include *antacids* (provide a direct alkaline buffer to control the pH of the gastric mucosa), *histamine blockers* (block parietal cell stimulation and secretion of hydrochloric acid), and *proton pump inhibitors* (work within the parietal cells to decrease the acidity of the acid produced). Mucosal enhancers (e.g., sucralfate) act directly on the mucosa to reduce the effects of acid secretion (Krumberger & Hammer, 1998).

Patient Outcome

Forty-eight hours following sclerotherapy of her bleeding gastric ulcer, Mrs. Hardin's condition deteriorates. Her WBC rises dramatically to 21,000. She becomes hypotensive and difficult to arouse. Her blood pressure decreases to 70/52. She is transferred to the intensive care unit, where intravenous vasopressor agents (i.e., dopamine) is started for blood pressure support. She is electively intubated and placed on mechanical ventilation. After 48 hours, her abdomen becomes distended and bowel sounds are absent. Blood cultures are positive for gram-negative rods supporting a diagnosis of gram-negative septicemia and shock. Antibiotics are being administered intravenously to treat or minimize septic complications. Dopamine and fluid resuscitation with normal saline is needed to support the blood pressure. Abdominal x-rays are taken and reveal distended bowel loops compatible with *paralytic ileus*. All oral foods and fluids are withheld, and an NG tube is inserted and attached to low wall suction in order to decompress the abdominal distention. The nurse monitors Mrs. Hardin's electrolyte levels closely. She requires potassium replacement to treat hypokalemia.

QUESTION

What assessment findings support the diagnosis of acute paralytic ileus?

ANSWER

Abdominal distention, absent bowel sounds, and distended loops of bowel seen with radiological examination support the diagnosis of adynamic or paralytic ileus. Paralytic ileus is a complication of septic shock. The decreased blood pressure and vasodilation that accompanies septic shock produce hypoperfusion to the bowel. This "low flow" state causes a reduction in the normal peristaltic activity of the GI tract, resulting in an obstruction. It is common for bowel sounds to be decreased or absent on auscultation of the abdomen. Gas and fluid accumulate above the obstructed segment of bowel and result in the intestinal distention (Krumberger & Hammer, 1998).

QUESTION

What nursing interventions are necessary when caring for a patient who has developed an adynamic paralytic ileus?

ANSWER

Maintain NPO status until bowel function returns. Until the patient can resume enteral feeding, an NG tube will need to be in place and attached to low wall suction in order to prevent gastric contents from entering the intestines and to rest the bowel. Hyperalimentation or total parenteral nutrition (TPN) may be required. As soon as bowel sounds return, the patient will need to be fed utilizing her GI tract. It is very important that the nurse observe for signs and symptoms that reflect perforation, ischemia, or necrosis of the bowel. These symptoms include rebound tenderness of the abdomen, increased pain and distention, increased WBC, and fluid and electrolyte imbalances (Krumberger & Hammer, 1998).

Pain and comfort relief measures are appropriate, as is frequent oral care.

Patient Outcome

Mrs. Hardin stabilizes hemodynamically. The dopamine is weaned off. Her bowel sounds return without any evidence of bowel necrosis. She is weaned off of mechanical ventilation and extubated. Oral feedings are reinitiated without any evidence of bowel obstruction. Her hematocrit remains stable, and her WBC returns to normal. She is discharged to home to reside with her daughter, with follow-up.

REFERENCES

Cello, J.P. (1995). Medical management of acute variceal hemorrhage. *Intern Surg* 80:82–86.

Hursch, C.G., & Caswell, D. (1999). Gastrointestinal disorders. In A. Gawlinski & D. Hamwi (eds.). *Acute care nurse practitioner: Clinical curriculum and certification review* (pp. 707–710). Philadelphia: W.B. Saunders.

Kee, J. (1999). *Handbook of laboratory and diagnostic tests with nursing implications* (5th ed.). Stamford: Appleton & Lange.

Krumberger, M.K., & Hammer, B. (1998). Gastrointestinal disorders. In M.R. Kinney, S.B. Dunbar, J.A. Brooks-Brunn, N. Molter, & J.M. Vitello-Cicciu (eds.), *AACN's clinical reference for critical care nursing* (4th ed.) (pp. 1033–1037). St Louis: C.V. Mosby.

Kuenzi, S.H., & Fenton, M.V. (1975, May). Crisis intervention in acute care areas. *Am J Nurs* 75:830–834.

Passaro, E. (1995). Gastrointestinal bleeding. In F.S. Bongard & D.Y. Sue (eds.), *Current critical care diagnosis and treatment* (2nd ed.) (pp. 562–575). Norwalk, CT: Appleton & Lange.

Thomas, C.L. (ed.). (1997). *Taber's cyclopedic medical dictionary* (18th ed.). Philadelphia: F.A. Davis.

PART VIII

Injury

MODULE 32

Complex Wound Management

Karen L. Johnson

This self-study module describes the anatomic structures and physiologic functions of the skin (Section One), physiologic events that occur when an alteration in skin integrity occurs (Section Two), factors that affect wound healing (Section Three), principles of wound management (Sections Four and Five), nursing assessment of and interventions for the patient with alteration in skin integrity (Section Six), and pressure ulcer prevention and treatment (Sections Seven & Eight).

To help determine your current level of understanding of this topic, the module begins with a pretest. Each section includes a set of review questions to help the learner evaluate his or her understanding of the section's content before moving on to the next section. It is suggested that the learner review those concepts answered incorrectly in the review questions before proceeding to the next section.

OBJECTIVES

Following completion of this module, the learner will be able to

1. Relate anatomic structures with physiologic functions of the skin.
2. State the three phases of wound healing.
3. Describe the events that occur in each phase of wound healing.
4. Define three methods of wound closure.
5. Recognize factors that affect the wound healing process.
6. Identify conditions that predispose a patient to develop a wound infection.
7. Identify criteria used to diagnose a wound infection.
8. State interventions that can be used to prevent and treat wound infections.
9. Describe the rationale for various treatment modalities used in wound management.
10. Identify the common clinical assessments made to evaluate wound healing.
11. Identify patients at risk for pressure ulcer development.
12. State interventions for the prevention of pressure ulcers.
13. Identify components of a pressure ulcer treatment program.

PRETEST

1. The layer of the skin that contains connective tissue, elastic fibers, blood vessels, and nerves is the
   A. epidermis
   B. dermis
   C. hypodermis
   D. subcutaneous tissue

2. The functions of the skin include all of the following EXCEPT
   A. regulation of body temperature
   B. production of vitamin D
   C. protection from the external environment
   D. production of calcium

3. The major events that occur during the proliferative phase of wound healing include all of the following EXCEPT
   A. hemostasis
   B. epithelialization
   C. granulation
   D. collagen cross-linking
4. The four cardinal signs of inflammation occur as a result of
   A. normal chemical and vascular events
   B. an infectious process
   C. bradykinins
   D. an increased number of white blood cells (WBCs)
5. Wounds that have significant contamination or significant tissue loss usually are not sutured. These wounds are left open to heal by the process of
   A. primary intention
   B. secondary intention
   C. delayed primary intention
   D. delayed secondary intention
6. Which of the following does not affect wound healing?
   A. age
   B. weight
   C. serum glucose of 450 mg/dL
   D. gender
7. Which of the following would not predispose a patient to developing a wound infection?
   A. susceptible host
   B. compromised wound
   C. infectious organism
   D. low hematocrit
8. A wound is considered to be infected when
   A. pus is present in the wound
   B. organisms elicit a host immune response
   C. the wound is found to be colonized
   D. yellow-green slough is present
9. All of the following are techniques to promote local wound healing EXCEPT
   A. application of a heat lamp
   B. debridement with scissors
   C. irrigation with normal saline
   D. application of dressings
10. A solution used for wound irrigation that aids in mechanical debridement but does not damage granulation tissue is
    A. Betadine (povidone–iodine)
    B. normal saline
    C. acetic acid
    D. hydrogen peroxide
11. A patient has an abdominal wound that is healing by secondary intention. On assessment of this wound, seropurulent drainage is noted from granulating tissue, with some necrotic tissue present. Which type of dressing would you select to remove the debris and necrotic tissue without causing harm to the granulation tissue?
    A. dry sterile dressing
    B. wet-to-dry dressing
    C. synthetic dressing
    D. hydrocolloid dressing
12. Pressure ulcer risk assessments can be made using the
    A. Brazen scale
    B. Braden scale
    C. Newton scale
    D. Norris scale
13. A pressure ulcer is defined as
    A. a sore on the skin over a bony prominence
    B. reactive hyperemia
    C. full-thickness skin loss with damage to muscle
    D. any lesion caused by unrelieved pressure resulting in damage of underlying tissue
14. Management of pressure ulcers may include all of the following EXCEPT
    A. systemic antibiotics
    B. management of tissue loads
    C. debridement
    D. operative repair

Pretest answers: 1. B, 2. D, 3. A, 4. A, 5. B, 6. D, 7. D, 8. C, 9. A, 10. B, 11. B, 12. B, 13. D, 14. A

GLOSSARY

Abrasion. Partial-thickness denudation of skin caused by friction or scraping

Avulsion. Full-thickness skin loss; wound edges cannot be approximated

Contusion. Injury to superficial tissues with disruption of blood vessels with extravasation into the skin

Debridement. Process of removing dead or foreign material from a wound

Dehiscence. The splitting open of wound edges

Delayed primary (tertiary) intention. Method of wound closure that uses a combination of primary and secondary intention

Dermis. Middle layer of skin, referred to as *true skin*

Endogenous. Arising from within the patient

Eschar. Hard, black, dehydrated tissue

Exogenous. Entering from the external environment

Exudate. Fluid produced by wounds

Laceration. Open wound causing incision or abrupt disruption of tissue

Primary intention. Method of wound closure using sutures or tape

Puncture wound. Deep, narrow, open wound resulting from penetrating or sharp objects

Secondary intention. Method of wound closure in which the wound is allowed to heal gradually, using the biologic phases of wound healing to fill in a cavity or defect

Slough. Moist, stringy, thick, yellow tissue that is dying

Susceptible host. Patient with some degree of local or systemic impairment of resistance to bacterial invasion

Wound. An alteration and disruption of the anatomic and physiologic functions of the skin

ABBREVIATIONS

E. coli. *Escherichia coli*

WBC. White blood cell

SECTION ONE: Anatomy and Physiology of the Skin

At the completion of this section, the learner will be able to identify the anatomic structures and physiologic functions of the skin.

The skin is a tough membrane covering the entire body surface. It is the largest organ of the body and is composed of three layers of tissue: the epidermis, the dermis, and the hypodermis or subcutaneous tissue. The epidermis is the outermost layer and contains epithelial cells. The middle layer, often referred to as the *true skin*, is the **dermis.** This layer contains connective tissue and elastic fibers, sensory and motor nerve endings, and a complex network of capillary and lymphatic vessels and muscles. From the dermis arise the appendages of the skin—hair, nails, sebaceous and sweat glands—which then penetrate the epidermis. The dermis lacks exact boundaries and merges with subcutaneous tissues containing blood vessels, nerves, muscle, and adipose tissue. The anatomy of the skin is depicted in Figure 32–1.

The epidermis contains epithelial tissue that is responsible for regeneration of the skin. This tissue is composed of cells that rapidly reproduce and regenerate through the process of epithelialization.

The various components of the dermis provide elements to protect and combat foreign materials and regenerate itself after exposure to the external environment. Connective tissue and elastic fibers provide strength and pliability to protect the internal environment. Nutrients are delivered to and cellular wastes are removed by the blood and lymphatic vessels. Nerve endings present within the dermis respond to cold, heat, touch, pain, and pressure.

The subcutaneous tissues store caloric energy in adipose tissue and assist in regulating the body temperature by acting as insulation, acting as a cushion against external forces, and providing the body with shape and sub-

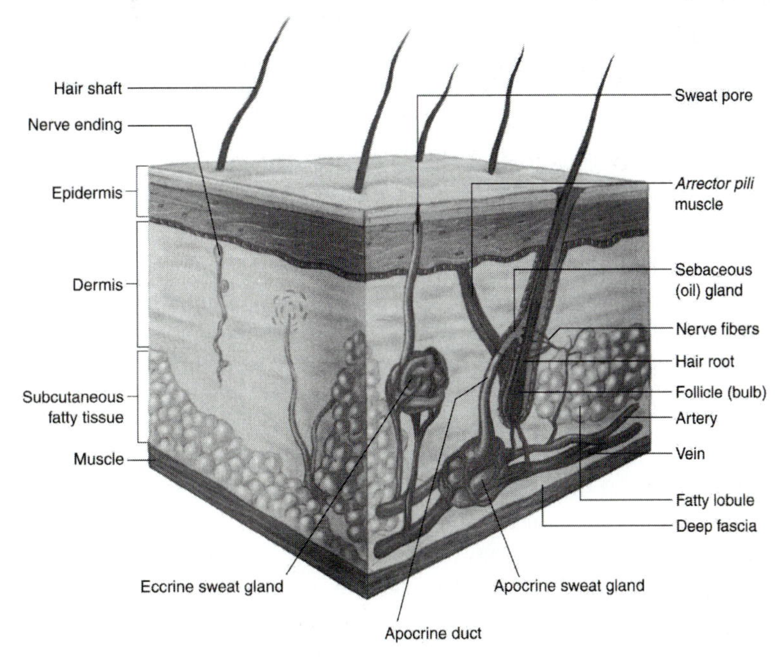

Figure 32–1. Anatomy of the skin. The skin is composed of three layers of tissue: the epidermis, dermis, and hypodermis. *(Reprinted by permission of Prentice Hall.)*

TABLE 32–1. PHYSIOLOGIC FUNCTIONS OF THE SKIN

Protection
Insulation
Sensation
Excretion
Communication
Preservation of internal fluids
Production of vitamin D
Storage for calories
Provision of shape and substance to the body

stance. A summary of the physiologic functions of the skin is shown in Table 32–1.

A **wound** creates an alteration and disruption of the anatomic and physiologic functions of the skin. A wound can be created intentionally, as with a surgeon's knife; by accidental trauma, such as a motor vehicle crash; or by chronic forces, such as in decubitus ulcer formation.

Terms used to describe injuries to the skin include **abrasion, avulsion, contusion, laceration,** and **puncture wound.**

Any wound interrupts the normal skin and tissue integrity and thus the normal physiologic functions of the skin. Healing begins at the moment of injury. The healing process is discussed in Section Two of this module.

In summary, the skin is composed of three layers. The outermost layer is the epidermis, which contains epithelial tissue. This tissue rapidly reproduces when injured through the process of epithelialization. The dermis is the middle layer and contains connective tissue, nerves, blood, and lymphatic vessels. The innermost layer is subcutaneous tissue containing adipose tissue that stores energy, regulates body heat, and acts as a cushion. The skin has more than 10 physiologic functions. A wound results in altered structure and function of the skin.

SECTION ONE REVIEW

1. Which of the following is NOT a layer of the skin?
   A. epithelial tissue
   B. epidermis
   C. dermis
   D. subcutaneous tissue
2. The components of the dermis are
   A. epithelial cells, subcutaneous tissue
   B. adipose tissue, subcutaneous tissue
   C. hair, nails, and sebaceous glands
   D. connective tissue, blood, and lymph vessels
3. The physiologic functions of the skin include
   A. secretion, production of vitamin C
   B. excretion, production of vitamin D
   C. storage of information, communication
   D. regulation of body temperature, storage of vitamin A
4. Wound healing begins
   A. within an hour after injury
   B. within 6 hours after injury
   C. at the moment of injury
   D. within 24 hours of injury

Answers: 1. A, 2. D, 3. B, 4. C

SECTION TWO: Wound Biology

At the completion of this section, the learner will be able to state the three phases of wound healing, describe the events that occur in each phase of wound healing, and define the three methods of wound closure.

A wound disrupts the skin's integrity and its physiologic mechanisms. On injury, the body immediately begins the process of restoring its integrity and the physiologic functions of the skin. A basic understanding of the wound healing process helps to assess, diagnose, plan, and evaluate nursing interventions for the patient with altered skin integrity.

Wound healing is a process that includes an integrated series of physiologic, cellular, and biochemical events that begin at the moment of injury. There are three phases of wound healing: (1) the inflammatory phase, (2) the proliferative phase, and (3) remodeling (Flynn, 1996).

Inflammatory Phase

The inflammatory phase occurs immediately after injury and lasts several days. This is a critical phase because the wound environment is being prepared for subsequent tissue development (Norris, Provo, & Stotts, 1990). The major events that occur in this phase are hemostasis and removal of cellular debris and infectious agents.

Immediately on injury, vascular and cellular events are initiated. Thromboplastin is released from injured cells, activating the clotting cascade. Platelets aggregate at the injury site to form a plug to seal a break in the vessel wall. The platelets also liberate growth factors essential in tissue development during the subsequent phase of healing (platelet derived growth factor, epidermal growth factor, etc.) (Flynn, 1996). A great deal of research currently revolves around the activities of these factors and other cytokines. Once hemostasis is achieved, the blood vessels dilate to bring needed nutrients, chemical, and WBCs to the injured area. WBCs quickly adhere to the endothelium and begin to control any bacterial contamination that has gained entry into the wound. Macrophages appear and begin to engulf and remove dead tissue. The chemical and vascular events that occur during the reaction phase of wound healing produce the four cardinal signs of inflammation: heat, redness, swelling, and pain (Fig. 32–2).

Proliferative Phase

The proliferative phase begins several days after injury and continues for several weeks. Major processes that occur during this phase are focused on building new tissue to fill the wound space. Major events that occur during this phase include epithelialization, collagen formation, granulation tissue formation, and contraction.

Epithelialization involves the migration of epithelial cells across a wound's surface. The cells rapidly undergo mitotic divisions and migrate along fibrin strands to reestablish layers of epithelium in an attempt to cover the defect. A moist environment enhances epithelialization. Epithelial cells cannot spread on a surface laden with debris or bacteria. Therefore, the wound healing process will be inhibited by the presence of debris or bacteria. The process of epithelialization serves to provide a barrier against the external environment and further bacterial invasion.

The proliferative phase provides strength to the healing wound. The dominant cells of this phase are fibroblasts. Fibroblasts produce collagen, the major component of new connective tissue. Fluid collections, hematomas, dead tissue, and foreign materials act as physical barriers to prevent fibroblast penetration. Therefore, removal of these materials is one of the primary goals of wound management (Section Five). The wound space fills with fiber bundles that enlarge and form a dense collagenous structure (the scar) that binds the tissues firmly together.

As the population of fibroblasts decreases, collagen fibers become dominant in the wound. Collagen cross-linking provides tensile strength to the wound. Collagen requires several nutrients and minerals for its synthesis. Thus, the nutritional status of the patient becomes very important during wound healing. This is discussed in greater detail in Section Three.

At the same time that epithelialization is occurring and collagen is forming, the formation of granulation tissue continues. The vascular endothelium proliferates, and a great deal of capillary budding appears. These buds give the new granulation tissue its characteristic pink-red color and appearance. As new granulation tissue fills in the wound, the wound margins begin to contract or pull together, and the surface area of the wound decreases.

Contraction of a wound occurs when the wound margins begin to pull toward the center of the wound to decrease the wound surface area. Shrinkage of the wound progresses from the wound's edges to heal open defects.

Remodeling

Usually, by the third week after a disruption in skin integrity, the wound has closed and the remodeling phase begins. Remodeling is the final repair process. This phase lasts 24 days to up to 2 years. Major events of this final phase include increased collagen reorganization and increased tensile strength. The final product of all the

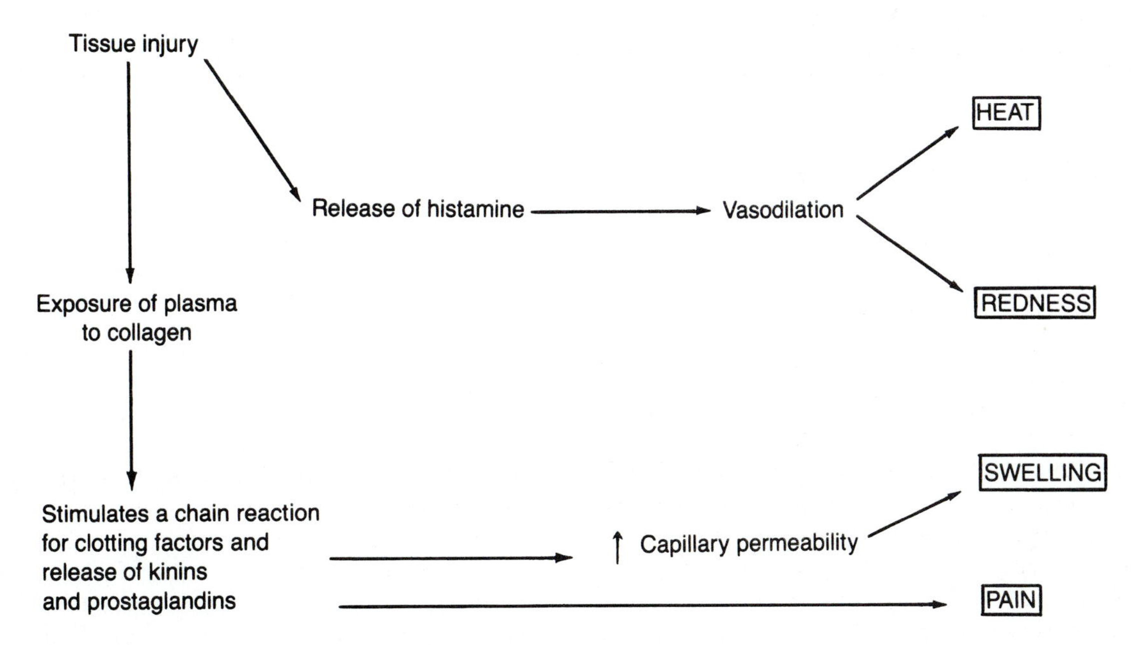

Figure 32–2. Basic inflammatory response to the four cardinal signs of inflammation. The chemical and vascular events that occur during the reaction phase of wound healing produce the four cardinal signs of inflammation.

events that occur during wound healing is the scar, which has covered the defect and restored the protective barrier against the external environment.

Methods of Wound Closure

The rate of wound healing differs depending on the method used to close the wound. The method used depends on the amount of tissue damage/loss and the potential for wound infection. Methods of wound closure include primary intention, secondary intention, and delayed primary intention (tertiary intention) (Fig. 32–3).

Primary intention refers to closing the wound by mechanical means, by either sutures or tape. This method is used when there is minimal tissue loss and skin edges are well approximated. Clean lacerations and most surgical incisions are closed using primary intention. The inflammatory phase resolves immediately, the proliferative phase is minimal, and the remodeling phase is complete with a thin scar.

Wounds that heal by **secondary intention** usually are large wounds in which there is significant tissue loss, damage, or bacterial contamination. These wound cavities heal gradually and use the biologic phases of wound healing to fill in the cavity or defect. Wounds healing by secondary intention include open abdominal wounds, dehisced sternal wounds, and stage III and IV pressure ulcers. These wounds require significantly more time to heal than do wounds healing by primary intention.

Tertiary intention (or **delayed primary intention**) is a method of wound closure that uses a combination of primary and secondary intention. The wound is left open for a short period of time, usually a few days, to allow edema and exudate to resolve. The wound is packed with dressings that are changed to remove any debris and is closed later by primary intention.

The expected outcome of the wound healing process is restoration of the skin and tissue integrity and its physiologic functions. The wound healing process depends on various factors that affect the efficiency and effectiveness of all events in the process. The next section discusses these factors.

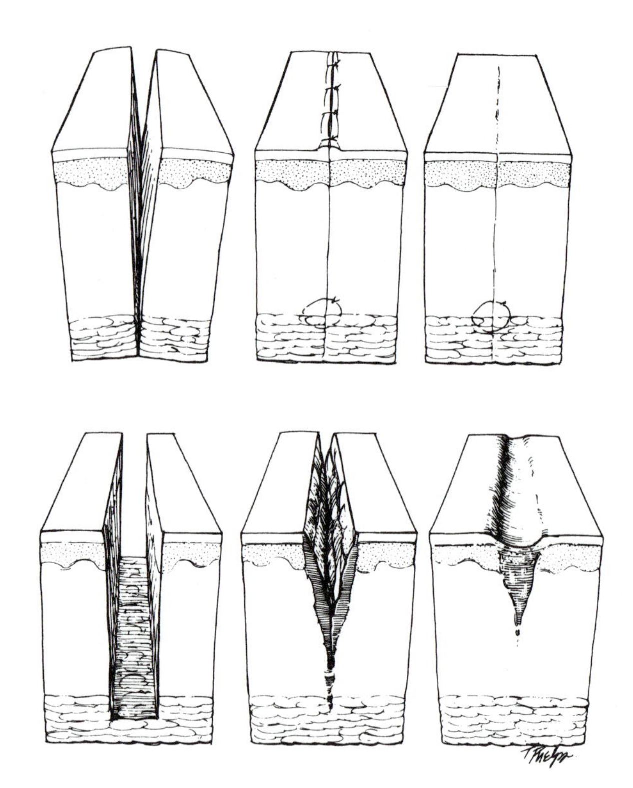

Figure 32–3. Methods of wound closure. Two methods of wound closure include primary intention **(A)** and secondary intention **(B)**. *(From Cardona, V.T., et al. [eds]. [1988].* Trauma nursing: From resuscitation through rehabilitation *[p. 275]. Philadelphia: W.B. Saunders.)*

In summary, wound healing is a complex process of events that begin at the moment of injury and continues for years after injury. There are three phases of wound healing. The first is the inflammatory phase, which lasts a few days. Hemostasis and removal of cellular debris and infectious agents are the goals of this phase. The second phase, which lasts several days, is the proliferative phase. Major events in this phase include epithelialization, collagen formation, formation of granulation tissue, and wound contraction. The final phase of wound healing, the remodeling phase, can last up to 2 years. During the final phase, collagen reorganization and increased tensile strength of the scar occur. The three methods of wound closure are primary, secondary, and tertiary intention. The rate of wound healing differs depending on the method used to close the wound. An understanding of the wound healing process helps to assess, diagnose, plan, and evaluate nursing interventions to facilitate the wound healing process.

SECTION TWO REVIEW

1. Heat, redness, swelling, and pain occur during which of the following phases of wound healing?

A. remodeling
B. contraction
C. proliferative
D. inflammatory

2. Epithelialization
   A. is enhanced by a moist environment
   B. is enhanced by a dry, sterile environment
   C. occurs to remove debris
   D. spreads on surfaces laden with debris
3. Fluid collections, hematomas, and dead tissue act as
   A. scaffolds for fibroblast proliferation
   B. barriers for fibroblast proliferation
   C. protective covers for new epithelial cells
   D. a moist environment to enhance epithelialization
4. An incision for a cholecystectomy usually would be allowed to heal by
   A. tertiary intention
   B. secondary intention
   C. primary intention
   D. delayed secondary intention
5. Delayed primary (tertiary) intention allows
   A. immediate resolution of the inflammatory phase
   B. edema and exudate to resolve
   C. gradual healing of the wound
   D. reorganization and cell differentiation for remodeling

Answers: 1. D, 2. A, 3. B, 4. C, 5. B

SECTION THREE: Factors That Affect Wound Healing

At the completion of this section, the learner will be able to state physiologic and environmental factors that affect wound healing.

Critically ill patients experience many risk factors that increase their vulnerability for wound complications. These include impaired oxygenation, nutritional status, age, preexisting disease, medications, and obesity. These risk factors increase the acutely ill patient's risk of delayed wound healing, development of wound infections, and wound dehiscence. It is a nursing challenge to provide the optimal environment that supports the patient's wound healing process.

Oxygenation/Tissue Perfusion

Many drugs and treatments have been investigated to accelerate healing. However, perfusion of injured tissue with well-oxygenated blood may be most important. A decrease in available oxygen to wounded tissues produces three major effects: (1) decrease in fibroblast reproduction rate, (2) decrease in the rate of epithelial cell reproduction, and (3) decrease in the rate of collagen synthesis and subsequently wound tensile strength (Norris, Provo, & Stotts, 1990). Many conditions can interfere with the delivery of oxygen to the wound (e.g., thrombosis, radiation, obesity, diabetes, cardiovascular disease, cigarette smoking, hypotension, hypothermia, and administration of vasoactive drugs). Significant blood loss, as frequently occurs in traumatically injured patients, results in hypovolemia, hypotension, and decreased tissue perfusion. Edema in the area of the wound may increase the diffusion distance between the capillary beds and the wound, causing a decrease in the delivery of oxygen and other nutrients to the wound (Flynn, 1996).

Nutrition

Adequate nutrition is a critical factor predisposing the acutely ill patient to immunocompetence and poor wound healing. It is essential to ensure that patients with wounds receive adequate nutritional support.

Metabolic processes involved in wound healing rely heavily on adequate nutritional substances. Physiologic and psychological stress, traumatic injury, and fever further increase the basal metabolic rate, demanding adequate nutritional reserves. Because of these demands, malnutrition in the critically ill patient is not uncommon. A sufficient amount of protein is one of the most important nutritional substances for wound healing. Protein is required for collagen synthesis, immune responses, formation of granulation tissue, and fibroblast proliferation. Glycolysis contributes the majority of the energy needed for restoring tissue integrity and fighting infection. Fats serve as building blocks for prostaglandins, which regulate cell metabolism, inflammation, and circulation. Vitamins and trace elements are necessary for numerous events in the tissue healing and rebuilding process.

Age

Aging affects almost every stage of wound healing and the wound healing process is markedly slower. In addition to the physiologic effects of aging, the elderly are more likely to have nutritional deficiencies and pulmonary or cardiovascular diseases that further diminish local oxygenation to wounds and immunologic resistance.

Diabetes

Wound healing in the patient with diabetes is compromised due to macrovascular and microvascular changes, poor glycemic control, and loss of sensation. These disease-associated changes result in impaired oxygenation and perfusion, slowed epithelialization and wound contraction, and impaired phagocytosis.

Medications

Steroid therapy, used to block the inflammatory component of many diseases, has a well known inhibitory effect on wound healing. Decreased protein synthesis, delayed development of granulation tissue, inhibition of fibroblast proliferation, and reduced epithelialization are effects of steroid administration. In addition, inhibition of the inflammatory response and the immunosuppressive actions of steroids make the patient more susceptible to developing a wound infection. Other medications that interfere with wound healing include chemotherapeutic agents, immunosuppressive drugs, and anticoagulants.

Obesity

The obese patient (weight > 20 percent ideal body weight) experiences an increased incidence of **dehiscence,** herniation, and infection (Flynn, 1996). Adipose tissue is poorly vascularized, which increases the risk of ischemia. Adipose tissue is difficult to suture, which makes the obese patient at risk to develop a wound dehiscence. A binder or split (pillow) to the incision can provide support during straining or coughing and take excess tension off the incision.

Blood Chemistries

Normal serum electrolytes enhance wound repair. Potassium is necessary for building proteins for wound repair. Phagocytosis is inhibited by elevated sodium and glucose levels. Oxygen is released more rapidly from oxyhemoglobin in slightly acidic environments. Wounds may heal more effectively in this type of local environment.

Moisture

The rate of epithelialization is enhanced in a moist, not dry, local wound environment. A wound bed is kept moist through the use of appropriate dressings. Ideally, the dressing will keep the wound surface moist without accumulation of excessive fluids that macerate the skin and allow bacterial proliferation (Makelbust, 1996).

Antibiotics and Infection

Traumatic wounds tend to be contaminated by the external environment. The administration of antibiotics greatly affects the outcome of healing. These two factors are so important to wound healing that they are discussed in greater detail in Section Four.

In summary, there are no medications or treatments to accelerate wound healing. There are conditions and factors known to affect the wound healing process. Perfusion of well-oxygenated blood to the wound is considered to be the most important factor affecting wound healing. It is important for the nurse to assess patients for any factor that may affect wound healing. Appropriate plans and nursing interventions must be instituted to manipulate as many variables as possible to promote efficient and effective wound healing.

SECTION THREE REVIEW

1. Small-vessel changes occur that impair tissue perfusion/ oxygenation with
   A. malnutrition
   B. elevated sodium levels
   C. diabetes
   D. steroid therapy
2. The most important nutritional substance for wound healing is
   A. glucose
   B. fat
   C. vitamins
   D. protein
3. Which of the following is NOT an effect of steroid therapy on wound healing?
   A. decreased protein synthesis
   B. proliferation of fibroblasts
   C. delayed development of granulation tissue
   D. reduced epithelialization
4. The most important factor that affects wound healing is
   A. preventing infection
   B. total parenteral nutrition
   C. perfusion of injured tissues with well-oxygenated blood
   D. potassium replacements
5. A moist wound environment
   A. enhances epithelialization
   B. macerates the skin
   C. promotes bacterial proliferation
   D. impedes epithelialization

Answers: 1. C, 2. D, 3. B, 4. C, 5. A

SECTION FOUR: Etiology, Diagnosis, and Prevention of Wound Infections

At the completion of this section, the learner will be able to identify conditions that predispose a patient to develop a wound infection, identify criteria used to diagnose a wound as being infected, and describe interventions that may be used in preventing and treating wound infections.

Infection is a common and very effective deterrent to effective wound healing. Any disruption of, or compromise to, the skin's integrity can result in infection, including physical trauma, operative and invasive procedures, and inadequate tissue perfusion. A wound infection develops when the body's defense mechanisms cannot eliminate the bacteria contaminating the wound or prevent further bacterial growth. Three elements predispose the patient to developing a wound infection: (1) a susceptible host, (2) a compromised wound, and (3) an infectious organism.

Susceptible Host

One of the major determinants of a subsequent infection after surgery or trauma is the patient's own ability to use defense mechanisms to resist the threat of infection. The patient who is a **susceptible host** has some degree of local or systemic impairment of resistance to bacterial invasion. Local impairment may be due to dead, foreign material or hematomas directly in the wound or some interference in blood supply to the area as a result of vascular disease. Systemic impairment of the patient's resistance may include diabetes, acute or chronic use of steroids, renal disease, malnutrition, cardiovascular disease, extremes of age, obesity, cancer, or the use of immunosuppressive therapies. These patients usually have some impairment in the acute inflammatory response or phagocytic mechanisms. Any patient with altered skin integrity has lost the major mechanical barrier blocking invasion by pathologic organisms and thus is a susceptible host.

Compromised Wound

A compromised wound is one that contains devitalized tissue. Devitalized tissue is tissue that has been separated from the circulation and the body's antimicrobial defenses. Bacteria proliferate on wounds that contain dead tissue, hematomas, or foreign material. Debridement of these materials is essential to prevent an environment conducive to bacterial growth.

Infectious Organism

Bacteria can contaminate any wound. Many different organisms are capable of initiating a wound infection. Organisms come from endogenous or exogenous sources. **Endogenous** sources arise from within the patient. Many organisms exist on and in the human body—on the skin, in the respiratory tract, and in the gastrointestinal and genitourinary tracts. Organisms in these areas are not pathogenic until they are released from their normal inhabitant sites and allowed to proliferate in a sterile area of the body. **Exogenous** organisms enter the body from the external environment when the skin barrier has been broken. The external environment may be the accident scene (for trauma patients) or the health care setting.

Infection

A differentiation in wound bacterial colonization and infection is necessary. Colonization of wounds refers to a large number of organisms loosely attached to devitalized tissue, but there is no movement of bacteria into viable tissue and no host immune response (Flynn, 1996). Infection is defined as the process by which organisms bind to tissue, multiply, invade viable tissue, and elicit a host immune response (Flynn, 1996). Wound infection alters all three phases of wound healing.

Diagnosis of Wound Infections

Wound infections range from superficial cases of cellulitis to deep-seated abscesses. A wound infection is suspected if the four cardinal signs of inflammation (heat, redness, swelling, and pain) exist at the wound site, along with an elevated WBC count and fever. However, many conditions may cause these symptoms, including the inflammatory phase of wound healing. In addition, drainage from a wound does not mean it is infected. The patient's overall condition and a positive wound culture are more definitive criteria to evaluate a wound for infection. Any drainage from a wound must be sent to the laboratory for culture and sensitivity testing and Gram stain. The culture and sensitivity testing will identify the specific organisms in the wound and antibiotic sensitivity of the organisms. The Gram stain characterizes the nature of the drainage and provides a rapid best guess as to the identity of the organism (gram-positive or gram-negative). The culture and sensitivity testing takes 24 to 72 hours for results, which are very reliable and specific. The Gram stain takes only several hours, but the results are not as specific.

Bacterial organisms contaminating wounds must be sensitive to the antibiotic administered. However, as previously stated, it may take up to 3 days to obtain this information. Thus, a knowledge of the likely wound contaminants and their established sensitivities is helpful in instituting prompt treatment. For example, organisms in the colon that have leaked into the peritoneum and are likely to cause infections in wounds in the abdomen are anaerobic organisms (*Bacteroides*, *Clostridium*, *Escherichia coli*), which respond to aminoglycosides.

Wound infections may not be apparent for several days postoperatively or after traumatic injury. When a wound infection is suspected, prompt and appropriate treatment should be instituted.

Prevention of Wound Infections

One of the greatest priorities in wound care is prevention of infection. Prevention of wound infections begins with recognition of the three elements that predispose the patient to a wound infection (susceptible host, compromised wound, infectious organism).

For elective surgical procedures, prevention begins preoperatively through skin preparation, mechanical and antibiotic bowel preparations, prophylactic administration of antibiotics, and sterile operative site draping. Intraoperatively, careful surgical technique minimizes injury, and aseptic technique prevents endogenous and exogenous sources of bacterial contamination.

For traumatically injured wounds, resuscitation and lifesaving measures often take priority over immediate treatment of wounds. Once the resuscitative phase is completed, prompt and proper management of the wounds decreases the likelihood of subsequent infection. It is not uncommon for traumatically incurred wounds to be filled with dirt, grass, glass, twigs, leaves, knives, bullets, or stool. Management of these wounds begins with cleansing of the wounds using high-pressure irrigation and debridement to remove bacteria and foreign debris from the wounds.

The importance of hand washing to prevent the transmission of infectious organisms was determined over a century ago. Hand washing is still considered one of the most important methods to prevent wound infections. This is especially important in critical care settings where susceptible hosts, compromised wounds, and infectious organisms are in close proximity to each other.

In summary, it is imperative that the nurse recognize the importance of nursing's role in preventing wound infections and preventing further bacterial proliferation in already infected wounds. Nursing plans and interventions should optimize the environment to promote wound healing. Each patient must be assessed as a susceptible host for pathogenic organisms, and interventions must be instituted to promote and safeguard the patient's ability to resist infection. Astute nursing assessments can identify a compromised wound. Measures can be taken to prevent the wound from being an ideal environment for bacterial invasion and proliferation. Plans for prophylactic interventions to reduce the infective risk can be made. Ongoing nursing assessments can detect signs of infection so that prompt and appropriate treatment can be instituted.

SECTION FOUR REVIEW

1. Which of the following would NOT predispose to the development of a wound infection?
   A. susceptible host
   B. exogenous organisms
   C. compromised wound
   D. infectious organism
2. Local impairment of resistance to bacterial invasion may be due to
   A. foreign material
   B. malnutrition
   C. cancer
   D. immunosuppressive drugs
3. Organisms from endogenous sources come from
   A. debris in the wound
   B. the accident scene
   C. the gastrointestinal tract
   D. the hospital setting
4. All of the following conditions must be present for a wound to be infected EXCEPT
   A. purulent drainage from a wound
   B. culture and sensitivity testing
   C. the four cardinal signs of inflammation
   D. temperature of 103°F

Answers: 1. B, 2. A, 3. C, 4. B

SECTION FIVE: Principles of Wound Management

The purpose of this section is to assist the learner in understanding treatment modalities and principles of wound management. At the completion of this section, the learner will be able to state the rationale for wound irrigation, debridement, and dressing changes and identify tube and drain placement and their indications for use in wound management.

Nursing has a major influence on the outcome of wound healing. Nurses have the opportunity to favorably manipulate certain environmental factors that promote wound healing (Makelbust, 1996). This includes local wound care, which includes irrigation, debridement, and selection of appropriate wound dressing materials.

Irrigation

The purpose of irrigating a wound is to remove debris and bacterial contamination by the pressure in a stream of fluid. The wound should be irrigated with a solution under pressure. It is not the volume of the solution used but the pressure exerted that removes debris and bacteria. Solution in a 30-mL syringe with a 19-gauge angiocath or needle can accomplish this. Wound irrigation with a bulb syringe or red rubber catheter is considered low-pressure irrigation, which is ineffective in removing foreign material (Makelbust, 1996). Irrigation can remove enough bacteria to cross the threshold to ineffective levels.

Normal saline is the most common solution used for wound irrigation. Antiseptic solutions (hydrogen peroxide, povidone–iodine) are controversial and may be cytotoxic and harmful to tissues (Makelbust, 1996). It is recommended that only physiologic agents, such as saline, be used so that tissue defenses are not suppressed by toxic agents (Bergstrom et al., 1994).

Debridement

Debridement is important to healing because the presence of foreign material fosters bacterial growth and inhibits formation of granulation tissue. Wound healing cannot take place until nonviable tissue is removed. Various methods of debridement exist: sharp, mechanical, chemical, and autolytic (Makelbust, 1996). Sharp debridment is the removal of necrotic areas using a scapel or scissors. This is usually done with a physician's order. Mechanical debridement is accomplished with moist dressing changes, irrigation, or whirlpool. Chemical debridement involves the use of topical enzymes that are applied to necrotic areas. Autolytic debridement involves the use of dressing materials (hydrocolloid wafer, Carrington gel gauze, etc.). When applied, these dressings allow endogenous enzymes in the wound to selectively liquefy necrotic tissue. Clinicians should select a debridement method most appropriate to the type of wound, the amount of necrotic tissue, the condition of the patient, the setting, and the clinician and the caregiver's experience (Makelbust, 1996).

Dressings

Dressings are placed over wounds for multiple purposes: debridement; protection from the external environment; provision of a physiologic environment conducive to wound healing; and to provide immobilization, support, comfort, information regarding quality and quantity of drainage, pressure, and absorption. The goal of using dressings in wound management is to provide a moist environment at the wound surface to optimize wound healing, prevent infection, and control wound drainage.

The purpose of the dressing and condition of the wound bed should determine the type of dressing used. As a wound changes, the dressing care should be modified. It is essential that the nurse reassess the patient's wound throughout the wound healing process to evaluate the effectiveness of the wound management plan.

Specific types of dressings and their care are summarized in Table 32–2. Wounds healing by primary intention require dressings that absorb exudate and protect the wound from trauma and contamination. Dry, sterile gauze dressings remain the gold standard for wounds healing by primary intention. The length of time a dressing is required for wounds healing by primary intention varies greatly (usually less than 3 days), although research demonstrates that wounds healing by primary intention are sealed within 72 hours after surgery in healthy patients.

Wounds healing by secondary or tertiary intention require dressing materials to provide a warm, moist, local wound environment conducive to wound healing, to debride necrotic tissue, to absorb exudate, and to protect the wound from further trauma and contamination. As noted in Table 32–3, a variety of dressings can be used, including alginates, hydrocolloids, and traditional moist gauze dressings. Solutions frequently used when dressing wounds are also listed in Table 32–3.

A broad assortment of additional interventions can be used with wound management, including electrical stimulation, ultrasound, pressure-relieving devices, nutritional support, hydrotherapy, and mattress overlays. Further research is needed to explore these interventions and their impact on patient outcomes.

Tubes and Drains

Various surgical tubes and drains are used whenever there is an actual or potential accumulation of fluid in naturally occurring or surgically created spaces. Drainage tubes can

TABLE 32–2. WOUND DRESSINGS

TYPE	INDICATION	CONSIDERATIONS
Wet-to-dry gauze		
Put on wet and remove dry	Use with wounds healing by secondary intention	No solution should be visibly dripping from the dressing as it is placed into the wound; this retards wound closure, increases bacteria, and macerates periwound skin
	Removes debris and necrotic materials from wounds; use as a debriding alternative for yellow wounds	Gauze touching wound surfaces should be a single layer; wounds with large amounts of exudate should be dressed with gauze with large interstices; as exudate decreases, gauze with small interstices should be used
	Provides moist wound environment	If gauze is removed too dry, newly formed granulation tissue may be disrupted
Wet-to-damp gauze		
Put on moist and remove moist	Use with wound healing by secondary intention	As above
	Use for mechanical debridement of red or yellow wounds	Packing material is soaked in a solution, wrung out until moist, and packed into the wound
	Provides moist wound environment	If packing sticks to tissue as it is removed, wet the packing with normal saline before removing it; this will preserve regenerating tissue
		Continuous moist dressings can be used for protection of red wounds, delivery of topical medications, or for autolytic debridement of yellow or black wounds
Dry dressings		
Put on dry and remove dry	Used with wounds healing by primary intention	Carefully remove the dressing so that the incision does not reopen
	Protects the wound during epithelialization	
	Can be used with heavily exudating red wounds	
Polyurethane films	Cutaneous wounds	Do not use with draining or infected wounds
	Minor burns	Change only if dressing leaks
	Abrasions	
	Donor sites	
	Protects partial-thickness red wounds	
Hydrocolloid	Protects granulation and epithelial tissue	Gellike substance becomes puslike in appearance and may even become odiferous; this should not become confused with the development of a wound infection
	Autolytic debridement of small, noninfected yellow wounds	Is water resistant and can adhere to uneven surfaces
		Do not use on documented or suspected infected wounds
		Change when it leaks or becomes dislodged
Alginates	Use on moderate to heavily exudating wounds	Alginates absorb secretions to form a gel that provides humidity and temperature conducive to wound healing
	Best suited for flat wounds	Use gentle irrigation with normal saline to remove the dressing

be classified into one of three categories: simple drains, closed suction drains, or sump drains (Amato, 1982). The categories and uses of drainage tubes are summarized in Table 32–4.

It is the nurse's responsibility to maintain the security, integrity, and patency of all tubes and drains.

In summary, nursing has a major influence on the outcome of wound healing through assessing the effectiveness of the wound management regimen. A wound management regimen may include debridement, irrigation, dressing changes, and placement of tubes and drains. Dressings are used in wound management for a multitude of purposes. The method of wound closure plays a large role in determining the type of dressing to be used in the regimen. Consideration must be made as to the solution to be used to irrigate, debride, or dress the wound. Various tubes and drains are used in wound management whenever there is an actual or potential accumulation of fluid.

TABLE 32–3. SOLUTIONS FOR WET-TO-DRY OR WET-TO-MOIST DRESSINGS

Normal saline	Most commonly used solution Aids in mechanical debridement Does not damage granulation tissue
Acetic acid	Used to treat *Pseudomonas* infections
Dakin's solution	Chlorine bleach compound; use in a weak solution Antiseptic that slightly dissolves necrotic tissue Can be used in dirty, malodorous wounds Can inhibit growth of granulation tissue
Betadine	Antiseptic that kills bacteria and fungi Used to pack dirty or infected wounds May damage granulation tissue and irritate periwound skin Use in diluted concentrations
Antibiotic solutions	Antibiotics in a solution that are applied topically Commonly used solutions are neomycin or bacitracin

TABLE 32–4. CATEGORIES AND USES OF DRAINAGE TUBES

CATEGORY	PURPOSE	EXAMPLES
Simple drains	Provide pathway to allow fluid to drain by gravity	Penrose, T-tube, gastrostomy tube, jejunostomy tube
Closed suction drains	Collapsible device attached to tube creates a negative pressure, allowing for continual removal of fluids	Jackson Pratt, Hemovac, Davol
Sump drains	Double-lumen drains; air enters drainage area and breaks the vacuum, displacing air and fluid into the outflow lumen; used in conjunction with wall suction	Salem Sump, Shirley Sump, Axion

Section Five Review

1. What size syringe would you select to irrigate a wound?
   A. 30-mL
   B. 50-mL
   C. 60-mL
   D. 100-mL
2. What type of dressing would be indicated to cover a wound healing by primary intention?
   A. dry
   B. wet-to-wet
   C. wet-to-dry
   D. polyurethane
3. The layer next to the wound in wet-to-dry dressings
   A. should adhere to the wound to prevent disruption of epithelial layers
   B. provides protection and strength in immobilizing the wound
   C. debrides the wound
   D. should be put on wet so the wound remains soupy
4. A solution used to treat *Pseudomonas* wound infections is
   A. Dakin's solution
   B. acetic acid
   C. Betadine (povidone–iodine)
   D. half-strength hydrogen peroxide
5. An example of a closed suction drain would be
   A. gastrostomy tube
   B. Salem Sump
   C. Penrose
   D. Hemovac

Answers: 1. A, 2. A, 3. C, 4. B, 5. D

SECTION SIX: Clinical Assessment of Wound Healing

At the completion of this section, the learner will be able to identify the common clinical assessments to evaluate wound healing.

In assessing wound healing, it is important to assess the patient's preexisting health problems, perform a physical assessment of the wound using inspection and palpation, and collect and evaluate objective data to assess the patient's tissue perfusion/oxygenation, immunologic, and nutritional status. Systematic assessment and comprehensive evaluation of both patient and wound provide a consistent method for assessing wound healing.

Preexisting Health Problems

In collecting the initial nursing database, it is important to assess the patient for diseases, conditions, and medications or treatments that may impair the healing process. This will assist in identifying patients at risk for delayed wound healing. It is important to assess for conditions that alter tissue perfusion/oxygenation and impair the body's resistance to infection.

Inspection

Wounds, suture lines, casts, pins, and surrounding skin integrity should be inspected for signs of infection, breakdown, and irritation. Inspect wounds to assess and evaluate the healing process and the effectiveness of wound care. Inspection should include at least the following components.

Measurement of the Wound

Measure and record the length, width, and depth of the wound. A diagram should be made in the nursing care plan for ongoing comparison of the healing process. The amount and depth of tissue loss and tunneling should be assessed, because this greatly influences the choice of treatment for wound management. Depth can be determined by inserting a sterile, cotton-tipped applicator into the deepest part of the wound and grasping the applicator where it meets the wound's edge. Irregular wound beds are difficult to measure accurately, so it is important to take measurements of depth and length from the same point each time. The same method of measurement should be used each time, with a consistent approach to documentation of such information.

Presence of Exudate or Drainage

Estimating the amount of blood and fluid loss allows for appropriate fluid and electrolyte replacement. The fluid produced by wounds is called **exudate,** which can consist of blood, serum, serosanguineous fluid, and leukocytes. Exudate bathes the wound continuously, keeping it moist, supplying nutrients, and providing the best conditions for migration and mitosis of epithelial cells and control of bacteria at the wound surface. Documentation of all wound drainage should include color, amount, consistency, and odor. Inspect the wound dressing as it is removed from the wound. If the dressing is too dry, reevaluate how moist the packing was at the time of insertion or increase the frequency of dressing changes.

Appearance of Wound Tissue

Wound color depends on the balance between granulation and necrotic tissue. Healing wounds should be pink or red, characteristic of granulation tissue. In the presence of moisture and bacteria, exudate and devitalized tissue are yellow or cream-colored and puslike in consistency (Cuzzell, 1990). This is **slough** tissue. Black or dark-brown color indicates the presence of **eschar,** which is thick, nonpliable necrotic tissue. Slough and necrotic tissue have a negative effect on wound healing because they prevent granulation and epithelialization. The ideal local wound environment should be free from slough and eschar and be moist with red-pink budding granulation tissue.

Inspection of Wound Edges

Inspect the wound for contraction (gradual healing from the edges to the center of the wound), and assess for gradual healing from the interior to the surfaces of deep wounds. Wound margins should not be erythematous or tender.

Skin Color

Using a bright light, observe the surrounding tissues for color. Compare the color with similar, uninjured areas. Distinguish erythema from ecchymosis by blanching the area. Areas of erythema will blanch, but areas of ecchymosis will not.

Palpation

Palpation of the wound and surrounding areas will assist in recognizing changes in size, consistency, moisture, and texture. To assess circulation into and from the wound, assess the proximal and distal pulses by palpation or by Doppler (auditory pulse). Proximal pulses demonstrate adequate circulation to the area. Distal pulses indicate that the wound is not interfering with distal circulation. Capillary refill time should be assessed and compared to the norm of < 2 seconds. Compare the skin temperature bilaterally. Sensorimotor assessment distal to the wound can be done by testing for discrimination between sharp and dull.

Assessment of Tissue Perfusion/Oxygenation

Adequate tissue perfusion/oxygenation is one of the most important factors to assess for in wound healing. Local and systemic factors that alter tissue perfusion and oxygenation should be assessed. Necrotic areas, debris, and foreign materials in the wound do not allow adequate local tissue perfusion/oxygenation. Adequate systemic tissue perfusion/oxygenation is dependent on a full blood volume, adequate arterial oxygen content, and an adequate cardiac output. Tissue perfusion/oxygenation can be assessed using invasive and noninvasive techniques. Noninvasive techniques include transcutaneous oximetry, assessment of capillary refill, skin temperature, and the presence of proximal and distal pulses around the wound. Invasive techniques may include hemodynamic readings, such as central venous pressure, cardiac output/cardiac index, arterial blood pressure, mean arterial pressure, pulmonary artery wedge pressure, and systemic vascular resistance. In addition, serum blood tests, including hematocrit and hemoglobin levels, should be monitored and assessed.

Assessment of Immunologic Status

An intact immunologic response to injury, regardless of the cause of injury, is a key factor in proper wound healing. The patient should be assessed for the three elements that predispose the patient to a wound infection: susceptible host, compromised wound, and infectious organism. Factors that cause local and systemic resistance of infection (Section Four) should be assessed. Compromised wounds containing devitalized tissue, hematomas, and debris should be debrided to prevent an environment conducive to bacterial proliferation. The patient should be assessed for sources of pathogenic organisms.

Assessment of immunologic status should include WBC, fibrinogen, body temperature, wound cultures, and serum antimicrobial levels.

The inflammatory phase of wound healing releases WBCs. It is not uncommon for patients with wounds to have elevated WBC counts during the initial phase of wound healing. Elevated WBCs in later phases of wound healing are more indicative of an infectious process.

Neutrophils are the primary cells involved in phagocytosis. Elevated neutrophil counts are indicative of an acute infection as mature and immature neutrophils are released in response to an increased need for phagocytosis. Neutrophils are essential in the presence of infection if wound healing is to occur.

Adequate amounts of fibrinogen are needed to convert to fibrin. This aids in localizing the infectious process by providing a matrix for phagocytosis.

Increased body temperature, regulated by the hypothalamic thermoregulatory system, is triggered by microorganisms, bacterial toxins and antigens, and the inflammatory process. Since fever is a manifestation of the inflammatory process and the infectious process, it is important to assess the patient's overall clinical picture for etiologic factors of the fever. Patients in a hypothermic state experience decreased tissue perfusion/oxygenation and decreased leukocyte activity.

Wounds suspected as being infected should be sampled, and the samples of wound tissue should be sent to the laboratory for Gram stain and culture and sensitivity testing. The nurse should be aware of all culture results.

Monitoring concentrations of antimicrobial agents in the blood can confirm therapeutic drug levels and determine toxicity. The best assessment of this can be made by drawing serum peak and trough samples, depending on the antimicrobial administered. The nurse must be aware of these protocols so that accurate therapeutic concentrations and toxicity can be assessed.

Assessment of Nutritional Status

The metabolic processes involved in wound healing rely on an adequate nutritional supply. Malnutrition affects the patient's ability to defend against pathogenic microorganisms. A complete and thorough nutritional assessment for all patients with altered skin and tissue integrity should be made. Nutritional assessment is discussed in detail in Module 22.

In summary, when assessing wound healing, it is important to assess the patient's preexisting health problems, oxygenation/perfusion, nutrition status, and immunologic status and to perform a physical assessment of the wound.

Section Six Review

1. In assessing wound healing, it is important to assess the patient's
   - A. past medical history
   - B. renal status
   - C. mental status
   - D. fluid and electrolyte balance
2. Physical examination of all wounds includes all of the following EXCEPT
   - A. inspection
   - B. palpation
   - C. auscultation
   - D. documentation
3. A noninvasive technique to assess tissue perfusion would be
   - A. mean arterial pressure
   - B. presence of proximal/distal pulses
   - C. systemic vascular resistance
   - D. hemoglobin levels
4. In early phases of wound healing, it is not uncommon for white blood cell counts to be
   - A. 10,000 to 20,000/mL
   - B. 20,000 to 40,000/mL
   - C. 5,000 to 10,000/mL
   - D. 40,000 to 50,000/mL
5. If a wound is suspected as being infected
   - A. the WBC and core temperature will be high
   - B. there will be exudate in the wound
   - C. antimicrobial levels should be drawn
   - D. wound cultures should be taken

Answers: 1. A, 2. C, 3. B, 4. B, 5. D

SECTION SEVEN: Pressure Ulcers: Prediction and Prevention

At the completion of this section, the learner will be able to identify patients at risk for pressure ulcer development and to describe interventions for the prevention of pressure ulcers.

Staging of Pressure Ulcers

The Panel for the Prediction and Prevention of Pressure Ulcers in Adults (1992) defined pressure ulcer as "any lesion caused by unrelieved pressure resulting in damage of underlying tissue." Pressure ulcers most frequently occur over bony prominences and are staged to classify the degree of tissue damage observed. The staging of pressure ulcers as defined by the Panel for the Prediction and Prevention of Pressure Ulcers in Adults (1992) is summarized in Table 32–5. Three important assessment limitations must be considered during the staging of pressure ulcers:

1. For patients with darkly pigmented skin, identification of stage I pressure ulcers may be difficult.
2. When eschar is present in a pressure ulcer, staging is not possible. Accurate staging cannot be made until the eschar has sloughed or the wound has been debrided.
3. It may be difficult to assess patients with orthopedic devices (casts) or support hose. Nursing assessments may fail to detect pressure ulcers. For patients with these devices, assess the skin under the edges of casts, determine whether casts should be altered to relieve pressure, remove support stockings to assess skin conditions, and be alert to patient complaints of pressure-induced pain.

TABLE 32–5. STAGING OF PRESSURE ULCERS

Stage I	Nonblanchable erythema of intact skin; the heralding lesion of skin ulceration. *Note:* Reactive hyperemia can normally be expected to be present for one half to three quarters as long as the pressure occluded blood flow to the area. This should not be confused with a stage I pressure ulcer.
Stage II	Partial-thickness skin loss involving epidermis and/or dermis. The ulcer is superficial and presents clinically as an abrasion, blister, or shallow crater.
Stage III	Full-thickness skin loss involving damage or necrosis of subcutaneous tissue that may extend down to, but not through, underlying fascia. The ulcer presents clinically as a deep crater with or without undermining of adjacent tissue.
Stage IV	Full-thickness skin loss with extensive destruction, tissue necrosis, or damage to muscle, bone, or supporting structures (e.g., tendon or joint capsule). *Note:* Undermining and sinus tracts may also be associated with stage IV pressure ulcers.

Risk Assessment Tools and Risk Factors

Acutely ill patients are at high risk for developing a pressure ulcer because they have decreased activity and are immobile due to surgical and diagnostic procedures, and the need to maintain various catheters (Boynton & Paustian, 1996). These risk factors are compounded in the face of altered sensation due to neurologic dysfunction or administration of drugs (sedatives, neuromuscular blocking agents, etc.).

Patients should be assessed for factors that increase the risk for developing pressure ulcers. These factors include immobility, incontinence, nutritional factors (inadequate dietary intake or impaired nutritional status), and altered level of consciousness. Patient risk factors should be assessed using a validated risk assessment tool such as the Braden Scale (Braden, 1989) or the Norton Scale (Norton, 1989). Pressure ulcer risk should be reassessed periodically and all assessments of risk should be documented. These risk predictor tools improve the ability to predict which patients will develop pressure ulcers so that preventive measures can be promptly instituted.

Skin Care and Early Treatment

The Panel for the Prediction and Prevention of Pressure Ulcers in Adults (1992) identified nine interventions that can be used to maintain and improve tissue tolerance to pressure in order to prevent injury. These interventions are listed in Table 32–6.

Mechanical Loading and Support Surfaces

The Panel for the Prediction and Prevention of Pressure Ulcers in Adults (1992) identified 11 interventions that can be used to protect against the adverse effects of external mechanical forces, such as pressure, friction, and shear. These interventions are listed in Table 32–7.

In summary, pressure ulcers most frequently occur over bony prominences and can be staged to classify the degree of tissue damage observed. Patients should be assessed on admission for their risk for pressure ulcer development using the Norton Scale or the Braden Scale. Patients at risk for pressure ulcer development should have prompt preventive interventions instituted. Skin care and early treatment should be instituted to maintain and improve tissue tolerance to pressure in order to prevent injury. Interventions should include measures to protect against the adverse effects of external mechanical forces.

TABLE 32–6. NURSING INTERVENTIONS TO MAINTAIN AND IMPROVE TISSUE TOLERANCE TO PRESSURE IN ORDER TO PREVENT INJURY

1. Complete a skin assessment daily on all individuals at risk, with particular attention given to bony prominences. Document findings.
2. Cleanse skin at time of soiling and PRN. Frequency of skin cleansing should be individualized according to need and/or patient preference. Avoid hot water, and use a mild cleansing agent that minimizes irritation and dryness of the skin. During the cleansing process, use care to minimize the force and friction applied to the skin.
3. Minimize environmental factors leading to skin drying, such as low humidity (less than 40%) and exposure to cold. Treat dry skin with moisturizers.
4. Avoid massage over bony prominences, as this may be harmful.
5. Minimize skin exposure to moisture due to incontinence, perspiration, or wound drainage. Underpads or briefs can be used.
6. Minimize skin injury secondary to friction and shear forces through proper positioning, transferring, and turning techniques. Friction injuries may be reduced by the use of lubricants (corn starch and creams), protective films (transparent film dressings and skin sealants), protective dressings (hydrocolloids), and protective padding.
7. Ensure adequate dietary intake of protein and calories. Nutritional supplements or support may be needed. If dietary intake remains inadequate and if consistent with overall goals of therapy, more aggressive nutritional intervention such as enteral or parenteral feedings should be considered.
8. Institute rehabilitation efforts aimed at mobility and activity, if consistent with the overall goals of therapy. Maintaining current activity level, mobility, and range of motion is an appropriate goal for most patients.
9. Monitor and document interventions and outcomes.

TABLE 32–7. NURSING INTERVENTIONS TO PROTECT AGAINST THE ADVERSE EFFECTS OF EXTERNAL MECHANICAL FORCES

1. Any bedridden patient assessed to be at risk for developing pressure ulcers should be repositioned at least every 2 hours if consistent with overall patient goals. Use a written schedule for systematic turning and repositioning.
2. Use positioning devices (pillows, foam wedges) for bedridden patients to keep bony prominences from direct contact with one another.
3. Completely immobile bedridden patients should have a care plan that includes the use of devices that totally relieve pressure on the heels (raising the heels off the bed). Do not use donut-type devices.
4. When the side-lying position is used, avoid positioning directly on the trochanter.
5. Limit the amount of time the head of bed is elevated and maintain the head of the bed at the lowest degree of elevation consistent with medical conditions and other restrictions.
6. Use lifting devices (trapeze or bed linen) to move (rather than drag) patients in bed who cannot assist during transfers and position changes.
7. Any patient assessed to be at risk for developing pressure ulcers should have a bed with a pressure-reducing device (foam, static air, alternating air, gel, or water mattresses).
8. Avoid uninterrupted sitting for any patient at risk for developing pressure ulcers. Reposition the patient, shifting the points under pressure at least hourly.
9. For chair-bound patients, the use of a pressure-reducing device (made of foam, gel, air, or a combination) is indicated. Do not use donut-type devices.
10. Positioning of chair-bound individuals should include consideration of postural alignment, distribution of weight, balance and stability, and pressure relief.
11. Include in the written care plan all positioning devices and schedules.

Section Seven Review

1. Nonblanchable erythema of intact skin could be staged as
   - **A.** stage I
   - **B.** stage II
   - **C.** stage III
   - **D.** stage IV
2. Nursing interventions to maintain and improve tissue tolerance to pressure in order to prevent injury include all of the following EXCEPT
   - **A.** treat dry skin with moisturizers
   - **B.** massage over bony prominences
   - **C.** minimize skin exposure to moisture by using underpads
   - **D.** use hydrocolloid dressings to reduce friction injuries
3. Pressure ulcer risk assessments should be made on
   - **A.** patients who are immobile
   - **B.** patients who have altered level of consciousness
   - **C.** patients who are incontinent
   - **D.** all patients
4. Which of the following interventions can be used to protect against the adverse effects of mechanical forces?
   - **A.** elevate the head of the bed continuously
   - **B.** reposition patients who are sitting at least every 4 hours
   - **C.** use lifting devices to move patients in bed
   - **D.** use donut-type foam devices for bedridden patients

Answers: 1. A, 2. B, 3. D, 4. C

SECTION EIGHT: Management of Pressure Ulcers

At the completion of this section, the learner will be able to identify the components of a pressure ulcer treatment program, including assessment of the patient and the pressure ulcer, management of tissue loads, ulcer wound management, management of bacterial colonization and infection, and operative repair of the pressure. Figure 32–4 is an overview of these activities related to pressure ulcer treatment.

Assessment

A systematic nursing assessment of the patient with a pressure ulcer provides the basis for planning and evaluat-

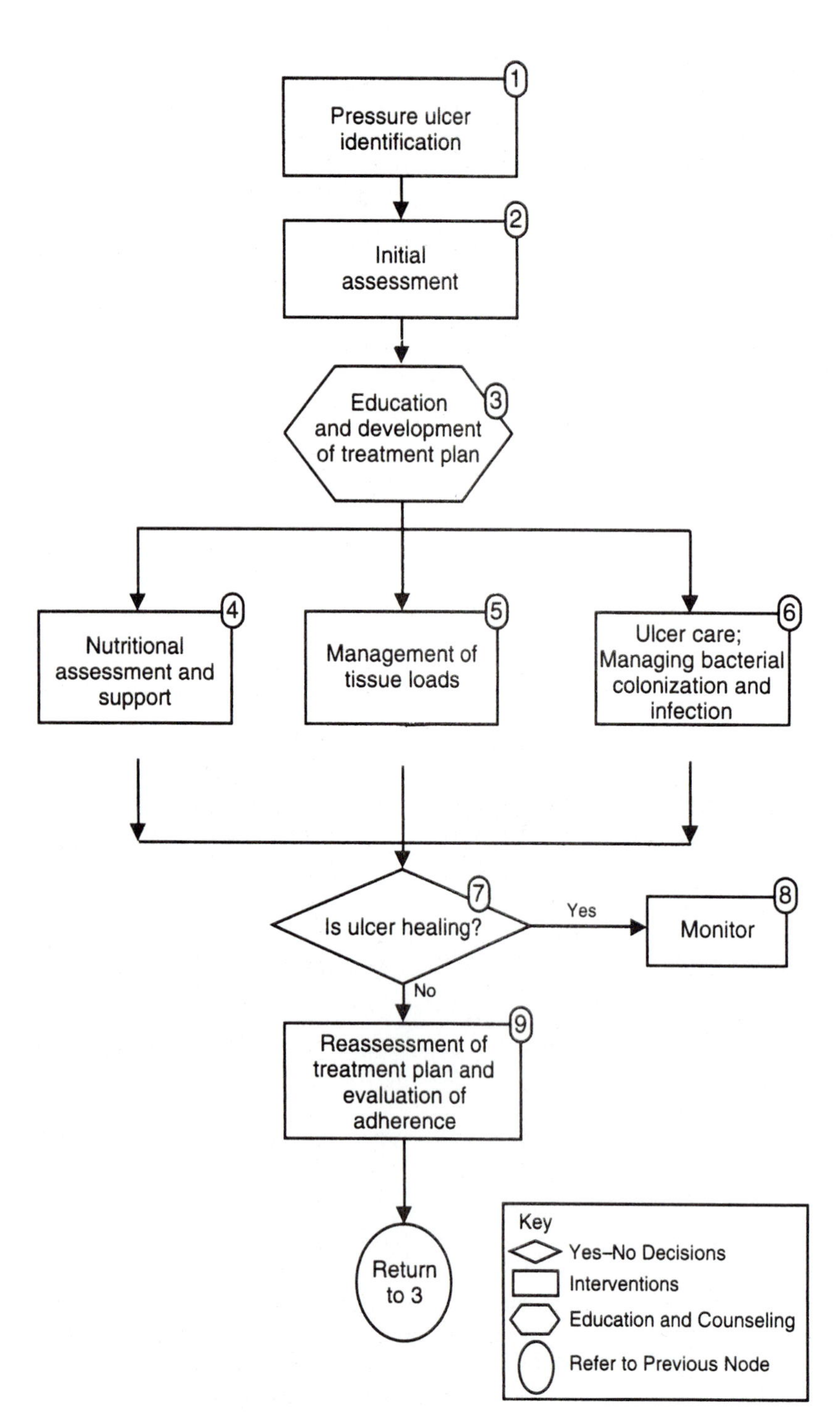

Figure 32–4. Overview of activities related to pressure ulcer treatment. (*From Bergstrom, N., Bennett, M.A., Carlson, C.E., et al. [1994]. Pressure ulcer treatment: Clinical practice guidelines. In* Quick reference guide for clinicians, *No. 15. Rockville, MD: U.S. Department of Health and Human Services, AHCPR Pub. No. 95-0653.*)

ing pressure ulcer treatment. This assessment should include psychosocial status, pain level, nutritional status, and physical health. Table 32–8 summarizes the assessment guidelines recommended for use with pressure ulcers (Bergstrom et al., 1994).

TABLE 32–8. NURSING ASSESSMENT OF A PRESSURE ULCER

1. Initial assessment of the pressure ulcer should include location, stage, size, sinus tracts, undermining, tunneling, exudate, necrotic tissue, and the presence or absence of granulation tissue and epithelialization.
2. Pressure ulcers should be reassessed at least weekly. If the patient's condition or the pressure ulcer's condition deteriorates, immediately reevaluate the treatment program.
3. Some evidence of pressure ulcer healing should be noted within 2 to 4 weeks. If no progress has been noted, reevaluate the treatment plan as well as adherence to the treatment plan and modify as needed.

Management of Tissue Loads

Tissue load refers to the distribution of shear, pressure, and friction on tissue. Nursing interventions should be instituted that reduce tissue loads in an effort to create an environment that promotes healing of the pressure ulcer and enhances soft tissue viability. The algorithm in Figure 32–5 was developed by Bergstrom and colleagues (1994) to guide clinical decisions on the management of tissue loads.

Management of tissue load begins with proper positioning techniques and support surfaces for patients while in bed. Avoid positioning patients on the pressure ulcer because this can delay healing. Positioning devices can be used to raise the pressure ulcer off the bed; however, few studies have documented the effects of ring cushions (donuts), and they should not be used. The care plan should include a repositioning plan that is designed to protect uninvolved areas. Patients placed on a pressure-reducing support surface must be regularly repositioned because ulcers can still develop.

When selecting a support surface for a patient, the nurse must consider the performance characteristics of the various products. A variety of support surfaces are available; however, research to date demonstrates that one support device is no better than the others. Table 32–9 summarizes the various classes of support surfaces and their ability to counteract forces that contribute to pressure ulcer development. After determining which forces might be increasing a patient's risk for pressure ulcer development, the nurse can use this table to select an appropriate support surface. Certain patient conditions warrant specific support surfaces. Patient characteristics to consider when selecting a support surface are summarized in Table 32–10.

Ulcer Care

Management of pressure ulcers includes debridement, wound cleansing, and dressing changes. Recommended management of ulcer care is summarized in Figure 32–6.

Debridement of pressure ulcers can proceed as recommended by Bergstrom and colleagues (1994):

1. When the need for removal of devitalized tissue is not urgent, sharp mechanical debridement or enzymatic or autolytic techniques can be used. If the need for debridement is urgent (progressive cellulitis or sepsis), sharp debridement should be used.
2. Use clean, dry dressings for 8 to 24 hours after sharp debridement associated with bleeding; then reinstitute moist dressings. Clean dressings may be used in conjunction with mechanical or enzymatic debridement techniques.
3. Heel ulcers with dry eschar need not be debrided if they do not have edema, erythema, fluctuance, or drainage. Assess these wounds daily to monitor for pressure ulcer complications requiring further debridement.
4. Prevent or manage pain associated with debridement as needed.

The process of cleaning a wound involves selection of a solution and the appropriate mechanical means to deliver the solution to the wound. Bergstrom and colleagues (1994) recommend the following:

1. Wounds should be cleaned at each dressing change, using minimal mechanical force when cleaning the ulcer with gauze, cloth, or sponges.
2. Normal saline is recommended for cleaning wounds.
3. Use enough irrigation pressure to cleanse the wound without causing trauma to the wound.
4. Whirlpool treatments are effective in cleansing pressure ulcers that contain thick exudate, slough, or necrotic tissue; the treatments should be discontinued when the ulcer is clean.

The condition of the pressure ulcer and the desired dressing function determine the type of dressing that should be used for a pressure ulcer. According to Bergstrom and colleagues (1994), the cardinal rule is to keep the ulcer tissue moist and the surrounding skin dry, which can be accomplished by the following:

1. Wet-to-dry dressings should be used only for debridement.
2. Use clinical judgment to select a type of moist dressing; current research demonstrates no difference in pressure ulcer healing outcomes related to type of moist wound dressing used.

3. Choose a dressing that controls exudate but does not desiccate the ulcer bed.
4. Eliminate wound dead space by loosely filling all cavities with dressing material and avoid over-packing the wound.
5. Monitor dressings applied near the anus because they are difficult to keep intact.

Managing Bacterial Colonization and Infection

Stage II, III, and IV pressure ulcers are likely to be infected. Adequate cleansing and debridement can prevent bacterial colonization from progressing into a clinical infection. Bergstrom and colleagues (1994) recommend the following:

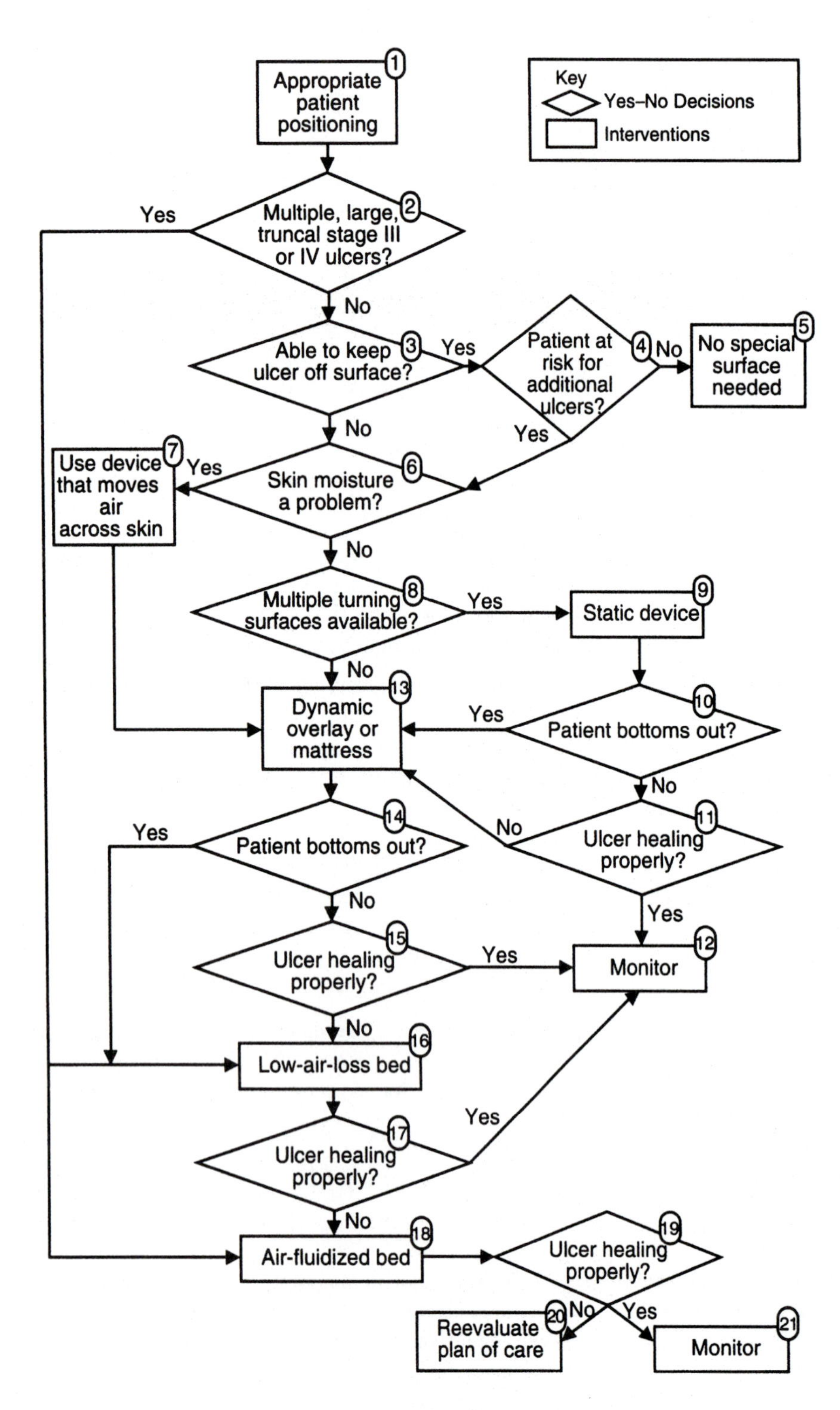

Figure 32–5. Algorithm to guide clinical decisions on the management of tissue loads. For explanation of "bottoms out" see Table 32–10. (*From Bergstrom, N., Bennett, M.A., Carlson, C.E., et al. [1994]. Pressure ulcer treatment: Clinical practice guideline. In* Quick reference guide for clinicians, *No. 15. Rockville, MD: U.S. Department of Health and Human Services, AHCPR Pub. No. 95-0653.)*

TABLE 32–9. SELECTED CHARACTERISTICS FOR CLASSES OF SUPPORT SURFACES

	SUPPORT DEVICES					
PERFORMANCE CHARACTERISTICS	AIR-FLUIDIZED	LOW-AIR-LOSS	ALTERNATING-AIR	STATIC FLOTATION (AIR OR WATER)	FOAM	STANDARD MATTRESS
Increased support area	Yes	Yes	Yes	Yes	Yes	No
Low moisture retention	Yes	Yes	No	No	No	No
Reduced heat accumulation	Yes	Yes	No	No	No	No
Shear reduction	Yes	?	Yes	Yes	No	No
Pressure reduction	Yes	Yes	Yes	Yes	Yes	No
Dynamic	Yes	Yes	Yes	No	No	No
Cost per day	High	High	Moderate	Low	Low	Low

From Bergstrom, N., Bennett, M.A., Carlson, C.E., et al. (1994). Pressure ulcer treatment: Clinical practice guideline. In Quick reference guide for clinicians, *No. 15. Rockville, MD: U.S. Department of Health and Human Services, AHCPR Pub. No. 95–0653.*

1. If purulence or a foul odor is detected, more frequent cleansing and debridement may be required.
2. Swab cultures should not be used to diagnose wound infections because all pressure ulcers are colonized. Needle aspiration of fluid or biopsy of ulcer tissue is recommended.
3. Topical antibiotics used should be effective against gram-positive, gram-negative, and anaerobic organisms. If the ulcer does not respond to topical antibiotic therapy after 2 weeks, soft tissue cultures should be performed and the potential for osteomyelitis should be evaluated. Systemic antibiotics are indicated in the event of bacteremia, advancing cellulitis, or osteomyelitis.
4. Topical antiseptics should not be used to reduce bacteria in wound tissue.
5. Pressure ulcers should be protected from exogenous sources of contamination.

TABLE 32–10. MATCHING PATIENT CHARACTERISTICS WITH SUPPORT SURFACES

Indication for pressure-reducing surface	Use if patient is at risk for further pressure ulcer development.
Indications for static support surfaces	Use if the patient can assume a variety of positions without bearing weight on a pressure ulcer and without "bottoming out." To assess for bottoming out, place outstretched hand with palms up under the overlay below the pressure ulcer or below the part of the body at risk for pressure ulcer development. If less than an inch of support material is felt, the patient has bottomed out and the support surface is inadequate.
Indications for dynamic support surfaces	Patient cannot assume a variety of positions without bearing weight on a pressure ulcer. Patient fully compresses the static support surface. Pressure ulcer does not show evidence of healing within 2 to 4 weeks.
Indications for low-air-loss and air-fluidized beds.	Patient has stage III or IV pressure ulcers on multiple turning surfaces. Patient bottoms out or fails to heal on a dynamic overlay or mattress. To control excess moisture on intact skin (follow manufacturer's instructions for the use of linens and pads so as to not obstruct air flow).

Operative Repair

Operative repair of pressure ulcers may be indicated when clean stage III or IV pressure ulcers do not respond to conventional guidelines (Bergstrom et al., 1994). Operative repair of pressure ulcer wounds may include direct closure, skin grafting, skin flaps, musculocutaneous flaps, or free flaps. Nursing care postoperatively must include interventions to promote wound healing. Pressure to the operative site should be minimized through the use of an air-fluidized, low-air-loss bed for at least 2 weeks (Bergstrom et al., 1994).

In summary, management of pressure ulcers begins with a systematic nursing assessment, management of tissue load through the use of proper positioning techniques and support surfaces for the patient in bed, pressure ulcer management using debridement, wound cleansing and dressing changes, managing bacterial colonization and infection, and possible operative repair.

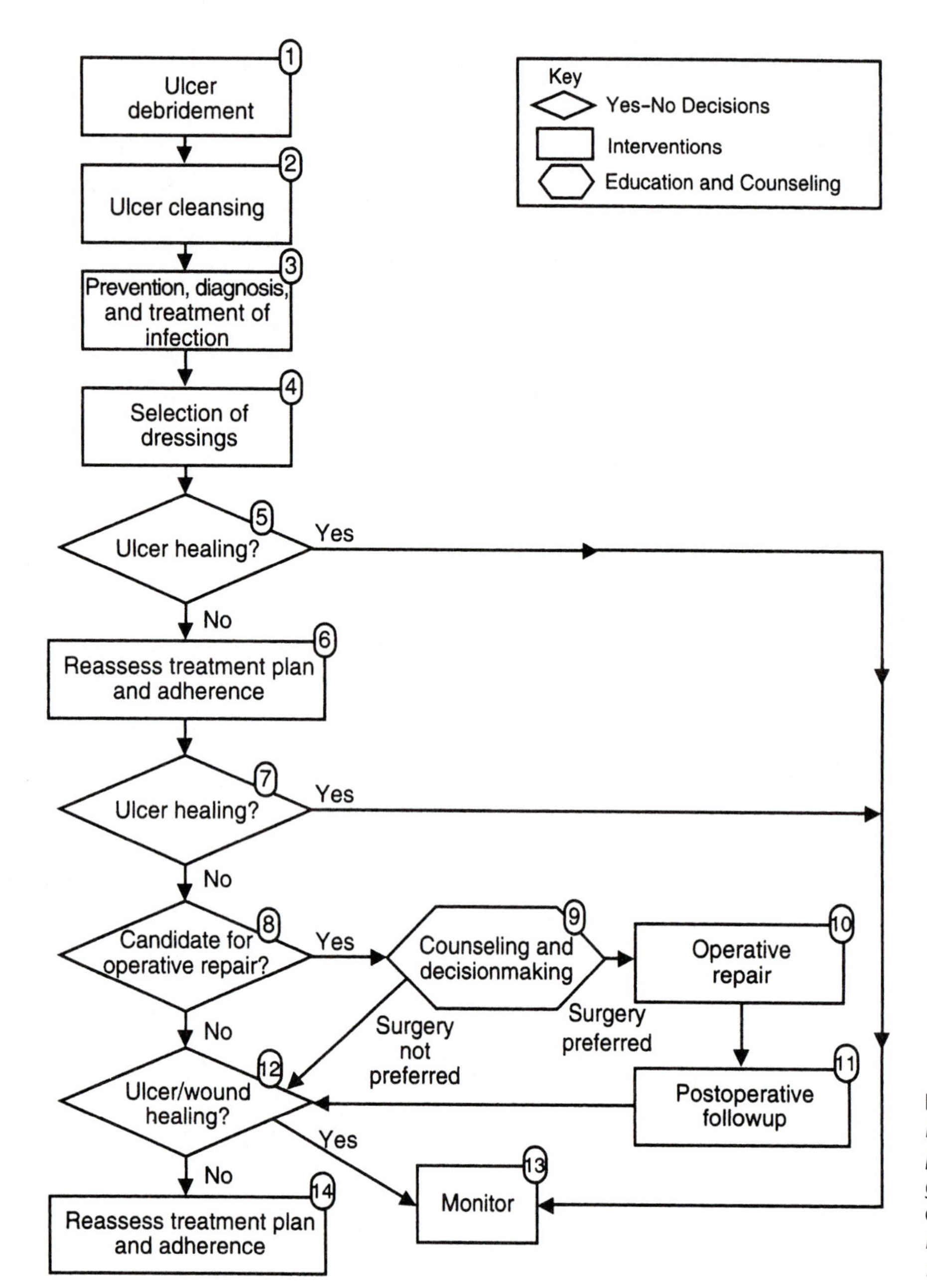

Figure 32–6. Management of ulcer care. (*From Bergstrom, N., Bennett, M.A., Carlson, C.E., et al. [1994]. Pressure ulcer treatment: Clinical practice guidelines. In* Quick reference guide for clinicians, *No. 15. Rockville, MD: U.S. Department of Health and Human Services, AHCPR Pub. No. 95–0653.)*)

SECTION EIGHT REVIEW

1. Pressure ulcer healing is usually evidenced
   A. in less than a week
   B. within 1 to 2 weeks
   C. within 2 to 4 weeks
   D. within 4 to 6 weeks
2. Which support surface should be used if a patient is at risk for further pressure ulcer development?
   A. pressure-reducing surface
   B. static support surface
   C. dynamic support surface
   D. low-air-loss surface
3. Which of the following treatments is recommended for cleansing pressure ulcers containing thick exudate, slough, and necrotic tissue?
   A. wet-to-dry dressing changes
   B. enzymatic debridement
   C. normal saline irrigation
   D. whirlpool treatments

4. Bacterial colonization can be prevented from progressing to a clinical infection by
   A. adequate wound cleansing
   B. adequate wound debridement
   C. adequate wound cleansing and debridement
   D. systemic antibiotics
5. Which of the following interventions is recommended if a pressure ulcer wound develops purulent drainage?
   A. swab the drainage for culture
   B. institute systemic antibiotics
   C. increase the frequency of wound cleansing and debriding
   D. institute topical antiseptics

Answers: 1. C, 2. A, 3. D, 4. C, 5. C

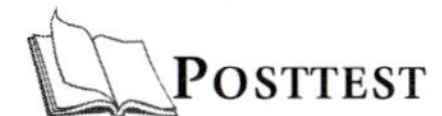

POSTTEST

1. Which of the following stores energy, assists in regulating the body temperature, acts as a cushion, and provides the body with shape and substance?
   A. dermis
   B. epidermis
   C. subcutaneous tissue
   D. hypodermis
2. Epithelialization
   A. occurs even in the presence of debris
   B. spreads on surfaces laden with bacteria
   C. occurs only in healthy tissue
   D. occurs within moments after injury
3. A patient has undergone a cholecystectomy. Most likely, his incision would be allowed to heal by
   A. primary intention
   B. secondary intention
   C. delayed primary (tertiary) intention
   D. delayed secondary intention
4. Of the factors that affect wound healing, which of the following has been found to be the most important?
   A. age
   B. normal serum potassium levels
   C. moisture
   D. adequate tissue perfusion
5. Prevention of wound infections can be accomplished by all of the following EXCEPT
   A. hand washing
   B. skin preparation
   C. mechanical bowel preparation
   D. use of acetic acid dressings
6. Topical enzymes applied to necrotic wounds is
   A. contraindicated
   B. a form of mechanical debridement
   C. a form of autolytic debridement
   D. a form of chemical debridement
7. Which of the following dressing materials should NOT be used for documented or suspected wound infections?
   A. wet-to-dry dressings
   B. hydrocolloid dressings
   C. wet-to-damp dressings
   D. wet-to-wet dressings
8. Acetic acid is a solution used with wet-to-dry dressings that may be used
   A. to promote vasodilation in the wound
   B. to treat *Pseudomonas* infection in the wound
   C. to slightly dissolve necrotic debris in the wound
   D. as a fast-acting broad-spectrum antimicrobial
9. Red-pink tissue with a budding appearance is characteristic of
   A. granulation tissue
   B. imminent wound infections
   C. poor tissue perfusion
   D. the inflammatory process
10. Moist, yellow, stringy tissue in a wound is
    A. a sign of epithelialization
    B. eschar
    C. slough
    D. granulation tissue
11. Friction injuries may be reduced by
    A. massage over bony prominences
    B. use of donut foam devices
    C. protective dressings (hydrocolloids)
    D. vigorous cleansing of soiled skin

12. Pressure ulcer wounds should be reassessed
   A. daily
   B. at least twice a day
   C. at least twice a week
   D. weekly

13. Which of the following repositioning schedules would be used for a patient placed on a pressure-reducing support surface?
   A. reposition until the patient "bottoms out"
   B. reposition the patient regularly
   C. turn no more frequently than needed
   D. the patient will not require repositioning

POSTTEST ANSWERS

Question	Answer	Section	Question	Answer	Section
1	C	One	8	B	Five
2	C	Two	9	A	Six
3	A	Two	10	C	Six
4	D	Three	11	C	Seven
5	D	Four	12	D	Eight
6	D	Five	13	B	Eight
7	B	Five			

REFERENCES

Amato, E.J. (1982). Gastrointestinal tubes and drains. *Crit Care Nurse* 2(6):50–57.

Bergstrom, N., Bennett, M.A., Carlson, C.E., et al. (1994). Pressure ulcer treatment: Clinical practice guidelines: In *Quick reference for clinicians*, No. 15. Rockville, MD: U.S. Department of Health and Human Services, AHCPR Publication 95–0653.

Boynton, P.R., & Paustian, C. (1996). Wound assessment and decision making options. *Crit Care Nurs Clin North Am* 8:125–139.

Braden, B.J. (1989). Clinical utility of the Braden Scale for predicting pressure sore risk. *Decubitus* 2(3):44–46, 50–51.

Cuzzell, J.Z. (1990). Choosing a wound dressing: A systemic approach. *AACN Clin Issues Crit Care* 1(3):566–577.

Flynn, M.B. (1996). Wound healing and critical illness. *Crit Care Nurs Clin North Am* 8:115–123.

Makelbust, J. (1996). Using wound care products to promote a healing environment. *Crit Care Nurs Clin North Am* 8:141–158.

Norris, S.O., Provo, B., & Stotts, N.A. (1990). Physiology of wound healing and risk factors that impede the healing process. *AACN Clin Issues Crit Care Nurs* 18:545–552.

Norton, D. (1989). Calculating the risk: Reflections on the Norton Scale. *Decubitus* 2(3):24–31.

Panel for the Prediction and Prevention of Pressure Ulcers in Adults. (1992). *Pressure Ulcers in Adults: Prediction and Prevention*. Clinical Practice Guideline, Number 3. AHCPR Publication No. 92: Rockville, MD: Agency for Health Care Policy and Research, Public Health Service, U.S. Department of Health and Human Services.

Module 33

Acute Burn Injury

Julia Fultz, Susan Wells, Darlene Welsh

This self-study module focuses on the three phases of burn injury: the resuscitative, acute rehabilitative, and long-term rehabilitative phases. The module is composed of 12 sections. Sections One through Three discuss the mechanisms of burn injury, classification of burns, and burn centers. Sections Four through Six discuss the systemic effects burn injury produces in the resuscitative phase. Section Seven discusses initial wound care and wound healing. Sections Eight through Eleven describe the acute rehabilitative phase of burn injury. Section Twelve discusses the long-term rehabilitation phase of burn care. Each section includes a set of review questions to help the learner evaluate his or her understanding of the section's content before moving on to the next section. All Section Reviews and the module Pretest and Posttest include answers. It is suggested that the learner review those concepts answered incorrectly in the review questions before proceeding to the next section.

OBJECTIVES

Following completion of this module, the learner will be able to

1. Describe the local effects of burn injury.
2. Classify burn wounds.
3. Describe the composition of a burn center.
4. Discuss the nursing care of a burn patient in the emergent phase of injury.
5. Discuss the nursing care of a burn patient in the acute phase of injury.
6. Discuss the nursing care of a burn patient in the rehabilitation phase of injury.

PRETEST

1. A burn wound that is white, painless, and leathery in texture describes a
   A. third-degree burn
   B. deep partial-thickness burn
   C. second-degree burn
   D. first-degree burn
2. Antibiotics are administered topically to burn patients primarily because
   A. they facilitate debridement
   B. burn wounds are ischemic
   C. they are soothing
   D. they are less costly
3. Of the following demographic groups, which is at highest risk for burn injury/death?
   A. Caucasians
   B. suburbanites
   C. women
   D. children
4. Single rooms with positive airflow are ideal in a burn unit because this arrangement promotes
   A. privacy
   B. noise reduction
   C. infection control
   D. adequate ventilation

5. Burn shock occurs during which phase of burn injury?
   A. rehabilitative phase
   B. emergent phase
   C. acute phase
   D. critical phase
6. To prevent paralytic ileus, a nasogastric tube should be inserted and continuous low wall suction applied to patients with burn surfaces
   A. > 10 percent
   B. < 15 percent
   C. > 20 percent
   D. > 25 percent
7. Upper airway edema usually peaks during which time period postinhalation injury?
   A. 24 to 48 hours
   B. 1 to 2 hours
   C. 4 to 8 hours
   D. 12 to 24 hours
8. Which medication can be used to promote cardiac contractility during fluid resuscitation in the burned cardiac patient?
   A. lidocaine
   B. metoprolol
   C. dopamine
   D. sodium bicarbonate
9. The most effective method for delivering pain medication during the emergent phase is
   A. orally
   B. subcutaneously
   C. intramuscularly
   D. intravenously
10. The burn patient should receive which diet, when feasible?
    A. high calorie, high protein
    B. high sodium, low cholesterol
    C. high fiber, low potassium
    D. high sodium, high potassium
11. Fluid resuscitation should be calculated for patients with ___ percent total body surface area burned.
    A. 10
    B. 15
    C. 20
    D. 30
12. During the acute phase, childlike behavior in the critically burned adult patient is
    A. abnormal
    B. a coping mechanism
    C. pathologic
    D. rare

Pretest answers: 1. A, 2. B, 3. D, 4. C, 5. B, 6. C, 7. A, 8. C, 9. D, 10. A, 11. C, 12. B

GLOSSARY

Allograft. Biologic dressings obtained from human donor. Usually a cadaver

Autografting. Transplanting tissue from another part of the patient's body

Bulla. A large blister or skin vesicle filled with fluid (plural, bullae)

Burn shock. Hypovolemic shock that develops secondary to fluid shifts occuring with burn injury

Carbon monoxide (CO). A colorless, tasteless, odorless, poisonous gas that is a byproduct of the combustion of organic materials

Carboxyhemoglobin. A compound formed by carbon monoxide and hemoglobin

Compartment syndrome. Pressure within a muscle compartment rises and exceeds microvascular pressure thereby interfering with cellular perfusion

Debridement. The removal of foreign material and nonviable tissue from a wound

Deep partial-thickness burn. Involves epidermis and more than one half of the dermis

Eschar. A tough, dry inelastic wound indicative of a full-thickness burn

Escharotomy. Surgical incision of the eschar and superficial fascia of a circumferentially burned limb or trunk in order to restore blood flow distal to the affected area

Fasciotomy. Incision in the fascia to restore blood flow to tissues

First-degree burn. Injury involves only epidermis (currently referred to as superficial partial-thickness burn)

Full-thickness burn. Destroys epidermis, dermis, and portions of subcutaneous tissues (formerly known as third- and fourth-degree burns)

Heterograft. Tissue transplanted from an animal of a different species, usually pigs for human recipients

Homograft. Tissue transplanted from another individual to be used as a biological dressing

Myocardial depressant factor. Humoral substance that exerts a negative inotropic effect on myocardial tissues

Myoglobin. Substance released from damaged muscle tissue

Myoglobinurea. The presence of myoglobin in the urine

Oxygen free radicals. Highly reactive oxygen-containing molecules that can damage healthy tissues

Partial-thickness burn. Involves epidermis, and the superficial layers of the dermis (formerly referred to as first- or second-degree burns)

Second-degree burn. Destroys epidermis and portions of the dermis (currently referred to as a partial-thickness burn)

Third-degree burn. Destroys epidermis, dermis, and portions of subcutaneous tissues (currently referred to as a full-thickness burn)

Xenograft. Tissue transplanted from an animal of a different species, usually pigs for human recipients

Abbreviations

CO. Carbon monoxide

GI. Gastrointestinal

MODS. Multiple organ dysfunction syndrome

TBSA. Total body surface area

SECTION ONE: Mechanisms of Burn Injury

At the completion of this section, the learner will be able to give an overview of burn injuries and describe the mechanisms of burn injury.

More than 1.25 million people are burned each year resulting in approximately 5,500 deaths per year. (Brigham & McLoughlin, 1996). The economic costs from burn injury recovery rise into the billions of dollars as do the social costs from days lost from work and physical and vocational rehabilitation. Most burn injuries occur in the home. Children and the elderly are most prone to burn injuries. The most frequent type of injury is a scald injury; however, the major cause of severe burn is flame injury.

Burn injury may occur from exposure to heat (flames, hot objects), caustic chemicals, radiation or electric current. The severity of the injury depends on the length of exposure, and temperature of the offending substance.

Thermal burns caused by exposure to flame or a hot object produce microvascular and inflammatory responses within minutes of the injury. The effects from these two responses can last from 2 to 3 days. Substances released by damaged cells increase vascular permeability, causing fluid, electrolytes, and proteins to leak into the interstitial space. An inflammatory response is initiated to inhibit bacterial contamination. The various inflammatory mediators also contribute to cell wall changes that permit intravascular fluid and proteins to leak into the interstitial spaces. Both of these responses contribute to burn edema formation.

Burn edema is usually limited to the injured tissues if the total body surface area (TBSA) involved is less than 25 percent. If the injury includes more than 25% TBSA, edema can occur in noninjured tissues also. The fluid shift from intravascular to interstitial spaces may cause a hypovolemic shock state. This hypovolemic shock state is frequently referred to as **burn shock.** Fluid loss by evaporation from the burn wound also contributes to the volume deficit.

Chemical burns are the result of exposure to acid, alkali or organic substances. The extent of injury is dependent on the concentration of the substance, the amount, the length of exposure, and the mechanism of chemical action (National Burn Institute, 1994; Rutan, 1998). An acid substance will cause an eschar type of wound resulting from a coagulation necrosis. The eschar prevents continued tissue damage beneath the layer of eschar. An alkali substance usually causes more tissue damage than an acid substance (given the same volume) because an alkali causes protein liquefaction producing a soupy wound, which allows for continued tissue damage into deeper structures (Rutan, 1998). Damage may continue to occur with alkali burns for several hours after exposure. Organic substances produce a thermal component and may be absorbed systemically producing renal and hepatic toxicity.

Inhalation of chemical substances can cause direct parenchymal lung injury. Absorption of a chemical through either the pulmonary system or through direct skin contact can cause systemic effect involving the pulmonary, cardiovascular, renal, and/or hepatic systems, producing injury.

Electrical burns result from the conversion of electrical energy into heat. The extent of thermal injury is dependent on the type of current, the pathway of current flow, local tissue resistance, and the duration of contact. All tissues are conductive to some extent but there are differences in the resistance to the current flow. For example, nerves and blood vessels are less resistant than bone. The more resistant a tissue is, the more heat the electricity will create as it passes through the tissue and therefore produce more damage. Electricity takes the path of least resistance once it makes contact with the body, therefore nerves and blood vessels are the path most likely taken through the body. Due to the internal damage that can be caused by electrical injuries, the severity of the burn is difficult to determine. In addition to the heat injury, contact with an electrical source can also cause tetanic muscle contractions severe enough to cause bone fractures or joint dislocations.

Electrical injury can be classified three ways. A true electrical injury occurs when electricity passes through the body. This usually results in an entrance wound, which is the point of electrical contact, and an exit wound, which is usually larger than the entrance wound. The second type of electrical burn is an arc burn, which results when electricity passes over the body externally. The injury is usually scattered over the body in what has been described as a "splashed on," spidery pattern (National Burn Institute, 1994). These burns are usually the result of lightning striking an object near the person and flashing over the person or from high tension current. The third type of electrical burn results from clothing igniting from sparks of electrical arcing, causing a true thermal burn.

Radiation burns result from radiant energy being transferred to the body resulting in production of cellular toxins. The effect is most rapidly evident on those cells that reproduce rapidly such as skin, blood vessels, intestinal lining, and bone marrow. The greater the exposure, the more significant the damage and the more types of cells affected. A radiation victim's injury usually results from radiation therapy or from an industrial or laboratory incident.

In summary, over 1.25 million Americans are burned every year, resulting in 5,500 fatalities. Burn injuries are the result of thermal, electrical, chemical, or radiation exposure. The causes and basic effects of each type of exposure has been discussed.

SECTION ONE REVIEW

1. Most burn injuries/deaths occur
   A. at the workplace
   B. in car accidents
   C. in plane crashes
   D. in the home
2. Fluid shifting from the intravascular to the interstitial spaces causes
   A. intravascular coagulation
   B. hypovolemic shock
   C. direct parenchymal injury
   D. bacterial contamination
3. Which burns are often more extensive than initially assessed?
   A. thermal burns
   B. inhalation burns
   C. acidic burns
   D. electrical burns
4. The type of burn where tissues are deeply penetrated and necrosis may continue to occur for several hours after injury is MOST likely a(n)
   A. acidic burn
   B. alkaline burn
   C. electrical burn
   D. flash burn

Answers: 1. D, 2. B, 3. D, 4. B

SECTION TWO: Burn Wound Assessment

At the completion of this section, the learner will be able to describe and calculate the extent of burn injury.

Burns are classified according to the depth of injury and the extent of body surface area involved. Burn depth has been traditionally described as **first-, second-,** or **third-degree** (see Fig. 33–1). Currently, burn wounds are more specifically differentiated as **partial-** or **full-thickness,** depending on the level of dermis and subcutaneous tissue involved (Table 33–1). The depth of the burn is often difficult to assess initially. Calculation of the extent of in-

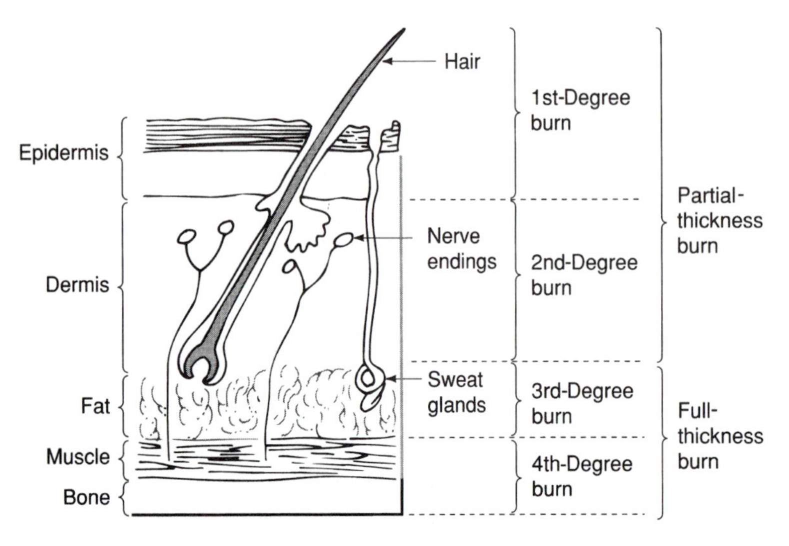

Figure 33–1. Anatomy of skin and depth of burn injury. (*From Rue, L.W., and Cioffi, W.G. [1991]. Resuscitation of thermally injured patients.* Crit Care Nurs Clin North Am *3(2):183.*)

TABLE 33–1. DESCRIPTION OF FIRST-, SECOND-, AND THIRD-DEGREE BURNS

DEGREE OF BURN	DESCRIPTION
First-degree burn	Involves epidermis only Skin is hot, red, painful, no blisters
Second-degree burn	Destruction of epidermis and portions of dermis
Partial-thickness	
Superficial partial-thickness	Involves destruction of the epidermis and damage to the superficial layers of the dermis; blisters, blanching, extreme pain are present; skin is red, mottled, and moist
Deep partial-thickness	Destruction of epidermis and deep dermal layers; skin is mottled, red/white, non-blanching, sensation to deep pressure
Third-degree burn Full-thickness	Destruction of epidermis, dermis, and portions of subcutaneous tissues; wound is white or charred, painless, and insensate; skin is leathery in texture. If bone and muscle destruction occur, may be termed fourth-degree

jury should be re-evaluated after the initial wound debridement and over the course of the ensuing 72 hours to accurately describe the wound. Wound conversion sometimes occurs when viable tissue becomes nonviable, thereby increasing the depth of the wound. Infection, hypothermia, and external pressure are common causes of wound conversion.

The extent of injury is expressed by the percentage of total body surface area (TBSA) burned. A commonly used guide in determining the extent of injury is the Lund and Browder Chart, which adjusts TBSA for age, as seen in Figure 33–2 (Lund & Browder, 1944). This is important as various pediatric patients' body parts are disproportionate to adults'. For example, a child's head is allowed a greater TBSA percentage than an adult's. To use the guide, one assesses all partial- and full-thickness burns and shades the figure accordingly. The percentage of each anatomic area involved is calculated, then all are totaled. For example, if an adult were to sustain a scald injury to the right lower arm and hand, his or her TBSA burned wound would be 5.5 percent.

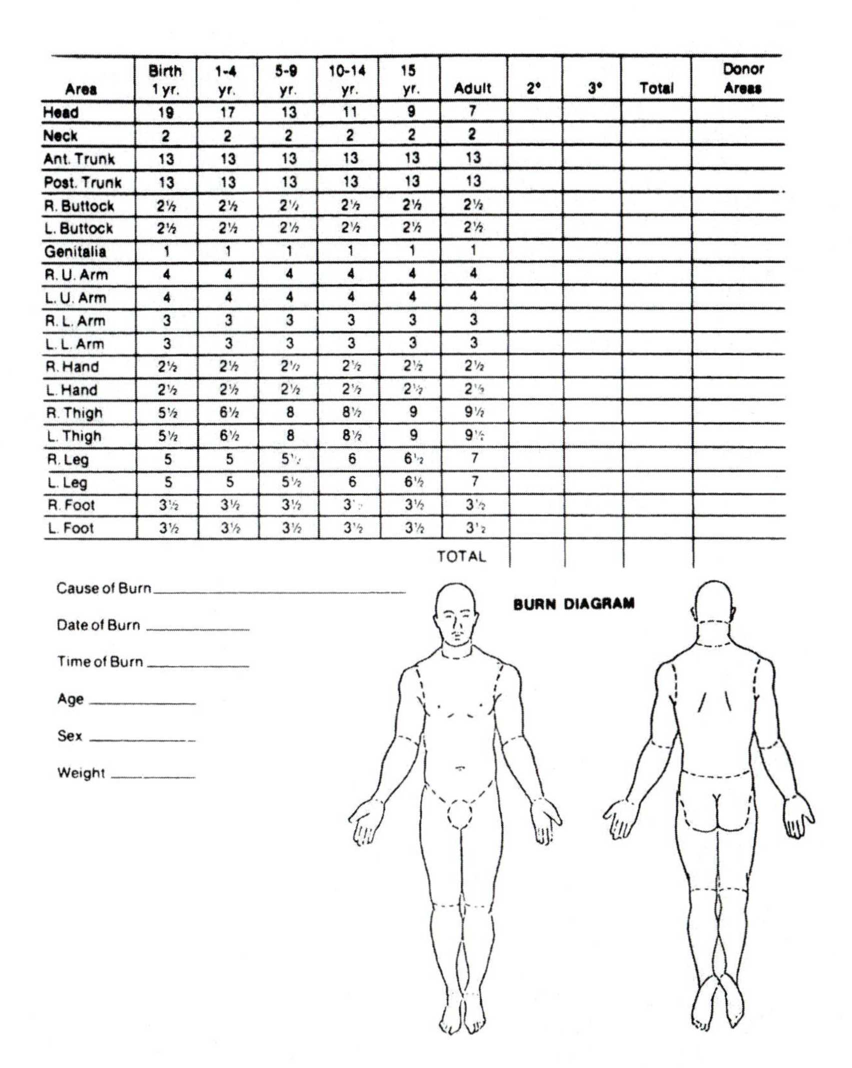

Area	Birth 1 yr.	1-4 yr.	5-9 yr.	10-14 yr.	15 yr.	Adult	2°	3°	Total	Donor Areas
Head	19	17	13	11	9	7				
Neck	2	2	2	2	2	2				
Ant. Trunk	13	13	13	13	13	13				
Post. Trunk	13	13	13	13	13	13				
R. Buttock	2½	2½	2½	2½	2½	2½				
L. Buttock	2½	2½	2½	2½	2½	2½				
Genitalia	1	1	1	1	1	1				
R. U. Arm	4	4	4	4	4	4				
L. U. Arm	4	4	4	4	4	4				
R. L. Arm	3	3	3	3	3	3				
L. L. Arm	3	3	3	3	3	3				
R. Hand	2½	2½	2½	2½	2½	2½				
L. Hand	2½	2½	2½	2½	2½	2½				
R. Thigh	5½	6½	8	8½	9	9½				
L. Thigh	5½	6½	8	8½	9	9½				
R. Leg	5	5	5½	6	6½	7				
L. Leg	5	5	5½	6	6½	7				
R. Foot	3½	3½	3½	3½	3½	3½				
L. Foot	3½	3½	3½	3½	3½	3½				
						TOTAL				

Cause of Burn __________

Date of Burn __________

Time of Burn __________

Age __________

Sex __________

Weight __________

BURN DIAGRAM

Figure 33–2. (From Rudolphs' Pediatrics, 20th ed. *K. Overby, © 1998. Permission granted by McGraw-Hill Companies.*)

Another method of evaluating burn injuries, especially those that are irregularly shaped or occur in patches, is to use the palmar surface of the patient's hand which represents approximately 0.5 percent of the patient's body surface area. For example, if a patchy burn to the torso includes four burned areas, each approximately the size of the patient's palm, the TBSA involved would be 2 percent.

In summary, burns are classified according to the extent of body surface area injured and their depth. Various charts and formulas are used to guide the estimation of the extent of injury.

SECTION TWO REVIEW

1. A patient received partial-thickness flash burns to his anterior chest, right arm, and perineum. The estimated extent of his injury according to the Lund and Browder Chart would be
   A. 50 percent
   B. 37 percent
   C. 28 percent
   D. 56 percent

2. White, charred, leathery-textured wounds are the result of
   A. third-degree or full-thickness burns
   B. first-degree burns
   C. deep partial-thickness burns
   D. superficial partial-thickness burns

Answers: 1. C, 2. A

SECTION THREE: Burn Centers

At the completion of this section, the learner will be able to discuss criteria for transfer of a patient to a burn center and to describe the unique structures, processes, and personnel that make up a burn center.

Burn Center Referral Criteria

Once the extent and depth of the burn injury has been classified, the severity of the injury must be evaluated using guidelines developed by the National Burn Institute (1994). Should a patient's injury meet any one of the criteria outlined in Table 33–2, the injury warrants immediate transfer to a burn center.

TABLE 33–2. BURN CENTER REFERRAL CRITERIA

- Second- and third-degree burns > 10 percent total body surface (TBSA) in patients < 10 or > 50 years of age
- Second- and third-degree burns > 20 percent TBSA in other age groups
- Second- and third-degree burns that involve the face, hands, feet, genitalia, perineum, or major joints
- Third-degree burns > 5 percent TBSA in any age group
- Electrical burns, including lightning injury
- Chemical burns
- Burn injury with inhalation injury
- Burn injury in patients with preexisting medical disorders that could complicate management, prolong recovery, or affect mortality
- Any patient with burns and concomitant trauma (e.g., fractures) in which the burn injury poses the greatest risk of morbidity or mortality. In such cases, if the trauma poses the greater immediate risk, the patient may be treated initially in a trauma center until stable before being transferred to a burn center. Physician judgment will be necessary in such situations and should be in concert with the regional medical control plan and triage protocols
- Hospitals without qualified personnel or equipment for care of children should transfer children with burns to a burn center with these capabilities
- Burn injury in patients who will require special social/emotional and/or long-term rehabilitative support, including cases involving suspected abuse
- Circumferential burns of an extremity and/or the chest

Structure of the Burn Unit

Patients in the burn unit are susceptible to infection because of altered resistance to microorganisms due to the presence of open wounds and immunosuppression. A model burn unit provides an environment that promotes isolation from pathogens and prevents infection. In the ideal unit, patients occupy single rooms that provide positive air flow. Reverse isolation techniques such as strict hand washing and the proper use of masks, gowns, gloves, and caps should be used by all personnel and visitors entering the unit. These techniques decrease the patient's risk for infection. Each patient room should contain individual controls for temperature and humidity and ample space for equipment and supplies.

The typical burn unit is equipped to provide standard intensive care unit (ICU) monitoring and ventilatory support. Hydrotherapy or whirlpool facilities are often located in burn units since patients may require hydrotherapy to promote wound healing.

Burn Team Members

Care of the critically injured burn patient is complex and requires a multidisciplinary approach. Burn team members include nurses, physicians (plastic and general surgeons), physical therapists, occupational therapists, dietitians, discharge planners, social workers, chaplains, and psychologists. Additional services are requested as needed.

In summary, the criteria for patient transfer to a burn center was presented. Burn centers are designed to treat patients experiencing burns using a multidisciplinary approach. Burn units are equipped to provide standard ICU monitoring, ventilatory support, hydrotherapy, and reverse isolation for those recovering from critical burn injury.

Section Three Review

1. Treatment of the critically burned patient is MOST efficient when the _______ approach is used.
   - **A.** systems
   - **B.** functional
   - **C.** multidisciplinary
   - **D.** authoritarian
2. The most common isolation technique used in burn units is
   - **A.** wound isolation
   - **B.** enteric isolation
   - **C.** respiratory isolation
   - **D.** reverse isolation

Answers: 1. C, 2. D

SECTION FOUR: Resuscitative Phase: Cardiopulmonary and Peripheral Vascular Effects

At the completion of this section, the learner will be able to discuss nursing care of the burn patient experiencing cardiopulmonary and peripheral vascular effects from burn injury. The resuscitative phase lasts from the time of injury to 48 to 72 hours postinjury. Burn shock with cardiovascular collapse can occur during this time period. Traumatic injuries such as head trauma, internal injuries, and fractures, that may occur concurrently with burn injuries, should be identified and treated early in this phase. Primary and secondary assessments for traumatic injury are completed on all burn patients (see Module 34 for the components of primary and secondary assessment of the trauma patient).

Cardiovascular

Adults with large burns may have heart rates between 110 and 125 beats/min, which is considered normal. Children may experience heart rates of 120 to 170 in the first 24 hours despite adequate urine output. Remember that children compensate for a decreased cardiac output by increasing their heart rate. Guarded evaluation of a child who has an elevated heart rate is mandatory. Blood pressure is not a reliable indicator of fluid status; however, a low mean arterial pressure (child ≤ 40 mm Hg, adult ≤ 65 mm Hg) may be indicative of the need for further evaluation of fluid status (Gordon & Goodwin, 1997; Gordon & Winfree, 1998).

Burns of more than 40 percent TBSA produce significant myocardial dysfunction. A decrease in myocardial contractility occurs and cardiac output falls within the first few minutes of injury, even prior to a decreased plasma volume. During the initial few hours, plasma volume drops, contributing to the decreased cardiac output. An increased peripheral vascular resistance accompanies decreased cardiac output. The causes of myocardial dysfunction in burn patients are not well understood, however there are several theories including the release of a substance from the burn wound itself called **myocardial depressant factor** (Kramer & Nguyen, 1996) and the release of **oxygen free radicals** from the ischemic myocardial tissues (Ahrens & Rutherford, 1993).

Administration of fluids dramatically improves the outcome of the burn patient. Fluid resuscitation will usually be initiated in adult patients with ≥ 20 percent TBSA involvement, in the elderly with ≥ 5 to 15 percent TBSA involvement, and in children with ≥ 10 to 15 percent TBSA involvement (Gordon & Winfree, 1998). Children and the elderly are less able to tolerate the stress of injury. Volume replacement must be implemented very carefully in children and the elderly because they are very sensitive to volume. Frequently, a pulmonary artery catheter will be used to monitor fluid status in the elderly.

Patients with thermal burns that involve a TBSA of ≥ 40 percent frequently experience hypovolemic shock or burn shock. Chemical and vasoactive mediators produced as a result of burn injury cause arterial constriction initially, followed by vasodilation and increased capillary permeability. Vasodilation in combination with increased capillary permeability is referred to as *a loss of capillary seal.* The loss of capillary seal leads to massive fluid and electrolyte shifts from intravascular spaces to the interstitium. Figure 33–3 illustrates fluid and protein loss as a result of increased capillary permeability. Hypovolemic shock is a complication of loss of capillary seal and other

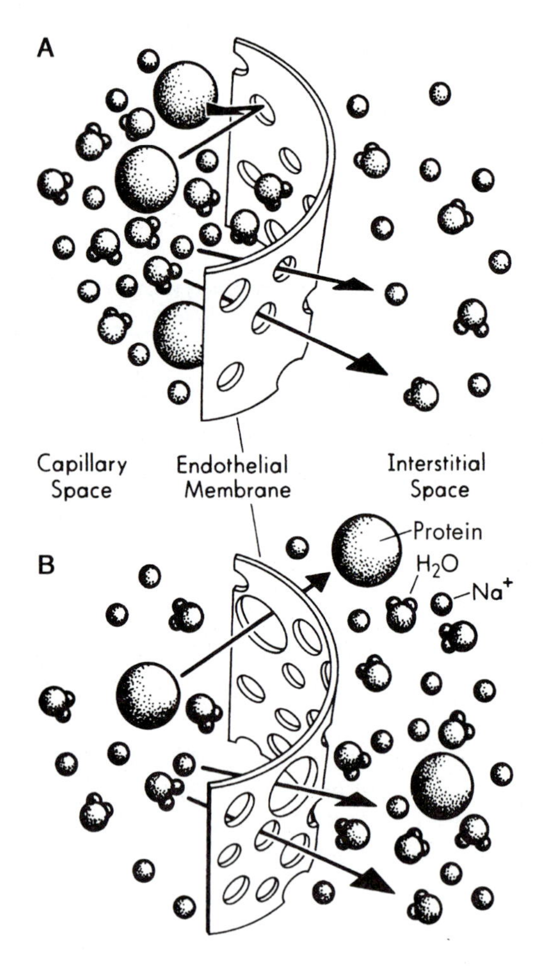

Figure 33–3. Changes in capillary permeability determines extravascular fluid levels. Note, under normal conditions **(A)** large molecules such as proteins are held in the capillary. When permeability of the capillary changes, such as in sepsis and ARDS, capillary permeability increases **(B)**. This allows proteins and other substances that normally control fluid movement to move into the interstitial space. The result is an increase in fluid outside the blood vessel.

factors. Although the exact mechanisms for vascular and fluid changes are not well understood, the capillary seal is usually restored at approximately 18 to 36 hours postinjury (Gordon & Winfree, 1998).

Restoration of intravascular volume by fluid resuscitation is a critical intervention for burn shock. The goal is to maintain vital organ perfusion without exacerbating tissue edema. The patient's physiologic responses, such as urine output, adequate vital signs, appropriate mentation, capillary refill, and peripheral pulses, will guide fluid administration efforts. The best determinant of adequate fluid resuscitation is urine output as long as the patient is not receiving a medication that will cause diuresis (e.g., diuretics or mannitol) or have glucosuria (glucose in the urine causes an osmotic diuresis).

Warmed Ringer's lactate is the fluid of choice for crystalloid fluid replacement. Fluids should be infused at a steady rate by two large-bore (14 to 16 gauge) intravenous (IV) catheters placed through unburned skin if possible. There are a number of formulas used to guide crystalloid fluid administration during the first 24 hours. Each formula will have to be modified according to the patient's response. One of the most frequent formulas used is the Parkland formula:

4 mL Ringer's lactate × TBSA % burned × pt weight (kg)

With the Parkland formula, one-half of the amount is infused over the first 8 hours postinjury. This is followed by the last half in the next 16 hours. For example, using the Parkland formula, a patient weighing 68 kilograms who experiences a 50 percent TBSA burn would require 6,800 mL of IV fluids over the first 8 hours postinjury with a subsequent infusion of 6,800 mL over the next 16 hours. Urinary output trends are monitored to determine the adequacy of fluid replacement. For adults and children weighing over 30 kg, a urinary output of 30 to 50 mL/hr is acceptable. In the child weighing less than 30 kg, 1 mL/kg/hr is the goal.

Fluid administration requirements will be altered under certain circumstances. Patients with inhalation injuries in conjunction with thermal burns will require increased amounts of fluid initially (up to 40 to 50 percent more) (Gordon & Winfree, 1998). Patients with electrical burns and associated trauma, extensive deep thermal burns, alcohol intoxication, those receiving delayed resuscitation (> 2 hours after the time of injury), or those with preexisting medical conditions (e.g., patients receiving diuretic therapy) may require increased amounts of fluid initially according to their physiologic response.

In addition to fluid resuscitation for the burn, children will need a maintenance dose of fluids to compensate for insensible water loss and to provide some glucose. Remember that children have limited glycogen stores and become hypoglycemic rapidly. Hypoglycemia must be considered in the child who is inconsolable or lethargic. For infants, the maintenance fluid should be 5% dextrose in 0.225% (¼) normal saline, and for children, the fluid should be 5% dextrose in 0.45% (½) normal saline.

The initial 24 hours of fluid therapy is aimed at maintaining vital organ perfusion and avoiding over- or underresuscitation. After the initial 24 hours postinjury, the goal shifts to restoring plasma volume and maintaining tissue perfusion. A solution containing glucose and a solution for colloid replacement (at a dose of 0.5 mL/kg/% TBSA) for patients with burns greater than 30 percent TBSA will be added to the fluid regiment. In adults the glucose containing solution is usually 5% dextrose in water (D_5W) and for children 5% dextrose in 0.45% normal saline is usually used (Gordon, 1997).

Patients who have been exposed to electrical currents are predisposed to cardiac dysrhythmias including sinus tachycardia, ST segment elevation, QT segment prolongation, ventricular ectopy, atrial fibrillation, a bundle branch block, ventricular fibrillation, and asystole (Cooper, 1998). Patients who experience lethal dysrhythmias from electrical or lightning contact (ventricular fibrillation or asystole) should receive aggressive resuscitation due to the frequency with which these patients can be successfully resuscitated. Cardiac monitoring should continue for at least 24 hours postinjury in cases in which patients having electrical contact do not seem to have any obvious injury.

Pulmonary

Alterations in pulmonary function can occur as part of the systemic response to burn injury or from direct inhalation injury. The systemic response to burn injury results in an increased systemic vascular resistance with a corresponding increase in pulmonary vascular resistance. This results in pulmonary edema from the increased capillary pressure and vasoconstriction of microcirculation. A decrease in pulmonary perfusion results in decreased diffusion of oxygen at the capillary level. Respiratory insufficiency can occur at two points postinjury; immediately during the resuscitation phase and 10 days to 2 weeks postinjury during the acute rehabilitation phase. Respiratory failure during the resuscitative phase is usually due to inhalation injury, and failure in the acute rehabilitation phase is usually due to infection (Rutan, 1998).

Circumferential full-thickness burns to the chest can also cause alterations in pulmonary function. Full-thickness burns result in **eschar** formation, which is a tough, dry, inelastic wound. If these eschar chest wounds are circumferential, the patient cannot adequately expand the chest to ventilate effectively and respiratory distress will develop. **Escharotomy** incisions are performed at the bedside to allow movement of the chest wall and to restore adequate ventilation. Third-degree burns are insensate except for perhaps the edges of the wound, so the procedure is done without anesthesia. The sites for chest escharotomy incisions are shown in Figure 33–4.

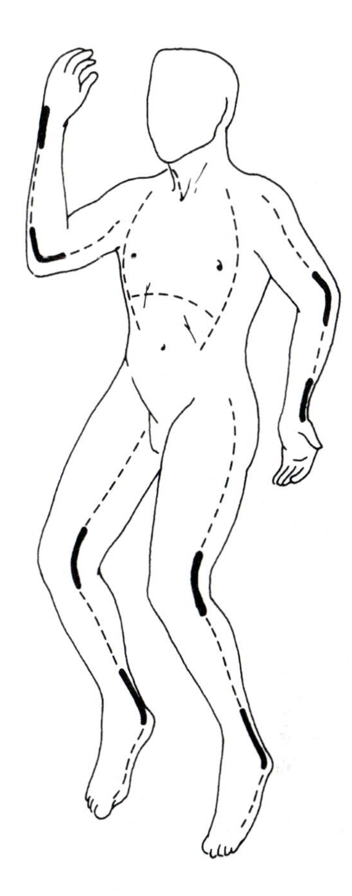

Figure 33–4. Preferred sites of escharotomy incisions. (*From Rue, L.W., & Cioffi, W.G. [1991]. Resuscitation of thermally injured patients.* Crit Care Nurs Clin North Am *3(2):181–189.*)

An inhalation injury should be suspected in the patient who presents with an altered level of consciousness or one who was within a confined space in a burning environment. It is imperative to obtain information regarding the circumstances of the fire during the initial assessment. Inhalation injury occurs from chemical and thermal mechanisms such as gases, toxic fumes, and/or steam. The clinical indicators of inhalation injury are listed in Table 33–3. The composition and amount of the inhaled substance correlates with the severity of the injury. For the purpose of this module, inhalation injury will be discussed in reference to upper airway injury (above the glottis), lower airway injury (below the glottis), and carbon monoxide (CO) injury.

Upper Airway Injury

Upper airway injury refers to an injury that is above the glottis (supraglottic) resulting from either heat or chemicals dissolved in water. Heat causes an immediate injury to the mucosa. Thermal burns from hot air are usually isolated to the supraglottic (as opposed to the infraglottic area) due to the ability of the nasopharynx to absorb the heat and a reflex closure of the glottic opening when exposed to heat. Evaluation of patients with upper airway burns may reveal facial burns, singed nasal hairs, erythema, swelling, tachypnea, dyspnea, hoarseness, a brassy cough or stridor, and ulceration, especially of the nasopharynx. Initial treatment for upper airway injury is humidified 100 percent oxygen by a snugly fitting nonrebreather mask. Careful observation is necessary to identify impending airway obstruction. Once the tissues start to swell, patients can rapidly experience an airway occlusion. Patients with

TABLE 33–3. CLINICAL INDICATORS OF INHALATION INJURY

- Facial burns with charred lips and tongue
- Carbonaceous sputum
- Wheezing or rhonchi on auscultation
- Stridor
- Cough
- Tachypnea
- Singed nasal hair
- Altered level of consciousness
- Injury in enclosed space
- History of flash burn
- Elevated carboxyhemoglobin levels
- Abnormal arterial blood gases

hoarseness, stridor, or pharyngeal burns should be intubated and transferred to a burn center. Upper airway edema peaks at 24 to 48 hours postinjury (Cioffi, 1998). If not contraindicated by concurrent trauma, the head of the bed should be elevated to help reduce edema. Circumferential burns to the neck can also cause airway obstruction due to edema. These patients will also require intubation.

Lower Airway Injury

There is an increased mortality in patients who have an inhalation component to their injury. Sixty to seventy percent of patients who die in burn centers have inhalation injuries (National Burn Institute, 1994). Lower airway injury (infraglottic) is usually due to toxic gases and chemicals contained in inhaled smoke. The inhaled smoke contains gaseous and chemical by-products of combustion. When these products come into contact with the pulmonary mucosa, a variety of things happen, such as irritation, an inflammatory reaction, or alkali or acid burns. The result is an ulceration of mucous membranes, edema, excessive secretions, a decreased ciliary action, bronchospasms, an inactivation of surfactant, and atelectasis, among other things. The end result is air flow obstruction causing hypoxia and pulmonary dysfunction. These patients develop respiratory failure and are prone to the development of pulmonary infections.

The onset of symptoms of lower airway injury is unpredictable. Patients with lower airway injury may present without symptoms to the emergency department. However, they also may present with the signs and symptoms listed for upper airway injury, in addition to a cough, carbonaceous (sooty) sputum, signs of hypoxia (agitation, anxiety, cyanosis, impaired mental status), chest tightness, flaring nostrils, grunting, crackles, rhonchi, or wheezing. If the potential for inhalation injury exists, the patient must be monitored closely for 24 hours postinjury (National Burn Institute, 1994). Diagnostic tests for determining the effects and extent of inhalation injury include arterial blood gases (partial pressure of oxygen may be normal initially), serial chest radiographs, fiberoptic bronchoscopy (visualizes tracheobronchial injuries), Xenon ventilation perfusion scan (identifies small airway and parenchymal injuries), and serum carboxyhemoglobin levels.

Treatment for lower airway injury is supportive. Any patient with the potential for inhalation injury must receive high-flow humidified oxygen (100 percent by nonrebreather mask). Patients with severe inhalation injuries or impending respiratory failure must receive high-flow humidified oxygen while preparations for endotracheal intubation are made. Nasal intubation is the preferred route for patients with burn injury. It allows for improved oropharyngeal suctioning and if the patient remains intubated for a long period of time, less glottic and subglottic stenosis has been noted due to decreased tube movement (Cioffi, 1998). A 7.5-mm endotracheal tube is preferable because it allows for passage of a fiber-optic bronchoscope.

One of the major goals of nursing care is superb pulmonary toilet. Ensuring that the patient does the coughing and deep breathing exercises, turning the patient, suctioning, chest physiotherapy, and pharmacologic interventions will help achieve this goal. Repeated assessments of respiratory status and accurate documentation for other caregivers is necessary. Ventilatory support will be tailored to each patient's needs, with the ultimate goal being improvement so that support is no longer needed. Ensuring that the endotracheal tube is secured appropriately is very important, especially in children under the age of 8 since the endotracheal tube will not have a cuff. Accidental displacement of an endotracheal tube in a patient with airway edema can have catastrophic results.

Carbon Monoxide Poisoning

Carbon monoxide poisoning is a chemical inhalation injury that has an action different than other chemicals that are inhaled. **Carbon monoxide (CO)** is a colorless, odorless gas that is a by-product of the combustion of organic material. CO is over 200 times more likely to bind to hemoglobin than oxygen, so it blocks the uptake of oxygen and causes hypoxia. Hemoglobin is saturated with CO rather than oxygen. The diagnosis of CO poisoning is made by obtaining a history of exposure to by-products of combustion, especially in an enclosed space, and by drawing a serum **carboxyhemoglobin** level (percentage of CO bound to hemoglobin). Signs and symptoms of CO poisoning result from tissue hypoxia and therefore will vary related to the degree the patient's hemoglobin is saturated with CO instead of oxygen. A serum carboxyhemoglobin level of up to 10 percent may be found in patients who are smokers or in those who live in urban environments. Mild symptoms of CO poisoning (serum level of 10 to 20 percent) include headache, confusion, and dyspnea on exertion. More severe symptoms (serum level of 20 to 40 percent) include vomiting, tachycardia, tachypnea, and hallucinations with eventual respiratory failure, coma, shock, and death (serum levels of 40 to 60 percent). The treatment for CO poisoning is simple—warmed, humidified, 100 percent oxygen by nonrebreather mask. In some cases, if the level of consciousness is decreased or if mandated by associated trauma, endotracheal intubation may be warranted. Serum carboxyhemoglobin levels are monitored, and the patient should remain on oxygen until the serum level is < 10 percent. Pulse oximetry may not be able to differentiate between hemoglobin saturated with oxygen and hemoglobin saturated with CO, so readings may be misleading.

Peripheral Vascular

Peripheral vascular assessment of each extremity occurs in the initial assessment and should be repeated every hour thereafter throughout the resuscitative phase. At this point, the capillary leak has stopped, capillary permeability has returned to normal, and edema should start to subside (Gordon & Winfree, 1998). Each extremity should be evaluated for color, temperature, pulses, capillary refill, sensation, pain, and motor movement. The best method for evaluating pulses is an ultrasonic flow meter (Doppler) (Gordon & Winfree, 1998; Jordan & Harrington, 1997). The extent of edema is related to the amount of fluid resuscitation. Increased pressure within the limb from edema can cause tissue ischemia. Elevating burned extremities above the level of the heart will help to decrease edema. Jewelry and constricting clothing should be removed as soon as possible. If **compartment syndrome** is suspected, the limb should not be elevated but kept at the level of the heart. Compartment syndrome occurs when the tissue pressure within a muscle compartment exceeds microvascular pressure causing an interruption in perfusion at the cellular level. It can occur from a crushing-type injury, trauma such as fractures, reperfusion of an ischemic extremity, or compression of an extremity such as that which occurs with third-degree circumferential burns and the subsequent underlying edema that occurs. Signs and symptoms include pain on passive stretching of the muscle, decreased sensation, weakness, swelling, and pain beyond what would be expected for the injury sustained. Treatment for a compartment syndrome is a **fasciotomy** or an escharotomy if the cause is circumferential third-degree burns (see Fig. 33–4).

A peripheral complication of deep electrical injuries is a thrombus in the venous system. Blood can enter the extremity but cannot leave, causing edema. Lightning injuries can result in a transient vasospasm producing a cold, blue, pulseless and mottled extremity. This is known as *keranoparalysis* and will usually clear within a few hours (Cooper, 1998).

In summary, cardiopulmonary and peripheral vascular complications occurring after burn injury include airway obstruction, diminished oxygenation, hypovolemia, impaired myocardial contractility, and tissue ischemia. Continuous assessment and treatment of cardiopulmonary and peripheral vascular complications promotes optimal patient recovery.

SECTION FOUR REVIEW

1. The resuscitative phase of burn injury occurs from the time of injury to
   A. 24 to 48 hours after injury
   B. 36 to 60 hours after injury
   C. 48 to 72 hours after injury
   D. 60 to 84 hours after injury
2. Critically burned patients are at high risk for which of the following complications during the resuscitative phase?
   A. burn shock
   B. neurogenic shock
   C. contractures
   D. myocardial infarction
3. Patients with > ___ percent TBSA burn may experience hypovolemic shock.
   A. 20
   B. 30
   C. 35
   D. 40
4. To detect compartmental syndrome in those with critical burns, assess for
   A. pain in extremity with exercise
   B. pain in extremity with passive movement
   C. contractures
   D. pallor in extremity
5. Calculate the fluid resuscitation requirements for Mr. Combs using the Parkland formula. Mr. Combs is status post 55 percent TBSA burn and weighs 75 kilograms. His requirements for the first 8 hours are
   A. 8,250 mL
   B. 16,500 mL
   C. 4,125 mL
   D. 12,375 mL

Answers: 1. C, 2. A, 3. D, 4. B, 5. A

SECTION FIVE: Resuscitative Phase: Neurologic and Cognitive Effects

At the completion of this section, the learner will be able to discuss nursing care of the patient experiencing neurologic and cognitive effects of burn injury and discuss pain management of the burn-injured patient.

Neurologic effects are common with electrical and lightning injury. Neurologic tissue offers low resistance to electrical currents and is easily damaged. The skull is the most common entry site for electrical current (Winfree & Barillo, 1997). Respiratory paralysis can occur and loss of consciousness is frequent especially with high-voltage injury although it is usually transient. Patients may experience confusion, exhibit a flat affect, be unable to concentrate and/or have short-term memory problems (Cooper, 1998). Seizures, headaches, peripheral nerve damage, and loss of muscle strength may be seen. Long-term or permanent numbness, prickling, tingling, heightened sensitivity, or paralysis may also occur. Spinal cord injuries can occur with high-voltage injuries. The onset of clinical manifestations may be acute or delayed and injury is usually permanent (Winfree & Barillo, 1997).

Burn injuries cause a number of physiological alterations that can impair cognition. In addition to electrical injuries altering the patient's thought process, hypoxia, hypercarbia, hypovolemia, cerebral edema, carbon monoxide, or trauma can also cause an altered level of consciousness. Each possible cause must be ruled out. A computed tomographic (CT) scan of the head may be needed to rule out an intracranial bleed. An initial neurologic examination should include pupillary response, reflexes, function of all extremities, and a scoring system to document the level of consciousness such as the Glasgow Coma Scale. Careful documentation of the assessment findings should occur so subsequent neurologic evaluations can be compared to the prior findings.

Burn injury cannot be discussed without attention being given to the pain that accompanies the injury. Full-thickness burns are usually insensate, except for the edge of the wound where partial-thickness injury exists. Partial-thickness burns are exceptionally sensitive and painful even to the effect of an air current passing over them. Pain and anxiety can hinder a patient's recovery, so the relief of pain and anxiety are critical. Burn patients typically experience two types of physical pain after injury: (1) chronic pain from damaged tissue, and (2) acute pain as a result of procedures such as wound care and physical therapy (Marvin, 1998). Anxiety contributes to the patient's perception of pain, so pharmacologic treatment must include an opiate and an anxiolytic to help alleviate both of these. Morphine sulfate and midazolam are usually the drugs of choice. Pain is very individualized and should be measured by the patient if possible, not assessed by the health care provider. A pain scale should be used to evaluate pain, and medication should be given on a schedule, not as a PRN dose. The intravenous route is preferred, as absorption from muscle is unpredictable due to vasoconstriction and edema.

Watkins and associates (1988) describe seven stages of psychological adaptation to burn injury. Patients move forward and backward through the stages of adaptation and they frequently overlap. Stages of psychological adaptation, patient response, and nursing interventions appropriate for patients and families are outlined in Table 33–4.

TABLE 33–4. STAGES OF PSYCHOLOGICAL ADAPTATION FOLLOWING BURN INJURY

ADAPTIVE STAGE	PATIENT RESPONSE	NURSING INTERVENTIONS
Stage 1: Survival anxiety		
Patient is concerned about survival; fear of death prevails	Tremulousness, easy startle response, difficulty concentrating or following instructions, tearfulness, poor cooperation with treatments, social withdrawal, silence	Educate patient regarding extent of burn injury and most likely course for recuperation. Allow time for verbalization of fears, give reality-based responses.
Stage 2: The problem of pain		
Burn injuries can be extremely painful; patients focus on pain relief in this stage	Increased reports of pain, frequent requests for analgesia, poor cooperation with treatments, demanding and dependent behaviors	Assess and treat pain with pharmacologic and nonpharmacologic interventions.
Stage 3: The search for meaning		
During this stage the patient searches for a logical, understandable explanation for the injury	Repeated recounts of events preceding and during injury	Provide nonjudgmental listening and discussion to assist patient with finding acceptable answers. This is called "validation." If the patient does not successfully complete stage 3, posttraumatic stress disorder can occur.
Stage 4: Investment in recuperation		
Patients in this stage focus on understanding and participating in treatments necessary for obtaining daily life skills such as walking, self-feeding, and grooming	Open interest in treatments; asks many questions; desires to complete tasks without assistance; high motivation; hostility if unsuccessful with tasks	Praise attempts for autonomous functioning. Orient to physical phenomena related to healing such as itching and decreased activity tolerance. Continue education on expected course of recovery.
Stage 5: Acceptance of losses		
Comprehension of long-term losses occur cognitively and emotionally	Sadness over losses exhibited by tearfulness, decreased appetite, social withdrawal, sleep disturbance, or anger	Allow time for discussion of feelings. Legitimize patient feelings (reassure that feelings are appropriate for loss). Encourage interactions with family and friends to provide evidence of worth despite injury. Depression can occur if acceptance does not take place.
Stage 6: Investment in rehabilitation		
Patients work on resuming own unique lifestyle	Interest in treatments; increased motivation; trial and error attempts to return to preburn functioning	Praise patient's efforts to adapt to injuries and manipulate environment to provide newer ways of functioning.
Stage 7: Reintegration of identity		
Assessment of the cumulative effects of burn injury helps the patient cognitively and affectively define postburn "self"	Verbalizes perceptions of how functioning has changed from preburn norm	Acknowledge patient's view of self. Refrain from forcing the staffs' expectations for those recovering from burn injury on patients.

Data from Watkins, P.N., Cook, E.L., May, S.R., & Ehleben, C.M. (1988). Psychological stages in adaptation following burn injury: A method for facilitating psychological recovery of burn victims. J Burn Care Rehab *9(4):376–384.*

Coping with a burn injury is complex and requires a multifaceted approach. Emotional support from family and friends can be very helpful to the patient. Distraction, imagery, self-hypnosis, information, and relaxation techniques can also help a patient to cope with the stress, pain, and anxiety that occurs. If the patient is a child, parents who are capable of support should be included in the nursing care plan. Crisis intervention counseling immediately following an event may have positive long-term effects for some patients. Frequently, patients will need counseling into the long-term rehabilitation phase.

In summary, neurologic difficulties experienced by burn patients during the emergent phase include altered levels of consciousness, acute pain, and suboptimal psychological adaptation. Nursing interventions to relieve pain and promote adaptation are important components of the nursing care plan.

SECTION FIVE REVIEW

1. In general, full-thickness burns are
   A. not painful
   B. mildly painful
   C. moderately painful
   D. extremely painful

2. During the survival-anxiety stage of psychological adaptation to burn injury (stage I), patients typically
   A. recount events preceding injury
   B. ask many questions
   C. fear death
   D. are highly motivated

Answers: 1. A, 2. C

SECTION SIX: Resuscitative Phase: Gastrointestinal/Metabolic and Renal Effects

At the completion of this section, the learner will be able to discuss nursing care of the patient experiencing gastrointestinal, metabolic, and renal effects of burn injury.

Gastrointestinal

Gastrointestinal (GI) dysfunction is directly related to the size of the burn injury. Complications include paralytic ileus, gastric dilation, constipation, and stress ulcers (Curling's ulcer). These complications all alter the GI system's ability to absorb and provide the body with needed nutrients. Gastric emptying and decompression should be accomplished with a gastric tube if the TBSA burned is ≥ 20 percent because decreased peristaltic activity causes gastric dilation and increases the risk of aspiration (Oman & Reilly, 1998; Edlich & Moghtader, 1998). Patients with significant burns are prone to stress ulcers. Treatment is preventative in nature utilizing antacids to neutralize gastric acids and a histamine receptor agonist to decrease the gastric acid production.

In addition to the absorption problems, the second effect burns have on the GI system has to do with the movement of bacteria from the intestines to other parts of the body. The intestinal mucosa loses the ability to contain bacteria within the intestinal lumen (increased permeability of the intestinal mucosa) in a phenomenon called *bacterial translocation*. This may be one mechanism by which multiple organ dysfunction syndrome (MODS) develops in burn patients (Rutan, 1998).

Metabolic

The metabolic changes that occur in the burn patient also are related to the extent of injury. Initially, metabolism is depressed. Within a few days, when capillary wall integrity is restored and the patient becomes hemodynamically stable, marked hormonal changes occur resulting in a hypermetabolic state. Patients experience an increase in cardiac output, oxygen consumption, carbon dioxide production, caloric requirements, energy consumption, heart rate, respiratory rate, and body temperature. This hypermetabolic state will remain until the wounds close.

Nutritional requirements are strongly influenced by the metabolic response. Adequate caloric intake is imperative for wound healing and maintaining the immune system. Multiple formulas exist for estimating caloric needs of burn patients. Energy requirements are assessed and formulas that calculate both energy and protein needs are used. Increased protein intake is needed to counteract the use of lean body mass and viscera as a source of protein in this hypermetabolic state (Gottschlich & Jenkins, 1998). Adequate intake can be evaluated by monitoring the patient's weight, caloric intake, and fluid intake and output. Laboratory tests can also aid in the evaluation. Serum albumin is indicative of the depletion of visceral proteins, urinary urea nitrogen reflects protein breakdown, and urinary creatinine assesses lean body mass. Immune function can be assessed (total lymphocyte count), and the severity of the hypermetabolic response can be evaluated (resting energy expenditure) (Gottschlich & Jenkins, 1998).

Renal

Oliguria and anuria can be seen in the initial phase of burn injury. As intravascular volume is depleted, urine output decreases to compensate for the fluid loss. With adequate fluid resuscitation, urine output will increase. Urine output is the most reliable single indicator of adequate volume resuscitation. Placement of a urinary catheter with a collection chamber that allows for hourly urine output measurements is mandatory. Adequate urine output is considered 30 to 50 mL/hr in an adult. Adequate urine output in a child weighing less than 30 kg is 1 mL/kg/hr. For a child over 30 kg, urine output should be 30 to 50 mL/hr, which is the same as for an adult. These formulas are valid only if there is no glucose in the urine (glucose prompts an osmotic diuresis so urine output will not be indicative of the adequacy of fluid resuscitation) and no diuretics have been given (Gordon & Winfree, 1998). Urine output is used to evaluate the adequacy of fluid resuscitation in conjunction with other assessment parameters indicative of fluid status such as level of consciousness, capillary refill, skin color and temperature, age-appropriate vital signs, and peripheral pulses.

If a patient has experienced muscle damage from exposure to an electrical current or a crush-type injury, the urine may be a red to reddish-brown color. This discoloration is due to **myoglobin** in the urine. Myoglobin is released from damaged muscle tissue and can clog the renal tubules, causing renal failure especially in the face of inadequate fluid resuscitation, shock, or acidosis. If myoglobin is present in the urine, to guide the effectiveness of fluid administration and to prevent myoglobinuric renal failure, an adequate urine output is considered to be 75 to 100 mL/hr in an adult or 2 mL/kg/hr in a child. This rate of urine output should be maintained as long as the pigment is present. In addition to increasing the amount of fluids administered, alkalinization of the urine will also promote clearance of myoglobin. The solubility of myoglobin increases in an alkaline environment, so maintaining alkaline urine will increase the rate of myoglobin clearance. By adding 50 mEq of sodium bicarbonate to each liter of intravenous fluids, a slight alkalinization of the blood is maintained (pH—7.45) and ensures that the urine is also alkaline (Cooper, 1998; National Burn Institute, 1994). An osmotic diuretic such as mannitol may be used to increase diuresis and promote the clearance of myoglobin.

In addition to myoglobin causing discoloration of the urine, hemoglobin released from damaged red blood cells can also cause a red to reddish-brown urine. It is difficult to distinguish myoglobin from hemoglobin by looking at the urine, so until laboratory tests confirm the presence of one or both of these substances, treat all red to reddish-brown discoloration of the urine as if it were myoglobin until proven otherwise. Both myoglobin and hemoglobin are excreted more readily if the urine pH is alkaline.

In summary, patients with burns are prone to developing stress ulcers and an ileus. Measures to prevent and treat these conditions must be taken. Patients require close monitoring to ensure they meet the adequate energy and protein needs that will promote wound healing and maintain an efficient immune system. Urine output is the best single indicator of the adequacy of fluid resuscitation and should be monitored hourly during the initial phase of burn care.

SECTION SIX REVIEW

1. A gastric tube should initially be placed in patients with TBSA burn of ≥ 20 percent to
   A. remove bacteria from the stomach
   B. prevent vomiting and aspiration of contents due to decreased peristaltic activity
   C. decrease gastric acid production
   D. supplement energy and protein needs
2. What is the expected hourly urine output of the patient in question 2?
   A. 12 mL/hr
   B. 18 mL/hr
   C. 24 mL/hr
   D. 36 mL/hr
3. In the presence of myoglobin in the urine, alkalinization of the urine will
   A. promote renal clearance of myoglobin
   B. promote hepatic clearance of myoglobin
   C. increase urine output
   D. concentrate the myoglobin so it can be removed more easily

Answers: 1. B, 2. C, 3. A

SECTION SEVEN: Overview of Wound Healing and Initial Wound Care

At the completion of this section, the learner will be able to discuss wound healing and describe the care of the burn wound in the resuscitative phase. Before reading this section, it may be helpful to review normal wound healing as it is outlined in Module 32.

Wound Healing

The cellular and biochemical events that occur during the healing of burn injuries are similar to those that occur in the healing of other wounds. The major difference is that the phases of wound healing in the burn occur more slowly and last longer. Wound healing begins immediately after the injury occurs with the inflammatory response. The inflammatory phase lasts approximately 2 weeks, extending into the acute rehabilitative phase; thus, overall wound repair is delayed. Once the inflammatory phase is finished, the proliferative phase of healing begins and lasts up to one month. During this phase, collagen synthesis, revascularization, and reepithelialization occur although at a slower rate than in wounds from other injuries. Collagen layers are not as organized as they are in other wounds, which contribute to excessive scar tissue. The maturation phase of wound healing follows proliferative phase and can last 6 to 18 months or longer depending on the wound. New collagen layers are placed, strengthening the wound, while old collagen layers are broken down. Excessive deposits of collagen during this time will produce hypertrophic scars that are characteristic of deep partial and full-thickness burns. Hypertrophic scars contract while maturing, which can lead to contractures. Wound contraction can produce both cosmetic and functional deformities.

Initial Wound Care During the Resuscitative Phase

The first step in caring for the burn wound is to ensure the burning process has stopped. Clothing, jewelry, belts, or anything containing heat is removed from the patient (adhered clothing or tar is left in place and cooled with water—removing it will cause further damage to the skin). Dry chemicals are brushed from the patient (taking care not to contaminate the caregiver) and as soon as possible, burned areas should be cooled and flushed with copious amounts of tepid water (chemical burns for 20 to 30 minutes or until the pain has stopped). All burn victims are considered trauma victims and are assessed using primary and secondary assessment guidelines (see Module 34). The initial assessment of the burn wound takes place in the secondary assessment after the head-to-toe evaluation has been completed. Burned extremities should be elevated above the level of the heart to decrease edema formation unless contraindicated by the presence of compartment syndrome. The head of the bed can also be elevated to reduce upper body and head edema if not contraindicated by trauma. Tetanus prophylaxis should be administered if necessary.

Initial care of the burn wound will depend on the severity. If the patient meets criteria for transfer to a burn center, the patient should be covered with a clean, dry sheet. Care must be taken to avoid hypothermia. If time permits, the wound can be gently cleansed with sterile saline or a mild soap. Creams or ointments should not be applied as removal of the substance will be necessary on arrival to the burn center to evaluate the wounds. This is a painful procedure, so unless directed to do so by the receiving physician, leave the wound clean and covered with a sheet. An escharotomy may need to be performed on a circumferential burn. Definitive care of the wound will begin once the patient has been admitted to the hospital, whether that is a burn center or a hospital with the ability to care for the burn injury effectively.

In summary, burn wounds heal much like other wounds except that the healing process is slower; therefore, each phase of healing takes longer.

Section Seven Review

1. Initial evaluation of burn wounds takes place
   - **A.** immediately upon arrival
   - **B.** at the end of the primary assessment
   - **C.** at the end of head-to-toe evaluation during the secondary assessment
   - **D.** on admission to the burn center

2. Burned extremities should be
   A. elevated above the level of the heart to decrease edema
   B. placed in a position of comfort according to the patient's wishes
   C. placed below the level of the heart to facilitate drainage of fluid
   D. wrapped tightly to help prevent edema of the extremity

Answers: 1. C, 2. A

SECTION EIGHT: Burn Wound Management

At the completion of this section, the learner will be able to describe burn wound management in the resuscitative phase and the acute rehabilitative phase.

The acute rehabilitative phase of burn care lasts from 2 to 3 days postinjury to discharge from the hospital when the wounds have closed. The goals of burn wound management include prevention/control of infection, preserve viable tissue, and promote wound closure with a minimal number of side effects. Interventions aimed at supporting these goals are wound cleansing, debridement, topical antimicrobial therapy, and wound closure. Wound care must be performed in a warm environment to prevent hypothermia. Strict aseptic technique and sterile supplies must be used and the patient should be in protective isolation. In addition, appropriate analgesia must be given prior to initiation of the wound care. The analgesia must be given time to take effect.

In-patient burn care begins with wounds being initially cleansed with water (known as hydrotherapy) and a mild soap to remove exudate and devitalized tissue. This can be accomplished (1) by showering if the patient is able, (2) by immersion in a tub if the burn is moderate in size, (3) by placing the patient on a table where the wounds are washed and rinsed with running water from spray hoses, or if these methods are contraindicated, (4) wounds can be cleaned while the patient is in bed. Body hair within 2.5 cm of the wound is shaved. Once the wound has been cleaned, it must be debrided. Wound **debridement** is the removal of debris and nonviable tissue from a wound (Carrougher, 1998).

Wound Debriding

Wound debridement can be achieved mechanically, chemically, or surgically. Mechanical debridement immediately follows wound cleansing. Debridement can be partially achieved through hydrotherapy. Another means of debriding the wound is by wet-to-dry or wet-to-moist dressings in which drainage, exudate, and necrotic debris are adhere to the dressing and are removed as the dressing is carefully removed (Carrougher, 1998). Mechanical debridement can also be achieved with sterile scissors and forceps. With all of these methods of mechanical debridement, care must be taken to avoid disrupting newly formed granulation tissue and/or epithelial buds in the healing wound. When utilizing wet-to-moist or wet-to-dry dressings, protection of the healing tissue is difficult, as the process removes anything adhered to the dressing including healthy tissue (Carrougher, 1998). Treatment of burn blisters, or **bullae,** is controversial. Fluid-filled blisters less than 2 cm in diameter are usually left intact. Blisters larger than 2 cm in diameter may be left intact, sterilely drained of fluid by aspiration, or opened and the loose skin removed, depending on the caregiver's preference. Some studies have found burn blister fluid may interfere with wound healing.

Chemical debridement involves the application of enzymatic or a fibrinolytic preparation to the burn wound to digest necrotic tissue and hasten eschar separation. These products work best in a moist environment within a specific pH range (Carrougher, 1998), and they have no antimicrobial properties.

Surgical debridement is accomplished under general anesthesia in the operating suite and usually takes place in three to five days following the injury as the resuscitative phase ends and hemodynamic stability and capillary seal has been achieved (Jordan & Harrington, 1997). There are two methods of burn wound excision: tangential excision and fascial excision. The method used is dependent on the depth and extent of burn. Tangential excision involves the shaving away of thin layers of eschar until viable tissue is exposed. This method gives a better cosmetic result; however, significant blood loss may occur causing hypovolemia. Fascial excision involves removing nonviable tissue down to the fascial or subcutaneous planes. It is often used for patients with a large component of full-thickness burns because it is less stressful. Fascial excision will not produce as good a cosmetic result as tangential excision will; however, if the injury is such that the patient will not survive the stress of tangential excision, fascial excision should be used (Jordan & Harrington, 1997).

Topical Antimicrobial Therapy

Application of the topical agent immediately follows wound cleansing and debridement. The goal of antimicrobial therapy is to keep bacterial proliferation to a minimum so it can be controlled by the body's own immune system until the wound has closed. Because burn wounds are avascular, topical administration of antimicrobials is the route of choice. The burn team physicians order the antimicrobial and its frequency and method of application. Application of the topical agent is performed by the nursing staff using meticulous sterile technique once or twice daily. Table 33–5 lists topical agents most frequently used explaining the advantages and disadvantages of each. The most frequently used topical antimicrobial is silver sulfadiazine 1 percent (Silvadene). Many burn centers will combine the use of silver sulfadiazine and mafenide acetate to obtain the benefits of both and minimize the side effects. Mafenide acetate (Sulfamylon) is usually applied during the day to obtain its eschar penetration capabilities. Mafenide acetate is painful after application, so it is applied during the day when the patient will be awake. Silver sulfadiazine is applied during the evening to allow the patient a more restful night.

Once the antimicrobial has been applied, an open or closed dressing technique will be utilized. The open method leaves the antimicrobial-covered wound open to air. The antimicrobial is reapplied if it gets removed with patient movement. The open approach allows for increased visualization of the wound, decreased bacterial growth, and greater joint mobility. Disadvantages include messiness, poor patient acceptance, and high risk for wound trauma and hypothermia. The closed method involves the application of gauze dressings over the antimicrobial agent. Proponents of this method argue its superiority because it assists with debridement and protects granulation tissue and fragile epithelial buds, while also decreasing the evaporative fluid loss from the wounds. Disadvantages to the closed method include fewer opportunities to evaluate the wound as it is covered except during dressing changes and decreased joint mobility due to bulky dressings.

Biologic, synthetic, and biosynthetic materials act as a skin substitute and can be used to temporarily cover a burn. The type used depends on the depth of the wound and the goal of therapy. Biologic dressings obtained from animals and are referred to as **xenografts** or **heterografts** (frequently pigs). Biologic dressings obtained from humans are called **allografts** or **homografts.** These grafts are used to cover clean, superficial partial-thickness burns; maintain a moist wound environment; protect the ungrafted wound; and test the receptivity of a wound to autografting (Carrougher, 1998; Jordan & Harrington, 1997). If an infection or necrotic tissue is present in the wound, the biologic dressing will not adhere to the wound. If the biologic dressing will not adhere, it is termed a failure and it is better to have failure of a biologic dressing rather than the failure of a valuable donor site autograft (Carrougher, 1998). Biologic dressings are occlusive, so they also help to reduce pain. The functions of temporary wound coverings are listed in Table 33–6.

Synthetic materials such as thin film dressings are used to cover donor sites and to protect clean small superficial wounds. These dressings are waterproof, transparent, reduce pain, and maintain moisture in the wound to promote healing. Examples include Opsite and Tegaderm (3M Medical Surgical Division, St. Paul, Minnesota).

TABLE 33–5. TOPICAL ANTIMICROBIALS

MEDICATIONS	ADVANTAGES	DISADVANTAGES
Neomycin ointment	Painless No allergic reaction Aesthetically pleasing Won't harm eyes	Only indicated for superficial partial-thickness facial burns and donor sites
Silver nitrate 0.5% solution	Excellent antibacterial spectrum including yeast and fungus No allergic reactions No pain	Poor penetration of eschar Discoloration of the wound makes wound evaluation difficult Messy May cause hyponatremia, hypochloremia, hypercalcemia
1% silver sulfadiazine (Silvadene, SSD)	Broad antimicrobial activity Minimal sensitivity Minimal allergic reaction Painless on application No systemic effects May be used with open or closed dressing technique	Reported enterobacterial resistance Partial penetration through full-thickness eschar Poor cartilage penetration Reported transient leukopenia
Mafenide acetate (Sulfamylon)	Excellent tissue, cartilage, and eschar penetration Excellent gram-negative coverage	5% allergic rate Painful for 15 to 30 minutes postapplication Inhibits carbonic anhydrase, resulting in metabolic acidosis Does not kill yeast

TABLE 33–6. FUNCTIONS OF TEMPORARY WOUND COVERINGS

- Decreases bacterial proliferation
- Prevents desiccation
- Controls heat loss
- Decreases protein loss in wound exudate
- Increases patient comfort
- Protects underlying structures
- Stimulates healing
- Prepares/tests wound bed for autografting

Data from Duncan, D.J., & Driscoll, D.M. (1991). Burn wound management. Crit Care Clin *3(2):199–200.*

Another type of synthetic dressing is called a composite dressing. This type of dressing is used on wounds that are producing an exudate or a graft site. They absorb exudate while maintaining a moist environment. An example is Lyofoam (Seton Healthcare Group, London, England).

The third type of dressing used to cover wounds is a biosynthetic dressing. These dressings are also used to cover clean superficial partial-thickness burns, meshed autografts, donor sites, and exudative wounds (Carrougher, 1998). Examples include Biobrane (Dow Hickam Pharmaceuticals, Inc., Sugar Land, Texas) and Curasorb (Kendall Co., Mansfield, Massachusetts; Kalginate, DeRoyal Wound Care, Powell, Texas).

Nursing care related to temporary wound coverings include the periodic application and removal of the dressing material. Dressings and the surrounding tissues should also be regularly inspected for dislodgment, suppuration, fluid accumulation, and cellulitis. Most of these complications can be prevented by stabilizing the temporary covering with gauze, keeping it dry, keeping out contamination, and preventing wound shearing.

Wound Closure

Superficial partial-thickness burns heal by spontaneous reepithelialization within 7 to 10 days. In contrast, full-thickness wounds will not reepithelialize and require skin grafting for closure. A large TBSA or deep partial-thickness burn will also be grafted as healing usually takes ≥ 14 days and will usually scar significantly.

Early excision and closure of burn wounds has several advantages; improved survival, reduction in the incidence of infection, reduced in-hospital stay, require less grafting, improved cosmetic results and better functional outcome. Once the wound has been excised, steps must be taken to close the wound. **Autografting** is the process of transplanting skin from one part of the body to fill in another part that has been injured, as in a burn wound. It is a method of permanent burn wound closure and utilizes either full-thickness or split-thickness skin grafts.

When the skin is removed down to the subcutaneous layer for grafting it is termed a *full-thickness skin graft.* Full-thickness skin grafts are used to cover areas that need the extra thickness and the durability it provides, such as the palm of the hand, or to cover a point that will be exposed to pressure, such as the elbow or the scapula. When removing skin for a full-thickness graft, the donor site becomes a full-thickness skin defect. This defect must be closed by either suturing or by using a split-thickness skin graft. Full-thickness grafting is used for small areas only.

Split-thickness skin grafts are not as thick as full-thickness grafts. The donor site is a partial-thickness skin defect that will heal within 10 to 14 days. A split-thickness skin graft can be used a sheet graft or as a meshed graft. Skin is harvested from a donor site, using an instrument called a dermatome. The sheet graft is taken from the donor site and placed on the recipient wound. To make a meshed graft, the skin is taken from the donor site, then expanded using a mesh dermatome. The mesh dermatome makes multiple small slits in the skin, giving it a netting type of appearance. A meshed graft is expanded to cover a larger area. Sheet grafts usually provide a better cosmetic appearance than meshed grafts, so they are usually used for conspicuous sites such as the face and hands (Mozingo, 1998).

Skin grafts adhere to the recipient site by the presence of serum between the two layers. Soon, a fibrin matrix forms, which better secures the graft to the donor site. Within 48 hours, the wound will take on a pink or red color, indicating graft vascularization has taken place (Mozingo, 1998).

Nursing care of the burn includes monitoring for infection. Signs of noninvasive wound infection include reddened wound edges, generalized wound discoloration, change in the color of the wound exudate, foul-smelling exudate, loss of a healed skin graft, and an increase in wound pain. Signs of more severe invasive infection include conversion of a partial-thickness injury to a full-thickness injury, early separation of eschar, small necrotic subcutaneous vessels, tenderness at the wound edges, and edema. Burn wounds are not always easy to evaluate, so surface wound culture and sensitivity tests are frequently done. A burn wound biopsy will be done if an infection is suspected.

In summary, the nursing care goals related to postoperative management of autografts are to prevent infection and maintain graft immobility. Interventions include elevation of the extremity, the use of splints and bed cradles, frequent linen changes and the encouragement of patient compliance. Immobilization of the patient can cause side effects such as decubitus ulcers, joint stiffness, and pulmonary problems. Early mobilization can help prevent these complications. Donor site defects are painful in the immediate postoperative period and require the administration of analgesics.

SECTION EIGHT REVIEW

1. Which topical antimicrobial has excellent eschar penetration?
   A. Neomycin ointment
   B. silver nitrate
   C. silver sulfadiazine (Silvadene)
   D. mafenide acetate (Sulfamylon)
2. A method of permanent burn wound closure is
   A. xenograft
   B. allograft
   C. autograft
   D. homograft
3. Which of the following types of burns will not require skin grafting?
   A. small, partial-thickness
   B. large, partial-thickness
   C. small, full-thickness
   D. large, full-thickness

Answers. 1. D, 2. C, 3. A

SECTION NINE: Acute Rehabilitative Phase: Nutrition

At the completion of this section, the learner will be able to describe nutritional support for burn patients during the acute rehabilitative phase of injury.

High-calorie, high-protein diets with vitamin and mineral supplements are recommended to replace protein losses and to promote wound healing in patients with critical burns (Gottschlich & Jenkins, 1998). During the acute rehabilitative phase, the patient is offered an oral diet when bowel function returns. Nurses in the burn unit closely monitor the patient's food intake with daily calorie counts. High-calorie, high-protein oral supplements that are made to meet the specific nutritional needs of the patient are encouraged. Meals can be more palatable if the patient's favorite selections can be provided from the dietary department or from home. Family members should be encouraged to join the patient for meals when possible. Patients should feed themselves with minimal assistance from family or staff to promote range of motion and independence. Assistive devices may be necessary for self-feeding and are provided by the burn team's occupational therapist. Patients who cannot take food orally require enteral feedings or total parenteral nutrition (TPN). Enteral feedings are preferred over TPN because there are fewer side effects. TPN is associated with a high incidence of infection and is reserved for patients who have GI ulceration or bowel ischemia, or in whom enteral feedings cannot meet the caloric requirements of the patient (Gottschlich & Jenkins, 1998). Dietitians collaborate with other members to monitor closely the patient's weight (without dressings), diagnostic tests reflective of nutritional status, and progression of wound healing in order to provide adequate nutritional support. Laboratory tests commonly used to assess the nutritional status of burn patients include serum electrolytes along with transferrin, prealbumin, cholesterol, triglyceride, ionized calcium, and magnesium levels. (See Module 27 for further information.)

In summary, during the acute phase of burn injury patients should receive oral high-calorie, high-protein diets when GI function returns. If an oral diet is not feasible, nutritional support should be maintained by enteral feedings or TPN.

SECTION NINE REVIEW

1. The diet of choice for burn patients is
   A. high fat, low carbohydrate
   B. low fat, high carbohydrate
   C. high protein, high calorie
   D. low protein, high calorie
2. The nurse can enhance the patient's nutritional status by
   A. always feeding the patient
   B. discouraging visitors
   C. withholding nutritional support until bowel sounds return
   D. encouraging family involvement in meal time

Answers: 1. C, 2. D

SECTION TEN: Acute Rehabilitative Phase: Psychosocial Needs

At the completion of this section, the learner will be able to describe expected behaviors, emotional status, and levels of pain for burn patients during the acute rehabilitative phase, and their related nursing actions.

Behavioral Changes

In addition to the physical recovery during this phase, emotional recovery must also continue. The ramifications of the injury will begin to be apparent to the patient and the response by the patient can be varied. The patient's ability to cope with the injury will be in part dependent upon past coping mechanisms the patient has learned. These mechanisms may be healthy or they may be dysfunctional. Problems most frequently experienced by burn patients include anxiety, fear, grief, depression, sleep problems, acute stress disorder, and aggressive or regressive behavior.

Psychological and emotional problems can be minimized by involving the patient in self-care soon after injury. Patients should participate in wound care, feeding, exercising, and administering medications as soon as they are physically and emotionally able to improve their self concept. Fear and anxiety as a result of burn injury can be reduced with repeated and consistent explanations in appropriate terms. Visitors can help encourage the depressed burn patient. Visits by recovered burn patients allow patients to discuss their concerns with nonmedical personnel who can offer practical advice on coping with burns. This can be arranged by contacting the national office of the Phoenix Society, a support group for burn survivors, at (800) 888-BURN.

Pain

During the acute rehabilitative phase of burn injury, patients generally experience decreasing levels of pain. However, pain continues to occur as chronic or background pain and as procedural pain. Procedures, surgery, or infection can delay the easement of pain. Interventions may vary depending on the duration and severity of pain. Patients achieve better pain control when they are given opportunities to choose interventions that work best for them. As the patient stabilizes and pain levels begin to decrease, oral analgesics are used with greater frequency. Methadone is commonly administered around the clock and supplemented as needed for episodic procedure-related discomfort. Nonpharmacologic interventions for pain control include but are not limited to biofeedback, hypnosis, relaxation therapy, and guided imagery. Thorough pain assessment should be conducted on a regular basis throughout the patient's recovery and the plan of care adjusted accordingly.

In summary, behavioral changes and pain are common concerns during the acute rehabilitative phase of burn injury. Continued education and support coupled with a combination of psychological and pharmacological support will assist the patient in coping with the effects of the burn injury. Thorough assessment coupled with consistent intervention can diminish these complications.

SECTION TEN REVIEW

1. Members of the Phoenix Society are
   A. burn nurses
   B. safety educators
   C. social workers
   D. burn survivors

2. During the acute rehabilitative phase of burn care, analgesics are administered with increasing frequency by the ____ route.
   A. intravenous
   B. intramuscular
   C. oral
   D. topical

Answers: 1. D, 2. C

SECTION ELEVEN: Acute Rehabilitative Phase: Physical Mobility

At the completion of this section, the learner will be able to describe the goals, interventions, and health professionals involved with promoting physical mobility during the acute rehabilitative phase of burn care.

Physical mobility problems during the acute rehabilitative phase of burn care are directly related to the healing wound itself and the therapeutic interventions necessary to maintain life and close the wound. During the resuscitative phase, excessive edema develops in the extremities, which impairs or precludes range of motion and results in fibrosis and soft tissue contracture. Later, this problem is compounded by the limitations placed on mobility in an effort to protect healing grafts from shearing and the patient's desire to assume a position of comfort, which is typically flexed. Therefore, the treatment goals related to physical mobility during the acute rehabilitative phase include:

- Maintenance of musculoskeletal, cardiopulmonary, and respiratory function
- Promoting wound healing
- Protection of healing skin grafts
- Prevention of contractures and soft tissue deformity
- Preserving and strengthening extremity function
- Scar management
- Achievement of maximum functional recovery
- Education of patient and family

The burn team members most involved in this process are the physical therapist (PT), occupational therapist (OT), and nursing staff. The OT/PTs develop a treatment plan, fashion appliances, and perform daily treatments. The role of the nursing staff is to integrate the treatment plan into their delivery of care and to provide assessment feedback to the OT/PTs. In addition, nurses play a pivotal role in gaining patient compliance as they have continuous contact with the patient and many opportunities to support the patient toward these rehabilitation goals.

Interventions to promote physical mobility during the acute phase of burn care employ many techniques and devices. Antideformity positioning should begin at the time of admission unless contraindicated by a complicating condition. Its use is imperative during the acute phase because it decreases scar contracture across flexor surfaces, which often compromises joint mobility and functional capacity (Table 33–7). Slings, splints, donuts, wedges, and footboards are some of the assistive devices used to maintain proper positioning.

Joint function is also preserved by active and passive range of motion exercises. When appropriate, continuous passive motion machines may be applied to lower extremities early in the acute phase. Mobility outcomes may actually be improved by the administration of analgesics prior to therapy and should be discussed with the patient.

Early total body mobilization is important due to the impact that upright positioning has on cardiopulmonary functioning. Patients are assisted out of bed and ambulated early in the acute phase after hemodynamic stabilization. It is important to apply compression wraps on lower extremities before getting the patient out of bed, in order to prevent venous stasis. If extremities are not

TABLE 33–7. ANTIDEFORMITY POSITIONING

BODY PART	SUPINE POSITION	PRONE POSITION
Head and neck	There should be no pillow allowed under the head to maintain at least a neutral head position. Slight extension of the neck is preferred.	A pillow is placed under the upper chest with a small roll under the forehead to maintain the neck position for ease of breathing.
Shoulders	Upper extremities should be placed so there is at least 90 degrees of abduction at the shoulders in neutral horizontal abduction. This position will assist in preventing anterior and posterior axillary banding.	Upper extremities should be placed in no more than 90 degrees abduction.
Elbows	Elbows should be fully extended. Patients will experience decreased personal independence in activities of daily living if the elbow is allowed to tighten in a flexed position. Flexion is easier to regain than extension owing to the greater strength of the flexor muscle groups.	Elbows may be moved from full extension to 40 degrees flexion for brief periods of time as a position change.
Ankles	Neutral position of dorsiflexion/plantar flexion and inversion/eversion should be maintained. Heels should be kept free from pressure. Use of a footboard is advisable.	A space should be maintained between the foot of the bed and the end of the mattress so that the feet may hang off the end of the bed in a neutral position at the ankle.
	SPECIAL CARE AREAS	
Wrist and hand	In supine or prone positions the hands should be splinted with 90 degrees flexion at the MCP joints with the fingers in full extension. The thumb web space should be preserved and the wrist held at 30 to 40 degrees extension. This functional positioning will prevent deformities which are difficult to treat and limit patient activities.	
Hips	In both supine and prone positions, the hips should be maintained in neutral or slight extension. Fifteen degrees of abduction is advisable. Prevention of hip flexion contractures is important to facilitate early ambulation.	

Adapted from Harden, N.G., & Luster, S.H. (1991). Rehabilitation considerations in the care of the acute burn patient. Crit Care Nurs Clin.North Am 3*(2):245–253.*

wrapped, the patient is at risk for capillary bed bleeding, which could cause autograft failure or delay donor-site healing. Venous pooling coupled with prolonged immobility also predisposes the patient to deep vein thromboses. Wrapping the extremities should continue until all wounds are healed and pressure garments are available.

In summary, the physical mobility needs of burn patients in the acute phase of burn injury are managed by an interdisciplinary team. Goals are focused on achieving maximum function without compromising wound closure. Methods used include antideformity positioning, range of motion, and total body mobilization.

SECTION ELEVEN REVIEW

1. Antideformity positioning prevents scar contracture across joints by placing them in
   A. adduction
   B. flexion
   C. extension
   D. hyperextension
2. Which nursing action is MOST important in the prevention of autograft failure secondary to capillary bed bleeding?
   A. applying compression wraps to extremities
   B. encouraging high vitamin K intake
   C. monitoring prothrombin time/partial thromboplastin time (PT/PTT) and INR lab values
   D. maintaining the patient on bedrest

Answers: 1. C, 2. A

SECTION TWELVE: Long-Term Rehabilitation Phase

At the completion of this section, the learner will be able to discuss nursing interventions related to physical conditioning, protection of new skin, scar management, and psychosocial adjustment during the rehabilitation phase of burn care.

Traditionally, the rehabilitation phase of burn care has been thought to begin at the time that all wounds were healed and continued throughout the patient's life span. From this paradigm it would seem that the rehabilitation phase would not fall into the realm of high-acuity nursing. However, it is important to recognize that preventive rehabilitation interventions actually begin during the resuscitative phase—which directly involves high-acuity nurses. In addition, the patient is frequently discharged directly from the burn unit, thereby placing the responsibility for discharge planning and teaching on the ICU nurse.

Interventions during the rehabilitation phase are focused on physical conditioning, care of healing skin, and support of psychosocial adjustment. Physical conditioning during the rehabilitation phase moves beyond range of motion exercises and begins to address aerobic endurance and muscle strength. This process begins in the burn unit but is mainly accomplished after discharge.

Interventions related to the care of healing skin include protection of newly formed epithelium, scar management, and prevention of joint contractures. The epithelium over healing burn wounds is extremely fragile. Daily skin care should include cleansing with a mild soap and generous application of a high-quality emollient. Products frequently used include vegetable shortening, cocoa butter, and Sween Cream™. Patients should be instructed to apply this emollient several times a day because their sebaceous glands have been destroyed in the burning and grafting process. The skin should also be protected from mechanical traumas such as shearing and pressure. Finally, patients should be instructed to protect their scar from sun exposure for 1 year or until the scar turns silvery white. If not, the scar will "tan" and remain permanently pigmented, leaving the patient with a less satisfactory cosmetic result.

Scar management is usually achieved by the wearing of compression garments (Fig. 33–5). These garments are usually custom made and costly. The constant pressure from the garment assists in the remodeling of irregular collagen into a more parallel pattern to improve both function and appearance. Because hypertrophic scars are also hypervascular, pressure therapy may also help to reduce local blood supply, thereby improving the scars' appearance (Pessina & Ellis, 1997). Patient compliance is difficult to obtain as the garments are hot, difficult to put on, and require continuous wearing (except when bathing). Compression garments are worn until scars are mature as evidenced by a flat, white, and avascular appearance, which is usually achieved in 12 to 18 months.

Patients with burn wounds over a joint are at risk for future joint contracture. Preventive measures include compression garments, night splinting, and range of motion exercises. Should a contracture and functional deficit occur, surgical intervention may be necessary to regain full mobility.

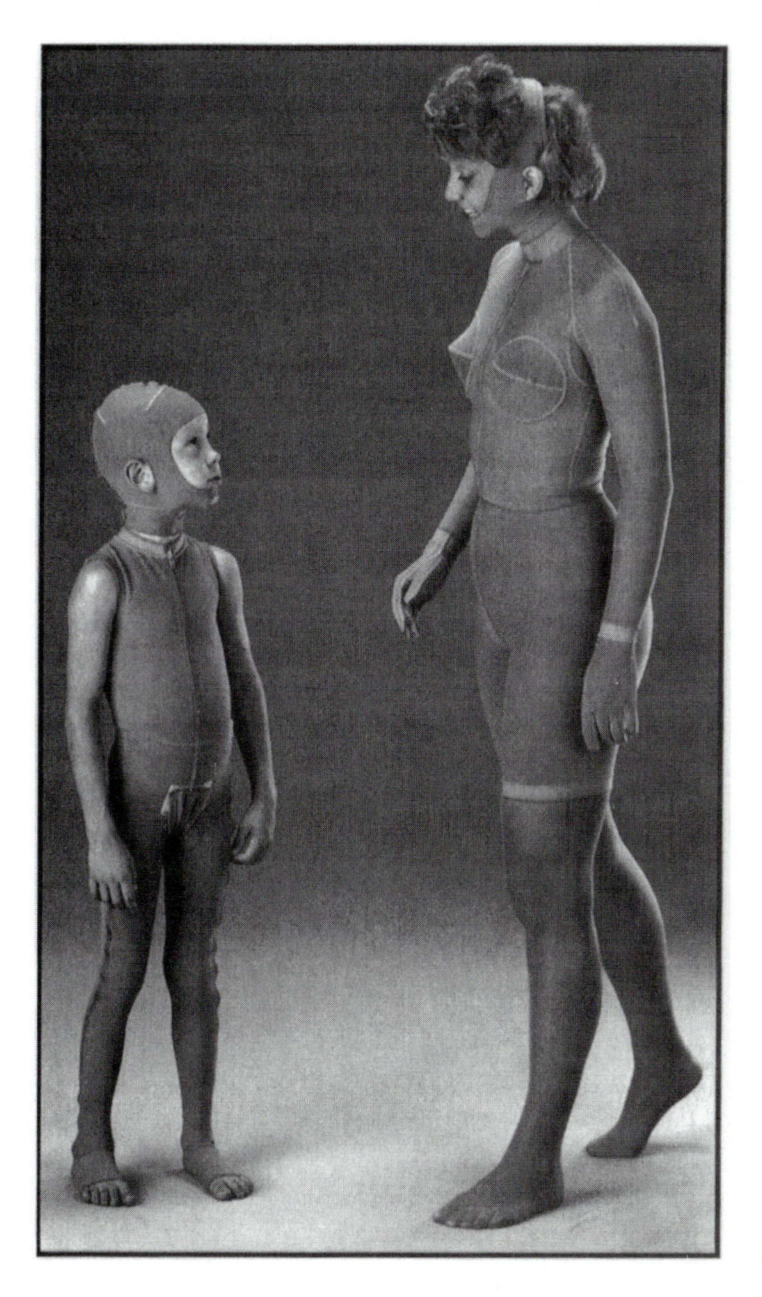

Figure 33–5. Jobst compression garments.

Psychosocial adjustment is a major task of the rehabilitation phase. During this time, patients begin to renew their interest in the outside world, invest in their rehabilitation, and reintegrate their identity. Burn unit nurses may witness some of these behaviors, but the majority of them occur after discharge. The burn team is challenged to find appropriate community resources for discharged patients as they adapt to postburn alterations in their appearance, level of physical functioning, and role concept. For example, patients with facial burns often struggle with their altered body image and have a difficult time resuming their preburn lifestyle. Therefore, it may be helpful to refer them to a licensed aesthetitian familiar with scar therapy and camouflage makeup techniques (Guzick, 1993). The Phoenix Society maintains a registry of these professionals and can assist with an appropriate referral.

In summary, the rehabilitation phase of burn care begins after all wounds are healed and continues for a lifetime. However, many rehabilitation-oriented interventions begin at the time of admission. Nursing care during this phase is focused on physical conditioning, care of healing skin, and support of psychosocial adjustment. The high-acuity nurse may not witness the resolution of these issues, as they often occur after discharge. However, it is the nurse's responsibility to provide patients with resources to facilitate their reentry into society.

SECTION TWELVE REVIEW

1. Rehabilitation interventions begin during which phase of burn care?
   A. resuscitative
   B. acute rehabilitative
   C. long-term rehabilitative
   D. transitional
2. Pressure garments improve immature scars by
   A. thinning hypertrophic epithelium
   B. remodeling irregular collagen
   C. reducing skin friction
   D. increasing arterial blood flow
3. In relation to psychological adjustment, which behavior is MOST likely to occur in the long-term rehabilitation phase?
   A. survival anxiety
   B. searching for meaning
   C. adaptation to severe pain
   D. reintegration of identity

Answers: 1. A, 2. B, 3. D

POSTEST

1. Using the American Burn Association's criteria, which of the following conditions would warrant admission to a burn center?
   A. full-thickness, less than 5 percent TBSA
   B. first-degree, 90 percent TBSA
   C. deep partial-thickness, entire face
   D. superficial partial-thickness, 10 percent
2. Painful wounds that blanch upon palpation and have large blisters are classified as
   A. full-thickness burns
   B. superficial partial-thickness burns
   C. deep partial-thickness burns
   D. first-degree burns
3. Which pulmonary tests are indicated to assess inhalation injury?
   A. electrocardiogram, thallium
   B. arterial blood gases, bronchoscopy
   C. serum potassium, sodium levels
   D. pulmonary angiograms, hemoglobin levels
4. Patients experiencing full-thickness burns involving the entire circumference of an extremity require frequent peripheral vascular checks to detect
   A. ischemia
   B. adequate wound healing
   C. arteriosclerotic changes
   D. hypothermia
5. Top treatment priorities during the resuscitative phase of care include
   A. obtaining lab work to assess pulmonary status
   B. flushing the skin with cool water for 60 minutes
   C. maintaining airway, breathing, and circulation
   D. starting intravenous fluids
6. Which data are most important to monitor during fluid resuscitation?
   A. hemoglobin
   B. blood pressure
   C. thirst
   D. urine output
7. Hypertrophic burn scars are caused by
   A. random layering of collagen
   B. delayed epithelialization
   C. wound ischemia
   D. exaggerated contraction
8. The most frequent medication given for relief of pain in the burn patient is
   A. midazolam
   B. meperidine
   C. methadone
   D. morphine sulfate
9. The hypermetabolic state of burn injury is characterized by
   A. decreased cardiac output, tachycardia
   B. increased cardiac output, increased oxygen consumption
   C. decreased caloric requirement, tachycardia
   D. increased heart rate, decreased carbon dioxide production
10. Which chemical substance usually causes more damage?
    A. acid
    B. organic
    C. alkali
    D. inorganic
11. Oral analgesics are most frequently used to control burn-injury pain
    A. during the acute rehabilitative phase
    B. during the resuscitative phase
    C. only after hospital discharge
    D. upon patient request

12. In a patient with upper torso and neck burns, which action is MOST likely to cause a functional contracture?

A. helping the patient to a position of comfort
B. discouraging pillows behind the head
C. encouraging self-care
D. hourly hyperextension neck exercises

POSTTEST ANSWERS

Question	Answer	Section	Question	Answer	Section
1	C	Two	7	A	Seven
2	B	Two	8	D	Five
3	B	Four	9	B	Six
4	A	Four	10	C	One
5	C	Four	11	A	Ten
6	D	Four	12	A	Eleven

REFERENCES

Ahrens, T., & Rutherford, K. (1993). *Essentials of oxygenation: Implications for clinical practice*. Boston: Jones & Bartlett.

Brigham, P.A., & McLoughlin, E. (1996). Burn incidence and medical care in the United States: Estimates, trends, and data sources. *J Burn Care Rehab 17*(2):95.

Carrougher, G.I. (1998). Burn wound assessment and topical treatment. In G.J. Carrougher (ed.), *Burn therapy and care*. (pp. 133–165). St. Louis: C.V. Mosby.

Cioffi, W.G. (1998). Inhalation injury. In G.J. Carrougher (ed.), *Burn therapy and care* (pp. 35–60). St. Louis: C.V. Mosby.

Cooper, M.A. (1998). Electrical and lightening injuries. In P. Rosen & R. Barker (eds.), *Emergency medicine concepts and clinical practice* (4th ed.) (pp. 1010–1022). St. Louis: C.V. Mosby.

Edlich, R.F., & Moghtader, J.C. (1998). Thermal burns. In P. Rosen & R. Barker (eds.), *Emergency medicine concepts and clinical practice* (4th ed.) (pp. 941–953). St. Louis: C.V. Mosby.

Gordon, M.D., & Goodwin, C.W. (1997). Burn management: Initial assessment, management, and stabilization. *Nurs Clin North Am 32* (2):237–249.

Gordon, M.D., & Winfree, J.H. (1998). Resuscitation after a major burn. In G.J. Carrougher (ed.), *Burn therapy and care* (pp. 107–132). St. Louis: C.V. Mosby.

Gottschlich, M.M., & Jenkins, M.E. (1998). Metabolic consequences and nutritional needs. In G.J. Carrougher (ed.), *Burn therapy and care* (pp. 213–232). St. Louis: C.V. Mosby.

Guzick, S.S. (1993). Skin care: Burn survivors case study part two. *Dermatol Nurs* 5(3):209–212, 236.

Jordan, B.S., & Harrington, D.T. (1997). Burn management: Management of the burn wound. *Nurs Clin North Am* 322(2):251–273.

Kramer, G.C., & Nguyen, T.T. (1996). Pathophysiology of burn shock and burn edema. In D.N. Herndon (ed.), *Total burn care*. Philadelphia: Saunders.

Lund, C.C., & Browder, N.C. (1944). The estimation of area of burns. *Surg Gynecol Obstet 79*:352–358.

Marvin, J.A. (1998). Management of pain and anxiety. In G.J. Carrougher (ed.), *Burn therapy and care* (pp. 167–183). St. Louis: C.V. Mosby.

Mozingo, D.W. (1998). Surgical management. In G.J. Carrougher (ed.), *Burn therapy and care* (pp. 233–248). St. Louis: C.V. Mosby.

National Burn Institute (1994). *Advanced burn life support manual*. Omaha: Author.

Oman, K.S., & Reilly, E.L. (1998). Initial assessment and care in the emergency department. In G.J. Carrougher (ed.), *Burn therapy and care* (pp. 89–106). St. Louis: C.V. Mosby.

Pessina, M.A., & Ellis, S.M. (1997). Burn management: Rehabilitation. *Nurs Clin North Am 32*(2):275–296.

Rutan, R.L. (1997). Physiologic response to cutaneous burn injury. In G.J. Carrougher (ed.), *Burn therapy and care* (pp. 1–33). St. Louis: C.V. Mosby.

Watkins, P.N., Cook, E.L., May, S.R., & Ehleben, C.M. (1988). Psychological stages in adaptation following burn injury: A method for facilitating psychological recovery of burn victims. *J Burn Care Rehab* 9(4):376–384.

Winfree, J., & Barillo, B. (1997). Burn management: Nonthermal injuries. *Nurs Clin North Am 32*(2):275–296.

Module 34

Trauma Assessment and Resuscitation

Julia Fultz, Pamela Stinson Kidd

This self-study module is intended to facilitate the learner's understanding of trauma. Focused attention is given to mechanism of injury for both blunt and penetrating trauma as an assessment factor to raise the learner's index of suspicion for certain injuries. The module is composed of 10 sections. Sections One through Four focus on mechanism of injury and kinematics of trauma. Section Five presents specific clinical and age-related variances that may mediate injury response. Sections Six and Seven focus on the trauma assessment and resuscitative principles based on primary and secondary assessments. Section Eight summarizes key points in the mediation of life-threatening injury related to trauma with a brief discussion about traumatic shock. Section Nine examines nursing care of the trauma patient, and Section Ten addresses trauma sequelae. Each section includes a set of review questions to help the learner evaluate his or her understanding of the section's content before moving on to the next section. All Section Reviews and the module Pretest and Posttest include answers. It is suggested that the learner review those concepts answered incorrectly in the review questions before proceeding to the next section.

Objectives

Following completion of this module, the learner will be able to

1. Define injury, potential mechanisms of injury, and risk factors that influence injury patterns.
2. Define the forces most often applied when considering the kinematics of blunt injury.
3. Define the forces most often applied when considering the kinematics of penetrating injury.
4. Describe the relationship between identified force eliciting an injury and suspected resultant injury pattern.
5. Apply clinical and age-related variances that may influence or mediate the host's response to injury.
6. Identify the clinical assessment format used to identify life-threatening injuries: the primary assessment.
7. Identify the clinical assessment format used to identify all injuries sustained: the secondary assessment.
8. Discuss the trimodal distribution of trauma-related mortalities and the importance of early recognition and intervention with traumatic shock.
9. Describe appropriate nursing care of the trauma patient.
10. Explain the relationship between trauma sequelae and the initial injury event.

Pretest

1. The most common cause of injury is
   A. falls
   B. motor vehicle crashes
   C. gunshot wounds
   D. near drowning

2. The typical profile of a trauma victim would be
   A. male, 15 to 24 years of age, intoxicated
   B. female, 15 to 24 years of age, intoxicated
   C. female, 24 to 32 years of age, intoxicated
   D. male, 24 to 32 years of age, not intoxicated

3. The most common force associated with blunt trauma is
   A. acceleration/deceleration
   B. compression
   C. shearing
   D. axial loading
4. The best definition of tensile forces is
   A. forces opposing one another across a plane
   B. squeezing/compartmentalization of tissue
   C. forces precipitating laceration, avulsion
   D. drawing out/extending tissue
5. The process of temporary displacement of tissue forward and laterally by a penetrating missile is
   A. tensile forces
   B. cavitation
   C. yaw
   D. tumbling
6. The extent of cavitation and tissue deformation produced by a missile is determined by
   A. yaw
   B. tumbling
   C. missile caliber and velocity
   D. all of the above
7. Secondary missiles often are created with penetrating trauma involving which two types of tissue?
   A. teeth and bone
   B. brain and soft tissue
   C. abdominal organs and vessels
   D. great vessels and brain
8. The most frequently seen pattern of injury for a pedestrian child hit by an automobile is
   A. fractures of femur, tibia, and fibula on side of impact
   B. fracture of femur, chest injury, and injury to contralateral skull
   C. pelvic fractures, compression fractures
   D. fractured spleen or liver, upper extremity fractures
9. Impairment of judgment occurs with blood alcohol content as low as
   A. 100 mg/dL
   B. 20 to 80 mg/dL
   C. 200 mg/dL
   D. 300 mg/dL
10. Cocaine usually manifests itself as a
    A. central nervous system (CNS) depressant
    B. sympathomimetic
    C. hallucinogenic
    D. antidepressant
11. When assessing a pediatric trauma patient, one must consider
    A. increasing frequency of multiorgan injuries
    B. decreasing frequency of multiorgan injuries
    C. decreased risk of hypothermia
    D. increased ability of the skeleton to absorb significant forces
12. The center of gravity in a child is considered to be the
    A. head
    B. pelvis
    C. lower extremities
    D. abdominal area
13. The immediate nursing intervention for the hypotensive pregnant trauma patient should be
    A. turning the patient to the right lateral decubitus position
    B. turning the patient to the left lateral decubitus position
    C. high-flow oxygen
    D. Trendelenburg position
14. Ordered priorities in the primary survey are
    A. disability, airway, breathing
    B. cervical spine immobilization, circulation, breathing
    C. hemorrhage, fractures, chest trauma
    D. airway, breathing, circulation, disability, and exposure
15. In maintaining the pediatric airway, all of the following are true EXCEPT
    A. the tongue is small and unlikely to cause airway obstruction
    B. the glottic opening is more anterior and cephalad
    C. the trachea is short and narrow
    D. hypoxemia is very poorly tolerated
16. In the early shock state (blood volume loss < 25 percent), the blood pressure usually will be
    A. normal
    B. slightly elevated
    C. slightly decreased
    D. markedly decreased
17. The distribution of trauma-related mortalities is
    A. modal
    B. bimodal
    C. trimodal
    D. quasimodal
18. The intra-abdominal organ most frequently associated with exsanguination is
    A. liver
    B. spleen
    C. small bowel
    D. colon
19. A patient with a left lower rib fracture may also have an associated injury of the
    A. liver
    B. heart
    C. spleen
    D. stomach

20. Which of the following contributes the greatest to complications posttrauma?
    A. hypoperfusion
    B. delay in supporting nutrition
    C. infection
    D. vasoconstriction

Pretest answers: 1. B, 2. A, 3. A, 4. D, 5. B, 6. D, 7. A, 8. B, 9. B, 10. B, 11. A, 12. A, 13. B, 14. D, 15. A, 16. A, 17. C, 18. A, 19. C, 20. A

GLOSSARY

Acceleration. An increase in the rate of velocity or speed of a moving body

Autocannibalism. The breakdown of skeletal muscle mass to provide nutrients during a hypermetabolic phase

Blast effect. Phenomenon of structure injury outside the direct missile path in penetrating injury

Blood alcohol concentration (BAC). Measurement of intoxication in mg/dL or g/dL; a BAC indicating legal intoxication is usually 100 mg/dL or 0.100 g/dL

Blunt trauma. Injury without interruption of skin integrity

Cavitation. Creation of a temporary cavity as tissues are stretched and compressed and displaced forward and laterally, creating a tract from a penetrating missile

Chance fracture. Distraction or tension fractures of the thoracolumbar spine, usually between L1 and L4

Compression. The process of being pressed or squeezed together with a resulting reduction in size or volume.

Contrecoup injury. Injury to parts of the brain located on the side opposite that of the primary injury

Coup injury. Injury to parts of the brain located on the side of primary injury

Crepitus. A grating sound heard on movement, as with ends of broken bone

Cribriform. The thin, perforated, medial portion of the horizontal plate of the ethmoid bone

Cricothyroidotomy. A surgical airway created by division and cannulation of the trachea between the cricoid and thyroid cartilage

Deceleration. A decrease in the rate of velocity or speed of a moving body

Disseminated intravascular coagulation (DIC). Syndrome initiated by the release of thrombin and characterized by initial coagulation that precipitates massive lysis of clots and hemorrhage

Exsanguination. The most extreme form of hemorrhage, with an initial loss of blood volume of 40 percent and a rate of hemorrhage exceeding 250 mL/min

Force. A physical factor that changes the motion of a body either at rest or already in motion

Injury. Resulting body damage from intentional (e.g., violence) or unintentional (e.g., falls) forces

Kinematics. The science or study of motion

Multiple organ dysfunction syndrome (MODS). Syndrome precipitated by hypoperfusion, usually occurs in a sequential format; lungs, liver, and renal and cardiovascular systems fail, respectively; may be associated with sepsis

Paradoxical pulse. A fall in the systolic blood pressure associated with inspiration due to decreased left ventricular filling because of increased intrathoracic pressure

Penetrating trauma. The result of the transmission of energy from a moving object into the body tissue as the object disrupts the integrity of the skin and the underlying structures.

Pericardial tamponade. Bleeding into the pericardial sac produced by blunt or penetrating trauma to the pericardium or the ascending aorta associated with decreased cardiac output

Sepsis. The systemic response to infection manifested by two or more of the following conditions: (1) temperature > 30°C or < 36°C; (2) heart rate > 90 bpm; (3) respiratory rate > 20 breaths/min or $PaCO_2$ < 32 mm Hg; and (4) WBC count > 12,000/mL or < 4,000/mL or > 10 percent immature (band) forms

Septic shock. Sepsis associated with hypotension despite adequate fluid resuscitation along with the presence of perfusion abnormalities that may include but are not limited to lactic acidosis, oliguria, or an acute alteration in mental status

Shearing. Structures sliding in opposite directions causing a tearing or degloving type injury

Subcutaneous emphysema. Distention of subcutaneous tissues by gas or air in the interstices

Subdural hematoma. Bleeding between the dural and arachnoid layers of the brain, usually venous in nature; classification based on time from injury to onset of symptoms: acute 24 to 72 hours, subacute 72 hours to 14 days, and chronic > 14 days (Thelan, Davie, & Urden, 1990)

Synergistic. The harmonious action of two agents, such as drugs, producing an effect that neither could produce alone or an effect that is greater than the total effects of each agent operating by itself

Tensile forces. Forces that cause tissues to stretch or extend

Tension pneumothorax. Collapse of a lung that leads to collection of inspired air into the pleural space that compresses the mediastinum and decreases ventilation of the unaffected lung and cardiac output

Tracheostomy. A surgical airway created by cutting into the trachea below the cricothyroid membrane

Tumble. The forward rotation of a missile around the center of mass (somersaulting)

Velocity. The speed of a moving object on a ratio of distance and time

Waddell's triad. A defined triad of injury associated with an automobile hitting a pedestrian

Yaw. Deviation of a missile from its straight path

ABBREVIATIONS

ARDS. Acute respiratory distress syndrome

ATP. Adenosine triphosphate

BAC. Blood alcohol concentration

CNS. Central nervous system

CO. Cardiac output

COPD. Chronic obstructive pulmonary disease

CPP. Cerebral perfusion pressure

CSF. Cerebrospinal fluid

CT. Computed tomography

CVP. Central venous pressure

DIC. Disseminated intravascular coagulation

F_{IO_2}. Fraction of inspired oxygen

ETOH level. Ethanol level

GCS. Glasgow Coma Scale

ICP. Intracranial pressure

MAP. Mean arterial pressure

MODS. Multiple organ dysfunction syndrome

mph. Miles per hour

MVC. Motor vehicle crash

NG. Nasogastric

Pa_{CO_2}. Partial pressure of carbon dioxide

Pa_{O_2}. Partial arterial pressure of oxygen

PEEP. Positive end-expiratory pressure

psi. Pounds per square inch

Sp_{O_2}. Peripheral oxygen saturation

SECTION ONE: Overview of the Injured Patient

At the completion of this section, the learner will be able to define injury, potential mechanisms of injury, and personal and environmental factors that influence injury patterns.

Understanding injury (or trauma as we often call it) will enable you to approach a patient in crisis with a level-headed, systematic plan based on your body of nursing knowledge surrounding the concept. Historically, injuries or accidents were viewed as a result of random chance that was beyond human control. Now, **injury** is viewed as an event with an identifiable cause via the interaction of energy and force with a recipient. The recipient may be an inanimate object, such as a car, or may be a human being. Webster identifies injury as "that which causes harm or damage, the damage, or hurt done." A definition of trauma is "any body injury caused by violence or other forces."

Injury results from acute exposure to energy, such as kinetic (motor vehicle crash [MVC], fall, bullet), chemical, thermal, electrical, ionizing radiation, or from a lack of essential agents, such as oxygen and heat (drowning and frostbite) (Waller, 1985). Motor vehicle crashes are the most common cause of injury, followed by falls. The injury occurs because of the body's inability to tolerate excessive exposure to the energy source. Effects of injury on the human body vary depending on the injuring agent. For the purposes of this module, the focus will be on two major categories of injury—blunt and penetrating.

Blunt trauma is considered injury without interruption of skin integrity. Blunt trauma may be life threatening because the extent of the injury may be covert, making diagnosis difficult. Blunt forces transfer energy causing tissue deformation. The nature of the injury is related to both the transfer of energy and the anatomic structure involved.

Penetrating trauma refers to injury sustained by the transmission of energy to body tissues from a moving object which interupts skin integrity, whereas blunt trauma produces tissue deformation by the transfer of energy.

Penetrating trauma produces actual tissue penetration and may also cause surrounding tissue deformation based on energy transferred by the penetrating object.

Because the transfer of energy occurs with both blunt and penetrating injury, deformation and displacement of body tissue and organs occurs with both forms of injury. Injury takes place as the structural limits of the organ are exceeded. Damage may be localized, such as hematoma formation, or systemic, as in shock states. The local response of the patient varies according to the organ involved. Additional examples are bone fractures, bleeding vessels, or tissue edema.

Injuries, like other diseases, do not occur at random. Identifiable risk factors are present that predispose individuals to certain injury patterns. A brief discussion of a few of these risk factors is presented.

Age

Injury is the leading cause of death in all Americans ages 1 through 44. The death rate from injury is highest for patients ≥ 75 years. The lowest injury death rate is for patients aged 5 through 14. The highest injury rate is for patients aged 15 through 24 because of their exposure to high-risk activities (including poor judgment with the use of alcohol, drugs, and driving practices). The highest homicide rate occurs among people between 20 and 29 years of age.

Gender

Injury rates are highest for 15- to 24-year-old males. The risk for males is 2.5 times that of females, possibly because of male involvement in hazardous activities.

Alcohol

The use and abuse of alcoholic beverages influence the likelihood of virtually all types of injury, even among young teenagers. Over 50 percent of all trauma is reported to occur in the presence of high **blood alcohol concentrations (BACs).** Approximately 30 to 40 percent of vehicular crashes can be associated with significant elevations in BAC. Thirty percent of individuals with gunshot wounds have a BAC of ≥ 0.03 g/dL. An increase in BAC is associated with an increase in the severity of injury.

Race, Income, Geography

Native Americans have the highest death rates from unintentional injury, African Americans have the highest homicide rates, and Caucasians and Native Americans have the highest suicide rates. An inverse relationship between income levels and death rates exists for blacks and whites. There is a higher unintentional injury rate in rural areas and a higher intentional injury rate in urban areas. Mechanisms of rural unintentional injuries commonly are MVCs, lightning, and chemical exposure. Urban intentional injuries usually are related to homicide attempts.

In summary, this section has discussed the definitions of trauma and injury and that these two terms are frequently interchangable. The two major categories of injury, penetrating and blunt, were discussed in addition to demographic information and its relationship to the occurrence of trauma. Injuries were discussed as events with identifiable causes, contrary to the public's view of injuries as accidents.

SECTION ONE REVIEW

1. The two major categories of injury are
A. chemical and thermal
B. fractures and burns
C. blunt and penetrating
D. MVCs and gunshot wounds

2. The death rate from injury is highest for patients
A. 24 to 42 years
B. 15 to 24 years
C. 5 to 14 years
D. ≥ 75 years and older

3. The highest injury rate occurs in which age group?
A. 15 to 24 years
B. 1 to 5 years
C. 24 to 32 years
D. ≥ 75 years

4. The risk for males versus females for injury is
A. 2.5 times lower
B. 2.5 times higher
C. 5 times higher
D. equal

5. Over _____ percent of all trauma is reported to occur in the presence of high BAC ratios.
A. 10
B. 25
C. 50
D. 75

Answers: 1. C, 2. D, 3. A, 4. B, 5. C

SECTION TWO: Kinematics of Blunt Trauma

At the completion of this section, the learner will be able to define the forces most often associated with blunt trauma and be able to apply the concepts to the clinical assessment of a patient with blunt trauma.

Force is a physical factor, the push or pull that changes the state of an object that is either at rest or already in motion. Injury resulting from force is related to the amount and speed (velocity) of energy transmission, the surface area to which the energy is applied and the elasticity of the tissues affected. The more slowly the force is applied, the more slowly energy is released, with less subsequent tissue deformation. The forces most often applied are acceleration, deceleration, shearing, and compression (American College of Surgeons Committee on Trauma [ACSCT], 1997a).

Acceleration is a change in the rate of velocity or speed of a moving body. The most significant determinant of the amount of injury sustained is velocity. As velocity increases, so does tissue damage due to the greater amount of energy present. The following example illustrates the concept of acceleration. On impact with a solid object (e.g., another car, brick wall, telephone pole), the driver is suddenly propelled forward. He experiences a sudden acceleration of body mass determined by the rate of speed at which he was traveling and his body mass. This relationship is reflected in the following formula.

$$\text{Body weight} \times \text{mph} = \text{psi of impact}$$

A person weighing 100 pounds, traveling at 35 mph, will hit at 3,500 pounds per square inch (psi). This is equivalent to jumping head-first from a three-story building!

Deceleration is a decrease in the velocity of a moving object. The same driver in the example given who is moving forward after hitting a solid object will experience a sudden deceleration after he comes into contact with the mass that impedes his forward (or backward) progression (e.g., the steering wheel, a tree, the road, or another passenger).

Shearing refers to injury resulting from two structures or two parts of the same structure, sliding in opposite directions causing a tearing or degloving type injury. For example, shearing forces are frequently the cause of spinal injury at the C7–T1 juncture because the mobile cervical spine attaches at that point to the relatively immobile thoracic spine. Shearing forces are often the cause of aorta tears (at the ligamentum arteriosum), splenic and renal injuries (at the pedicle junctures), and liver, brain, or heart injuries. These structures have a relatively immobile section connected to a relatively mobile section and are therefore subject to shearing forces.

Compression is the process of being pressed or squeezed together with resulting reduction in volume or size. For example, sudden acceleration or deceleration during an MVC can cause compression of the heart and lung parenchyma between the posterior and anterior chest wall. The small bowel may be compressed between the vertebral column and the lower part of the steering wheel or an improperly placed seat belt. The bowel may rupture. The same mechanism can cause compression of the liver causing it to burst.

Acceleration and deceleration injuries are most common with blunt trauma. An example of this mechanism of injury is injury to the thoracic aorta. Typically, MVCs and falls from 20 feet or higher precipitate stretching, bowing, and shearing in major vessels, such as the aorta. Aortic damage may occur to any or all layers of the vessel wall (intima, media, adventitia). The aortic vessel wall can tear, dissect, rupture, or form an aneurysm immediately or at any time postinjury. Shearing damage occurs in the vessels when deceleration occurs at a different rate than other internal structures. For example, the relatively mobile ascending aorta continues to move after the relatively stationary descending aorta (held in place by the ligamentum arteriosum, the spine, the parietal pleura, and the intercostal arteries) has stopped moving. A shearing injury occurs from the two sections of the aorta moving at different speeds. One is still moving (ascending aorta) while the other has stopped (descending aorta).

Other injuries associated with blunt trauma forces are head injuries (think about the movement of the brain inside the skull with acceleration, deceleration, and shearing **coup injury**), spinal cord injuries (the cervical spine is predisposed to shearing and acceleration/deceleration because of its instability and poor support, since it is weakest at cervical vertebrae 5, 6, and 7), fractures (from shearing and compression), and abdominal injuries (abdominal organs, especially the spleen and liver, are very vascular, and trauma patients may exsanguinate from shearing and disruption of major vessels supplying these areas).

Tissue responsiveness to applied forces varies, creating characteristic limits of the tissues' ability to withstand the forces of acceleration, deceleration, compression, and shearing. Tissue deformation is generally the result of tensile forces or shear forces. **Tensile forces** cause tissues to stretch and extend. Tensile strength of a specific tissue is the greatest longitudinal stretch or stress it can withstand without tearing apart. Joint dislocations, muscle sprains and strains, are frequently the result of tensile forces. Tensile forces are also the cause of **contrecoup** brain injuries. Brain tissue is pulled away from the skull with the initial alteration in motion due to acceleration or deceleration.

Tissue, organ, and systemic responses to the forces applied with blunt trauma often present a complex interrelationship of potential injury manifestation. Trauma patients with similar mechanisms of injury typically have different combinations of organ and systemic injury based on individual variances in ability to withstand the forces applied. A myriad of potential injury combinations, manifestations, and outcomes exists, prompting the clinician to approach the patient in a systematic fashion.

In summary, this section identified different types of forces related to blunt injury. A brief discussion of how tissues respond to forces was presented.

Section Two Review

1. Acceleration is a change in the rate of velocity or speed of a moving body. As velocity increases, tissue damage
   A. decreases
   B. increases
   C. remains constant
   D. cannot be determined
2. A decrease in the velocity of a moving object is
   A. acceleration
   B. deceleration
   C. compression
   D. shearing
3. Structures slipping in opposite directions to each other is a force known as
   A. acceleration
   B. deceleration
   C. compression
   D. shearing
4. The process of being pressed or squeezed is known as
   A. acceleration
   B. deceleration
   C. compression
   D. shearing
5. Forces that cause tissues to stretch are known as
   A. tensile
   B. shearing
   C. mass
   D. compression

Answers: 1. B, 2. B, 3. D, 4. C, 5. A

SECTION THREE: Kinematics of Penetrating Trauma

At the completion of this section, the learner will be able to define the forces most often reflected during assessment of penetrating injury and apply the concepts to the clinical assessment of a patient with penetrating trauma.

Penetrating trauma is the result of the transmission of energy from a moving object into body tissues as the object disrupts the integrity of the skin and the underlying structures. The amount of kinetic energy transmitted by the object has a direct relationship to the amount of tissue damage. As tissue and/or organ penetration occurs, the severity of injury is dependent on the structures damaged by the transmission of energy. A penetrating object can be most anything—a knife, a bullet, buckshot, an arrow, a stick, a metal rod, a fork, a gear shift, and so on.

The amount of kinetic energy available to be transmitted to tissues is dependent on the surface area of the point of impact, the density of the tissue, and the velocity of the projectile at the time of impact (ACSCT, 1997a). Weapons are usually classified by the amount of energy they are capable of producing; low-energy weapons include knives, arrows, or any type of hand missile; medium-energy weapons include handguns and some rifles; and high-energy weapons include hunting rifles and shotguns.

Low- to medium-energy missiles travel below 2,000 feet per second. The injury sustained usually results from the missile contacting the tissue. Typically, damage is localized to those structures directly in the missile's path. However, special consideration must be given when injury occurs where body cavities lie in close proximity to one another. This principle is of critical importance when considering the close proximity of the thoracic and abdominal cavities, especially with injuries occurring near the diaphragm, which offers very little resistance to the penetrating agent. Penetrating injuries to the chest below the nipple line anteriorly, the sixth rib laterally, or the inferior point or the scapula posteriorly may involve both intrathoracic and abdominal structures. The right diaphragm may rise as high as the fourth intercostal space and the left diaphragm to the fifth intercostal space (the right hemidiaphragm is slightly elevated by the liver) during maximum expiration, rendering the contents of the abdominal cavity exposed to injury with lower chest trauma (Fig. 34–1). During maximum inspiration, the diaphragm recedes as low as the sixth intercostal space at the midclavicular line and the eighth intercostal space at the midaxillary line. Although stab wounds and impalement wounds are considered low-velocity injuries, the potential extent of damage should not be underestimated.

If the offending weapon is impaled in the body, it is critical that the object be left in place and protected from further movement until definitive surgical intervention is available. Protective padding can be placed around the object, such as gauze rolls or abdominal pads, or a protective device such as a plastic cup can be secured around the protruding handle of objects such as knives or the end

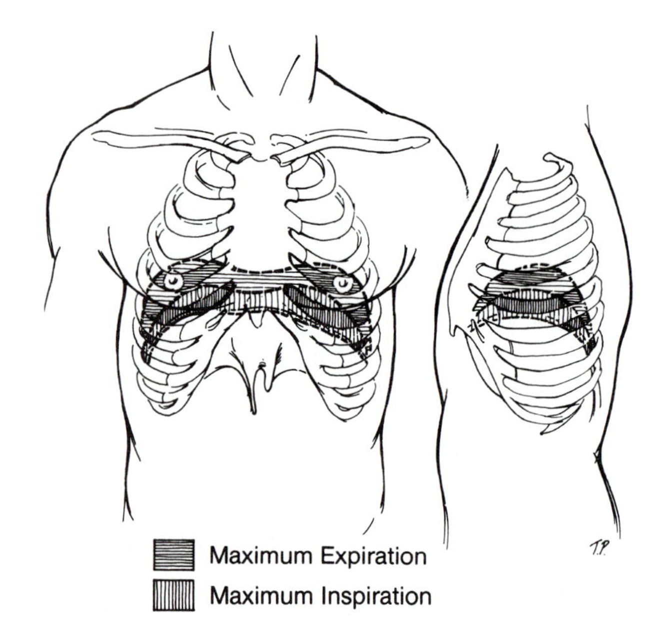

Figure 34–1. Diaphragmatic excursion during the respiratory cycle. Injury to lower chest or upper abdomen can occur, with penetrating injury dependent on the phase of the respiratory cycle and the site of injury. (*From Cardona, V.A., et al. [eds]. [1994].* Trauma nursing from resuscitation through rehabilitation, *[p. 120]. Philadelphia: W.B. Saunders.)*

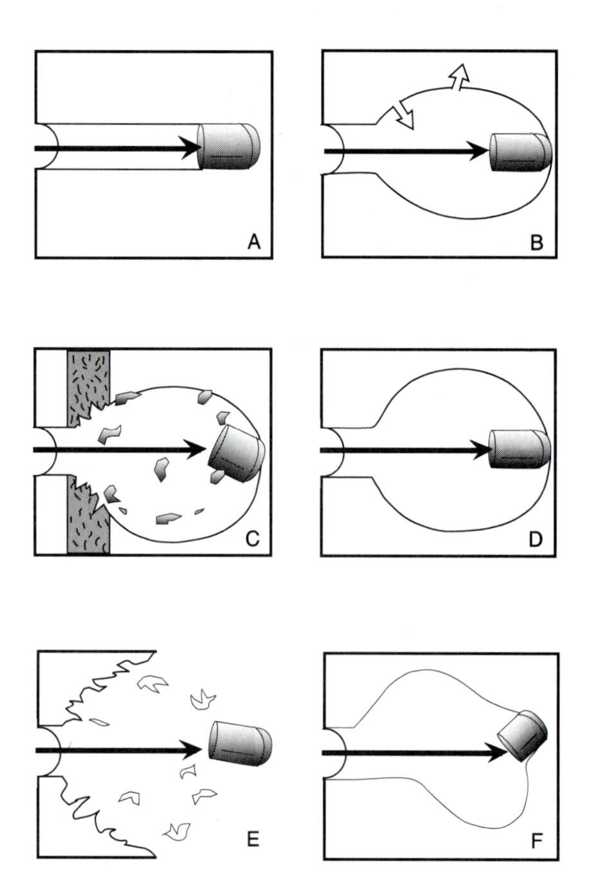

Figure 34–2. Patterns of tissue injury secondary to gunshot wounds. **A.** Low velocity, small entrance, and exit wounds. **B.** Higher velocity, cavitation present with energy dispersion outward from missile path (blast effect). **C.** Same velocity as in B but with penetration of bone and greater blast effect due to projections of bone being spread through tissue. **D.** Higher velocity than in B or C with greater cavitation effect, small entrance and exit wounds. **E.** Same velocity as in D, but person or extremity hit is thinner resulting in large exit wound. **F.** Asymmetrical cavitation as bullet begins to yaw and tumble.

of a stick or metal rod. Impaled objects may actually be controlling hemorrhage from damaged structures and removal may precipitate exsanguination.

High-energy missiles are those that travel greater than 2,000 feet per second. At higher velocities, a tremendous amount of tissue destruction can occur due to forces transmitted to the tissues by the missile. High-energy missiles (also referred to high-velocity missiles) transmit more kinetic energy, creating an intense blast result within the tissues. As the missile penetrates the tissue, the transmission of kinetic energy displaces tissues forward and laterally to form a temporary cavity. The process of cavity formation is called **cavitation** (Fig. 34–2). The degree of cavitation is directly related to the amount of kinetic energy transmitted to the tissues, which in turn is determined by the **velocity** of the missile. The size of the cavity may be up to 30 times the diameter of the missile (ACSCT, 1997a). Tissue surrounding the missile tract is exposed to tensile (stretching), compressing, and shearing forces, which produce damage outside the direct path of the missile. Vessels, nerves, and other structures that were not directly damaged by the missile may be affected. The phenomenon of structure injury outside the direct missile path is referred to as a **blast effect.** Higher-velocity missiles will produce more serious injury owing to the destructive process of cavitation and blast effect to surrounding tissue and organs.

Another concept to consider when evaluating the forces that can injure a patient is the missile's trajectory. Consider a missile moving in stable flight toward the host (for our purposes, the patient). The missile passes from air into human tissue, which is several hundred times denser than air. As the missile passes into the tissue, the surrounding environment changes and precipitates an instability of the missile. The unstable missile may yaw, tumble, deform, fragment, or any combination of these actions.

Yaw is the deviation of a missile either horizontally or vertically about its axis. **Tumble** is the action of forward rotation around the center of a mass (somersaulting) (Figs. 34–3 and 34–4). The action of yawing and/or tumbling increases the surface area of the missile as it impacts the body (side of the missile versus the point of the missile). This creates a larger entrance wound. It also allows for increased energy transfer to the surrounding tissues, creating a larger area of tissue destruction. Higher-

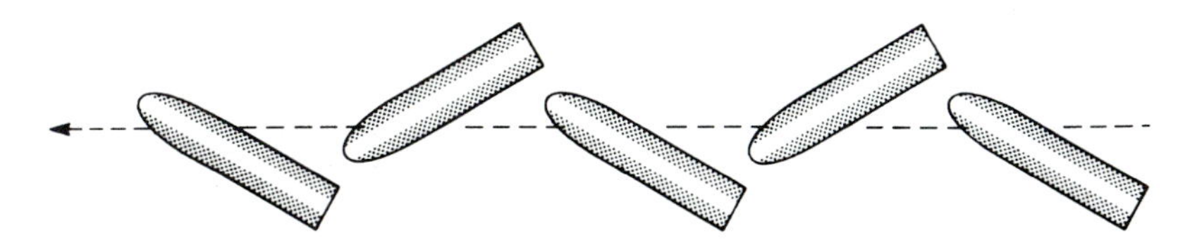

Figure 34–3. Yawing is the deviation of a bullet in its longitudinal axis from the straight line of flight. (*From Swan, K.G., & Swan, R.C. [eds]. [1989].* Gunshot wounds: Pathophysiology and management, *2nd ed. [p. 13]. St. Louis: Mosby-Year Book.*)

velocity missiles have a greater propensity for yaw and tumble.

Another principle to consider when analyzing the effects of penetrating injury is the creation of secondary missiles by the pentrating object. A missile or its fragments may impart sufficient kinetic injury to dense tissue, such as bone or teeth, to create highly destructive secondary missiles. These secondary missiles may take erratic, unpredictable courses, resulting in additional injury. Secondary missiles also may be created by fragmentation of the primary missile. Thus, the anticipated missile path may be compounded, complicated, or enhanced by tissue damage precipitated by a secondary missile.

An evaluation of the wounds caused by the missile is necessary, noting the location, size, shape, if there is any foreign substance on the surrounding tissue such as a black powder, and if the wound is actively bleeding. If there are two wounds, noting the location of each only gives the clinician a hint of the trajectory the missile may have taken if the same missile caused both wounds. Missiles usually take the path of least resistance, so the path the missile followed may not be a straight line between the two wounds. Entrance wounds are usually smaller than exit wounds. However, the characteristics of a wound are dependent on the forces causing the injury such as velocity, cavitation, and blast effect. A summary of the effects of these forces on a wound are depicted in Figure 34–2. Identifying which wound is the entrance and which is the exit is not necessary and should be left to experienced personnel. Identifying the wounds as wound one and wound two will suffice. The presence of two wounds does not necessarily mean one is an entrance and one is an exit wound. They may be two entrance wounds from two separate missiles. Not all medium- and high-energy penetrating injuries have a resulting exit wound because the missile may remain inside the body.

In summary, this section has reviewed the kinematics of penetrating injury. Velocity, cavitation, yaw, and tumbling were reviewed for their influence on ultimate injury of structures. Critical application of these concepts will maximize the clinician's ability to evaluate penetrating traumatic injury based on mechanism.

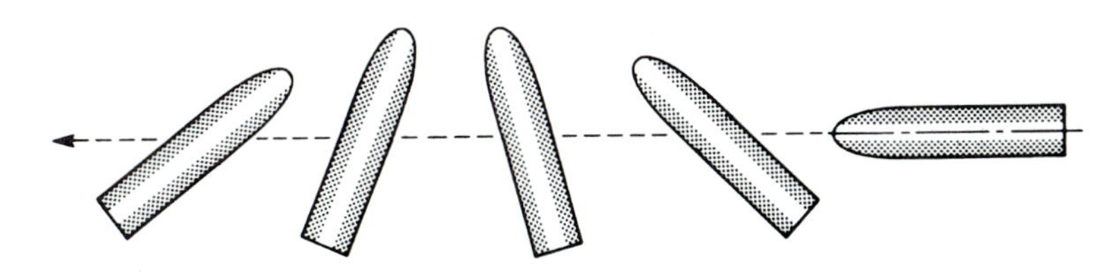

Figure 34–4. Tumbling is the action of forward rotation around the center of mass. (*From Swan, K.G., & Swan, R.C. [eds]. [1989].* Gunshot wounds: Pathophysiology and management, *2nd ed. [p. 13]. St. Louis: Mosby-Year Book.*)

SECTION THREE REVIEW

1. As a missile penetrates, the tissue is temporarily displaced forward and laterally, creating a tract. This process is known as
   A. velocity
   B. yaw
   C. tumbling
   D. cavitation
2. Cavitation demonstrates a(n) ____ relationship with the amount of kinetic energy transmitted to tissue.
   A. inverse
   B. direct
   C. insignificant
   D. diagonal
3. The phenomenon of structure injury outside the direct missile path is referred to as
   A. cavitation
   B. blast effect
   C. yaw
   D. tumbling

4. Yaw and tumble will _____ the area of tissue destruction precipitated by a missile.
   A. decrease
   B. increase
   C. minimize
   D. not affect
5. A patient has an impaled knife in the upper abdomen. You should immediately
   A. remove the knife and apply pressure
   B. manipulate the knife to facilitate assessment of injured organs
   C. stabilize the knife without removal and minimal manipulation
   D. leave the knife alone

Answers: 1. D, 2. B, 3. B, 4. B, 5. C

SECTION FOUR: Translating Principles of Mechanism of Injury

At the completion of this section, the learner will be able to translate mechanism of injury into potential injury patterns manifested by the patient for both blunt and penetrating injuries.

Certain mechanisms result in predictable injury patterns. Thus, the history of the event preceding the injury should elicit an increased index of suspicion for certain combinations of injured structures. Some commonly seen injuries resulting from blunt and penetrating trauma and their injury mechanism are listed in Table 34–1. This table addresses pedestrian/motor vehicle injuries (Fig. 34–5), motor vehicle driver and passenger injuries, fall injuries, and missile injuries.

An example illustrating the importance of the application of mechanism of injury follows. A 21-year-old male, unrestrained driver hits another vehicle head on (Fig. 34–6). Traveling speed was in excess of 95 mph. Both the steering wheel and windshield were broken. A high index of suspicion must be maintained for the following injuries:

1. Potential intracranial injury, due to the high rate of speed and shattered windshield

TABLE 34–1. COMMONLY SEEN INJURIES

MECHANISM OF INJURY	POTENTIAL STRUCTURE INJURY
Pedestrian hit by automobile	
Adult (**Waddell's triad**, Fig. 34–5)	Fractures of femur, tibia, and fibula on side of impact; ligamental damage to impacted knee; mild contralateral head injury
Child (Waddell's triad)	Fractures of femur, chest injury, contralateral head injury
Unrestrained driver (Fig. 34–6)	Head and/or facial injury, fractures of ribs, sternum with underlying myocardial or pulmonary contusion, cervical spine fractures, laryngotracheal injuries, spleen, liver, small bowel injuries, posterior fracture–dislocation of hip, femur fractures
Unrestrained front seat passenger	Head and/or facial injuries, laryngotracheal injuries, posterior fracture–dislocation of femoral head, femur/patellar fractures
Restrained driver (lap and shoulder harness)	Contusions of structures underlying harness (i.e., pulmonary contusion, contusion of small bowel)
Restrained passenger (lap belt only)	Flexion/distraction fractures (**Chance fractures**), especially lumbar vertebrae (L1–4), duodenal injuries, cervical spine injuries
Fall injuries	Compression fractures of lumbosacral spine and calcaneus fractures; fractures of radius/ulna, patella if victim falls forward
Vehicular ejection	Multiple injuries, especially head and cervical spine injuries. *Injury risk increases by 300 percent when ejection occurs*
Low-velocity impalement	Local tissue/organ disruption, little or no cavitation
High-velocity missile, short missile path	Entrance wound larger than missile caliber; large ragged exit wound with cavitation
High-velocity missile, long missile path	Entrance wound larger than missile caliber; exit wound slightly larger than or equal to missile caliber; extensive cavitation (blast effect to deep structures absorbing lost kinetic energy)
High-velocity missile hitting bone or teeth	Entry wound larger than missile caliber; possibly no exit wound with missile fragmentation; secondary missile injury in unpredictable, erratic pattern

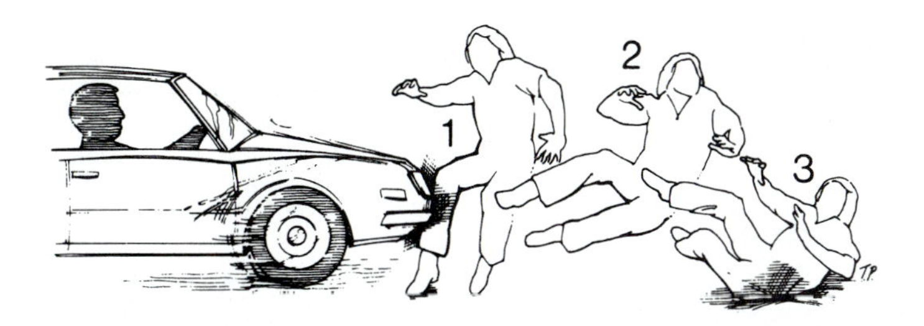

Figure 34–5. Waddell's triad in adult pedestrians. Impact **(1)** with the bumper or hood and lateral rotation **(2)** produce injury to the upper or lower leg and contralateral skull **(3)**. (*From Cardona, V.A., et al. [eds]. [1994].* Trauma nursing from resuscitation through rehabilitation *[p. 107]. Philadelphia: W.B. Saunders.*)

2. Potential cervical vertebrae injury, due to suspected acceleration/deceleration at a high rate of speed and the broken windshield
3. Potential intrathoracic injuries, due to the broken steering wheel—suspect rib fractures, myocardial and pulmonary contusions, great vessel injury
4. Potential intra-abdominal injuries, due to the broken steering wheel and acceleration/deceleration mechanism; injuries could include splenic/liver lacerations, small bowel injuries, great vessel injuries
5. Potential long-bone fractures, especially femur fractures or posterior hip fracture—dislocation, because of impact of knees with dashboard
6. Potential multiple skin lacerations, avulsions, punctures from the patient impacting various parts of the vehicle interior

In summary, the importance of mechanism of injury in anticipating an injury pattern has been stressed in this section. Both blunt and penetrating injuries were addressed.

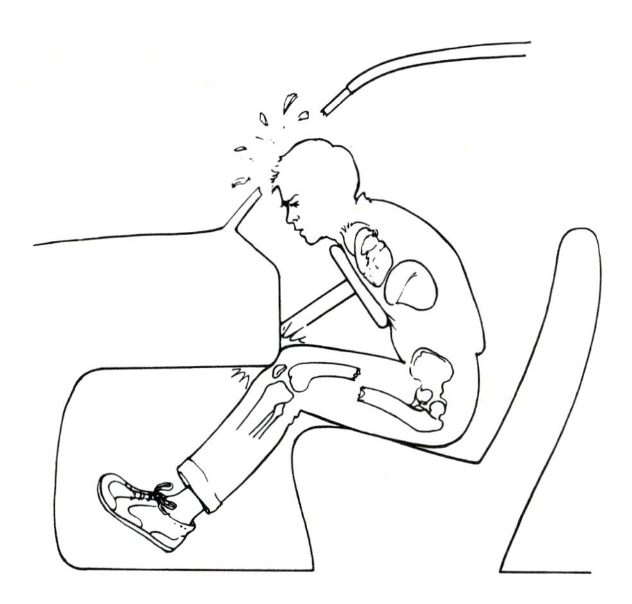

Figure 34–6. Unrestrained driver in motor vehicle crash may sustain injuries to the cranium, face, sternum, ribs, myocardium, lung parenchyma, cervical vertebrae, spleen, liver, small bowel, pelvis, and lower extremities. (*Reproduced from Baylor College of Medicine*).

SECTION FOUR REVIEW

1. **Waddell's triad** is a characteristic injury pattern exhibited by
   A. unrestrained driver in MVC
   B. unrestrained passenger in MVC
   C. victims of gunshot wounds
   D. pedestrians injured by vehicular contact
2. A restrained passenger (lap belt only) may exhibit flexion/distraction fractures of which area of the vertebral column?
   A. cervical
   B. lumbar
   C. thoracic
   D. sacral
3. The intra-abdominal organ injury usually associated with a Chance fracture is the
   A. liver
   B. duodenum
   C. colon
   D. spleen
4. A restrained (lap and shoulder harness) occupant involved in an MVC can receive what types of injuries from the restraints?
   A. pulmonary contusions
   B. lumbar fractures
   C. femur fractures
   D. facial injuries
5. Which of the following is true?
   A. vehicular ejection increases the risk for potential injury
   B. vehicular ejection decreases the risk for potential injury
   C. vehicular ejection is not related to the risk for potential injury
   D. vehicular ejection is associated with seat belt use

Answers: 1. D, 2. B, 3. B, 4. A, 5. A

SECTION FIVE: Mediators of Injury Response

At the completion of this section, the learner will be able to state some clinical conditions that could mediate the patient's response to injury. These include underlying medical conditions, drug ingestion, and physiologic alterations based on age and body size.

Underlying Medical Conditions

Underlying medical conditions are extremely important to identify when considering the patient's physiologic and hemodynamic response to trauma. The most commonly encountered conditions include chronic obstructive pulmonary disease (COPD), heart disease, and underlying cerebral insufficiency, such as with brain attacks (stroke). These conditions or the medication used to control their effects may alter the physiologic response to trauma. The patient with COPD who sustains a minor pulmonary contusion related to blunt trauma may require prompt, life-saving intubation because of the alteration in the ventilation-perfusion ratio and effects on the resilience of affected lung tissue. Beta blockade used for coronary artery disease to minimize oxygen demands by the heart could prevent a normal response to hypovolemia (i.e., tachycardia). The patient with a head injury who has had a stroke in the past may experience an altered level of consciousness, difficulty in communication, or sensorimotor dysfunction due to the stroke and not due to the acute head injury. Eliciting a complete medical history is crucial during the initial assessment. Table 34–2 lists common medical conditions that increase risk for injury.

Drug Ingestion

The high incidence of alcohol as a contributing factor to injury has already been demonstrated. How is injury affected by alcohol ingestion? The most common effect is the inability to establish clearly a baseline level of consciousness. As a CNS depressant, the effects of alcohol on the brain are concentration dependent. The most sensitive tool for evaluation of brain injury is level of consciousness. Therefore, alcohol involvement is a critical consideration.

Blood alcohol concentration (BAC) is a measurement of intoxication. Measurement is conducted in milligrams per deciliter or grams per deciliter, varying from institution to institution. Legal intoxication in most states is 100 mg/dL or 0.100 g/dL. However, impairment of judgment occurs at a level of 50 mg/dL or 0.05 g/dL. A history of alcohol use should be obtained, since a degree of tolerance ensues with frequent alcohol ingestion. The effects of alcohol on motor, sensory, and memory functions are summarized here (McCabe & Hassan, 1988).

Alcohol (Ethanol) Concentration (mg/dL)	Effects
20 to 80	Impairment of judgment, thought processes, reaction time, suppression of inhibition
100 (legal intoxication)	Further impairment of judgment, increased reaction time, decreased motor control

TABLE 34–2. COMMON MEDICAL CONDITIONS THAT INCREASE RISK FOR INJURY

MEDICAL CONDITION	MECHANISM OF INCREASED RISK	ETIOLOGY OF INCREASED RISK
Diabetes mellitus	Altered level of consciousness	Hypoglycemia Hyperglycemia
Seizures	Altered level of consciousness	Hitting head or face Fracture extremity Fall into path of vehicle
Cardiovascular disease	Altered level of consciousness	Syncope
Peripheral vascular disease	Altered sensory input	Orthostatic hypotension Dysrhythmias Myocardial infarction Stroke Transient ischemic attack Neuropathies
Substance abuse	Altered level of consciousness Altered sensory input Altered thought process	Altered judgment Altered reflexes Unconsciousness
Psychiatric illness	Altered thought process	Depression Suicidal ideation Self-destructive behavior

Kidd, P. & Sturt, P. (1995). Mosby's emergency nursing reference. *St. Louis: C.V. Mosby.*

200 to 300	Gross intoxication evident ataxia, diplopia, vomiting
300 to 400	Stuporous, hypothermic, amnesic
400 to 500	Death may result from respiratory arrest

The concomitant use of alcohol and other CNS depressants (e.g., barbiturates, opiates, sedative–hypnotics) may result in potentiation of each drug's effects, creating a **synergistic** effect.

CNS stimulants, such as cocaine, also can alter the level of consciousness in the injured patient. Cocaine use mimics and intensifies a sympathetic stimulation or the fight-or-flight response in the patient. Notably, increase in heart rate and blood pressure occur along with vasoconstriction, dilated pupils, tremors, excitability, and restlessness. Ventricular dysrhythmias, tachypnea, or Cheyne–Stokes respirations may occur with large doses. Neurologically, mental status changes range from anxiety to acute paranoid psychosis. Seizure activity also may occur after cocaine ingestion (McCabe & Hassan, 1988).

You can begin to appreciate the difficulty in obtaining a baseline level of consciousness when the patient is intoxicated with alcohol or other drugs that cloud his or her sensorium. Table 34–3 lists common medications that increase injury risk.

Age-Related Variances in Children

Age-related variances are especially important in the pediatric population. The injured child possesses unique characteristics that should be considered during your initial assessment. The primary mechanism of injury to children in the United States is blunt trauma. Automobiles cause the most significant injury to children, who suffer as passengers, pedestrians, and bicyclists. Falls, MVCs, pedestrian injuries, and burns account for 75 percent of the unintentional injuries children experience (Haley, 1998). The most common injuries sustained by children requiring admission to a trauma center are head trauma, followed in frequency by fracture of the extremities and

TABLE 34–3. COMMON MEDICATION CLASSES THAT INCREASE RISK OF INJURY

MEDICATION CLASS	ETIOLOGY OF INCREASED RISK OF INJURY
Antidiabetics	Hypoglycemia
Antiseizure	Depressed level of consciousness
Antihypertensives	Syncope Orthostatic hypotension
Antidysrhythmias	Hypotension Bradycardia Dysrhythmias
Antihistamines	CNS depression
Antineoplastics	Anemia
Antipsychotics	Extrapyramidal symptoms Hypotension Dysrhythmias
Barbiturates	CNS depression
Benzodiazepines	CNS depression
Diuretics	Hypovolemia Hypotension Electrolyte imbalances
Narcotics	CNS depression
Thyroid hormone	Thyroid storm

Kidd, P., Sturt, P., & Fultz, J. (2000). Mosby's emergency nursing reference. *2nd ed. St. Louis: C.V. Mosby.*

injury to the torso (Eichelberger, 1991). Trauma to children will frequently result in multisystem injury due to the mechanism of injury usually being blunt in nature and the anatomic characteristics of children. The priorities of care for a child are the same as for an adult; however, the following unique aspects must be considered during the initial assessment.

Size and Shape

Smaller physical size is the most obvious difference between children and adults. The applied energy from trauma dissipates over the smaller mass of the child, resulting in greater force over a smaller area. The smaller body mass results in more compact internal structures resulting in a higher frequency of multi-organ damage.

Circulation

The normal circulating blood volume of a child is 8 to 9 percent of the body weight (80 to 90 mL/kg) and is small when compared to the volume of an adult, which is 7 percent of body weight (70 mL/kg) (ACSCT, 1997b). Thus, blood loss considered negligible in an adult can produce shock in a child. Despite a smaller blood volume and a heart that has a limited functional capacity, children can compensate for volume loss better than an adult. This is due in part to a child's cardiac output being almost entirely dependent on heart rate. A child experiencing volume loss will respond with tachycardia and peripheral vasoconstriction. Blood pressure is maintained until volume loss reaches 25 percent. Keeping the vasoconstriction in mind, if a child presents with cool, mottled extremities and delayed capillary refill, volume loss is very likely the cause even if the blood pressure is adequate (Haley, 1998).

Skeleton

The child's skeleton is incompletely calcified, meaning the bones are more pliable and porous. This characteristic means the bones are able to withstand significant amounts of energy without fracturing. However, damage to the underlying structures still occurs, such as the presence of a pulmonary contusion without overlying rib fractures. Spinal cord damage can occur without spinal fractures due to the same mechanism. The elasticity of the child's developing bones requires significant stress for fracture.

Surface Area

Children have a large body surface area (BSA) in comparison to weight. There are two implications of the relatively large BSA to weight ratio in children: (1) increased susceptibility to dehydration due to greater insensible water loss and (2) increased risk of hypothermia from increased conductive and corrective heat losses. This factor is of crucial importance in a child less than 6 months of age, who lacks the insulation of subcutaneous fat and the involuntary shivering mechanism of older children (Rogers, 1998). Maintaining body heat is of primary importance in children.

Other Considerations

RENAL FUNCTION. Renal function in children < 1 year of age is immature. The kidneys cannot concentrate urine well, so fluids are not readily reabsorbed if circulatory volume loss occurs (Rogers, 1998).

ALTERATION IN CENTER OF GRAVITY. The center of gravity is in the umbilicus in an infant whereas in the adult it is the symphysis pubis. A higher center of gravity in infants and children in conjunction with the relatively large head size in relation to the body, leads to an increased frequency of head trauma.

SENSITIVITY TO HYPOXIA. The child's CNS is exquisitely sensitive to hypoxia. Hypoxia is very poorly tolerated in the pediatric population. Children have increased metabolic rates so they require increased amounts of oxygen.

MEDIASTINUM MOBILITY. The mediastinum is not well fixed in the child, resulting in wide swings of the heart and great vessels during trauma.

In children who die soon after injury, the primary mechanisms causing death are airway compromise, hypovolemic shock, and CNS damage. All of these mechanisms impair adequate tissue perfusion, precipitating a shock state. Prompt recognition and intervention for the aforementioned life-threatening conditions are addressed in later sections. The reader is referred to Module 36 for additional pediatric considerations.

The Pregnant Patient

The pregnant trauma patient presents unique aspects of care that must be considered carefully.

Anatomic Changes

Anatomic rearrangement as pregnancy progresses is inevitable and may cause confusion in physical diagnosis. Depending on the gestational size of the uterus, different patterns of injury may occur to the mother as well as to the fetus. The liver and spleen of the gravid patient are compacted, or confined to a space that is continuously decreasing in size. As energy is dissipated via the uterus to these organs, a predisposition for organ rupture is evident. A decrease in lower esophageal sphincter tone from the influence of progesterone, results in reflux and predisposes the pregnant patient to aspiration. The bladder, attached to the lower uterus, concomitantly rises out of the pelvis as the pregnancy progresses, increasing the bladder's vulnerability to injury. Diaphragmatic elevation causes a decrease in residual lung volume, ventilatory reserve, and PaO_2. Minute ventilation increases by 40 percent, with increasing tidal volume and diaphragmatic excursion. These changes result in chronic respiratory alkalosis, with $PaCO_2$ averaging 30 mm Hg. The pregnant patient experiences an increased oxygen consumption rate and has less oxygen reserve; therefore, hypoxia can occur quickly (ACSCT, 1997c).

Hemodynamic Changes

After the tenth week of pregnancy, cardiac output is increased by 1.0 L to 1.5 L/min. A high-output, low-resistance hemodynamic state is characteristic in pregnancy. Plasma volume increases 50 percent between 10 and 30 weeks. Maternal heart rate increases by 10 to 15 bpm throughout pregnancy, with a slight increase in stroke volume. Blood pressure is usually 5 to 15 mm Hg lower (systolic and diastolic) due to hormonal influences during the second trimester but returns to normal as the patient approaches term (ACSCT, 1997c). An important fact to remember is that some women experience profound hypotension when placed in the supine position (especially during the third trimester). This is known as the vena cava syndrome and is caused by the enlarged uterus compressing the inferior vena cava against the spinal column, decreasing venous return and preload. The hypotension can be relieved by turning the patient to the left lateral decubitus position or by manually shifting the weight of the uterine contents to the left.

Blood Volume and Composition

The pregnant trauma patient responds very differently to physiologic stress than the nonpregnant patient. Because of the hypervolemic state associated with pregnancy, a 30 to 35 percent (1,200 to 1,500 mL) blood loss may occur in a pregnant patient before signs and symptoms of hypovolemia occur. A physiologic anemia results in pregnancy as plasma volume increases by 50 percent and red blood cell volume increases by only 35 percent. Late in pregnancy, the hemoglobin may have fallen to 10.5 to 11 g and the hematocrit to 31 to 35 percent. The white blood cell count increases during pregnancy (15,000 to 18,000/mm^3) and during labor may be as high as 25,000/mm^3. White blood cell counts are valuable when evaluating abdominal trauma (ACSCT, 1997c).

The pregnant trauma patient exhibits a hypercoagulation state. Clotting factors VII, VIII, IX, and fibrinogen levels are increased. Circulating plasminogen activator decreases. Bleeding, clotting, and prothrombin times are not altered (Manley, 1993). (See Module 37 for additional considerations.)

The Elderly Patient

Physiologic changes associated with aging (ages 65 and older), such as delayed reaction times, disturbances of gait and balance, diminished visual acuity, and hearing loss may predispose the elderly to traumatic injury (see Module 38). Also, age-related deterioration in body systems alters the elderly trauma victim's response to injury and increases his or her susceptibility to complications. Respectively, falls, motor vehicle crashes, pedestrian versus automobile crashes, and penetrating trauma are the four most common mechanisms of injury in this age group.

Chronic Disease States

The elderly may have chronic disease states that could exacerbate or compound the trauma. Common underlying medical conditions include COPD, coronary artery disease, diabetes mellitus, congestive heart failure, hypertension, and conditions leading to diminished neurologic acuity (e.g., stroke and carotid insufficiency). The patient not only may have a chronic medical condition but also could be treated with a polypharmaceutical regimen that may affect the response to a traumatic injury.

Deterioration in Body Systems

Age-related deterioration in body systems is a normal process. The deterioration is noted most often in the cardiorespiratory, neurologic, and musculoskeletal systems. Cardiorespiratory effects include decreased distensibility of blood vessels, increased systolic blood pressure and systemic vascular resistance, increased vascular resistance, decreased coronary blood flow, decreased cardiac output, decreased respiratory muscle strength, limited chest expansion, and decreased number of functioning alveoli. These alterations combine to reduce greatly the ability to sustain adequate tissue perfusion and oxygenation. Mild anemia is also common in this age group and potentiates alterations in oxygenation by limiting oxygen transport capabilities (DeMaria, 1993). Neurologic changes associated with aging include short-term memory loss and reduced cerebral blood flow. Preexisting neurologic conditions such as senility, dementia, and Alzheimer's disease may significantly affect evaluation of the patient's neurologic status. Head injuries are common in the elderly. A high index of suspicion, awareness of the patient's preexisting neurologic status, and frequent, thorough neurologic assessments are necessary to avoid detrimental delays in diagnosis and intervention.

Osteoporosis and decreasing muscle mass contribute to the high incidence of fractures in the elderly. Normal aging processes diminish blood supply to the skin and result in delayed healing of soft tissue injuries. This reduction of blood supply also predisposes the elderly trauma patient to the development of decubitus ulcers. Prolonged backboard times and undue pressure from traction devices and splints should be avoided (Stamatos, 1994; Stubbs et al., 1994).

Difficulties during the initial assessment related to normal aging may present themselves to the clinician. Because of the decline in gag and cough reflexes, airway integrity may be difficult to maintain. Detection of shock may be difficult because of the propensity toward hypertension. Thus, normal blood pressures actually may indicate low perfusion states in the elderly.

Multiple factors affecting evaluation of the elderly trauma patient have been discussed. The following example illustrates these concepts. A 72-year-old male is involved in an MVC. He has a previous history that includes myocardial infarction and hypertension and currently is taking Inderal. A syncopal episode precipitated the MVC. The patient arrives with a blood pressure of 105/60, heart rate 65, and initial hematocrit 25 percent. A CT scan of the abdomen reveals a complex splenic laceration. Although the patient was in hypovolemic shock, the tachycardia usually associated with the shock state was prevented by the beta blockade and the diminished cardiorespiratory responsiveness.

In summary, this section has addressed individualizing the patient's response to injury based on a variety of factors. Age-related variances across the life span were discussed briefly.

SECTION FIVE REVIEW

1. Alcohol use in the trauma patient acts as a CNS
   A. stimulant
   B. depressant
   C. vasoconstrictive agent
   D. vasodilator
2. Cocaine use in the trauma patient acts as a CNS
   A. stimulant
   B. depressant
   C. vasodilator
   D. vasoconstrictor
3. Impairment of judgment occurs with a blood alcohol content of _____, whereas legal intoxication in most states is considered a blood alcohol content of _____.
   A. 50 mg/dL, 100 mg/dL
   B. 10 mg/dL, 100 mg/dL
   C. 100 mg/dL, 150 mg/dL
   D. 300 mg/dL, 400 mg/dL
4. A child's cardiac output is almost entirely dependent on
   A. stroke volume
   B. heart rate
   C. blood pressure
   D. vasoconstriction
5. The most common injury to a child precipitating admission to a trauma center is
   A. pulmonary contusion
   B. head injury
   C. rib fractures
   D. femur fractures
6. The normal blood volume for a child is _____ percent of body weight compared to that of an adult, which is _____ percent of body weight.
   A. 7 to 8, 8
   B. 7 to 8, 6
   C. 8 to 9, 7
   D. 9 to 10, 7
7. In children, the injury pattern of internal organ damage without overlying bony fracture is related to
   A. an incompletely calcified, resilient skeleton
   B. diminished body surface area
   C. increased elastic connective tissue
   D. increased fat
8. The immediate nursing intervention for a pregnant woman in her third trimester who is hypotensive after an MVC is
   A. administering vasopressors
   B. colloid transfusion
   C. turning the patient to the left lateral decubitus position, maintaining immobilization
   D. placing the patient in Trendelenburg
9. Increasing progesterone levels causing smooth muscle relaxation may elicit esophageal reflux in the pregnant woman. Thus, a predisposition to _____ may occur.
   A. aspiration
   B. increased gastric motility
   C. difficulty in intubation
   D. gastritis
10. After the tenth week of pregnancy, cardiac output is increased by _____ L/min.
    A. 0.5 to 1.0
    B. 1.0 to 1.5
    C. 1.5 to 2.0
    D. 2.0 to 2.5
11. A 24-year-old female, 7 months pregnant, victim of an MVC, has arrived. Her initial hematocrit is 31 percent. You should
    A. check fetal heart tones
    B. check for vaginal bleeding
    C. anticipate transfusion
    D. consider this normal
12. Hypotension may not be a reliable sign of shock in the elderly because
    A. the elderly patient may be taking vasodilators for hypertension
    B. coronary blood flow increases with aging
    C. reflux tachycardia occurs
    D. systemic vascular resistance decreases in aging

Answers: 1. B, 2. A, 3. A, 4. B, 5. B, 6. C, 7. A, 8. C, 9. A, 10. B, 11. D, 12. A

SECTION SIX: Trauma Assessment and Resuscitation: Primary Assessment

At the completion of this section, the learner will be able to identify the specific clinical assessment format used to determine the effects of injury.

Because of the unpredictable effects of trauma-related injury on the patient, you must develop a rapid, systematic approach to assessing each patient to ensure that no effects of injury will be overlooked. Remember, trauma should never be approached as a unisystem disease but a multisystem disease. If one body system is injured, you must ensure that no other body system has been adversely affected. Thus, a rapid systematic approach to assessment with establishment of management priorities is essential.

Trauma presents a myriad of potentially life-threatening injuries. The life-threatening injuries must be evaluated quickly, with immediate intervention. The trauma assessment is divided into three phases: primary assessment, resuscitation, and secondary assessment.

The primary assessment and resuscitation are the focus of this section. The purpose of the primary assessment is to identify life-threatening conditions and intervene appropriately. Primary assessment is done via the A, B, C, D, and E approach, as outlined here:

- **A—Airway** (with cervical spine immobilization). Ensure that the patient has an open airway.
- **B—Breathing.** Is the patient breathing? Are respirations effective? Does the patient need assistance via Ambu-bag or mechanical ventilation?
- **C—Circulation.** The trauma patient is at very high risk of hypovolemic shock from acute blood loss and third spacing of fluid with soft tissue damage. You must identify hypovolemia quickly and search for the etiology.
- **D—Disability.** Do a quick neuroexamination of the patient's level of consciousness and motor function.
- **E—Exposure and Evacuation.** The patient should be completely undressed to provide for visualization of external causes of injury. If the severity of the patient's injury exceeds the capability of the hospital, consider transport of the patient to a definitive care facility.

Each of the components of the primary assessment is explored in detail to ensure that you have all the information necessary to approach the multiply injured patient using critical thinking and problem-solving strategies. Pediatric variances in approach are addressed under each heading.

Airway and Cervical Spine

The goal of airway management is optimization of ventilation and oxygenation, with cervical spine protection. The first step in the primary assessment of a trauma patient is assessment for the patency of the patient's airway. An injury to the cervical spine should always be assumed in the patient with multisystem trauma, especially in the patient with an injury above the clavicle. Excessive manipulation of the head, face, or neck, precipitating hyperextension or hyperflexion of the cervical spine, may convert a fracture without neurologic manifestations into a fracture–dislocation with spinal cord contusion, laceration, compression, or transection. Therefore, cervical immobilization should be ensured when airway assessment occurs.

Potential causes of airway obstruction include the tongue falling back into the oropharynx, obstructing the airway; blood, vomitus, secretions, or foreign objects obstructing the airway; fractures of the facial bony structures; or crushing injuries of the laryngotracheal tree. You should be alerted to actual or potential airway obstruction based on the following symptoms:

- Dyspnea
- Diminished breath sounds despite respiratory effort
- Dysphonia (hoarseness, stridor)
- Dysphagia
- Drooling

Airway management techniques range from simple positional maneuvers to complex surgical procedures. During all maneuvers, it is critical that the cervical spine be maintained by inline immobilization with the head in the neutral position. Cervical spine immobilization can best be achieved by manual inline axial traction by a caregiver or by a hard cervical collar, a lateral immobilization device (commercial variety), disposable head blocks, or towel rolls on either side of the patient's head, and tape across the patient's forehead, securing the head to the backboard. This prevents forward flexion, hyperextension, and lateral rotation of the cervical spine. Sandbags are no longer an acceptable means of lateral cervical immobilization due to the increased application of lateral pressure to the cervical spine if turning or tilting of the backboard becomes necessary.

The first, and most simple, maneuver to attempt in opening the airway is a chin lift or modified jaw thrust, maintaining the head in a neutral position. This maneuver may very well open the airway adequately and allow ventilation to take place. The pediatric airway is easily obstructed, especially in the child with an altered level of consciousness. As in the adult, loss of muscle tone in the oral pharynx results in the tongue falling posteriorly, causing airway obstruction. In comparison to an adult, the following pediatric considerations apply in regard to airway management.

- The child's tongue is proportionately larger and is housed in a smaller oral cavity.
- The glottic opening is more anterior and cephalad.
- The trachea is short and narrow.
- Children < 12 months of age are obligatory nose breathers. Nasal passages must remain clear unless an artificial airway is provided.

Along with the modified jaw thrust/chin lift, the airway can be suctioned for debris, secretions, blood, or vomitus. An oropharyngeal or nasopharyngeal airway may be used to facilitate airway maintenance.

The oropharyngeal airway should be used only in patients who are unconscious and have no gag reflex. Using this airway in a conscious patient may precipitate gagging, vomiting, and potential aspiration. Improper placement of the oropharyngeal airway actually may cause airway obstruction. The nasopharyngeal airway also may be used to facilitate airway integrity in the conscious victim with an intact gag reflex.

If the aforementioned procedures are inadequate in establishment of an airway, more aggressive measures must be taken. The patient should be hyperventilated with a bag-valve-mask with 100 percent oxygen. A frequent complication of hyperventilation with this technique is gastric distention. Increased risks secondary to the distention include vomiting, aspiration, and diaphragmatic impingement. After a definitive airway has been secured, placement of a gastric tube will decompress the stomach. If enough help is available, pressure applied over the cricoid cartilage will compress the esophagus and help prevent gastric insufflation.

Endotracheal intubation can be achieved either orally or nasally. Nasotracheal intubation is preferred in the injured patient, since hyperextension of the neck is minimized. However, a patient must have spontaneous respiratory effort for placement of the tube. With the nasotracheal method, the tube should be advanced during the inspiratory effort when the epiglottis is open. Orotracheal intubation is necessary when the patient is apneic or a cribriform plate fracture is suspected, as with basilar skull fractures. With fractures of the **cribriform** plate, the nasally inserted endotracheal tube could pass into the cranial vault, injuring brain tissue. Should orotracheal intubation be necessary, absolute and vigilant care must be taken to avoid hyperextension of the cervical spine.

After intubation is achieved, breath sounds anteriorly and laterally should be auscultated to confirm tracheal intubation. The clinician also should ausculate over the epigastrium for gurgling sounds to help rule out an esophageal intubation, which would be lethal in the acute trauma situation. Tube displacement may occur during transport, especially in children under eight years old, since the endotracheal tubes used are uncuffed, thereby more mobile. Right mainstem bronchus intubation occurs occasionally if the endotracheal tube is passed too far into the trachea. The right mainstem bronchus is straighter than the left as it branches from the trachea, facilitating passage of the tube into its lumen. Repeated assessment of breath sounds in any intubated patient, adult or pediatric, is a crucial nursing action.

The only indication for creating a surgical airway is inability to intubate the trachea. Inability to intubate the trachea may result from edema of the glottis, larynx fracture, severe oropharyngeal hemorrhage, or gross instability of the midface. A surgical airway can be achieved by a needle cricothyroidotomy, surgical cricothyroidotomy, or tracheostomy. Surgical **cricothyroidotomy** is performed by making an incision through the cricothyroid membrane and into the trachea. Surgical cricothyroidotomy is not recommended for children less than 12 years of age because the cricoid cartilage is only circumferential support to the upper trachea. Thus, tracheostomy must be performed should a surgical airway become necessary (ACSCT, 1997d).

Tracheostomy must be considered in the child less than 12 years of age and in the patient with suspected laryngeal trauma. Symptoms of laryngeal injury include tenderness, hoarseness, **subcutaneous emphysema,** and intolerance of the supine position. The supine position is poorly tolerated by these patients because on assuming the position, the airway will collapse where the laryngeal injury has occurred. With the patient sitting upright, an open airway is maintained even though the larynx is injured.

Aggressive airway management is critical in the trauma population. Assurance of airway integrity is the priority in the primary assessment, with techniques ranging from a simple modified jaw thrust to a complex surgical procedure. The clinician must be ready for anything to ensure optimal patient management. Remember, however, that airway integrity does not ensure adequate ventilation. The airway must be opened and secured, and then ventilation can be addressed.

Breathing

The next step in the primary assessment is to address the adequacy of ventilation in the injured patient. The primary goal of ventilation is to achieve maximum cellular oxygenation by providing an oxygen-rich environment. Thus, all trauma patients should receive high-flow oxygen during the initial evaluation.

Breathing should be evaluated by the look, listen, and feel parameters. Look to detect the presence of respiratory excursion, listen for breath sounds, and feel for breathing. Positive pressure ventilation may be required in some patients and can be provided in a number of ways: mouth-to-mask, bag-valve-mask, or positive pressure ventilator.

Confirmation of the adequacy of ventilation is best achieved by obtaining an arterial blood gas determination or continuous monitoring of end-tidal carbon dioxide and arterial oxygen saturation by noninvasive measures. If arterial blood gases are inadequate, the airway should be reevaluated, and the patient should be evaluated for the presence of pneumothorax, hemothorax, hemopneumothorax, or **tension pneumothorax.** Tube thoracostomy would be indicated for any of these conditions, since they are all considered life threatening. Refer to Module 35 for assessment guidelines in evaluating these clinical conditions.

Circulation

The third step in the primary assessment after airway and breathing have been adequately addressed is circulation. Inadequate circulation is manifested as shock. Shock is a clinical state characterized by inadequate organ perfusion and tissue oxygenation (ACSCT, 1997b).

Assessment for adequate circulation should include palpating for strength, rate, rhythm, and symmetry of carotid, radial, femoral, and pedal pulses. Skin temperature also should be evaluated, as should capillary refill centrally and peripherally. Mucous membranes can be inspected as well. The adequacy of tissue perfusion is reflected sensitively by the patient's level of consciousness.

Successful treatment of shock depends on early recognition, controlling obvious hemorrhage, and aggressive fluid resuscitation to prevent the development of hypotension. Intravenous (IV) access is critical for volume infusion. Two large-bore IVs should be established (16 gauge or larger in adults, 18 gauge or larger in children), and crystalloid administration should ensue promptly. Warm lactated Ringer's solution is the solution of choice for adults and children. Lactated Ringer's solution can be infused at a wide-open rate in the adult to infuse 1 to 2 L. If the adult shows no signs of improvement after 2 L, crystalloid infusion should continue and blood infusion should be initiated. Children should be bolused at 20 mL/kg of body weight. If the child shows no improvement, a second bolus can be administered at 20 mL/kg of body weight. If signs of shock persist, a 10 mL/kg bolus of packed red blood cells can be transfused. A failure of adults or children to respond to crystalloid and blood infusion indicates rapid surgical intervention is required (ACSCT, 1997b).

Remember that the early signs of shock are subtle in children. Normal blood volume in the child varies from 8 to 9 percent, or 80 to 90 mL/kg body weight. A small volume loss for an adult can precipitate shock in the child. Early shock from acute blood loss of up to 25 percent of blood volume (20 mL/kg body weight) generally is well tolerated in healthy children. Signs and symptoms based on shock stages in children are as follows (ACSCT 1997e; Haley, 1998).

Shock Stage	Signs and Symptoms
Mild shock Blood volume loss < 25 percent	Mild tachycardia; cool, clammy, mottled skin, normal blood pressure (> 80 mm Hg systolic), dyspnea, tachypnea, agitation, lethargy, or hypotonia
Moderate shock Blood volume loss > 25 percent	Significant tachycardia, decreasing pulse pressure (< 20 mm Hg), cyanosis, cool extremities, prolonged capillary refill (longer than 2 seconds)
Severe shock Blood volume loss > 50 percent	Profound hypotension, vasoconstriction, coma, anuria, cyanosis, and pallor

Recognition of the site of blood loss is critical in the mediation of shock. Blood volume loss in quantities enough to produce a shock state can occur in one or more of the following five areas:

1. *Chest*. In the adult, 2.5 L of blood can be lost in each hemothorax. Thus, a total of 5 L can be lost inside the chest, which would be the total blood volume of a 70-kg person.
2. *Abdomen*. As much as 6 L of blood can be lost via intraperitoneal bleeding from damaged organs or vessels.
3. *Pelvis and retroperitoneum*. An unstable pelvic fracture, especially those involving the posterior elements of the pelvis, can precipitate liters of blood loss. A patient actually may exsanguinate from an unstable pelvic fracture involving posterior bony elements.
4. *Femur fractures*. For each femur fracture, 500 to 1,000 mL of blood can be lost.
5. *External hemorrhage*. Bleeding wounds are a consideration especially in children. A scalp laceration particularly requires proper hemostasis, since it can lead to a shock state in young children.

Of the causes of early postinjury deaths in the hospital that are amenable to effective treatment, hemorrhage is predominant. The most common cause of shock in the injured patient is hypovolemia resulting from acute blood loss. Fluid resuscitation is the fundamental treatment for hypovolemic shock until definitive surgical intervention is available to treat the site (or sites) of injury.

Disability

After airway, breathing, and circulation are managed adequately, the fourth step is evaluation for neurologic disability. The purpose of the neurologic examination in the primary assessment is to establish quickly the patient's level of consciousness and pupillary size and reaction.

The patient's level of consciousness can quickly be determined by the AVPU method.

- A—Alert
- V—Responds to verbal stimulation
- P—Responds to painful stimulation
- U—Unresponsive

A more detailed examination should be included in the secondary survey.

Exposure

At this point in the primary assessment, the patient should be completely disrobed in preparation for the secondary assessment. Cold ambient temperatures of resuscitation areas, large volumes of room temperature IV fluids and cold blood products, wet clothing, and exposure all predispose the trauma patient to hypothermia. Careful attention to heat conservation measures cannot be overemphasized.

In summary, this section has given you a broad overview of the primary assessment conducted during the initial phase of trauma evaluation. Special considerations for children were presented.

SECTION SIX REVIEW

1. The following are true concerning the pediatric airway EXCEPT
   A. the glottic opening is more anterior and cephalad
   B. the trachea is short and narrow
   C. the child's tongue is proportionately smaller and usually has little to do with airway integrity
   D. cervical spine immobilization requires meticulous attention
2. Contraindications to the use of an oropharyngeal airway include
   A. consciousness/presence of gag reflex
   B. unconsciousness
   C. absence of gag reflex
   D. questionable airway integrity
3. A frequent complication of hyperventilation is
   A. vomiting
   B. increased airway pressures
   C. gastric distention
   D. increased pulmonary compliance
4. Your patient has just been intubated for progressive respiratory failure. On ausculation of breath sounds, you note present breath sounds in right lung fields and absent breath sounds in left lung fields. You should anticipate the cause as
   A. right mainstem intubation
   B. esophageal intubation
   C. tension pneumothorax
   D. pericardial effusion
5. The surgical airway of choice in the child < 12 years of age who has severe facial fractures and bleeding is
   A. tracheostomy
   B. cricothyroidotomy
   C. orotracheal intubation
   D. nasotracheal intubation
6. High-flow oxygen should be used for all of the following groups of trauma patients EXCEPT
   A. acute respiratory failure
   B. normal respiratory rate, systolic blood pressure of 90 mm Hg
   C. hemopneumothorax
   D. patient with COPD and an isolated ankle injury
7. When bolusing the injured child with a crystalloid solution, the initial bolus should be
   A. 10 mL/kg
   B. 20 mL/kg
   C. 50 mL/kg
   D. 1 L

Answers: 1. C, 2. A, 3. C, 4. A, 5. A, 6. D, 7. B

SECTION SEVEN: Trauma Assessment and Resuscitation: Secondary Assessment

This section outlines the components of the secondary assessment during the initial trauma evaluation. At the completion of this section, the learner should have an understanding of the components of the secondary assessment and of the suggested format for conducting the secondary assessment.

The secondary assessment should begin only after the primary assessment is completed and all immediately life-threatening injuries have been addressed. A head-to-toe approach is usually adopted, with thorough examination of each body system. A critical point to remember is that if the patient becomes hemodynamically unstable at any point during the secondary assessment, you should immediately return to the primary assessment format (A, B, C, D, and E) to troubleshoot the problem. A summary of key points in the secondary assessment has been adapted in Table 34–4 from the American College of Surgeons Committee on Trauma Advanced Trauma Life Support Course Provider Manual (1997f).

At the completion of the secondary assessment, you must remember that the trauma patient demands repeated reevaluation so that any new signs or symptoms are not overlooked. Other life-threatening problems may appear, or exacerbation of previously treated injuries may occur (such as tension pneumothorax, **pericardial tamponade,** or intracranial bleeding). Continuous monitoring of vital signs and urine output is critical. Urine output should be maintained at 50 mL/hr for the adult and 1 mL/kg/hr for children as an indicator of adequate tissue perfusion.

In summary, this section has outlined the format for the secondary assessment to be conducted during initial assessment and resuscitation of the trauma patient. Key criteria for evaluation were identified in each area to facilitate assessment parameters.

TABLE 34–4. KEY POINTS IN THE SECONDARY ASSESSMENT

SURVEYED SYSTEM	EVALUATED CRITERIA
Head	Complete neurologic examination using a tool, such as the Glasgow Coma Scale (GCS), reevaluation of pupillary size and reactivity, inspection, palpation of cranium for lacerations, fractures, contusions, hemotympanium, cerebrospinal fluid leakage, edema, etc.
Maxillofacial	Assessment for facial fractures via inspection, palpation for open fractures, lacerations, mobility/instability of facial structures
Cervical spine/neck	Inspection and palpation of neck anteriorly (maintaining cervical spine immobilization) and palpation anteriorly and posteriorly for pain, **crepitus,** bony stepoffs indicating fracture–dislocation, neck vein distention, and tracheal deviation
Chest	Inspection for paradoxical movement, flail segments, open chest wounds, ecchymosis; palpation for rib fractures, subcutaneous emphysema, respiratory excursion, sternal fractures; auscultation for quality, equality of breath sounds, presence of adventitious sounds; auscultation of heart sounds for quality, extra heart sounds, murmurs, or pericardial friction rubs possibly indicating pericardial effusion
Abdomen	Inspection and auscultation before palpation to prevent precipitation of misleading bowel sounds by manual manipulation; abdomen inspection for abrasions, contusions, lacerations, distention; auscultation for bowel sounds in four quadrants, bruits, and breath sounds; light and deep palpation precipitating a painful response may indicate intraperitoneal bleeding and should be quickly attended
Pelvis, perineum, genitalia	Pelvis inspection for deformation and palpation for stability Perineum and genitalia inspection for bleeding at the meatus, hematoma, vaginal bleeding, lacerations Rectal examination to evaluate rectal wall integrity, presence of blood, position of prostate, presence of palpable pelvic fractures, and quality of sphincter tone
Musculoskeletal	Visual evaluation of extremities for contusions or deformities; palpation of all extremities for tenderness, crepitation, or abnormal range of motion, which may raise index of suspicion for fracture; all peripheral pulses should be evaluated, and capillary refill, skin color, temperature rechecked
Back	All patients should be logrolled with careful attention to spinal immobilization to afford the clinician a full view of the patient's posterior surfaces, including neck, back, buttocks, and lower extremities; these areas should be carefully inspected and palpated to detect any area of injury
Complete neurologic examination	Motor and sensory evaluation of the extremities and reevaluation of the patient's GCS score and pupils; any evidence of paralysis or paresis should prompt immediate immobilization of the entire patient if not already done

Section Seven Review

1. During the secondary assessment, your patient becomes hemodynamically unstable. You should immediately
   A. stop the secondary assessment and reinstitute the primary assessment
   B. finish the secondary assessment, looking for potential etiologies of instability
   C. start at the beginning of the secondary assessment
   D. reevaluate patency and flow rates of IVs
2. The purpose of the secondary assessment is to
   A. identify and intervene with life-threatening injuries
   B. identify the existence of all injuries
   C. facilitate treatment of airway and breathing
   D. assess response of resuscitative interventions
3. The complete and immediate immobilization of the entire patient should take place with the following findings during secondary assessment
   A. inability to establish airway
   B. tense, distended abdomen
   C. Glasgow Coma Scale score ≤ 8
   D. evidence of paralysis or paresis
4. Presence of abdominal pain on light or deep palpation in the injured patient usually indicates
   A. gastritis
   B. presence of intraperitoneal blood
   C. pelvic fracture
   D. intracerebral pathology
5. Rectal examination should be done to evaluate all of the following EXCEPT
   A. rectal wall integrity
   B. presence of blood
   C. bladder injury
   D. palpable pelvic fractures

Answers: 1. A, 2. B, 3. D, 4. B, 5. C

SECTION EIGHT: Trauma Mortality and Traumatic Shock

At the completion of this section, the learner will be able to describe the trimodal distribution of trauma-related mortalities and how time-elapsed postinjury will affect your clinical assessment. A brief discussion of traumatic shock and exsanguination is presented.

Trauma Deaths

Twenty percent of trauma-related mortalities are considered preventable in the United States today. This is an astounding statistic in an age of modern technology with the myriad of life-saving interventions we use. When plotted on a graph, trauma-related mortalities exhibit a trimodal distribution; that is, death from trauma has three peak periods of occurrence. The first peak occurs within minutes of the injury. These deaths usually result from injuries to the brain, upper spinal cord, heart, aorta, or other major blood vessel. The second peak occurs within 2 hours of injury, and death usually is related to subdural or epidural hematomas, hemopneumothorax, ruptured spleen, lacerated liver, fractured femurs, or other injuries resulting in significant blood loss. The third peak occurs days to weeks after the injury and usually results from complications of sepsis or multiple organ failure (ACSCT, 1997g).

How does the knowledge of this distribution affect your clinical practice? Again, this knowledge can empower you to anticipate the needs of the patient based on time from injury and physiologic manifestation of the injury. If you receive a patient within minutes of injury or perhaps you are the first responder as a flight nurse, what are the life-threatening injuries that may cause death in this time frame? Has the patient experienced brain stem compression or laceration resulting in respiratory center dysfunction? Perhaps the patient has experienced atlanto-occipital dislocation and severe spinal cord contusion or transection, or perhaps the heart or great vessels have been lacerated, transected, or disrupted. What assessment and intervention must be performed to mediate these injuries?

An unstable female patient arrives within 30 minutes of injury. What conditions must you appreciate clinically to anticipate a life-threatening situation? Epidural or **subdural hematoma** (What is her level of consciousness?), hemopneumothorax (What is her respiratory effort? How are her lung sounds? Will a chest tube be necessary?), ruptured spleen or lacerated liver (Does she have a tense and painful abdomen? Is she hypotensive with no signs of obvious blood loss?), or fractured femur (Is her leg painful, with an obvious fracture?).

Perhaps you are in the critical care environment with a patient 2 weeks after his injury. If he is experiencing multiple organ dysfunction or sepsis, what could be the precipitating factors or contributing factors to his condition? Was he overhydrated during the first 24 to 48 hours and acute respiratory distress syndrome (ARDS) has ensued? Did he have a missed intra-abdominal injury predisposing him to sepsis?

Shock from Trauma

Mortality from trauma may result from what is considered a preventable cause. One of the most frequently encountered clinical states in the injured patient is traumatic shock. Because of the frequency of traumatic shock, a brief discussion of hemorrhagic shock ensues. You should refer to Module 10 for an in-depth examination of the cellular tissue, organ, and system response to shock.

The most common cause of shock in the injured patient is hypovolemia resulting from acute blood loss. Acute blood loss can occur externally, as with lacerations, open fractures, avulsion injuries, or amputations, or internally within a body cavity, as with bleeding into the chest cavity, abdominal cavity, retroperitoneum, or soft tissue. (Section Six of this module has a discussion of potential sites of blood loss in large enough quantities to precipitate shock.)

As with most body systems dysfunction, a general pattern of body compensatory mechanisms occurs in response to hemorrhagic shock in an effort to stabilize the unstable body system. Remember, shock is basically a cellular derangement, and all cells usually are affected when a shock state is encountered.

As blood loss continues in the injured patient, the compensatory mechanisms become more pronounced and eventually fail, precipitating severe problems with tissue perfusion, unless prompt recognition and intervention are conducted. A small volume of blood (approximately 10 percent of total blood volume) can be removed without significant effect on mean arterial pressure (MAP) or cardiac output. With blood loss exceeding 10 percent, decreased venous return precipitates a decreased cardiac output and, thus, a decreased MAP. Should 35 to 40 percent of total blood volume be lost, both cardiac output and MAP fall to zero (Vary & Linberg, 1988).

The body maintains a regional distribution of blood flow in hemorrhage with greater than 10 percent loss of blood volume. The body selectively shunts blood away from nonvital tissue to critical, vital organs, such as the heart and brain. If left untreated for any length of time, the shock state will progress until it becomes refractory to any treatment.

Exsanguination is the most extreme form of hemorrhage. There is an initial loss of 40 percent of the patient's blood volume, with a rate of blood loss, or a rate of hemorrhage, exceeding 250 mL/min. If uncontrolled, the patient may lose 50 percent of the entire blood volume in 10 minutes (Asensio, 1990).

Most injuries precipitating exsanguination are from penetrating trauma. An identifiable cluster of organs and organ systems with a high incidence of exsanguination has been identified (Asensio, 1990).

I. Heart
II. Abdominal vascular system
  A. Arterial system
    1. Abdominal aorta
    2. Superior mesenteric artery
  B. Venous system
    1. Inferior vena cava
    2. Portal vein
    3. Liver

Resuscitation of the exsanguinating patient rests on the intensified basic principles of circulation management. IV access must be established quickly with adequate, large-bore catheters. The preferred fluid for resuscitation of the exsanguinating patient is warm lactated Ringer's solution (ACSCT, 1997b). In the patient experiencing hemorrhage shock, the red cell mass is likely to be reduced by 50 percent, and the plasma space may be reduced to 35 percent. For adequate resuscitation to ensue, both plasma and interstitial fluid spaces must be replenished by the most appropriate electrolyte solution, lactated Ringer's solution (Asensio, 1990).

Transfusion of blood ideally should occur after the initial infusion of 2 to 4 L of lactated Ringer's solution. O-negative blood should be used during initial resuscitation until type-specific or crossmatched blood becomes available. In male patients, O-positive blood can be given during resuscitation as the Rh factor will not cause the adverse effects (Rh sensitization) that it may in females of childbearing age. Controversy continues about the use of packed red blood cells versus whole blood versus other component therapy.

Other adjuncts are available in the acute phase of resuscitation of the exsanguinating patient. Rapid infusion devices are available and can deliver large amounts of crystalloid and colloid incredibly quickly. The use of autotransfusion devices in major chest injury may facilitate resuscitative efforts, especially in those patients with large hemothoraces.

Emergency department open resuscitative thoracotomy also may be used to manage the exsanguinating patient, especially if exsanguination is suspected to be related to injury to the great vessels (i.e., aorta) or the heart.

Critical analysis during the primary assessment and quick recognition of traumatic shock are essential skills in the resuscitative phase of trauma. The 20 percent of preventable trauma-related mortalities can be mediated with improved prehospital and hospital care in the provision of highly skilled clinicians who can evaluate the injured patient rapidly and effectively.

In summary, the process of trauma assessment can be refined and polished with the knowledge of clinical conditions that cause deaths in our trauma population. Nursing can play a key role in mediating the preventable deaths from trauma that continue to plague our modern society.

Section Eight Review

1. _____ percent of trauma-related mortalities are considered preventable.
   A. 10
   B. 20
   C. 30
   D. 50
2. Trauma-related mortalities exhibit a _____ distribution.
   A. modal
   B. bimodal
   C. trimodal
   D. bell-shaped
3. The second mode occurs within 2 hours postinjury and may be attributed to all of the following EXCEPT
   A. sepsis
   B. ruptured spleen
   C. liver laceration
   D. hemopneumothorax
4. The third mode occurs within days to weeks postinjury and usually can be attributed to
   A. exsanguination
   B. multiple organ dysfunction/sepsis
   C. brain stem compression
   D. atlanto-occipital dislocation
5. The most common cause of shock in the injured patient is
   A. hypovolemia
   B. cardiogenic
   C. neurogenic
   D. sepsis
6. The three organs and organ systems most commonly associated with exsanguination are
   A. heart, liver, abdominal vasculature
   B. lung, brain, heart
   C. brain, kidney, spleen
   D. kidney, abdominal vasculature, lung
7. The crystalloid of choice for infusion in the exsanguinating patient is
   A. normal saline
   B. Lactated Ringer's solution
   C. D_5W
   D. hypertonic saline

Answers: 1. B, 2. C, 3. A, 4. B, 5. A, 6. A, 7. B

SECTION NINE: Nursing Diagnoses Associated with Traumatic Injury

At the completion of this section, the learner will be able to cluster patient symptoms and derive appropriate nursing diagnoses.

If a traumatic injury is suspected, the nurse should focus on assessing the symptoms most commonly associated with life-threatening conditions. These symptoms include ineffective breathing, altered blood pH, hypotension, distended neck veins, decreased urine output, and a change in level of responsiveness. The nursing diagnoses associated with these symptoms include: ineffective breathing patterns, impaired gas exchange, altered airway clearance, fluid volume deficit, altered urinary elimination, and alteration in cerebral tissue perfusion. Table 34–5 links associated injury patterns.

Ineffective Airway Clearance, Ineffective Breathing Pattern, and Impaired Gas Exchange

In the trauma patient, airway is always assessed first and necessary interventions made. The airway may be compromised if the patient has a depressed mental status. The gag reflex may be absent, and foreign bodies may be present in the oropharynx. A partially obstructed airway will be noisy. Snoring, gargling, or wheezing may be present. If the airway is obstructed, it should be reopened using a manual maneuver (chin lift maneuver if cervical spine injury has not been ruled out), immediately suctioned, and an oral or nasopharyngeal artificial airway placed. Oral or nasotracheal intubation is another method of securing a patent airway. Facial trauma may produce copious amounts of bleeding, and skeletal integrity of the face may be disrupted. The performance of a cricothyroidotomy (surgical airway) is preferred to obtain a patent airway in a patient with massive facial injuries. Direct trauma to the airway may occur from blunt larnygotracheal injuries. These patients are unable to tolerate a supine position, are hoarse, have subcutaneous emphysema, and are tender over the tracheal area. A tracheostomy is the best method of securing an airway in these patients.

Ineffective breathing patterns are associated with tracheobronchial and thoracic injuries. The chest is observed for bruising, open wounds, and symmetry of chest wall movement. Open wounds are evaluated further by logrolling the patient and inspecting the posterior surface. No chest wall movement and the presence of abdominal breathing may indicate a cervical cord lesion. The patient's respiratory rate should be noted, as should the degree of breathing effort. Paradoxical movement of the chest (inward motion of a segment of the chest during inhalation and outward motion of the same segment with expiration) indicates multiple rib fractures and a flail segment. The patient with a large flail segment may require intubation and mechanical ventilation or pain control therapy to prevent respiratory acidosis and to promote tissue oxygenation. The chest area is palpated to detect the presence of subcutaneous emphysema, rib/sternum tenderness, or defects. Auscultation detects the presence of breath sounds bilaterally in the primary survey. Gross differences in breath sounds are an important finding, since it usually indicates a pneumothorax or hemothorax. A more detailed pulmonary assessment is performed during the secondary assessment. High flow oxygen is administered to trauma patients before obtaining arterial blood gas results. A nonrebreathing mask or a bag-valve-mask device with an oxygen reservoir may be used depending on the patient's responsiveness level. Pulse oximetry and end-tidal carbon dioxide measurement (if the patient is intubated) may provide additional data regarding oxygenation before arterial blood gas analysis.

Aerobic metabolism is dependent on saturation of hemoglobin with oxygen. The patient's PaO_2 must be > 60 mm Hg on room air, respiratory rate must be between 12 and 24, and tidal volume must be 10 mL/kg to ensure aerobic metabolism (Thelan, Davie, & Urden, 1990). The trauma patient may experience respiratory acidosis as a result of a partially obstructed airway, ineffective breathing patterns, or impaired circulation. Intubation with mechanical ventilation may be necessary to correct the acid–base imbalance. Fluid resuscitation with warm lactated Ringer's solution may facilitate compensation due to the solution's buffering abilities.

TABLE 34–5. SENTINEL INJURY AND ASSOCIATED INJURY PATTERN

- *First rib fracture:* Heart/great vessel injury (subclavian vein and artery), CNS injury (head/neck)
- *Scapula fracture:* Brachial plexus, pulmonary contusion, great vessel, CNS injury
- *Sternal fracture:* Blunt cardiac injury, great vessel, pulmonary contusion
- *Right lower rib fractures:* Liver lacerations
- *Left lower rib fractures:* Spleen lacerations

Kidd, P., Sturt, P., & Fultz, J. (2000). Mosby's emergency nursing reference. *2nd ed. St. Louis: C.V. Mosby.*

Fluid Volume Deficit

Peripheral vasoconstriction may artificially elevate blood pressure readings even though central arterial pressures are low. This is a short-acting compensatory mechanism. The value of clustering assessment data is to prevent misdiagnosis by focusing on one symptom while ignoring others. It is very important to monitor the trauma patient's blood pressure and at the same time assess neck veins, responsiveness level, and urine output.

Hypotension in the trauma patient usually is related to hypovolemia. Hypovolemia may result from internal bleeding or uncontrolled external bleeding. Fractures and lacerations of abdominal organs are frequent sources of bleeding in the trauma patient. For example, a fractured femur may result in 1 to 2 L of blood loss (Rea, 1995). However, hypotension may be related to factors that inhibit cardiac output (CO) or the loss of peripheral vascular resistance. The two most frequently encountered conditions associated with restriction of CO are cardiac tamponade and tension pneumothorax. In cardiac tamponade, hypotension occurs in response to decreased CO. A tear in the pericardium produces bleeding into the pericardial sac. The increased pressure prohibits filling of the ventricles and decreases stroke volume. The increased pericardium pressure also impedes coronary blood flow. Myocardial ischemia results and further decreases CO. Lung parenchymal injury from chest trauma may produce a tension pneumothorax. As atmospheric air enters the pleural cavity through the injury site, the lung on the affected side collapses while mediastinal contents and the trachea are pushed away from the injury site. The pressure placed on the great vessels inhibits venous return. Thus, the neck veins become distended.

Both cardiac tamponade and tension pneumothorax are life-threatening conditions that require immediate treatment. Blood in the pericardial sac is removed by pericardiocentesis. Insertion of a chest tube and covering the open chest wound (if present) with an impermeable dressing are appropriate interventions for the patient with a tension pneumothorax.

Hypotension also may occur in patients with spinal cord injuries who develop spinal shock. In spinal shock, the patient's blood pressure may be < 70 mm Hg due to a loss of sympathetic tone that occurs secondary to transection of the spinal cord. The parasympathetic nervous system is unopposed, so peripheral vasodilation and bradycardia occur. Bradycardia is the key assessment finding that helps to differentiate spinal shock from hypovolemia. However, the patient may also be hemorrhaging but is unable to compensate by increasing the heart rate. Atropine and/or intravenous fluids are administered to increase the pulse rate high enough to perfuse core organs. Fluid resuscitation is appropriate for a patient with spinal cord injury who is hypotensive as internal trauma cannot be ruled out initially. However, caution must be taken to avoid causing pulmonary edema. For the patient with an isolated spinal cord injury, if a fluid challenge does not resolve the hypotension, careful administration of a vasopressor may be considered (ACSCT, 1997h).

The presence of a radial pulse indicates an arterial pressure of 80 mm Hg. A pressure of at least 70 mm Hg is required for palpation of a femoral or brachial pulse. If a cartoid pulse can be palpated, the pressure is at least 60 mm Hg (Rea, 1995). The nurse can discriminate hypotension resulting from hypovolemia from that associated with increased pericardial pressure by assessing for the presence of a **paradoxical pulse.** The systolic blood pressure will fall more during inspiration if tension pneumothorax or cardiac tamponade exists. In these conditions, the increased thoracic pressure from inspiration further decreases left ventricle filling and results in blood backing up into the right heart so CO is compromised. If a central venous pressure (CVP) catheter or pulmonary arterial catheter is in place, the CVP reading will be elevated due to increased right atrial filling with decreased emptying. A CVP reading of greater than 15 cm H_2O is significant. Jugular venous distention will be present. Hypotension resulting from hypovolemia will be associated with flat neck veins. The value of capillary refill as an assessment parameter of hypovolemia has been questioned. However, normal capillary refill is 2 seconds in the adult male and children, 2.9 seconds in the adult female, and 4.5 seconds in the elderly (Schriger & Baraff, 1988). Allowances should be made if the extremity is hypothermic, since capillary refill will be delayed. Decreased pedal pulses and pale or mottled skin also may be present.

Altered Urinary Elimination

The kidneys receive 20 percent of the CO, and the kidneys may reflect decreased CO earlier than other organs. In most circumstances, decreased or absent urine output in the trauma patient will indicate decreased core perfusion from an extrarenal cause. When MAP falls below 50 to 70 mm Hg, antidiuretic hormone (ADH) is released. ADH is a potent vasoconstrictor and it promotes renal water reabsorption. Urine output is an excellent clinical indicator of tissue perfusion. The adult trauma patient should maintain an hourly urine output of at least 25 to 30 mL to ensure adequate core circulation. In rate situations, the renal artery may be lacerated from a fall or an abrupt deceleration injury. The patient will show signs of hypovolemia, with flat neck veins and hypotension. The patient usually will be anuric.

Altered Cerebral Tissue Perfusion

A change in responsiveness in the trauma patient may be related to numerous factors. In the presence of hypovolemia, cerebral blood flow decreases, resulting in stupor, unconsciousness, and eventually failure of subconscious mental processes, including vasomotor control and respiration. The more highly specialized the tissue, the more vulnerable it is to hypoxemia. Cortical functions are lost first with cerebral hypoxia. Cerebral hypoperfusion is present when the systolic blood pressure is below 60 mm Hg. Hypoxia, hypoglycemia, and drug use also may impair responsiveness. Since a change in responsiveness may be present from cerebral injury or from systemic causes, clustering of assessment data is helpful. Responsiveness generally is evaluated at the same time that pupillary size and reaction and motor response are assessed. If a spinal cord injury is present, the patient may not be able to respond to commands even if the patient comprehends. It is important to document the stimulus used to elicit a motor response, the exact response, and bilateral differences. The use of a standardized scale, such as the Glasgow Coma Scale (GCS) (refer to Module 17) can facilitate monitoring of neurologic status and improve communication among multiple health care providers.

Airway protection is of major concern in a patient with decreased responsiveness. An oral or nasopharyngeal airway is inserted to maintain airway patency. Unconscious patients should be intubated endotracheally. Oxygen administration is necessary in a patient with decreased responsiveness to promote cerebral oxygenation.

Focused Assessment Findings and Nursing Diagnoses

Life-threatening conditions produce characteristic symptoms that the nurse can identify. The following cluster of data strongly suggests the presence of a life-threatening injury:

- Noisy airway
- Absent breath sounds
- Deviated trachea
- Flat or distended neck veins
- Paradoxical chest movement
- Open chest wound
- Subcutaneous emphysema
- Hypotension
- Decreased responsiveness
- Decreased urine output

Nursing diagnoses that pertain to the trauma patient can be clustered in the same manner as the assessment data. Clustering around the ABCs of airway, breathing, and circulation will assist the nurse in prioritizing nursing care.

- *Ineffective airway clearance* related to obstruction or cognitive impairment
- *Ineffective breathing pattern* related to tracheobronchial or chest wall injury, decreased area for gas exchange or pain
- *Impaired gas exchange* related to ventilation–perfusion imbalance or decreased hemoglobin
- *Decreased cardiac output* related to impairment of venous return or myocardial injury
- *Altered tissue perfusion* related to an imbalance between cellular oxygen demands and supply
- *Fluid volume deficit* related to hemorrhage or extravasation (i.e., burns)

In summary, certain symptoms can clue the nurse to suspect a life-threatening condition in a patient with multiple injuries. Appropriate nursing diagnoses address airway, breathing, and circulation impairment.

SECTION NINE REVIEW

Mary W is admitted into the emergency department following an assault where she was beaten in the face and head. She has a large amount of facial edema, both eyes are swollen shut. She has broken teeth and blood in her mouth. Mary follows commands but does not verbalize a response to questions. Breathing pattern is rapid and noisy. Questions 1 through 3 pertain to Mary.

1. Based on Mary's history, which of the following interventions should be performed first?
   A. open the airway and clear the oral pharynx
   B. the application of 100 percent oxygen by mask
   C. obtain arterial blood gases
   D. insert an intravenous catheter
2. Her arterial blood gases reflect respiratory acidosis. The acidosis is MOST likely related to
   A. ineffective breathing pattern
   B. pain
   C. partially obstructed airway
   D. head injury
3. Mary loses consciousness. The nurse should prepare for which of the following first?
   A. CT scan of the head
   B. endotracheal intubation or surgical airway placement
   C. placement of a second IV line
   D. placement of a nasogastric tube

Answers: 1. A, 2. C, 3. B

SECTION TEN: Trauma Sequelae

At the completion of this section, the learner will be able to link complications posttrauma with the physiology of the traumatic injury and preexisting risk factors.

As discussed in Section Eight, trauma deaths occur in three peaks. The first peak is within the first hour postinjury, and the major causes of death are massive bleeding secondary to great vessel tears and head injuries. The second peak occurs during the initial hours postinjury during the resuscitation phase. Deaths in this phase generally are attributed to internal bleeding. The final peak of trauma-related deaths occurs days to weeks after the injury event. Infection is the major cause of death in the final phase.

The primary responsibility of the nurse caring for a trauma patient in this final phase is in the area of prevention and surveillance. Treatment of trauma sequelae is controversial and primitive, since research in this area is still in its infancy as compared with trauma resuscitation research. Therefore, the goal of nursing care is to prevent that which you may not be able to treat adequately once it is present. Major medical complications in the trauma patient are sepsis/septic shock, **multiple organ dysfunction syndrome (MODS), disseminated intravascular coagulation (DIC),** and acute respiratory distress syndrome (ARDS).

Injury Event

Several types of injuries predispose the trauma patient to complications. Table 34–6 summarizes injuries and their associated sequelae. Thoracic trauma may produce massive hemorrhage in addition to disruption in the lung parenchyma. Thus, the thoracic trauma patient is at high risk for DIC and ARDS. Abdominal trauma increases the likelihood of hemorrhage and infection. Orthopedic trauma predisposes the patient to pulmonary emboli and prolonged immobility, which may compound the effect on gas exchange. Head injuries also may result in prolonged immobility plus local tissue destruction. The physiologic complications of trauma are intimately related. It is common for a patient to have a combination of these disorders. Although the etiologies of these conditions may differ slightly, the result is the same: inadequate oxygen delivery to the tissue. For this reason, it is important to keep in mind when reading Table 34–6 that the patient may be at higher risk for one of these disorders because of the initial injury, but, in reality, any one of and more than one of these conditions may occur.

TABLE 34–6. TRAUMATIC INJURIES AND ASSOCIATED SEQUELAE

CONDITION	PATHOPHYSIOLOGY	COMPLICATION
Thoracic trauma		
Great vessel tears	Hemorrhage	DIC
Hemothorax	Decreased gas exchange	ARDS
Tension pneumothorax	Decreased gas exchange	ARDS
Open pneumothorax	Disruption in skin integrity	Sepsis
Abdominal trauma		
Perforation of intestine	Extravasation of gastrointestinal contents into peritoneum	Sepsis
Liver/splenic laceration	Hemorrhage	DIC
Orthopedic trauma		
Femur/pelvis fracture	Hemorrhage	DIC
Long-bone fractures	Disruption of fat-containing tissue, increased flow of fat globules in microcirculation	ARDS
Open fractures	Disruption in skin integrity	Sepsis

Hypoperfusion

Hypoperfusion is a precursor to all of the complications discussed in this section. In sepsis and MODS, the hypoperfusion may be distributional and secondary to vasodilation and not actual loss of volume. In DIC, hypoperfusion occurs because of diffuse hemorrhage and destruction of red blood cells as they become trapped in fibrin strands. Increased aleveolar capillary permeability as well as overzealous fluid resuscitation predispose the patient to ARDS. The treatment of hypovolemic shock previously has focused on improving systems (i.e., preload and contractility). The nurse should view hypovolemia from a cellular perspective to appreciate the cellular changes that predispose the trauma patient to complications.

Poor cellular perfusion results in a shift to anaerobic metabolism. Anaerobic metabolism is an inefficient system, since two adenosine triphosphate (ATP) molecules are created for energy use, per molecule of glucose used, as compared to 38 ATP with aerobic metabolism. Anaerobic metabolism increases the production of acids as waste products. This increased acid (such as lactic acid) produces a chemical insult that triggers the inflammatory/immune response, which activates other systems (refer to Module 11 for more information). The humoral immunity system is activated to produce vasodilation and to increase capillary permeability. Initially, this is a local response to enhance tissue repair. Cellular immunity is activated to eliminate wastes from the dying hypoxic cells. The cellular immunity system includes polymorphonuclear granulocytes, monocytes, and lymphocytes. Other biochemical substances are activated. These substances include but are not limited to oxygen free radicals, tumor necrosis factor, and interleukins. The purpose of these substances is to facilitate the humoral and cellular immunity systems and to serve as transporters and mediators in cellular reactions. Overall, their net response is vasodilation.

Inflammatory/Immune Response

The functions of a local inflammatory/immune response are:

- Improvement of oxygen supply and decrease of oxygen demand at the cellular level
- Redistribution of circulatory blood volume to injured area
- Correction of metabolic alterations
- Killing of microorganisms

The inflammatory/immune response is intended to be protective for the patient. If the local response becomes systemic (through what is yet an unknown process), the process is no longer compensatory but becomes pathologic. Tissue destruction continues because of massive vasodilation. Hypoperfusion produces cellular death. (If enough cells die, organs die [MODS], and the patient dies.)

The trauma patient must be assessed for risk factors associated with a malfunction of the compensatory inflammation/immune response. Table 34–7 summarizes the risk factors and the rationale for their association with complications posttrauma. The nurse should suspect the presence of complications in the older, malnourished patient with a history of chronic illness as well as the younger, healthy patient who has sustained massive injuries and has had a delay in initial treatment.

Sepsis

Sepsis is the presence of microorganisms in the blood. **Septic shock** is the physiologic response to microorganisms in the blood that results in hemodynamic instability.

TABLE 34–7. RISK FACTORS ASSOCIATED WITH COMPLICATIONS POSTTRAUMA

RISK FACTOR	RATIONALE
Elderly	Decreased production of lymphocytes may increase susceptibility to infection Decreased microcirculation may impair cellular oxygen delivery
Malnutrition (obesity, chronic illness, alcoholism)	Decreased available protein to produce immunoglobulins and cells
Systolic blood pressure < 80 mm Hg (massive transfusion greater than 6 L within 6 hours of injury)	Hypovolemia decreases cellular oxygen supply and results in compensatory vasoconstriction that further destroys cells
Large wounds, burns	Destruction of skin as first defense against infection Increased capillary permeability in an attempt to provide nutrients and remove wastes from injured areas
Previous history of organ transplants (immunosuppression therapy) or chronic use of antibiotics	Inability to initiate local inflammatory response allows for microorganism invasion and ultimately systemic infection Decreased sensitivity to medications used for microorganism resistance
Prolonged time between injury and treatment (exact time is unknown but longer than 1 hour has been associated with increased morbidity and mortality)	Delayed volume resuscitation results in additional cellular death Delayed wound debridement results in higher microorganism invasion

A pathogen is identified in the body from cultures. The pathogens may be part of the patient's normal flora or may be present in the external environment. Gram-negative and gram-positive bacteria, viruses, and fungi can produce sepsis. There are several portals of entry for these microorganisms. Table 34–8 summarizes these entry points. Gram-negative bacteria produce endotoxins that cause direct cellular damage in addition to the release of vasoactive proteins (humoral response) that result in vasodilation, increased capillary permeability, and activation of the clotting cascade. Although other microorganisms may not produce endotoxins, other vasoactive substances are released through a yet to be confirmed mechanism. In some situations, the patient exhibits the symptoms of sepsis but the cultures are negative. Most clinicians believe that a microorganism is present but not in a sufficient cluster to produce a positive finding. The patient's white cell count may be elevated because of the total number of microorganisms.

Septic shock (or sepsis) is characterized by two different phases: high output and low output. Both phases are related to a systemic response to microorganisms that produces cellular damage. The high-output phase is the body's initial response to massive vasodilation. The patient's skin is warm and flushed (similar to that seen in neurogenic shock, another condition due to vasodilation from unopposed parasympathetic stimulation). Most patients will be tachypneic, which leads to respiratory alkalosis. Fever is usually present. The systemic vascular re-

TABLE 34–8. COMMON PORTALS OF ENTRY OF MICROORGANISMS

ENTRANCE POINT	PREDISPOSING AGENT
Urinary tract	Urinary catheters Suprapubic tubes Cystoscopic examination
Respiratory tract	Endotracheal tubes Tracheostomy tubes Mechanical ventilation Suctioning Inhalation therapy Aspiration
Gastrointestinal tract	Peritonitis Abdominal abscess Cirrhosis Ascites Peptic ulcers
Skin	Surgical wounds Burns Traumatic injury Intravenous catheters Intra-arterial catheters Invasive monitoring Decubitus ulcers

Adapted from Dolan, J. (1991). Critical care nursing: Clinical management through the nursing process. *Philadelphia: F.A. Davis.*

sistance is low and the CO is high, since afterload is diminished. Hypotension may result from inadequate preload due to decreased venous return. As preload decreases, CO ultimately will decrease, and the patient enters the second phase of septic shock. During this phase, the sympathetic nervous system attempts to enhance compensation. Tachycardia, peripheral vasoconstriction, and decreased urine output occur in an attempt to restore core circulation. The patient will have a low CO reading, a high systemic vascular resistance level, and decreased preload (central venous pressure) if the patient has a pulmonary arterial catheter in place. The signs can be detected in the patient even if pulmonary arterial readings are unavailable. The patient is cold, diaphoretic, oliguric, and nonresponsive to verbal stimuli. Failure to mount a fever or to increase the white cell count are poor prognostic signs. For more information, refer to Module 10.

Acute Respiratory Distress Syndrome

ARDS is characterized by the presence of bilateral pulmonary infiltrates, a pulmonary capillary edge pressure of 18 mm Hg (in the absence of left ventricular dysfunction), and a PaO_2/FIO_2 ratio of ≤ 200, regardless of the amount of positive end-expiratory pressure (PEEP) (Morris, 1996). Increased pulmonary capillary permeability results in pulmonary edema and impaired gas exchange. Pulmonary hypertension stimulates the synthesis of thromboxane. Thromboxane produces regional vasoconstriction in the lungs. Pulmonary shunting occurs in response to ventilation–perfusion mismatches. The trauma patient is vulnerable to ARDS because of volume resuscitation and untreated hypoxia related to direct thoracic injury or indirect thoracic injury, such as that from aspiration.

Multiple Organ Dysfunction Syndrome

A persistent perfusion deficit, inflammation, and infection are related to the occurrence of MODS. The hypermetabolism eventually results in a phenomenon referred to as **autocannibalism.** Skeletal muscle mass is used as a nutritional source (Kimbrell, 1996). Both muscle wasting and an associated peripheral neuropathy with skeletal muscle denervation have been associated with mechanical ventilator dependency (Morris, 1996). For more information, refer to Module 11.

Disseminated Intravascular Coagulation

DIC is an exaggeration of a normal response. Normal clotting is a localized reaction to injury, whereas DIC is a systemic response. The healthy individual maintains a balance between clot formation and lysis. In trauma, both the extrinsic and intrinsic pathways of coagulation may be stimulated. Head injury can precipitate the release of tissue thromboplastin (extrinsic pathway). Hypoxia and acidosis also stimulate the extrinsic pathway. Crush injuries, burns, and sepsis result in blood cell injury as well as platelet aggregation (intrinsic pathway). For more information, refer to Module 11 and Module 23.

Assessment and Nursing Diagnosis

Posttrauma complications are related to hypoperfusion and decreased oxygen delivery to the cells. These conditions may coexist, and one may be the precursor to another. There are numerous physiologic relationships among the conditions. Figure 34–7 illustrates these relationships. The complement cascade is initiated as a normal response to microorganism invasion. Granulocyte aggregation is stimulated, resulting in slowing of microcirculation. Tissue hypoxia and cellular death occur. Thus, activation of the complement cascade also initiates MODS. Gram-negative sepsis can initiate both fibrinolysis and coagulation, linking sepsis with DIC. In MODS and sepsis, alveolar type II pneumocytes are destroyed by endotoxins. Thus, surfactant is diminished and a ventilation-perfusion mismatch occurs, resulting in the development of ARDS. An astute nurse assesses for symptoms that are common to all these conditions and relies on laboratory testing to confirm which disorder is present.

Complications may occur at any time in the postinjury phase. It should be clear from this discussion why baseline laboratory and diagnostic data are so important in the trauma patient. With these data, the nurse is able to monitor for subtle changes that indicate that a complication is occurring. The following assessment data would indicate the presence of a posttrauma complication:

- Elevation of WBC count
- Fever
- Change in characteristics of wound drainage (foul odor, thick, and colored)
- Inability to tolerate movement, nursing procedures (e.g., decreasing SpO_2, PaO_2)
- Decreasing level of responsiveness (related to decreased oxygenation or increased serum ammonia levels)
- Decreased urine output
- Diaphoresis
- Cool, mottled skin
- Presence of bleeding (melena, hemoptysis, hematemesis, petechiae, hematuria)
- Changing trends in vital signs/hemodynamic readings (e.g., elevated CO, decreased SVR)

Nursing diagnoses that pertain to the trauma patient can be clustered mainly into the two broad areas of ventilation and perfusion.

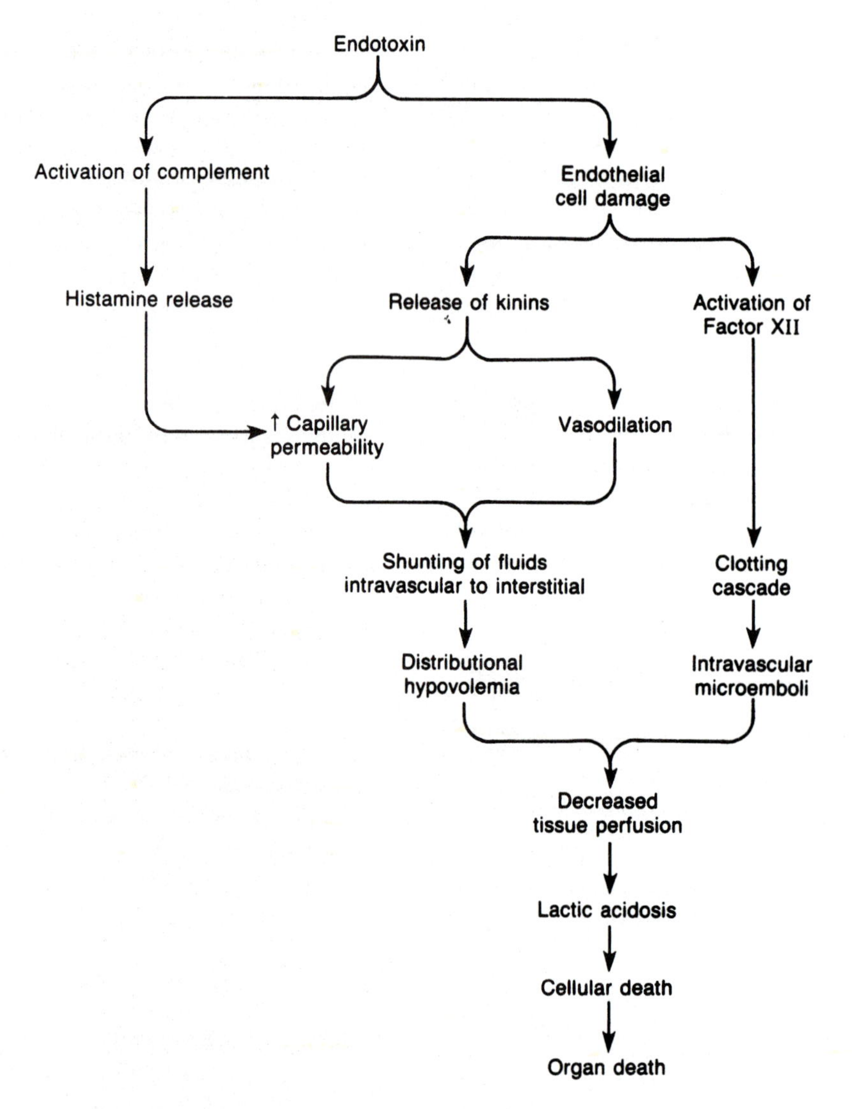

Figure 34–7. Interrelationship between multiple organ dysfunction, acute respiratory distress syndrome, disseminated intravascular coagulation, and sepsis. (*From Dolan, J. [1991].* Critical care nursing: Clinical management through the nursing process. *Philadelphia: F.A. Davis.*)

Ventilation

- *Impaired gas exchange* related to increased capillary permeability and decreased surface area for gas exchange or obstruction in pulmonary capillary perfusion
- *Ineffective breathing patterns* related to decreased skeletal muscle mass and denervation
- *Ineffective airway clearance* related to fatigue and artificial airway placement with mechanical ventilation

Perfusion

- *Fluid volume deficit* related to vasodilation, bleeding, or interstitial fluid shift
- *Decreased tissue perfusion* related to capillary obstruction and vasodilation
- *Increased cardiac output* related to catecholamine excretion and decreased systemic vascular resistance
- *Decreased cardiac output* related to decreased vascular volume

Additional nursing diagnoses would include:

- *Altered urinary elimination patterns* related to obstruction (microemboli and myoglobin) of renal blood flow and tissue necrosis
- *Altered nutrition: Less than body requirements* related to catecholamine release, activation of inflammatory response resulting in a hypermetabolic state, and decreased or absent oral intake
- *Risk of infection* related to open wounds, invasive procedures, surgical incisions, debilitated state, and altered nutrition

Interventions for Posttrauma Complications

Nursing and collaborative interventions for the trauma patient experiencing complications are addressed in Module 11.

In summary, hypoperfusion related to hemorrhage, direct vessel injury, and interstitial fluid shifting initiates the sequence of events for posttrauma complications. The hypoperfusion initiates the inflammatory process. Nursing care centers on supporting ventilation and perfusion.

Although this section has emphasized physical manifestations of posttrauma complications, psychosocial aspects should not be ignored. The reader is referred to Module 11 for additional information. Patients who have complications posttrauma remain in the critical care unit for prolonged periods and are susceptible to sensory disturbances. Quality-of-life issues need to be considered by the patient and the family. Extensive rehabilitation may be necessary to regain skeletal muscle mass and neurologic function. The family's standard of living may decrease because of financial factors related to change in the role of the patient as well as health care costs.

SECTION TEN REVIEW

Sam W was pinned underneath his tractor for 1 hour before being extricated and transported to the hospital for treatment. He has open fractures of both legs and abdominal tenderness. Questions 1 through 3 pertain to Sam.

1. What risk is associated with this delay in treatment?
   - A. he will not be able to produce the same number of immunoglobulins
   - B. he will have a higher microorganism count due to delay in wound debridement
   - C. he is at higher risk for antibiotic resistance
   - D. he will be unable to mount a local inflammatory response
2. Because of his crush injury, DIC may occur due to
   - A. activation of the intrinsic pathway via platelet aggregation
   - B. activation of the extrinsic pathway via thromboplastic release
   - C. a high microorganism count
   - D. long-bone injury
3. All of the following nursing diagnoses would be appropriate for Sam EXCEPT
   - A. *Risk for infection*
   - B. *Decreased peripheral tissue perfusion*
   - C. *Risk for fluid volume deficit*
   - D. *Risk for trauma*
4. Which of the following statements best describes the relationship between ARDS and MODS?
   - A. decreased ventilation leads to decreased tissue oxygenation and cellular death
   - B. pulmonary edema produces a fluid volume deficit and hypoperfusion of tissues
   - C. organ death releases endotoxins that kill pulmonary epithelial cells
   - D. increased carbon dioxide retention stimulates peripheral vasodilation and hypoperfusion of tissue

Answers: 1. B, 2. A, 3. D, 4. A

POSTTEST

1. Typically, a trauma patient has which demographic profile?
   - A. 15 to 24 years, male, using alcohol, lower income level
   - B. 24 to 32 years, male, using alcohol, upper income level
   - C. 15 to 24 years, female, using alcohol, lower income level
   - D. 15 to 24 years, male, no alcohol involvement, lower income level
2. What are the four forces that must be considered in assessment of injury?
   - A. acceleration, mass, axial loading, deceleration
   - B. shearing, compression, impact, axial loading
   - C. acceleration, deceleration, shearing, synergistic
   - D. acceleration, deceleration, shearing, compression
3. The coup and contrecoup injury is an example of application of _____ and _____ forces, respectively.
   - A. shear, tensile
   - B. tensile, shear
   - C. compression, axial loading
   - D. acceleration tensile
4. As penetration of tissue occurs with penetrating trauma, tissues are temporarily displaced forward and laterally, creating a temporary cavity. This process is called
   - A. tumbling
   - B. yaw
   - C. blast effect
   - D. cavitation

5. The extent of cavitation and tissue deformation is most determined by
   A. yaw
   B. velocity
   C. blast effect
   D. tissue density
6. The higher the velocity of the missile, the greater the propensity for
   A. yaw
   B. tumble
   C. cavitation
   D. all of the above
7. A patient is admitted to your unit with a stab injury to the right sternal border, fifth intercostal space. Injury must be considered to the abdomen as well as to the thorax because
   A. the left diaphragm can rise as high as the fourth intercostal space during maximum expiration
   B. the right diaphragm can rise as high as the fourth intercostal space during maximum expiration
   C. the diaphragm recedes to the eighth intercostal space during maximum inspiration at the midclavicular line
   D. the diaphragm recedes to the sixth intercostal space during maximum inspiration at the midaxillary line
8. Which of the following best describes the injury pattern associated with a pedestrian (child) hit by an automobile?
   A. fractured femur, tibia, fibula on side of impact
   B. compression fractures of lumbosacral spine
   C. high cervical fractures and head injuries
   D. fracture of femur, chest injury, and injury to contralateral skull as child is thrown on impact
9. An injury pattern unique to the restrained passenger with lap belt only is
   A. pulmonary contusion
   B. cervical fractures
   C. flexion/distraction fractures of lumber vertebrae
   D. femur fractures
10. Trauma victims who have ingested cocaine before arrival may exhibit a sympathomimetic presentation. Clinical signs may include
    A. tachycardia, dilated pupils, tremors, elevated blood pressure
    B. tachycardia, constricted pupils, tremors, elevated blood pressure
    C. bradycardia, hypotension
    D. dilated pupils, hypotension, bradycardia
11. With pediatric trauma victims, multisystem injury is the rule rather than the exception. This is due to
    A. size and shape of the child
    B. skeleton of the child
    C. surface area of the child
    D. all of the above
12. Hypothermia is critically important in trauma patients less than 6 months of age because
    A. they lack subcutaneous fat and involuntary shivering mechanism
    B. they poorly metabolize brown fat to conserve heat
    C. their body surface area facilitates heat conservation
    D. involuntary shivering is the only available mechanism for heat conservation
13. The metabolic derangement typically seen in the pregnant trauma patient is
    A. respiratory alkalosis
    B. respiratory acidosis
    C. metabolic alkalosis
    D. metabolic acidosis
14. The IMMEDIATE nursing intervention for a pregnant woman in her third trimester who is hypotensive after an MVC is
    A. vasopressors
    B. colloid transfusion
    C. turning the patient to the left lateral decubitus position, maintaining immobilization or leftward uterine displacement manually
    D. Trendelenburg position
15. The first three components of the primary assessment are
    A. airway, circulation, cervical spine control
    B. airway, breathing, circulation
    C. circulation, cervical spine control, breathing
    D. breathing, disability, circulation
16. Airway considerations in the pediatric trauma victim include all of the following EXCEPT
    A. the child's tongue is proportionately larger and housed in a smaller oral cavity
    B. the glottic opening is more anterior and cephalad
    C. the trachea is short and narrow
    D. it is easier to intubate the left mainstem bronchus rather than the right
17. Nasotracheal intubation should be avoided in any patient where a cribriform plate fracture is suspected because
    A. the technique is extraordinarily difficult
    B. the cranial vault becomes vulnerable, and the tube could be passed into the brain tissue
    C. vocal cord visualization is difficult
    D. cervical spine injury is unlikely
18. All of the following may indicate injury to the larynx EXCEPT
    A. tenderness
    B. hoarseness
    C. subcutaneous emphysema
    D. preference for the supine position

19. The purpose of the secondary assessment is to
    A. identify and intervene with life-threatening injuries
    B. identify the existence of all injuries
    C. facilitate treatment of airway and breathing
    D. assess response to resuscitative interventions
20. Any injured patient in a shock state should be evaluated for the most common etiology of traumatic shock, which is
    A. hypovolemic
    B. cardiogenic
    C. neurogenic
    D. sepsis
21. Which of the following suggests the presence of a life-threatening injury?
    A. hypotension
    B. crepitus of the lower extremity
    C. rapid respiratory rate
    D. open shoulder wound
22. Which of the following interventions during the trauma resuscitation phase would increase the risk of the patient developing ARDS as a complication of trauma?
    A. administration of 6 L/min of oxygen via nonrebreather mask
    B. prolonged supine positioning of the patient on a backboard
    C. administration of IV lactated Ringer's solution at 500 mL/hr
    D. performance of endotracheal suctioning

POSTTEST ANSWERS

Question	Answer	Section	Question	Answer	Section
1	A	One	12	A	Five
2	D	Two	13	A	Five
3	A	Two	14	C	Five
4	D	Three	15	B	Six
5	B	Three	16	D	Six
6	D	Three	17	B	Six
7	B	Three	18	D	Six
8	D	Four	19	B	Seven
9	C	Four	20	A	Eight
10	A	Five	21	A	Nine
11	D	Five	22	C	Ten

REFERENCES

American College of Surgeons Committee on Trauma. (1997a). Biomechanics of injury. In *Advanced trauma life support course manual* (pp. 345–366). Chicago: American College of Surgeons.

American College of Surgeons Committee on Trauma. (1997b). Shock. In *Advanced trauma life support course manual* (pp. 87–107). Chicago: American College of Surgeons.

American College of Surgeons Committee on Trauma. (1997c). Trauma in pregnancy. In *Advanced trauma life support course manual* (pp. 313–323). Chicago: American College of Surgeons.

American College of Surgeons Committee on Trauma. (1997d). Airway and ventilatory management. In *Advanced trauma life support course manual* (pp. 59–72). Chicago: American College of Surgeons.

American College of Surgeons Committee on Trauma. (1997e). Pediatric trauma. In *Advanced trauma life support course manual* (pp. 289–311). Chicago: American College of Surgeons.

American College of Surgeons Committee on Trauma. (1997f). Initial assessment and management. In *Advanced trauma life support course manual* (pp. 21–58). Chicago: American College of Surgeons.

American College of Surgeons Committee on Trauma. (1997g). Course overview. In *Advanced trauma life support course manual* (pp. 9–19). Chicago: American College of Surgeons.

American College of Surgeons Committee on Trauma. (1997h). Spine and spinal cord trauma. In *Advanced trauma life support course manual* (pp. 215–230). Chicago: American College of Surgeons.

Asensio, J.A. (1990). Exsanguination from penetrating injuries. In R.F. Buckman & L.N. Manro (eds.), *Trauma quarterly—Difficult problems in urban trauma, Part II* (pp. 1–25). Rockville, MD: Aspen.

DeMaria, E.J. (1993). Evaluation and treatment of the elderly trauma victim. *Clin Geriatr Med* 9(2):461–471.

Eichelberger, M.R. (1991). Pediatric trauma. In D.D. Trunkey & F.R. Lewis (eds.), *Current therapy of trauma* (3rd ed.) (pp. 21–39). St. Louis: C.V. Mosby.

Haley, K. (1998). Multiple trauma management. In T.E. Soud & J.S. Rogers (eds.), *Manual of pediatric emergency nursing* (pp. 487–510). St. Louis: Mosby.

Kimbrell, J. D. (1996). Alterations in metabolism. In V.H. Secor (ed.), *Multiple organ dysfunction and failure* (pp. 148–163). St. Louis: C.V. Mosby.

Manley, L.K. (1993). Trauma in pregnancy. In J.A. Neff & P.S. Kidd (eds.), *Trauma nursing* (pp. 499–525). St. Louis: C.V. Mosby.

McCabe, P.E., & Hassan, E. (1988). The trauma patient with a history of substance abuse. In V.A. Cardona, P.D. Hurn, P.J. Mason, A.M. Scanlon-Schlipp, & S.W. Veise-Berry (eds.), *Trauma nursing from resuscitation through rehabilitation* (pp. 759–784). Philadelphia: W.B. Saunders.

Morris, M.T. (1996). Adult respiratory distress syndrome. In V.H Secor (ed.), *Multiple organ dysfunction and failure* (pp. 167–195). St. Louis: C.V. Mosby.

Rea, R.E. (ed.). (1995). Epidemiology and mechanism of injury. In R.E. Rea (ed.), *Trauma nursing core course association manual* (3rd ed.) (pp. 43–71). Chicago: Emergency Nurses Association.

Rogers, J.S. (1998). Unique characteristics of children. In T.E. Soud & J.S. Rogers (eds.), *Manual of pediatric emergency nursing* (pp. 443–469). St. Louis: C.V. Mosby.

Schriger, D., & Baraff, L. (1988). Defining normal capillary refill: Variation with age, sex, and temperature. *Ann Emerg Med 17*:932–935.

Stamatos, C. (1994). Geriatric trauma patients: Initial assessment and management of shock. *J Trauma Nurs 1*:45–54.

Stubbs, H., Knudson, M.M., Lieberman, J., Morris, J.A., & Cushing, B.M. (1994). Mortality factors in geriatric blunt trauma patients. *Arch Surg 129*(4):448–453.

Thelan, L., Davie, J., & Urden, L. (1990). *Textbook of critical care nursing*. St. Louis: C.V. Mosby.

Vary, T.C., & Linberg, S.E. (1988). Pathophysiology of traumatic shock. In V.A. Cardona, P.D. Hurn, P.J. Mason, A.M. Scanlon-Schilpp, & S.W. Veise-Berry (eds.), *Trauma nursing from resuscitation through rehabilitation* (pp. 127–159). Philadelphia: W.B. Saunders.

Waller, J.A. (1985). *Injury control: A guide to the causes and prevention of trauma*. Lexington, MA: D.C. Heath.

Module 35

Nursing Care of the Patient with Multiple Injuries

Pamela Stinson Kidd

This module is designed to integrate the major points discussed in Modules 32 through 34. Principles from Part III (Cellular Oxygenation) will also be applied. This module summarizes relationships between key concepts and assists the learner in clustering information to facilitate clinical application. The module is divided into parts. Content is applied in an interactive learning style. The learner is encouraged to identify nursing actions based on an assessment of a patient in a case study format. Consequences of selecting a particular action are discussed, and the rationale for correct actions is presented. The first part of the module addresses assessment of the trauma patient and interpretation of laboratory data. Development of nursing diagnoses and supporting data follows next. The last part focuses on nursing management of a patient experiencing sequelae associated with tramatic injury. The module ends with a summary of nursing priorities in caring for a patient with traumatic injuries.

Objectives

Following completion of this module, the learner will be able to

1. Identify relationships among traumatic injury patterns, trauma assessment and resuscitation issues, and complications associated with immobility and traumatic wounds.
2. Cluster assessment data to formulate nursing diagnoses associated with traumatic injury.
3. Appraise a traumatically injured patient's status based on a nursing assessment.
4. Identify priorities in nursing care for a patient with traumatic injuries.
5. Explain the relationship between trauma resuscitation and complications following traumatic injury.
6. Explain rationale for nursing actions that prevent complications associated with traumatic injuries.

Glossary

Acute respiratory distress syndrome (ARDS). Noncardiogenic pulmonary edema precipitated by increased pulmonary alveolar-capillary membrane permeability; fluid shifts from intravascular space into pulmonary interstitium; lung compliance is decreased related to destruction of alveolar epithelial cells (types I and II) that produce surfactant

Ectopy. Extra heart beat initiated by a focus other than the sinoatrial node

Multiple organ dysfunction syndrome (MODS). Syndrome precipitated by hypoperfusion, usually occurs in a sequential format; lungs, liver, renal and cardiovascular system fail, respectively; may be associated with sepsis

ABBREVIATIONS

ARDS. Acute respiratory distress syndrome

CO. Cardiac output

CPP. Cerebral perfusion pressure

CSF. Cerebrospinal fluid

CT. Computed tomography

CVP. Central venous pressure

FIO_2. Fraction of inspired oxygen

ETOH level. Ethanol level

GCS. Glasgow Coma Scale

ICP. Intracranial pressure

MAP. Mean arterial pressure

MODS. Multiple organ dysfunction syndrome

MRI. Magnetic resonance imaging

MVC. Motor vehicle crash

NG. Nasogastric

$PaCO_2$. Partial pressure of carbon dioxide

PaO_2. Partial pressure of oxygen

PEEP. Positive end-expiratory pressure

SpO_2. Oxygen saturation (via pulse oximetry)

TPN. Total parenteral nutrition

CASE STUDY

PAM K, A PATIENT WITH DECREASED LEVEL OF CONSCIOUSNESS

You are the nurse assigned to admit Pam K from the postanesthesia recovery unit. Pam was transported to the emergency department by the aeromedical service. You have been informed by the postanesthesia nurse that Pam K was involved in a motor vehicle crash (MVC). She was an unrestrained driver and was ejected from the vehicle. She was diagnosed with a subdural hematoma by CT scan of the head. She was taken to the operating suite, where the hematoma was drained and an intraventricular catheter was placed. Pam's intraventricular sensor was placed at the end of the craniotomy procedure. She is being mechanically ventilated. Pam is unable to ask questions about procedures, but she can feel and hear. She was awake and obeyed commands. The nurse must explain what to expect during procedures to patients receiving neuromuscular blocking agents. Because of the injury and the potential use of a neuromuscular blocking agent, it may be impossible to determine exactly what the patient can process cognitively. Pam is 25 years old. Her medical history is positive for seizures. She takes Dilantin 100 mg bid. She is being admitted with a diagnosis of closed head injury.

QUESTION

Because Pam was an unrestrained driver who was ejected from the vehicle, she is at risk for what injury?

A. compression fracture of the lumbar sacral spine
B. cavitation injuries
C. cervical spine injuries
D. small bowel contusion

ANSWER

The correct answer is C. Injury risk increases 300 percent when ejection occurs. Cervical spine injuries are frequently associated with head injuries. Lumbar–sacral fractures are most frequently associated with falls. Cavitation injuries occur from penetrating trauma from missiles. Small bowel contusions are associated with restrained drivers.

QUESTION

Because of Pam's past medical history for seizures, what additional information do you need?

ANSWER

You want to know when her last seizure was. Was she taking her medication as scheduled? It is possible that a seizure caused the MVC. You should check her admission lab work to see if a Dilantin level was obtained. Because of her head injury and her seizure susceptibility, you must monitor her closely to prevent further injury since she may seize. It would be prudent to check her admission orders to see if anticonvulsant medication was ordered.

The Initial Appraisal

On entering Pam's intensive care unit (ICU) room, you notice that she is overweight. A bulky gauze dressing is wrapped around her head. There is blood on the dressing over her forehead region.

You note that Pam is intubated and on a mechanical ventilator. In report, you were told that Pam was initially an 8T on the Glasgow Coma Scale (GCS) before going to the operating suite. She tried to push the emergency department nurse's hand away when she was starting an intravenous (IV) line. She opened her eyes to her name. Her neurologic status later deteriorated. She has a peripheral IV line of 0.45 percent normal saline running in her right hand. She has an intraventricular intracranial pressure (ICP) monitoring device. A nasogastric (NG) tube is in place. All extremities are in soft restraints. She has numerous abrasions over her body, and there is no active external bleeding. There are no signs of acute distress at present.

Question

The best reason for Pam's receiving an NG tube in the emergency department is that

A. stress ulcers are common in head-injured patients
B. Pam may be neuromuscularly paralyzed and, if so, cannot eat
C. spontaneous emesis is common in the head-injured patient
D. it facilitates endotracheal intubation

Answer

The correct answer is C. Spontaneous emesis is common in the head-injured patient, particularly in the first 30 to 60 minutes postinjury. If Pam vomits and aspirates, she may develop aspiration pneumonia and ultimately **acute respiratory distress syndrome (ARDS).** Both of these conditions decrease oxygen diffusion and ultimately decrease cerebral oxygenation.

Focused Trauma Assessment

You complete a head-to-toe assessment, keeping in mind your initial appraisal and the report you obtained from the postanesthesia nurse.

Head and Neck. Her neck veins are full but not distended. She has a bulky head dressing in place. The chart states that she had a 3-cm laceration of her right forehead that was sutured in the operating suite. Pam does not open her eyes, but she is tugging at her restraints. She has a 7T GCS score at present. She has an intraventricular catheter in place. No drainage is noted in the drainage bag. ICP is 15 mm Hg. C waves are present. Her number 7.5 endotracheal (ET) tube is anchored firmly and connected to the ventilator. Her NG tube is anchored and connected to low wall suction.

Chest. Because Pam was ejected from the vehicle, you know that her mechanism of injury was severe enough to produce chest and abdominal injuries. Since Pam is on the ventilator, her airway and breathing are being controlled. Breath sounds are auscultated bilaterally, indicating that the ET tube is positioned correctly. No open chest wound or subcutaneous emphysema is noted. Ventilator settings are mode, assist/control; rate, 20; tidal volume, 750 mL; FIO_2, 40 percent. Her chest expansion is equal bilaterally. She is in normal sinus rhythm. At present, Pam's blood pressure is being monitored by an external cuff device. It is 100/70 mm Hg. Her pulse is 96, temperature 99.0°F rectally.

Abdomen. Her abdomen is soft, without bowel sounds. There is no response when her abdomen is palpated.

Pelvis. Pam has a urinary catheter in place with a urine meter collection device. Her hourly urine output is 65 mL.

Extremities. There are no signs of external bleeding. She has a 7-cm-long, 2-cm-wide, deep-thickness laceration of her right thigh that was irrigated, sutured, and covered with a dry sterile dressing. No blood is noted on the dressing. In report, you were told that the wound was grossly contaminated with pavement debris and dirt. Her circulation is being supported by one peripheral IV line. A solution of 0.45 percent normal saline is infusing at 50 mL/hr through a 14-gauge IV catheter in her right antecubital space. The site is patent.

Posterior. Posterior breath sounds are auscultated per ventilator cycle. No abrasions or expanding flank mass is noted.

You review her emergency department chart to identify historical data and diagnostic tests that were performed and their findings. These data will help you in planning her nursing care in the intensive care unit. You note that Pam vomited at the scene per ground emergency medical services report before the arrival of the medical team.

The following laboratory studies were performed in the emergency department:

- Arterial blood gas (ABG)
- Complete blood count (CBC) with differential
- Serum electrolyte profile with glucose
- Type and screen
- Serum ethanol level
- Serum osmolality
- Lactic acid level
- Prothrombin and partial thromboplastin times (PT/PTT)
- Dilantin level

The following radiographic studies were performed:

- Cervical spine films
- AP and lateral chest films
- Computed tomographic (CT) scan of the head and abdomen

QUICK REVIEW

What is the rationale for ordering these tests in a trauma patient?

ABG (normal values: pH, 7.35 to 7.45; PCO_2, 35 to 45; PO_2, 75 to 100; HCO_3, 24 to 28; base excess, −2 to +2). In hypovolemic shock, metabolic acidosis results (for assistance in interpreting arterial blood gases, refer to Module 6). In Pam's case, baseline ABGs provide ventilatory data to use in determining ventilator settings. Her last set of gases were pH, 7.45; PCO_2, 35; PO_2, 96; HCO_3, 25; SpO_2, saturation 100 percent.

CBC (normal values—female: Hgb, 12 to 16 g/dL; Hct, 36 to 46 percent; WBC, 5,000 to 10,000 mL; platelets, 150,000 to 400,000 mL). The CBC provides baseline measurement of fluid loss. The hemoglobin will decrease after hemorrhage. The hematocrit will increase, indicating hemoconcentration. The WBC count may be slightly elevated due to tissue damage. A decreased platelet count will prolong clotting. Pam's hemoglobin is 11 g/dL. Her hematocrit is 47 percent. Her WBC count is 9,000, and her platelets are 300,000. These values may be indicative of hypovolemia, or they may be related to a chronic anemia.

Serum electrolyte panel (normal values: K, 3.5 to 5.3 mEq/L; Na, 135 to 145 mEq/L; Ca, 9 to 11 mg/dL; Cl, 95 to 105 mEq/L; glucose, 80 to 120 mg/dL). Potassium levels may increase in the trauma patient due to tissue injury and hypoxia. Hyponatremia may be present if a large amount of cellular damage has occurred because sodium moves into the cell as potassium moves out. Calcium may accumulate at the injury site, producing hypocalcemia. Chloride will usually decrease, since it combines with sodium. Hyperglycemia (blood sugar is usually > 120 and < 200 mg/dL) is associated with traumatic injury due to the release of corticosteroids and catecholamines. All of Pam's electrolyte values are within normal limits.

Type and screen. This is used to determine blood compatibility in case blood volume replacement is needed. Pam is typed as O+.

Serum ethanol level. Alcohol can produce vasodilation and hypotension. A change in responsiveness may be associated with ethanol use. Pam's ethanol (ETOH) level is 100 mg/dL, indicating positive use. This level is considered a legally intoxicated level in most states. It is not high enough to produce massive vasodilation.

Serum osmolality (normal value: 280 to 300 mOsm/kg H_2O). This is an indication of body fluid concentration. If fluid loss has occurred, serum osmolality is increased. Pam's serum osmolality level is 300 mOsm/kg H_2O. She may have lost some volume.

Lactic acid (normal value: 8.1 to 15.3 mg/dL). Lactic acid accumulation is directly related to cellular hypoxia and may increase before hypotension and decreased urine output occurs (Kee, 1995). An elevated lactic acid level indicates acidosis. Pam's lactic acid level is normal.

PT/PTT (normal values: PT, 11 to 15 seconds; PTT, 60 to 70 seconds). These are ordered to provide baseline data on the patient's ability to clot in case hemorrhaging occurs. Pam's clotting times are normal.

Dilantin level (normal value: 10 to 20 mg/mL). Pam's Dilantin level was 18 mg/mL. It is within normal limits, suggesting Pam has been compliant with her medication. This decreases the likelihood that a seizure precipitated the MVC.

Cervical spine films. Spinal cord injuries are accompanied by head injuries in 19 percent of cases (Swain, Grundy, & Russell, 1985). To rule out a cervical spine fracture, all seven cervical and T1 vertebrae must be visualized on the film. Head and spinal cord injuries are more likely to be present when the patient has been ejected from a vehicle, as in Pam's case. Pam's spinal films were negative.

AP and lateral chest films, abdominal CT scan. Head trauma rarely occurs alone. Thoracic and abdominal injuries frequently are associated with head injuries. Pam's films are negative. This is important, since there was a report of emesis at the scene. However, an aspiration pneumonia will not be readily apparent on chest x-ray initially.

Head CT scan. This is the procedure of choice in the initial assessment of the head-injured patient. Noncontrast scanning is used most frequently for the head unless a tumor is suspected. MRI is not feasible for the initial assessment of the trauma patient because of the metal associated with stabilization equipment and the length of time required for the procedure. Pam's head CT scan revealed a small, acute subdural hematoma without mass effect. Her injury was classified as moderate, since she does not respond spontaneously and she does not obey motor commands. The neurosurgeon decided to operate and relieve the hematoma.

Development of Nursing Diagnoses

Clustering Data

You have just completed your head-to-toe assessment and are ready to list the appropriate nursing diagnoses for Pam. To cluster the data, look for abnormals found during the assessment. Pam's major symptom at this time is her decreased responsiveness. This symptom can initiate the cluster of critical cues.

Cluster 1. *Subjective data.* Involved in MVC as unrestrained driver ejected from the car.

Objective data. GCS score on arrival 8T, 7T at present. ICP monitoring device in place. Craniotomy for draining of subdural hematoma. Present ICP measurement is 15 mm Hg. C waves present. Normal Dilantin level.

Pam's decreased responsiveness is related to numerous factors. The primary injury to her head as well as the secondary cerebral edema contribute to her decreased responsiveness. The anesthesia used during the craniotomy procedure and the alcohol she drank before the MVC are also contributing factors. Hypovolemia, hypoglycemia, or hypoxia does not appear to be a factor at this time based on laboratory analysis.

Cluster 2. *Subjective data.* Report that Pam vomited at the scene.

Objective data. Chest film clear. ABGs suggest borderline respiratory alkalosis. No adventitious breath sounds noted. Several invasive tubes present: IV line, intraventricular catheter, ET tube, NG tube, and urinary catheter. Repair of two contaminated lacerations. Surgical incision from craniotomy. WBC, 9,000.

Cluster 3. *Subjective data.* Unrestrained, ejected driver in MVC.

Objective data. Hgb, 11 g/dL. Hct, 47 percent. Serum osmolality, 300 mOsm/kg H_2O. Blood pressure, 100/70 mm Hg. Pulse, 96 normal sinus rhythm (NSR). No active bleeding noted. Abdomen soft and appears nontender.

It is important to look at the pattern of laboratory data instead of isolated findings. At first glance, it may appear that Pam is losing volume because of her low hemoglobin and high hematocrit. An adult head trauma patient cannot be hypotensive due to blood loss from a closed head injury (ACSCoT, 1997). Thus, other sources of bleeding should be suspected. Since her abdominal CT scan and chest films were normal, internal bleeding has initially been ruled out. External sources of bleeding, such as lacerations, may be the culprit. In Pam's case, she has a 3-cm laceration of the forehead. The bleeding was controlled by application of a pressure dressing in the field. She also has a 7-cm long, 2-cm wide, and 2-cm deep laceration to the right thigh that was bleeding. This laceration may have produced the decreased hemoglobin, although it is not likely. Changes in hemoglobin and hematocrit related to active bleeding usually require hours to manifest postinjury. Her serum osmolality is borderline high and could be related to hydration status before injury. Since Pam's other laboratory values are within normal limits, she is probably not hypovolemic. Her decreased hemoglobin may be related to a chronic condition, such as menstruation. However, if Pam had been hypovolemic, which method of fluid resuscitation would have been preferred?

Question

Hypovolemia associated with a closed head injury is treated by

- **A.** volume replacement with lactated Ringer's solution
- **B.** combination therapy with lactated Ringer's solution and mannitol
- **C.** use of whole blood
- **D.** autotransfusion

Answer

The correct answer is A. The priorities of care of the closed head-injured patient is restoration of circulating blood volume in hopes of maintaining cerebral perfusion (Bullock et al., 1999). Mannitol is administered to euvolemic patients in combination with fluid resuscitation. Small doses of mannitol (0.25 to 1 g/kg) decrease ICP rapidly, is shorter acting, and has less effect on electrolyte management (Vos, 1994). Since cerebral perfusion pressure (CPP) is dependent on the mean arterial pressure (MAP) as well as ICP, hypovolemia must be corrected. Fluid should be administered if the systolic blood pressure is less than 90 mm Hg. Two large-bore IV lines should be initiated, and 2 L of lactated Ringer's solution should be given. If Pam's hemoglobin or hematocrit demonstrated a deficit of 20 percent, O+ (Pam's blood type) packed cells would be given. In these cases, a pulmonary arterial catheter should be placed. The placement of a pulmonary arterial catheter provides data that can be used to determine the minimal amount of fluid that needs to be administered to maintain the MAP and thus CPP. (Calculation of CPP is discussed in Module 17.)

Based on the obtained data, the following nursing diagnoses are appropriate for Pam:

- *Altered tissue perfusion: Cerebrovascular* related to cerebral edema
- *Risk for fluid volume deficit* related to undetected concomitant injuries
- *Risk for infection* related to intraventricular catheter, lacerations, aspiration, and placement of invasive tubes

Desired patient outcomes (DPOs) for Pam would include:

1. ICP returns to 10 mm Hg
2. PaO_2 remains > 80 torr
3. PCO_2 remains between 30 and 35 mm Hg
4. Maintain CPP at a level > 70 mm Hg
5. GCS improves to 11T
6. No drainage is noted in CSF drainage bag while catheter is patent
7. Absence of A and B ICP waves

8. Urine output remains > 30 mL/hr
9. Negative cultures (wound, blood, sputum, urine)
10. Temperature < 100°F rectally
11. WBC < 10,000 mL

Based on Pam's available data, additional nursing diagnoses pertain to her case even if they are not a priority at this time.

- *Body image disturbance* related to shaving of head, forehead, and thigh laceration
- *Risk for disturbance in role performance* related to hospitalization and neurologic deficit
- *Pain* related to surgical incision and ejection from vehicle

Development of the Plan of Care

Nursing interventions will be based on activities that will help Pam meet her DPOs. They will consist of collaborative interventions that are both multidisciplinary and interdisciplinary. Independent interventions are activities that are within the scope of nursing practice and do not require a physician's order.

Collaborative Interventions Related to Decreased Level of Consciousness

1. *Diuretic therapy*. A mannitol IV bolus of 0.25 g/kg is ordered PRN for ICP greater than 20 mm Hg. A one-time dose of furosemide (Lasix) 60 mg intravenous push (IVP) is also ordered for ICP > 20 mm Hg.

QUESTION

Mannitol is a hyperosmolar agent. It is used in a head-injured patient to

A. promote renal perfusion
B. enhance renal excretion of drugs
C. correct acid–base imbalances
D. promote cerebral tissue fluid movement

ANSWER

The correct answer is D. Mannitol can lower ICP and increase cerebral blood flow. The effectiveness of mannitol has long been debated in the literature. Mannitol may remove water from normal brain tissue rather than the injured tissue. The net effect is decreased ICP, but the long-term effects of dehydration of normal brain tissue are unknown. The drug is most effective when administered by bolus than by continuous IV drip. This drug further decreases ICP by reducing total body volume and inhibiting cerebrospinal fluid (CSF) production. Furosemide (Lasix) may be administered in conjunction with mannitol (as in Pam's case).

2. *Neuromuscular blocking agent*. An order for vecuronium 0.1 mg/kg IVP initially, followed by 0.015 mg/kg 40 minutes later and PRN was written.

QUESTION

Vecuronium is ordered for a head-injured patient because it

A. stimulates smooth muscle contractions
B. prevents muscular depolarization
C. promotes spinal cord impulse transmission
D. prevents apnea

ANSWER

The correct answer is B. Vecuronium (Norcuron) is a neuromuscular blocking agent. This agent prevents acetylcholine from binding with nicotinic receptors, and muscular contraction is blocked. It produces paralysis of skeletal muscles, including those necessary for ventilation. The patient is able to see, feel, and hear but is unable to move or speak. Pam will still require sedation and pain relief. Ideally, the patient is sedated and receives pain medication before administration of the neuromuscular blocking agent. Since she is endotracheally intubated, her airway is secured. Once the neuromuscular blocking agent is administered, the patient is unable to ventilate without external support. The major adverse reaction of these agents is prolonged paralysis after the medication has ceased to be administered. Electrolyte abnormalities and fever increase the likelihood of prolonged paralysis (Shlafer & Marieb, 1989). Thus, the nurse must monitor vital signs and laboratory values closely. Vecuronium will keep Pam from fighting the ventilator and treatment and helps to ensure that she will receive adequate cerebral oxygenation. Pam will require another CT scan to monitor the size of the subdural hematoma, motion artifact will be eliminated, and the obtained films may be clearer and easier to interpret.

3. *Anticonvulsant therapy*. A loading dose of 10 mg/kg of IV phenytoin is usually given prophylactically for seizures. Since Pam's Dilantin level is therapeutic, she will receive Dilantin 100 mg IV every 8 hours.

QUESTION

A nursing implication associated with phenytoin administration is

A. administer phenytoin in D_5W
B. phenytoin is poorly soluble

C. phenytoin metabolizes quickly and should be administered over 2 minutes
D. phenytoin produces hypertension

Answer

The correct answer is B. Phenytoin should not be mixed with other drugs or solutions (including dextrose solutions) because it is poorly soluble and may produce a precipitate. It should be administered in a large-bore IV line, and the line should be flushed with saline postadministration. The dose should be given slowly, at a rate of ≤ 50 mg/min. Rapid administration may produce hypotension and cardiovascular collapse. Pam is receiving phenytoin because it inhibits the spread of seizure activity and depresses brain stem centers responsible for seizures. Seizure activity would further decrease Pam's cerebral perfusion and increase cerebral oxygen demands. However, if Pam did not have a history of seizures, Dilantin would most likely still be ordered. It is effective in preventing early (within 7 days after the event) posttrauma seizures (Bullock et al., 1999).

The following additional collaborative interventions have not been ordered for Pam at this time but may be necessary if Pam's neurologic status deteriorates.

4. *Fluid restriction*. Fluid may be restricted from 900 to 2,500/day to decrease the potential for cerebral edema (Hickey, 1992). As used in Pam's case, 0.45 percent normal saline is the preferred IV solution, since this concentration decreases the likelihood of cerebral edema. The patient's serum osmolality is used to titrate fluid volume. The head-injured patient's serum osmolality should be maintained between 305 and 315 mOsm/L (Walleck, 1989).
5. *Glucocorticosteroids*. There is great controversy concerning the effect of steroids in the management of a patient with a head injury. Latest research does not show an improvement in outcomes associated with corticosteroid use. They are hypothesized to stabilize the cell membranes, thus improving cerebral blood flow and ultimately restoring autoregulation (refer to Module 17 for further discussion of autoregulation). Steroids also may produce negative effects because of their immunosuppression function. Since Pam had a grossly contaminated wound and a surgical procedure, she may be predisposed to infection. Steroids may not be the best choice of therapy for her.
6. *Barbiturate therapy*. High-dose barbiturates may be administered to reduce cerebral metabolism and cerebral blood flow by inducing coma. Although this therapy is effective in reducing ICP, it does not decrease mortality. Barbiturates are used in cases of uncontrolled intracranial hypertension that has not responded to conventional therapy. Narcotic sedation and neuromuscular blocking agents may be better choices in controlling agitation and decreasing ICP.

Independent Nursing Interventions

The nurse can make independent interventions that focus on the identified nursing diagnoses.

1. *Positioning*. Pam should be positioned with her head elevated 30 to 45 degrees and in straight alignment. This promotes venous drainage and cerebral blood flow. Hip flexion should be avoided, since this can increase ICP. Research has demonstrated that position changes can increase ICP significantly if the patient's baseline ICP is > 15 mm (Parsons & Wilson, 1984). At least 15 minutes should be allowed between position changes to prevent accumulative increases from ICP (Mitchell, Ozuna, & Lipe, 1981).
2. *Suctioning*. Pam will require suctioning because she is being ventilated mechanically. The patient should be hyperoxygenated first, and the suctioning should be confined to 10 seconds. Manual hyperventilation should be extended after the third suctioning. Patients with ICP measurements < 20 mm Hg can be suctioned safely (Parsons, Peard, & Page, 1985). Suctioning increases ICP on the average of 12 mm Hg above the baseline level (Reimer, 1989).
3. *Interaction*. In 1981, Bruya noticed that the patient's ICP dropped when the family approached the patient or touched the patient's arm. Family visits have been associated with decreases in ICP (Hendrickson, 1987). Other studies did not show a decrease in ICP, but family visits have not been associated with increases in ICP (Prins, 1989). Conversation about the patient or directed to the patient without touching the patient has been related to increases in ICP (Mitchell & Mauss, 1978). Therefore, the nurse caring for Pam should touch her while speaking and encourage visits by her family.
4. *Nutrition*. The head-injured patient is hypermetabolic and hypercatabolic. Nutritional interventions should be initiated in the acute phase of treatment and may take the form of total parenteral nutrition (TPN) or early nasointestinal or gastrojejunostomy feedings. Although the physician will order the nutritional route and solution, the nurse must ensure that the feeding is administered correctly. Feeding by some route should be

initiated by the end of the first week post closed head injury (Bullock et al., 1999). The nurse must treat the feeding as an essential component of the patient's therapy and be meticulous about its administration.

In summary, independent nursing interventions for Pam include the following:

1. Keep the head of the bed elevated 30 to 45 degrees.
2. Keep Pam's head in straight alignment and prevent hip flexion.
3. Administer nutritional therapy as ordered.
4. Suction PRN, monitoring ICP waveform and reading during the procedure. Complete the procedure within 10 seconds. Hyperoxygenate and hyperventilate before each suctioning pass and after the final pass for a longer time period.
5. Allow family visitation and interaction.
6. Use touch when talking to the patient.
7. Monitor ICP readings and waveforms and ventricular drainage.
8. Monitor effects of drug therapy.
9. Maintain accurate intake and output records.
10. Prevent increase in ICP:
    - Decrease stimulation.
    - Allow at least 15 minutes between nursing interventions.
    - Prevent constipation and increases in intra-abdominal pressure.
    - Drain CSF as indicated per physician order.

QUESTION

Which of the following would indicate that Pam was experiencing increased ICP during range of motion exercises?

A. decreased Spo_2 according to pulse oximetry
B. stimulation of low pressure alarm on the ventilator
C. presence of B waves on the pressure monitor
D. a 10 mm Hg drop in blood pressure

ANSWER

The correct answer is C. B waves indicate increased ICP and are associated with decreased responsiveness. They occur before A waves. A waves indicate severe increased ICP. The ventilator low pressure alarm indicates that the machine is not meeting any resistance from the patient's lungs, indicating an air leak or disconnection of the artificial airway from the ventilator system. A drop in blood pressure or oxygen saturation may be related to perfusion changes and not be associated with changes in ICP.

Pam's plan of care is developed and ready to be executed. Her progress will be monitored at regular intervals to evaluate the effects of the various therapeutic actions. If progress is not noted toward attainment of Pam's desired patient outcomes, her plan may need revision, examining alternative interventions that may be more effective.

Nursing Care of the Patient Experiencing a Posttrauma Complication

Pam has made considerable progress. The intraventricular catheter was removed 48 hours postsurgery. She is extubated and on nasal cannula at 2 L/min. Pam is alert and oriented, with a GCS score of 15. Her NG tube was discontinued. A peripheral IV line is in her left hand, and D_5W 0.45 percent normal saline is infusing at 100 mL/hr. Her urinary catheter is still in place because she gets fatigued and dyspneic at times when placed on the bedpan. Gentamicin 100 mg q6h was ordered today because her WBC has increased to 14,000, and she has a fever of 100.6°F orally. Pam is to be moved out of the unit to the general trauma floor today as soon as the bed is ready. It has been 6 days since her injury.

QUESTION

Which of the following events could place Pam at the highest risk for development of posttrauma complications?

A. craniotomy
B. history of aspiration
C. intraventricular catheter
D. immobility

ANSWER

The correct answer is B. Although all of these factors increase Pam's risk for complications, aspiration places her at the highest risk for several reasons. The introduction of foreign substances in the lung fields precipitates an inflammatory response. Initiation of the inflammatory response with increased capillary permeability can produce ARDS and pulmonary edema. She has required anesthesia and mechanical ventilation. Anesthesia and mechanical ventilation prevent Pam from coughing and clearing her own airway. Coughing would be a compensatory mechanism for managing the inflammation from the aspiration. She is dependent on suctioning. In addition, suctioning can introduce pathogens. Even though Pam's chest film is clear at present, patchy infiltrates may develop later.

As the nurse caring for Pam, you are notified that the floor bed will be ready in 45 minutes. You go to Pam's bedside to relay the message. Pam is lethargic and diaphoretic. She responds appropriately when stimulated by shaking. Her GCS score is 14. Her blood pressure is 90/66 mm Hg by the automatic external blood pressure cuff device. Her extremities are warm, and her skin is flushed. You suspect that her blood sugar may be a little low, since Pam's oral intake has been poor. Before performing a fingerstick and checking her blood glucose, you obtain a full set of vital signs. These measurements will provide a basis from which to evaluate the effect of subsequent nursing interventions.

Pam's heart rate is 106, her blood pressure is 90/66 mm Hg, oral temperature is 101.6°F, and her respirations are 28. Before proceeding further with the assessment, you put down the head of Pam's bed. You scan her nursing record and note that her blood pressure was 126/86. Her blood pressure has changed and may indicate a perfusion abnormality. You perform a fingerstick to obtain a blood glucose measurement. While waiting for the results, you keep speaking with Pam, who remains alert. Her blood glucose is 150 mg/dL by visual determination. You have ruled out the hypothesis of hypoglycemia. The remaining potential causes of hypotension in Pam's case are hypovolemia or an alteration in blood volume distribution.

You notify the physician about the change in Pam's status. The physician requests the following interventions:

- D_5W 0.45 percent normal saline IV at 150 mL/hr
- Electrocardiogram (ECG)
- ABGs
- Cefotaxime (Claforan) 2 g intravenous piggyback (IVPB) q8h
- Stat CBC; electrolyte panel
- 200-mL fluid bolus STAT
- Blood cultures before antibiotic administration
- Acetaminophen 325 mg orally q4h for fever > 101°F orally

QUESTION

Which of these orders is of the highest priority to implement based on Pam's condition?

A. administer the fluid bolus
B. administer the cefotaxime
C. obtain ECG
D. obtain CBC and electrolytes

ANSWER

The correct answer is A. You administer the fluid bolus. Blood for the CBC and electrolyte panel can be obtained later, since another antibiotic has been ordered regardless of the results. The hemoglobin and hematocrit levels will be helpful in assessing blood loss as a potential source of the hypotension. However, Pam needs to have her hypotension treated immediately to prevent decreased cerebral perfusion. If she responds to the fluid bolus, hypovolemia is the origin of her hypotension. It is possible that a dysrhythmia may be producing decreased CO. However, she is in sinus tachycardia, without **ectopy,** on the cardiac monitor. Although Pam has healing wounds that may be infected, an alteration in perfusion has taken precedence. The antibiotic can be initiated later.

After these interventions are performed, you reassess Pam's vital signs.

- Heart rate = 100
- Blood pressure = 72/60 mm Hg
- Respirations = 18

Pam is easily aroused, but she is less alert. Her blood pressure has not improved with position change or IV fluid bolus. The ECG confirms that Pam is in sinus tachycardia. The test results are as follows

CBC	
WBC = 22,000/mL	(normal range 4,500 to 10,000/mL)
RBC = 4.0 × 10^6/L	(normal range, 4.0 to 5.0 × 10^6/L)
Hgb = 15 g/dL	(normal range, 12 to 15 g/dL in females)
Hct = 46 percent	(normal range 36 to 46 percent in females)
Electrolyte panel	
Sodium (Na) = 144 mEq/L	(normal range, 135 to 145 mEq/L)
Potassium (K) = 4.0 mEq/L	(normal range, 3.5 to 5.3 mEq/L)
Chloride (Cl) = 104 mEq/L	(normal range, 95 to 105 mEq/L)
Calcium (Ca) = 8.8 mg/dL	(normal range, 9 to 11 mg/dL)
Glucose = 142 mg/dL	(normal range, 80 to 120 mg/dL)

QUESTION

Which of the following reasons best explains Pam's lack of response to the fluid bolus?

A. her blood volume is adequate
B. the source of her problem is decreased cardiac contractility
C. her hypotension may be related to vasodilation
D. she is actively bleeding

ANSWER

The correct answer is C. This is a tough question, since all the answers in certain situations are correct. Pam's CO is not adequate, as evidenced by her decreased responsiveness. Decreased CO may be related to an actual decreased blood volume, decreased contractility, or redistribution (vasodilation) of an adequate blood volume. In each situation, her stroke volume would be low, and her heart rate is increasing to maintain CO. It is possible that Pam may be so volume depleted that 200 mL does not restore preload to a level to maintain CO. However, at this point in her hospitalization, internal bleeding is unlikely unless a stress ulcer has developed. Since her skin is warm and flushed, you should suspect vasodilation. During hypovolemic shock, vasoconstriction occurs, making the skin cool and clammy. The elevated WBC is consistent with the presence of infection. The high-normal hemoglobin is reflective of dehydration. The high-normal sodium and chloride levels are consistent with dehydration/fluid shifts. The elevated glucose level may be related to infection. The ECG validates the increased heart rate, but it also indicates that myocardium is not ischemic from lack of oxygen or decreased contractility, since there are no T or ST changes, blocks, or changes in amplitude of the complexes.

You call the physician and notify her of the laboratory results, Pam's blood pressure postfluid bolus, and her decreased responsiveness. The decision is made to keep Pam in the intensive care unit. The physician arrives and orders a dopamine drip at 4 mg/kg/minute to be titrated until the systolic blood pressure remains at 90 mm Hg. The decision is made to intubate Pam and place her on the ventilator because her oxygen saturation continues to drop, and her ABG results were pH, 7.29; $PaCO_2$, 49; PaO_2, 68; HCO_3, 29. Pam has had 40 mL of urine output in the last hour. She is less responsive, and she reacts to pain by withdrawing. Her GCS score is 8T. She has the ECG pattern shown in Figure 35–1.

QUESTION

This pattern is

- **A.** atrial tachycardia
- **B.** normal sinus rhythm
- **C.** sinus tachycardia
- **D.** atrial flutter

ANSWER

The correct answer is C. Sinus tachycardia is defined as greater than 100 bpm. The sinoatrial node is serving as pacemaker, as indicated by the uniformity in the P wave configuration. In Pam's case, this is a compensatory effort to maintain an adequate CO.

QUESTION

Pam's blood gas results indicates that she is in

- **A.** respiratory acidosis
- **B.** respiratory alkalosis
- **C.** metabolic acidosis
- **D.** mixed acidosis

ANSWER

The correct answer is A. Pam is in respiratory acidosis because her pH is low, her $PaCO_2$ is high, and her bicarbonate is high.

Focused Nursing History

You review Pam's chart to identify her course of illness. You recall that Pam was not hypotensive in the field; but she did aspirate before her arrival at the hospital. Pam's first day in the intensive care unit was uneventful. She had one episode of increased ICP—18 mm Hg—that lasted 2 minutes after she was suctioned. No A or B waves were noted. The intraventricular catheter was pulled 48 hours after insertion. She was weaned from the ventilator without difficulty the third day of her admission. Pam did not complain of dyspnea and had one episode of her oxygen saturation dropping to 80 percent when she tried to use the bedpan and missed. Her bed had to be changed, and the procedure fatigued her. She complained of difficulty using the incentive spirometer. Last night, the nurse noted medium crackles in her right lower lung fields. Today's morning chest film detected small patchy infiltrates in her right lung fields with questionable areas in her left lung fields. The radiologist questioned the beginning of ARDS but stated that it was unlikely based on her ease of weaning. Antibiotic therapy was initiated by the physician in response to the chest film and the increased WBC. Pam's fever also began today.

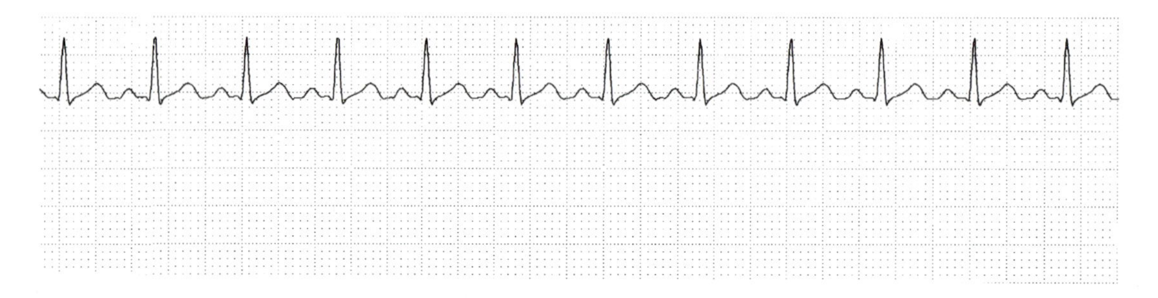

Figure 35–1.

The Systematic Bedside Assessment

Because of the change in Pam's status, you initiate a head-to-toe assessment.

HEAD AND NECK. Pam responds to pain by withdrawing. She is intubated. Her ventilator settings are FIO_2 80 percent, tidal volume 750 mL, rate 20, and mode assist/control. No venous distention is noted. Her neck veins are one-third filled at an angle of 30 degrees.

CHEST. Coarse crackles are auscultated bilaterally, with the right being greater than the left. Breath sounds are diminished in the lower lung fields. Pam's pulse oximeter finger reading is SpO_2 of 90 percent. S_1 and S_2 are auscultated. No extra heart sounds or murmurs are noted. Heart rate is 110. Her blood pressure is 84/60 mm Hg after initiation of the dopamine drip.

ABDOMEN. Pam's abdomen is soft and supple. Bowel sounds are present in all four quadrants. Her liver area is nontender, and the liver border is nonpalpable.

PELVIS. Pam has voided 40 mL in the last hour. It is dark amber, and the specific gravity is 1.019.

EXTREMITIES. Pam is flushed, and her skin is warm. She is diaphoretic. Pam's right thigh wound is draining nonodorous yellow liquid. Her scalp incision and facial laceration are not draining. Her capillary refill is 2 seconds. Peripheral pulses are palpable in all extremities.

POSTERIOR. No sacral edema is present. Posterior breath sounds are diminished in bilateral bases, and coarse rales are noted, with the right greater than the left.

Development of Nursing Diagnoses

Clustering Data

You have just completed your head-to-toe assessment and are ready to develop nursing diagnoses. To cluster your data, focus on abnormal findings found during the assessment. Pam's major symptoms at this time are decreased blood pressure, impaired gas exchange, and decreased responsiveness.

CLUSTER 1. *Subjective data.* History of aspiration in the field before arrival at the hospital. Charted episodes of dyspnea on exertion and decreased oxygen saturation.

Objective data. Decreased oxygen saturation. Elevated temperature. Blood sugar elevated. Elevated WBC. Patchy infiltrates noted on chest film. Course crackles noted bilaterally on auscultation. Presence of respiratory acidosis. Right thigh wound draining yellow material.

QUESTION

Based on these data, which of the following nursing diagnoses would you select as being the priority for Pam?

A. decreased cardiac output
B. fluid volume deficit
C. risk of infection
D. impaired gas exchange

ANSWER

The correct answer is D. All these diagnoses are appropriate. However, airway and breathing always take priority. Vasoactive substances and catecholamines are released in response to cellular damage from bacteria. Vasoactive substances increase capillary permeability, producing extravasation of volume into the pulmonary interstitium. The hyperglycemia is characteristic of a hypermetabolic state seen in activation of the inflammatory/immune response. **Multiple organ dysfunction syndrome (MODS)** may not be manifested until later in the hospitalization. It may be preceded by infection or sepsis and ARDS. Any stimulus that precipitates hypoperfusion or the release of endotoxins can initiate MODS. It is too early to determine whether Pam will experience MODS. However, her clinical changes are indicative of ARDS. She may need the addition of PEEP or pressure support to maintain tissue oxygenation and overcome the ventilation–perfusion mismatch. If PEEP is used, a decreased CO may result from the increased intrathoracic pressure decreasing cardiac filling and, thus, ejection.

DPOs for Pam would include:

1. Improved or clear breath sounds
2. Absence of fever
3. WBC within normal limits
4. Oxygen saturation > 95 percent, ABG within normal limits
5. GCS score of 15
6. Clear chest film

Additional data clusters pertain to Pam's case. Nursing diagnoses are formulated after data are clustered and patterns are identified.

CLUSTER 2. *Subjective data.* As stated in Cluster 1.

Objective data. Responds to painful stimuli with withdrawing. Sinus tachycardia is noted. Decreased blood pressure, and no increase noted with fluid bolus. Presence of fever, hyperglycemia, and elevated WBC. Blood culture pending. Draining wound in right thigh. Negative jugular venous distention. Hgb 15 g/dL, Hct 46 percent.

The same data may support multiple nursing diagnoses. This cluster includes some of the data in the first cluster. The cluster supports the diagnosis of *Fluid volume deficit.* Pam's symptoms are related to an alteration in fluid volume. The fluid volume deficit in Pam's case is probably related to endotoxins released from bacteria secondary to her wound and pulmonary infection. This would account for her tachycardia, fever, and hypotension. Urinary output is adequate, which suggests that CO is within normal limits. Pam's cerebral perfusion may be poor because of her decreased responsiveness, or her responsiveness level may be related to hypoxia. Because the data are conflicting, direct measurement of Pam's CO is desirable. CO may be decreased from massive vasodilation in response to endotoxins. The physician will most likely insert a pulmonary artery catheter to obtain direct CO (and hemodynamic) measurements. However, her hypotension clearly indicates a fluid volume deficit. Pam does appear to have an active infection that will require treatment, but this will be treated in conjunction with her fluid deficit.

DPOs for Pam would include:

1. Systolic blood pressure > 90 mm Hg
2. Decreased wound drainage and size
3. Heart rate 60 to 100
4. GCS score of 15
5. Urine output of ≥ 30 mL/hr maintained
6. Decreased wound drainage and wound size

Based on the preliminary data already collected on Pam, there are sufficient data to support the following additional nursing diagnoses:

- *Infection* related to aspiration, wounds, and invasive procedures
- *Skin integrity, impaired: Actual* related to wound infection, right thigh
- *Mobility, impaired: Physical* related to decreased responsiveness, fatigue, and ventilator
- *Risk for altered urinary elimination patterns* related to antibiotic use, decreased renal blood flow

Treatment goals for Pam will focus on increasing her oxygen supply and delivery to the tissue by improving ventilation and perfusion. These goals should be reflected in the nursing diagnoses and DPOs on the nursing care plan. For example, improving ventilation is addressed in the nursing diagnosis *Impaired gas exchange*. Accomplishment of this goal will be measured in criteria, such as patient's SpO_2 will be greater than 95 percent.

DEVELOPMENT OF A PLAN OF CARE

Recall that several collaborative and nursing interventions for posttrauma complications are discussed in Module 11, since inflammation is common to both medical and "surgical" (trauma) conditions. Thus far, antibiotics and vasopressor therapy have been initiated. Independent nursing interventions appropriate for Pam are:

1. Promote ventilation and oxygenation:
   - Suction PRN aseptically, hyperoxygenating and hyperventilating before each attempt.
   - Pace nursing activities and monitor patient's SpO_2.
   - Turn patient at least every 2 hours if SpO_2 does not drop.
2. Provide nutritional support:
   - Consult with physician concerning preferred nutritional route.
   - Administer supplement on time and without interruption.
   - Provide oral care at least every shift to promote oral intake as soon as possible.
   - Monitor weight daily; maintain intake and output record.
3. Prevent increased oxygen demand:
   - Promote wound healing by completing dressing changes on time and aseptically.
   - Provide pain relief and comfort with back rubs, conversation, and distraction.
   - Treat fever with prescribed agent; monitor temperature closely.
4. Assess for and prevent bleeding:
   - Use gentle force when completing mouth care and dressing changes.
   - Monitor for hematuria.
   - Monitor laboratory values (PT, platelets).
   - Test all drainage for the presence of blood.
5. Prevent infection:
   - Monitor for indications of infection (laboratory data, wound drainage, secretions).
   - Administer antibiotics as prescribed.
   - Monitor peak and trough antibiotic levels.
   - Culture any new drainage per physician order.
6. Surveillance:
   - Monitor vital sign trends.
   - Monitor ventilation trends (ABGs, SpO_2, ventilatory effort in relation to mechanical ventilator).
   - Monitor trends in intake and output, daily weight.

Pam's plan of care is now ready to be executed by the ICU nurse. Her progress will be examined at regular intervals to evaluate the effects of various therapeutic actions. If progress is not being noted toward attainment of her DPOs, Pam's plan of care may need to be revised.

Summary

This module has addressed the nursing care of a patient with multiple injuries. Concepts from the related modules, Trauma Assessment and Resuscitation, Complex Wound Management, Consciousness, and Multiple Organ Dysfunction Syndrome, have been applied in a case study approach. It is impossible to address specifically each traumatic injury and associated complication a nurse may encounter in the clinical setting. However, these problems can be managed by applying basic principles. These principles can be classified around assessing and treating the etiology of the patient's altered airway clearance, ineffective breathing patterns, impaired gas exchange, hypotension, distended neck veins, decreased urine output, or change in level of responsiveness. A case study was used to illustrate the relationship between traumatic injury and posttrauma complications. Nursing care responsibilities associated with the initial traumatic injury as well as the development of a posttrauma complication were discussed. Review questions were integrated throughout the module to encourage application of material and assimilation of content.

REFERENCES

American College of Surgeons Committee on Trauma. (1997). Shock. In *Advanced trauma life support course manual* (pp. 87–107). Chicago: Author.

Bruya, M. (1981). Planned periods of rest in the intensive care unit: Nursing care activities and intracranial pressure. *J Neurosurg Nurs 13*:184–194.

Bullock, R., et al. (1999). Guidelines for the management of severe head injury. *J Neurotrauma* 13:639–734.

Hendrickson, S. (1987). Intracranial pressure changes and family presence. *J Neurosci Nurs 19*(1):14–17.

Hickey, J. (1992). *The clinical practice of neurological and neurosurgical nursing* (3rd ed.). Philadelphia: J.B. Lippincott.

Kee, J. (1995). *Laboratory and diagnostic tests with nursing implications* (4th ed.). Norwalk, CT: Appleton & Lange.

Mitchell, P., & Mauss, N. (1978). Relationship of patient–nurse activity to intracranial pressure variations: A pilot study. *Nurs Res 27*:4–10.

Mitchell, P., Ozuna, J., & Lipe, H. (1981). Moving the patient in bed: Effects on intracranial pressure. *Nurs Res 30*:212–218.

Parsons, L., Peard, A., & Page, M. (1985). The effects of hygiene interventions on the cerebrovascular status of closed head injured persons. *Res Nurs Health* 8:173–181.

Parsons, L., & Wilson, M. (1984). Cerebrovascular status of severe closed head injured patients following passive position changes. *Nurs Res 33*(2):68–75.

Prins, M. (1989). The effect of family visits on intracranial pressure. *West J Nurs Res 11*:281–297.

Reimer, M. (1989). Head injured patients: How to detect early signs of trouble. Nursing 1989, 34–41.

Shlafer, M., & Marieb, E. (1989). *The nurse, pharmacology, and drug therapy*. Redwood City, CA: Addison-Wesley.

Swain, A., Grundy, D., & Russell, J. (1985). ABCs of spinal cord injury: At the accident. *Br Med J 291*:1558–1560.

Vos, H. (1994). Neurologic therapeutic management. In L. Thelan, J. Davie, L. Urden, & M. Lough (eds.). *Critical care nursing: Diagnosis and management*, 2nd ed., pp. 544–555. St. Louis: C. V. Mosby.

Walleck, C. (1989). Controversies in the management of the head injured patient. *Crit Care Clin North Am 1*:67–74.

PART IX

LIFE SPAN: SPECIAL NEEDS

MODULE 36

Nursing Care of the Acutely Ill Pediatric Patient

Sharon Barton, Deborah Dobbelhoff, Paula Vernon-Levett

The self-study module is written at the core knowledge level for the novice nurse who is caring for acutely ill patients. This module is designed to apply and supplement pathophysiologic concepts already discussed in previous modules in relation to the pediatric patient. The focus of the module is on maturational aspects of the child's anatomy and physiology that not only predispose children to certain pathophysiologic disorders but are responsible for the way they respond to illness. The five parts of the module cover the following topics: ventilation; perfusion; cognition/perception; metabolism/thermoregulation; immunocompetence; and psychosocial considerations. A pretest precedes the module. Each part includes a set of review questions to help the learner evaluate his or her understanding of the section's content before moving on to the next part. All Part Reviews and the module Pretest and Posttest include answers. It is suggested that the learner review those concepts answered incorrectly in the review questions before proceeding to the next part.

OBJECTIVES

Following completion of this module, the learner will be able to

1. Describe the unique anatomic and physiologic characteristics of the child's respiratory system.
2. Classify the most common etiologies of respiratory failure during infancy and childhood according to the dominant functional abnormality.
3. Identify clinical manifestations of acute respiratory failure observed in the infant and child.
4. Describe the nursing management of a child with acute respiratory failure.
5. Describe the most common etiologies of circulatory failure in the child.
6. List the clinical manifestations of circulatory failure in children.
7. Describe specific interventions used to manage a child with circulatory failure.
8. Discuss the unique anatomic and physiologic characteristics of the immature central nervous system.
9. List the most common types of neurologic dysfunction in children.
10. Describe the key components of the neurologic examination of the child with altered mental status.
11. Discuss the nursing management of the neurologically impaired child.
12. Describe the nursing management of a child with altered fluid and electrolytes.
13. Discuss the nursing management of a child with altered nutritional status.
14. Identify regulatory mechanisms of heat balance.
15. Discuss the nursing management of altered heat balance.
16. Identify age-related factors and situational stressors that alter the immune response of the acutely ill child.

17. State treatment strategies to prevent infection and augment host defenses in the child.
18. Discuss age-related stressors and reactions to hospitalization.
19. List specific methods to reduce the negative effects of hospitalization.

PRETEST

Refer to the following case study to answer questions 1 through 5.

Amanda is a 4-year-old girl brought to the emergency department after aspirating a piece of hot dog in her trachea. She has a respiratory rate of 60, decreased breath sounds in her lower lobes, inspiratory stridor, use of accessory muscles, and supraclavicular retractions. Her mucous membranes, nailbeds, and sclera are bluish in color.

1. What is the underlying dominant respiratory abnormality?
   A. obstructive lung disease
   B. restrictive lung disease
   C. ineffective gas transfer from decreased alveoli
   D. ineffective gas transfer from central nervous system depression
2. Based on the above data, which of the following nursing diagnoses would you select as being appropriate in Amanda's care?
   A. *Ineffective airway clearance*
   B. *Altered cardiac output: Decreased*
   C. *Potential for infection*
   D. *Altered tissue perfusion: Cerebral*

Noninvasive efforts to remove the hot dog were unsuccessful. A bronchoscopy was ordered. During the procedure, Amanda's arterial oxygen saturation decreased acutely to 40 percent, her heart rate dropped to 60, and she had a respiratory arrest. The hot dog piece was removed.

3. What intervention should be performed first?
   A. intubation
   B. bag-valve-mask ventilation with FIO_2 1.0
   C. passive flow of oxygen
   D. chest compressions
4. If Amanda requires chest compressions, what is the correct compression/ventilation ratio?
   A. 5:1
   B. 10:1
   C. 15:2
   D. 10:2

Amanda recovers nicely. Later in the day, Amanda's parents have to leave the hospital. Amanda becomes very upset, crying and yelling for her parents.

5. What nursing intervention would most likely reduce Amanda's anxiety?
   A. using a clock to explain when her parents will return
   B. bringing her favorite teddy bear to the bedside
   C. developing a contract with Amanda to negotiate visitation
   D. explaining to Amanda she will have no play time if she continues crying

Refer to the following case study to answer questions 6 through 11.

Johnny is a 2-month-old, 5-kg infant admitted to the intensive care unit with a 3-day history of fever. On admission, he is lethargic and minimally responsive to noxious stimuli. Vital signs are temperature 103.1°F (39.5°C), heart rate 180, respiratory rate 80, blood pressure 50 by palpation. Extremities are cool and pale in color. Lungs are clear to auscultation.

6. What patient order should be initiated first by the nurse?
   A. intravenous (IV) line insertion
   B. supplemental oxygen
   C. synchronized cardioversion
   D. acetaminophen administration
7. Based on the above data, which of the following nursing diagnoses would you select as being appropriate in Johnny's plan of care?
   A. *Ineffective airway breathing*
   B. *Altered nutrition: Less than body requirements*
   C. *Fluid volume deficit*
   D. *Self-care deficit*

Peripheral IV line insertion has been attempted at least three times in 5 minutes without success.

8. Access to the circulation should be attempted by which of the following routes?
   A. central cannulation
   B. cutdown cannulation
   C. intraosseous cannulation
   D. arterial cannulation

Access to the circulation is successful. The patient becomes unresponsive. The heart rate is 190, and the blood pressure is no longer palpable. Femoral pulses are faint.

9. How much fluid should Johnny receive as a bolus?
   A. 5 mL
   B. 25 mL
   C. 50 mL
   D. 300 mL

10. What type of IV solution should you prepare for fluid resuscitation?
    A. lactated Ringer's solution
    B. 5 percent dextrose in water
    C. 5 percent dextrose in 0.2 normal saline
    D. albumin

Another bolus of fluid is given. Johnny's vital signs are stabilized. A urinary catheter is inserted for urine output monitoring.

11. What should be the normal urine output per hour for Johnny?
    A. 20 mL
    B. 30 mL
    C. 10 mL
    D. 2 mL

Refer to the following case study to answer questions 12 through 15.

Ricky, an 18-month-old child, is brought to the intensive care unit (ICU) with a history of fever for 2 days, irritability, loss of appetite, and lethargy. Vital signs are temperature 101.3°F (38.5°C), heart rate 180, respiratory rate 50, and blood pressure 80/60. Breath sounds are clear, urine culture is negative, white blood count (WBC) is 20,000. Ricky also has a petechial rash. A lumbar puncture is performed. Results are cloudy appearance, WBC 604/mL, protein 110 mg/100 mL, Gram stain positive for gram-negative cocci.

12. If Ricky is not treated quickly, which of the following pathophysiologic processes is most likely to develop?
    A. decreased perfusion from cardiogenic shock
    B. decreased perfusion from septic shock
    C. increased intracranial pressure (IICP)
    D. hypoxemia from central nervous system (CNS)-induced pulmonary edema

Ricky is diagnosed with bacterial meningitis.

13. Which of the following pathogens is most likely the cause?
    A. *Escherichia coli*
    B. *Neisseria meningitidis*
    C. respiratory syncytial virus (RSV)
    D. *Pseudomonas aeruginosa*
14. Which of the following nursing interventions has the highest priority?
    A. administer broad-spectrum antibiotics
    B. assess airway and breathing
    C. administer medications to prevent hypotension
    D. hyperventilate with an Ambu bag
15. Which of the following interventions would most likely be needed following the administration of lorazepam (Ativan) for status epilepticus?
    A. bag-valve-mask ventilation
    B. isotonic fluid bolus 20 mL/kg
    C. naloxone (Narcan) administration
    D. dopamine (Intropin) administration

Refer to the following case study to answer questions 16 through 19.

Christine is a 3-year-old girl admitted to the ICU with a 3-day history of vomiting and diarrhea. Vital signs are temperature 98°F, respiratory rate 40, heart rate 170, blood pressure 84/40. Additional clinical symptoms include pale skin color, loss of skin elasticity, dry mucous membranes, capillary refill of four seconds, and irritability. She has not voided for 7 hours. Prehospital weight is not known. Present weight is 17 kg. CBC is normal, glucose normal, serum electrolytes are Na^+ 138, K^+ 3.4, Cl^- 102.

16. What best describes her current status?
    A. compensated shock
    B. decompensated shock
    C. hyponatremic dehydration
    D. stable
17. What would initial treatment for Christina be?
    A. assure stability of airway, administer 100% oxygen
    B. assist with lumbar puncture
    C. offer rehydrating preparation by mouth
    D. obtain IV access and bolus with 20 cc/kg normal saline or lactated Ringer's
18. After receiving 340 cc of normal saline over 15 minutes, Christina's exam is as follows: RR 40, HR 160, BP 85/40, capillary refill 3 seconds, color slightly improved, mucous membranes still dry, irritability still present. What action is indicated at this time?
    A. another 20 cc/kg normal saline bolus
    B. start vasoactive IV medicine to improve perfusion
    C. no action, monitor closely
    D. prepare to assist with intubation
19. If Christine normally weighs 19 kg, what percentage of weight loss does she have?
    A. 8
    B. 2
    C. 20
    D. 10

Questions 20 and 21 do not refer to Christine.

20. An infant's level of immunoglobulins is lowest between
    A. 4 and 6 years of age
    B. 4 and 5 months of age
    C. 2 and 3 weeks of age
    D. 2 and 5 years of age
21. Low levels of immunoglobulin E (IgE) place the young child at increased risk for
    A. pyogenic infections
    B. bacterial respiratory infection
    C. parasitic infection
    D. overwhelming sepsis

Refer to the following case study to answer questions 22 and 23.

Cathy is a 2½-year-old girl admitted to the ICU for antibiotics to treat severe pneumonia. She is intubated.

22. What intervention would best help decrease her anxiety?
    A. administer paralytic drugs (neuromuscular blocking agents)
    B. allow her to have her favorite toy
    C. encourage a parent to stay with her
    D. allow her to draw pictures

Cathy's IV catheter needs to be changed.

23. What nursing intervention would best help her deal with this procedure?
    A. use deep sedation for IV insertion
    B. use distraction and simple directions when inserting the IV
    C. encourage her to be involved in the procedure
    D. prepare her by using a doll the day before

Question 24 does not pertain to Cathy.

24. Which of the following nursing interventions would be most effective in a patient with elevated ICP?
    A. maintaining neutral head position
    B. maintaining the head of the bed at 40 degrees
    C. applying hypothermia mattress
    D. placing patient in Trendelenburg position

Pretest answers: 1. A, 2. C, 3. A, 4. B, 5. A, 6. D, 7. B, 8. B, 9. C, 10. C, 11. C, 12. B, 13. B, 14. C, 15. B, 16. A, 17. A, 18. A, 19. B, 20. B, 21. C, 22. C, 23. B, 24. A

GLOSSARY

Bradycardia. An abnormally slow heart rate

Tachycardia. An abnormally high heart rate

Tidal volume. Volume of air that is inhaled and exhaled during normal breathing

Ventilation–perfusion mismatch. An abnormality in the distribution of the ventilation and perfusion of the gas-exchanging units

ABBREVIATIONS

ABG. Arterial blood gas

BMR. Basal metabolic rate

BSA. Body surface area

CBF. Cerebral blood flow

CNS. Central nervous system

CO. Cardiac output

CPP. Cerebral perfusion pressure

CSF. Cerebrospinal fluid

CT. Computed tomography

CVC. Central venous catheter

CVP. Central venous pressure

EEG. Electroencephalogram

GCS. Glasgow Coma Scale

Hct. Hematocrit

Hgb. Hemoglobin

ICP. Intracranial pressure

kcal. Kilocalorie

LOC. Level of consciousness

MRI. Magnetic resonance imaging

$Paco_2$. Partial pressure of carbon dioxide

Pao_2. Partial pressure of oxygen

PAOP. Pulmonary artery output pressure

PCWP. Pulmonary capillary wedge pressure

PVR. Pulmonary vascular resistance

RDA. Recommended dietary allowances

SCIDS. Severe combined immunodeficiency syndrome

Spo_2. Peripheral arterial saturation of oxygen

SBP. Systolic blood pressure

SVo_2. Venous saturation of oxygen

SVR. Systemic vascular resistance

TBI. Traumatic brain injury

VENTILATION

SECTION ONE: Maturational Anatomy and Physiology

At the completion of this section, the learner will be able to describe unique anatomic and physiologic characteristics of the child's respiratory system.

Respiratory disorders producing respiratory distress or failure are the most common admitting diagnoses in the pediatric intensive care unit. To understand the nursing assessment and the nursing care of a pediatric patient with acute respiratory failure, one must first have a basic understanding of the unique anatomic and physiologic characteristics of the immature respiratory system. The focus of this section is to discuss briefly developmental aspects of the respiratory system.

Even though the term newborn's lungs are capable of immediate function at birth, growth of the lungs continues for several years. Growth occurs primarily from an increase in the size of the conducting airways and from an increase in the number of bronchioles and alveoli. There also are a number of other significant anatomic and physiologic differences in the immature respiratory system (Table 36–1). Consequently, the young child has a predisposition to respiratory dysfunction, as well as limited respiratory reserve.

In summary, the child's respiratory system is not only quantitatively different but also is qualitatively different, predisposing children to acute respiratory failure. Knowledge of the anatomic and physiologic differences can assist in early recognition and management of acute respiratory failure.

TABLE 36–1. ANATOMIC AND PHYSIOLOGIC CONSIDERATIONS OF THE IMMATURE RESPIRATORY SYSTEM

ANATOMY	CLINICAL SIGNIFICANCE
Small airway diameter	Airway obstruction increases airway resistance in infant to a greater degree than in adult: Infant airway is only one-fourth the diameter of the adult airway; easily obstructed
Larynx higher in the neck Epiglottis is U-shaped, large Vocal cords short	Difficult to visualize, the pharynx to the glottis for endotracheal intubation
Large tongue	Easily obstructed
Cricoid cartilage narrowest portion of the airway	Use uncuffed ET tube; tape ET securely
Small lower airways	Predisposition to obstruction and atelectasis from mucus, blood, pus, edema
Decreased number of alveoli and surface area	Decreased diffusion and increased shunting
Cartilaginous thoracic cage	Less bony structure to support, more likely to have retractions
Diaphragm primary muscle of respiration	Respiratory function compromised with gastric distention, abdomen distended
PHYSIOLOGY	**CLINICAL SIGNIFICANCE**
Large body surface area, immature thermostatic control	Likely to have hypothermia causing decreased oxygen consumption and metabolic rate
Metabolic rate twice the adult rate	More likely to become hypoxic with altered respiratory function

SECTION TWO: Etiologies

At the completion of this section, the learner will be able to classify the most common etiologies of respiratory failure during infancy and childhood according to the dominant functional abnormality.

Respiratory failure is a state in which the respiratory system is unable to deliver adequate oxygen to or remove carbon dioxide from the circulation in order to meet the demands of the body. As noted previously, children are predisposed to respiratory failure because of the unique anatomic and physiologic features of their immature respiratory system. In addition, a number of respiratory disorders can impair the child's ability to adequately oxygenate or ventilate or both. The purpose of this section is to describe common etiologies of acute respiratory failure in children:

- Obstructive lung disease
- Restrictive lung disease
- Primary ineffective gas transfer

All three functional derangements may be present in isolation or in combination. However, all three groups have a common final pathway of the mismatching of ventilation and perfusion in the lung. Consequently, hypoxemia, hypercarbia, and acidosis develop.

Obstructive Lung Disease

Airway obstruction is a common cause of respiratory failure in children. Whether the obstruction is acute or chronic, partial or complete, there is increased resistance to flow. If the obstruction is complete or if the child cannot compensate for a partial obstruction, a **ventilation–perfusion mismatch** develops, resulting in hypoxemia and hypercarbia. Table 32–2 lists the most common causes of obstructive lung disease during infancy and childhood.

Restrictive Lung Disease

Restrictive lung disease also can cause respiratory failure in children. The main functional alteration is impaired lung expansion from loss of lung volume, decreased distensibil-

TABLE 36–2. CAUSES OF OBSTRUCTIVE RESPIRATORY DISEASE IN CHILDREN

	SPECIFIC DISEASE CONDITIONS	
SITE OF DISTURBANCE	Newborn and Early Infancy	Late Infancy and Childhood
Upper airway		
Anomalies	Choanal atresia, Pierre Robin syndrome, laryngeal web, tracheal stenosis, tracheomalacia, vascular ring	Tracheal stenosis, vocal cord paralysis, vascular ring, laryngotracheomalacia
Lower airway		
Anomalies	Bronchostenosis, bronchomalacia, lobar emphysema	Bronchostenosis, lobar emphysema, aberrant vessels
Aspiration	Meconium, mucus, vomitus	Foreign body, vomitus
Infection	Pneumonia, pertussis, respiratory syncytial virus	Laryngotracheitis, epiglottis, peritonsillar or retropharyngeal abscess, bronchiolitis, pneumonia, respiratory syncytial virus
Tumors	Hemangioma, cystic hygroma, teratoma	Hemangioma, teratoma, hypertrophy of tonsils and adenoids
Allergic or reflex	Larynogospasm from local irritation (intubation) or tetany	Laryngospasm from local irritation (aspiration, intubation, drowning) or tetany, allergy, smoke inhalation, asthma, bronchospasm

ity of lung tissue, and chest wall disturbance. Regardless of the cause, there is inadequate aeration of the alveoli, whereas pulmonary blood flow is normal (intrapulmonary shunt). Table 36–3 lists the most common causes of restrictive lung disease during infancy and childhood.

Ineffective Gas Transfer

The last group of respiratory dysfunction producing respiratory failure is primary ineffective gas transfer. Specific disease conditions resulting in ineffective gas transfer can result from pulmonary diffusion defects or from CNS respiratory depression. With pulmonary diffusion defects, gas transfer between alveoli and pulmonary capillaries is blocked by abnormal tissue. Respiratory depression produces a decrease in total minute ventilation (i.e., a reduction in respiratory rate, **tidal volume,** or both). Table 36–4 lists the most common causes of primary inefficient gas transfer during childhood.

In summary, any condition that impairs oxygenation or ventilation when compensatory mechanisms are inadequate will result in respiratory failure.

SECTION THREE: Clinical Manifestations

At the completion of this section, the learner will be able to identify clinical manifestations of acute respiratory failure observed in the infant and child.

Clinical manifestations of acute respiratory failure in children are extremely variable and nonspecific. Consequently, clinical findings must be correlated with diagnostic findings. To be able to recognize signs and symptoms of impending respiratory failure, one must first have an understanding of normal respiratory parameters during childhood. This section compares and contrasts normal and abnormal findings of the respiratory examination.

TABLE 36–3. CAUSES OF RESTRICTIVE RESPIRATORY DISEASE

	SPECIFIC DISEASE CONDITIONS	
SITE OF DISTURBANCE	Newborn and Early Infancy	Late Infancy and Childhood
Parenchymal		
Anomalies	Agenesis, hypoplasia, lobar emphysema, congenital cyst, pulmonary sequestration	Congenital cyst
Atelectasis	RDS	Thick secretions, foreign body
Infection	Pneumonia	Pneumonia, cystic fibrosis, bronchiectasis
Alveolar rupture	Pneumothorax (spontaneous or iatrogenic), interstitial emphysema	Trauma, asthma
Others	Pulmonary hemorrhage, pulmonary edema, bronchopulmonary dysplasia	Pulmonary edema, lobectomy, chemical pneumonitis, pleural effusion, near-drowning, ARDS
Chest wall		
Muscular	Diaphragmatic hernia, eventration, edema	Muscular dystrophy, botulism, Guillain-Barré, tetanus
Skeletal malformations	Hemivertebrae, absence of ribs	Kyphoscoliosis, hemivertebrae, absence of ribs
Others	Abdominal distention	Obesity, flail chest

TABLE 36–4. CAUSES OF PRIMARY INEFFICIENT GAS TRANSFER

SITE OF DISTURBANCE	SPECIFIC DISEASE CONDITIONS
Pulmonary diffusion defect	
Increased diffusion path between alveoli and capillaries	Pulmonary edema, pulmonary fibrosis, collagen disorders, *Pneumocystis carinii* infection, sarcoidosis
Decreased alveolocapillary surface area	Pulmonary embolism, sarcoidosis, pulmonary hypertension, mitral stenosis, fibrosing alveolitis
Inadequate erythrocytes and hemoglobin	Anemia, hemorrhage
Respiratory center depression	
Increased cerebrospinal fluid pressure	Cerebral trauma, traumatic cerebral injury during birth, intracranial tumors, central nervous system infection (meningitis, encephalitis, sepsis)
Excess central nervous system depressant drugs	Maternal oversedation, overdosage with barbiturates, morphine, or diazepam, deliberate ingestion
Excessive chemical changes in arterial blood	Severe asphyxia (hypercapnia, hypoxemia)

Adapted from Chernik, V., & Kendig, T. (1998). Kendig's disorders of the respiratory tract in children. *Philadelphia: W.B. Saunders.*

TABLE 36–5. SIGNS AND SYMPTOMS OF INCREASED WORK OF BREATHING

CLINICAL FINDING	CLINICAL SIGNIFICANCE
Inspiratory stridor	Upper airway obstruction between the supraglottic space and lower trachea
Prolonged expiration with wheezing	Bronchial and bronchiolar obstruction
Grunting	Premature glottic closure during expiration, an attempt to increase functional residual capacity
Nasal flaring	Enlarges anterior nasal passages and reduces upper and total airway resistance
Chest wall retractions (intracostal, subcostal, suprasternal)	Increased negative intrapleural pressure during inspiration with high airway resistance
Use of accessory muscles (older child), head bobbing (infant)	Upper airway obstruction
Paradoxical breathing	Premature/newborn: extremely compliant rib cage; infant/toddler: respiratory muscle fatigue and impending respiratory arrest

Respiratory Rate

Respiratory rate normally decreases with age, with the greatest normal variation during the first 2 years of life (Wong, 1999). Approximate averages of breaths/min during infancy and childhood are

Newborn	< 40
1 year old	30
18 years old	16 to 18

An abnormally fast respiratory rate (tachypnea) can be seen in children with increased anxiety, fever, anemia, pain, exertion, and conditions producing decreased lung compliance.

Tachypnea is often the first sign of respiratory distress in the young child, especially when it is associated with increased work of breathing (Table 36–5). Tachypnea is the body's attempt to maintain a normal pH by eliminating excess carbon dioxide via the lungs. Tachypnea without associated signs of respiratory distress (see Table 36–6), quiet tachypnea, usually is due to nonrespiratory causes, such as disorders producing metabolic acidosis or due to congenital heart disease.

TABLE 36–6. RESPIRATORY DISTRESS CLINICAL DATA

Heart rate	Tachycardia Bradycardia (infant) Tachycardia leading to bradycardia (child)
Respiratory rate	Tachypnea Newborn > 60 2 months–2 years > 30 2–12 years > 30 > 12 years > 20
Respiratory effort	Nasal flaring, expiratory grunt, paradoxical breathing, chest retractions, inspiratory stridor, wheezing
Color	Pale, dusky leading to cyanotic
Auscultatory finds	Variable: absent or diminished breath sounds, adventitious breath sounds
Level of consciousness	Altered or depressed
Pulse oximetry	< 95%
Arterial blood gases	With loss of compensation: decreased PaO_2 and/or increased $PaCO_2$

Source: Curley, M., Smith, J., & Maloney-Harmon, P. (1996). Critical care nursing of infants and children. *Philadelphia: W.B. Saunders.*

An abnormally slow respiratory rate (bradypnea) or absent respiratory rate (apnea) can occur with CNS depression, extreme fatigue, and hypothermia. Bradypnea is a very ominous sign in a child who is acutely ill and usually hallmarks an impending respiratory arrest.

Respiratory Mechanics

After assessing the rate and rhythm of breathing, one should look at respiratory mechanics to determine whether there is increased work of breathing. Specific signs and symptoms of increased work of breathing in the child and their clinical significance are listed in Table 36–5.

Color

Cyanosis is a very late and insensitive indicator of acute respiratory failure. It refers to a bluish color, which is due to an absolute amount of reduced hemoglobin (Hgb) in capillary blood. Clinically detectable cyanosis is dependent on arterial oxygen saturation (SaO_2) and total circulating hemoglobin concentration. Depending on the amount of hemoglobin, clinical cyanosis will occur at different levels of arterial oxygen saturation. For example, a child with polycythemia (hematocrit > 60 percent) will show clinical signs of cyanosis before a child with anemia because of an increase in the number of unsaturated red blood cells. It is important to recognize cyanosis from a respiratory origin, as a sign of inadequate oxygenation.

Pulse Oximetry

Pulse oximetry is used to provide continuous noninvasive monitoring of respiratory status. Pulse oximetry has many advantages. It provides a continuous readout. It is noninvasive. The oximeter requires no calibration. Pulse oximetry is considered a useful adjunct to cardiovascular monitoring (Curley, Smith, & Maloney-Harmon, 1996).

Arterial Blood Gases

Arterial blood gases (ABGs) are a widely used clinical method to evaluate acute respiratory failure in children. Normal ABG values are listed in Table 36–7. The use of pulse oximetry and end-tidal CO_2 for the intubated child have greatly reduced the need for invasive blood draws for arterial blood gas.

SvO_2 Monitoring

Pulmonary artery catheters allow for continuous monitoring of mixed venous oxygen saturation (SvO_2). SvO_2 can also be obtained from a central venous catheter (CVC). A CVC line should never be tourniqueted for obtaining an SvO_2 specimen. A decreased SvO_2 indicates the child is extracting and depleting oxygen from tissue. SvO_2 monitoring also allows the clinician to assess the child's tolerance to treatment and physical care activities. A decrease in SvO_2 can indicate that the child has been physiologically stressed. A decreasing SaO_2 combined with increasing SvO_2 is an ominous sign of impending cell death, while an increasing SaO_2 combined with decreasing SvO_2 indicates cell viability (Curley, Smith, & Maloney-Harmon, 1996).

TABLE 36–7. NORMAL ARTERIAL BLOOD GAS VALUES IN CHILDREN

	INFANTS	SCHOOL-AGE	ADOLESCENCE
HCO_3	19–23 mEq/L	22–24 mEq/L	23–25 mEq/L
PCO_2	30–34 mm Hg	35–41 mm Hg	38–44 mm Hg
PO_2	80–100 mm Hg	80–100 mm Hg	80–100 mm Hg
pH	7.36–7.42	7.37–7.43	7.35–7.41

In summary, a key factor in reducing mortality and morbidity from a respiratory arrest is early recognition of signs and symptoms of respiratory failure. Table 36–6 summarizes the early signs and symptoms of respiratory compromise. These signs and symptoms coupled with diagnostic information provide the database to guide respiratory management.

SECTION FOUR: Nursing Management

At the completion of this section, the learner will be able to describe the specific steps in managing a child with acute respiratory failure.

The specific interventions needed to manage a child with altered respiratory function are based on clinical data. For the child with mild respiratory distress, only comfort measures may be required. At the opposite end of the continuum with total respiratory arrest, complete cardiopulmonary resuscitation may be required. This section presents guidelines for managing a child with altered respiratory function.

On the basis of a rapid respiratory assessment, the child should be categorized into one of three groups:

1. Mild respiratory distress (stable)
2. Impending respiratory failure (unstable)
3. Respiratory arrest

The goals of emergency airway management are to anticipate and recognize respiratory problems and to support and replace those functions that are compromised or lost. Oxygen at the highest possible concentrations should be administered to all seriously ill or injured patients with respiratory insufficiency, shock, or trauma. Use of airway adjuncts to deliver the oxygen is dependent on the severity of the respiratory problem. In the spontaneously breathing patient, a simple oxygen mask can be used. It can deliver 35 to 60 percent oxygen with a flow rate of 6 to 10 L/min. Oxygen delivery systems should be selected from least to most invasive. The next oxygen delivery system is a partial rebreather mask, with a nonrebreather mask being the next option. The next level of invasiveness is the oxygen hood or tent followed by use of a nasal cannula, insertion of an oral airway or nasopharyngeal airway. For respiratory arrest, the approach to treatment is described in Figure 36–1.

The goal in treating the child with respiratory distress is to minimize oxygen demand while correcting the underlying disease process. The first nursing intervention to implement is opening the airway. Infants should be placed in a sniffing position, and older children should be allowed to determine their own position of comfort. Second, maximize tidal volume by elevating the head of bed. This position prevents abdominal organs from impinging on the diaphragm and the thoracic cavity. Third, maximize oxygenation by administering supplemental oxygen via an age-appropriate delivery system. Finally, provide interventions to minimize oxygen demand. For example, withhold feedings or administer them through a nasogastric tube, minimize environmental stress, and maintain normothermia. The oxygen demand in children is usually reduced when children are allowed to be comforted by family members.

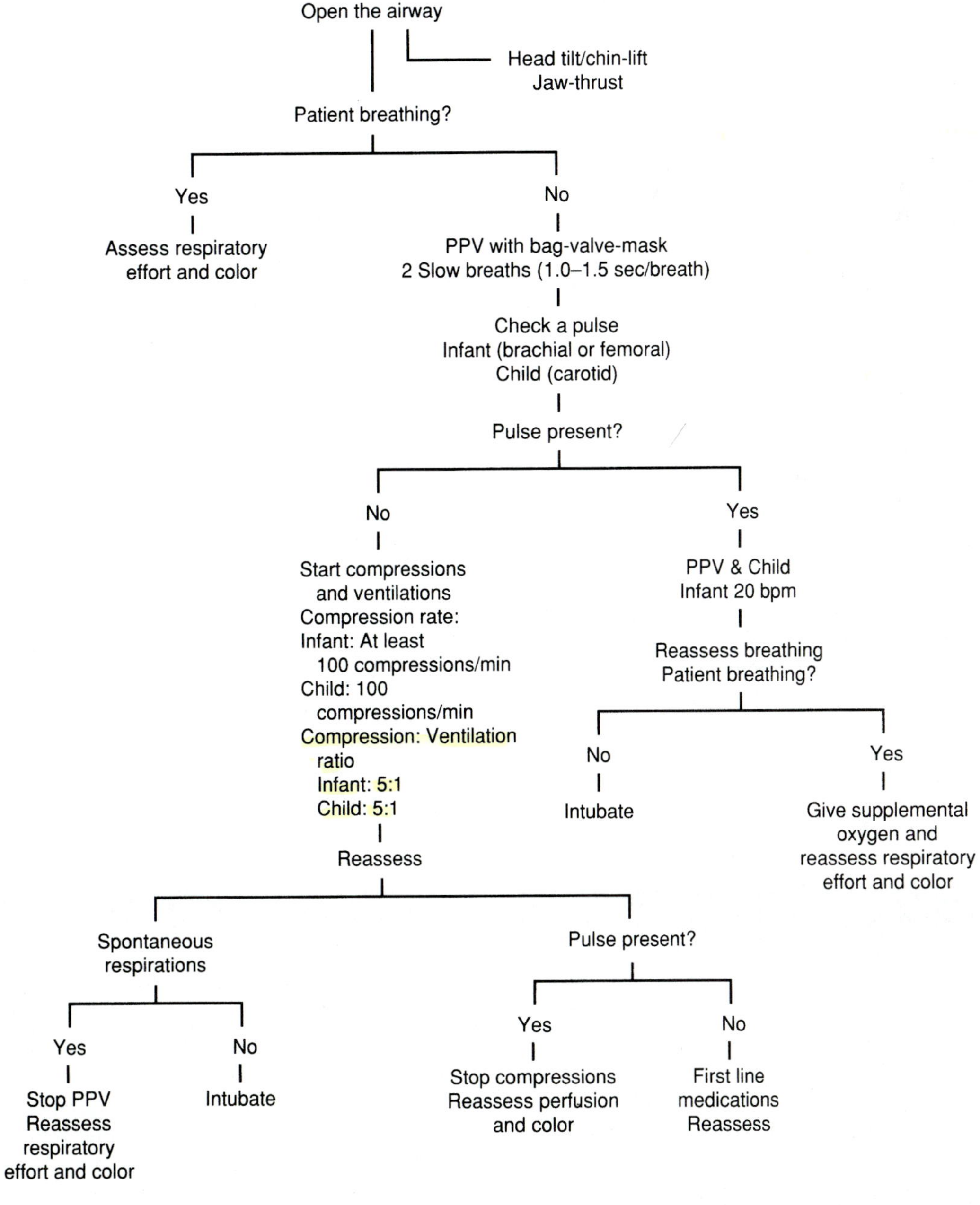

Figure 36–1. Management of respiratory failure. PPV, positive pressure ventilation; bpm, breaths per minute.

In patients with respiratory failure or arrest, more aggressive management is required to stabilize the patient. The goal is to restore ventilation and oxygenation to prevent ensuing cardiac asystole. Figure 36–1 outlines a systematic approach to the emergent management of respiratory failure or arrest.

A number of oxygen delivery systems can be used in children. The selection of a system is based on patient tolerance of the device, patient minute ventilation, and oxygen concentration needed. In general, a patient with acute respiratory failure or impending respiratory arrest requires the highest concentration of oxygen available. Therefore, high flow oxygen masks that can reliably deliver high oxygen concentrations should be used. Table 36–8 provides equipment guidelines for airway resuscitation in the infant and child.

The role of the nurse during intubation is to ensure the child is continuously monitored and assessed for decompensation. The two parameters that are of concern during intubation are the heart rate and oxygen saturation. Prior to intubation, the child may be given drugs for relaxation. The use of a narcotic or benzodiazapene in conjunction with a fast-acting paralytic agent or a short-acting anesthetic agent may assist the physician in ease of intubation. The child is ventilated with a bag-valve-mask device until the child is well saturated and the heart rate is optimal. During intubation, vagolytic bradycardia may occur. Atropine IV push may be required to increase the heart rate. After the endotracheal tube is placed, it is taped to prevent movement. Placement can be assured through a variety of means. The tube will "fog" with condensation, a CO_2 indicator will change color in the presence of CO_2. Breath sounds will be equal bilaterally, and heart rate and oxygen saturation will be stable. A chest x-ray confirming placement is definitive. Post-airway stabilization care of the ventilated child includes continuous monitoring of vital signs, including oxygen saturation and end-tidal CO_2. The child may require sedation or the use of restraints to avoid dislodgement of the tube. The endotracheal tube should be monitored for placement by marking the placement depth in centimeters relative to the child's teeth or gums. This should be charted at the time of insertion and assessed frequently. Patency of the tube is attained through suctioning. The child should be oxygenated before suctioning if suctioning causes a reduction in oxygen saturation that does not return quickly to baseline. The use of normal saline lavage should be limited to situations where secretions cannot be removed due to thickness without thinning.

In summary, regardless of the cause of a respiratory failure or arrest and the age of the child, the management steps are the same: (1) airway, (2) breathing, and (3) circulation. Attention to these basic steps can significantly improve survival and minimize hypoxic brain damage.

TABLE 36–8. EQUIPMENT GUIDELINES ACCORDING TO AGE AND WEIGHT

	AGE (50TH PERCENTILE WEIGHT)				
EQUIPMENT	Neonate (2.5–4.0 kg)	6 Months (7.0 kg)	1–2 Years (10–12 kg)	5 Years (16–18 kg)	8–10 Years (24–30 kg)
Airway—oral	Infant/small (0)	Small (1)	Small (2)	Medium (3)	Medium/large (4/5)
Breathing					
Self-inflating bag	Infant	Child	Child	Child	Child/adult
O_2 ventilation mask	Newborn	Infant/child	Child	Child	Small adult
Endotracheal tube	3.0–3.5 (uncuffed)	3.5–4.0 (uncuffed)	4.0–4.5 (uncuffed)	5.0–5.5 (uncuffed)	5.5–6.5 (cuffed)
Laryngoscope blade	1 (straight)	1 (straight)	1–2 (straight)	2 (straight or curved)	2–3 (straight or curved)
Suction	6	8	8	10	12
Nasal or orogastric tube (F)	5–8	8	10	10–12	14–18

Adapted from Chameides, L., & Hazinski, M.F. (1997). Pediatric advanced life support *(pp. 4–15). Dallas: American Heart Association.*

VENTILATION REVIEW

1. The infant is predisposed to upper airway obstruction because of a(n)
   A. decreased number of alveoli
   B. immature thermostatic control
   C. increased metabolic rate
   D. small airway diameter
2. The dominant functional disturbance with obstructive lung disease is
   A. increased resistance to airflow
   B. impaired lung expansion
   C. a primary diffusion defect
   D. impaired respiratory control mechanism
3. Clinically detectable central cyanosis is dependent on
   A. arterial oxygen saturation and blood pressure
   B. arterial oxygen saturation and hemoglobin concentration

C. partial pressure of oxygen and hemoglobin concentration
D. partial pressure of carbon dioxide and hemoglobin concentration

4. Chest wall retractions in the young child are produced from
   A. premature glottic closure during expiration
   B. constriction of the anterior nasal passages
   C. increased negative intrapleural pressure during inspiration
   D. diaphragmatic muscular spasms
5. An initial intervention for a child experiencing mild respiratory distress is
   A. endotracheal intubation
   B. elevating the head of the bed
   C. positive pressure ventilation
   D. administration of a mild sedative
6. A 1-year-old known asthmatic patient presents with a respiratory rate (RR) of 60, pale, mild-to-moderate nasal flaring, and substernal retracting, coarse wheezes bilaterally. The child's condition would best be assessed as
   A. mild respiratory distress
   B. respiratory arrest
   C. normal RR and work of breathing for this age group
   D. impending respiratory failure
7. A 3-month-old infant with RSV is in severe respiratory distress with RR 80, copious thick secretions, increased work of breathing, and cyanosis. What would be the immediate intervention?
   A. offer the infant a bottle to calm the infant down
   B. call for a stat chest x-ray
   C. perform bag-valve-mask ventilation
   D. provide 100 percent blow-by oxygen, suction the infant's secretions, and anticipate possible intubation
8. If a child's heart rate and oxygen saturation do not improve with bag-valve-mask ventilation, what intervention should be performed?
   A. obtain a chest x-ray and continue with bag-valve-mask ventilation
   B. perform blind sweep of her mouth for any residual pieces of hot dog
   C. perform abdominal thrust
   D. prepare equipment for assisting the physician in intubation

Answers: 1. D, 2. A, 3. B, 4. C, 5. B, 6. D, 7. D, 8. D

PERFUSION

SECTION FIVE: Maturational Anatomy and Physiology

At the completion of this section, the learner will be able to discuss the unique characteristics of the immature cardiovascular system.

The specific role of the cardiovascular system in the child is to deliver adequate amounts of oxygen and nutrients to body tissue and organs. However, the cardiovascular system is not fully mature at birth and matures over time. The functional differences between the neonatal and adult cardiovascular systems are, for the most part, directly related to transitional circulation. At birth, when the infant begins to breathe, placental circulation is eliminated, and fetal shunts close. Consequently, hemodynamic and anatomic changes take place. The ductus venosus and the ductus arteriosus normally constrict and become nonfunctional. The foramen ovale establishes a functional closure in response to increased left-sided heart pressure. These three fetal shunts are usually eliminated within the first days of life, and adult circulatory patterns are established.

In contrast to the normally rapid closure of fetal shunts, there are some anatomic and hemodynamic changes that occur more gradually. Pulmonary vascular resistance (PVR) drops precipitously after birth from an increase in the diameter of the pulmonary arteries. A further decrease in PVR occurs as the medial muscle layer of the pulmonary arteries continues to thin over the first 2 to 8 weeks of life. Normal adult values of PVR are present at about 2 months of age.

Left ventricular muscle mass and ECG voltage increase over time and correspond to increasing left ventricular workload as systemic vascular resistance increases. Sympathetic innervation is incomplete at birth, suggesting vagal predominance for the first weeks of life (Hazinski & van Stralen, 1990). Table 36–9 summarizes the key maturational changes of the cardiovascular system and their clinical significance.

In summary, the immature cardiovascular system is anatomically and physiologically different. Clinical assessments and management are directly affected by these maturational differences, requiring age-appropriate modification.

SECTION SIX: Etiologies of Shock

At the completion of this section, the learner will be able to describe the most common etiologies of shock in the child.

TABLE 36–9. MATURATIONAL CHANGES OF THE CARDIOVASCULAR SYSTEM

ANATOMY	CLINICAL SIGNIFICANCE
Closure of fetal shunts	Decreased mixing of pulmonary and systemic blood; increased $Sa{O_2}$
PVR decreases Decreased RV workload Decreased RV dominance on ECG	Normal PVR 1st week of life: 8–10 units/m² BSA > 6 weeks of life: 1–3 units/m² BSA
SVR increases Increased LV workload LV wall thickness increases LV dominance on ECG	Normal SVR < 12 months: 10–15 units/m² BSA 12–18 months: 20–30 units/m² BSA
PHYSIOLOGY	**CLINICAL SIGNIFICANCE**
Fetal Hgb replaced with adult Hgb	Oxyhemologlobin dissociation curve shifts to the right
Cardiac output (L/min)	Increases with age Newborn: 0.8–1.0 L/min 5 year-old: 2.5–3.0 L/min 10-year-old: 3.8–4.0 L/min
Cardiac index (CI)	Child's CI is slightly higher than adults Child: 3.5–4.5 L/min/m² BSA
Heart rate	As stroke volume increases, heart rate decreases
Sympathetic innervation of the heart	Incomplete at birth; vagal effects may dominate during first weeks of life
Myocardial contraction	May be less in the newborn due to less contractile tissue per unit of myocardium

PVR, pulmonary vascular resistance; SVR, systemic vascular resistance; SaO_2, arterial oxygen saturation; BSA, body surface area; Hgb, hemoglobin.

Shock is present when poor cardiovascular function results in inadequate perfusion to organs. When cells cannot receive life-sustaining substrate or remove waste, anaerobic metabolism occurs causing cellular damage. Death can occur immediately from cardiovascular collapse or later from multiple organ dysfunction (Chameides & Hazinski, 1997).

Shock can be classified by etiology, its effect on blood pressure, or its effect on cardiac output. By etiology, the three types of shock are hypovolemic, septic, and cardiogenic. Hypovolemic shock is the most common form of shock in children. Common causes are diarrhea, inadequate intake, burns, and trauma.

Septic shock is caused when an infectious organism triggers a host response that compromises cardiovascular function, systemic perfusion, and oxygen delivery and utilization. Septic shock is characterized by increased capillary permeability and shifting of fluid into the extracellular space. More than one-third of children hospitalized in intensive care for more than 3 weeks will develop a nosocomial infection that can lead to sepsis and septic shock. Good hand washing is of great importance to prevent this complication.

Cardiogenic shock occurs when impaired myocardial function significantly compromises cardiac output. It is seen most commonly after cardiac surgery or in conjunction with cardiomyopathy (Hazinski, 1992).

Shock Characterized by Its Effect on Cardiac Output

Hypovolemic shock is commonly associated with low cardiac output. Hypovolemic shock activates the sympathetic nervous system compensatory mechanisms to divert blood flow from the skin, mesenteric, and renal circulation to the heart and brain. Signs of low cardiac output are tachycardia and normal or low blood pressure (late sign). Other signs are cool, mottled skin; delayed capillary refill; poor-quality or absent pulses; decreased urine output; irritability; and lethargy (Chameides & Hazinski, 1997).

Septic shock can be associated with a high cardiac output state. The cardiac output is unevenly distributed, however, resulting in poor perfusion to some tissue beds. These ischemic areas generate lactic acid, leading to acidosis and inappropriate blood flow distribution. Symptoms include warm extremities, normal capillary refill, bounding pulses, wide pulse pressure, normal urine output, and mild mental confusion. For this reason, cardiac output should not be evaluated as low or high but rather as adequate or inadequate.

Finally, shock may also be characterized as compensated or decompensated. When compensated shock is present, blood pressure is normal, although signs of inadequate perfusion are present. Decompensated shock occurs when hypotension develops.

A quick assessment can determine the adequacy of cardiovascular function. The assessment includes vital signs and systemic perfusion. After a patent airway is assured, the assessment progresses to circulation. (See Box on facing page and Table 36–10 for normal heart rate and for blood pressure values for children). Heart rate is used

TABLE 36–10. NORMAL BLOOD PRESSURE RANGES

AGE	SYSTOLIC PRESSURE (MM HG)	DIASTOLIC PRESSURE (MM HG)
Neonate (1 month)	85–100	51–65
Infant (6 months)	87–105	53–66
Toddler (2 years)	95–105	53–66
School age (7 years)	97–112	57–71
Adolescent (15 years)	112–128	66–80

Blood pressure tables taken from the 50th to 90th percentile ranges of the ages noted; extrapolated from graphs. *Adapted from Horan, M.J. (Chairman). (1987). Report of the Second Task Force on Blood Pressure in Children 1987.* Pediatrics *79:5–7. Reproduced by permission of* Pediatrics, *vol. 79, p. 57, copyright © 1987.*

to assess the adequacy of cardiac output. Cardiac output is the product of heart rate and stroke volume (the amount of blood pumped with each heartbeat). The child with impaired circulation cannot increase stroke volume to increase cardiac output. The child can increase heart rate to increase cardiac output. A child commonly develops **tachycardia** as a response to stressors. Anxiety, fear, fever, pain, as well as hypoxia, hypercapnia, hypovolemia, and cardiac impairment may all result in tachycardia.

Bradycardia is an early sign of hypoxemia in an infant but a late and ominous sign of hypoxemia in a child. Children usually compensate for inadequate cardiac output by increasing, not decreasing, their heart rate. The normal heart rate limits for children depend not only on age and physiologic status but on the emotional state as well. In general, the normal ranges of pulse when the child is awake are:

Newborn	100 to 180
1 year	100 to 160
2 years	80 to 110
4 years	70 to 110
> 8 years	65 to 110

Unlike the adult, life-threatening dysrhythmias in children often are a secondary response to hypoxemia and acidosis. Once hypoxemia and acidosis are corrected, normal sinus rhythm usually resumes and is maintained. For emergency assessment and management, pediatric dysrhythmias are classified into one of three groups based on heart rate:

1. Tachydysrhythmias
2. Bradydysrhythmias
3. Disorganized or absent rhythms

Table 36–11 summarizes the most common dysrhythmias seen in children and their clinical significance.

Blood Pressure

Blood pressure is determined by cardiac output and systemic vascular resistance. Normal blood pressure (Table 36–10) can be maintained despite a fall in cardiac output. Children compensate for the fall in cardiac output by increasing heart rate, vasoconstriction, and increasing myocardial contractility. When these compensatory mechanisms fail, hypotension develops and decompensated shock occurs. Cardiac arrest is imminent. Mild hypotension in a child at risk for vascular collapse must be treated immediately.

In a pediatric trauma victim with blood loss, the circulating blood volume should be estimated. Neonates should have 85 cc/kg blood volume, infants 80 cc/kg blood volume, and children 75 cc/kg of circulating blood volume. A rapid blood loss of as little as 5 to 10 percent of circulating blood volume can be significant for an infant or child. Hypotension usually does not occur until a 25 percent blood loss occurs because of the child's compensatory mechanisms (Chameides & Hazinski, 1997).

Systemic Perfusion

Early compensated shock must be recognized because tachycardia is nonspecific and hypotension is a late and ominous sign. Early compensated shock can be recognized by evaluating the presence and strength of peripheral pulses and by determining the quality of end-organ perfusion.

Assessment of Pulses

The carotid, axillary, brachial, radial, femoral, and pedal pulses should be palpable in healthy children. If a child has a weaker peripheral pulse in relation to a central pulse, this can be an early sign of decreased cardiac output. Pulse volume is related to pulse pressure (the difference between systolic and diastolic blood pressure).

TABLE 36–11. PEDIATRIC RHYTHM DISTURBANCES

CLASSIFICATION	ETIOLOGY	CLINICAL SIGNIFICANCE
Tachyarrhythmias	Sinus tachycardia	Related to physical/emotional stress
	Supraventricular tachycardia (SVT)	Usually caused by a reentry mechanism
	Ventricular tachycardia	Usually related to underlying structural heart disease or prolonged QT interval Other causes include poisons, medications, hypoxia, acidosis, electrolyte imbalance
Bradyarrhythmias	Sinus bradycardia	Most common terminal rhythms with cardiopulmonary arrest
	Sinus node arrest with escape beats	
	Atrioventricular blocks	
Absent or disorganized rhythms	Asystole	Terminal rhythm with cardiopulmonary arrest
	Ventricular fibrillation (VF)	Uncommon rhythm in children
	Electromechanical dissociation (EMD)	Exact mechanism unknown, may result from tension pneumothorax, cardiac tamponade, hypovolemia, severe acidosis, hypoxemia

When pulse pressure narrows and the pulse feels thready, cardiac output is decreased. In contrast, a wide pulse pressure and a bounding pulse indicate early septic shock with high cardiac output. An absent central pulse should be treated as cardiac arrest.

Assessment of Quality of End-Organ Perfusion

SKIN PERFUSION. End-organ perfusion can be determined by assessing the blood flow to the skin, brain, and kidneys. Evaluate blood flow to the skin through touch and appearance. Under normal conditions, a child who is adequately perfused should feel warm to the touch. When cardiac output is decreased, a line will be felt between warmness and coolness. This line ascends toward the trunk. Capillary refill also assesses the quality of skin perfusion. Capillary refill should be < 2 seconds when the extremity is elevated above heart level. A prolonged capillary refill can indicate shock, fever, or cold temperatures.

Under normal conditions, infants and children should be pink on nonpigmented surfaces. Mottling, paleness, and peripheral cyanosis indicate poor perfusion. When vasoconstriction occurs as a compensatory response to increase cardiac output, skin will be gray or ashen in a newborn and very pale in an older child.

BRAIN PERFUSION. The quality of brain perfusion can be assessed quickly through use of the modified Glasgow Coma Scale. Assess the child by determining level of alertness. Is the child awake, responsive to pain, responsive to voice, or unresponsive? For more in-depth neurological assessment, see Section Nine of this module.

KIDNEY PERFUSION. Normal urine output for children is 1 to 2 cc/kg/hr. A low urine output indicates poor cardiac output and poor perfusion. A Foley catheter may be necessary to accurately determine urine output.

In summary, circulatory failure represents inadequate perfusion of tissue. The clinical manifestations of circulatory failure result from compensatory mechanisms and end-organ dysfunction. The key to a successful outcome is early recognition and treatment of impending circulatory failure.

SECTION SEVEN: Treatment of Shock

At the completion of this section, the learner will be able to describe specific interventions used to manage a child with circulatory failure.

The primary goal in treatment of circulatory failure is to restore normal blood flow and maximize oxygen delivery to organs. The interventions depend on the specific functional shock state and the degree of cardiovascular dysfunction.

Priorities of management of patients in shock include adequate oxygen by providing 100 percent O_2 with an appropriate airway adjunct; continuous monitoring of vital signs and O_2 saturations; establishing vascular access; fluid support; and pharmacological interventions.

Vascular Access

Vascular access must be established to ensure fluid and drug administration. It can be very difficult to establish vascular access in children with cardiovascular impairment. Peripheral venipuncture is the first route to try. Shock or cardiopulmonary arrest may make peripheral access difficult. In these cases, larger peripheral veins such as the femoral, median cubital, or saphenous can be used. If peripheral access is unsuccessful and an experienced practitioner is available, central access may be attempted. Femoral venous access is preferred because it does not interfere with health care providers who may be at the head of the child providing airway management. Each facility must develop its own protocol for attempts at venous access in children. Numerous, repetitive, unsuccessful attempts to establish venous access cause unnecessary delay in treatment. Vascular access is required for fluid resuscitation although some medications (LANE—lidocaine, atropine, naloxen, and epinephrine) can be given via endotracheal tube. Intraosseous access is recommended for children under 6 years of age when peripheral venous access cannot be established rapidly. It provides a safe and reliable method for the administration of fluids, medications, and blood products. Insertion can be achieved in 30 to 60 seconds. The intraosseous site is on the proximal tibia about 1 to 3 cm below the tibial tuberosity. Onset of action of drugs delivered intraosseously is comparable to venous access (Chameides & Hazinski, 1997). Onset of action of drugs is enhanced by adequate normal saline flush between drugs. Intraosseous access is contraindicated in the presence of a fracture in the pelvis or femur proximal to the tibia or in the tibial bone itself.

Fluid Administration

The two most common etiologies of shock in the child are hypovolemia and sepsis. Both of these forms of shock require volume resuscitation. Once vascular access is obtained, the nurse should assist with rapid infusion of fluids (20 cc/kg) to establish intravascular volume. The specific type of fluid to use is controversial. The American Heart Association recommends a balanced crystalloid solution (normal saline or lactated Ringer's) for first-line volume expansion. Crystalloid fluid remains in the intravascular system for a short time. This may require boluses of up to five times the deficit to restore volume. Each bolus should be administered rapidly, in less than 20 minutes (Chameides & Hazinski, 1997). This is well tolerated in children with no underlying disease. A child with health deficits such as underlying cardiac or pulmonary conditions may not be able to tolerate the increased fluid volume. Colloids (synthetic colloid or blood products) remain in the intravascular system hours longer than crystalloids. Crystalloids should be used as a first line for fluid replacement, with colloids a second line because of the increased cost, less availability, and potential for allergic reaction.

Every child receiving fluid resuscitation must be continuously reassessed. This is accomplished through monitoring of vital signs, O_2 saturation, and quality of end-organ perfusion.

Medications

In addition to volume expansion, medications may be indicated to improve myocardial contractility, to correct metabolic acidosis, to correct hypoxemia, and to improve cardiac rate and rhythm (Chameides & Hazinski, 1997). Oxygen should be administered in the highest available concentration to the unstable child. Table 36–12 lists the first-line medications used in pediatric cardiopulmonary resuscitation. After each intervention, the nurse should reassess the patient's clinical response (e.g., vital signs and systemic perfusion). Continuous infusions of medications also may be used to support blood pressure and maintain CO.

In summary, definitive management of circulatory failure depends on the etiology. Most often, etiology can be determined based on physical examination and history. The most common form of shock in children is hypovolemic or sepsis. Nursing management is based on early recognition of signs and symptoms of shock, assisting with venous access and volume expansion, and continuous reassessment.

TABLE 36–12. DRUGS USED IN PEDIATRIC ADVANCED LIFE SUPPORT

DRUG	DOSAGE (PEDIATRIC)	REMARKS
Adenosine	0.1–0.2 mg/kg Maximum single dose: 12 mg	Rapid IV bolus
Atropine sulfate[a]	0.02 mg/kg	Minimum dose: 0.1 mg Maximum single dose: 0.5 mg in child, 1.0 mg in adolescent
Bretylium	5 mg/kg; may be increased to 10 mg/kg	Rapid IV
Calcium chloride 10%	20 mg/kg	Give slowly
Dobutamine hydrochloride	2–20 μg/kg/min	Titrate to desired effect
Dopamine hydrochloride	2–20 μg/kg/min	α-Adrenergic action dominates at ≥ 15–20 μg/kg/min
Epinephrine for bradycardia[a]	IV/IO: 0.01 mg/kg (1:10,000, 0.1 mL/kg) ET: 0.1 mg/kg (1:1000, 0.1 mL/kg)	
Epinephrine for asystolic or pulseless arrest[a]	**First dose:** IV/IO: 0.01 mg/kg (1:10,000, 0.1 mL/kg) ET: 0.1 mg/kg (1:1000, 0.1 mL/kg) IV/IO doses as high as 0.2 mg/kg of 1:1000 may be effective. **Subsequent doses:** IV/IO/ET: 0.1 mg/kg (1:1000, 0.1 mL/kg) Repeat every 3–5 min IV/IO doses as high as 0.2 mg/kg of 1:1000 may be effective.	
Epinephrine infusion	Initial at 0.1 μg/kg/min Higher infusion dose used if asystole present	Titrate to desired effect (0.1–1.0 μg/kg/min)
Lidocaine[a]	1 mg/kg	
Lidocaine infusion	20–50 μg/kg/min	
Naloxone[a]	If ≤ 5 years old or ≤ 20 kg: 0.1 mg/kg If > 5 years old or > 20 kg: 2.0 mg/kg	Titrate to desired effect
Prostaglandin E_1	0.05–0.1 μg/kg/min	Monitor for apnea, hypotension, hypoglycemia
Sodium bicarbonate	1 mEq/kg/dose or 0.3 × kg × base deficit	Infuse slowly and only if ventilation is adequate

[a] For ET administration, dilute medication with normal saline to a volume of 3 to 5 mL and follow with several positive-pressure ventilations.
Source: Chameides, L., & Hazinski, M.F. (1997). Textbook of pediatric advanced life support. *Dallas: American Heart Association.*

PERFUSION REVIEW

1. What vital sign is used to differentiate compensated shock from decompensated?
   A. blood pressure
   B. heart rate
   C. capillary refill
   D. respiratory rate
2. What type of shock is associated with a high cardiac output?
   A. septic
   B. hypovolemic
   C. anaphylactic
   D. cardiogenic
3. What is the first-line drug of choice for pulseless arrest in a child?
   A. epinephrine
   B. lidocaine
   C. glucose
   D. sodium bicarbonate
4. In the child, the most common functional shock state is
   A. obstructive
   B. cardiogenic
   C. hypovolemic
   D. transport
5. An early sign of compensated shock in children is
   A. hypotension
   B. bradycardia
   C. tachycardia
   D. absent femoral pulse
6. The recommended first-line IV fluid for hypovolemic shock in children is
   A. lactated Ringer's solution
   B. dextrose 5 percent in water
   C. dextrose 5 percent with 0.2 percent normal saline
   D. fresh frozen plasma
7. If a peripheral IV line insertion has been attempted for 10 minutes without success in an infant, access to the circulation should be attempted next by which of the following routes?
   A. central cannulation
   B. cutdown cannulation
   C. intraosseous cannulation
   D. arterial cannulation
8. After receiving one bolus of crystalloid solution, an infant's vital signs are the following: heart rate 180, respiratory rate 60, blood pressure 50 by palpation. The infant remains cool and pale. The next action is
   A. rebolus with 20 cc/kg of crystalloid solution
   B. begin CPR
   C. administer epinephrine
   D. continue to monitor

Answers: 1. A, 2. A, 3. A, 4. C, 5. C, 6. A, 7. C, 8. A

COGNITION/PERCEPTION

SECTION EIGHT: Maturational Anatomy and Physiology

At the completion of this section, the learner will be able to discuss the unique anatomic and physiologic characteristics of the immature CNS.

Accurate assessment and management of CNS disorders in children is complicated by the fact that CNS development is incomplete at birth. In fact, for the first 3 years of life, CNS maturation continues at the same rate as in utero. Because the immature CNS is qualitatively and quantitatively different from the adult's CNS, it is commonly believed that it may respond to injuries differently. This section discusses the unique features of the immature CNS.

A number of developmental differences of the immature CNS not only predispose the young child to traumatic brain injury but also are responsible for specific types of characteristic brain injuries. Table 36–13 summarizes the key development differences of the immature CNS. Postnatal myelination, glial cell growth, dendritic arborization, and increased synaptic connections are responsible for the rapid increase in head size and weight. The child's brain weight is approximately 70 percent of adult weight at 4 years of age and 90 percent at 6 years of age. The child's relatively large head, as well as limited supporting neck muscles, predisposes him or her to traumatic brain injury with multiple trauma. In addition, because the skull is thin and pliable, it offers less protection against external trauma.

Adequate cerebral blood flow (CBF) is critical for normal cellular function of the brain. Factors that control CBF (e.g., $PaCO_2$, cerebral perfusion pressure [CPP]) have been studied extensively in animals and in adults, but comparable research does not exist for newborns and infants. Because of the physiologic differences among newborns, infants, and adults, mechanisms that control CBF in the adult may not hold true for the young child.

TABLE 36–13. UNIQUE FEATURES OF THE IMMATURE NERVOUS SYSTEM

Myelinization	Within the CNS, myelinization progresses most rapidly in the first postnatal year and is complete by the second decade of life
Glial cell population	Cell members increase into third year of life
Dendritic arborization and synaptic connection	Occur primarily in the first and second postnatal years
Brain weight	Increases from 25% of adult weight at birth to 70% of adult weight at 4 years of age
Skull	Thin and pliable at birth with unfused suture lines (independent floating plates) Orbital roofs and floors of middle fossa smooth
Water content of cortical and white matter	Decreases from 87% and 89% at birth to 85% and 78% during first decade
Cerebral blood flow	Normal values are not known for infants and young children
Cerebrospinal fluid (CSF)	Normal volume production is not known for infants and young children A few white blood cells present in CSF; higher concentration of glucose and protein in CSF

Adapted from Vernon-Levett, P. (1991). Head injuries in children. Crit Care Nurs Clin North Am 3:412.

In summary, there are significant anatomic and physiologic differences of the CNS between young children and adults. CNS growth occurs at a very rapid rate for the first few years of life. Age-related differences in the CNS must be considered when assessing and managing a child with neurologic dysfunction.

SECTION NINE: Neurologic Exam

At the completion of this section, the learner will be able to describe the key components of the neurologic examination of the child with altered mental status.

Effective nursing management of the neurologically impaired child is based on initial and serial neurologic assessments. As described in Section Nine of this module, the infant's CNS is structurally and functionally different than the older child's and adult's CNS. For these reasons, the neurologic examination of the infant varies from that of the older child and the adult. Differences in the neurologic examination do not vary in terms of the process but in terms of findings. The purpose of this section is to describe the key components and significant findings of the rapid neurologic assessment of the child with impaired CNS function. Diagnostic data used to assess the child with status epilepticus, traumatic brain injury (TBI), and CNS infection are described.

Regardless of age, the clinical manifestations of neurologic dysfunction are related to the degree and duration of CNS hypoperfusion (relative or actual). Neurologic dysfunction with corresponding assessments is on a continuum. A child with a severe primary TBI may be in unresponsive coma, whereas a child with a slow-growing intracranial tumor may have progressive signs of increased ICP. A complete neurologic examination may be inappropriate, impractical, and too time consuming for all patients. However, there are key components of the neurologic assessment that must be completed for every patient: patient history, vital signs, level of consciousness, motor function, pupil signs, and brain stem function.

Patient History

The patient history can provide valuable information regarding the patient's baseline neurologic development, diagnosis, and prognosis. Pertinent history information should be individualized to the age, condition, and disposition of the child. For a traumatic injury or an acute event, the sequence of events before the injury or episode is important. For more gradual deterioration, the chief complaint and related assessments are critical to diagnosis and management. Table 36–14 lists additional pertinent history information that needs to be obtained on admission.

Vital Signs

Vital signs often are nonspecific and need to be correlated with coexisting disease states. Temperature may be abnormally elevated due to infection, drug intoxication, shock, and intracranial bleeding. It may also be low in the newborn with immature thermostatic control or a preexisting infection. Abnormal patterns of breathing associated with pathologic lesions may be difficult to differ-

TABLE 36–14. PERTINENT HISTORY INFORMATION

Infant	Maternal history Age, previous births, prepartum and intrapartum course, exposure to drugs and infections Neonatal history Feeding, sucking, and crying patterns; presence of apnea, cyanotic spells, infection, jaundice, or seizures; Apgar score Developmental milestones Motor Infantile reflexes Verbal Medical history Psychiatric history
Child (> 2 years)	Developmental milestones Motor Verbal Medical history Psychiatric history

entiate in the child. Respiratory assessment should include rate and description of the pattern of breathing. Abnormal cardiac rhythms usually are transient. However, symptomatic bradycardia often is a late sign of increased ICP. Another late and inconstant sign of increased ICP is an increase in systolic pressure, with a widened pulse pressure. ↑S ↓D

Level of Consciousness

Consciousness is a state of awareness of self and environment. An altered level of consciousness (LOC) results from disease states that significantly alter functioning of the cerebral hemispheres, the reticular activating system, or both. The range of LOC may vary from minor alterations to unresponsive coma. The Glasgow Coma Scale (GCS) is a widely used neurologic assessment tool to grade the depth of coma by standardizing assessments. It consists of three sections, each of which measures a separate function of LOC: arousability, mentation, and motor function. The GCS has one main disadvantage in infants: it cannot accurately assess preverbal infants. As a result, a number of institutions and individuals have modified the GCS. Table 36–15 is an example of a modified GCS for infants.

Motor Function

Motor functions can be assessed easily in the older child by using the categories outlined in the GCS. In the infant, motor function must be compared with developmental milestones and age-appropriate primitive reflexes. For example, a positive Babinski response is an abnormal finding in the older child and adult but a normal finding in the 6 month old.

TABLE 36–15. MODIFIED COMA SCALE FOR INFANTS

ACTIVITY	BEST RESPONSE	SCORE
Eye opening	Spontaneous	4
	To speech	3
	To pain	2
	None	1
Verbal	Coos and babbles	5
	Irritable cries	4
	Cries to pain	3
	Moans to pain	2
	None	1
Motor	Normal spontaneous movements	6
	Withdraws to touch	5
	Withdraws to pain	4
	Abnormal flexion	3
	Abnormal extension	2
	None	1

From Holbrook, P. (1993). Textbook of pediatric critical care. *Philadelphia: W.B. Saunders, © 1993.*

Pupil Signs

The integrity of the brain stem and the depth of coma can be further assessed by examining the pupils. As in the adult, the child's pupils are evaluated for size, reactivity, and shape. Abnormal findings and their clinical significance are essentially the same in the child as in the adult.

Brain Stem Function

In addition to pupil signs, brain stem function should be further assessed. For the comatose child, brain stem function is limited to assessment of the corneal reflex, the oculocephalic response, the oculovestibular response, and abnormal spontaneous eye movements. The presence of abnormal findings has the same clinical significance for the child as for the adult. Refer to Module 17 for additional information.

Meningeal Irritation Signs

If meningitis is suspected, the presence of meningeal irritation should be assessed. Kernig's sign may be present and is elicited by placing the child supine with the hips flexed and passively extending the leg at the knee. With significant meningeal irritation, the child may resist and complain of back pain. Brudzinski's sign produces involuntary flexion of the knees and hips with passive flexion of the child's neck when supine. Signs of meningeal irritation may be less specific or unreliable in the infant. However, the infant may have paradoxical irritability: comforting the child by holding him may paradoxically produce more irritability.

Intracranial Pressure

Normal ICP in newborns is 0.7 to 1.5 mm Hg; in infants it is 1.5 to 6.0 mm Hg, and in children, it is 3.0 to 7.5. ICP is age dependent (Curley, Smith, & Maloney-Harmon, 1996). In infants with open fontanels and unfused cranial sutures, clinical signs of increased ICP are less acute and more nonspecific than in the older child. Table 36–16 lists the signs and symptoms of increased ICP in children.

Clinical evidence of increased ICP may not be present until significant increases in ICP have occurred. The most precise means of assessing changes in ICP and evaluating the effectiveness of pressure reduction therapy is with continuous ICP monitoring. A number of invasive ICP monitoring devices are available, all of which have advantages and disadvantages. The most common sites for ICP monitoring are intraventricular, subdural, epidural, and parenchymal. Newer fiber-optic monitoring devices can be placed in several common sites for ICP monitoring.

TABLE 36–16. SIGNS AND SYMPTOMS OF INCREASED INTRACRANIAL PRESSURE[a]

Infants < 2 years of age	Lethargy
	Poor feeding
	Poor suck
	Bulging, tense anterior fontanel
	Increased head circumference
	Irritability
Older child	Nausea
	Vomiting
	Anorexia
	Headache
	Papilledema (chronic increased intracranial pressure)
	Alteration in level of consciousness
	Visual disturbances
	Lethargy
	Third nerve palsy (transtentorial herniation)
	Sixth nerve palsy (diffuse increased intracranial pressure)

[a] Clinical manifestations vary and depend on how rapidly cerebral hypertension develops.

Cerebral Perfusion Pressure

CPP is calculated as the numerical difference of the mean arterial pressure (MAP) and the mean ICP with both transducers referenced to the ear canal with the patient flat (Rosner, Rosner, & Johnson, 1995). Normal CPP has not been determined in children. However, evidence indicates that a pressure above 50 mm Hg is necessary for adequate cerebral perfusion. CPP less than 40 mm Hg because of cerebral hypertension or systemic hypotension is a cause for concern (Curley, Smith, & Maloney-Harmon, 1996).

Neurodiagnostic Evaluation

To assist with the clinical evaluation of the neurologically impaired child, several neurodiagnostic techniques may be used. A lumbar puncture for CSF analysis is a commonly used procedure in children with suspected CNS infection. CSF values in a child with bacterial meningitis include:

- Cloudy appearance
- WBC count > 500/mL
- Protein > 100 mg/100 mL
- Glucose < ½ to ⅓ blood glucose
- Gram stain/culture: positive
- Polymorphonuclear leukocytes predominate

Signs and symptoms of increased ICP (focal neurologic deficits, papilledema, altered LOC) contraindicate a lumbar puncture.

The use of skull radiographs in evaluating traumatic brain injury has been under much debate in recent years (Marshall et al., 1990). In most situations, computed tomography (CT) remains the procedure of choice with a head injury < 72 hours old (Snow et al., 1986). Magnetic resonance imaging (MRI) is superior to CT in imaging the posterior fossa, spinal cord structures, small vascular lesions, and most brain tumors (Marshall et al., 1990). Electroencephalography (EEG) may be used as an adjunct to the clinical examination in situations of seizures or to establish absence of brain waves. The indications, use, and interpretation of EEG findings are similar for children and adults.

In summary, the key components of the neurologic assessment are the same regardless of age. However, the evaluation process should be adapted to the developmental level and conditions of the child. It is essential that the examiner be able to distinguish between age-appropriate normal findings and subtle abnormal changes in neurologic function. Early detection of subtle changes with prompt treatment can improve outcome.

SECTION TEN: Nursing Management

A number of injuries and disease processes can adversely affect the CNS. This section discusses the most common forms of severe neurologic dysfunction in children: status epilepticus, traumatic brain injury, and CNS infection. Defining terms and pathogenesis of each disorder are described. At the completion of this section, the learner will be able to discuss the nursing management of the neurologically impaired child.

The first steps in managing a child with acute neurologic dysfunction are related to the ABCs (airway, breathing, and circulation). Hypoxia or hypotension may invalidate the neurologic assessment. Airway patency, adequacy of breathing, and perfusion must be assessed and supported if necessary. Elective intubation may be required for airway protection and controlled hyperventilation. Once oxygenation, ventilation, and circulation are adequate, attention may be directed to treating the underlying neurologic disorder. The focus of this section is to describe the management of a child with status epilepticus, TBI, and CNS infection.

Status Epilepticus

Seizures are described as abnormal electrical impulses originating from the cerebral cortex. Status epilepticus is defined as a continuing series of seizures without regaining full consciousness between seizures or one continuous seizure lasting approximately 30 minutes. The cause of status epilepticus in children is approximately 30 percent idiopathic and 60 to 70 percent symptomatic (Delgado, 1990). The majority of symptomatic cases are from hyperthermia (febrile seizures) and CNS infection. Less common causes of seizures include trauma, metabolic derangement, drug intoxication, and acute anoxia. Although the cause of status epilepticus may vary, the common final pathway of uncontrolled electrical activity is anoxia and cellular death.

The goals in treating a child with status epilepticus are threefold: maintenance of adequate CBF, controlling seizure activity, and treatment of systemic abnormalities. Adequate CBF can be maintained with adherence to the basic principles of the ABCs. When a child is in status epilepticus, the nurse should be prepared to protect the patient from physical injury, prevent aspiration by turning the patient's head to the side, and maximize oxygenation by administering oxygen. Hypoglycemia is a common finding, precipitating a seizure in the young infant. Therefore, a rapid glucose approximation (using a glucose meter) should be obtained as soon as feasible. Usual laboratory tests are ABG, electrolytes including calcium and blood urea nitrogen (BUN), and a urine specimen for toxicology.

There are no universally accepted guidelines for the selection or order of administration of anticonvulsants. However, a number of general principles are considered by the health care team when selecting appropriate drug therapy:

1. The IV route is preferred.
2. Long-acting medications must follow short-acting medications for maintenance.
3. Respiratory depression should be expected and easily controlled.

Nurses should be aware of the commonly used anticonvulsants to control seizures, as well as their side effects. For example, respiratory depression is a common side effect with many anticonvulsants. Therefore, nurses should always be prepared to assist with airway protection and supportive ventilation. Table 36–17 lists commonly used anticonvulsants to control seizures in children.

As the seizure is being controlled, it is also important to control systemic abnormalities (e.g., hypoglycemia, hyperthermia, hypoxemia) that may have caused or resulted from the seizure.

Traumatic Brain Injury

TBI is one of the leading causes of mortality and morbidity in children. TBI in children is different from TBI in adults in several important ways: mechanism of injury, specific types of injury, and response to injury. The most common cause of TBI in infancy is falls. The older child is more often injured from a motor vehicle–related accident as a passenger, pedestrian, or cyclist.

Specific types of TBI commonly are classified according to chronologic events. CNS damage that can be attributed directly to forces at the moment of impact are primary injuries. CNS damage that develops as a consequence of the primary injury is referred to as a secondary injury. Secondary TBI most often has a common final pathway of raised ICP, which is an important feature determining outcome. Table 36–18 summarizes the most common forms of primary and secondary head injuries in children.

Although the exact mechanisms are not understood, the immature CNS responds to injury differently in children. The overall incidence of diffuse bilateral cerebral swelling and subsequent increased intracranial pressure (increased ICP) is much higher in children compared to adults. The incidence of focal brain injury is lower in children compared to adults (Bruce et al., 1981).

Because of the relatively low incidence of intracranial lesions in children with TBI, most injuries are nonoperable. The most common secondary injury in children is diffuse bilateral cerebral swelling. Consequently, aggressive medical management to control increased ICP is the guiding principle for treating TBI in children. Table 36–19 lists the independent and collaborative nursing interventions to control increased ICP. As a general rule,

TABLE 36–17. INITIAL ANTICONVULSANTS TO CONTROL STATUS EPILEPTICUS

DRUG	DOSE	RATE OF ADMINISTRATION	TIME TO EFFECT	SIDE EFFECTS
Rapid-acting agents				
Lorazepam 2 mg/mL	0.03–0.1 mg/kg × 4, 20 minutes apart, maximum dose 4 mg	1 mg/min	2–3 minutes; 60–90 minutes for peak effect	Drowsiness, confusion, ataxia
Diazepam (undiluted) (used less frequently)	Begin 0.25 mg/kg IV and titrate to effect; maximum dose 10 mg	< 1 mg/min	1–2 minutes	Respiratory depression; thrombophlebitis
Midazolam	0.075 mg/kg IV 0.150 mg/kg IM			Same as above; respiratory arrest
Longer-acting agents				
Phenytoin 50 mg/mL; dilute in normal saline 1:10	10–15 mg/kg	20–50 mg/min	10 minutes	Heart block; hypotension
Phenobarbital 130 mg/mL	10 mg/kg up to 30 mg/kg	30 mg/min	10–12 minutes	Respiratory depression; hypotension

From Blumer, J.L. (1990). A practical guide to pediatric intensive care *(p. 231). Chicago: Mosby-Year Book; and Hazinski, M. (1992).* Nursing care of the critically ill child. *Chicago: Mosby-Year Book.*

TABLE 36–18. COMMON HEAD INJURIES IN CHILDREN

Primary	Minor
	Caput succedaneum[a]
	Cephalohematoma[a]
	Scalp laceration
	Scalp contusion
	Cerebral laceration
	Moderate/severe
	Concussion
	Contusion
	Skull fractures
	Simple linear
	Basilar
	Depressed
	Growing[a]
	Diffuse axonal injury
Secondary	Moderate/severe
	Expanding intracranial lesions
	Diffuse cerebral edema

[a] Usually limited to infancy.

TABLE 36–19. NURSING MANAGEMENT TO ASSURE ADEQUATE CEREBRAL PERFUSION

Independent nursing interventions	HOB neutral
	Position head in midline
	Hyperventilate with bag-valve-mask; for acutely ↑ ICP, be careful to avoid ↓ in arterial blood pressure and central perfusion pressure
	Preoxygenate and hyperventilate before suctioning
	Maintain normothermia
	Organize nursing care to minimize patient stimulation
Collaborative nursing interventions	Maintain patent airway
	Administer supplemental oxygen to keep Pao_2 > 80–90 mm Hg
	Administer diuretics as ordered
	Administer anticonvulsants as ordered for seizure control
	Administer barbiturate therapy as ordered; monitor serum levels, neurologic status, and hemodynamic status
	Consider administering neuromuscular blocking agent to induce pharmacological paralysis
	Drain CSF as ordered to maintain ICP
	Administer vasopressors to keep MAP elevated to sustain CPP

the least invasive therapy to control increased ICP should be initiated first. Once increased ICP is controlled, the last intervention to be initiated or the most invasive intervention should be discontinued while continuously monitoring ICP.

CNS Infections

The most common type of CNS infection during childhood is meningitis (inflammation of the meninges), and it is almost always bacterial in origin. The highest incidence occurs in infants less than 1 year of age. In newborns, the most common pathogens producing acute bacterial meningitis are group B streptococci, *Escherichia coli*, and *Listeria monocytogenes*. Between 2 months and 12 years of age, the primary offending pathogens include *Streptococcus pneumoniae*, and *Neisseria meningitidis*.

Invasion of the meninges most often results from bacteremia from a distant site of infection, such as the upper respiratory tract. Less frequently, it may develop as a consequence of direct pathogenic invasion from penetrating trauma, surgical procedures, or paranasal infections. If the bacterial infection is left untreated or progresses rapidly throughout the CNS, irreversible damage or death usually results from increased ICP.

The goal in treating bacterial meningitis is early recognition, early administration of antimicrobials, and control of systemic effects. Early diagnosis and treatment are dependent on the neurologic assessment discussed in Section Nine. The selection of antimicrobials is based on the most likely pathogens for a given age group. Until CSF culture results are known, broad-spectrum antibiotics are used for all suspected cases of meningitis. Advanced cases of meningitis also may cause abnormal systemic effects, such as hypotension, hyperthermia, and IICP. Immediate attention must be given to supporting circulation and controlling IICP or decreased CPP.

Viral Encephalitis

Viral encephalitis is an acute inflammation of the brain and meninges. The most common viruses causing encephalitis are herpes simplex and arboviruses. Viral growth begins outside the brain and spreads to the CSF through the circulation or passively through the blood–brain barrier.

Clinical manifestations are similar to those of meningitis. However, the patient may show signs of changes in behavior. Agitation, seizures, headache, fever, and changes in LOC. Treatment includes anticonvulsants, analgesics, and antiviral therapy (Curley, Smith, & Maloney-Harmon, 1996).

In summary, the most common CNS disorders seen in the acutely ill child include status epilepticus, TBI, and CNS infection. Status epilepticus is usually a symptom of an underlying problem, TBI produces characteristic head injuries in young children, and meningitis occurs most often in the infant. Initial management of the child with an acute neurologic disorder is based on maintaining adequate cerebral blood flow by focusing on the ABCs. Beyond resuscitation, therapy should be directed to controlling systemic effects and correcting the primary disorder.

COGNITION/PERCEPTION REVIEW

1. Which of the following statements best explains why the young child may be predisposed to traumatic brain injury?
   A. cerebral blood flow is lower in the child, which alters sensory and motor function
   B. the ratio of brain weight to body weight is greater in the child
   C. the skull thickness is greater in the child
   D. cranial nerve function is incomplete, altering motor function and balance
2. The best description of a positive Kernig's sign is
   A. involuntary flexion of the knees and hips with passive flexion of the child's neck
   B. resistance and complaints of pain with passive flexion of the lower leg while supine with hips flexed
   C. resistance and complaints of back pain with passive extension of the leg at the knee while supine with hips flexed
   D. increased irritability while holding the child
3. Intracranial hypertension following traumatic brain injury is more common in children than adults because
   A. there is a higher incidence of focal brain injury in children
   B. loss of autoregulation is more common in children
   C. diffuse bilateral cerebral edema is more common in children
   D. children do not respond as well to osmotic diuretics
4. Bacterial meningitis most often results from
   A. direct penetrating trauma to the CNS
   B. spina bifida
   C. a paranasal infection
   D. bacteremia from a distant site of infection

Refer to the following case study to answer Questions 5 through 8.

Melanie, an 18-month-old child, is brought to the ICU after being an unrestrained passenger in an MVC. Vital signs are temperature 98.6°F (37°C), heart rate 80, respiratory rate 12, and blood pressure 150/50 mm Hg. Breath sounds are clear, urine culture negative, WBC 20,000. She has pupil asymmetry.

5. If Melanie is not treated quickly, which of the following pathophysiologic processes may develop?
   A. decreased perfusion from cardiogenic shock
   B. decreased perfusion from hypovolemic shock
   C. increased ICP
   D. hypoxemia from CNS-induced pulmonary edema
6. A CT scan reveals diffuse intracranial edema. What might you expect?
   A. placement of an ICP monitoring device
   B. surgery to relieve the edema
   C. anticonvulsants
   D. antibiotics
7. Why would you want to maintain Melanie's blood pressure at an elevated level?
   A. to maintain adequate CPP
   B. to avoid tachycardia
   C. to diminish blood loss
   D. to keep her GCS score stable
8. If Melanie's ICP cannot be lowered, what actions might be needed to maintain adequate CPP?
   A. elevate the head of the bed
   B. keep her awake as much as possible
   C. use pressor drugs to elevate blood pressure
   D. bring her favorite stuffed animal from home
9. Which of the following nursing interventions has the highest priority in a child?
   A. administer broad-spectrum antibiotics
   B. administer oxygen
   C. administer medications to prevent hypertension
   D. maintain IV access
10. Which of the following interventions would most likely be needed following the administration of lorazepam for status epilepticus?
    A. bag-valve-mask ventilation
    B. isotonic fluid bolus 20 mL/kg
    C. naloxone administration
    D. dopamine administration

Answers: 1. B, 2. C, 3. C, 4. D, 5. C, 6. A, 7. A, 8. C, 9. B, 10. A

METABOLISM/THERMOREGULATION

SECTION ELEVEN: Fluid and Electrolytes

At the completion of this section, the learner will be able to describe nursing management of a child with alteration in fluid and electrolytes.

Altered fluid and electrolyte balance is more common in the young child than in the adult. Acutely ill children are at even greater risk because of compromised compensatory mechanisms. Fluid and electrolyte disturbances can be classified into one of three groups: dehydration, water intoxication, and third space fluid shifts. The group that is most characteristic of disturbances seen in children is dehydration. This section focuses on the management of three forms of dehydration after a brief discussion of developmental considerations and calculations of fluid and electrolyte requirements.

Homeostasis

Fluid and electrolyte intake and output vary daily, but volume and composition of body fluids are maintained within a narrow therapeutic range. Organs that are responsible for fluid and electrolyte homeostasis are the kidneys, heart and blood vessels, pituitary gland, adrenal glands, parathyroid gland, hypothalamus, and lungs.

Because of anatomic and physiologic differences in the child, regulatory mechanisms are less efficient in maintaining balance. Young children are predisposed to fluid and electrolyte imbalances for various reasons. Table 36–20 summarizes the developmental considerations of fluid and electrolyte balance and their clinical significance.

Management Principles

Dehydration is a very common form of fluid loss in the infant and young child. Children compensate for dehydration initially by increasing heart and respiratory rates. If the dehydration goes untreated, the child decompensates and is at risk for hypovolemic shock. Once the blood pressure begins to drop, the child is moving into decompensated shock and circulatory failure.

Initial management of dehydration with circulatory failure is the same for all types of fluid and electrolyte loss: rapid expansion of the extracellular space. Beyond resuscitation, replacement therapy differs depending on the amount and type of dehydration.

Nurses play an important role during all phases of rehydration therapy. They should be able to assess the circulatory status, approximate the degree of dehydration, and evaluate response to therapy. Preparation and calculation of parenteral fluids also are vital to patient care. Monitoring right-sided heart pressure and urine output is an important nursing responsibility.

TABLE 36–20. FLUID AND ELECTROLYTE BALANCE: DEVELOPMENTAL CONSIDERATIONS

ANATOMIC DIFFERENCE[a]	CLINICAL SIGNIFICANCE
Greater percentage of extracellular water	More prone to fluid loss with illness
Greater percentage of water per unit of weight	Fluid requirements are greater than in adult
Greater body surface area per unit of weight	Greater loss of fluids, electrolytes, and body heat with exhaled air and through skin evaporation and radiation
Renal tubules immature, with smaller surface area	Diminished response to ADH; inefficient absorption and excretion of electrolytes
Renal nephrons have relatively short loops	Inefficient concentration of urine; increased water loss
PHYSIOLOGIC DIFFERENCE[a]	**CLINICAL SIGNIFICANCE**
Metabolic rate is twice the adult rate per unit of weight	Greater fluid exchange rate per day; less reserve of fluid; urea excretion (necessary for urine concentration) is low because infants are in a high anabolic state for growth; more prone to hypoglycemia
Low glycogen stores	More prone to hypoglycemia

From K. Overby, Rudolph's Pediatrics *© 1998 McGraw-Hill.*

[a] Anatomic and physiologic differences are seen primarily in the infant and young child.

Fluid and Electrolyte Replacement Therapy

Many acutely ill children are totally dependent on parenteral replacement therapy to maintain fluid and electrolyte balance. The two determinants of replacement therapy are maintenance and deficit fluids. Maintenance fluids represent ongoing normal physiologic losses, and deficit fluids represent abnormal fluid losses before initiation of therapy.

Because of the narrow margin of safety when administering parenteral fluids to infants and young children, nurses should always double check calculations for infusion rates. Several methods are used to calculate daily maintenance fluid needs. Table 36–21 illustrates a commonly used method to calculate maintenance fluids as determined by body weight.

The following is an example of how to calculate daily maintenance fluids for a child who weighs 24 kg.

$$\text{First } 10 \text{ kg} = 10 \times 100 \text{ mL} = 1{,}000 \text{ mL}$$
$$11\text{–}20 \text{ kg} = 10 \times 50 \text{ mL} = 500 \text{ mL}$$
$$4 \text{ kg} = 4 \times 25 \text{ mL} = 100 \text{ mL}$$
$$\text{Total fluids in 24 hours} = 1{,}600 \text{ mL}$$

Replacement therapy for deficit fluids is based on the degree of dehydration. This can be determined by calculating the percentage of weight loss when the pre-illness weight is known. The steps for calculating the percentage of weight loss follow.

TABLE 36–21. DAILY MAINTENANCE FLUID NEEDS

BODY WEIGHT (kg)	FLUID REQUIREMENT/24 h
For each kg ≤ 10 kg	100 mL/kg/24 hr
For each kg, 11–20 kg	1000 mL/kg for first 10 kg + 50 mL/kg for kg 11–20
For each kg > 20 kg	1500 mL/kg for first 20 kg + 25 mL/kg for kg 21–30

Adapted from Curley, M., Smith, J., & Maloney-Harmon, P. (1996). Critical care nursing of infants and children. *Philadelphia: W.B. Saunders.*

1. Subtract the child's current weight (kg) from the pre-illness weight (kg)
   Example: Pre-illness weight = 10 kg
   Current weight = 9 kg
   Difference = 1 kg
2. Divide the weight loss (step 1) by the pre-illness weight
   Example: 1 kg/10 kg = 0.10
   Percentage of weight loss = 10%

For each 1 percent of weight loss, 10 mL/kg of fluid have been lost. In the example shown, an infant with a 10 percent weight loss has a fluid loss of 100 mL/kg ($10 \times 10 = 100$). Total fluid deficit is determined by multiplying the pre-illness weight by the milliliters per kilogram of fluid loss. Therefore, 100 mL/kg (fluid loss) is multiplied by 10 kg (pre-illness weight) to give a total fluid deficit of 1,000 mL. Deficit fluids must be added to maintenance fluids to determine the total amount of replacement therapy. If pre-illness weight is not known, clinical assessment data should be used to estimate the percentage of dehydration (Table 36–22).

The type of parenteral fluid to use for replacement therapy is determined by sodium, potassium, and glucose requirements. Sodium and potassium requirements are based on calorie requirements per kilogram of body weight. Established ranges for sodium are 3 to 4 mEq/kg/24 hr and for potassium are 2 to 3 mEq/kg/24 hr. Normal glucose requirements are 200 to 400 mg/kg/24 hr.

In summary, almost all acutely ill children require parenteral fluid and electrolyte therapy. Regulatory mechanisms that control fluid and electrolyte homeostasis are less efficient in infants and young children. Developmental differences underscore the importance of accurate calculation and replacement of fluid and electrolyte therapy.

SECTION TWELVE: Nutrition

At the completion of this section, the learner will be able to discuss the nursing management of a child with altered nutritional status.

Nutrition is defined as the process by which food is converted into living tissue. This process is dependent on normal physiologic functioning of ingestion, digestion, transportation, use, and excretion of nutrients. The purpose of this section is twofold: (1) to discuss how age-related factors and disease states affect the process of nutrition, and (2) to discuss nursing management of the child with increased nutritional needs.

Developmental Considerations

Unlike adults, children normally have an increased basal metabolic rate (BMR) and subsequent increased nutritional needs to support rapid growth and development. In addition, the infant has an immature digestive tract, making absorption and use of nutrients less efficient. Gastric emptying time is increased, and peristalsis is more rapid in the infant, causing less reabsorption of water. As a consequence, infants' stools usually are watery and occur more frequently than at other periods of life. Reverse peristalsis may also occur during infancy, contributing to frequent regurgitation. Digestion of all fats is not possible until approximately 1 year of age because of composition and secretion of bile and pancreatic lipase. Beyond infancy, gastrointestinal function is similar in children and adults.

Because infants have a relatively large body surface area and less subcutaneous fat, they are more prone to hypothermia. The process to increase heat production also increases glucose consumption and caloric needs. Section Thirteen provides a more detailed description of this process.

TABLE 36–22. CLINICAL ASSESSMENT DATA: DEGREES OF DEHYDRATION

AREA OF ASSESSMENT	MILD Infant 5% Loss Children 3% Loss	MODERATE Infant 10% Loss Children 6% Loss	SEVERE Infant 15% Loss Children 9% Loss
Thirst	Thirsty	Thirsty	May be unresponsive to thirst
Anterior fontanel	Normal	Sunken	Very sunken
Skin	Pale, cool	Grayish	Cool, pale to cyanotic, mottled
Blood pressure	Normal	Normal or decreased	Less than 90 mm Hg in a child
Pulse	Slightly increased or normal	Increased, weak	Tachycardia (rapid, thready, feeble)
Skin turgor	Decreased	Loss of elasticity	Very poor (pinch retracts very slowly) (> 2 sec)
Mucous membranes	Normal to dry	Dry	Dry, cracked
Eyes	Normal	Somewhat depressed	Grossly sunken
Tears	Present	Decreased	Absent
Urine output	Decreased	Oliguria	Greatly diminished or absent
Behavior	Normal, alert, possibly some restlessness	Irritable, restless or lethargic	Hyperirritable to lethargic, limp

Adapted from Curley, M., Smith, J., & Maloney-Harmon, P. (1996). Critical care nursing of infants and children. *Philadelphia: W.B. Saunders.*

Normal Nutritional Requirements

Specific energy needs vary somewhat among children and depend on four factors: BMR, body activity, caloric loss in excreta, and dynamic action of food. The approximate kilocalorie (kcal) expenditure for each of these processes in the infant is listed (Shayevitz & Weissman, 1992).

BMR first year of life	70 kcal
Body activity and growth during childhood	20 kcal
Caloric loss in excreta	10 kcal
Dynamic action of food	5 kcal
TOTAL CALORIC EXPENDITURE	105 kcal

The three nutrients that contribute energy value (calories) are proteins, carbohydrates, and fats. Recommended dietary allowances (RDAs) have been published by the Committee on Food and Nutrition of the National Research Council. These guidelines make recommendations for daily intake of calories, proteins, vitamins, and minerals. Protein and caloric requirements per kilogram of body weight are highest during infancy and gradually decline throughout the childhood years. There are no specific RDAs for fats and carbohydrates. The average American diet supplies an adequate amount of these nutrients. For additional information on normal nutritional requirements, the learner should review Module 22.

Alteration in Nutritional Requirements

Nutritional metabolism in a delicate balance between anabolism (physical growth of tissue) and catabolism (breakdown of tissue for energy). Stress factors are commonly used to estimate caloric needs of critically ill children. Recent research indicates these factors may be too high. Research using an indirect calorimetry method to measure resting energy expenditure found lower energy expenditure estimates. Clinical response to feeding is the best indicator of caloric needs (Curley, Smith, & Maloney-Harmon, 1996).

Nutritional Management

The goals of nutritional management in the acutely ill child are to supply enough nutrients to maintain basal metabolic energy requirements, promote normal growth, and promote tissue repair.

The first step toward these goals is identifying the patient at risk. The nurse is an important member of the nutritional support team and assists with the nutritional assessment. Table 36–23 summarizes the key components of the nutritional assessment. Once the acutely ill child at risk has been identified, nutritional repletion can begin. The two modes of delivering nutrients are enteral and parenteral routes.

The preferred route of administration of nutrients is enteral. The enteral route provides more normal and homeostatic metabolism than parenteral routes and is essential for the maintenance of normal structure and function of the small intestine (Shayevitz & Weissman, 1992). It is also associated with a lower incidence of infection compared with a parenteral route.

TABLE 36–23. SUMMARY OF METHODS OF NUTRITIONAL ASSESSMENT

Measurement of height and weight
Skinfold thickness
Arm muscle size
Creatine-height index
Total body potassium-height index (more useful for research than clinical practice)
Urea nitrogen excretion
Plasma proteins
Cellular immunity

From Rogers, M.C. (1992). Textbook of pediatric intensive care *(p. 949). Baltimore: Williams & Wilkins. © 1992.*

There are numerous enteral formulas on the market. The nutritional team must consider the given osmolality and composition of the formula when selecting a product to meet the patient's individual needs. Continuous delivery of duodenal or jejunal feedings is preferred to intermittent delivery to avoid bowel distention, fluid and electrolyte shifts, and diarrhea (Mahan & Arlin, 1992).

Patients who cannot tolerate enteral feedings or require additional nutritional support may benefit from supplementary or total nutritional support. The composition of parenteral nutritional support is individualized to the patient. Children on TPN support need frequent close monitoring of electrolytes, glucose, and liver enzymes.

Regardless of the type and method of nutritional support, nurses need to assist the nutrition team by maintaining accurate records of height and weight, caloric intake, and feeding tolerance. Second, nurses must be familiar with hospital procedures for enteral and parenteral nutrition. Third, nurses need to minimize the child's energy expenditure by limiting environmental stress.

In summary, nutritional needs of the acutely ill child are increased significantly. Nutritional baseline assessment therapy must be initiated early in the patient's hospital course to maintain an anabolic state. Nutritional therapy must consider the child's increased basal energy needs, growth needs, and tissue repair needs.

SECTION THIRTEEN: Thermoregulation

At the completion of this section, the learner will be able to identify regulatory mechanisms of heat balance and discuss the nursing management of heat imbalance.

In the healthy individual exposed to normal seasonal temperatures, core temperature remains constant, within ±1°F (Guyton, 1987). A number of regulatory mechanisms within the body maintain a balance between heat production and heat balance. It is the purpose of this section to discuss regulation of heat balance in the healthy and acutely ill child.

Methods of Heat Loss

Heat is being produced in the body and transferred to the environment continually. The four main methods of heat loss are radiation, evaporation, conduction, and convection. Radiation is responsible for most heat exchange and refers to the transfer of heat by infrared rays. Evaporation represents the second largest method of heat loss and occurs with the vaporization of liquid from the body. Only minute amounts of heat are lost by conduction, which represents a transfer of heat between two objects along a temperature gradient. Heat loss by convection occurs when body heat is conducted to the air and then removed by air currents.

Methods of Heat Production

Heat production is determined by the basal metabolic rate (BMR), shivering thermogenesis, and chemical thermogenesis. BMR is a term used to express the rate of heat liberation with cellular chemical reactions under basal conditions. The primary motor center for shivering is located in the posterior hypothalamus. When stimulated, this center transmits impulses that increase tone of the skeletal muscle. After a critical level, shivering begins with an increase in heat production. The young infant cannot shiver to generate heat and is dependent on metabolic processes to maintain heat balance. Chemical thermogenesis, also referred to as nonshivering thermogenesis, produces heat from oxidative metabolism of brown fat. Newborns have brown fat in the interscapular space and mediastinum and around the kidneys. For the first weeks of life, it is a very important factor in thermogenesis. However, brown fat supply is limited, and the cold stressed infant can quickly deplete stores and become hypothermic.

In addition, increased consumption of glucose and oxygen to metabolize brown fat may produce acidosis, hypoxemia, and hypoglycemia. Figure 36–2 illustrates the physiologic consequences of cold stress in the neonate.

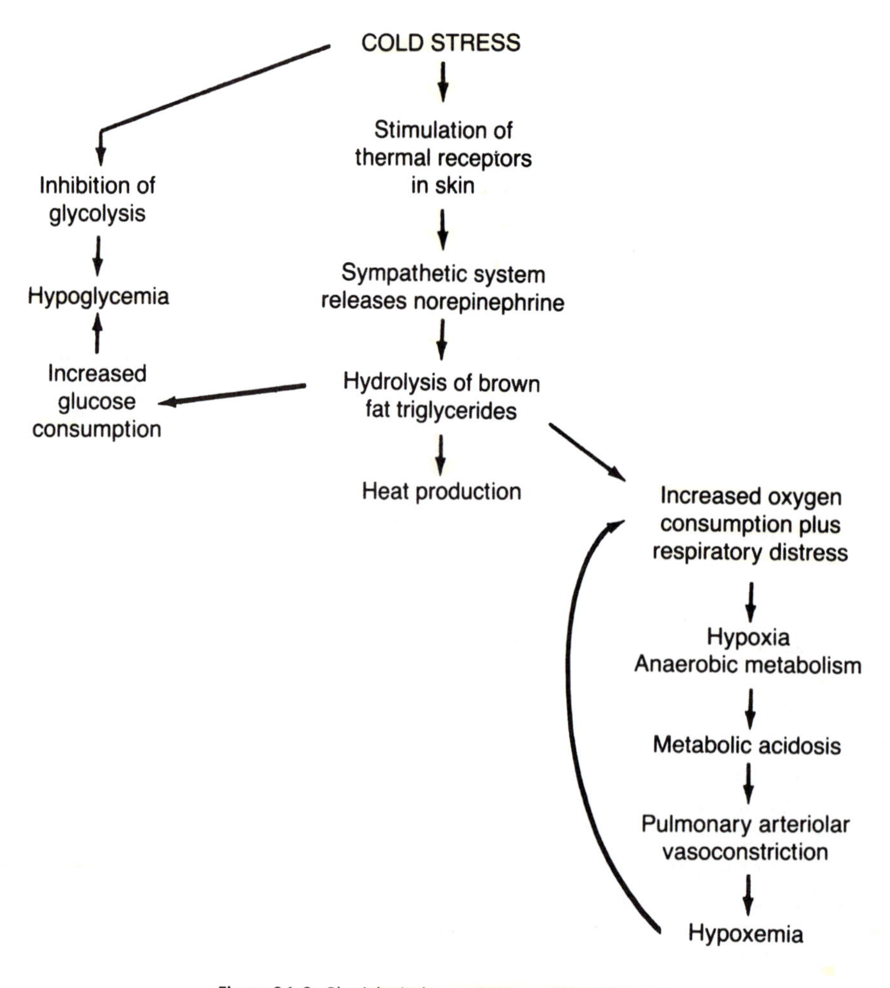

Figure 36–2. Physiological consequences of hypothermia.

Regulatory Mechanisms

When an individual is exposed to a cold or hot state, there are several regulatory mechanisms that attempt to maintain normal body temperature. Figure 36–3 illustrates the neuroendocrine mechanisms of temperature control.

Hypothermia

Core temperature below 95°F (35°C) usually are considered significant, and thermoregulatory mechanisms are activated (Curley, Smith, & Maloney-Harmon, 1996). Uncontrolled severe hypothermia causes significant alterations in normal physiologic processes. Most notable of these are lethal dysrhythmias, apnea, and coma. Neonates are at risk for developing hypothermia because of their relatively large body surface area and limited brown fat stores. Acutely ill children also are at risk because of impaired physiologic function, poor nutritional reserves, and pharmacologic agents. Trauma, submersion injuries, and drug intoxication are common etiologies producing hypothermia.

Management of hypothermia is aimed at preventing further heat loss and restoring normothermia. Children should be kept warm and dry at all times and kept in a neutral thermal environment. Drafts from windows and air conditioners should be eliminated. Blood for transfusions and supplemental oxygen should be warmed before administration. For severe hypothermia (e.g., submersion injury), the child must be handled with care because of ventricular irritability. To restore normal body temperature, rewarming methods must be used. These include radiant warmer, heating pads, warmed blankets, and head covering. Multiple methods of rewarming are generally more effective than a single method. Rewarming must be gradual, usually not > 1°C per hour. Rapid rewarming can increase oxygen consumption in tissues with limited perfusion and can produce apnea in infants (Hazinski, 1992). Table 36–24 summarizes three methods of rewarming.

Hyperthermia

Hyperthermia refers to a condition when the body temperature exceeds the usual normal range. Factors in the

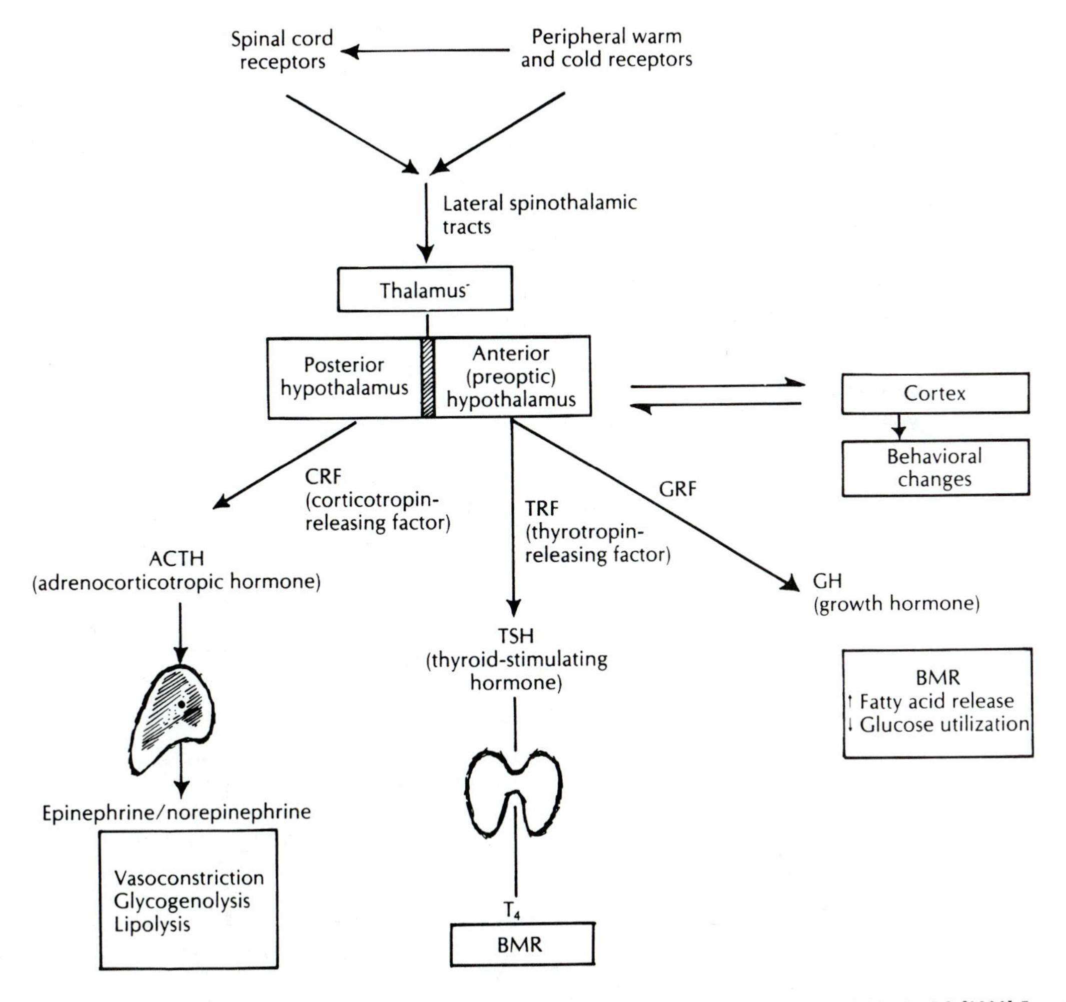

Figure 36–3. Neuroendocrine mechanisms of temperature control. BMR, basal metabolic rate. (*From Levin, D.L., & Morriss, F.C. [1990].* Essentials of pediatric intensive care *[p. 177]. St. Louis: Quality Medical Publishing.*)

TABLE 36–24. METHODS OF REWARMING

Passive external rewarming[a]	Endogenous thermogenesis (e.g., blankets) Slowest, least invasive method Prevent further heat loss
Active external rewarming[a]	Application of conductive and radiant rewarming devices (e.g., infant warmers, radiant warming beds, heating pads, warm blankets) Used for mild hypothermia Variable rate of rewarming
Active central rewarming	Rewarming occurs internally (e.g., warm IV or peritoneal fluids, warm inspired gases, mediastinal lavage) Most invasive Optimal rate of rewarming is not known

[a] Problems associated with external rewarming include shock secondary to peripheral vasodilation and burns from poorly perfused areas.

child such as fever, malignant hyperthermia, or heat-related illnesses may produce hyperthermia. External factors contributing to hyperthermia include environmental heat and accidental overheating (Curley, Smith, & Malnoney-Harmon, 1996). Common etiologies that produce hyperthermia in children include infectious states, CNS injuries, and pharmacotherapeutics.

The treatment of fever unrelated to a hyperthermic syndrome is controversial. It is believed that the elevated temperature may support the body's normal defense against invading pathogens. Treatment usually is indicated when symptoms produced by the fever are not tolerated well by the child (e.g., dehydration, tachypnea, tachycardia). When treatment is indicated, general modes of therapy include passive and active external cooling and the use of antipyretics. Acetaminophen and ibuprofen are used more often than aspirin because of fewer side effects, shorter duration of action, and aspirin's association with Reye's syndrome.

In summary, the balance of heat production and heat loss in the body is controlled by a number of neuroendocrine regulatory mechanisms. The acutely ill child is at risk for developing alterations in temperature regulation because of a large surface area/volume ratio and a debilitated state. The neonate is at further risk because of limited brown fat stores and limited subcutaneous fat. Alteration in heat balance needs to be prevented or controlled to prevent further impairment of the acutely ill child.

METABOLISM/THERMOREGULATION REVIEW

Refer to the following case study to answer questions 1 through 6.

A 3-year-old girl admitted to the ICU with a 3-day history of vomiting and diarrhea. Vital signs are temperature 102.2°F (39°C), respiratory rate 40, heart rate 110, blood pressure 74/40 mm/Hg. Additional clinical symptoms include pale skin color, loss of skin elasticity, dry mucous membranes, and irritability. She has not voided for 4 hours. Prehospital weight is not known. Present weight is 17 kg. CBC is normal, glucose normal, serum electrolytes are Na^+ 138, K^+ 3.4, Cl^- 102.

1. What type of fluid would be used to rehydrate the child?
   A. dextrose 10%
   B. dextrose 5% in 0.45% NS
   C. dextrose 5% in 0.45% NS with 40 mEq KCL
   D. packed red blood cells
2. Based on clinical symptoms, what degree of dehydration does the child have?
   A. mild
   B. moderate
   C. severe
   D. none
3. Based on these data, which order would you initiate first?
   A. chest radiograph
   B. IV line insertion
   C. urinary catheter insertion
   D. blood culture
4. What is the hourly maintenance fluid requirement for the child (based on hospital weight)?
   A. 26 mL
   B. 56 mL
   C. 10 mL
   D. 88 mL
5. Based on the child's temperature, what is the percentage of increase in caloric requirements?
   A. 12
   B. 24
   C. 20
   D. 10
6. The enteral route is preferred over the parenteral route for nutrition repletion because
   A. minerals are absorbed most efficiently through the small intestine
   B. there is a lower incidence of infection
   C. amino acids cannot be administered parenterally
   D. glucose is metabolized less efficiently in parenteral form

7. Cold stress can indirectly cause
   A. hyperglycemia from decreased glucose consumption
   B. hypoxemia from pulmonary arteriolar vasoconstriction
   C. decreased oxygen consumption
   D. hyperglycemia from stimulation of glycolysis
8. A potential complication of active external rewarming for hypothermia is
   A. hyperthermia
   B. respiratory distress
   C. hypotension
   D. hypoglycemia
9. The neonate is predisposed to hypothermia because of
   A. increased body surface area
   B. decreased CO
   C. decreased myelination of cortical centers
   D. increased respiratory rate

Answers: 1. B, 2. B, 3. B, 4. B, 5. B, 6. B, 7. B, 8. C, 9. A

IMMUNOCOMPETENCE

SECTION FOURTEEN: Risk Factors

At the completion of this section, the learner will be able to identify age-related factors and situational stressors that alter the immune response of the acutely ill child.

Infections are a common problem seen in the pediatric ICU. They may develop as a primary disorder or may be a secondary complication of another illness. The very fact that the child is admitted to an intensive care unit places him or her at risk for altered immune function. In addition to environmental risk factors, the child also may have an altered immune response from a preexisting disease state. Infancy compounds the risk factors because of the immaturity of the immune system. The purpose of this section is to discuss developmental aspects and situational stressors that place the child at risk for developing an infection.

Developmental Immunity

In the past, it was believed that the newborn had very little immunologic function. Today, we know that many areas of immune expression are present at birth, and other areas are acquired with age. An understanding of the developmentally immature immune system helps to explain the infant and child's predilection for characteristic infections. Developmental aspects of immune function are discussed in terms of first-line defense, nonspecific immunity, and specific cellular and humoral immunity.

The first line of defense against invasion by pathogens is barriers, mechanical and chemical. Intact skin is a mechanical barrier and normally prevents penetration of microorganisms. The newborn's skin is different than the adult's in terms of reduced thickness and durability. The stratum corneum is present in reduced amount in the newborn, resulting in increased skin permeability. However, it rapidly develops and is adequate by 2 weeks of age (Rosenthal, 1989).

Chemical barriers refer to secretions that assist in host defense. Specific types of chemical barriers include acidic surface secretions, gastric secretions, and urine. In the infant, there is diminished sweat production, resulting in decreased secretion of bactericidal and fungicidal substances. Surface secretion of IgA, which helps prevent attachment of pathogenic organisms, may be reduced in the gastrointestinal tract of the infant (Rosenthal, 1989; Tribett, 1989).

If mechanical or chemical barriers are altered or bypassed, pathogenic invasion can occur, and an inflammatory response is triggered. The second line of host defense is nonspecific defenses, which include phagocytic cells, the complement system, and chemical mediators. Table 36–25 summarizes specific areas of immaturity of nonspecific mechanisms of host defense and their clinical significance.

When natural and nonspecific defense are unsuccessful in eradicating or containing pathogens, an acquired immune response is triggered. Humoral immunity (B cell function) is primarily responsible for synthesis of im-

TABLE 36–25. DEVELOPMENTAL ASPECTS OF NONSPECIFIC MECHANISMS OF HOST DEFENSE

HOST DEFENSE	DEFICIENCY	CLINICAL SIGNIFICANCE
Phagocytes	Diminished motility, adherence, and chemotaxis in newborn	May contribute to decreased ability to localize infection
	Reduced stores of neutrophils per kilogram	Neutrophils are depleted with repeated infections or with an overwhelming infection
Complement	Complement proteins are 60–80% of normal adult levels; serum complement reaches adult levels between 3 and 6 months of age	Low levels may contribute to the neonate's afebrile and reduced leukocytosis response to infection Opsonization and chemotactic activity is deficient in the newborn compared with the adult

munoglobins. In the newborn, absolute numbers of B cells are present, but the actual synthesis of some types of immunoglobulins is limited. Table 36–26 lists the levels of immunoglobulins present at birth and when mature levels are obtained (Rosenthal, 1989). Passive transplacental transfer of IgG occurs in the last trimester. Newborns have adult serum levels of IgG at birth, but levels gradually fall over the first 4 months of extrauterine life. The infant's level of immunoglobulins is lowest at approximately 4 to 5 months of age, when passive immunity is decreasing and active immunity is still deficient (Rosenthal, 1989).

Age-specific cell-mediated function (T cell function) is less well understood than humoral immunity. However, it is known that in normal newborns, T cells are present in approximately the same quantity as in adults. T cells also respond to antigens to which the mother has been sensitized. Newborn T cells do, however, have decreased function in terms of gamma-interferon secretion, which activates macrophage function (Rosenthal, 1989).

Situational Risk Factors

In addition to developmental factors, there are also situational factors that place the acutely ill child at risk for infection. Invasive procedures that bypass epithelial barriers (e.g., IV lines, urinary catheter, inhalation therapy equipment) are the mainstay of intensive care therapy. Unfortunately, they predispose the host to opportunistic infections. Surgical trauma and burn trauma also affect immune function by altering skin barriers. Some pharmacologic agents used pre-, intra-, and postoperatively alter immune function. For example, nitrous oxide depresses bone marrow function. The child's preexisting health status may alter the immune response and function.

Anatomic defects frequently also are associated with opportunistic infections. Children with cardiac defects may develop subacute and acute bacterial endocarditis. Urinary tract obstructive lesions have a significant incidence of gram-negative enteric infections. Congenital dermal abnormalities of the craniospinal axis that communicate with the CNS can cause a lethal infection. Other acquired conditions such as acquired immune deficiency syndrome (AIDS), severe combined immunodeficiency syndrome (SCIDS), cancer, and transplant recipients can increase the incidence and seriousness of infections.

In summary, although newborns are not completely devoid of immunologic function at birth, they are deficient in many areas. Nonspecific and acquired immunity become functional at various ages from birth to adolescence. Age-specific infections may be predicted, and prevention measures can be developed. Situational stressors of the intensive care environment, as well as therapeutic measures, also can place the child at risk. An understanding of risk factors can help the nurse develop surveillance measures and management strategies when caring for the acutely ill child.

SECTION FIFTEEN: Nursing Management

At the completion of this section, the learner will be able to state treatment strategies to prevent infection and augment host defenses in the child.

Acutely ill children are at risk for developing opportunistic infections because of a developmental predisposition and situational stressors that alter immune function. They are subjected to invasive procedures and immunosuppressive agents and reside in a location with many other patients. Nurses must consider these risk factors when developing a therapeutic plan to care for the child. The goal of therapy is to prevent or minimize infection by limiting exposure to pathogens, by early detection and monitoring of infection, and by augmenting host defenses. The first part of this section describes measures to prevent infection, followed by a discussion on augmentation of host defenses.

TABLE 36–26. IMMUNOGLOBULINS: FUNCTION, LEVELS, AND CLINICAL SIGNIFICANCE

IG	FUNCTION	% OF ADULT LEVEL AT BIRTH	CLINICAL SIGNIFICANCE OF LOW LEVEL	AGE MATURE LEVEL ATTAINED
IgM	First to be formed after antigen stimulation Serologic defense	10	Risk for overwhelming sepsis	1–2 years
IgD	Unknown	Small amount		1 year
IgG	Guards tissue from bacteria	110[a]	Risk for pyogenic infection, especially pulmonary	4–10 years
IgA	Defends mucosal surfaces/secretions	Small amount or none	Risk for viral and bacterial infection at mucosal surfaces, especially respiratory and sinusitis	6–15 years
IgE	Triggers immediate hypersensitivity (type I)	Small amount	Risk for parasitic infection	6–15 years

[a] Crosses placenta

Adapted from Rosenthal, C.H. (1989). Immunosuppression in pediatric critical care patients. Crit Care Nurs Clin North Am 1:779.

Prevention of Infection

One of the first steps in preventing infection is early detection. In the infant and young child, clinical manifestations often are nonspecific and variable. Diagnostic criteria to confirm sepsis in the newborn are limited. WBC count with bacterial disease may be low, normal, or elevated, and erythrocyte sedimentation rate and C-reactive protein also are relatively insensitive. Therefore, clinical assessment data must be correlated with the patient's history and laboratory data. If suspicion of infection exists, blood, urine, and CSF cultures should be obtained (Ackerman, 1996).

In the older infant and child, clinical manifestations and laboratory tests are more specific and diagnostic. Specific signs and symptoms depend on whether the infection is localized or systemic. Table 36–27 lists possible immunologic clues seen with altered immune function.

Limiting exposure to pathogens can help prevent infection. The importance of hand washing and strict adherence to isolation policies need no explanation. A clean environment, including room, equipment, and supplies, is critical. Liberal visitation of the child's family is important in the pediatric intensive care unit. However, visitation of the immunocompromised patient should be restricted to the immediate family, and they should adhere to isolation policies. Children and families should be questioned about prior and current use of antibiotics. Antibiotic resistance is becoming common due to individual overuse and misuse of antibiotics and the prevalence of "hidden antibiotics" from agricultural use. As a result, children may develop potential lethal infections that cannot be treated with available antibiotics.

TABLE 36–27. IMMUNOLOGIC PHYSICAL ASSESSMENT FINDINGS

SYSTEM	ASSESSMENT FINDINGS
Neurosensory/motor	Visual changes, headaches/migraines, deafness, ataxia, tetany, altered level of consciousness, diminished cranial nerve function (blink, tear, cough, gag)
Respiratory	Wheezing and crackles, cough, rhinitis, hyperventilation, bronchospasm, altered rate and depth
Cardiovascular	Hypotension, tachycardia, arrhythmias, vasculitis, anemia, pale skin and mucous membranes
Gastrointestinal	Hepatosplenomegaly, dyspepsia, colitis, vomiting/diarrhea (chronic), altered bowel sounds, protuberant abdomen
Skin/hygiene	Breaks in skin integrity, palpable lymph nodes, dermatitis, purpura, urticaria, altered temperature, diminished turgor, dehydration, oral lesions
Mobility/comfort	Tender and swollen joints, muscle weakness, limited range of motion, fever and chills, decreased activity
General factors	Poor nutritional status, age

Adapted from Curley, M., Smith, J., & Maloney-Harmon, P. (1996). Critical care nursing of infants and children. *Philadelphia: W.B. Saunders.*

Augmentation of Host Defenses

Host defenses may be augmented by maintaining physical and chemical barriers, providing adequate nutrition, reducing psychologic stress, and maintaining comfort. The importance of maintaining the body's first line of defense is discussed in Section Fourteen, and the importance of adequate nutrition is discussed in Section Twelve. Prolonged or uncontrolled psychologic stress may result in depression of some components of the immune system (Schindler, 1985).

Specific measures to maintain epithelial integrity (e.g., skin, oral, respiratory, urinary, bowel surfaces) are outlined in Table 36–28. Nurses should take an active role in providing nutritional support, as outlined in Section Twelve. Stress reduction techniques must be individualized to the age of the child. The learner should refer to Section Seventeen for a more in-depth discussion of this topic. Finally, the source of discomfort must be identified and eliminated. Analgesics must be individualized in terms of route, selection, and dosage. Noxious procedures must be minimized.

In summary, acutely ill patients in the pediatric intensive care unit are at risk for developing infection. The goals of nursing management are prevention and augmentation of host defenses. Prevention is accompanied with close surveillance and monitoring and limiting exposure to potential pathogens. Augmentation of host defenses includes maintaining physical and chemical barriers, nutritional support, reduction of stress, and relieving discomfort.

TABLE 36–28. ALTERATION IN SKIN BARRIERS: METHODS TO REDUCE INFECTION

Establish guidelines for invasive monitoring

IV therapy
- Use sterile technique for IV insertion
- Secure IV catheters to prevent mechanical trauma to vessels
- Do not prepare insertion site with acetone or betadine
- Check IV site frequently

Maintain adequate patient fluid intake

Promote activity

Reposition patient frequently

Use sterile technique with airway suctioning

Promote normal urinary and bowel elimination

Maintain appropriate nutrition

IMMUNOCOMPETENCE REVIEW

1. The infant's level of immunoglobulins is lowest between
   A. 4 and 6 years of age
   B. 4 and 5 months of age
   C. 2 and 3 weeks of age
   D. 2 and 5 years of age
2. Because complement protein levels in the infant are 60 to 80 percent of normal adult levels, in which of the following areas of the immune system is the infant most deficient?
   A. ability to localize infections
   B. ability to increase leukocytes in response to an infection
   C. ability to increase neutrophil stores
   D. ability to form immunoglobulins
3. Low levels of IgE place the young child at increased risk for
   A. pyogenic infections
   B. bacterial respiratory infection
   C. parasitic infection
   D. overwhelming sepsis
4. The best nursing intervention to prevent the transfer of pathogens is
   A. hand washing
   B. strict adherence to isolation
   C. bathing the patient frequently
   D. good nutrition

Refer to the following case study to answer questions 5 and 6.

Suzanne is a 4-year-old girl admitted to the ICU following open heart surgery. Postoperative monitoring devices include a right atrial catheter, radial artery catheter, and urinary catheter. On postoperative day 3, she is diagnosed with a urinary tract infection.

5. The most likely cause of the urinary tract infection is
   A. oliguria from decreased renal perfusion
   B. prophylactic antibiotics
   C. radial artery cannulation
   D. indwelling urinary catheter
6. Suzanne's immune function has been significantly altered because of
   A. low levels of IgD
   B. low levels of IgM
   C. low levels of complement proteins
   D. altered skin barriers

Answers: 1. B, 2. B, 3. C, 4. A, 5. D, 6. D

PSYCHOSOCIAL FACTORS

SECTION SIXTEEN: Impact of Hospitalization

At the completion of this section, the learner will be able to discuss age-related stressors and reactions to hospitalization.

Children often are admitted to the intensive care unit in an acute state without advance preparation. In general, childhood responses to hospitalization do not vary significantly between pediatric general and intensive care units. However, the family reaction to an ICU hospitalization is often overwhelming. Furthermore, hospital-related stressors are more similar than dissimilar and are characteristically age dependent. In addition to age, the child's understanding of and reaction to hospitalization depends primarily on personality, parent–child relationship, previous separation, and characteristics of illness and treatment. On the other hand, the frequency of stressors often is greater in the ICU, which may intensify the child's response. The purpose of this section is to describe age-related stressors and reactions commonly experienced by the hospitalized child.

Separation Anxiety

Separation from one's parents is a major stressor during infancy throughout the preschool years. Infants and toddlers have limited internal coping abilities and depend on significant others as their main source of coping. Three distinct stages of separation have been described in the infant: protest, despair, and detachment (Bowlby, 1969). Reactions during the protest stage include crying, screaming for a parent, and inconsolable behavior. If separation continues, the infant goes through a stage of despair. The infant is depressed from a sense of hopelessness, demonstrated by decreased activity, no crying, and withdrawal from others. The last stage is one of detachment or denial. This is a confusing stage and often is misinterpreted by health care professionals. The child outwardly appears content, but in reality, he or she emotionally detaches from the parents to avoid the emotional pain of wanting them. These stages are not always apparent in the acutely ill child who has limited ability to express emotion overtly. A hospitalized child who always acts passive is a cause for worry.

Toddlers and preschoolers also experience tremendous stress when separated from their parents, but they react to this stressor differently than the infant. Toddlers are able to verbalize their displeasure with pleas for their parents to stay. They may also react with temper tantrums and uncooperative behavior. Preschoolers normally can tolerate brief periods of separation from their parents. However, stress of illness and hospitalization may alter usual mechanisms of coping, and preschoolers may demonstrate reactions to separation. In general, their reactions are less intense than those seen in toddlers. Reactions include whimpering, repeatedly making requests for parents, repeatedly asking when parents will visit, and refusing to cooperate with activities and care. Preschoolers are magical thinkers. They think of illnesses and treatments as a form of punishment. When children show less overt reactions to separation, they may refuse to eat, withdraw, be uninterested in toys, or sleep excessively (Wong, 1999).

Older children generally do much better with separation from their parents, but the stress of hospitalization usually increases their desire for parental guidance. Older children have developed some coping strategies and have developed support systems and relationships outside their immediate family. When alone, they may complain of boredom, isolation, and loneliness.

Loss of Control

The infant's reactions to and the effects of loss of control are not well understood. However, the older infant normally likes to explore the environment and is physically quite active. When immobilized or restricted to a bed, infants demonstrate generalized dislike by, for example, crying and screaming. A very quiet or overly cooperative infant is a cause for concern.

Toddlers are struggling for autonomy. Therefore, any obstacle that restricts their behavior or desires will result in negativism, for example, noncompliance and temper tantrums. The toddler is struggling with self-control, which is maintained by ritualistic behavior. The hospital environment is foreign and alters the child's usual routines. Reaction to disrupted routines is principally regression, for example, asking for a bottle or wetting the bed when previously toilet-trained.

The preschooler's thought processes are characterized by egocentricity, magical thinking, and preconceptual logic. They feel all-powerful and omnipotent. In the hospital setting, where many restrictions exist, the child's self-power is threatened, and self-control is lost. Reactions to loss of control include behaviors of protest, despair, detachment, aggression, and regression. Hospital routines and equipment may be especially frightening to the preschooler.

Older children may be characterized as industrious and independent. They are increasingly able to view situations objectively. They question their own perceptions, as well as those of others. When they are unable or not allowed to make decisions about their care, they feel a loss of independence and privacy. They also fear what they do not understand. Usual reactions of loss of control include frustration, hostility, and depression.

Fear of Bodily Injury and Pain

Procedures or physical disabilities that cause pain or fear of bodily injury are also experienced by the hospitalized child. Effects of and reactions to fear of bodily injury are not known in the preverbal infant. The infant responds to pain with generalized rigidity, followed by thrashing of extremities, crying, facial expression of discomfort, alteration in heart rate and respiratory rate, and physical resistance (older than 6 months). Pain should be assessed using a scale such as the neonatal Infant Pain Scale (Wong, 1999).

The toddler has a poor concept of body boundaries and may react as intensely to intrusive procedures as painful ones. Preschoolers have concerns about the integrity of their bodies. For example, they fear they will exsanguinate with cuts and needle punctures. They also have fears of castration and mutilation. The toddler and preschooler react to painful injuries or fear of bodily injury with physical aggression and uncooperative behavior (Betz, Hunsberger, & Wright, 1994). Pain in a toddler or preschooler should be assessed using a valid and reliable pain scale developed specifically for children.

Older children have fears not only of bodily injury but also of disabilities (real or imagined) that will make them different and, therefore, rejected by their friends. They are beginning to understand the need for procedures and may request why the procedure is needed, especially if it is painful. In general, the older the child, the more cooperative he or she usually is with painful procedures. They try to act brave. If they are distressed about a procedure or are experiencing pain, they usually will communicate their concerns verbally. Older children can use a faces pain scale or a visual analog scale (Wong, 1999).

In summary, regardless of the inpatient setting, the hospitalized child may have very specific age-related stressors. These stressors can be categorized into three groups: separation, loss of control, and fear of bodily injury and pain. Depending on the age of the child and other significant variables, the child's reaction to these stressors may be predicted and controlled.

SECTION SEVENTEEN: Nursing Management of Stressors

At the completion of this section, the learner will be able to list specific methods to reduce the negative effects of hospitalization.

When a child who is acutely ill is admitted to the intensive care unit, her emotional needs frequently are given low priority. Once her condition is stabilized, she becomes increasingly more aware of the environment. Stressors are apparent to the child, and negative reactions may occur. Nursing care should encompass management of both physiologic and emotional stressors. The purpose of this section is to discuss nursing management that minimizes negative reactions to hospitalization. Specific age-related interventions are discussed in terms of separation anxiety, loss of control, and fear of bodily injury and pain.

Separation Anxiety

The intensive care environment is normally loud, hectic, frightening, and intimidating. For all age groups, it is extremely important to have liberal visitation to minimize separation anxiety. Most pediatric ICUs recognize the importance of parental presence and have instituted open visitation including rooming in for parents or guardians. If the ICU has limited visitation, the family needs a schedule of visiting times. Nursing flexibility is encouraged to meet the needs of the family and child. Whenever possible, the nurse should involve family members in patient care. Family involvement often reduces the child's separation anxiety, and the family member feels more in control. Using consistent caregivers also is important. It allows the child to develop a trusting relationship with a surrogate parent (Wong, 1999). Table 36–29 lists additional age-specific interventions to minimize separation anxiety.

Loss of Control

Feelings of loss of control can be minimized by limiting physical restrictions, preparing for procedures, maintaining routines, and maintaining a level of independence. Immobilizing the child for procedures is often unavoidable. However, whenever possible, the nurse should attempt to gain cooperation first to prevent restraining or allow the parent to hold a child to reduce anxiety during procedures. Anticipatory preparation is not always possible. When time and patient condition permit, age-appropriate preparation should be done. Promoting independence can be accomplished by allowing the child to participate in self-care, allowing the child to make decisions about care, and maintaining rituals and daily routines when possible (Wilson & Broome, 1989). Table 36–30 lists age-specific interventions to minimize feelings of loss of control.

Fear of Bodily Injury and Pain

Interventions to reduce fear of bodily injury vary depending on the age of the child and previous experiences. It is frequently not possible to prepare a child for an ICU admission. In cases in which a child has an anticipated admission as in cardiac surgery, the child should be prepared beforehand. Parents can be oriented to the environment and procedures. They can help their child adapt as the child's condition improves. For pain management, assessment is important for recognizing pain and for evaluating the effectiveness of interventions. Several assessment tools have been developed specifically for children to help quantify assessments (Hester, 1993). For relieving pain, nonpharmacologic and pharmacologic management may be used. Table 36–31 lists specific interventions to minimize fears of bodily injury and reduce the pain experience.

TABLE 36–29. ANXIETY RELATED TO SEPARATION: NURSING INTERVENTIONS

INFANT	TODDLER/PRESCHOOLER	SCHOOL AGE
Consistent caregiver	Consistent caregiver	Consistent caregiver
Encourage parents to stay	Encourage parents to stay	Encourage parents to stay
Promote cuddling, holding when patient condition permits	Talk about parents frequently Place pictures of family members at bedside Allow sibling visitation when possible Explain when parents will return in terms of significant events (e.g., lunch, dinner) Encourage child to talk about family members	Talk about parents frequently Place pictures of family members at bedside Allow sibling and peer visitation when possible Use a clock to explain when parents will return Encourage child to talk about family members
Encourage family to make tape recordings of family voices	Encourage family to make tape recordings of family voices telling favorite stories or singing a favorite song	
Allow infant to visualize parents face during procedures	Encourage expression of loneliness Encourage family to bring personal items Be honest Accept regressive behavior	Encourage expression of loneliness Encourage family to bring personal items Be honest Regressive behavior is usually absent

TABLE 36–30. POWERLESSNESS RELATED TO ENVIRONMENT: NURSING INTERVENTIONS

INFANT	TODDLER	PRESCHOOLER	SCHOOL AGE
Maintain normal routine as much as possible	Maintain normal routine as much as possible Allow to wear own pajamas Allow choices Promote self-care	Maintain normal routine as much as possible Allow to wear own pajamas Allow choices Promote self-care	Maintain normal routine as much as possible Allow to wear own pajamas or clothing Allow choices Promote self-care
Use analgesics and distraction and parental contact to minimize restraints		Maintain privacy	Maintain privacy Allow input when scheduling nursing care
	Accept ritualistic behavior Avoid questions inviting a "no" answer	Accept ritualistic behavior	Develop contracts to negotiate scheduling of nursing care

TABLE 36–31. PAIN RELATED TO INJURY AND/OR PROCEDURES: NURSING INTERVENTIONS

INFANT	TODDLER	PRESCHOOLER	SCHOOL AGE
Use restraints only when necessary	Use restraints only when necessary Use the least intrusive procedure when possible (e.g., axillary instead of rectal temperature)	Use restraints only when necessary Use the least intrusive procedure when possible (e.g., axillary instead of rectal temperature)	Use restraints only when necessary Use the least intrusive procedure when possible (e.g., axillary instead of rectal temperature)
Allow parents to hold or be present with procedures	Allow parents to hold or be present with procedures	Allow parents to hold or be present with procedures	Allow parents to hold or be present with procedures
Keep procedure brief	Explain procedure just before performing if possible	Explain procedures before performing if possible	Explain procedures before performing if possible
Comfort during and after procedure	a. Use simple concepts b. Explain to child how to act (e.g., "hold leg still") c. Explain procedure shortly before it begins d. Allow expression of feelings (e.g., crying) e. Use distraction	a. Explain to child he or she did not cause procedure and is not being punished b. Encourage expressions of anger through play c. Explain how procedure will feel d. Allow expression of feelings (e.g., crying) Suggest ways to maintain control during a procedure (e.g., deep breathing) "blowing out candles" e. Use distraction	a. Use correct medical terminology b. Allow more time for teaching (than younger children) c. Explain functioning of equipment d. Allow time for questions Suggest ways to maintain control during a procedure (e.g., deep breathing, distraction, relaxation) Provide privacy from peers during procedure
Assess pain Signs and symptoms Neonatal Infant Pain Scale	Assess pain Faces pain scale	Assess pain Numeric pain scale Color pain scale Descriptive pain scale, faces	Assess pain Numeric pain scale or visual analog Color pain scale Descriptive pain scale, faces
Manage pain Encourage holding, cuddling Rock in wide rhythmic arc Repeat one or two words softly	Manage pain Encourage holding, cuddling Rock in wide rhythmic arc Repeat one or two words softly Distract with play	Manage pain Encourage holding, cuddling Help assume comfortable position Help with slow breathing and relaxation (e.g., limp doll) Distract with play	Manage pain Encourage holding, cuddling Help assume comfortable position Help with slow breathing and relaxation (e.g., limp doll) Distract with television, radio, etc.
Administer analgesics as ordered; assess effectiveness	Administer analgesics as ordered; assess effectiveness	Administer analgesics as ordered; assess effectiveness	Administer analgesics as ordered; assess effectiveness

In summary, children have age-specific reactions to their hospital experience. Despite the stresses normally associated with the intensive care unit, nurses can develop specific strategies to minimize negative reactions. Age-specific interventions to reduce separation anxiety, feelings of loss of control, and fears of bodily injury and pain have been described.

PSYCHOSOCIAL REVIEW

1. The three stages of separation anxiety in the infant are
   A. protest, despair, detachment
   B. protest, regression, detachment
   C. depression, despair, detachment
   D. protest, despair, aggression
2. The preschooler's behavior is best characterized as
   A. negative and ritualistic
   B. egocentric and magical
   C. industrious and independent
   D. quiet and modest
3. Children from which of the following age groups would most likely want a bandage for a cut or venipuncture?
   A. infant
   B. toddler
   C. preschooler
   D. school age

Cathy is a 2½-year-old girl admitted to the intensive care unit with epiglottitis. She is intubated and started on antibiotics. Restraints are necessary to prevent Cathy from extubating herself. Her parents are allowed to visit her every hour for 5 minutes.

4. What intervention would be most helpful to prevent feelings of loss of control?
   A. maintain a clock at the bedside
   B. encourage her to make her own bed
   C. minimize change in normal daily routines
   D. obtain a psychiatric consult

Answers: 1. A, 2. B, 3. C, 4. C

POSTTEST

1. The young infant is predisposed to respiratory dysfunction because of which of the following anatomic and physiologic features?
   A. relatively small tongue
   B. narrow vocal cords
   C. small airway diameter
   D. small body surface area
2. Initial signs of respiratory distress in the child are usually manifested by which of the following?
   A. unresponsive
   B. tachycardia
   C. perioral cyanosis
   D. bradypnea
3. Intracostal retractions in the infant are produced by
   A. narrowing of the nasal passages during expiration
   B. respiratory muscle fatigue
   C. premature glottic closure during expiration
   D. increased negative intrapleural pressure during inspiration

Refer to the following case study to answer questions 4 and 5.

Sally is a 9-month-old child who is brought to the emergency department with the following history: fever for 8 hours and difficulty breathing. Clinical data: pale, respiratory rate 60, protruding tongue, temperature 103°F (39.5°C), intercostal retractions.

4. Considering Sally's clinical presentation, which of the following orders should be initiated first?
   A. IV access
   B. chest radiograph
   C. blood culture
   D. oxygen
5. Based on these data, which of the following nursing diagnoses would you select as being appropriate in Sally's plan of care?
   A. *Fluid volume deficit*
   B. *Ineffective airway clearance*
   C. *Altered tissue perfusion: Renal*
   D. *Impaired physical mobility*

Refer to the following case study to answer questions 6 through 9.

Carlos is a 4-year-old boy admitted to the pediatric ICU following an MVC (unrestrained passenger). Clinical data: blood pressure 80/58 mm Hg, heart rate 120, respirations 32. Peripheral pulses slightly diminished. Hct 30 percent and Hgb pending. Pulse oximeter 98 percent. Serum electrolytes normal. CT scan is positive for abdominal bleeding. Weight is 20 kg.

6. Based on these data, which of the following nursing diagnoses would you select as being appropriate in Carlos's care?
   A. *Impaired gas exchange*
   B. *Altered cardiac output: Decreased*
   C. *Fluid volume deficit*
   D. *Ineffective airway breathing*

Carlos is placed on a cardiac monitor, and a urinary catheter is inserted. The one peripheral IV catheter in the left arm is infiltrated and is discontinued. An indirect blood pressure reading is 74/40 mm Hg and the heart rate is 140.

7. Which of the following orders should be initiated first?
   A. IV access
   B. dopamine continuous infusion
   C. serum Hct and Hgb
   D. arterial line setup

IV access is successful.

8. What parenteral solution would you most likely prepare for Carlos's volume replacement?
   A. 5 percent dextrose in water
   B. 0.9 percent normal saline
   C. 5 percent dextrose in 0.25 percent normal saline
   D. 25 percent albumin
9. How much fluid would Carlos most likely receive as a bolus?
   A. 100 mL
   B. 40 mL
   C. 400 mL
   D. 500 mL
10. Central nervous system development is greatest during which of the following ages of life?
    A. 5 to 10 years
    B. birth to 3 years
    C. 15 to 25 years
    D. consistent throughout life
11. Which of the following is considered to be a secondary traumatic brain injury?
    A. skull fracture
    B. scalp laceration
    C. diffuse axonal injury
    D. epidural hematoma
12. CSF values for a child with bacterial meningitis would most likely include
    A. protein < 50 mg/100 mL
    B. WBC > 500/mL
    C. negative Gram stain
    D. glucose > ⅓ serum glucose

Refer to the following case study to answer questions 13 and 14.

Maria is a 3-year-old girl admitted to the pediatric ICU 2 days previously with a diagnosis of bacterial meningitis. She has been on antibiotics since admission. On the third day of admission, Maria has a generalized seizure.

13. Which of the following nursing interventions would you perform first?
    A. administer oxygen
    B. prepare an anticonvulsant
    C. call the doctor
    D. administer a fluid bolus

Lorazepam (Ativan) is administered. Heart rate is 102, respirations 18 and shallow, blood pressure 102/70 mm Hg.

14. Based on Maria's postseizure status, what complication should be anticipated?
    A. hypotension
    B. apnea
    C. hypertension
    D. heart block
15. Which of the following is a physiologic response to cold stress in the newborn?
    A. hypoxemia
    B. hypernatremia
    C. hypotension
    D. hyperglycemia
16. The treatment of a moderate increase in body temperature is controversial because
    A. lowering body temperature too quickly may cause a seizure
    B. increased body temperature improves perfusion
    C. the elevated temperature may support the body's normal defense against invading pathogens
    D. antipyretics may cause hypotension in children

Refer to the following case study to answer questions 17 through 22.

Bobby is a 3-month-old infant diagnosed with tetralogy of Fallot (ventricular septal defect and severe right ventricular outflow obstruction). He has been taking digoxin (Lanoxin) and furosemide (Lasix) since diagnosis. He is admitted to the hospital for elective cardiac surgery. Heart rate is 160, respirations 52 (at rest), blood pressure 72/50 mm Hg. The liver is enlarged. He has circumoral cyanosis, nasal flaring, grunting, and intercostal retractions.

17. Bobby has a poor perfusion from what type of shock?
    A. hypovolemic
    B. septic
    C. compensated
    D. cardiogenic
18. Which of the following orders should be initiated first to improve Bobby's oxygenation?
    A. chest radiograph
    B. oxygen administration
    C. CBC, Hgb, and Hct determination
    D. postural drainage

Bobby's surgery is successful in correcting his heart defect, and he is admitted to the pediatric intensive care unit for postoperative management. Monitoring devices include right atrial pressure line, right radial arterial line, two peripheral venous lines, a mediastinal chest tube, and a urinary catheter. He is intubated and has assist volume ventilation.

19. Bobby is most at risk for infection because of
    A. a low perfusion state
    B. alteration in skin barriers
    C. abnormal WBC formation
    D. high levels of IgM

After 12 hours, Bobby is weaned off the ventilator and extubated. However, Bobby's $Paco_2$ level progressively increases over the next 24 hours, as well as his work of breathing. While waiting for a decision to reintubate, Bobby has a respiratory arrest.

20. What nursing intervention would you perform first?
    A. assemble intubation kit
    B. chest compressions
    C. ventilate with an Ambu bag
    D. administer oxygen

21. Bobby requires ventilatory support via an endotracheal (ET) tube. What size ET tube would you have available?
    A. 4.0 cuffed
    B. 3.5 uncuffed
    C. 5.0 uncuffed
    D. 2.5 uncuffed

Bobby's cardiopulmonary status eventually stabilizes. His invasive lines are removed, except for one peripheral IV line. He is transferred to the floor.

22. Which of the following nursing interventions would be most effective in limiting Bobby's anxiety related to hospitalization?
    A. promote cuddling by parents
    B. encourage visitation of grandparents
    C. place pictures of family members in his crib
    D. talk about parents frequently

POSTTEST ANSWERS

Question	Answer	Section	Table/Figure	Comment
1	C	One	Table 36–1	
2	B	Three	Table 36–7	
3	D	Three	Table 36–5	
4	D	Four		The patient had an actual loss of adequate ventilation related to airway obstruction from the swollen epiglottis. The clinical data represent defining characteristics of the nursing diagnosis.
5	B	Four		
6	C	Two		The crash has produced an actual loss of intravascular volume. The normal blood pressure indicates that the patient is compensating for the volume deficit by increasing heart rate and by peripheral vasoconstriction (decreased peripheral pulses). Therefore, CO still remains within the normal range. CO will decrease if bleeding continues and compensatory mechanisms become exhausted.
7	A	Seven		
8	B	Seven		
9	C	Seven		
10	B	Eight		
11	D	Nine	Table 36–19	
12	B	Nine		
13	A	Ten		
14	B	Ten		
15	A	Thirteen	Figure 36–4	
16	C	Thirteen		
17	C	Six		
18	B	Seven		
19	B	Fourteen		
20	C	Four	Figure 36–1	
21	B	Four	Table 36–8	
22	A	Seventeen	Table 36–35	

REFERENCES

Ackerman, A.D. (1996). Conditions that predispose the critically ill child to infection. In M.C. Rogers (ed.), *Textbook of pediatric intensive care* (pp. 789–842). Baltimore: Williams & Wilkins.

Betz, C.L., Hunsberger, M.M., & Wright, S. (1994). *Family centered nursing care of children*. Philadelphia: W.B. Saunders.

Bowlby, J. (1969). Patterns of attachment and contributing conditions. In J. Bowlby (ed.), *Attachment and loss* (pp. 331–350). New York: Basic Books.

Bruce, D.A., Alavi, A., Bilaniuk, L., Dolinskas, C., Obrist, W., & Uzzell, B. (1981). Diffuse cerebral swelling following head injuries in children: The syndrome of "malignant brain edema." *J Neurosurg* 54:170–178.

Chameides, L., & Hazinski, M.F. (1997). *Textbook of pediatric advanced life support*. Dallas: American Heart Association.

Curley, M., Smith, J., & Maloney-Harmon, P. (1996). *Critical care nursing of infants and children*. Philadelphia: W.B. Saunders.

Delgado, M.R. (1990). Status epilepticus. In D.L. Levin & F.C. Morriss (eds.), *Essentials of pediatric intensive care* (pp. 59–63). St. Louis: Quality Medical Publishing.

Guyton, A.C. (1987). *Human physiology and mechanism of disease* (4th ed.). Philadelphia: W.B. Saunders.

Hazinski, M.F. (1992). *Nursing care of the critically ill child* (2nd ed.). St. Louis: C.V. Mosby.

Hazinski, M.F., & van Stralen, D. (1990). Physiologic and anatomic differences between children and adults. In D.L. Levin & F.C. Morriss (eds.), *Essentials of pediatric intensive care* (pp. 5–17). St. Louis: Quality Medical Publishing.

Hester, N.O. (1993). Pain in children. *Ann Rev Nurs Res* *11*:105–142.

Mahan, L.K., & Arlin, M. (1992). *Krause's food, nutrition and diet therapy* (8th ed.). Philadelphia: W.B. Saunders.

Marshall, S.B., Marshall, L.F., Vos, H.R., & Chestnut, R.M. (1990). *Neuroscience critical care*. Philadelphia: W.B. Saunders.

Rosenthal, C.H. (1989). Immunosuppression in pediatric critical care patients. *Crit Care Nurs Clin North Am 1*:775–785.

Rosner, M., Rosner, S., & Johnson, A. (1995). Cerebral perfusion pressure: management protocol and clinical results. *J Neurosurg 83*:949–962.

Schindler, B. (1985). Stress, affective disorders and immune function. *Med Clin North Am* 69:585–597.

Shayevitz, J.R., & Weissman, C. (1992). Nutrition and metabolism in the critically ill child. In M.C. Rogers (ed.), *Textbook of pediatric intensive care* (pp. 943–978). Baltimore: Williams & Wilkins.

Snow, R.B., Zimmerman, R.D., Gandy, S.E., & Deck, D.F. (1986). Comparison of magnetic resonance imaging and computed tomography in the evaluation of head injury. *Neurosurgery 18*:45–52.

Tribett, D. (1989). Immune system function. *Crit Care Nurs Clin North Am 1*:725–740.

Wilson, T., & Broome, M.E. (1989). Promoting the young child's development in the intensive care unit. *Heart Lung 18*:274–280.

Wong, D.L. et al. (1999). *Whaley and Wong's nursing care of infants and children* (6th ed.). St. Louis: C.V. Mosby.

Module 37

Nursing Care of the Acutely Ill Obstetric Patient

Laurie Giovanitto, Michelle Wermes Renneker

The self-study module is written for the nurse who has basic knowledge of the critically ill patient. The focus of the module is the physiologic changes that occur with pregnancy and the unique needs of the acutely ill pregnant patient. The module consists of 14 sections. The first section focuses on the normal physiologic changes in pregnancy. The second section pertains to monitoring of the pregnant patient and the fetus. The third section discusses altered ventilation. Sections Four, Five, and Six addresses perfusion-related conditions. Sections Seven and Eight discusses shock states. Sections Nine and Ten discuss altered metabolism. Special conditions of pregnancy are discussed in Sections Eleven, Twelve, and Thirteen. The final section examines basic neonatal resuscitation. Each section includes a set of review questions to help the learner evaluate his or her understanding of the section's content before moving on to the next section. All Section Reviews and the module Pretest and Posttest include answers. It is suggested that the learner review those concepts answered incorrectly in the review questions before proceeding to the next section.

Objectives

Following completion of this module, the learner will be able to

1. Describe the normal pathophysiologic changes in pregnancy that lead to alteration in perfusion, ventilation, and metabolism.
2. Identify changes in fetal heart rate pattern, probable causes, and appropriate nursing interventions.
3. Identify factors that contribute to alterations in ventilation in a pregnant patient.
4. Identify an obstetric patient in shock and the underlying factors that predispose to shock.
5. Identify potential problems that can develop in the obstetric patient and her fetus as a result of diabetes.
6. Identify factors that contribute to alterations in perfusion in the obstetric patient.
7. Identify signs and symptoms of preterm labor.
8. List potential complications of the fetus with maternal drug use.
9. Describe the nursing interventions taken during an emergency delivery.
10. Describe the nursing interventions provided during neonatal resuscitation.

Pretest

1. The system most affected by pregnancy is the
   A. gastrointestinal (GI) system
   B. renal system
   C. cardiovascular system
   D. respiratory system

2. The second stage of labor involves
   A. consistent regular uterine contractions
   B. descent and rotation of the fetal head
   C. delivery of the placenta
   D. complete dilation
3. A nonstress test (NST) involves
   A. an amniotomy and placement of internal monitors
   B. application of external monitors
   C. inducing uterine contractions
   D. test dose of IV terbutaline
4. Signs of preeclampsia include
   A. hematuria
   B. blurry vision
   C. hyporeflexis
   D. hyperglycemia
5. Nursing care of a preeclamptic inpatient involves all of the following EXCEPT
   A. evaluating level of consciousness
   B. placing the patient in the Trendelenburg position
   C. infusing magnesium sulfate ($MgSO_4$)
   D. assessing deep tendon reflexes (DTRs)
6. HELLP syndrome (hemolysis, elevated liver enzymes, low platelets) is a complication of
   A. hypertension in pregnancy
   B. premature labor
   C. amniotic fluid embolus
   D. hypotension in pregnancy
7. Disseminated intravascular coagulation (DIC) occurs in obstetrics in association with
   A. primagravida
   B. fetal diabetes
   C. abruptio placentae
8. A complete previa is implantation of the placenta
   A. partially covering the cervical os
   B. on the anterior wall of the uterus
   C. covering the cervical os
   D. completely avoiding the cervical os
9. A cause of uterine rupture is
   A. uterine infection
   B. Pitocin infusion
   C. prolonged vaginal bleeding
10. A laboring patient experiencing obstetric complications requires
   A. no IV
   B. a 16- to 18-gauge IV
   C. a 22-gauge IV
   D. at least two IV accesses
11. Gestational diabetes occurs due to
   A. an unhealthy diet
   B. the diabetogenic effects of pregnancy
   C. drug abuse
   D. drug withdrawal
12. Premature labor is defined as all of the following EXCEPT
   A. documented cervical change with uterine contractions every 5 to 8 minutes after 20 weeks' gestation but before 37 completed weeks' gestation
   B. cervical dilatation of 2 cm or more after 20 weeks' gestation but before 37 completed weeks' gestation
   C. cervical effacement of 80 percent after 20 weeks' gestation but before 37 completed weeks' gestation
   D. positive vaginal bleeding with cramps after 20 weeks' gestation but before 37 completed weeks' gestation
13. A drug use history should be obtained
   A. at the first prenatal visit on every patient
   B. only if the patient has not completed high school
   C. only if the patient admits to drug use
   D. only if the patient presents complaining of uterine contractions
14. If a prolapsed umbilical cord is noted the nurse should
   A. place the patient in knee–chest position
   B. apply oxygen at 1 to 2 L/min per mask
   C. place the patient on her left side
15. Chest compressions should be initiated on a neonate if the heart rate is
   A. 100/bpm
   B. 60 to 100/bpm and rising
   C. below 80/bpm
   D. above 100/bpm with acrocyanosis present

Pretest answers: 1. C, 2. B, 3. B, 4. B, 5. B, 6. A, 7. C, 8. C, 9. B, 10. B, 11. B, 12. D, 13. A, 14. A, 15. C

Glossary

Accelerations. Increase in FHR by 15/bpm lasting for 15 seconds occurring with or without uterine contractions

Acme. The peak of the uterine contraction

Acrocyanosis. Cyanosis of the extremities

Amniocentesis. Transabdominal puncture of the amniotic sac, using a needle and a syringe, in order to collect a sample of amniotic fluid

Amniotomy. Artificial rupture of the fetal membranes

Antepartum. Before the presence of labor

Anti-TPO antibodies. Antibodies that form in response to thyroglobulin and thyroperoxidase

Baseline fetal heart rate. The range of the FHR between uterine contractions, normal range 120 to 160/bpm, without periodic FHR changes

Bradycardia. Prolonged baseline FHR below 120/bpm lasting > 10 minutes

Cesarean section. Delivery of a fetus through an incision in the abdominal wall and the wall of the uterus

Chorioamnionitis. Inflammation of the membranes that cover the fetus

Clonus. Spasmodic alternation of muscular contractions and relaxation

Cryoprecipitate. Precipitate formed from the serum of patients with chronic disease and stored at 4°C

Cyanosis. Bluish discoloration of the skin due to decreased amounts of oxygen in the blood

Decidua. A name given to the endometrium of the uterus during pregnancy

Decidua basalis. The part of the decidua that unites with the chorion to form the placenta

Diplopia. Double vision

Dystocia. Prolonged, painful, or otherwise difficult labor and delivery resulting from mechanical factors relating to either uterine dysfunction, inadequate pushing, or abnormalities of maternal pelvis, birth canal, or fetal development, position and presentation

Early deceleration. Decelerations in FHR beginning at the onset of a contraction and returning to baseline by the end of the contraction, related to head compression

Endometrium. The mucous membrane lining the inner surface of the uterus

Fetus. The baby in utero from the fifth week of gestation until delivery

Fundus. Top portion of the uterus

Gestational age. The age of the product of conception between the first day of the last normal menstrual period and birth of the baby, measured in weeks

Hemolysis. Destruction of red blood cells with liberation of hemoglobin and diffusion into surrounding fluid

Hydramnios (polyhydramnios). Amniotic fluid in excess of 1.5 L

Hyperreflexia. Increase in deep tendon reflexes (DTRs) that is associated with central nervous system irritability in preeclampsia/eclampsia recorded on a scale from 0 (absent) to 4+. Usually elicited in lower extremities

Hypovolemia. An abnormally decreased volume of liquid (plasma) circulating in the body

Lanugo. Fine, downy hair that covers the fetus

Late decelerations. Decelerations in fetal heart rate either beginning after the onset or at the acme of the contraction with a slow recovery to the baseline after the end of the contraction, related to uteroplacental insufficiency

Macrosomia. Birth weight equal to or greater than 90th percentile for gestational age and sex

Multiparity. Condition of having borne more than one child

Myometrium. Muscular wall of the uterus

Nuchal cord. Condition in which the umbilical cord is wrapped around the fetal neck

Obstetric laceration. Tearing of cervical, vulvar, vaginal, periurethral, or rectal tissue during childbirth

Parity. The number of births greater than 20 weeks' gestation, including live and stillborn births

Periodic FHR. Variations of the FHR above or below the baseline, acceleration, and deceleration

Postpartum. Referring to six-week period following childbirth

Retained placenta. Pieces of the placenta remaining adhered to the uterine wall

Scotomata. Islandlike blind gaps in the visual field

Supine hypotension. Condition resulting when a pregnant patient lies in a supine position producing decreased venous return to the heart, decreasing CO and causing a sudden drop in blood pressure

Term. A pregnant woman between 37 and 40 weeks' gestation

Thrombocytopenia. Abnormal decrease in the number of blood platelets

Tocolytic therapy. Use of medication to halt preterm labor

Tummy grip. An elastic material used to hold the instruments of the external fetal monitor in place on the patient's abdomen

Uterine irritability. Condition in which the uterus responds excessively to stimuli

Valsalva's maneuver. The bearing down activity performed during a bowel movement and during the second stage of labor with pushing

Variability. Fluctuations in baseline FHR due to beat-to-beat changes obtained by use of a fetal scalp electrode

Variable deceleration. Sudden drop in FHR, U, V, or square shape in appearance, usually with quick recovery to baseline, related to cord compression

Vernix. A sebaceous deposit covering the fetus

ABBREVIATIONS

AFP. Alpha-fetoprotein

ALT. Alanine aminotransferase

ARDS. Acute respiratory distress syndrome

AST. Aspartate aminotransferase

BTBV. Beat-to-beat variability

BUN. Blood urea nitrogen

CT. Computed tomography

CNS. Central nervous system

CO. Cardiac output

COP. Colloid oncotic pressure

CVP. Central venous pressure

CVS. Chorionic villus sampling

DIC. Disseminated intravascular coagulation

DKA. Diabetic ketoacidosis

DTR. Deep tendon reflexes

EFW. Estimated fetal weight

FHR. Fetal heart rate

FSE. Fetal scalp electrode

GDM. Gestational diabetes mellitus

GFR. Glomerular filtration rate

GI. Gastrointestinal

GTT. Glucose tolerance test

Hct. Hematocrit

HELLP. Hemolysis, elevated liver enzymes, and low platelets

Hgb. Hemoglobin

HPL. Human placental lactogen

IUFD. Intrauterine fetal demise

IUGR. Intrauterine growth retardation

IUPC. Intrauterine pressure catheter

KHB. Kleihauer–Betke

L/S. Lecithin/sphingomyelin

LOC. Level of consciousness

MAHA. Microangiopathic hemolytic anemia

$MgSO_4$. Magnesium sulfate

MVC. Motor vehicle crash

NST. Nonstress test

PAC. Pulmonary artery catheter

PAP. Pulmonary artery pressure

PAWP. Pulmonary artery wedge pressure

PE. Pulmonary embolus

PT. Prothrombin time

PTT. Partial thromboplastin time

RDS. Respiratory distress syndrome

SAB. Spontaneous abortion

SVR. Systemic vascular resistance

Toco. Tocodynamometer

TPO. Thyroperoxidase

UOP. Urine output

US. Ultrasound

UTI. Urinary tract infection

SECTION ONE: Normal Physiologic Changes in Pregnancy

At the completion of this section, the learner will be able to identify normal physiologic changes specific to the pregnant female.

Cardiovascular System

Changes that occur in the cardiovascular system during pregnancy are so significant and extensive that this system is described as hyperdynamic. The maternal hemodynamics adapt to meet the demands of pregnancy and the growing fetus. See Table 37–1 for hemodynamic values and blood volume changes.

The Heart

During pregnancy, there is an increase in blood volume (40 to 45 percent) and cardiac stroke volume resulting in myocardial hypertrophy and increased cardiac filling. The end result is a 10 percent (75 mL) increase in cardiac volume.

End-diastolic volume is increased owing to the thickening of the ventricular wall. This thickening is the result of the upward pressure from the diaphragm caused by the enlarged uterus. The point of maximal impulse is therefore higher due to displacement of the heart.

The first heart sound is more pronounced. This occurs between 12 and 20 weeks' gestation and is maintained until approximately 2 to 4 weeks' **postpartum.** Systolic murmurs are common. Mammary flow murmurs (mammary souffles) are normal and usually are heard over the breasts. These sounds result from increased blood flow throughout the vessels of the breast.

Maternal heart rate increases 10 to 15 beats per minute during the second trimester and remains at that rate until delivery.

Cardiac Output

Cardiac output (CO) increases 30 percent to 50 percent in pregnancy. The increase in CO in pregnancy is the result of an increase in both heart rate and stroke volume. CO will also vary according to maternal position. A **term** patient in the supine position has a decreased CO due to obstruction of the inferior vena cava and aorta by the enlarged uterus and decreased venous blood return to the heart (Cunningham, Gant, MacDonald, et al., 1997). Therefore, a lateral recumbent position is encouraged during labor to promote venous return. Although historical studies show

TABLE 37–1. CHANGES IN SELECTED HEMODYNAMIC, BLOOD AND URINE LABORATORY VALUES DURING PREGNANCY

HEMODYNAMIC VALUES	NONPREGNANT	PREGNANT
Cardiac output (L/min)	4–7	5–10
Heart rate (bpm)	70	80
Central venous pressure (mm Hg)	2–10	No change
Mean arterial pressure (mm Hg)	86–93	90–96
Systemic vascular resistance (dynes/second/cm^{-5})	800–1,200	600–900
Stroke/volume (mL/beat)	65	75
Left ventricular stroke work index (g × m × m^{-2})	33–50	42–54
Pulmonary artery pressure (mm Hg)	20–30/5–15	No change
Pulmonary artery wedge pressure (mm Hg)	6–12	No change
Pulmonary vascular resistance (dynes/second/cm^{-5})	20–120	15–90
BLOOD VALUES		
Leukocytes (per cm^3)	4,500–10,000	5,000–18,000
Hemoglobin (g/dL)	12–16	10–13
Hematocrit (%)	36–46	32–42
Fibrinogen (mg/dL)	200–400	400–500
Blood urea nitrogen (mg/dL)	5–25	4–12
Creatinine (mg/dL)	.67	.46
Sodium (mEq/L)	135–145	132–140
Ionized calcium (mEq/L)	2.2–2.5	4–5
URINE VALUES		
Creatinine clearance (mL/min)	85–135	150–200
Glucose	Negative	May be present as pregnancy increases, must be monitored closely
Protein (mg/dL/24 hr)	0–5	No change, increase may suggest complication

Sources: Kee, J.L. (1991). Laboratory and diagnostic tests with nursing implications. *3rd ed. St. Louis: C.V. Mosby; Harvey, C. (1991).* Critical care obstetrical nursing *[p. 21]. Rockville, MD: Aspen; Dunn, P. (1990). Assessing a pregnant woman after trauma.* Nursing '90. *20:53–57; and Clark, S.L., et al. (1989). Central hemodynamic assessment of normal term pregnancy.* Am J Obstet Gynecol 161:*1439.*

increased CO in the left lateral position, recent studies suggest equal increases while in the right lateral position.

During labor, CO increases 15 to 45 percent, increasing during each stage of labor and owing to the repeated performance of the Valsalva maneuver during pushing. After delivery, the increased blood volume that circulated to the placenta is now shifted back into the maternal bloodstream. This shifting of blood volume produces a dramatic increase in CO as soon as 5 minutes postpartum. At 1 hour postpartum, the cardiac output is 13 percent higher than nonpregnant values.

With a cesarean section, the increases in CO that accompanies performance of **Valsalva's maneuver** during pushing is eliminated. Along with the approximate blood loss of 1000 mL, autotransfusion is reduced causing fewer hemodynamic changes. However, a cesarean section does not prevent the normal increase in CO after delivery.

Blood Pressure

Blood pressure falls in the first trimester, as early as 7 weeks, reaches its lowest levels in the second trimester, and then returns to the patient's prepregnant level at term. The average decrease is 3 to 5 mm Hg systolic and 5 to 10 mm Hg diastolic.

Systemic Vascular Resistance

The placental vascular bed is a low-resistance system that utilizes a large amount of the maternal CO. Uterine vessels increase in size, thereby decreasing resistance and allowing an increase of blood flow to the uterus.

This vasodilation is the result of increased production of progesterone. Progesterone relaxes smooth muscles, including muscular walls and blood vessels, thus reducing systemic vascular resistance (SVR). With decreased venous resistance and increasing peripheral blood flow, venous stasis and pooling occurs.

Regional Blood Flow

The uterus receives approximately 10 percent to 20 percent of the cardiac output, which is facilitated by the decreased resistance of the uteroplacental circulation (Harvey, 1991). Similarly, blood flow increases in other organ systems.

The blood flow to the kidneys increases 25 to 50 percent by the middle of the second trimester (Creasy & Resnik, 1999). This increase occurs as early in pregnancy as six weeks. There is also an increase in mammary blood flow. The newly visible veins are evidence of this, along with enlargement of the breasts (Harvey, 1991). Increased blood flow to the skin, cervix, and vagina is also seen. Vascular proliferation and dilation are probably the result of estrogen effects (Creasy & Resnik, 1999). Edema of the skin, subcutaneous tissue, vulva, and legs occurs because of a combination of venous pooling and altered permeability of vascular tissue.

Respiratory System

The maternal respiratory system is extremely important for the maintenance of fetal oxygenation during pregnancy (Harvey, 1991). A relative hyperventilation of pregnancy begins in the first trimester and increases 15 to 25 percent by term gestation. Other respiratory changes that occur with pregnancy are:

- *Pulmonary vascular bed:* pulmonary vascular resistance may be decreased

- *Arterial blood gases:* decreased PCO_2 related to an increased respiratory rate and slight increase in pH
- *Oxygen consumption:* increases (32 to 58 mL/min) due to the decrease in vital capacity (Creasy & Resnik, 1999)
- *Lung volume:* increased tidal volume; alveolar ventilation is increased related to a rapid respiratory rate

Pregnancy has been called a state of chronic respiratory alkalosis because of the increase in oxygen consumption and vital capacity and a fall in $PaCO_2$ (Table 37–2).

Dyspnea is a common complaint of pregnant women, starting in the second trimester. Breathlessness increases on exertion. However, if a patient complains of shortness of breath at rest it may be more than just a normal complaint of pregnancy. Pathologic causes should be ruled out, such as severe anemia, pulmonary edema, pulmonary embolism, acidosis, **hydramnios,** and cardiac problems.

Renal System

Renal function undergoes profound changes with pregnancy. The kidneys need to make up for the increased metabolic and circulatory requirements of the pregnant woman and the waste products of the fetus.

The size of the kidney increases due to hypertrophy and hyperemia. The ureters dilate by midpregnancy in more than 80 percent of women with the effects greater on the right. It is thought that this effect is the result of compression by the uterus and ovarian vein plexus. Also, by term the enlarging uterus forces the bladder forward and upward and the bladder becomes concave rather than convex. The length of the urethra increases. Pressure from the presenting part of the fetus can block drainage of blood and lymph from the base of the bladder, causing edema and making the pregnant women more prone to urinary tract infections (UTIs).

Blood flow through the kidneys increases 25 to 50 percent with pregnancy. The glomerular filtration rate (GFR) and renal plasma flow increase. As a result, the renal clearance of many substances is elevated during pregnancy with a corresponding decrease in serum levels (Harvey, 1991). (See Table 37–1.)

TABLE 37–2. VENTILATORY MEASURES: PREGNANT VERSUS NONPREGNANT

	NONPREGNANT	PREGNANT
Respiratory rate (breaths/minute)	12–20	20–30
Tidal volume (mL/kg)	6–7	8–10
Minute ventilation (mL/minute)	5–10	7–25
Oxygen consumption (mL/minute)	173–311	249–331
Arterial Po_2 (mm Hg)	90–105	104–108
Venous Po_2 (mm Hg)	38–40	27–32
Arterial pH	7.35–7.40	7.40–7.45

Adapted from Dunn, P. (1990). Assessing a pregnant women after trauma. Nursing '90. *20:53–57.*

Sodium retention is normal in pregnancy. This increase does not affect maternal electrolyte balance, but is necessary to meet the needs of the fetus. Table 37–1 lists common electrolyte changes in pregnancy.

The incidence of glycosuria increases as pregnancy advances. This increase is due to an increase in GFR and the kidneys' inability to keep up with reabsorption. As a result excess glucose is excreted in the urine. This makes urine glucose levels an unreliable tool for monitoring diabetes in pregnancy. Although glycosuria is considered somewhat normal in pregnancy, it must be differentiated from gestational diabetes.

Protein in the urine is never normal although you may see an increase due to the increased GFR. An amount over 250 mg/dL is considered abnormal during pregnancy. Causes include preeclampsia, renal disease, and UTI.

Gastrointestinal System

Changes in the function of the GI system are mainly due to increased levels of progesterone and estrogen, causing decreased gastric motility, and mechanical compression from the growing uterus (i.e., the stomach is misplaced).

The side effects of these changes are evidenced by:

- Increase in appetite
- Nausea and vomiting (especially in first trimester)
- Heartburn, resulting from relaxation of the lower esophageal sphincter, constipation, bloating, and flatulence (as a result of decreased GI motility)
- Bleeding gums
- Increase in salivation

Hepatic System

The liver does not change in size or morphology in a normal pregnancy. However, there is a change in liver function tests. For example, hemodilution of pregnancy lowers the serum concentration of albumin and other proteins.

Gallstones occur more frequently in pregnancy due to accumulation of cholesterol crystals, which result from slow emptying. High progesterone levels cause decreased gallbladder contractility.

Central Nervous System

Headache is a common symptom associated most frequently with tension, depression, and migraine. In pregnancy, headache is rarely associated with a life-threatening condition and is the most common neurologic complaint. In most situations, the cause is unknown unless there is a head injury, allergy, hypertension, or inflammation present. The broad categories headaches are divided into are vascular, muscular, and pathologic. The differentiation of these headaches includes ruling out causes like alcohol and caffeine consumption, trauma, and abuse of prescription and nonprescription medications. It also requires detailed headache histories, including frequency, severity, location, duration, and what activity or conditions cause, exacerbate, or relieve the headache. With tension headaches, the most common type in pregnancy, muscular contractions of the neck and back lead to chronic, daily headaches that worsen throughout the day, and are most acute in the neck (Feller & Franko-Filiposie, 1993). Migraine headaches are vascular headaches that are the next most frequent headache in pregnancy. They occur twice as often in women during child-bearing years and show an association with changing estrogen levels. The steady elevated estrogen levels seen after the first trimester usually are related to a decrease in migraine episodes. These headaches are moderate to severe, throbbing, may have an aura or prodromal period, and are associated with slow onset, duration up to 72 hours, photophobia, phonophobia, and nausea. Normal levels of activity exacerbate symptoms as does fatigue, stress, missing meals, change in sleep patterns, and weather changes. Headache seen with severe preeclampsia is most likely a vascular headache. Vasospasms are the most likely causative factor (Cunningham, Gant, MacDonald, et al., 1997). Pathologic headaches include those associated with trauma or brain tumors. Pain that is deep-seated, dull, worsens with exercise, includes nausea and vomiting or is severe with sudden onset may be associated with brain tumor, cerebral hemorrhage, thrombi, or meningitis. Treatment of nonpathologic headaches relies on mild analgesics/sedatives (acetaminophen, codeine, Fioricet), relaxation and biofeedback exercises, and eliminating triggers (caffeine, fasting, stress, lack of sleep). Headaches that suggest further study include severe headache of sudden onset; headaches that interfere with sleep; headaches associated with physical exertion; headaches associated with changes in sensorium or vision, seizures, numbness/tingling, loss of control of part of the body; and headaches associated with changes in intellect (Creasy & Resnik, 1999).

Dizziness during early pregnancy is also a common complaint. Dizziness may result from dehydration, peripheral vasodilation, hypotension, or possibly hypoglycemia.

Numbness in the arms and hands can occur if lumbar lordosis is exaggerated. Posture is very important in preventing circulation problems. Flexion of the head and neck and slumping shoulders puts pressure on the ulnar and median nerves, causing aching, numbness, and weakness of the arms. The incidence of carpal tunnel syndrome increases with pregnancy, due to swelling and pressure on the median nerve. Numbness in the legs and feet is due to pressure on the femoral veins and nerves from the enlarging uterus.

In summary, the increased blood volume during pregnancy contributes to a greater CO. Decreased systemic vascular resistance exists; therefore, blood pressure drops in the first two trimesters. P_{CO_2} drops due to an increased respiratory rate as the fetus enlarges and diaphragmatic excursion decreases. The GFR increases in pregnancy while GI motility decreases. Numbness of all extremities may occur as pressure increases on the ulnar, median, and femoral nerves.

SECTION ONE REVIEW

1. In pregnancy, blood volume increases
   A. 10 percent
   B. 20 to 25 percent
   C. 40 to 45 percent
   D. 50 to 60 percent
2. Myocardial hypertrophy in pregnancy
   A. results from an increase in blood volume
   B. results from mitral valve prolapse
   C. is accompanied by a decrease in cardiac filling
   D. is abnormal
3. The supine position in a pregnant patient
   A. increases CO
   B. causes obstruction of the inferior vena cava
   C. increases venous return to the heart
   D. relieves stress to the fetus
4. Glycosuria occurs as pregnancy progresses due to
   A. an increase in GFR
   B. decreased blood flow to the kidneys
   C. renal disease
   D. renal trauma
5. Changes in the GI system are due to
   A. an increase in progesterone and estrogen
   B. decreased exercise
   C. poor diet
   D. decreased fluid intake
6. Gallstones occur more frequently with pregnancy due to
   A. accumulation of calcium crystals
   B. slow emptying
   C. an increase in gallbladder contractility
   D. greater liver activity

Answers: 1. C, 2. A, 3. B, 4. A, 5. A, 6. B

SECTION TWO: Maternal and Fetal Monitoring

At the completion of this section, the learner will be familiar with the stages of labor, applications of external and internal monitors, and assessment of the fetal monitor tracing.

Stages of Labor

The First Stage

The first stage of labor begins with the onset of regular contractions and culminates when the cervix has reached full dilation.

The first stage of labor consists of two phases. The first, latent labor, also called early labor, consists of regular uterine contractions until the active phase. Women are usually not admitted to the hospital in latent labor. Unfortunately for the patient, latent labor can continue for several days. Though the contractions are strong enough to keep the woman from sleeping, they are not strong enough to dilate the cervix quickly. The active phase usually begins at 3 to 4 cm with a more rapid rate of cervical dilation and effacement.

Cervical effacement is thinning of the cervix. In the nullipara, effacement usually occurs prior to dilation. In the multipara, it usually accompanies dilation.

The Second Stage

The second stage of labor consists of descent and rotation of the fetal head. In the past, the second stage of labor was considered a separate entity; however, descent and rotation frequently occur prior to complete dilation.

The Third Stage

The third stage of labor is defined as the time from the delivery of the infant to the delivery of the placenta. In several references, the third stage also includes 1 hour after delivery during the recovery period. This is the time most frequently associated with postpartum hemorrhage and other complications related to childbirth.

External Monitoring

External monitoring is important in any pregnant patient to evaluate fetal heart rate (FHR) and uterine contractions. External monitoring is used most frequently in the latent phase of labor. If labor progresses efficiently and without complications, it is continued through the active phase. However, in the case of a nonviable baby or fetus under 20 weeks, it is sometimes eliminated due to difficulty in maintaining tracing. Uterine activity may be monitored.

Ultrasound Transducer

An ultrasound transducer consists of a device that is applied to the maternal external abdominal wall by way of a turning grip, and transmits a high-frequency sound wave to assess FHR. Although this device is easy to apply and can be used prior to **amniotomy,** its disadvantage is that it is not always accurate and does not allow assessment of beat-to-beat variability (BTBV). Patient movement, fetal movement, and fetal hiccups interfere with transmission, and the fetal tracing may be compromised by frequent breaks in the tracing.

Tocodynamometer (Toco)

A toco, also an external device, is attached to the maternal abdominal wall, over the uterine fundus. The toco records tightening of the fundus during a contraction via a pressure sensitive "button" in the center of the toco. The contraction is displayed on the monitor recorder. The toco is useful in detecting contraction frequency but is useless for assessing the intensity of the contractions. For example, in obese patients contractions may not display even though the patient is having strong contractions. To evaluate intensity of the contraction more accurately, the nurse can palpate the contractions by placing a hand on the fundus. Table 37–3 lists steps in applying external fetal monitors.

Internal Monitoring

Fetal Scalp Electrode (FSE)

The FSE detects FHR by attaching a small stainless steel spiral electrode to the fetal presenting part, avoiding the fontanels, face, and genitalia. FSEs are the most accurate method of obtaining FHR. They also depict accurate BTBV. It is placed after amniotomy and secured to the mother by an EKG pad. It is not affected by maternal or fetal movements.

Intrauterine Pressure Catheter (IUPC)

The IUPC is made of soft plastic. It is inserted through the cervical opening into the uterus. The IUPC transmits the exact pressure changes exerted by uterine contractions and during uterine rest and is therefore the most accurate method for evaluating whether contractions are adequate for labor to progress. The uterine resting tone is the pressure between contractions. The IUPC also allows use of an amnioinfusion. Figure 37–1 shows placement of the FSE and IUPC.

To measure adequacy of contractions using an IUPC the nurse measures montevideo units. This is performed by counting the units of a contraction from the uterine resting tone to the peak of each contraction in a 10 minute period. Adequate labor and contractions are exhibited when the montevideo units are above 200 units.

Fetal Evaluation Tests

Nonstress Test (NST)

An NST is performed to determine fetal well-being. It consists of applying external monitors to detect FHR and

TABLE 37–3. APPLICATION OF THE FETAL MONITOR

EQUIPMENT NEEDED	PREPARATION OF EQUIPMENT	NURSING INTERVENTIONS
Fetal monitor	Plug fetal monitor into wall outlet	Explain importance of fetal monitoring to patient
Monitor paper	Check monitor paper Plug ultrasound transducer into outlet on front of monitor	Elevate head of bed 15–30° if possible
Ultrasound transducer	Plug tocodynamometer into outlet in front of monitor	Establish left uterine displacement by placing a wedge under the patient's right hip or turning patient to (L) lateral position Assess fetal position through modified Leopold's maneuvers
Tocodynamometer	Turn monitor on and press record button Check monitor paper speed, time, and date	Apply conductive jelly to ultrasound transducer and place transducer on abdomen; adjust transducer location until a strong FHR is heard and is recording on the monitor strip
Two monitor straps or tummy grip		Maintain ultrasound in place by straps or cover with tummy grip
Conductive jelly		Locate the fundus (the top) of the uterus Place the toco and secure with straps or cover with tummy grip Zero the toco by pressing the zero button (varies depending on type of machine) Adjust sound as desired Record on the monitor strip patient's name, hospital number, date, time, and RN signature; this is a legal document and part of the medical records

uterine activity for a 20- to 30-minute period. The patient is positioned in a lateral or semi-Fowler's position.

A reactive NST is obtained if there are at least two FHR accelerations noted within a 20-minute period, with FHR baseline within normal limits and long-term variability noted. Boundaries of a reactive NST may vary from facility to facility but at the least must include two accelerations in 20 minutes of 15 bpm over 15 seconds. A reactive NST is positively correlated with survival of fetus an additional 7 days in 99 percent of cases (Creasy & Resnik, 1999).

If a nonreactive NST is obtained the nurse should

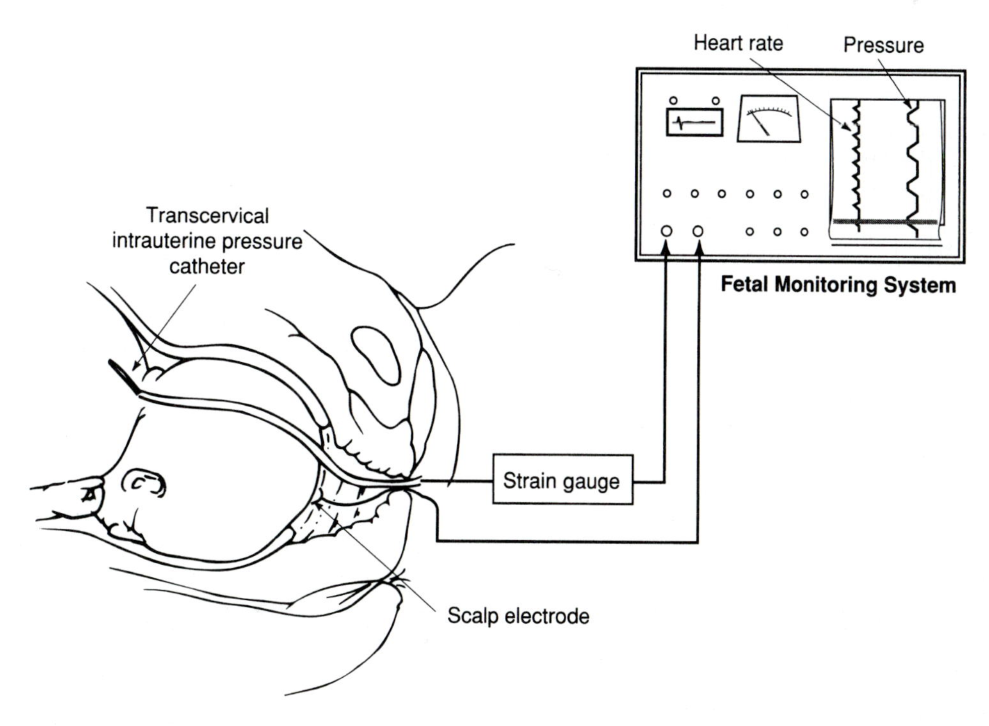

Figure 37–1. The fetal heart rate monitor, showing direct application, with fetal scalp electrode and intra-amniotic catheter. *(From Creasy, R., & Resnick, R. [1994].* Maternal-fetal medicine: Principles and practice, *3rd ed [p. 304]. Philadelphia: W.B. Saunders.)*

rule out any factors affecting the NST and repeat the test before any other interventions are implemented. Factors that could affect the results of an NST include fetal sleep patterns, maternal drug therapy, and cigarette smoking. Smoking a cigarette within 1 hour of an NST can cause a nonreactive NST. This occurs due to increased placental resistance that results from smoking (Cunningham, Gant, MacDonald, et al., 1997). If the NST is nonreactive or equivocal (one acceleration in 20 minutes, accelerations less than 15 bpm for 15 seconds) further testing may be warranted in the form of prolonged external monitoring, a repeat NST, or a contraction stress test (CST).

Contraction Stress Test (CST)

A CST is performed to determine fetal tolerance to the stress of labor. An external monitor is applied. A baseline strip of 10 minutes is obtained prior to the induction of contractions. An IV should be started, recognizing the potential for immediate intervention being required.

There are two methods of obtaining a CST: nipple stimulation and oxytocin infusion. Nipple stimulation is carried out by manual nipple stimulation with a warm washcloth. Stimulation is limited to 2 minutes, with 5-minute intervals between stimulation to prevent hyperstimulation (Creasy & Resnick, 1999). Once three adequate contractions of at least one minute's duration are noted in a 10-minute period, stimulation is discontinued.

Oxytocin infusion involves infusing Pitocin via infusion pump at 1 U/min, increasing infusion 1 unit every 15 minutes until three contractions are noted in a 10-minute period.

A negative CST result consists of no late decelerations with an FHR within normal limits. It is associated with the same survival rates as reactive NSTs.

A positive CST result consists of persistent late decelerations and possible decreased variability.

A suspicious CST consists of intermittent late decelerations or variable decelerations. Problems with interpreting CSTs results from inadequate recording of contractions and/or FHR. An unsatisfactory CST results from either overstimulation of the uterus, lack of adequate contraction frequency, or poor tracing.

Management of Changes in Fetal Heart Rate

Decreased Variability

Before managing decreased **variability** (fluctuation in **baseline FHR**), the nurse should first try to determine the underlying cause. Remember that any alteration the patient may experience directly affects the fetus (Fig. 37–2).

First, determine the **gestational age** of the **fetus.** Prior to 28 weeks' gestation, decreased variability is expected due to an immature fetal brain stem; thus, no interventions are necessary. Second, are there any congenital

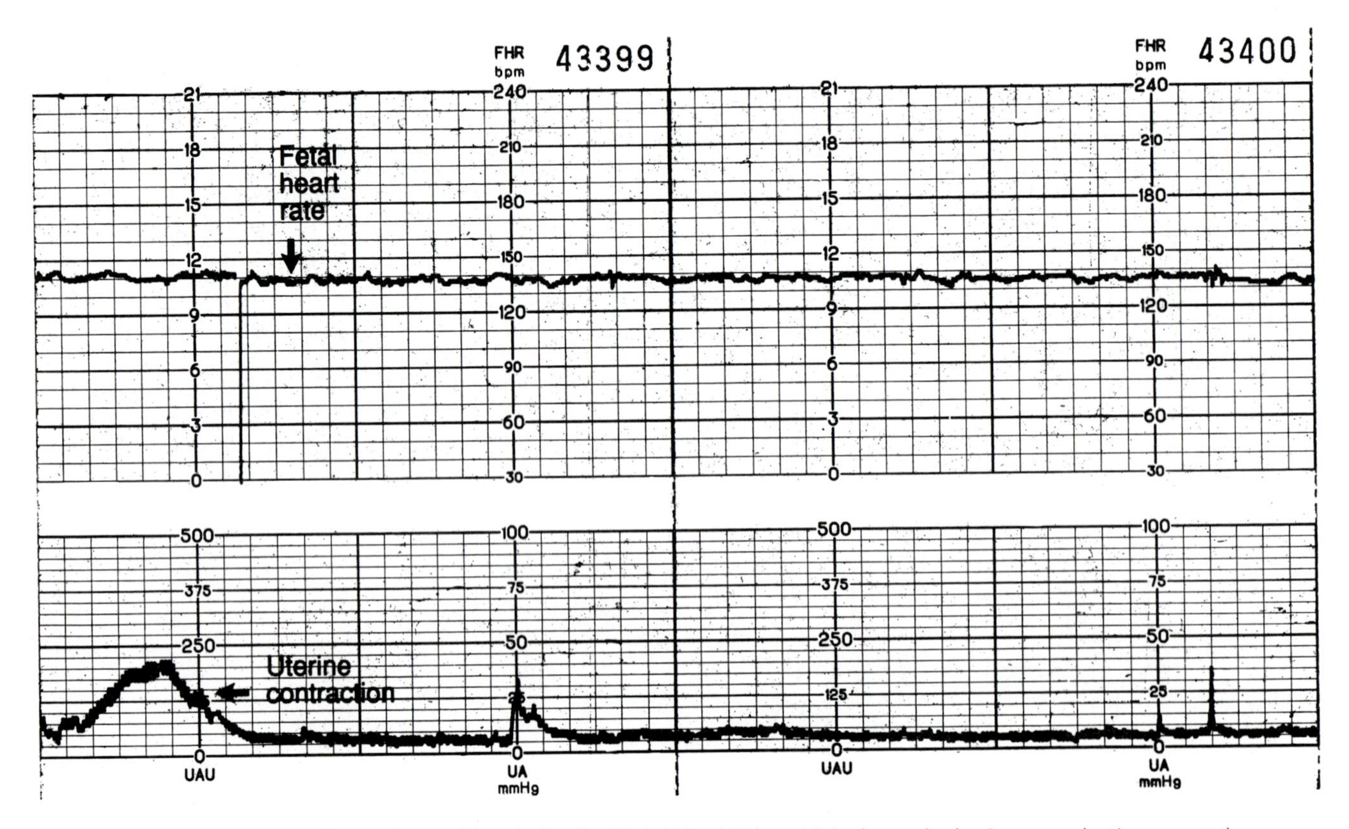

Figure 37–2. Decreased FHR baseline variability. The baseline FHR is 140 to 145 bpm. Minimal to no decelerations or accelerations are noted. *(From Kidd, P., & Wagner, K. [1992].* High acuity nursing: Preparing for practice in today's health care settings *[p. 559]. Norwalk, CT: Appleton & Lange.)*

anomalies? If so, intervention may not be indicated. Third, has the patient received any medications? $MgSO_4$, sedatives, tranquilizers, and narcotics will decrease variability. Variability will eventually increase dependent on the medications duration of action. Fourth, was variability previously normal? Review the entire fetal monitor strip. The nurse may see patterns of increased and decreased variability, which may be cycles of fetal sleep. This is an example of long-term variability for which no intervention is needed. Fifth, assess the patient's breathing patterns. Hyperventilation causes maternal respiratory alkalosis, reducing P_{CO_2} and increasing pH. Encourage the patient to take slow deep breaths. Sixth, is long-term variability decreased with evidence of a change in FHR baseline? This may be indicative of hypoxia and fetal distress; further fetal evaluation is necessary. Notify the physician. Apply oxygen at 8 to 10 L/min. If the patient is not in a lateral recumbent position, reposition her. Increase IV fluids. Explain these interventions in a simple reassuring manner to the woman and her supportive other.

Although external fetal monitoring is not accurate in evaluating BTBV it does reflect changes in long-term variability. If the patient's membranes are intact, a vibroacoustic stimulator, a handheld mechanism that vibrates and produces a noise equivalent to approximately 80 decibels, may be used to evaluate fetal response. It is applied to the external maternal abdomen over the fetal head for 3 to 5 seconds. If accelerations are noted, no further evaluation is needed. However, if there is no response or decelerations are noted, further evaluation and intervention are indicated.

Further evaluation may require an amniotomy and application of an FSE. If decreased variability remains consistent, the nurse or physician may attempt fetal scalp stimulation. This is accomplished by vigorously rubbing the top of the fetal head during a digital exam. Positive fetal scalp stimulation is evidenced by an acceleration. If no response is noted a fetal scalp blood sample is obtained for pH. This is done by making a small puncture in the fetal scalp. A pH of ≤ 7.20 requires consideration of delivery or may be repeated 30 minutes later before delivery is sought. The route of delivery depends on the patient's dilation status. For example, if the patient is at 4 cm and remote from vaginal delivery, cesarean section is indicated. If the patient is completely dilated and fetal station is low, forceps or a vacuum-assist device may be applied to expedite delivery.

Accelerations

Accelerations are indicative of fetal well being and are reflective of normal oxygenation. No interventions are required (Fig. 37–3).

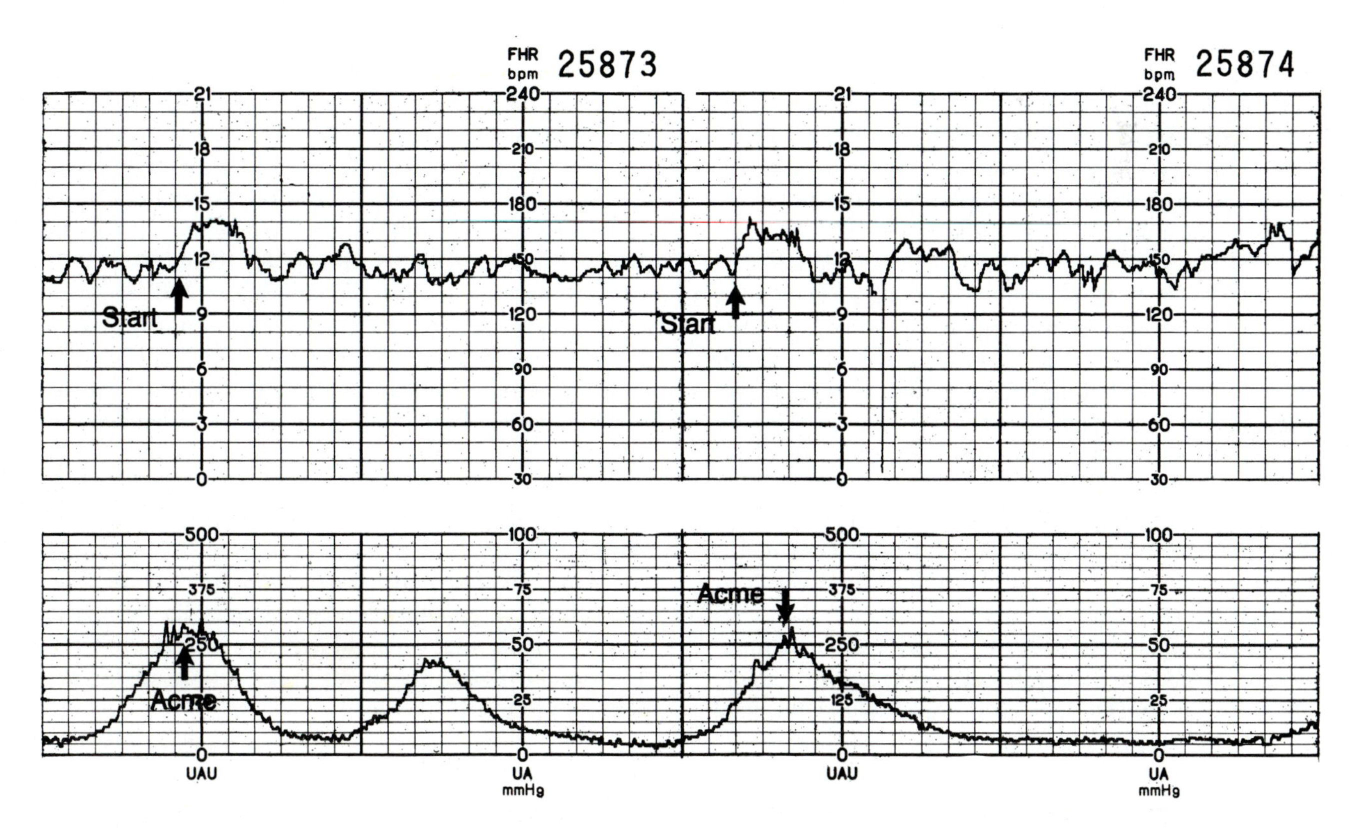

Figure 37–3. FHR accelerations. The baseline FHR is 140 to 155 bpm, with accelerations to 160 to 170 bpm at the acme of the contraction. This tracing is termed "reactive" and is very reassuring. *(From Kidd, P., & Wagner, K. [1992].* High acuity nursing: Preparing for practice in today's health care settings *[p. 555]. Norwalk, CT: Appleton & Lange.)*

Early Decelerations

Early decelerations are caused by head compression (Fig. 37–4). A sudden onset of early decelerations may be indicative of descent of the fetal head. At the onset of early decelerations, a digital exam is indicated to determine cervical dilation and station. Delivery may be imminent and the nurse should be prepared for delivery. Early decelerations are benign and require no interventions.

Variable Decelerations

Variable decelerations result from vagal stimulation and in response to cord compression usually in the first stage of labor or head compression in late second stage of labor (Fig. 37–5). These decelerations vary in shape, depth, and duration with each contraction. The onset and return are usually abrupt. Mild to moderate variable decelerations last < 60 seconds and fall no lower than 60 bpm. An occasional variable deceleration with quick recovery occurs in a premature fetus or a patient with premature ruptured membranes. No intervention is needed. Persistent and deep variable decelerations, under 100 bpm lasting longer than 30 seconds, result in hypoxia and many interventions may be used to resolve these decelerations.

Quick and easy remedies that can be implemented by the nurse include assessing for prolapsed umbilical cord and changing the patient's position. Oxygen may be applied; however, it is a supportive measure and will not help resolve decelerations. If variable decelerations are persistent and do not resolve with position change the physician should be notified. If an IUPC is not being used the physician may insert one and order an amnioinfusion. An amnioinfusion involves infusing warmed normal saline through a double-lumen IUPC. The fluid is warmed to prevent cold stress to the fetus. If your facility does not use a double-lumen IUPC, a second IUPC may be inserted. A single-lumen IUPC will not register contractions while an amnioinfusion is running. The theory behind the use of an amnioinfusion is to "float" the cord. With the absence of fluid, as in a patient whose membranes are ruptured, the umbilical cord drops with gravity into the lower segment of the uterus; when the uterus contracts, the cord is compressed between the side of the uterus and the fetus. The nurse may see a minimal increase in uterine resting tone due to an increase in fluid. The amnioinfusion is first infused at a bolus rate ordered by a physician and then slowed to 150/mL/hr. Remember to maintain warm fluid.

Any variable that does not resolve with amnioinfusion may be due to a **nuchal cord.** Other type of cord occlusions may include bandelero cords around the fetal body and shoulder; extremity cord, true knots in the cord; occult cord prolapse; or any combination. A nuchal cord may be seen on the fetal monitor strip as a W-shaped variable, as seen in Figure 37–5. This type of variable is usually seen with rapid descent and pushing. The only intervention to resolve this type of variable is delivery.

Late Decelerations

Late decelerations are caused by uteroplacental insufficiency (Fig. 37–6). They may occur as single entities in the absence of contractions or persistently with contractions. Late decelerations with contractions may be an indication of fetal intolerance to labor.

A single, spontaneous, late deceleration requires prolonged monitoring for fetal well-being, but aggressive interventions are not required.

If late decelerations are persistent (occurring with ≥ 50 percent contractions), prompt interventions are necessary. The nurse should reposition the patient, administer oxygen, increase the rate of IV fluids, and notify the physician immediately. If the patient is receiving Pitocin, the drip should be discontinued. Though Pitocin has a short half-life, terbutaline 0.25 mg subcutaneously may be ordered to halt contractions to allow time for the fetus to recover. If late decelerations continue, amniotomy is performed and an FSE is placed to evaluate variability and fetal scalp stimulation. If variability is absent and scalp stimulation is negative, a fetal scalp pH is obtained. Further decisions are based on the pH results. For example, if the patient is laboring and dilation is advanced and pH is within normal limits (7.29 to 7.33), labor may continue with continual monitoring and periodic pH checks. If the pH is below 7.24 and the patient is in early labor, a cesarean may be indicated for fetal intolerance to labor.

Moderate Bradycardia

Moderate bradycardia, 100 to 110 bpm, may be due to a change in the maternal condition (Fig. 37–7). However, what may be considered moderate bradycardia in one fetus, may be the FHR baseline in another. Always compare the FHR to previous FHR strips. Maternal conditions that may change the FHR baseline are drugs, hypotension, and respiratory changes. Before interventions are taken, the nurse should evaluate FHR for variability and accelerations. If these are present, the fetus is tolerating the change in baseline. If these signs are not present, the nurse should intervene by changing the patient's position, placing the bed in the Trendelenburg position, applying oxygen, increasing IV fluids, and notifying the physician. Correcting maternal condition is warranted; once the patient's condition is stabilized, the FHR usually returns to its previous baseline.

If marked bradycardia is noted (99 bpm), prompt interventions are required. Marked bradycardia can occur after a vaginal exam, placement of a urinary catheter, from umbilical cord compression, hypertonic uterine activity, or placental abruption.

Bradycardia occurring after a vaginal exam or placement of a urinary catheter can occur for two reasons: (1) the patient is usually in a supine position, tilting the uterus back and compressing the vessels supplying oxygen to the placental–fetal compartment, and (2), vagal stimulation of the fetus due to a change in the fetal environ-

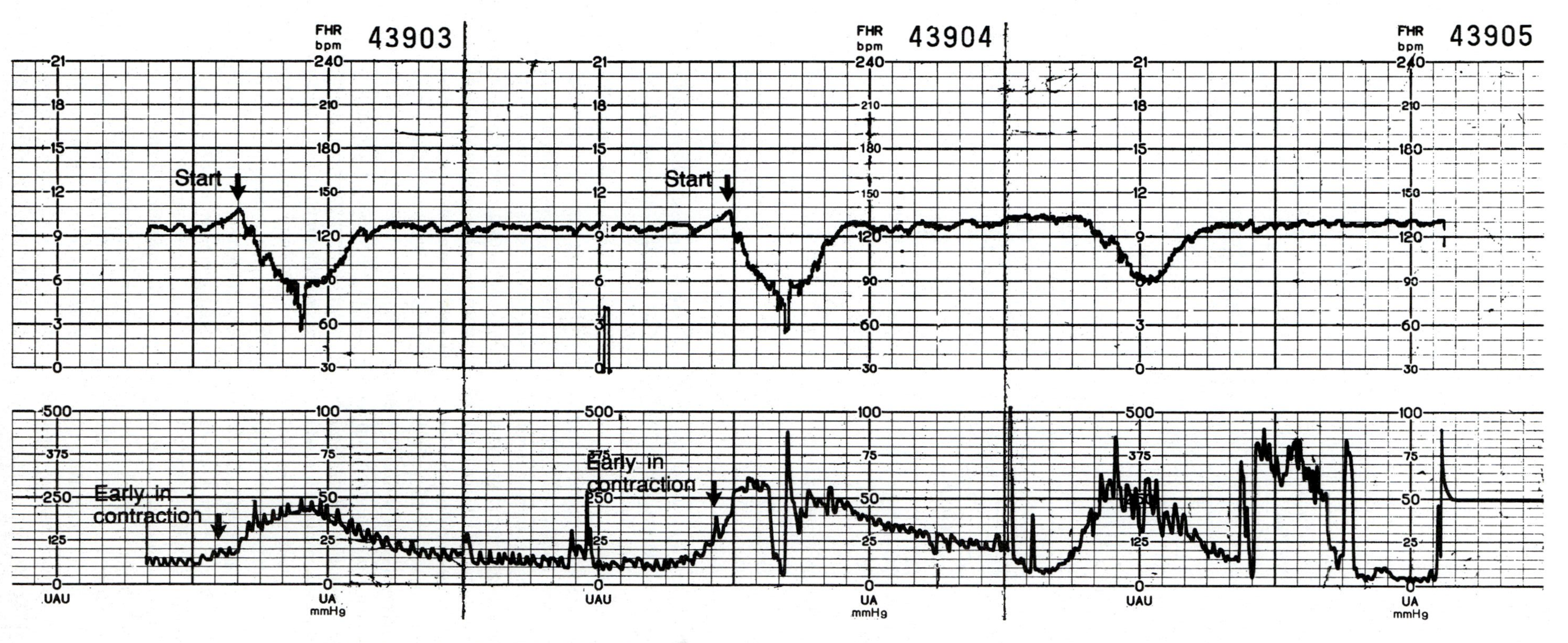

Figure 37–4. Early FHR decelerations. The baseline FHR is 125 to 130 bpm. The deceleration starts early in the contraction and fully recovers after the contraction ends (it mirrors the contraction). *(From Kidd, P., & Wagner, K. [1992].* High acuity nursing: Preparing for practice in today's health care settings *[p. 556]. Norwalk, CT: Appleton & Lange.)*

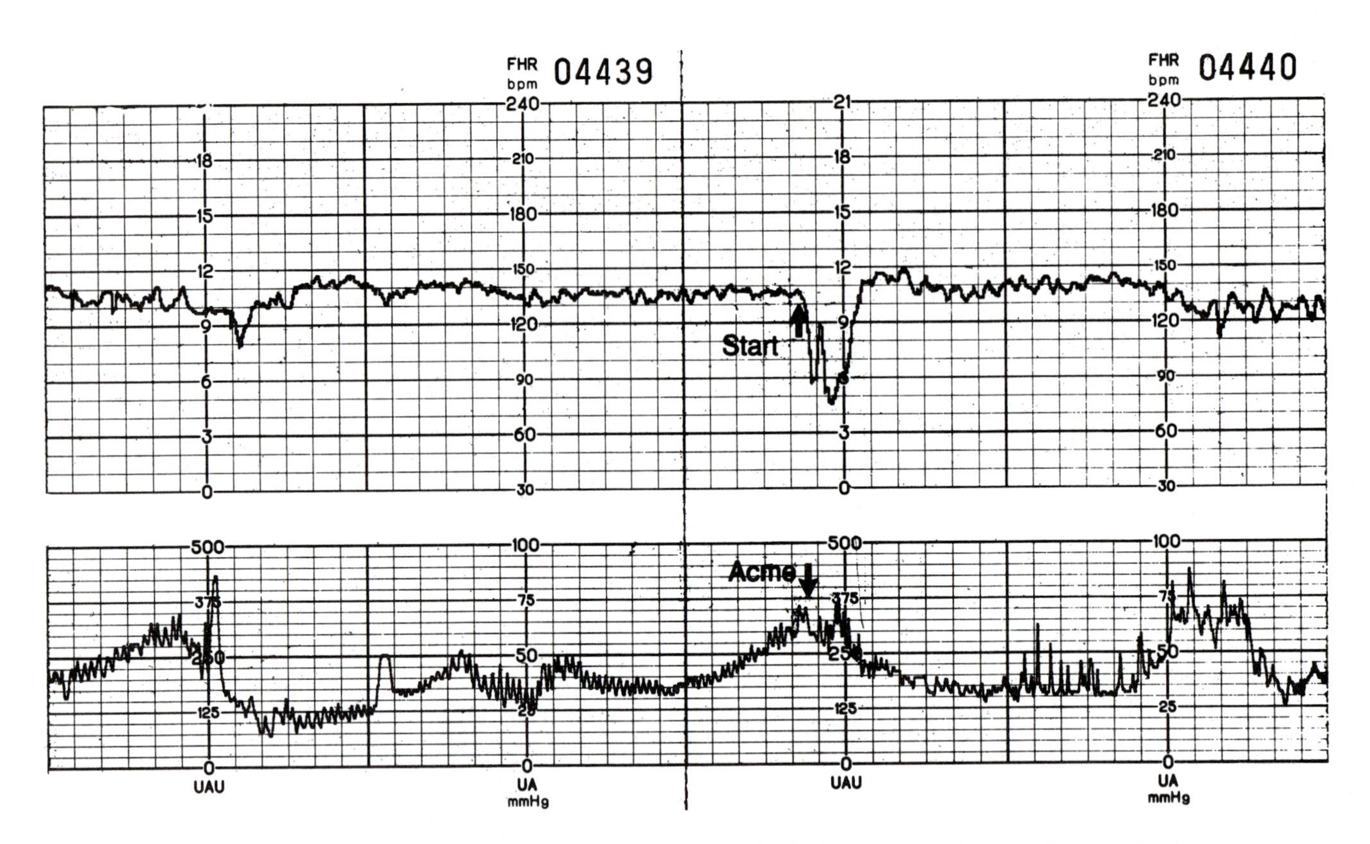

Figure 37–5. Variable FHR decelerations. The baseline FHR is 140 to 155 bpm. The deceleration starts as the contraction approaches the acme and is fully recovered to baseline after the contraction is over. *(From Kidd, P., & Wagner, K. [1992].* High acuity nursing: Preparing for practice in today's health care settings *[p. 557]. Norwalk, CT: Appleton & Lange.)*

ment. Emptying a distended maternal bladder allows the fetal head to descend rapidly, which is not always tolerated by the fetus. In both cases, changing the patient's position generally resolves bradycardia.

If bradycardia occurs spontaneously, the nurse should perform a vaginal exam to rule out a prolapsed cord. The patient's position should be changed, oxygen applied, fluid bolus begun, and Pitocin discontinued, if infusing. The nurse next evaluates the maternal condition and corrects hypotension and hypertonic uterine activity. Hypertonic uterine activity is either a uterine contraction lasting longer than 90 seconds or several contractions with little uterine rest in between. Hypertonic contractions are usually associated with Pitocin infusion but can also be associated with placental abruption. Terbutaline will be given 0.25 mg subcutaneously to halt uterine activity. Amniotomy with FSE placement will be implemented, if not already done. Fetal scalp stimulation will also be attempted. The patient may be placed in the knee–chest position. If bradycardia continues despite interventions for longer than approximately 10 minutes, an emergency **cesarean section** will be performed.

Bradycardia may also occur within minutes before vaginal delivery due to rapid descent. If the patient is unable to push effectively and deliver baby promptly, forceps or vacuum-assist device will be applied.

New Trends in Fetal Assessment and Fetal Oxygen Saturation Monitoring

External fetal monitoring (EFM) is now utilized in about 98 percent of laboring women in the United States (Simpson, 1998). Although EFM has been proven to be safe and effective, there have been studies recently revealing conflicting evaluations of FHR patterns among health care providers, contributing to a higher risk of cesarean birth. Essentially, this means a significant percentage of cesarean births may not be necessary for ensuring good fetal outcome. Fetuses demonstrating "non-reassuring" FHR patterns are not always intolerant to labor. The development of alternative methods of fetal surveillance has been in process. One method currently under multicenter study with Food and Drug Administration (FDA) guidance is fetal oxygen saturation monitoring. The goal is to accurately identify fetuses compromised by the labor process and in need of emergent delivery (Simpson, 1998). Oxygen saturation monitoring is commonly used in intensive care unit (ICU), operating room (OR), and postanesthesia care unit (PACU) settings. It is a reflection of the percentage of arterial oxygen that is bound to hemoglobin (oxyhemoglobin). The measurement of oxygen saturation means of measurement is possible because oxyhemoglobin absorbs more infrared light while deoxyhemoglobin absorbs more

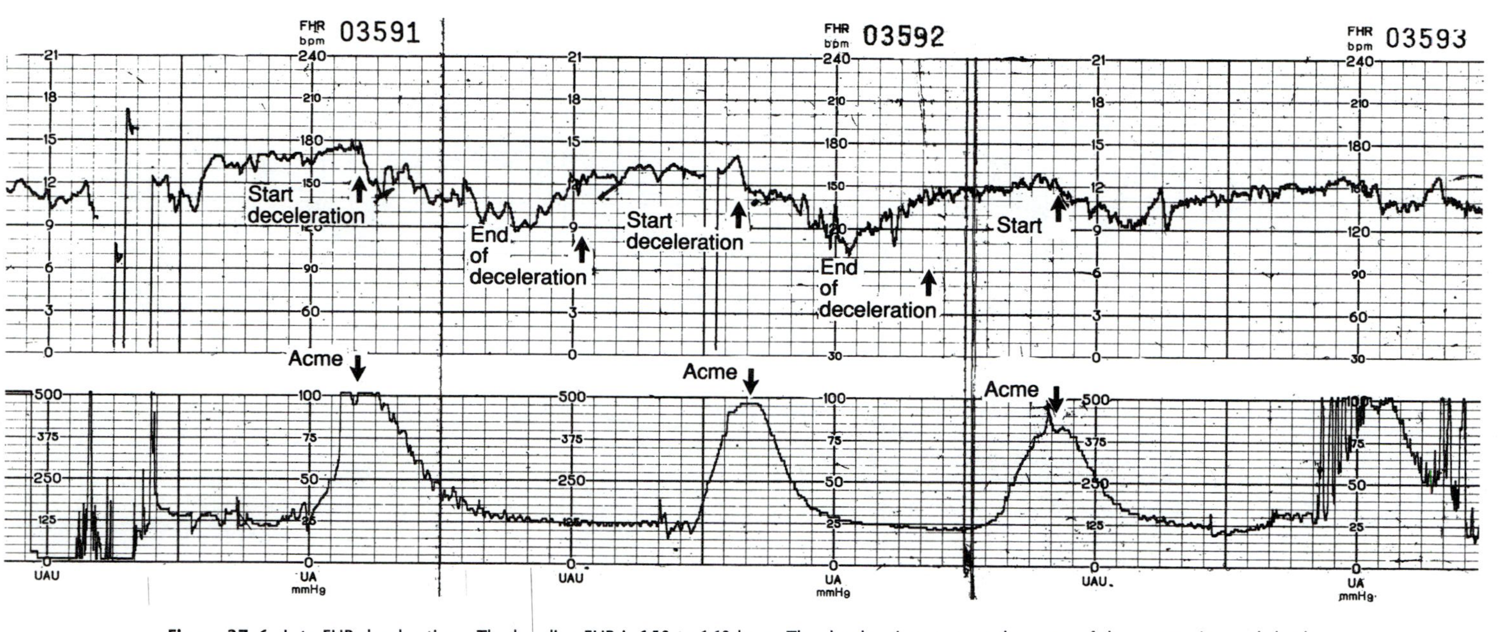

Figure 37–6. Late FHR decelerations. The baseline FHR is 150 to 160 bpm. The deceleration starts at the acme of the contraction and slowly returns to baseline. *(From Kidd, P., & Wagner, K. [1992].* High acuity nursing: Preparing for practice in today's health care settings *[p. 558]. Norwalk, CT: Appleton & Lange.)*

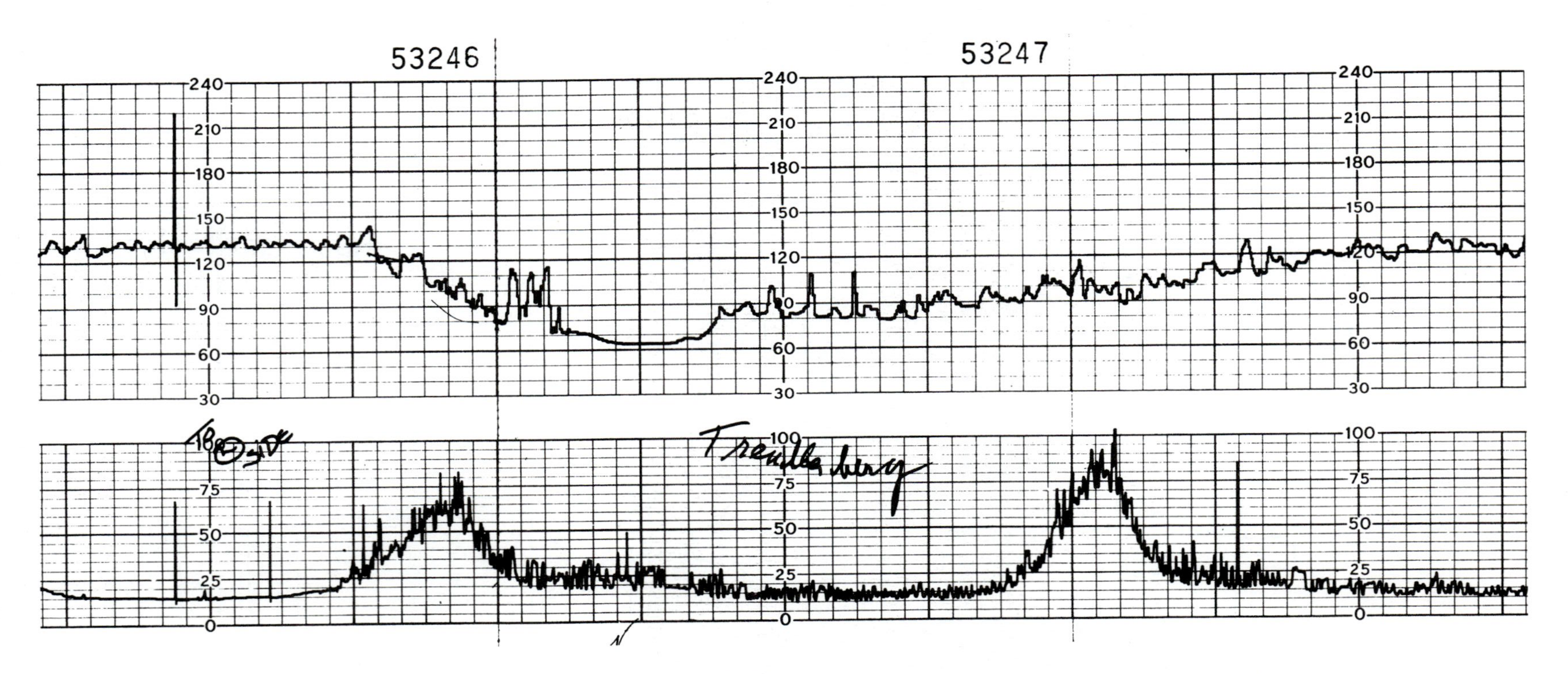

Figure 37–7. Baseline 125–135 bpm. Presence of good variability following the prolonged deceleration suggests the fetus was able to tolerate the stress. *(From Rabello, Y., & Lapidus, M. [1992].* Fundamentals of electronic fetal monitoring *[p. 71]. Wallingford, CT: Corimetrics Medical Systems, Inc.)*

red light. The saturation monitor is able to measure these values and display a percentage. New techniques in saturation monitors have allowed development of reflectance oximetry with the two light-emitting diodes (infrared and red) and the photo detector aligned side by side instead of opposing each other (transmission oximetry). The resulting flat sensor can be inserted into the uterus after rupture of membranes and placed against the fetal cheek or temple. Currently, it is known that fetal oxygen saturation (30 to 70 percent) differs from that of adults (95 to 100 percent). Determining the level at which fetal compromise occurs is part of this ongoing research. Thirty percent seems to be the critical point, suggesting that levels above 30 percent are supportive of fetal tolerance to labor. Over the next few years, use of oxygen saturation monitoring may become a routine adjunct to EFM helping us to refine our understanding of what constitutes fetal compromise.

In summary, the nurse must be prepared for any situation, responding quickly and implementing appropriate interventions in the presence of fetal distress. Correctly interpreting fetal monitor strips is imperative in order not to overlook distress. Remember, the fetus is a patient too.

Section Two Review

1. The first stage of labor begins
   A. with the loss of the mucus plug
   B. with the onset of regular contractions
   C. at 40 weeks' gestation
   D. with rupture of the fetal membranes
2. The active phase of labor includes
   A. cervical dilation at 1 cm
   B. pushing
   C. cervical dilation at 3 to 4 cm
   D. complete effacement of the cervix
3. The nurse who notes acceleration of the FHR should
   A. do nothing; this is an indication of a healthy fetus
   B. place the patient in the Trendelenburg position
   C. apply oxygen for supportive measures
   D. notify the physician
4. A sudden onset of early decelerations requires
   A. application of oxygen
   B. a digital exam
   C. placing the patient in the knee–chest position
   D. injecting terbutaline to halt contractions
5. An amnioinfusion is
   A. used in the presence of variable decelerations
   B. an infusion of cooled normal saline
   C. infused through an IV catheter
   D. removal of amniotic fluid
6. If marked bradycardia occurs, the nurse should
   A. place the patient supine
   B. defibrillate the patient
   C. begin a fluid bolus and apply oxygen
   D. perform cardiac massage

Answers: 1. B, 2. C, 3. A, 4. B, 5. A, 6. C

RESPIRATORY

SECTION THREE: Acute Pulmonary Complications

At the completion of this section, the learner will be familiar with the most common pulmonary insults in pregnancy and how to care for a pregnant patient experiencing such insults.

Pulmonary Edema

Etiology

Pulmonary edema is usually classified as cardiogenic or noncardiogenic. The incidence of pulmonary edema is difficult to determine because it is usually classified as a complication of another underlying disease in pregnancy. A third theory of etiology of pulmonary edema is a decrease in colloid oncotic pressure (COP). COP is the pressure exerted by the protein fraction of the blood that opposes capillary hydrostatic pressure and helps to keep fluid within the vessels.

Pathophysiology

Cardiogenic pulmonary edema results as the left ventricle is unable to empty its contents completely and efficiently. This causes dilation of the ventricle. As it continues, pressure in the pulmonary veins and arteries increases. If untreated, the hydrostatic pressure of the fluid becomes greater than that of the pressure exerted by the COP and this forces fluid into the interstitial spaces and alveoli, decreasing gas exchange.

Noncardiogenic pulmonary edema results from increased pulmonary capillary permeability. The cause is a direct injury that damages the alveolar capillary membrane. Once permeability is altered, fluid shifts into the interstitial spaces and alveoli. The result of noncardiogenic is the same as cardiogenic pulmonary edema; decreased gas exchange and hypoxemia.

The third theory postulated for a decrease in COP is similar to cardiogenic pulmonary edema except that the heart is functioning normally. The results are the same.

Clinical Manifestations

The symptoms vary depending on the severity. Patients often complain of shortness of breath, dyspnea, and tachypnea. On auscultation of the lungs, coarse crackles and rhonchi may be heard or the lungs may sound normal. A chest x-ray may appear normal, have patchy infiltrates, or be completely opaque (indicative of fluid in the interstitial spaces). In severe cases, the patient produces pink, frothy sputum.

Management

Management of pulmonary edema is supportive in nature. The patient's anxiety due to difficulty of breathing can be treated with morphine sulfate. Oxygen saturations should be maintained above 90 percent. Arterial blood gases should also be evaluated periodically. If PaO_2 drops below 60 mm Hg and oxygen saturations drop below 90 percent, oxygen therapy should be initiated. These patients may require intermittent positive pressure ventilation or mechanical ventilation depending on severity.

Continuous fetal monitoring is imperative. In the presence of fetal distress, intervention must be taken. In the absence of fetal distress, once the patient shows signs of improvement, the fetus will recover without any adverse effects.

The type of pulmonary edema must be determined prior to drug therapy. Placement of a pulmonary artery catheter (PAC) can help in identifying the cause by obtaining pressures in the heart.

Drug therapy differs greatly from author to author. Lasix is used very conservatively. Antibiotics are normally ordered prophylactically. Drugs used should decrease SVR, increase CO, and maintain urine output. A renal dose of dopamine may be ordered to maintain renal perfusion.

Amniotic Fluid Embolism

Etiology

The most common factors attributing to amniotic fluid embolus are advanced maternal age, multiparity, macrosomia, Pitocin induction, hypertension, and precipitous labor. Other causes have been reported in association with abruption and intrauterine fetal distress (IUFD).

Pathophysiology

It is difficult to determine the exact pathophysiology of amniotic fluid embolism because of the acute nature and the fact that subsequent death occurs 86 percent of the time within 2 hours following the initial insult (Creasy & Resnick, 1999). It is theorized that the primary event is characterized by severe pulmonary hypertension resulting from amniotic fluid in the lung. This elevated pressure leads to right heart failure and hypoxia. In patients who survive the initial event, left ventricular failure occurs with normal right ventricular function and severe pulmonary edema.

Amniotic fluid embolism results in disseminated intravascular coagulation (DIC) as the fibrinolytic system is activated.

Clinical Manifestations

The symptoms usually occur immediately after delivery. The patient develops acute respiratory distress, shock out of proportion to blood loss, chills, shivering, sweating, and possible seizures. Pink, frothy sputum may also be present. Diagnosis is made usually by autopsy. Aspiration of blood from the pulmonary artery will contain fetal cells, **lanugo, vernix,** or meconium.

Management

The first step in managing amniotic fluid embolism is to maintain oxygenation by intubation and mechanical ventilation; in most cases, cardiopulmonary resuscitation (CPR) is necessary. A PAC is placed to evaluate hemodynamic status. Drug therapy is controversial and may vary from physician to physician. Blood products are used to correct DIC.

Acute Respiratory Distress Syndrome (ARDS)

Etiology

ARDS is the response of the pulmonary system to a physiologic insult or series of insults to the integrity of the human body. These insults may result from the trauma of a motor vehicle crash or hemorrhage postoperatively or with sepsis. In association with pregnancy, ARDS can be a final and fatal result of obstetric complications. Complications that predispose to ARDS are aspiration, DIC in preeclampsia, eclampsia, abruptio placentae, IUFD, amniotic fluid embolus, hemorrhagic shock, pyelonephritis, and sepsis. The apparent frequency of pregnancy as an underlying cause of ARDS in women may relate to the physiologic changes caused by pregnancy.

Pathophysiology

As stated earlier, ARDS results from an underlying disease process. The initial insult to the lungs causes damage to the alveolar capillary membrane. This increases permeability and fluid leaks from vessels into the interstitium, causing further damage and interference with surfactant production. The lungs become stiff and difficult to ventilate. As the damage progresses, fluid in the lungs increases, decreasing lung volume. Intrapulmonary shunting begins, which affects oxygen transfer to the blood, causing severe hypoxemia. As this process progresses, intubation and mechanical ventilation is necessary to maintain oxygenation. The mortality rate in ARDS remains 50 to 60% (Creasy & Resnik, 1999). Death usually occurs from myocardial ischemia. See Table 37–4 for the phases of ARDS.

Clinical Manifestations

The patient with ARDS presents with severe hypoxemia despite high inspired oxygen concentration (Creasy & Resnick, 1999). Accompanying hypoxemia, the patient will experience dyspnea, tachypnea, and cyanosis. On assessment diffuse, fine crackles are auscultated. Chest x-ray reveals bilateral infiltrates.

Management

Management of ARDS is supportive. Supplemental oxygen alone is not effective and intubation and mechanical ventilation is implemented to maintain PaO_2 at 60 mm Hg. The use of positive end-expiratory pressure (PEEP) between 5 and 35 cm H_2O may aid in forcing fluid from the lung into the pulmonary circulation. A PAC is placed, initially to rule out any cardiac abnormalities, and then for observation of pulmonary artery pressure (PAP) and CO.

Treatment is focused on correcting the underlying cause. Vasoactive drugs, inotropes, and steroids are often used. Fluid balance is crucial. If the patient is hypovolemic, albumin or blood may be administered, with the end goal of maintaining CO and oxygenation.

Pulmonary Embolism (PE)

Etiology

Although a PE is not an obstetric condition, it is the leading obstetric-related cause of postpartum death. Pulmonary embolus during pregnancy occurs with roughly the same incidence antenatally and postnatally (Creasy & Resnik, 1999). The increased risk over nonpregnant women is 5.5 times greater. The incidence increases with maternal age, **multiparity,** obesity, and with decreased ambulation after delivery. The incidence in pregnancy is associated with the hypercoagulable state and venous stasis.

Pathophysiology

PE occurs by the migration of thrombi most commonly formed in the legs. The clot migrates to the pulmonary circulation and lodges in a vessel of the same size. The blockage prevents blood flow to the area distal to the clot. Unoxygenated blood recirculates peripherally, resulting in hypoxemia.

Clinical Manifestations

The classic symptoms of pulmonary embolus are dyspnea and tachypnea. Table 37–5 lists frequently encountered symptoms of PE.

Pulmonary embolism in a pregnant woman affects not only the patient but also the fetus. Once the patient is stabilized, the fetus tends to recover with no long-term effects.

Multiple small emboli can mimic one large embolus. If at least 50 percent of the pulmonary arterial system is blocked, the clinical picture may mimic a myocardial infarction. The signs and symptoms produced may include hypotension, syncope, or seizures.

Management

Oxygen therapy is crucial to maximize oxygen delivery to the fetus if the embolism is an **antepartum** event. The PaO_2 should be maintained at 70 mm Hg (Creasy & Resnik, 1999). Bedrest for 5 to 7 days in association with Demerol or morphine for pain and anxiety is indicated. Heparin is the most common drug used in the treatment of antepartum and intrapartum PE because it does not cross the placental barrier. It is usually administered intravenously. Laboratory values are monitored closely, and

TABLE 37–4. FINDINGS IN ACUTE RESPIRATORY DISTRESS

PHASE	PHYSICAL FINDINGS	SYMPTOMATOLOGY
Phase I Initial injury phase	None to minimal Usually adequate arterial oxygenation	Hyperventilation with resultant metabolic acidosis
Phase II Latent period	Minor auscultatory and radiographic evidence of pulmonary disease Progressive formation of alveolar and interstitial edema Hyaline membrane formation begins	Decreased lung compliance Increased intrapulmonary shunting of blood
Phase III Acute respiratory failure	Bilateral lung involvement on radiography Diffuse abnormalities noted on auscultation Alveolar septum 5–10 times thicker than normal	Marked dyspnea, tachypnea, and hypoxemia Worsening lung compliance and intrapulmonary shunting Endotracheal intubation and mechanical ventilation
Phase IV Irreversible respiratory failure/lung damage	Intra-alveolar fibrosis and fibroblastic infiltrates of alveolar septum mask original structure and appearance of lungs	Severe and refractory hypoxemia Intrapulmonary shunts in excess of 30% Hypercapnia Metabolic and respiratory acidosis

Adapted from: Hankins, G.D.V. et al. (1991). Acute pulmonary injury and respiratory failure during pregnancy. In Critical Care Obstetrics *(2nd ed.), pp. 340–370. Blackwell Scientific Publications, Boston.*

TABLE 37–5. SIGNS AND SYMPTOMS OF PULMONARY EMBOLISM

Tachypnea
Dyspnea
Pleuritic pain
Apprehension
Cough
Tachycardia
Hemoptysis
Temperature (< 37°C)

Modified from Sasahara, A.A., Sharma, G.V.R.K., Barsamian, E.M., et al. (1988). Pulmonary thromboembolism. JAMA 249:2945. Copyright 1988, American Medical Association.

the patient should be observed closely for any signs of hemorrhage, which is the largest risk of heparin therapy. Protamine sulfate should be at the bedside to reverse the anticoagulation effect of heparin.

Coumadin is primarily used in the postpartum period. The same risks of hemorrhage apply with Coumadin therapy. In the acute phase, oxygen is applied per mask. In the case of a large embolus, intubation may be needed until the clot is dissolved.

Surgery is rarely needed since anticoagulation therapy is usually effective. If the embolus is so large that surgery is required, the patient often dies within an hour of the insult.

In summary, in all cases of respiratory insults the nurse's goal is to maintain adequate oxygenation and perfusion. The nurse should assess patients frequently for respiratory rate, breath sounds, and overall condition. Notify the physician of any subtle changes in status.

SECTION THREE REVIEW

1. The most common factors attributing to amniotic fluid embolus include
   A. young maternal age
   B. nulliparity
   C. precipitous labor
2. A patient with ARDS requires
   A. supplemental oxygen via face mask
   B. no intervention in pregnancy
   C. intubation and mechanical ventilation
   D. placing the patient in the knee–chest position
3. A PE occurs in the postpartum period due to
   A. young maternal age
   B. obesity
   C. short labor
   D. hemorrhage
4. The drug of choice used in treating PE in the antepartum and intrapartum period is
   A. heparin
   B. Coumadin
   C. aspirin
   D. tissue plasminogen activator

Answers: 1. C, 2. C, 3. B, 4. A

PERFUSION

SECTION FOUR: Hypertension in Pregnancy

At the completion of this section, the learner will be able to differentiate the classifications of hypertension in pregnancy and will be able to recognize signs and symptoms of preeclampsia and how to care for a preeclamptic patient.

Hypertension in pregnancy presents a challenge for both the medical and nursing team. Management of the hypertensive patient demands meticulous observation. Treatment depends on the severity. Maternal and fetal risks must be weighed in choosing appropriate management. Hypertension in pregnancy complicates 7 to 10 percent of all pregnancies. Apart from being the most common medical complication of pregnancy, hypertension is one of the major causes of maternal and perinatal morbidity and mortality in the United States. Between 1987 and 1990, 256 of a total 1,453 maternal deaths in the United States directly resulted from high blood pressure in pregnancy (van Beek, 1998).

Hypertension in pregnancy can lead to multisystem damage and failure, with pathologic changes noted in the brain, kidney, liver, and cardiovascular system as well as altered uteroplacental perfusion.

Definition

The term *toxemia* was used in the past to include all hypertensive disorders in pregnancy. However, a more specific classification was necessary to differentiate the severity of clinical findings and physiologic changes.

The American College of Obstetricians and Gynecologists (Creasy & Resnick, 1999) developed a classification system to help physicians and nurses to identify the best patient treatment. This classification is as follows:

- Chronic hypertension
- Preeclampsia–eclampsia
- Preeclampsia superimposed on chronic hypertension
- Transient hypertension (PIH)

Chronic Hypertension

Chronic hypertension is blood pressure > 140/90 mm Hg that is present prior to 20 weeks' gestation or before pregnancy. Hypertension diagnosed during pregnancy that persists after the 42nd day postpartum is also classified as chronic hypertension (Creasy & Resnik, 1999).

Preeclampsia–Eclampsia

Preeclampsia is an increase in blood pressure of at least 30 mm Hg systolic or 15 mm Hg diastolic as compared to a blood pressure prior to 20 weeks; edema; and/or proteinuria. The elevation of blood pressure must be present at two intervals taken 6 hours apart. If previous blood pressure is unknown, a value of 140/90 is considered diagnostic for preeclampsia. Proteinuria is greater than 0.1 g/L (1 to 2+ on urine drip) in a random specimen or 0.3 g/L in a 24-hour period. Edema is characterized by an acute onset and measured by weight gain of ≥ 5 pounds in 1 week.

Preeclampsia has mild and severe types. Severe preeclampsia is defined as a blood pressure elevated at 160/110 mm Hg on two occasions at least 6 hours apart with bedrest, proteinuria ≥ 5 g in a 24-hour specimen, oliguria (≤ 500/mL in 24 hours), headache (especially frontal), hyperreflexia, scotomata and other visual disturbances, epigastric pain, and finally pulmonary edema or cyanosis (Creasy & Resnick, 1999). Table 37–6 provides a summary of the signs and symptoms of preeclampsia.

Eclampsia is preeclampsia with seizures present.

TABLE 37–6. SIGNS AND SYMPTOMS OF PREECLAMPSIA–ECLAMPSIA

Cerebral	Headache Dizziness Tinnitus Drowsiness Change in respiratory rate Tachycardia Fever
Visual	Diplopia Scotomata Blurred vision Amaurosis
Gastrointestinal	Nausea Vomiting Epigastric pain Hematemesis
Renal	Oliguria Anuria Hematuria Hemoglobinuria

From Creasy, R., & Resnick, R. (1999). Maternal–fetal medicine: Principles and practice, *4th ed., [p. 838]. Philadelphia: W.B. Saunders.*

Preeclampsia Superimposed on Chronic Hypertension

Preeclampsia superimposed on chronic hypertension is diagnosed in a patient with a history of chronic hypertension who develops proteinuria or generalized edema with an additional increase of 30 mm Hg systolic and 15 mm Hg diastolic.

Transient Hypertension

Transient hypertension is diagnosed by an increase in blood pressure in pregnancy after 20 weeks or in the first 24 hours postdelivery with no other signs of preeclampsia. Pregnancy-induced hypertension (PIH) would fall under this definition.

Etiology

Preeclampsia has no known cause. It is known, however, that damage to the endothelium, which triggers vasospasm, is directly linked to preeclampsia. Histopathologic findings also reveal the incidence of early placental ischemia (van Beek, 1998). Epidemiologic findings indicate that it occurs more often in first pregnancies. Socioeconomic status does not seem to be a predisposing factor; however, it is more common in women who receive little or no prenatal care, which may be related to low income. Variables associated with preeclampsia include extremes of age (under 20 and over 35); race, particularly blacks; obesity; immune and nonimmune fetal hydrops; hydatidiform mole; and pregnancy states associated with a large placenta (i.e., diabetes and multiple gestation).

Physiologic Changes

Hypertension in pregnancy is associated with damage in any or all of the following systems: renal, uteroplacental, pulmonary, hepatic, and central nervous system. Preeclampsia also alters the amount of circulating blood volume and is responsible for multiple hematologic changes and cardiac function. Damage to organ systems results from poor tissue perfusion (hypoxia) that occurs secondary to profound vasospasm. Vasospasm, in turn, increases peripheral vascular resistance and causes elevation of blood pressure.

Renal System

Pregnancy causes a normal 40 to 50 percent increase in plasma blood flow by approximately the 30th week. Renal plasma blood flow and the GFR are increased approximately 30 to 50 percent in the first trimester. Proteinuria develops as a result of a glomerular lesion caused by hypercoagulability. The lesion causes ischemic damage to the renal lumen.

With preeclampsia, there is a decrease in plasma volume, renal plasma flow, and GFR. Uric acid, creatinine, and blood urea nitrogen (BUN) serum levels rise especially in association with severe preeclampsia. A serum uric acid level of ≥ 4.5 mg/dL is indicative of preeclampsia. Oliguria may occur in severe preeclampsia as a result of movement of intracellular fluid to the extracellular space. Table 37–7 lists normal lab values in pregnancy.

The patient's urine may appear amber due to hematuria as a result of increased red blood cell destruction. Acute tubular necrosis with short-term renal failure may also occur. The renal effects of preeclampsia are usually reversible.

Uteroplacental System

In normal pregnancy, the uteroplacental blood vessels and spiral arteries are dilated to provide adequate perfusion to the uterus and fetus. With preeclampsia, uteroplacental perfusion is decreased due to vasospasm, decreased circulating volume, vasospasm of spiral arteries, and possible lesions from damage to the endothelium. As a result of decreased perfusion to the uterus and fetus, a preeclamptic patient has an increased chance of intrauterine growth retardation (IUGR), oligohydramnios, and intrauterine fetal demise (IUFD).

Pulmonary System

The pulmonary system may be affected by the fluid changes that occur with preeclampsia. Colloid oncotic pressure (COP) normally decreases with pregnancy. In the presence of preeclampsia, COP decreases even further due to damaged vessels, worsening both generalized and pulmonary edema.

Hepatic System

Liver damage is also related to vasospasm and vascular changes related to preeclampsia. The changes are so great that ischemia, necrosis, and even hemorrhagic necrosis can occur. This is a medical emergency. Patients who present with signs and symptoms of preeclampsia and/or complain of right upper quadrant pain or epigastric pain should have liver enzyme levels evaluated, in particular alanine transaminase (ALT), for the presence of liver damage. ALT levels should be evaluated until delivery and, if necessary, a CT scan of the liver should be obtained to rule out rupture in women experiencing epigastric and shoulder pain.

TABLE 37–7. NORMAL LABORATORY VALUES IN PREGNANCY

Hemoglobin	10–12 g/dL
Hematocrit	32–40%
Plasma blood volume	Up by 40–50%
Glomerular filtration rate	Up by 30–50%
Uric acid	4.5 mg/dL
BUN	12 mg/dL
Creatinine	0.8 mg/dL
Creatinine clearance	150–200 mL/min
SGOT	35 mg/dL (may vary between labs)
Colloid oncotic pressure	23 mm Hg

Adapted from Harvey, C. (1991). Critical care obstetrical nursing *(p. 56). Rockville, MD: Aspen.*

Central Nervous System

Cerebrovascular resistance appears to be increased with preeclampsia. Autoregulation of cerebral blood flow seems impaired in preeclampsia as well. The mechanisms accounting for this alteration in cerebral blood flow are not well understood. It is known that central nervous system complications from preeclampsia are **scotomata** (seeing spots), **diplopia** or blurry vision, and headaches unrelieved by medications. Seizure activity occurs in eclampsia antepartally, intrapartally, or postpartally as long as 10 to 14 days after delivery. It is preceded by severe headache, usually frontal in origin (Cunningham, Gant, MacDonald, et al., 1997). **Hyperreflexia** and **clonus** are also common.

Hematologic System

As discussed earlier, plasma blood volume normally increases 40 to 45 percent with pregnancy. With preeclampsia, the circulating volume decreases. The decrease in circulating volume is not clearly understood but is attributed to vasospasm and vasoconstriction associated with hypertension in pregnancy.

Hemoconcentration occurs as a result of fluid shifts to the extravascular space. Hemoglobin (Hgb) and hematocrit (Hct) normally decrease with pregnancy, however with hypertension they may increase. The degree of hemoconcentration can be used as an indicator of the severity of the disease process of preeclampsia.

Thrombocytopenia, a complication associated with preeclampsia, results from damage, caused by vasospasms to the vascular endothelium to which platelets adhere. A patient's platelet count decreases, increasing the risk of hemorrhage during delivery.

Patients with severe preeclampsia also seem at risk for developing DIC. The patient will begin to bleed from IV sites, puncture sites, or surgical incisions. There will be a decrease in fibrinogen levels, an increase of fibrin degradation or fibrin split products; and a prolonged partial thromboplastin time (PTT) and/or prothrombin time (PT). Whether this is due to DIC or a localized coagulation change is being debated (Creasy & Resnik, 1999). DIC will be discussed in further detail in the next section.

Cardiovascular System

In normal pregnancy, CO increases 50 percent and total peripheral resistance decreases. However, blood pressure remains normal or slightly decreased. With preeclampsia, CO remains the same or slightly lower compared with a normal pregnant patient. Vasoconstriction and vasospasm, as a result of preeclampsia, increases total peripheral resistance, which seems to be responsible for the elevation in blood pressure since blood pressure is the product of both CO and total peripheral resistance. Table 37–8 compares severity of symptoms.

Management

Antepartal (Home)

In women with mild to moderate hypertension and trace to 1+ proteinuria, outpatient management is reasonable. Close follow-up requires bedrest with blood pressure and protein checks by a home health nurse daily as well as once or twice weekly office visits to include fetal evaluation. If evidence of fetal compromise or worsening maternal status is noted, hospitalization is required.

Antepartal (Hospital)

If delivery is indicated by worsening maternal parameters (increased blood pressure, increased proteinuria, headache, fetal growth retardation), antepartal management then depends on gestational age. If gestational age is beyond 32 weeks, delivery is accomplished as fetal well-being is more assured. Prior to 32 weeks, bedrest, careful maternal and fetal observation, and administration of glucocorticoids (betamethasone 12 mg IM × 2, 12 to 24 hours apart) are initiated. This approach attempts to give the fetus an additional 48 to 72 hours for enhancement of fetal lung maturity prior to delivery. Rapid maternal deterioration indicates imminent delivery is the wisest course of action. Minimizing fetal and maternal morbidity and mortality is the ultimate goal of any prolongation of pregnancy affected by preeclampsia.

Intrapartal

Magnesium sulfate ($MgSO_4$) is the drug of choice for preventing eclamptic seizures. $MgSO_4$ slows or blocks neuromuscular and cardiac conducting system transmission, decreasing smooth muscle contractility and depressing CNS irritability. The results include a desired anticonvulsant effect and undesirable effects such as decreased uterine and myocardial contractility, depressed respirations, and interference with cardiac conduction. These effects occur at different magnesium levels, which may also differ from person to person. Magnesium levels should be checked every 24 hours and PRN. Because $MgSO_4$ is excreted by the kidney, decreased urine output can lead to magnesium toxicity. The therapeutic range for serum magnesium levels is 4 to 8 mg/dL.

Nursing assessment is crucial. The nurse should check blood pressure (with the patient in the left lateral position, using nondependent arm each check), urine output (UOP) with protein dips, deep tendon reflexes (DTRs), and level of consciousness (LOC) hourly. A 24-hour urine for protein may be ordered. Breath sounds should be auscultated prior to $MgSO_4$ bolus as a baseline, preferably on admission, and at least every 8 hours during infusion. A urinary catheter should be placed with urometer collection for accurate output with periodic specific gravity checks. Remember, $MgSO_4$ is excreted by the kidney. If UOP decreases, the risk for magnesium toxicity increases. Rates of $MgSO_4$ infusion need to be titrated accordingly. If the patient complains of chest pain or shortness of breath, DTRs become absent, or respirations fall below 12, the infusion is stopped immediately and the physician notified. Calcium gluconate should be placed at the bedside and may be used as an antagonist if magnesium toxicity occurs.

TABLE 37–8. PREGNANCY-INDUCED HYPERTENSION: INDICATIONS OF SEVERITY

ABNORMALITY	MILD	SEVERE
Diastolic blood pressure	< 100 mg Hg	110 mm Hg or higher
Proteinuria	Trace to 1+	Persistent 2+ or more
Headache	Absent	Present
Visual disturbances	Absent	Present
Upper abdominal pain	Absent	Present
Oliguria	Absent	Present
Convulsions	Absent	Present (eclampsia)
Serum creatinine	Normal	Elevated
Thrombocytopenia	Absent	Present
Hyperbilirubinemia	Absent	Present
Liver enzyme elevation	Minimal	Marked
Fetal growth restriction	Absent	Obvious
Pulmonary edema	Absent	Present

From Cunningham, F.G., Gant, N.F., McDonald, P.C., et al. (1997). Williams Obstetrics. *20th ed. New York: McGraw Hill (p. 695).*

Postpartal (Hospital)

Although progress of the disease process of preeclampsia halts following delivery, the maternal condition does not return to prepregnancy norms immediately. Within the first 48 hours after delivery, the risk of eclamptic seizures almost entirely abates. Rare exceptions to this can occur as long as 2 weeks postdelivery. $MgSO_4$ therapy is continued for 24 hours postdelivery or longer in selected cases. Maternal diuresis is generally recognized as an indication of resolution of preeclampsia. Hypertension usually resolves within 6 weeks.

Use of $MgSO_4$ postdelivery can cause an increase in postpartal uterine atony. $MgSO_4$ is a uterine relaxant drug, hence its value in preterm labor. In the newly delivered woman, however, it can increase the incidence of postpartum hemorrhage. Careful attention to vaginal bleeding and frequent assessment for uterine atony while postpartum $MgSO_4$ therapy continues is needed to assure maternal well-being. Use of oxytocin and prostaglandins (Hemabate 250 μg) will successfully prevent most uterine atony. Prostaglandins are relatively contraindicated in patients with cardiovascular disease and asthma.

Prior to infusion of $MgSO_4$, a 16- to 18-gauge IV will be inserted. A main line of an isotonic crystalloid will be ordered by the physician and should infuse via infusion pump. These patients are at high risk for pulmonary edema, so strict intake and output is imperative. Preeclamptic patients are fluid restricted for this reason. Total fluids are maintained at 100 to 150 mL/hr. $MgSO_4$ is infused by pump and should be connected by a Y connector to the main line below an antireflux valve to prevent backflow and to ensure accurate infusion. $MgSO_4$ is initially ordered by a physician as a 4- to 6-g bolus over 20 to 30 minutes (a rate of no more than 150 mg/min), then at 2 to 3 g/hr. During a bolus, the patient may complain of flushing, a metallic taste, nausea, or burning at the IV site as normal responses. During hourly infusion, the patient will appear listless, complain of achiness and nausea, and often vomit. Due to these responses, the patient is usually ordered an NPO or clear liquid diet. Always prepare your patient for what to expect prior to infusion to alleviate anxiety. $MgSO_4$ is usually continued for 12 to 24 hours after delivery. Though you normally see the physiologic changes of preeclampsia reversed after delivery, the patient is still at risk for exacerbation and seizures as long as 6 weeks postpartum. Close observation is still required.

Fetal monitoring is imperative in the preeclamptic patient. Continuous fetal monitoring is required due to the stress of hypertension on the fetus. Compromise of blood flow to the uteroplacental unit places the fetus at risk for fetal intolerance to labor and fetal distress. $MgSO_4$ usually cause a decrease in FHR variability, complicating the task of fetal assessment.

In the presence of oliguria, urinary output < 25 to 30 mL for 2 consecutive hours, a conservative fluid challenge, 200 to 500 mL, may be ordered. The nurse should auscultate breath sounds before and after the fluid challenge. Diuretics are rarely used in preeclampsia unless pulmonary edema is present. Diuretics decrease circulating volume in an intravascular system that is already depleted, decreasing perfusion to placenta and fetus even further. When used, diuretics are dosed very conservatively.

If an eclamptic seizure occurs, the nurse's role is to protect the patient from injury. Ensure adequate oxygenation and minimize aspiration. A physician should be notified immediately. Valium may be given to control seizure activity in doses of 10 to 30 mg. An $MgSO_4$ bolus and increase in infusion rate may be ordered. Arterial blood gases are obtained. FHR variability usually decreases and late decelerations may occur. Once the patient is stabilized, the focus shifts to facilitating delivery.

Antihypertensive Agents

Antihypertensives are not routinely used in preeclamptic patients. However, due to the risks of persistent elevated diastolic pressures > 110 mm Hg, such as seizure, cardiovascular accident, or intracranial bleeding, they may be necessary to stabilize the patient. The effects of a sudden drop in blood pressure on the fetus should be considered prior to administration.

Hydralazine is the most widely used antihypertensive in treating severe preeclampsia. Hydralazine has two major benefits relevant to pregnant women. Vasodilation with hydralazine increases CO. This promotes uterine blood flow and minimizes the hypotensive effect on the fetus. Important side effects of hydralazine are headache and epigastric pain, which, if not known by the nurse, may appear to be worsening symptoms of preeclampsia.

Hydralazine is rarely ineffective; however, nifedipine, another vasodilator, may also be used to lower blood pressure rapidly. Remember that continuous fetal monitoring is imperative. The fetus exists in an intrauterine environment already compromised by decreased intravascular volume and generalized vasospasms. A sudden drop in maternal blood pressure may lead to changes in FHR resulting from decreased CO with resultant decreased placental oxygenation. The nurse should anticipate fetal distress and be ready to respond.

Labetalol is also a common drug used to lower blood pressure. Unlike hydralazine and nifedipine, labetalol does not decrease afterload, which puts into question its advantage in managing cardiac failure associated with preeclampsia. See Table 37–9 for dosages and mechanisms of actions of these drugs and others.

TABLE 37–9. DRUGS FOR TREATMENT OF HYPERTENSIVE EMERGENCIES

	TIME COURSE OF ACTION						
DRUG	Onset	Maximum	Duration	IM	DOSAGE IV	INTERVAL BETWEEN DOSES	MECHANISM ACTION
Hydralazine	10–20 min	20–40 min	3–8 hr	10–50 mg	5–25 mg	3–6 hr	Direct dilatation of arterioles
Trimethaphan camsylate	1–2 min	2–5 min	10 min	—	IV solution, 2 gm/L; IV infusion rate, 1–5 mg/min		Ganglionic blocker
Sodium nitroprusside	1/2–2 min	1–2 min	3–5 min	—	IV solution, 0.01 gm/L; IV infusion rate, 0.2 to 0.8 mg/min		Direct dilatation of arterioles and veins
Labetalol	1–2 min	10 min	6–16 hrs	—	20–50 mg	3–6 hr	Alpha- and beta-adrenergic blocker
Nifedipine	5–10 min	10–20 min	4–8 hrs	—	10 mg orally; no IV solution	4–8 hr	Calcium channel blocker

From Creasy, R., & Resnick, R. (1999). Maternal–fetal medicine: Principles and practice, *4th ed. (p. 860). Philadelphia: W.B. Saunders.*

Mode and Timing of Delivery

Delivery is the only "cure" for preeclampsia. The effects of preeclampsia are totally reversible after delivery. If maternal well-being were the only consideration, all preeclamptic patients would be delivered as soon as signs and symptoms developed. The goal of treatment of preeclampsia is to stabilize the patient to prolong gestation for reduction of perinatal morbidity and mortality.

Vaginal delivery is preferred over a cesarean delivery, due to the added stress of surgery on the preeclamptic patient. If vaginal delivery is chosen, induction will be carried out aggressively. Fetal monitoring is very important in determining fetal tolerance to labor. The fetus of a preeclamptic patient is stressed from the beginning. This is one positive aspect of preeclampsia. Due to the stress on the fetus, fetal lungs tend to mature at an earlier age. As mentioned earlier, steroids may be given to accelerate fetal lung maturity. If given, induction will be delayed 36 to 48 hours to allow the drugs to be effective. Fetal lung maturity will be discussed in further detail in another section.

In summary, the range and severity of the effects of preeclampsia and hypertension on the patient and the fetus depend greatly on how early the complication is diagnosed. Once a patient is known to have hypertension in any way, precautions are taken to protect the patient and fetus. Bedrest and frequent prenatal checks are prescribed with periodic laboratory assessments. With any worsening in condition, as seen in lab results or patient appearance and complaints, and noted changes in fetal growth and development, prompt intervention is taken. Normally, these patients are treated early in the disease process with minimal lasting effects noted. In patients who receive little or no prenatal care, extensive complications arise, resulting in higher rates of morbidity and mortality.

SECTION FOUR REVIEW

1. CNS complications related to preeclampsia include
   A. scotomata
   B. blindness
   C. flaccid neck
   D. headache relieved with medication
2. With preeclampsia, plasma blood flow
   A. increases
   B. redistributes to the kidneys
   C. is affected by vasospasm and vasoconstriction
   D. redistributes to the brain
3. Infusion of $MgSO_4$ involves
   A. a 20-gauge IV
   B. a main line of an isotonic crystalloid
   C. a baseline cardiac assessment
   D. a rapid infusion rate
4. As a result of $MgSO_4$, the nurse should suspect changes in the FHR, including
   A. decreased variability
   B. early decelerations
   C. variable decelerations
   D. asystole
5. The most widely used antihypertensive in treating hypertension in pregnancy is
   A. nifedipine
   B. labetalol
   C. hydralazine
   D. $MgSO_4$
6. The only cure for preeclampsia is
   A. infusion of blood components
   B. delivery
   C. infusion of $MgSO_4$
   D. hyperoxygenating the mother

Answers: 1. A, 2. C, 3. B, 4. A, 5. C, 6. B

SECTION FIVE: Hematologic Complications in Pregnancy

At the completion of this section, the learner will be able to define HELLP syndrome and DIC and will know appropriate interventions when caring for patients with these disorders.

HELLP Syndrome

Definition

HELLP syndrome occurs in up to 15 percent of patients experiencing hypertension in pregnancy (Crosby, 1991). It is a combination of hemolytic anemia, elevated liver enzymes (transaminases), and low platelets (Weinstein, 1982). HELLP usually occurs in the third trimester, but occasionally is seen as early as the 20th week or as late as the postpartum period and can be present without hypertension (Creasy & Resnick, 1999).

Clinical Manifestations

Hematologic abnormalities include a decrease in Hct, abnormal erythrocyte forms, increased levels of fibrin degradation products, reduced levels of antithrombin III, and microangiopathic hemolytic anemia with DIC. The platelet count falls below $100 \times 10^9/L$ (100,000 mL). Aspartate transaminase (AST) usually remains below 1,000 IU/L. Indirect bilirubin and creatinine are often elevated as well (Creasy & Resnick, 1999). PT, and PTT, and fibrinogen levels are frequently normal.

The patient may present with epigastric pain with normal or only mildly elevated blood pressure and no proteinuria.

Pathophysiology

HELLP is a result of vasospasm in the microvasculature and increased capillary permeability associated with preeclampsia.

Microangiopathic hemolytic anemia (MAHA) occurs when red blood cells are fragmented as they pass through the fibrin-obstructed blood vessels (Harvey, 1991). Due to elevated levels of free fatty acids and decreased serum albumin associated with hypertension, there is a pathologic alteration in cell membranes causing red blood cell **hemolysis** (Shannon, 1987). MAHA is diagnosed by a low haptoglobin level. Haptoglobin is a plasma protein that binds with free hemoglobin.

Histologic changes occur in pregnant patients with hypertension. Fibrin and thrombin in the hepatic sinusoid cause areas of focal necrosis and subscapular hemorrhages (Shannon, 1987). ALT and AST are elevated, indicating liver dysfunction.

Thrombocytopenia occurs as a result of vasospasm damaging the vascular endothelium. Platelets adhere to vessel walls, decreasing the platelet count. Table 37–10 lists criteria for diagnosis.

Management

In patients with HELLP, delivery is mandatory. Aggressive movement toward delivery depends on the severity and gestational age. If the patient is stable, a vaginal delivery is possible. Transfusion may be indicated with a patient whose platelet count is less than 50,000 mL.

The patient will be placed on a $MgSO_4$ infusion. All precautions discussed with preeclampsia should be implemented. A second IV access should be obtained. Antihypertensive therapy is aggressive when diastolic pressure reaches ≥ 110 mm Hg. These patients may require invasive hemodynamic monitoring and an arterial line. Laboratory values will be checked frequently. If any deterioration occurs, a cesarean section may be indicated. Although vaginal delivery is preferred, some authors advocate cesarean delivery if the platelet count begins to fall below 50,000/mL. Close fetal monitoring is imperative. The fetus is at high risk of intrauterine asphyxia.

TABLE 37–10. CRITERIA FOR DIAGNOSIS OF HELLP SYNDROME

AST (SGOT) > 50 IU/L
LDH > 180 IU/L
Platelet count < 100,000
Hemolysis is present

Adapted from Creasy, R., & Resnick, R. (1999). Maternal–fetal medicine: Principles and practice, *4th ed. Philadelphia: W.B. Saunders.*

Postdelivery, the resolution of thrombocytopenia is delayed with a continued decrease in platelet count, continuing up to as long as 72 hours. This places these patients at risk for delayed postpartum hemorrhage.

Disseminated Intravascular Coagulation

Definition

DIC is thought to be a syndrome rather than a disease. DIC is a disturbance of the coagulation mechanism. In obstetrics, DIC is seen in association with abruptio placentae, AFE (amniotic fluid embolism), preeclampsia, retained dead fetus syndrome, gram-negative sepsis, and saline abortion. (For more information concerning DIC, refer to Module 11.)

Pathophysiology

As part of another disease entity acting as a trigger, DIC results in disruption of the coagulation mechanism. This disruption is caused by a consumption of plasma factors, including platelets, fibrinogen, prothrombin, factor V and factor VIII, and the production of anticoagulants by the fibrinolytic system. Replacement of plasma factors and platelets, which are needed for clot formation, is not unlimited. Availability of clotting factors in the circulating blood volume is compromised, which may result in severe bleeding. The fibrinolytic system is activated, producing fibrin degradation products that further interfere with the coagulation mechanism.

Another result of DIC is clots found in the microcirculation. These clots can cause ischemia of multiple organs.

Diagnosis

Diagnosis is made by routine screening tests for coagulation. The platelet count is decreased and progressively falls. Fibrinogen level is low. Fibrin degradation products are elevated. The PT and PTT may be normal, prolonged, or shortened. Shortening of PT and PTT occurs early when excess amounts of factor V and X are in the circulation. Subsequent consumption of clotting factors lead to prolonged PT and PTT.

Management

The most important step in treating DIC is treating the underlying disease process. However, in obstetrics this may involve termination of pregnancy. Shortly after delivery, coagulation abnormalities generally return to normal (plasma factors in 24 hours and platelets 5 to 7 days after DIC ceases).

These patients frequently require invasive hemodynamic monitoring to determine need for volume replacements. Vital signs should be monitored closely, and the nurse should be on the alert for subtle signs of bleeding.

Transfusion is usually required. Fresh whole blood or packed red blood cells and fresh frozen plasma are used most often. **Cryoprecipitate** may be given in fluid-restricted patients. It contains fibrinogen and other clotting factors in a smaller volume. Platelets should be administered if the patient's platelet count falls below 50,000 mL.

UOP should be monitored closely as an indicator of poor perfusion. If UOP falls below 30 mL/hr, a physician should be notified.

SECTION FIVE REVIEW

1. HELLP syndrome results from
   A. vasospasm in the microvasculature
   B. a decrease in capillary permeability
   C. illicit drug use
   D. drug withdrawal

2. The most important step in treating DIC includes
   A. treatment of the underlying disease process
   B. transfusion
   C. monitoring UOP
   D. monitoring blood pressure frequently

Answers: 1. A, 2. A

SECTION SIX: Hemorrhagic Complications in Pregnancy

At the completion of this section, the learner will be able to determine different causes of hemorrhage in pregnancy and the nurse's role in caring for patients experiencing hemorrhage and shock.

Placenta Previa

Definition

Placenta previa is defined as an implantation of the placenta in the lower segment of the uterus below the presenting part of the fetus. There are three types of previa depending on the relationship of the placenta to the cervical os.

- *Placenta previa*—implantation of the placenta covering the cervical os
- *Marginal placenta previa*—implanted placenta reaching 2 to 3 cm from the cervical os
- *Low-lying placenta*—placenta that is uncertain in relationship to cervical os or a previa found prior to onset of third trimester (Creasy & Resnik, 1999)

Etiology

The actual cause of placenta previa is not known. It has been theorized that damage to the **endometrium** may play a role, which would explain why there is an increased incidence in patients with multiple cesarean sections and multiparity.

The incidence of placenta previa is roughly one in 200 to 250 births. It occurs more frequently in multiparous women. An early diagnosis of a previa may change as the pregnancy progresses. The relationship of the placenta to the cervical os changes as the uterus grows. In approximately 5 percent of women diagnosed with second trimester previa, 90 percent will resolve by term (Creasy & Resnik, 1999).

Diagnosis and Clinical Manifestations

The classic diagnosis of placenta previa includes the sudden onset of painless bleeding in the second or third trimester. In the past, previa was thought to be absent of abruption and uterine contractions; however, in approximately 10 percent of cases there is an abruption—a separation of the implanted placenta from the uterine wall—and in one of four cases, contractions are present. If the patient is contracting the incidence of future abruption increases.

The absence of bleeding throughout pregnancy does not rule out a previa. Bleeding may not occur until the onset of labor in approximately 10 percent of affected pregnancies (Creasy & Resnik, 1999).

An ultrasound should be done in all patients with bleeding. The position of the placenta is ascertained and a diagnosis made. Also, if the cervical os is opened, a gentle speculum exam with adequate lighting can be used to find the source of bleeding and to determine the presence of a previa. Digital vaginal exams are contraindicated due to manipulation of the cervix that could cause further bleeding. Evaluation of cervical dilatation is obtained visually with a sterile speculum.

Management

Any patient suspected of having a placenta previa who is actively bleeding should be hospitalized and placed on bedrest. A 16- to 18-gauge IV should be inserted whether or not IV fluids are needed. Maintaining venous access is very important.

Patients with mild to moderate bleeding are placed on expectant management with continuous fetal monitoring. The nurse will assess hourly sanitary pad counts and evaluate bleeding, noting color and amount. If a pad is saturated in 1 hour, a physician is notified. Intermittent blood replacement may be indicated for maternal and fetal stability. Expectant management is used in cases of immature fetal lung. If the patient's bleeding slows significantly and the patient is without contractions, intermittent monitoring and bathroom privileges may be ordered.

Hgb and Hct are checked periodically to evaluate the patient's stability. Once the patient reaches 32 weeks, an **amniocentesis** may be performed every 7 to 10 days to determine fetal lung maturity. If the mother is RH negative, Rhogam administration is indicated.

Mode and Timing of Delivery

In cases of severe bleeding, delivery is imminent regardless of gestational age or fetal lung maturity.

In the majority of cases, delivery is performed by cesarean section. Vaginal delivery in the operating room in marginal previa may be attempted, but if bleeding increases, a cesarean section is performed.

Complications

Abnormal implantation of the placenta in placenta previa may be complicated by trophoblastic invasion of the placenta beyond normal limits. This gives rise to placenta accreta, a condition which is 10 to 25 percent more common in women with one prior cesarean section and over 50 percent in women with two or more cesarean sections. If the accreta is more invasive, it gives rise to placenta increta (into the myometrium) or placenta percreta (through the myometrium to the serosa or even to the bladder or other abdominal organs). Presence of an accreta increases the risk of both postpartum hemorrhage from retained placental tissue and uterine atony and hysterectomy (Creasy & Resnik, 1999).

Abruptio Placentae

Definition

Abruptio placentae is separation of a normally implanted placenta before the birth of the fetus. The diagnosis is usually made during the third trimester but can be diagnosed after the 20th week. This is a life-threatening condition for both patient and fetus.

Incidence and Etiology

There is not one unifying cause of abruptio placentae. Past pregnancy complications seem to play a part in the chances of having an abruption and in turn produce more complications in future reproduction.

Trauma to the abdomen has caused abruption but only in a minority of cases. An abruption may occur within 24 hours of abdominal trauma. These women should be hospitalized for at least 24 hours for continuous fetal monitoring. A Kleihauer–Betke (KHB) test should be performed for the presence of fetal cells in the maternal blood.

Another, albeit infrequent, cause is a short umbilical cord or uterine anomaly. Delivery by cesarean section in the preceding pregnancy also increases risk.

Hypertension—either chronic or pregnancy-induced—increases the risk of abruption. Maternal vascular disease resulting from hypertension has been an underlying cause of 50 percent of cases of abruptio placentae that were extensive enough to cause fetal death (Creasy & Resnick, 1999).

Cigarette smoking during pregnancy is associated with an increase in abruption. Smoking more than 10 cigarettes a day has been correlated with decidual necrosis on examination of the placenta. Premature rupture of membranes and its association with early subchorionic hemorrhage increase frequency of abruption (Cunningham, Gant, MacDonald, et al., 1997).

Cocaine abuse is also associated with an increase in abruption, especially in the past several years. This is related to the vasoactive properties of cocaine (Creasy & Resnick, 1999). As many as 10 percent of these women may end pregnancy close to term as a result of abruption.

Pathophysiology

Abruptio placentae is initiated by bleeding into the **decidua basalis.** The source of bleeding is small arteries in the basal layer of the **decidua** that are pathologically altered and then rupture. As the bleeding occurs a hematoma may form and expand, causing further separation. On gross inspection of the placenta, a clot is noted in a cup-shaped depression on the maternal side of the placenta. This represents a risk to the fetus due to decreased surface area for exchange of respiratory gases and nutrients.

The severity of abruption can be mild to severe. The initial insult may be limited or it may continue and cause complete abruption.

Clinical Manifestations

The classic symptoms of abruptio placentae are vaginal bleeding, abdominal pain, uterine contractions, and uterine tenderness. Not all of these symptoms need to be present for a diagnosis of abruption. For example, if the abruption is concealed, bleeding may not be obvious. Increased fundal heights and abdominal girth may reflect bleeding. The amount of visible bleeding may not indicate the severity of the abruption. Vaginal bleeding associated with abruption is usually dark red and nonclotting but may also appear serosanguinous.

The patient may complain of a sudden onset of abdominal pain that is sharp and severe. However, pain may not be present or it may be confused with uterine contractions.

On an external toco, uterine contractions may not accurately register. An IUPC will show more frequent contractions than a normal labor pattern with increased uterine resting tone.

Evidence of maternal **hypovolemia** beyond what is expected by estimated blood loss is also an indicator. Fetal distress or fetal death also reflects a loss of a large portion of villous exchange areas.

The diagnosis is based on ruling out all other causes of vaginal bleeding. Complications that can be confused with abruption are **chorioamnionitis,** appendicitis, pyelonephritis, or uterine rupture.

Management

Any patient suspected of having abruptio placentae should be hospitalized immediately. Vital signs may appear normal and be misleading due to the presence of underlying hypertension. Postural changes may not occur until a large amount of intravascular volume is lost. Vital signs should be reassessed at least every 15 minutes. If the mother is Rh negative, Rhogam administration is indicated and may necessitate more than one vial if the maternal exposure is more than 30 cc of fetal blood, (Cunningham, Gant, MacDonald, et al., 1997).

If the fetus is still alive an external fetal monitor should be applied to evaluate fetal well-being and signs of distress along with a toco to assess uterine contractions. Fetal distress will appear on an external fetal monitor as absent variability and/or late decelerations.

A 16- to 18-gauge IV should be placed, and preferably a second large-bore IV access initiated in case transfusion is necessary. The initial infusate ordered may be normal saline, lactated Ringer's, or plasmalyte.

The patient's initial Hgb and Hct may be misleading. If the values are decreased from prenatal values, transfusion should be anticipated.

Mode and Timing of Delivery

Once a patient is stabilized, a plan for delivery is established. The mode and timing of delivery are imperative. Factors influencing delivery are based on condition and gestational age of the fetus, condition of the patient, and dilation of the cervix (Creasy & Resnick, 1999).

If there is no evidence of fetal distress in an immature fetus and the abruption is determined to be mild, an expectant management course may be instituted, allowing time for steroids to aid in fetal lung maturity. (Corticosteroid therapy will be discussed in a later section.) **Tocolytic therapy** may be initiated if uterine contractions are present as long as stable maternal hemodynamics are demonstrated. The nurse's role in expectant management of abruptio placentae includes continuous fetal monitoring; frequent vital signs; assessment of vaginal bleeding, contractions, and abdominal tenderness; and placement of a urinary catheter for accurate intake and output evaluation.

If the abruption is considered moderate to severe delivery is induced. If the patient is stable and there are no signs of fetal distress, a vaginal delivery may be attempted. If vaginal delivery is chosen, an amniotomy is performed. This procedure reduces extravasation of blood into the myometrium and entry of thromboplastic substances into the maternal circulation, may stimulate labor, and allows placement of internal monitors. Internal monitors allow for accurate fetal assessment. Pitocin may be ordered to augment uterine activity. Pitocin should be used cautiously due to the risk of overstimulation of the uterus and extension of the abruption. Pitocin should be used cautiously until internal monitors are in place, particularly with abruptio placentae. The IUPC gives a reliable measurement of uterine resting tone. Increased uterine resting tone may indicate advancement of abruption, which may require a cesarean section. If the fetus demonstrates definite signs of distress an immediate cesarean section is performed. In the case of fetal death, vaginal delivery is attempted to minimize maternal morbidity.

Complications that can occur with abruptio placentae include hemorrhagic shock, DIC (more common with the presence of fetal demise), ischemic necrosis of distant organs, and fetal complications. Fetal complications include IUGR and congenital anomalies. There may be significant fetal bleeding resulting in fetal anemia and transient coagulopathy (Harvey, 1991).

Uterine Rupture

Definition and Etiology

Uterine rupture is one of the most dangerous complications in pregnancy. Maternal mortality is approximately 50 percent, while perinatal mortality is approximately 75 percent (Creasy & Resnick, 1999).

There are two types of uterine rupture. In the first, incomplete rupture, the rupture does not extend through the uterus into the peritoneum. In the second, complete rupture, the rupture extends through the entire thickness and into the peritoneal cavity. Uterine rupture also differs from uterine scar dehiscence. With uterine rupture, there is extravasation of part or all of the fetus into the peritoneum as well as fetal distress and maternal bleeding. With uterine scar dehiscence, separation does not include the peritoneum and retains the fetus in the uterine cavity (Cunningham, Gant, MacDonald, et al., 1997). Low transverse uterine scar dehiscence is not associated with maternal mortality and has low maternal morbidity, as well as low perinatal morbidity and mortality. This supports trials of labor for women with low transverse uterine scar dehiscence being safe (Cunningham, Gant, MacDonald, et al., 1997).

Causes of uterine rupture may be classified into traumatic rupture (by violent or obstetric causes), spontaneous rupture before or during labor, or a combination of both etiologies (Table 37–11).

The most common etiologic factor is a past cesarean section or a previous uterine incision. Other causes may include oxytocin use, placental abnormalities, uterine trauma (use of forceps), precipitous or prolonged labor, multiparity, and advanced maternal age.

Clinical Manifestations

Classic signs of uterine rupture are sudden, sharp, abdominal pain that may abate or be referred to the chest from blood collected under the diaphragm, fetal distress, vagi-

TABLE 37–11. CLASSIFICATION OF CAUSES OF UTERINE RUPTURE

UTERINE INJURY OR ANOMALY SUSTAINED BEFORE CURRENT PREGNANCY	UTERINE INJURY OR ABNORMALITY DURING CURRENT PREGNANCY
1. Surgery involving the myometrium	1. Before delivery
Cesarean section or hysterotomy	Persistent, intense, spontaneous contractions
Previously repaired uterine rupture	Labor stimulation—oxytocin or prostaglandins
Myomectomy incision through or to the endometrium	Intra-amnionic instillation—saline or prostaglandins
Deep cornual resection of interstitial oviduct	Perforation by internal uterine pressure catheter
Metroplasty	External trauma—share or blunt
2. Coincidental uterine trauma	External version
Abortion with instrumentation—curette, sounds	Uterine overdistention—hydramnios, multiple pregnancy
Sharp or blunt trauma—accidents, bullets, knives	2. During delivery
Silent rupture in previous pregnancy	Internal version
3. Congenital anomaly	Difficult forceps delivery
Pregnancy in undeveloped uterine horn	Breech extraction
	Fetal anomaly distending lower segment
	Vigorous uterine pressure during delivery
	Difficult manual removal of placenta
	3. Acquired
	Placenta increta or percreta
	Gestational trophoblastic neoplasia
	Adenomyosis
	Sacculation of entrapped retroverted uterus

From Cunningham, F.G., Gant, N.F., McDonald, P.C. et al. (1996). Williams Obstetrics *20th ed. New York: McGraw Hill (p. 773).*

nal bleeding, and shock. As in abruption, bleeding may not be evident and uterine contractions may continue. Patients interviewed after recovering from uterine rupture complain of a sensation of tearing, diaphragmatic or suprapubic pain, anxiety, restlessness, weakness, and dizziness (Harvey, 1991).

Management

Prevention is very important in the management of uterine rupture. A patient attempting vaginal birth after having a previous low transverse uterine incision for cesarean delivery should be closely observed. An intrauterine pressure catheter is required for safe uterine contraction monitoring. The use of cesarean section instead of allowing a breech delivery or high forceps, and discouragement of fundal pressure (pushing on patients' abdomen), have decreased the risk of uterine trauma.

Mode and Timing of Delivery

Many times, uterine rupture is not diagnosed until uterine exploration after delivery. Uterine exploration is usually performed in cases of cesarean section, breech delivery, cervical lacerations, forceps delivery, delivery in which fundal pressure was used, postpartum bleeding, and any delivery of a uterus that was overdistended (e.g., polyhydramnios, **macrosomia**). Nursing management includes close assessment of vital signs, progression of labor, fetal heart rate, and the onset of maternal symptoms.

An ultrasound may be used to diagnose rupture. Fetal extremities outside uterine boundaries and abnormal position of intraperitoneal air supports diagnosis of rupture.

A cesarean section is often necessary for safe delivery and uterine repair. Fetal distress is the usual precipitating factor.

Postpartum Hemorrhage

Definition

Postpartum hemorrhage is defined arbitrarily as blood loss > 500 mL following delivery. Hemorrhage occurs most often 1 hour after delivery. This is why the recovery period after delivery starts after the delivery of the placenta, with close observation of fundal height and bleeding for at least 1 hour. However, delayed postpartum hemorrhage can occur weeks after delivery. Postpartum hemorrhage remains a leading cause of maternal deaths and accounts for more than half of all hemorrhagic mortality (Creasy & Resnik, 1999).

Pathophysiology

Placental separation occurs by cleavage along the plane of the decidua basalis (Creasy & Resnick, 1999). The separation is usually complete two contractions after delivery but can take up to 30 minutes to separate. Once the placenta separates, the **myometrium** contracts, compressing the vessels that were supplying the placenta. If this does not occur severe bleeding will result.

Etiology and Clinical Manifestations

The three most common causes of postpartum hemorrhage are uterine atony, lacerations, and retained products of conception.

Uterine atony occurs when the myometrium fails to contract and compress the vessels supplying blood flow to the placenta. This is manifested by a soft, boggy uterus and excessive bleeding.

Obstetric lacerations can occur from a spontaneous vaginal delivery but are more frequent when forceps or a vacuum-assist device are used. The **fundus** is firm, but rules out uterine atony. The bleeding will appear bright red.

Retained placenta may occur with a prolonged third stage. It usually occurs when manual removal is necessary. After delivery, all placentas should be examined to be sure the placenta is intact. A retained fragment of the placenta or fetal membranes interferes with uterine contractility, allowing excessive blood loss from the uterus. Additionally, delayed hemorrhage can occur late in the postpartum period.

Management

After delivery of the placenta, the recovery period begins. The nurse should immediately take vital signs and assess fundal height and firmness and bleeding. With uterine atony, the fundus will feel soft and boggy and bleeding will be excessive. Fundal massage should be implemented. If massage is ineffective pharmacologic agents should be used (Table 37–12). Pitocin 20 U/L will normally be ordered to run at bolus rate, 1 L over 1 to 2 hours. An additional liter of Pitocin 20 U/L will often be run at 100 to 150 cc/hr. If uterine atony is present, a third liter is often given but further administration of Pitocin is contraindicated. Other measures should be instituted. If pharmacologic measures are ineffective, surgical treatment is implemented. Uterine exploration bimanually and/or curettage for retained products of conception usually stops bleeding without need for hysterectomy. Uterine tamponade (packing of the uterine cavity or inflation of a urinary catheter balloon) has also been successful in controlling uterine hemorrhage (Creasy & Resnik, 1999; Marcovici & Scoccia, 1999).

With lacerations, the nurse will note excessive bleeding with a firm fundus. First, bladder distention should be ruled out. Bladder distention will displace the uterus up and to the right, causing increased bleeding. Once the bladder is emptied the fundus will return to midline and bleeding will slow. When bladder distention is ruled out, a physician should be notified and a complete examina-

TABLE 37–12. COMMON PHARMACOLOGIC AGENTS USED TO TREAT POSTPARTUM UTERINE ATONY

AGENT	ACTION	DOSAGE/ROUTE	ONSET/DURATION OF ACTION	SIDE EFFECTS	PRECAUTIONS
Oxytocin (Pitocin)	Causes phasic uterine contractions by acting on the myofibrils of the uterine muscle	IV: 10–40 units/L of fluid; most commonly added to LR, D_5LR, or NS; run at 200–300 mL/hr; for rapid infusion, use 20 U/L to run at 10 mL/min or 200 mU/hr IM: 10 units	IV: onset 1 min IM: onset 3–7 min Duration: IV 30–60 min IM: 2–3 hr	Hypotension with rapid administration of undiluted bolus; water intoxication with prolonged administration especially over periods of > 24 hr	Bolus administration is never used due to hypotension and cardiac arrhythmias that may result Used cautiously if cyclopropane anesthesia or vasoconstrictive drugs are administered
Ethylergonovine maleate (Methergine)	Ergot alkaloid that causes sustained titanic uterine contractions	IVP: 0.2 mg infused slowly over 60 sec IM: 0.2 mg q 2–6 hr PO: 0.2 mg q 6 hr for up to 7 days	IV: onset immediately IM: onset 2–5 min PO: onset 5–15 min Duration: IV: 45 min IM: > 45 min, < 3 hr PO: 3 hr	Hypertensive episodes	Contraindicated in hypertensive disease states such as poorly controlled chronic hypertension, preeclampsia, and eclampsia
15-Methyl PGF_2-alpha (carboprost tromethamine—Prostin, Hemabate)	Increases uterine muscle tone, causes strong uterine contractions, acts as any prostaglandin	IM: 0.25 mg (250 μg) given as often as q 15 min up to a maximum dose of 2 mg (8 doses); 0.25 mg may be given intramyometrially by the obstetrician	Onset is variable but peak effect usually occurs in 15–30 min	Nausea, vomiting, diarrhea, headache, transient pyrexia, chills, transient diastolic hypertension	Used alone; not combined with other prostaglandins or with oxytocin May cause transient diastolic hypertension, which is more pronounced in preeclampsia and eclampsia, contraindicated in asthma due to potential for pulmonary airway and vascular constriction Contraindicated in SLE
PGE_2 (Dinoprostone)	Acts as any prostaglandin (see above)	PR: 20 mg q 2 hr	Onset is variable	Vomiting, diarrhea, headache, transient pyrexia, chills, transient diastolic hypertension	Contraindicated in hypertensive states

LR, lactated Ringer's; D_5LR, lactated Ringer's with 5% dextrose; NS, normal saline; SLE, systemic lupus erythematosus

Adapted from Cunningham FG, MacDonald FC, Gant NF, et al. (1997). *Williams obstetrics* (20th ed). Stamford, CT: Appleton & Lange; American College of Obstetricians and Gynecologists. (1997). Technical bulletin #235 *Hemorrhagic shock*, Washington, DC; Harvey C. (1991). *Critical care obstetrical nursing*. Gaithersburg, MD: Aspen; and Simpson K, Creehan P. (1996). *Perinatal nursing*. Philadelphia: Lippincott.

tion of the lower genital tract should be completed. Lacerations are repaired if > 2 cm; lacerations < 2 cm are repaired if the patient is actively bleeding.

The nurse should continue vital sign and fundal assessments during all procedures.

In summary, placenta previa, abruptio placentae, uterine rupture, and postpartum hemorrhage are considered serious hemorrhagic conditions in pregnancy. The nurse must monitor the mother for signs of hypovolemia (decreased LOC, decreased B/P, decreased UOP, acidosis). The fetus must be monitored for adequate oxygenation by assessment of baseline and heart rate variability and decelerations in response to contractions. In the cases of significant abruptio and uterine rupture, immediate cesarean section is indicated.

SECTION SIX REVIEW

1. Placenta previa involves
   A. separation of the implanted placenta from the wall of the uterus
   B. immediate delivery
   C. implantation of the placenta covering the cervical os
   D. premature labor
2. Causes of abruptio placentae include
   A. severe trauma to the abdomen
   B. nulliparity
   C. smoking < 10 cigarettes a day
   D. underweight mother
3. Symptoms of uterine rupture may include
   A. abdominal pain, vaginal bleeding, shock
   B. mild uterine contractions
   C. severe back pain and pelvic pressure
   D. leakage of amniotic fluid vaginally
4. Postpartum hemorrhage occurs most frequently due to
   A. uterine contractions
   B. rapid labor
   C. retained placenta parts
   D. clotting disorder

Answers: 1. C, 2. A, 3. A, 4. C

SHOCK STATES

SECTION SEVEN: Shock in Pregnancy

At the completion of this section, the learner will be able to identify a pregnant patient in shock and will know the appropriate nursing interventions when caring for a patient in shock.

Definition and Pathogenesis

Shock results when the patient's functional intravascular blood volume is below the capacity of the body's vascular bed. This results in decreasing blood pressure followed by decreased tissue perfusion. If untreated, resulting cellular acidosis and hypoxia lead to end-organ tissue dysfunction and death. The major type of shock in pregnancy is hemorrhagic or hypovolemic shock.

TABLE 37–13. ETIOLOGIES OF OBSTETRIC HEMORRHAGE[a]

ETIOLOGY	INCIDENCE PER DELIVERY
Late pregnancy	
Abruptio placentae	1:120
Placenta previa	1:200
Toxemia-associated	1:20
Delivery and postpartum	
Cesarean section	1:6
Obstetric lacerations	1:8
Uterine atony	1:20
Retained placenta	1:160
Uterine inversion	1:2300
Placenta accreta	1:7000

[a] Obstetric hemorrhage is usually defined as an acute blood loss in excess of 500 mL.
Modified from American College of Obstetricians and Gynecologists. (1984). Hemorrhagic shock *(p. 1). ACOG technical bulletin 82. Washington, DC: Author.*

Etiology and Incidence

Obstetric hemorrhage is the leading cause of maternal death. Postpartum hemorrhage accounts for more than 50 percent of all hemorrhagic obstetric deaths (Creasy & Resnick, 1999). Table 37–13 lists causes and incidence of obstetric hemorrhage. Concealed hemorrhage, found with pelvic fracture and abruptio placentae, is often undetected, resulting in an extremely large blood loss. In a nonpregnant patient, a loss of 15 to 20 percent of blood volume will result in clinical signs of shock. In a pregnant patient, approximately 20 to 25 percent loss of blood volume must occur before clinical signs are present. Table 37–14 lists clinical staging of hemorrhagic shock by volume of blood loss.

TABLE 37–14. CLINICAL STAGING OF HEMORRHAGIC SHOCK BY VOLUME OF BLOOD LOSS

SEVERITY OF SHOCK	FINDINGS	% BLOOD LOSS
None	None	Up to 15–20
Mild	Tachycardia (< 100 beats/min) Borderline mild hypotension Peripheral vasoconstriction	20–25
Moderate	Tachycardia (100–120 beats/min) Hypotension (80–100 mm Hg) Restlessness Oliguria	25–35
Severe	Tachycardia (> 120 beats/min) Hypotension (< 60 mm Hg) Altered consciousness Anuria	> 35

From Creasy, R., & Resnick, R. (1999). Maternal–fetal medicine: Principles and practice, *4th ed. (p. 909). Philadelphia: W.B. Saunders.*

TABLE 37–15. INDICATIONS FOR BLOOD COMPONENT REPLACEMENT THERAPY

BLOOD COMPONENT	INDICATION FOR USE
Whole blood	Active bleeding and > 25% blood volume loss or active bleeding and > 4 units RBC used
Red blood cells (RBC)	Hypovolemia and decreased oxygen-carrying capacity or > 15% blood volume loss or hematocrit < 24%
Platelets	< 20,000 or surgery and < 50,000 platelets
Fresh-frozen plasma (FFP)	Coagulation deficiencies with PTT > 60, PT > 16, or specific factor deficiency
Cryoprecipitate	Hemophilia A, von Willebrand's disease, decreased fibrinogen, or factor XIII deficiency

From Creasy, R., & Resnick, R. (1999). Maternal–fetal medicine: Principles and practice, *4th ed. (p. 910). Philadelphia: W.B. Saunders.*

Management

The two goals in management of hemorrhagic shock are blood volume replacement and treatment of the underlying cause of hemorrhage.

Stabilization of the patient takes first priority before any other definitive therapy is begun. The nurse should immediately assess blood pressure, character and rate of pulse and respirations, skin color, temperature, urine output, and mental status. This assessment should be continued every 15 to 30 minutes until the patient is stabilized. A large-bore, 14- to 18-gauge IV should be infusing. A second IV site should also be started for blood component replacement (Table 37–15). Laboratory values should be obtained for typing and crossmatching along with Hct and bleeding times. An arterial line may be required to facilitate frequent assessment of laboratory values. During shock, peripheral venous access is limited due to vasoconstriction (shunting blood away from the peripheral to the central circulation).

Evaluation of oxygen saturation is started. If the patient becomes dyspneic, oxygen should be applied at 6 to 8 L/min per face mask and arterial blood gases obtained. If oxygen therapy is ineffective the patient may need intubation and mechanical ventilation.

A urinary catheter is inserted with a urometer collection device. A decrease in UOP is a good indicator of core hypovolemia, hemodynamic status, and changes.

If hemorrhagic shock occurs before delivery, continuous fetal monitoring is imperative. Frequently, the first signs of hemorrhagic shock will be demonstrated as fetal distress. The loss in blood volume shunts blood from the uterus to other vital organs, resulting in decreased oxygen perfusion to fetus; late decelerations and decreased variability will be noted. Use of Trendelenburg position will increase perfusion to the core organs and uterus while stabilization measures are being instituted (Creasy & Resnik, 1999).

Once the patient is stabilized, the cause of hemorrhagic shock is treated and corrected. Invasive hemodynamic monitoring via a PAC may be used to assess the patient's hemodynamic status and for monitoring replacement therapy. The patient in shock will exhibit a decreased central venous pressure (CVP), pulmonary artery pressure (PAP), and pulmonary artery wedge pressure (PAWP) values. Cardiac output will initially appear normal. If untreated, eventually the myocardium no longer pump blood effectively and CO will decrease. Death occurs with an extreme drop in CO, which leads to intravascular collapse. Refer to Table 37–1 for normal hemodynamic values in pregnancy.

In summary, the goals in treating maternal hypovolemic shock are restoring blood volume through intravenous fluid (IVF) and/or transfusion and stopping the cause of hemorrhage.

Section Seven Review

1. Shock in pregnancy occurs as a result of
   - **A.** decreased blood volume below the capacity of the body's vascular bed
   - **B.** fetal death
   - **C.** an increase in blood volume and decrease in CO
   - **D.** peripheral vasodilation

2. Care of a patient in shock includes
   A. low flow oxygen
   B. evaluation of vaginal discharge
   C. continuous fetal monitoring

Answers: 1. A, 2. C

SECTION EIGHT: Trauma in Pregnancy

At the completion of this section, the learner will be able to discuss the physiologic changes associated with trauma and care of the pregnant trauma patient.

Etiology and Epidemiology

Trauma is a leading cause of death in women of childbearing years. The most common causes of trauma are motor vehicle crashes, assaults, and suicide. The incidence of trauma is increasing owing to (1) the growing trend for women to remain actively employed during pregnancy, (2) an increase in hazardous jobs for women, and (3) a more violent society.

Physiologic Alterations

There are great physiologic and anatomic changes associated with pregnancy. These changes affect the pregnant patient's response to trauma and the management of the pregnant trauma patient.

As discussed earlier, by term, there is an increase in blood volume of 30 to 40 percent. Due to the increase in blood volume the total loss of a pregnant patient will be much greater than that of a nonpregnant patient requiring greater replacement volumes. The pregnant patient will not show signs of shock as early as a nonpregnant patient. The pregnant patient at term may also be able to maintain hemodynamic stability longer at the expense of the fetus.

Supine positioning of the term pregnant trauma patient can significantly decrease blood return to the heart, affecting CO and causing hypotension and loss of consciousness. Repositioning the patient laterally will displace the uterus and correct **supine hypotension.**

When assessing vital signs, remember that by midpregnancy maternal blood pressure falls and heart rate increases 15 percent. What might be signs of shock in a nonpregnant patient are normal physiologic changes in a pregnant patient. It is important to obtain the patient's prenatal record to compare findings with their pregnant baselines.

The genitourinary tract is the organ system most affected by trauma. The uterus, which is normally protected by bony structures, becomes a prominent abdominal organ by 12 weeks' gestation. Due to the normal increase of blood flow to the uterus in pregnancy, injury to this organ adds additional risk of hemorrhage. The bladder is also at risk for trauma owing to its displacement by the enlarging uterus.

Hematologic changes also must be considered. Pregnancy is a state of hypercoagulability, which may increase the risk of thrombosis formation after injury. DIC is also prevalent with severe trauma. Knowledge of normal laboratory values of pregnant versus nonpregnant women is important for treating a pregnant patient. Table 37–16 lists physiologic changes of pregnancy and their relationship to trauma

Blunt Trauma

Severe blunt trauma is most frequently attributed to motor vehicle crashes (MVCs). Maternal death from MVCs usually results from head trauma and/or intra-abdominal hemorrhage. Other causes of blunt trauma include assault and battery and falls.

Mild trauma generally causes no significant sequelae for mothers and fetus. Though the uterus is no longer protected by the bony prominences of the pelvis, it is protected by the fluid-filled amniotic sac.

Severe blunt abdominal trauma has adverse consequences in pregnancy. The leading cause of fetal death is maternal death. Other effects on the fetus, some of which may result in neonatal morbidity, include skull fractures and intracranial hemorrhage. Abruptio placentae can cause poor placental–fetal oxygen exchange, leading to fetal morbidity and mortality. Abruption is most likely to occur within 48 hours of the trauma. If uterine rupture occurs, fetal mortality is 100%.

Management

A pregnant patient presenting with abdominal trauma is assessed immediately. Vital signs are assessed along with FHR and characteristics. These findings are compared with the patient's prenatal record if possible. Signs and symptoms of abruption and premature labor are assessed and may be manifested by vaginal bleeding, **uterine irritability** or contractions, pain, and leaking of amniotic fluid. Laboratory values, including CBC, fibrinogen, type and cross, and KHB, should be drawn. An ultrasound may be performed to assess fetal well-being.

TABLE 37–16. TRAUMATIC INJURY DURING PREGNANCY

SYSTEM	PREGNANCY-INDUCED PHYSIOLOGIC CHANGES	TREATMENT IMPLICATIONS
Cardiovascular	Increased blood volume Increased heart rate Increased cardiac output Decreased systemic vascular resistance (SVR) Decreased mean arterial pressure (MAP)	Compensatory mechanisms mask signs of shock 30% of volume must be lost before reflected by clinical parameters Supine positioning worsens fluid volume loss due to aortic/vena caval compression from uterus
Respiratory	Increased tidal volume Increased oxygen consumption Decreased functional residual capacity Compensated metabolic alkalosis (decreased $PaCO_2$, decreased serum bicarbonate)	Arterial blood gases in pregnancy differ from normals, potential for acidosis if nonpregnant values are used to guide treatment Decreased serum bicarbonate
Gastrointestinal	Displacement of abdominal organs Decreased gastric motility Increased esophageal reflux	Pain perception and location altered For anesthesia purposes, pregnant woman is always considered as having a "full stomach" (high risk for aspiration) Bowel sounds fainter
Renal	Increased blood flow to renal system Ureters and urethra dilated Bladder displaced	Urinary stasis increases risk of ascending urinary tract infections, risk of sepsis with untreated pyelonephritis Bladder more vulnerable to injury
Reproductive	Uterus enlarged Increased pelvic vascularity Vascular placenta	Bleeding may be concealed as in abruption or uterine rupture Progression of abruption from small to severe may occur over 24 hours Blood loss may be massive with uterine injury Potential for fetal loss

Adapted from de Swiet M. (ed). (1995). Diseases of the respiratory system. In *Medical disorders in obstetric practice* (3rd ed.). Cambridge, MA: Blackwell Science; Harvey KJ. (1991). *Critical care obstetrical nursing.* Gaithersburg, MD: Aspen; and Clark SL, Cotton DB, Hankins G, Phelan J. (1991). (2nd ed.) *Critical care obstetrics,* Chapters 11 and 25. Boston: Blackwell Scientific Publications.

In summary, in pregnancy blood pressure decreases and heart rate increases, making vital signs less helpful in monitoring shock. Deviations from prenatal vital signs are significant. Hypercoagulability promotes thrombosis and may decrease peripheral blood flow. The GU system and abdomen are most often affected by trauma.

SECTION EIGHT REVIEW

1. Positioning a pregnant trauma patient in a supine position
   A. can cause los of consciousness
   B. is an appropriate nursing intervention
   C. increases CO and is necessary to stabilize patient
   D. increases venous flow to the heart
2. Severe blunt abdominal trauma in pregnancy
   A. is the leading cause of fetal death
   B. produces no adverse complications to the fetus
   C. occurs more frequently in early pregnancy
   D. is extremely rare

Answers: 1. A, 2. A

METABOLISM

SECTION NINE: Diabetes Mellitus in Pregnancy

At the completion of this section, the learner will have a good understanding of the effects of diabetes on pregnancy, changes in insulin requirements, complications to both the mother and the fetus, and management of pregnancy complicated by diabetes.

There are two types of diabetes in pregnancy. The first type is diabetes diagnosed prior to pregnancy (preexisting diabetes), and the second type is diabetes diagnosed during pregnancy (gestational diabetes). Further classification of diabetes by White has diabetes categorized by the age of onset and presence of vascular complications (Table 37–17). Diabetes is also classified as type I, insulin dependent, and type II, non–insulin-dependent, diabetes. In both cases, if left untreated maternal and fetal morbidity and mortality increase greatly. Congenital anomalies are up to 4 times more common and macrosomia with its attendant birth injuries is 10 times more common in diabetic pregnancy (Creasy & Resnik, 1999). Both classes of diabetes require meticulous care

TABLE 37–17. CLASSIFICATION OF DIABETES

CLASS	AGE OF ONSET	DURATION (YEARS)	COMPLICATIONS
A (gestational)	Any	Any	Usually none, but always susceptible during subsequent pregnancies
B	Over 20	< 10	None
C	10–19	10–19	None
D	Before age 10	> 20	Benign retinopathy
F	Any	Any	Nephropathy
H	Any	Any	Arteriosclerotic heart disease
R	Any	Any	Proliferative retinopathy
T	Any	Any	After renal transplantation

in the antepartum and intrapartum periods to improve pregnancy outcomes.

During the past several decades, advances in care of the individual with diabetes in general, as well as in fetal surveillance and neonatal care, have continued to improve outcomes in most diabetic pregnancies to near that of the general population (American Diabetes Association [ADA], 1993).

Pathophysiology

Pregnancy normally produces a diabetogenic effect. During pregnancy, the woman is in a state of hyperinsulinemia, secondary to the effects of progesterone, estrogen, and HPL. The increase in these hormones causes a progressive increase in resistance by maternal tissues to maternal insulin. This in turn stimulates B cell hyperplasia, which increases insulin production. The anabolic effects of insulin result in disposition of subcutaneous fat and fat cell hypertrophy, the purpose of which may be to provide fuel stores for use later in pregnancy (Harvey, 1991).

As pregnancy progresses increased tissue resistance continues. Human placental lactogen (HPL) is an insulin antagonist. HPL, along with other placental hormones, including progesterone, cortisol, and prolactin, opposes the action of insulin and promotes maternal lipolysis. The outcome of the hormonal changes causes rapid storage of fuels while a woman is eating and insulin antagonism and accelerated metabolism while fasting. Because of the diabetogenic effects of pregnancy, gestational diabetes mellitus (GDM) develops in some women. In early pregnancy, a type I diabetic's insulin requirements decrease due to hyperinsulinemia. In latter pregnancy, insulin requirements increase due to insulin resistance. In a type II diabetic, diet and nutrition should be altered somewhat during early pregnancy to control caloric intake and total insulin requirements. The rate of HPL production is directly related to placental mass and as pregnancy progresses postprandial glucose levels increase and the fasting blood glucose level falls.

Screening and Diagnosis

When a pregnant patient presents with preexisting diabetes, an HbA1c (glycosylated hemoglobin) is drawn. This test expresses an average of the circulating glucose for 4 to 6 weeks prior to time the blood is drawn. It is a very useful tool for assessing the patient's metabolic control in early pregnancy, the critical period of organogenesis (ADA, 1993). If these results reveal poor metabolic control, there is an increased incidence of congenital anomalies and spontaneous abortion (SAB). Ideally, any woman with preexisting diabetes or a history of gestational diabetes will seek preconceptual counseling. This allows early monitoring and control of glucose levels.

Nondiabetic patients are first screened for GDM between 24 and 28 weeks' gestation. The test includes ingestion of 50 g oral glucose; 1 hour later, a fingerstick blood sugar is performed. This test is administered without regard to time of day or interval since last meal. If the glucose level is below 140, GDM is ruled out. If the glucose level is above 140, a 100-g 3-hour glucose tolerance test (GTT) is performed. For 3 days prior to the 3-hour GTT, the woman is instructed to eat 150 g of carbohydrate each day as part of her usual meals (see Table 37–18). After a fasting serum glucose level is drawn, the patient ingests 100 g of a glucose solution. Fasting serum glucose levels are then drawn at 1, 2, and 3 hours. If two or more of these levels meet or exceed threshold values, the diagnosis of GDM is made (Table 37–19).

TABLE 37–18. CARBOHYDRATE FOOD CHOICES: 30 G

2 slices white bread
⅔ cup cooked rice
1 cup cooked noodles
2 corn tortillas
8 oz apple juice
6 oz grape juice
8 oz orange juice
2 small bananas

Jones, M.W., & Stone L.C. (1998). Management of the woman with gestational diabetes mellitus. J Perinat Neonat Nurs 11(4):13–24.

TABLE 37–19. DIAGNOSTIC CRITERIA FOR GESTATIONAL DIABETES[a]

Fasting	≥ 105 mg/dL (5.8 mM)
1 hr	≥ 190 mg/dL (10.6 mM)
2 hr	≥ 165 mg/dL (9.2 mM)
3 hr	≥ 145 mg/dL (8.1 mM)

[a] Two or more values must be met or exceeded.
From the American Diabetes Association. (1993). Medical management of pregnancy complicated by diabetes *(p. 81). Alexandria, Virginia: Author.*

Monitoring

Perinatal

In addition to self-monitoring at home by the patient, including fingerstick blood sugars and urine ketone testing, women with diabetes will be monitored very closely by their physician. They can expect weekly or biweekly appointments.

Women with diabetes will have various laboratory studies done throughout pregnancy owing to the vascular changes of diabetes. A thyroid panel should be done as a baseline and then monitored serially depending on the results. A clean-catch dipstick urinalysis will be obtained at each visit to evaluate protein, ketones, and white blood cells. If positive, further tests will be completed to rule out UTI or preeclampsia. A fingerstick blood glucose level will be done and compared with the patient's home testing. As mentioned earlier, HbA1c levels will be drawn every 4 to 6 weeks to evaluate the patient's overall diabetic control. Observation of other diabetic-related complications is imperative. A 24-hour urine should be completed every trimester for creatinine clearance and total protein. If nephropathy is present, the patient will be referred to a nephrologist. A baseline retinal examination should also be performed and repeated if changes are noted.

Fetal Monitoring

As discussed earlier, poor diabetic control in early pregnancy can result in congenital anomalies and SAB. Therefore, it is important to keep close surveillance of fetal development. In addition, diabetes in pregnancy increases the rate of third-trimester stillbirth. This is especially true with poor glucose control and the resulting fetal macrosomia (Jones & Stone, 1998).

Establishing correct fetal age is important not only to determine the due date but also to plan various tests and evaluations as the pregnancy progresses. Between 7 and 10 weeks' gestation, the crown–rump length of the fetus can be measured, yielding 95 percent confident limits of 64.7 days for one measurement. If multiple measurements are taken, the accuracy increases (ADA, 1993).

Alpha-fetoprotein (AFP), a fetal product found in amniotic fluid and the maternal circulation, is present in higher concentrations when an open fetal neurological defect occurs and in low concentrations with chromosomal complications. This test is most accurate at 16 weeks' gestation. Though this test has high false-positive rates, it can help determine whether further testing is necessary with an amniocentesis or level II ultrasound (US).

Genetic testing may be ordered if the maternal serum AFP is elevated, if there is a family history that includes high genetic risk, or if advanced maternal age (> 35 years) is a factor.

The most common method of genetic testing is obtaining fluid via amniocentesis. Fetal cells are separated from the fluid and grown in tissue for chromosome analysis. The result takes 2 to 4 weeks, which can be agonizing to the expectant parents.

Chorionic villus sampling (CVS) is another method of obtaining tissue for genetic testing. This procedure involves taking a biopsy of the placenta in utero. Though this procedure is fairly new and is performed only in high-risk centers, it has many advantages. It can be performed as early as 8 to 10 weeks and the results only take a couple of days.

Though these tests can reveal significant information to both the patient and the physician, there are great risks that should be discussed with the woman and her supportive other. These risks include premature labor, fetal injury, rupture of membranes, and pregnancy loss.

As discussed earlier, ultrasound is used to establish dating and to rule out fetal anomalies. It is also a useful tool in assessing fetal size and weight. A baseline US is performed at about 24 weeks. Ultrasonography is usually performed in the third trimester to rule out macrosomia and IUGR.

After 28 weeks, women are instructed to perform daily fetal kick count assessments. Decreased fetal movement is associated with fetal distress. A fetal kick count requires the patient to record fetal movements during a certain time period each day. If criteria for fetal kick counts is not met the patient is instructed to notify her physician for further evaluation.

Another useful tool for evaluating fetal well-being is the NST. NSTs are performed weekly to biweekly depending on diabetic control. The physician may begin NSTs as early as 28 weeks but definitely after 34 weeks' gestation.

Delivery for diabetic women depends on quality of glucose control and normal results of fetal testing measures (US, kick counts, NSTs). Those women exhibiting good glucose control, however, will have fetal lung maturity screening by amniocentesis between 36 and 38 weeks with the goal of expeditious delivery as soon as fetal lung maturity is demonstrated (Creasy & Resnik, 1999). Evaluation of fetal lung maturity involves quantification of certain components of amniotic fluid. The L/S ratio (lecithin/sphingomyelin) of amniotic fluid at 35 weeks (in a noncomplicated pregnancy) is 2.0 or greater as one approaches term. The risk of RDS in a normal pregnancy is low beyond 35 weeks, therefore the risk of RDS is low with an L/S value of at least 2.0. In some complicated pregnancies (diabetes and RH isoimmunization), L/S alone does not ensure fetal lung maturity. In those cases, an additional test is used. Surfactant contains phospholipids; therefore, as fetal lungs mature, these lipids increase in amniotic fluid. Another phospholipid, PG (phosphatidylglycerol), appears at the time of normal lung maturity (usually about 35 weeks). Presence of PG eliminates the risk of neonatal respiratory distress syndrome (RDS) and is a more reliable predictor of RDS than the L/S ratio.

Insulin Requirements during Pregnancy

Insulin requirements during pregnancy change drastically from stage to stage due to great metabolic alterations.

In early pregnancy and toward the end of the first trimester, insulin requirements drop 10 to 20 percent of the dosage taken prior to conception (ADA, 1993). This is mainly due to loss of glucose to the fetus.

The diabetogenic effects of pregnancy begin at approximately 18 to 24 weeks' gestation. At this time, insulin requirements gradually increase as the patient switches from glucose-based to lipid-based energy economy from circulating fats or stored adipose tissue, sparing glucose for fetal growth (ADA, 1993).

In late pregnancy, basal insulin levels are higher than normal prepregnant levels and eating produces a twofold to threefold greater outpouring of insulin. The increase in plasma insulin is opposed by HPL, prolactin, estrogen, and progesterone production. During this period, insulin requirements gradually increase to as much as double the dose of insulin needed before pregnancy.

Human insulins are the least immunogenic of all insulins and should be used exclusively during pregnancy. Various insulin preparations may be used in combination to achieve optimal glycemic control. The proper use of insulin requires an understanding of the factors that affect its absorption, disposal, and action. See Table 37–20 for the most commonly used types of insulin.

During pregnancy, the type I diabetic is encouraged to check fingerstick blood glucose up to eight times a day and to maintain an accurate record of patterns. Insulin should not be adjusted in response to one or every glucose measurement that lies outside the target range but should be based on the patient's overall pattern. For example, a patient who is continually experiencing elevated blood glucose during the late afternoon should not react by taking supplemental insulin before dinner and risking hypoglycemia later in the evening. Instead, the patient should increase her morning insulin the next morning or increase a short-acting dose of insulin at noon.

Patient compliance is crucial for optimal maternal and fetal well-being. HbA1c levels are useful, but, unfortunately, the results are available only after the fact and after the damage is done. Meticulous record keeping by the patient and close monitoring by the physician enables quick reaction to and treatment of diabetic trends. Many institutions have incorporated an educator into the perinatal health care term. This individual educates the patient

TABLE 37–20. TYPES OF INSULIN[a]

TYPE	SOURCE	ONSET	PEAK	DURATION
Short acting				
Humulin R (Lilly)	Human	15–30 min	Hours 2–4	6–8 hr
Velosulin-H (Novo Nordisk)	Human	30 min	Hours 1–3	8 hr
Novolin R (Novo Nordisk)	Human	30 min	Hours 2½–5	6–8 hr
Novolin R Penfill (Novo Nordisk)	Human	30 min	Hours 2½–5	6–8 hr
Intermediate acting				
Humulin (Lilly)	Human	1–3 hr	Hours 6–12	18–24 hr
Humulin NPH (Lilly)	Human	1–2 hr	Hours 6–12	18–24 hr
Novolin L (Novo Nordisk)	Human	2½ hr	Hours 7–15	22 hr
Novolin N (Novo Nordisk)	Human	1½ hr	Hours 4–12	24 hr
Novolin NPH Penfill (Novo Nordisk)	Human	1½ hr	Hours 4–12	24 hr
Long acting				
Humulin U (Lilly)	Human	4–6 hr	Hours 8–20	24–28 hr
Premixed				
Humulin 70/30 (Lilly)	Human	30 min	Hours 2–12	24 hr
Humulin 50/50 (Lilly)	Human	30 min	Hours 2–12	24 hr
Novolin 70/30 (Novo Nordisk)	Human	30 min	Hours 2–12	24 hr
Novolin 70/30 Penfill (Novo Nordisk)	Human	30 min	Hours 2–12	24 hr
Mixtard H 70/30 (Novo Nordisk)	Human	30 min	Hours 4–12	24 hr

[a] Based on information from manufacturers. Duration and peak actions may differ from one individual to the next.

Modified from the American Diabetes Association. (1993). Medical management of pregnancy complicated by diabetes *(p. 61). Alexandria, Virginia: Author.*

on diet, exercise, and insulin requirements and acts as an overall resource person to the patient. Many times, the nurse is the mediator between the patient and the physician.

Insulin Requirements during Labor

The insulin requirements for all diabetic patients at the onset of labor is zero, although glucose requirements are constant (ADA, 1993). Jovanovic and Peterson (1982) have developed a protocol for meeting the glucose needs of active labor. The goal is to maintain glucose concentration between 70 and 90 mg/dL (ADA, 1993).

These following paragraphs summarize these protocols for induction of labor, active labor, and scheduled cesarean section.

Induction of Labor and Active Labor

On the evening before elective induction, the usual bedtime dose of intermediate-acting insulin may be given. On the morning of induction, insulin is withheld and an IV infusion of normal saline is started. Once active labor commences, with persistent adequate contractions, fluids are changed to 5 percent dextrose and infused at a rate of 125 mL/hr. Fingerstick blood glucose levels should be monitored hourly by the nurse. If the patient's glucose level falls below 60 mg/dL, the infusion rate should be doubled for the subsequent hour. If the patient's glucose level rises above 140 mg/dL, 2 to 4 U of subcutaneous or intravenous short-acting insulin can be given to maintain glucose between 70 and 90. However, if this is ineffective and to avoid constant swings of glucose levels, an insulin drip of 1 to 2 U/hr of short-acting insulin may be ordered.

Elective Cesarean Section

With elective cesarean section, the bedtime dose of intermediate-acting insulin may be given on the morning of the surgery. Normal saline is initially started but as stated before if glucose levels drop below 60 mg/dL, a dextrose solution will be started. If glucose levels rise above 140, subcutaneous or IV insulin can be given or an insulin drip started. This insulin infusion should be stopped immediately before surgery.

Although these protocols are useful in providing adequate care and management of glucose control, care should ultimately be based on the patient's own glucose levels, and trends and treatment should be individualized accordingly.

Gestational diabetic patients rarely require insulin during labor. The goal of management is to maintain glucose levels between 70 and 120 mg/dL (ADA, 1993). Hourly fingersticks are continued. IV fluids are started with a 5 percent dextrose solution at a rate of 100 mL/hr. However, if a fluid bolus is required for anesthesia purposes or fetal distress, the nurse should change fluids to a nonglucose solution. After the bolus the fluids should be changed back. If glucose levels rise and subcutaneous insulin is required and ineffective, an insulin drip may be started at 1 U/hr and adjusted according to hourly glucose levels. The insulin drip should be stopped immediately before delivery and in most cases is not necessary after delivery.

Complications Associated with Diabetes

Neonatal Complications

Infants of diabetic patients have increased morbidity and mortality rates due to maternal disease. The normal neonate is in transitional glucose homeostasis (Cowet, 1991). The fetus is dependent on the mother for glucose transfer in utero, and maintenance of glucose homeostasis may be a problem. The neonate must maintain a balance between glucose deficiency and excess. The development of homeostasis results from balance between substrate availability and developmental hormonal, sympathomimetic, and enzymatic systems (Cowet, 1991). With diabetes, this process is further complicated by great fluctuations in maternal glucose levels, making neonatal glucose homeostasis even more difficult to achieve.

Many factors influence neonatal morbidity in diabetic patients. Severe morbidity has been associated more frequently in patients with longer duration of maternal diabetes, lesser gestational age at birth, increased rates of cesarean section, and a higher frequency of preeclampsia.

MACROSOMIA, BIRTH INJURY, AND ASPHYXIA. In poorly controlled diabetics macrosomia may occur. This presents many possible complications, particularly if macrosomia was not detected prior to delivery. Vaginal delivery may be very difficult with subsequent shoulder dystocia and resultant birth injury and/or asphyxia. Injury to the brachial nerve plexus can lead to obvious nerve injury. If the phrenic nerve is affected, diaphragmatic paralysis occurs. Organomegaly is also associated with diabetes. Hemorrhage can occur specifically in the liver and adrenal glands. The cause of asphyxia is unclear but is associated with macrosomia. Asphyxia has diverse consequences and may affect respiratory, renal, and CNS function acutely (ADA, 1993). Table 37–21 lists the most common potential birth injuries.

CONGENITAL ANOMALIES. The etiology of the increased frequency of congenital anomalies among infants of diabetic mothers is unclear. Several theories have been proposed:

- Hyperglycemia, either preconceptional or postconceptional
- Hypoglycemia
- Uteroplacental vascular disease
- Genetic predisposition

TABLE 37–21. POTENTIAL BIRTH INJURIES IN INFANTS OF DIABETIC MOTHERS

- Abdominal organ injury
- Brachial plexus injuries
- Cephalohematoma
- Clavicular fracture
- Diaphragmatic paralysis
- External genitalia hemorrhage
- Facial palsy
- Ocular hemorrhage
- Subdural hemorrhage

From the American Diabetes Association. (1993). Medical management of pregnancy complicated by diabetes *(p. 95). Alexandria, Virginia: Author.*

With poor metabolic control in the early weeks of pregnancy, when organogenesis occurs, and when most patients are unaware that they are pregnant, data supports the preconceptional and early postconceptional theory.

The most frequent types of malformations found in infants of diabetic mothers involve the CNS, cardiovascular, genitourinary, gastrointestinal, and skeletal systems. These malformations are broken down and listed according to system.

Central Nervous System
- Anencephaly
- Meningocele
- Microcephaly

Cardiovascular System
- Transposition of the great vessels
- Ventricular septal defect
- Coarctation of the aorta
- Single ventricle
- Hypoplastic left ventricle
- Persistent patent ductus arteriosus
- Pulmonic stenosis

Genitourinary System
- Renal agenesis
- Multicystic kidneys
- Double ureters
- Hydronephrosis

Gastrointestinal System
- Anorectal atresia
- Small left colon
- Tracheoesophageal fistula
- Duodenal atresia
- Hirschsprung's disease

Skeletal System
- Sacral hypoplasia
- Sacral agenesis
- Hypoplastic limbs

All these malformations can be present either alone or in combination with other complications.

Respiratory Distress. Respiratory distress, including RDS, is frequently associated with infants of diabetic mothers. Neonatal RDS is caused by hyaline membrane disease and develops because of lung immaturity. The risk of RDS occurs more frequently in births less than 38 weeks' gestation. The incidence of RDS has decreased over the years due to better assessment of fetal lung maturity leading to deliveries at later gestational ages.

Maternal Complications

Diabetic Ketoacidosis (DKA). DKA, a condition of maternal acidosis and associated with dehydration, carries a risk of fetal death in utero. Some studies have shown the risk of fetal death as high as 50 percent.

DKA is associated with infections (respiratory, urinary, soft tissues), poor maternal compliance with treatment, and with undiagnosed GDM. Diagnosis includes hyperglycemia in the presence of serum ketones. The pathophysiology relates to the lack of insulin, which causes hyperglycemia, which in turn causes osmotic diuresis (with its attendant fluid and electrolyte imbalance) (Creasy & Resnik, 1999).

DKA occurs more frequently before the third trimester. The woman requires aggressive treatment, including hydration, insulin, potassium, and other electrolytes. With fetal monitoring, fetal distress is noted. A cesarean section may be indicated but is usually delayed to stabilize the patient. A cesarean section performed on a patient in DKA carries a higher maternal mortality rate. Usually, once the patient is stabilized, fetal well-being improves as well.

Preterm Labor. Although preterm labor is not a risk directly associated with diabetes, it does present particular problems involving management.

Beta-sympathomimetics, the most commonly used tocolytics, have beta-adrenergic agonist properties that cause rapid and extreme increases in maternal glucose levels, which can lead to DKA. Maternal hyperglycemia, hypokalemia, and pulmonary edema occur secondary to alveolar capillary leakage, electrocardiographic abnormalities, tachycardia, and other problems.

Another problem that presents with preterm labor is the use of steroids to accelerate fetal lung maturity. Steroids can further exacerbate hyperglycemia.

Although they do present problems with management and maintaining metabolic control, tocolytics and steroids are not completely contraindicated in patients with diabetes. The patient will require close glucose monitoring and in most cases an insulin drip.

If no attempt is made to halt preterm labor, an infant born with respiratory distress will result.

Timing and Mode of Delivery

In the past, all diabetic patients were delivered at some arbitrary number of weeks before term to lessen the likelihood of unexplained fetal death and to lessen the risk of complications associated with macrosomia and shoulder **dystocia.**

Due to medical advances in antepartum testing, delivery is avoided and pregnancy continued until closer to term. With weekly or biweekly NSTs, fetal well-being is monitored. A US can be performed to evaluate fetal growth, and timing of delivery can be based on estimated fetal weight (EFW). An amniocentesis can be performed to determine fetal lung maturity. The type of delivery depends greatly on the EFW. If the fetus is large (over 8 lb, 12 oz), pelvic studies may be completed to determine if fetal size compared with pelvic outlet will permit vaginal delivery as an option. This decision is complicated further by inaccuracies of EFW by US up to 10 percent. Some physicians attempt vaginal delivery but quickly move toward cesarean section if failure to progress or failure to descend occurs. If EFW is greater than 9 lb 14 oz, a cesarean section may be scheduled to prevent stress on mother and fetus from attempted labor and vaginal delivery.

In summary, due to all potential complications associated with maternal diabetes, diabetic patients should be referred to a facility that is equipped to manage all these complications, particularly one with a neonatal intensive care unit.

The latest advances in medicine and its ability to maintain maternal metabolic states diminishes but does not eradicate the increased perinatal and neonatal mortality and morbidity of diabetic pregnancy.

Section Nine Review

1. Gestational diabetes is diagnosed
   - **A.** in the first trimester
   - **B.** between 24 and 28 weeks of gestation
   - **C.** after the baby is born
   - **D.** with an elevated nonfasting 1-hour glucose tolerance test
2. Patients with diabetes require
   - **A.** close fetal monitoring
   - **B.** bed rest
   - **C.** insulin
   - **D.** oral hypoglycemia agent
3. Poor diabetic control in early pregnancy can result in
   - **A.** fetal congenital anomalies
   - **B.** underweight fetus
   - **C.** ARDS
   - **D.** maternal blindness
4. Insulin requirements during pregnancy
   - **A.** diminish greatly throughout pregnancy
   - **B.** change drastically throughout pregnancy
   - **C.** remain the same throughout pregnancy
   - **D.** are met by decreasing glycogen metabolism
5. An AFP
   - **A.** is performed at approximately 27 weeks' gestation
   - **B.** is performed to detect fetal size
   - **C.** has a high false-positive rate
   - **D.** to confirm congenital defect
6. Macrosomia resulting from maternal diabetes
   - **A.** can cause fetal birth injuries
   - **B.** causes congenital defects
   - **C.** causes maternal hyperglycemia
   - **D.** can cause DIC
7. Preterm labor accompanied with diabetes
   - **A.** requires no intervention
   - **B.** is directly related
   - **C.** is encouraged to avoid complications associated with a macrosomic fetus
   - **D.** requires close observation of maternal glucose levels due to the hyperglycemic effects of medications used to halt preterm labor

Answers: 1. B, 2. A, 3. A, 4. B, 5. C, 6. A, 7. D

SECTION TEN: Thyroid Disease in Pregnancy

At the completion of this section, the learner will have an understanding of the effects of thyroid disease on pregnancy and management of pregnancy complicated by thyroid disease.

Normal Thyroid Physiology

The thyroid gland, which normally weighs 15 to 25 grams in adults, is responsible for production and secretion of T_3 (L-triiodothyronine) and T_4 (L-thyroxine). Free thyroid hormone (amount of which is controlled by a relationship between the thyroid, pituitary, and hypothalamus) enters cells causing conversion of T_4 to T_3. T_3 (about four times more potent than T_4) then controls metabolism by a combination of gene expression and protein synthesis (Creasy & Resnik, 1999). Iodine is required to synthesize hormones. After ingestion, iodine is converted to iodide in the small intestine to facilitate absorption. Iodide is then carried into the thyroid gland (iodine trapping). Production of T_3 and T_4 are also regulated by TSH. TSH accelerates all steps involved in production of thyroid hormone. Elevated T_3 and T_4 levels effectively instruct the pituitary to decrease TSH production. T_3 and T_4, which are bound to serum proteins, are secreted at levels of 30 μg (T_3) and 90 μg (T_4) daily. T_3 has a short half-life of 1 day of 1 week. (This means it takes 5 or 6 weeks for a change in levothyroxine dose to reach equilibrium.) The liver and kidney are highly sensitive to thyroid hormone. In addition, the kidney is responsible for excretion of iodine, the total excreted in pregnancy being twice the prepregnancy rate. TSH is structurally related to human chorionic gonadotropin (hCG), which causes stimulation of thyroid hormone production normally in pregnancy. Thyroxin-binding globulin (TBG), which binds 75 percent of thyroid hormone, increases in amount due to elevated estrogen levels found in pregnancy as well. It has been hypothesized that these increases in early pregnancy may be significant for early fetal development. (Any thyroid hormone required for fetal development before 10 to 12 weeks has to come from the mother. Additionally, all fetal iodine comes directly from maternal supplies.) With the increased thyroid binding of pregnancy, total T_3 and T_4 levels are increased (free T_3 and T_4 remain stable until late pregnancy when they decrease about 30 percent). Evaluation of thyroid function in pregnancy is, therefore, best evaluated by use of a free T_4 level and third-generation TSH assay. Hyperthyroidism (thyrotoxicosis) has elevated free T_4 levels and suppressed TSH. Hypothyroidism has decreased free T_4 levels and elevated TSH.

Hyperthyroidism in Pregnancy

Pathophysiology

The incidence of hyperthyroidism in pregnancy is 2/1,000 pregnancies. Signs and symptoms mimic normal pregnancy effects including vomiting; fatigue; anxiety; emotional lability; warm, diaphoretic skin; heat intolerance; and wide pulse pressure. Hyperthyroidism resembles the increased metabolic state normally found in pregnancy. (Normal basal metabolism rises 15 to 20 percent between the fourth and eighth months of gestation.) Other signs not common in pregnancy that appear with thyrotoxicosis are weight loss, onycholysis (loosening of the nails) and maternal pulse over 100 bpm that does not respond to Valsalva's maneuver. Goiter or exophthalmos may be present. Graves' disease is responsible for 95 percent of the cases of pregnancy-related hyperthyroidism (Diehl, 1998). Laboratory abnormalities seen in thyrotoxicosis, especially Graves' disease, are mild increased calcium levels, decreased magnesium levels, mild neutropenia, normochromic normocytic anemia, and elevated liver function tests (alkaline phosphatase, transaminases, and bilirubin). Although Graves' disease is the most common cause of thyrotoxicosis in pregnancy, it is important to note that about 50 percent of women with gestational trophoblastic disease have laboratory evidence of hyperthyroidism. In these cases, hCG levels > 1,000 times normal can be present; hCG has a TSH-like effect on the thyroid gland.

Treatment of Hyperthyroidism

Treatment should ideally occur preconceptually for women with thyrotoxicosis. Inadequate treatment results in a higher incidence of minor fetal anomalies, preterm delivery, perinatal mortality, preeclampsia, and maternal congestive heart failure. Mode of treatment is directed at maintaining the maternal thyroxine level in a high normal/slightly elevated range to prevent fetal or neonatal hypothyroidism. Radioactive iodine is always contraindicated due to concentrated fetal thyroid uptake after about 10 weeks' gestation. PTU (propylthiouracil) is the drug of choice starting with a dose of 100 to 150 mg q8h up to 900 mg/day. The action of this drug is through inhibition of thyroid hormone synthesis. Maximum effect takes 6 to 8 weeks until all stored hormone is depleted. Clinical improvement may begin as early as 1 week after beginning therapy. When the woman becomes "euthyroid," the dosage is reduced or may be discontinued beyond 32 to 36 weeks' gestation to prevent fetal/neonatal hypothyroidism. Alternative drug therapy may include carbamazole (methimazole is the metabolite) dosed at 20 to 40 mg/day. Beta-blockers (Inderal dosed at 20 to 40 mg up to TID and atenolol 50 to 100 mg daily) can be used for short-term control of the annoying symptoms of hyperthyroidism. Potassium iodide (SSKI) can be used for short-term treatment of severe thyrotoxicosis or impending thyroid storm.

Thyroid Storm

In the presence of unrecognized or poorly controlled thyrotoxicosis a life-threatening condition called thyroid storm can occur. Hyperthermia (temperatures > 41°C/105.8°F), diarrhea, and congestive heart failure associated with altered mental status occurs. It is more likely to occur as a response to a factor such as infection, labor, or cesarean section. Thyroid storm is an obstetric emergency. Treatment is with either PTU or methimazole (thioamide drugs) orally, sodium iodine orally or IV, and if needed dexamethasone (which blocks conversion of T_4 to T_3).

Hypothyroidism in Pregnancy

Hypothyroidism occurs in one of 1,600 to 2,000 deliveries (Creasy & Resnik, 1999). It is also difficult to identify in pregnancy as decreased exercise tolerance, lethargy, intolerance to cold, muscle cramps or muscle weakness, some weight gain (inability to lose weight when dieting is a common sign in nonpregnant women), and constipation can be associated with pregnancy. Hoarse voice, brittle nails, and dry skin are also present. Hypothermia and slowed heart rate as well as carpal tunnel syndrome may be seen. Gestational hypertension, preeclampsia, low birth weight, stillbirth, and placental abruption are more common with hypothyroidism than with euthyroid states. Primary hypothyroidism is associated with elevation of TSH levels and depression of T_4. If the T_4 is normal with an elevated TSH, subclinical hypothyroidism may exist and is often associated with autoantibodies—a state common in pregnancy. Secondary hypothyroidism has a normal or low TSH and a low free T_4. It is also referred to as pituitary hypothyroidism. Laboratory abnormalities in hypothyroidism are anemia (mild, normochromic, normocytic), slightly elevated liver function tests, serum cholesterol and serum carotene, and modestly elevated creatine phosphokinase. Women with type I diabetes are at particular risk; in conjunction with levothyroxine replacement, insulin requirements may increase.

Causes of Hypothyroidism in Pregnancy

Hashimoto's thyroiditis is an autoimmune disorder, which causes most pregnancy-related cases of hypothyroidism in the United States. It is called chronic lymphocytic thyroiditis or autoimmune thyroiditis. It occurs in up to 10 percent of women in their childbearing years. Anti-TPO (thyroperoxidase) and anti-thyroglobulin antibodies characterize the disease. Autoimmune thyroiditis may also be found alongside autoimmune disorders such as myasthenia gravis, pernicious anemia, diabetes mellitus, and Addison's disease. Goiter may be present, yet as many as 75 to 80 percent of these women are euthyroid. The remaining 20 to 25 percent have either overt or subclinical disease. Treatment of Graves' disease by thyroidectomy or radioactive iodine is the second leading cause of hypothyroidism in pregnancy. Iodine deficiency is a rare cause of hypothyroidism in the United States where iodine-enriched foods are normally consumed.

Treatment of Hypothyroidism

Levothyroxine is the treatment of choice with dosage replacement ranging from 0.1 to 0.15 mg/day. The dosage is increased every four weeks until the TSH is low normal. In those women in whom hypothyroidism predates pregnancy, TSH levels should be checked during the first, second, and early third trimesters. Postdelivery, doses are returned to prepregnancy levels and the TSH is rechecked 6 to 8 weeks postpartum.

Postpartum Thyroiditis

Silent thyroiditis or that occurring in women following pregnancy is generally transient and often goes undiagnosed. It occurs in two phases, and has an association with anti-TPO and antithyroglobulin antibodies. Up to 7 percent of postpartum women may develop postpartum thyroiditis. As many as 80 percent of these affected women are euthyroid by 3 to 5 months following the hypothyroid phase. Permanent hypothyroidism may develop in 10 to 30 percent of women who develop postpartum thyroiditis. Progression of the disease begins at 2 to 3 months postpartum with symptoms of thyrotoxicosis followed several months later by onset of hypothyroidism and often depression. Interestingly, treatment of the hypothyroidism can alleviate some cases of postpartum depression. Although no cause-and-effect relationship has been established, there is evidence that depression occurs more commonly in women who have postdelivery hypothyroidism.

Postpartum laboratory values reflect presence of antimicrosomal antibodies in conjunction with abnormal free T_4 and TSH values. For confirmation, if needed, a short-lived low radioactive iodine (^{123}I) thyroid uptake scan can be done. Breast-feeding must be stopped for no less than 48 hours posttest (Creasy & Resnik, 1999). Treatment is symptomatic in nature when necessary. If hypothyroid symptoms become problematic, levothyroxine can be given. This should be withdrawn gradually at 1 year postpartum. Assessment focuses on ascertaining if hypothyroidism is permanent. For those women experiencing early postpartal symptoms without goiter, there is a greater likelihood of permanent hypothyroidism. Thyrotoxicosis symptoms require only temporary treatment with beta blockers. Follow-up in women experiencing postpartum thyroiditis is required due to the increased risk (as much as 25 percent) for recurrence after further pregnancies and for permanent hypothyroidism.

Fetal/Neonatal Hypothyroidism

Fetal/neonatal hypothyroidism may result in cretinism. Secondary to maternal deficiency of iodine, thyroid hormone levels are decreased in mother and fetus. This syndrome is manifested by significant mental retardation, deaf mutism, spasticity, and other signs. Maternal hypothyroidism in pregnancy is associated not only with creatinism but also with higher rates of stillbirth, perinatal mortality, and congenital anomalies. Congenital deficiency of thyroid hormone from reasons other than iodine deficiency also results in neurological deficits. If neonatal hypothyroidism is unrecognized at birth (possibly from thyroid dysgenesis or a congenital thyroid malfunction) and not treated, by 3 months of age neurological development is already hindered. These children experience significant developmental delay.

Fetal/Neonatal Effects of Maternal Thyroid Disease

Fetal thyrotoxicosis occurs in only 1 percent of pregnancies complicated by either Graves' disease or Hashimoto's thyroiditis. The disease is associated with FHR above 160 bpm, IUGR, advanced bone age, and craniosynostosis.

Evaluation of pregnancies with thyroid disease is required and all these signs are evident on ultrasound. Maternal TSH levels five times normal are also more common in the presence of congenital thyrotoxicosis. Fetal thyrotoxicosis is treated by keeping the mother euthyroid. Neonatal thyrotoxicosis is treated as in adults.

SECTION TEN REVIEW

1. Thyroid hormone
   - **A.** transports T_3 and T_4 to the small intestine
   - **B.** has a half-life of 1 week
   - **C.** accelerates production of TSH
   - **D.** is controlled by a relationship among the thyroid, pituitary, and hypothalamus
2. Thyroid storm is
   - **A.** untreated hypothyroidism in pregnancy
   - **B.** untreated or poorly controlled hyperthyroidism
   - **C.** associated with hypothermia and infection
   - **D.** associated with creatinism
3. Hypothyroidism may include an autoimmune component in
   - **A.** Hashimoto's thyroiditis and postpartum thyroiditis
   - **B.** iodine deficiency
   - **C.** Graves' disease
   - **D.** radioactive iodine therapy

Answers: 1. D, 2. B, 3. A

SPECIAL CONDITIONS

SECTION ELEVEN: Premature Labor

At the completion of this section, the learner will have a good understanding of premature onset of labor (POL) and delivery as well as medications used in treating POL and inducing lung maturity.

Preterm labor and delivery is a significant cause of perinatal morbidity and mortality. The advances in treatment modalities and the introduction of neonatal intensive care units have improved but not eliminated complications associated with preterm labor.

Definition

Preterm labor is defined as uterine contractions prior to 37 weeks' gestation with a documented cervical change. Preterm birth occurs prior to 37 weeks' but after 20 weeks' gestation. A birth prior to 20 weeks is considered an abortion.

Epidemiology and Etiology

Some studies have shown an increase of POL in women of lower socioeconomic status. This may be associated with poor prenatal care and nutritional status. POL is more common in women who weigh less than 50 kg at conception and who demonstrate poor weight gain in pregnancy. The incidence of preterm labor is higher in women under 20 years of age, not only for the first pregnancy but even the second and third. Childbearing beginning after the age of 35 has an increased incidence of POL. Once a woman has experienced one preterm birth, the risk increases with subsequent pregnancy. Incompetence of the cervix due to an inherent defect, which can lead to preterm delivery, is relatively rare (Creasy & Resnick, 1999). Cervical incompetence has been associated with a history of previous induced abortion. Preterm labor is also associated with uterine anomalies and the presence of large fibroid tumors. A number of studies have shown a correlation between preterm labor and women who maintain stressful, strenuous, and physically demanding employment. Systemic infections, such as bacterial pneumonia or acute appendicitis with sepsis, increase uterine activity, and endotoxins stimulate myometrial activity (Creasy & Resnick, 1999). Vaginal infections such as bacterial vaginosis (*Gardnerella vaginalis*, mixed anaerobes, and genital mycoplasms) and GBS (Group B streptococcus) have been implicated (Mahlmeister, 1996; Pastore et al., 1999). Diabetes is an underlying cause of preterm labor if polyhydramnios and/or macrosomia develops, causing overdistention of the uterus. Approximately 30 percent to 50 percent of multiple gestations end in delivery prior to 37 weeks for the same reason. See Table 37–22 for a summary of risk factors associated with premature labor.

Clinical Manifestations

The symptoms of premature labor are often so subtle many patients are not aware of them until labor and cervical dilation are far advanced or rupture of membranes occurs.

Early symptoms include:

- Uterine contractions (frequently painless)
- Menstrual-like cramps

TABLE 37–22. RISK FACTORS FOR PRETERM LABOR

Major
Trauma in pregnancy, hypovolemia
Multiple gestation
Diethylstilbestrol (DES) exposure
Uterine anomaly
Cervix dilated > 1 cm at 32 weeks
Second trimester abortion × 2
Previous preterm delivery
Previous preterm labor with term delivery
Abdominal surgery during pregnancy
History of cone biopsy
Cervical shortening < 1 cm at 32 weeks
Uterine irritability
Minor
Febrile illness
Bleeding after 12 weeks
History of pyelonephritis
Cigarettes more than 10/day
Second trimester abortion × 1
More than two first-trimester abortions

- Constant backache
- Pelvic pressure
- Increased vaginal discharge
- Blood-stained vaginal discharge

These symptoms may be misperceived by care providers as well and overlooked as normal common complaints of pregnancy.

Diagnosis

Diagnosis of preterm labor is difficult to make (Table 37–23). Often the patient will present with contractions and no other signs and symptoms. In this case, the patient will be admitted to the hospital for continuous fetal and toco monitoring and reexamined periodically per digital exam. A urinalysis will be obtained along with vaginal and endocervical cultures to rule out any type of infection. Once diagnosis is made and if no maternal or fetal contraindications are present, labor inhibition is attempted.

TABLE 37–23. CRITERIA FOR DIAGNOSIS OF PRETERM LABOR

	Gestation 20–37 weeks	
	and	
	Documented uterine contractions (4/20 min, 8/60 min)	
	and	
Ruptured membranes	*or*	Intact membranes
		and
		Documented cervical change
		or
		Cervical effacement of 80%
		or
		Cervical dilatation 2 cm

From Creasy, R., & Resnick, R. (1994). Maternal–fetal medicine: Principles and practice, *3rd ed. (p. 503). Philadelphia: W.B. Saunders.*

Management

Prior to initiating pharmacologic treatment for premature labor, maternal and fetal contraindications must be examined (Table 37–24). IV hydration is first attempted in patients with minimal to no cervical dilation along with bed rest and subcutaneous doses of terbutaline. Once a patient has a documented cervical change these noninvasive attempts are discontinued and more aggressive treatment begins. Table 37–25 lists frequently used tocolytics.

In summary, all of these tocolytic agents have certain drawbacks and adverse side effects. These effects must be weighed prior to administration. Their success is based on early diagnosis of premature labor and administration under close surveillance with continuous fetal monitoring in a specialized perinatal center.

Ritodrine, terbutaline, and $MgSO_4$ are the first-line drugs and are used more frequently due to the minimal and reversible side effects to the fetus (Viamontes, 1996). Indocin or nifedipine are used if the other tocolytics are ineffective in inhibiting premature labor.

Induced Lung Maturity

Most infants do not have mature lungs until approximately 36 weeks' gestation, although only approximately 50 percent of infants born at 30 weeks' gestation have

TABLE 37–24. CONTRAINDICATIONS TO USE OF TOCOLYTICS

Absolute contraindications
Severe PIH
Severe abruptio placentae
Severe bleeding from any cause
Chorioamnionitis
Fetal death
Fetal anomaly incompatible with life
Severe fetal growth retardation
Relative contraindications
Mild chronic hypertension
Mild abruptio placentae
Stable placenta previa
Maternal cardiac disease
Hyperthyroidism
Uncontrolled diabetes mellitus
Fetal distress
Fetal anomaly
Mild fetal growth retardation
Cervix more than 4–5 cm dilated
Bag of water bulging through cervix
Gestational age > 34 weeks

TABLE 37–25. FREQUENTLY USED TOCOLYTICS

DRUG	ACTION	ADMINISTRATION	SIDE EFFECTS	NOTES
β-mimetic agents				
Ritodrine HCl (Yutopar) Terbutaline Sulfate (Brethine)	1. Sympathomimetic that stimulates β_2-receptors.	1. Ritodrine is administered via infusion pump as a secondary line. The initial rate is 0.1 mg/min. The dose is increased at 10- to 30-minute intervals. The infusion rate is titrated according to uterine activity or until adverse maternal effects are noted. Once uterine activity is slowed or stopped, the infusion is slowed until the lowest inhibitory rate is established.	1. Maternal: Tachycardia, hypotension, hypokalemia, palpations, tremors, nausea, vomiting, headache, arrhythmia, nervousness, jitteriness, anxiety, malaise, chest pain, circulatory overload, elevations in glucose and insulin levels, widening pulse pressure. 2. Fetal: Tachycardia 3. Neonatal: Hypoglycemia, ileus, congestive heart failure, supraventricular tachycardia.	1. The infusion should be stopped if pulse reaches 130/bpm. Terbutaline dose should not be given if pulse is over 120/bpm. The pulse should be rechecked every half hour and then given when pulse is below 120/bpm. Neither should be given if systolic pressure is below 80 mm Hg. 2. Controlled diabetic patients need close monitoring for elevations in glucose levels.
	2. Stimulation of β_2-receptors inhibits the contractility of the uterine smooth muscle. 3. This drug has cardiovascular and bronchial effects as well.	2. Terbutaline is given SQ at 0.25 mg and may be repeated every 20 minutes × 2 additional doses. After the initial SQ dose, it is given orally 2.5 to 5 mg every 3 to 4 hours. May be given as continuous infusion by pump. IV doses start at 4 to 5 micrograms/min with increases of 5 to 10 μg every 20 min up to a maximum of 25 μg/min.	Antidote: Propranolol HCl (Inderal)	3. Any baby born to a mother who received tocolytics in pregnancy (from 34 weeks to term) needs close glucose monitoring after birth.
Calcium Antagonists				
Magnesium Sulfate ($MgSO_4$)	1. Neuromuscular blocking agent. 2. Anticonvulsant that prevents or controls convulsions by blocking neuromuscular transmission and decreasing the amount of acetylcholine liberated by the motor nerve impulse, therefore acting as a CNS depressant. 3. Tocolytic effect through enhancement of uterine blood flow and directly affecting myometrial contractility.	1. $MgSO_4$ is administered as a secondary line by infusion pump. Initially given with a 4 to 6 gm bolus, at a rate not to exceed 150 mg/min, then 2 to 4 gm per hour.	1. Maternal: Drowsiness, flushing, sweating, nausea and vomiting, sinus congestion, constipation, lethargy, blurry vision, depressed or no reflexes, respiratory depression, circulatory collapse, respiratory/cardiac arrest 2. Fetal: decreased variability, lower fetal heart rate baseline, diminished fetal breathing movements. 3. Neonate: Respiratory depression, hypotonia, sleepiness, poor cry and suck. Contraindications: 1. Renal failure 2. CNS depression 3. Respiratory complications Antidote: 1. Calcium gluconate	1. Absence of DTRs is considered therapeutic. If DTRs are noted, notify physician but usually no other interventions are necessary unless the patient becomes short of breath, complains of chest pain, or is unresponsive. If these occur turn infusion off immediately. 2. $MgSO_4$ levels are obtained every 6 to 8 hours: interventions are based on assessment of patient's status.

TABLE 37–25. FREQUENTLY USED TOCOLYTICS *(continued)*

DRUG	ACTION	ADMINISTRATION	SIDE EFFECTS	NOTES
Prostaglandin Synthetase Inhibitors				
Nifedipine	1. Inhibits the influx of calcium ions through the cell membranes, primarily affecting the calcium channels, decreasing smooth muscle contractility	1. Nifedipine is given as a loading dose of 10 mg sublingually or orally every 20 to 30 minutes times four doses and then 10 to 20 mg every 2 to 4 hours.	1. Maternal: Vasodilation, flushing, headache, and nausea. 2. Fetal: Decreased uterine blood flow, decreasing fetal arterial PO_2 and pH. 3. Neonate: None known	1. The peak effects of nifedipine occur in 30 to 60 minutes and even sooner in sublingual doses. 2. When administering, the nurse should obtain vital signs at least every 15 minutes for sudden decreases in blood pressure. 3. Nifedipine is often given with terbutaline, alternating the two every 2 hours. This is a fairly new modality and the patient should be monitored in the hospital at least during the first few days.
Indomethacin (Indocin)	1. Depresses synthesis of prostaglandins by inhibiting the cyclooxygenose enzyme necessary for the conversion of arachidonic acid to various prostaglandins. Prostaglandins promote uterine activity by increasing myometrial gap junctions and by stimulating an increase in cellular calcium. Spontaneous contractions are abolished by the addition of Indocin (Creasy and Resnick, 1994).	1. Indocin is first administered with a 50 mg to 100 mg rectal suppository as a loading dose and then given orally 25 mg every 6 hours. 2. Due to possible complications, Indocin is only given over a 48-hour period.	1. Maternal: Gastrointestinal effects if not taken with food, headaches, dizziness, depression, psychosis (if taken over a long period), increased risk of postpartum hemorrhage. 2. Fetal: Constriction of the ductus arteriosus in utero, oligohydramnios, development of small kidneys. 3. Neonate: Pulmonary hypertension due to the constriction of the ductus arteriosus. Necrotizing enterocolitis, intracranial bleeding, broncho-pulmonary dysplasia. Contraindications: 1. Asthma. 2. Coagulation disorders. 3. Hepatic and renal insufficiency. 4. Peptic ulcers. 5. ASA sensitivity. 6. Gestational age greater than 32 weeks.	1. The constriction of the ductus arteriosus is not seen in fetus' under 27 weeks and the effects are seen more frequently as gestational age progresses.

RDS. The incidence of RDS increases as gestational age decreases, but occasionally 24- to 25-week fetuses have functional lung maturity. Spontaneous early lung maturity has been associated with stress-induced maturation that can be maternal, placental, or fetal in origin. See Table 37–26 for a summary of pregnancy-related conditions associated with induced lung maturation.

Lung immaturity has been associated with the absence of hormonal stimuli. In the presence of hormonal stimuli agents such as corticosteroids, hormones accelerate lung maturation. See Table 37–27 for hormonal stimuli agents and their effects.

Prior to administering corticosteroids, efforts are made to delay delivery at least 24 hours and hopefully up

TABLE 37–26. PREGNANCY-RELATED CONDITIONS AND LUNG MATURATION

Delayed maturation
- RH isoimmunization
- Diabetes

Accelerated maturation

Fetal conditions
- Smaller or anemic member of twins

Placental conditions
- Chorioamnionitis (related to prolonged premature rupture of membranes)
- Placental infarction

Maternal conditions
- Chronic renal disease
- Pregnancy-induced hypertension (in some cases)
- Sickle cell disease
- Heroin addiction
- Hyperthyroidism

to 72 hours after administration of therapy to allow treatment to be effective.

In summary, premature labor may go undetected due to subtle symptoms. Several factors are associated with premature labor including, but not limited to, poor nutrition, low body weight, previous premature birth, previous induced abortion, and physically demanding work. Initially, subcutaneous terbutaline and IV hydration is administered to stop labor. Infant lung maturity varies with premature labor. In some situations, stress induces maturation. In cases of immaturity, corticosteroids may be given to induce maturity.

TABLE 37–27. INDUCED LUNG MATURATION BY HORMONAL STIMULI

DRUG	ACTION	ADMINISTRATION	SIDE EFFECTS	NOTES
Corticosteroids	1. Corticosteroids induce lung maturation by increasing gas exchange surface area as reflected by lung volume measurements. They also influence lung structural proteins 2. Corticosteroids also decrease the development of pulmonary edema, patent ductus arteriosus, intraventricular hemorrhage, and necrotizing enterocolitis, and induce kidney tubular maturation. 3. The overall effect of the use of corticosteroids is a decrease of approximately 50 percent of respiratory distress and fetal death.	1. Corticosteroids are administered by IM injection of 12 mg times two doses 12 to 24 hours apart. This may be repeated weekly if threat of preterm delivery remains.	1. There have been no consistent documented side effects of corticosteroids.	

SECTION ELEVEN REVIEW

1. Causes of preterm labor include all of the following EXCEPT
   - A. drug abuse
   - B. age
   - C. cervical incompetency
   - D. previous cesarean section
2. Common symptoms of preterm labor include
   - A. cramping, backache, increased vaginal discharge
   - B. headache
   - C. proteinuria
   - D. decreased UOP
3. When administering terbutaline, inform the patient of side effects she may experience, such as
   - A. euphoria
   - B. tachycardia
   - C. hypertension
   - D. hypoglycemia
4. Indocin is usually given
   - A. after 27 weeks' gestation
   - B. as a loading dose of 50 to 100 mg rectally
   - C. as a first choice in treating preterm labor
   - D. intravenously
5. Induced lung maturity is used
   - A. under 36 weeks' gestation
   - B. only if the patient has used marijuana
   - C. only if the patient is in active labor
   - D. to prevent a spontaneous abortion
6. Side effects of corticosteroids include
   - A. maternal hypertension
   - B. no side effects have been noted
   - C. constriction of the patent ductus arteriosus
   - D. tachycardia

Answers: 1. D, 2. A, 3. B, 4. B, 5. A, 6. B

SECTION TWELVE: Drug Use in Pregnancy

At the completion of this section, the learner will understand the effects of drug use in pregnancy on the woman and her fetus.

The use of illicit drugs during pregnancy has received widespread attention over the past 10 years. Though the knowledge of drug use and the effects on pregnancy has grown, prevalence and use of drugs has also grown. Socially acceptable drugs, alcohol, and tobacco, which are more widely used than illegal drugs, contribute to perinatal complications as well.

Screening

Studies support that there are no specific epidemiologic boundaries of drug use and that it affects all socioeconomic groups. Due to these factors all patients should be screened at the first prenatal visit. Developing a screening system requires consultation with both legal advisors and social service employees to determine liability, individual's rights and local reporting statutes.

The most common mode of screening is testing the patient's urine. The major disadvantage of urine drug screening is that it only detects relatively recent use rather than long-term use. The metabolites of alcohol are detectable for only 8 hours and amphetamines, cocaine, and LSD are detectable for only 24 to 72 hours following use. Opiates can be detected 24 to 48 hours after use. Marijuana and benzodiazepine metabolites are present for 1 to 4 weeks after use.

Once an initial drug screen is obtained, further testing is appropriate if certain factors and complications arise. Table 37–28 lists criteria for further urine drug testing.

TABLE 37–28. CRITERIA FOR URINE DRUG SCREENING

Physical appearance and demeanor
- Altered mental status
- Pupils extremely dilated or constricted
- Track marks/abscesses in extremities
- Inflamed or indurated nasal mucosa

Obstetric (past or present)
- Preterm labor/preterm delivery
- Low-birth-weight infant
- Intrauterine growth restriction
- Premature rupture of membranes
- Placental abruption
- Fetal death
- Unexplained congenital anomalies
- Suspected neonatal withdrawal symptoms
- Absent or erratic prenatal care

Medical
- AIDS/HIV infection
- Cellulitis
- Cirrhosis
- Endocarditis
- Hepatitis
- Pancreatitis
- Pneumonia
- Sexually transmitted diseases

Social
- Illicit drug use by partner
- Incarceration
- Prostitution
- Domestic violence

Modified from Chasnoff, I.J. (1987). Perinatal effects of cocaine. Contemp Obstet Gynecol *29:164.*

Alcohol

Alcohol, which metabolizes to acetaldehyde, has been a recognized terratogen for centuries. By 1973, a characteristic pattern of anomalies was identified and described. Fetal alcohol syndrome (FAS) is a constellation of characteristics that includes neurologic abnormalities, facial and cranial abnormalities, and growth restriction both prenatally and postnatally (see Table 37–29).

By 1980, the USFDA recommended that alcohol not be used in pregnancy. Unfortunately women continue to drink alcohol during pregnancy. In fact, the Centers for Disease Control and Prevention (CDC) conducted a telephone survey (CDC, 1997) which encompassed all 50 states and demonstrated an increase in alcohol use from 12.4 percent in 1991 to 16.3 percent in 1995. This is after numerous reports of the dangers of alcohol as the leading cause of mental retardation and FAS (Creasy & Resnik, 1999).

Cocaine

Cocaine comes from the leaves of the *Erythroxylon coca* plant. Cocaine inhibits reuptake of neurotransmitter substances, such as dopamine and norepinephrine, at the presynaptic nerve terminals. Maternal effects include tachycardia, hypertension, and increased circulating catecholamines (Ritchie & Green, 1985).

TABLE 37–29. CRITERIA FOR FETAL ALCOHOL SYNDROME

1. *Prenatal and/or postnatal growth restriction; failure to thrive* (weight, length, and/or head circumference < 10th percentile)
2. *Central nervous system involvement* includes signs of neurologic abnormalities (irritability in infancy and hyperactivity during childhood), development delay, hypotonia, or intellectual impairment (mild to moderate mental retardation)
3. *Characteristic facial dysmorphology* (at least 2 of 3)
   a. Microcephaly (head circumference < 3rd percentile)
   b. Microphthalmia and/or short palpebral fissures
   c. Poorly developed philtrum, thin upper lip (vermilion border), and flattening or absence of the maxilla

Metabolism of the drug is by the action of plasma and hepatic cholinesterases. Plasma cholinesterase may be diminished in pregnancy and this may lead to an accumulation of cocaine and an increased risk of toxicity. The cardiovascular effects are worsened with pregnancy possibly owing to the presence of progesterone, which increases metabolism of cocaine to a biologically active variant called norcocaine.

Fetal Complications

Congenital anomalies occur more frequently in patients who use cocaine in pregnancy. Theoretically, this is due to an interruption of placental blood supply during use, followed by deformation and destruction of embryonic structures. The most common include the extremities and the genitourinary, cardiovascular, and central nervous systems.

The incidence of placental abruption occurring in women who use cocaine during pregnancy has been cited. Abruption occurs due to the hypertensive effects of cocaine when associated with preeclampsia.

A decrease in fetal weight has also been associated with cocaine use. The decrease is independent of maternal weight gain but directly related to cocaine itself. This effect is related to the vasoconstrictive properties of cocaine and a decrease in uterine blood flow and uteroplacental circulation.

Preterm labor and delivery is directly related to cocaine use. The specific mechanism is not understood but it is thought that cocaine increases contractility of the myometrium.

The effects on the neonate include higher incidence of neurobehavioral abnormalities including sleeping patterns, feeding problems, hypertonia, and tremors, low birthweight, and sudden infant death syndrome (SIDS).

Opiates

Opiates are organic substances such as morphine and codeine that come from the Papaver somniferum poppy. "Opioids" are synthetic narcotics such as heroin, meperidine, fentanyl, propoxyphene, and methadone.

Fetal Complications

No association has been made between opiate exposure and congenital anomalies in the fetus. However, a neonatal withdrawal disorder called neonatal abstinence syndrome (NAS) occurs in two thirds of all neonates exposed to opiates (Stone, 1971). NAS is generally evident 3 to 5 days after delivery, usually after the woman and baby have been discharged from the hospital. Clinical findings of NAS are summarized in Table 37–30.

IUGR is associated with opiate use in pregnancy. This has been thought to result from decreased fetal growth hormone concentration and chronic fetal hypoxemia from opiate withdrawal in utero.

Methadone use in pregnancy has not been proven to eradicate the adverse effects of opiate use but does have several advantages. Scheduled doses of methadone prescribed by a physician have decreased the patient's risk of human immunodeficiency virus (HIV) infection and acquired immune deficiency syndrome (AIDS), hepatitis, and subacute bacterial endocarditis. It also decreases the pattern and reoccurrence of withdrawal, which has been associated with fetal hypoxemia, hypertension, bradycardia, and IUFD.

TABLE 37–30. CHARACTERISTICS OF FETAL ALCOHOL SYNDROME

Physical Characteristics
Underweight and underheight for age
Microcephaly
Micro-opthalmia
Flattened nasal bridge with short nose
Thin upper lip
Cognitive Characteristics
Impaired mental development (e.g., performance on test scores)
Impaired language development
Delayed fine and gross motor skills

Marijuana

The active ingredient of marijuana is tetrahydrocannabinol. Side effects of marijuana use include mild tachycardia, a slight increase in arterial pressure, and general euphoria. The onset of these effects is 30 to 60 minutes, with a duration of action of 3 to 5 hours.

Fetal Complications

The generalized fetal effects of marijuana use in pregnancy may include congenital anomalies, particularly limb growth and decrease in birthweight and length. These effects seem to be associated with marijuana use but have not been conclusive in most studies.

Amphetamine and Methamphetamine

Amphetamine and methamphetamine are sympathomimetic amines. Use of these substances causes an increase in the release of neurotransmitters from the presynaptic terminal. The result is stimulation of the sympathetic nervous system.

Fetal Complications

Low birthweight and decreased length due to decreased uterine blood flow and fetal hypoxemia have been associated with use. The most significant effect of amphetamine use involves the CNS. Cerebral ischemia, infarction, and intraventricular hemorrhage occur more frequently in neonates of women who use amphetamines. These neonates often have smaller head circumferences as compared to neonates of nonusers. Congenital anomalies and preterm labor have not been associated with amphetamine use in pregnancy.

In summary, women who use drugs in pregnancy require frequent prenatal visits and intensive counseling regarding the implications of their substance abuse. If possible, rehabilitation should be initiated. A social service referral will be made with follow-up visits and possibly placement for the baby in foster care until the mother is drug free.

SECTION TWELVE REVIEW

1. Fetal alcohol syndrome is
   A. found only in binge drinking
   B. acquired after birth
   C. the leading cause of mental retardation
   D. reversible
2. Cocaine use during pregnancy
   A. decreases fetal weight
   B. can cause placental previa
   C. can cause postterm labor
   D. can cause postpartum hemorrhage
3. Methadone given during pregnancy
   A. decreases the risk of maternal HIV infection
   B. obliterates any congenital anomalies
   C. is not considered a drug in pregnancy
   D. prevents fetal withdrawal
4. A patient with a positive urine drug screen requires
   A. frequent prenatal visits
   B. no IV pain medicine during labor
   C. imprisonment
   D. fetal electronic monitoring

Answers: 1. C, 2. A, 3. A, 4. A

SECTION THIRTEEN: Emergency Delivery

At the completion of this section, the learner will have basic knowledge of what to do during emergency delivery.

Precipitous Delivery

Definition

Precipitous (< 3 hours) labor and delivery may result from abnormally low resistance of the soft parts of the birth canal or from abnormally strong uterine and abdominal contractions (Cunningham, MacDonald, & Gant, 1989). Precipitous labor is also a risk for multiparous patients and for women with preterm labor due to small fetal size.

Clinical Manifestations

A patient with precipitous labor will present with advanced cervical dilation and effacement, after a short period of uterine contractions. If crowning of the fetal head is not evident, a digital exam is performed to determine whether the membranes are ruptured. With rapid cervical dilation, many patients are unaware of rupture of membranes. A small amount of fluid leakage may result, but fetal descent into the birth canal blocks the escape of fluid. As a result, meconium may not be evident until after the delivery of the baby. Preterm deliveries under 34 weeks are rarely complicated by meconium. If fluid is not seen by the nurse and the patient is over 34 weeks, suction equipment should be readily available for delivery.

Management

In the situation of precipitous delivery, there is limited time to prepare for delivery. In many facilities every area—emergency departments, triage, and patient rooms—are equipped with precipitous delivery packs.

These packs include:

1. Sterile drape (to carry infant to warmer)
2. Sterile hemostats (4)
3. Blunt scissors (in case episiotomy is needed)
4. Cord scissors
5. Bulb suction
6. Large basin (for placenta)

In many situations, the nurse is the only person available to deliver the baby. The steps taken in an emergency delivery are as follows:

1. Place the patient in the lateral position and encourage the patient to breathe through the contractions instead of pushing, to allow more time to prepare for delivery.
2. Get help from another nurse and try to notify a physician. One nurse must be available for the baby and one for the patient.

3. Have a neonatal resuscitation bag and oxygen supply available. Suction equipment is also needed.
4. A vaginal delivery is not a sterile procedure. If time allows, prep the patient's perineum with Betadine or Hebiclens scrub.
5. Wash your hands and glove.
6. Once the perineum begins to bulge with the crowning head, maintain gentle but steady pressure to the perineum to prevent tearing and explosion of the fetal head from the perineum. Have the patient push with contractions, gently easing back the perineum.
7. Once the head emerges, encourage the patient to pant or blow through contractions to allow suctioning of the mouth and nose. If meconium-stained fluid or skin is noted, deep suctioning is required. Suction the mouth first. If the nose is suctioned first it may elicit a reflex gasp of fluids into the lungs.
8. Before delivering the body, feel around the baby's neck for the umbilical cord. If present, try to reduce the cord over the baby's head. If unreducible, clamp cord with two hemostats approximately 1 inch apart and cut in between the clamps. Unwind the cord from the baby's neck.
9. By this time, the baby's head will restitute—turn to face right or left. If necessary, have the patient push with a steady but gentle push. Place fingers under chin and around neck, gently guiding the head in a downward motion to deliver the anterior shoulder, then in an upward motion to deliver the posterior shoulder. The rest of the body will deliver quickly, so maintain a steady hold on the baby.
10. Maintain the baby at the level of the placenta or above. If the baby is held below the level of the placenta, maternal–fetal transfusion can occur, causing fetal polycythemia. Conversely, fetal anemia can occur if the infant is held above the level of the placenta.
11. Clamp and cut the cord as discussed in Step 8.
12. The delivery of the placenta usually occurs within two contractions after delivery of the baby. The placenta should be examined to ensure it is intact. If time allows, an IV can be started in between delivery of the baby and the placenta for Pitocin 20/1 L infusion to clamp down the uterus and prevent excessive bleeding.
13. If an IV is not started, Pitocin 10 U can be administered IM.

Prolapsed Umbilical Cord

A prolapsed cord occurs when the umbilical cord presents prior to the presenting parts of the fetus. A prolapse occurs after rupture of the membranes. This necessitates emergency delivery due to fetal distress from profound compression of the cord. A vaginal delivery is not indicated.

Clinical Manifestations

A prolapsed cord is usually noticed first by fetal monitoring. A quick drop in FHR is caused by compression of the cord. Prolonged bradycardia with decreased variability leads to fetal distress. The cord may be visually obvious or felt on digital exam. In some situations an occult cord prolapse may occur and is characterized by variable decelerations that become severe with loss of variability and prolonged return to baseline. Though less dramatic than an obvious prolapse, emergency delivery is required for fetal survival.

Management

Once a prolapsed cord is diagnosed, the nurse should follow these steps.

1. Place the patient in the knee–chest position and adjust the bed in the Trendelenburg position.
2. Administer high flow oxygen at 10 L/min per nonrebreather mask.
3. Get help and notify the obstetrician and the anesthsiologist. At least three nurses are needed to prepare the patient for an emergency cesarean delivery.
4. A vaginal exam is done and a hand is applied to the fetal presenting part to alleviate pressure on the cord and palpate pulsation of the cord to document FHR.
5. Start a 16- to 18-g IV and infuse a nondextrose infusion at a bolus rate.
6. Place a urinary catheter, and if time permits clamp it, and instill 200 to 300 mL of sterile baby formula or sterile water to distend the bladder, pushing the fetus up and alleviating pressure on the cord.
7. Move the patient to the operating room in the knee–chest position.
8. Once in the OR, place the patient in lateral tilt and apply an external fetal monitor.
9. While the anesthesiologist is preparing the patient for general anesthesia, shave the patient's abdomen from the umbilicus down, including approximately 1.5 inches of pubic hair.
10. Prepare the abdomen with either a betadine or alcohol scrub.
11. When the physicians are ready to make the incision, unclamp the urinary catheter.
12. Be sure a pediatrician is available for delivery.

In summary, emergency deliveries are frightening for both the patient and the nurse. The nurse should maintain a calm voice and provide reassurance to the patient and her family. Try to explain what is happening in simple terms and reinforce that patient compliance is imperative. Time is of the essence. All of the previous steps should be carried out quickly, in a matter of minutes. Good team work between physicians and the nursing team helps the process run smoothly.

SECTION THIRTEEN REVIEW

1. A patient presents to the triage area contracting every 2 to 3 minutes, with FHR baseline in the 120s and early decelerations noted. The patient states, "The baby is coming." The nurse should
   A. complete a digital exam
   B. apply oxygen at 8 to 10 L/min
   C. tell the patient to push
   D. complete the patient's history before intervening
2. It is determined that the patient is completely dilated. The nurse should
   A. tell the patient to hold her breath until the physician comes
   B. place the patient in a lateral position and encourage her to breathe through her contractions
   C. prepare for IV terbutaline
   D. administer IV Pitocin
3. The perineum begins to bulge and crowning of the fetal head is noted. The nurse should
   A. attempt to push the fetal head back into the vagina
   B. tell the patient to push, applying pressure to the perineum
   C. place an FSE
   D. place the patient in the knee–chest position
4. After the head delivers, the nurse should
   A. suction mouth and then nose
   B. immediately tell the patient to push to deliver the body
   C. cut the cord
   D. administer oxygen

Answers: 1. A, 2. B, 3. B, 4. A

SECTION FOURTEEN: Neonatal Resuscitation

At the completion of this section, the learner will have basic knowledge of neonatal resuscitation.

In most facilities, a pediatrician is available to attend deliveries, especially in high-risk situations, but many times neonatal distress is not anticipated. Thus, the nurse should be experienced in neonatal resuscitation.

Situations in which a pediatrician should be present at delivery include

- Cesarean delivery
- Preeclampsia and use of $MgSO_4$
- Maternal diabetes
- Maternal fever
- Presence of meconium-stained fluid
- Premature fetus
- Fetal distress
- Known fetal anomaly
- Forcep delivery
- Lack of prenatal care

Steps in a neonatal resuscitation are as follows.

Prevent Heat Loss

As soon as a baby is delivered, the nurse should place the infant in a preheated radiant warmer in the Trendelenburg position to promote drainage of fluid. Quickly dry off the infant's head and body to remove amniotic fluid and prevent evaporative heat loss.

After drying off the infant, be sure to remove the wet towels. Presently, it is common practice to place the infant on the mother's abdomen immediately after birth to promote bonding between infant and mother. This is done only if there are no known complications. In this situation, to prevent heat loss, place the infant directly on the patient's skin. Dry the infant with preheated towels and cover the infant with a dry, warm blanket.

Open the Airway

Once the infant is warm and dry, the next step is to ensure an open airway. The infant should be positioned on his or her back or side in the Trendelenburg position with the neck slightly extended.

The mouth and nose should be suctioned. Turning the baby's head to the side can facilitate drainage into the mouth rather than the posterior pharynx.

Provide Tactile Stimulation

Normally, drying and suctioning of the infant is enough stimulation to induce cry and respirations. If the infant is not breathing after drying and suctioning, additional tactile stimulation is needed. If the baby is on the patient's abdomen, remove the infant and place in radiant warmer.

Appropriate methods of tactile stimulation are slapping or flicking the soles of the feet or rubbing the infant's back. However, if these methods are not effective after a few seconds and the infant remains apneic, bag-and-mask ventilation should be initiated.

Evaluating the Infant (Apgar Scoring)

During the resuscitation process, Apgar scores are assigned at 1 and 5 minutes after birth. Apgar scoring involves evaluating heart rate, respirations, muscle tone, reflex irritability (cry), and color (Table 37–31). A decreased heart rate and poor ventilation will directly affect all the other aspects of Apgar scoring.

After drying, suctioning, and providing tactile stimulation, the infant should be evaluated, first evaluating respiratory effort. If respiratory effort is present, evaluate the infant's heart rate. If the heart rate is above 100 bpm, evaluate color. Once the infant's respirations and heart rate improve significantly, the skin should begin to turn pink. However, **cyanosis** can occur even though heart rate is above 100 bpm and respirations are adequate. In this case, there is enough oxygen to sustain respirations and heart rate but not enough oxygen to fully oxygenate the infant. Oxygen must be provided.

Free-Flow Oxygen

Free-flow oxygen involves blowing oxygen over the infant's nose so that the infant breathes oxygen-enriched air. Free-flow oxygen is appropriate for infants with spontaneous, adequate respirations who sustain heart rate over 100 bpm but have persistent cyanosis.

Free-flow oxygen involves either holding the end of the oxygen tubing approximately one-half inch from the nares or holding an oxygen mask over the nose and mouth and providing a high concentration of oxygen, at least 80 percent.

Once the infant becomes pink, the oxygen should be gradually withdrawn until the infant can remain pink on room air. This can be accomplished by gradually decreasing the concentration of oxygen being administered, evaluating the infant's response with each decrease.

An infant with **acrocyanosis** does not require free-flow oxygen. Acrocyanosis is caused by a combination of a cool environment and an initially sluggish circulation.

TABLE 37–31. DETERMINATION OF APGAR SCORE

	POINTS		
Sign	0	1	2
Heart rate	Absent	Slow (< 100 bpm)	> 100 bpm
Respirations	Absent	Slow/irregular	Good crying
Muscle tone	Flaccid	Some flexion of extremities	Active motion
Reflex irritability	None	Grimace	Vigorous cry
Color	Pale blue	Body pink with blue extremities	Completely pink

Bag-and-Mask Ventilation

Bag-and-mask ventilation is appropriate if the infant is apneic after the initial steps of resuscitation or if the respirations are not adequate enough to sustain heart rate above 100 bpm.

The first step in providing bag-and-mask ventilation is selecting the appropriate equipment. These steps should be completed prior to delivery whether or not neonatal distress is anticipated so there is no delay in providing ventilation. Obtain the bag and mask and attach them to the oxygen source. Select a mask of the correct size, which can be determined prior to delivery by gestational age. Check bag and mask for proper functioning. Once it is determined that bag-and-mask ventilation is needed, check the infant's position. The neck should be slightly extended. Form a seal between the mask and the infant's face, covering both the nose and the mouth. Give the initial breath at a higher pressure of 30 to 40 cm H_2O, and then decrease pressure to 15 to 20 cm H_2O with every breath following, at a rate of 40 breaths per minute (premature infants may require higher ventilatory pressures secondary to lung immaturity and noncompliance).

After the infant has been ventilated for 15 to 30 seconds, check the heart rate. If the heart rate is above 100 bpm and the infant has spontaneous respirations, discontinue bag-and-mask ventilation and provide gentle tactile stimulation by rubbing the back or chest. If the heart rate is 60 to 100 bpm and increasing, continue ventilation. If the heart rate is 60 to 100 bpm and not increasing, continue ventilation and check the adequacy of ventilation. Is there a tight seal? Is the chest moving properly? If the heart rate is below 80 bpm, begin chest compressions.

Chest Compressions

Chest compressions consist of rhythmic compressions of the sternum that compress the heart against the spine, increasing the intrathoracic pressure and circulating blood to vital organs. Chest compressions are always accompanied by ventilations so that the blood being circulated is oxygenated.

Chest compressions are applied by placing two fingers over the lower third of the sternum. Draw an imaginary line between the infant's nipples and place fingers directly below this line. Be sure to avoid pressing on the xiphoid.

With fingers, apply enough pressure to compress the chest one-half to three-fourths inch and then release to allow refilling of the heart. Repeat compressions 120 times per minute. After 30 seconds of compressions, the heart rate should be checked and then rechecked periodically until the heart rate is above 80 bpm. Once the heart rate is above 80 bpm, chest compressions can be discontinued and ventilation continued until the heart rate is above 100 bpm and the infant is breathing spontaneously. If the heart rate continues to be below 80 bpm and ventilation is still required over a prolonged period, intubation and medications should be initiated.

A 10-minute Apgar score may be assessed to determine the effectiveness of resuscitation.

In summary, neonatal resuscitation is frightening for both the parents and the nurse, especially if neonatal distress was not anticipated. Be sure to provide the patient with a separate support person, such as a nurse, for reassurance and updates on the infant's status during the resuscitation process. It is important to remain calm and provide the patient with honest and accurate updates. For an overview, see Figure 37–8 for a summary of the steps of neonatal resuscitation.

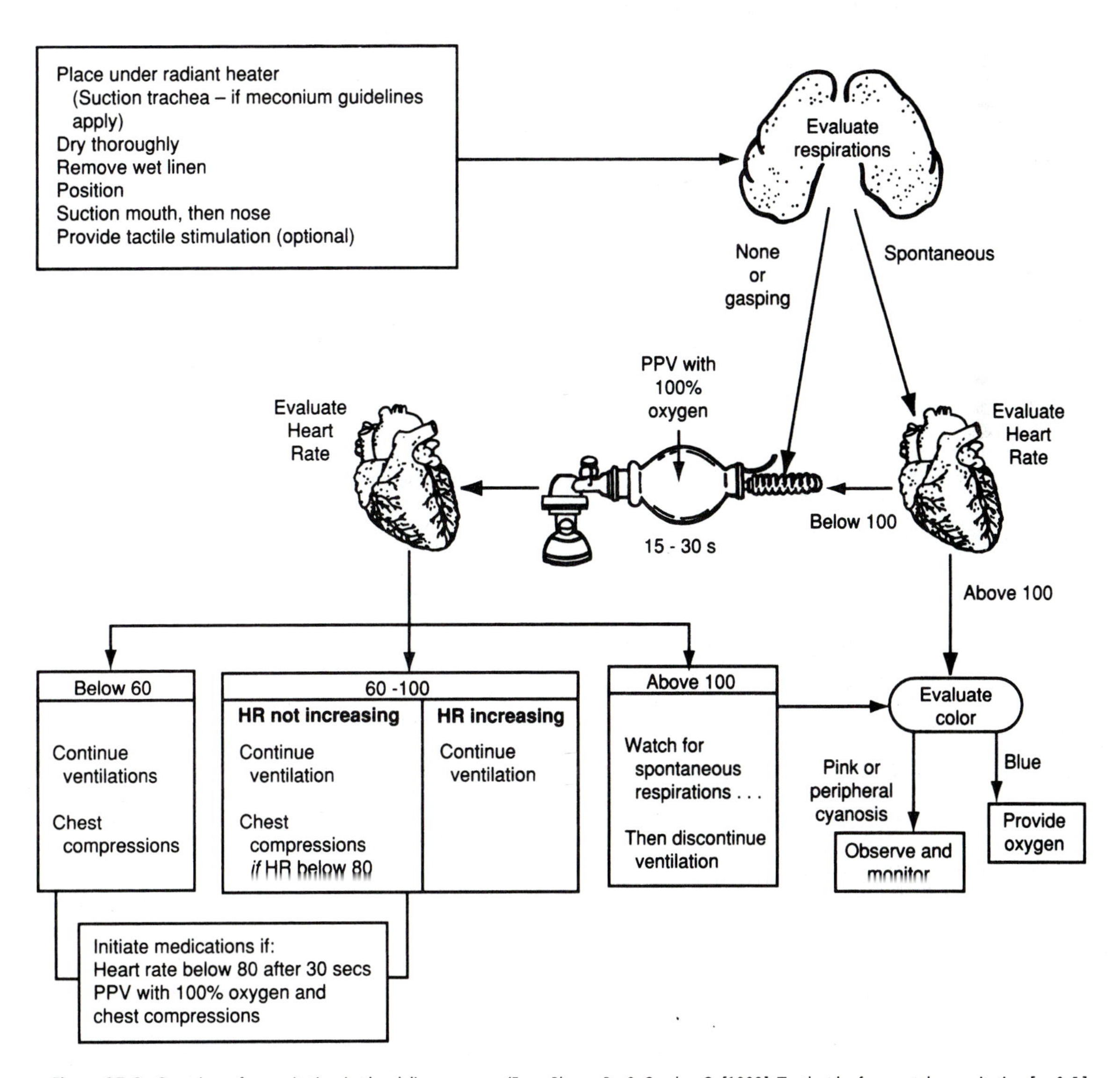

Figure 37–8. Overview of resuscitation in the delivery room. *(From Bloom, R., & Cropley, C. [1993].* Textbook of neonatal resuscitation *[p. 0-5.] Dallas: American Heart Association of Pediatrics.)*

SECTION FOURTEEN REVIEW

1. A baby is delivered and placed on the mother's abdomen. The nurse should
   A. do nothing and allow time for immediate bonding
   B. immediately suction mouth and nose and dry the infant thoroughly, removing wet towels
   C. apply free-flow oxygen
   D. slap the baby's bottom
2. The infant is not crying and is cyanotic. The nurse should do all of the following EXCEPT
   A. place the infant in a radiant warmer
   B. provide tactile stimulation
   C. suction the infant
   D. place the baby on the mother's breast
3. The baby has spontaneous respirations and a pulse above 100 bpm but still appears cyanotic. The nurse should
   A. begin bag-and-mask ventilation
   B. begin chest compressions
   C. apply free-flow oxygen
   D. defibrillate the baby
4. Chest compression should be started if
   A. the infant's heart rate is 100 bpm
   B. the infant's heart rate is below 80 bpm
   C. the infant's heart rate is 60 to 100 bpm and increasing
   D. acrocyanosis is present

Answers: 1. B, 2. D, 3. C, 4. B

POSTTEST

1. Maternal heart rate increases in pregnancy
   A. 10 to 15 bpm
   B. 40 bpm
   C. during the first trimester
   D. during the third trimester
2. Normal GI side effects associated with pregnancy include
   A. nausea and vomiting, constipation, and heartburn
   B. chest pain and rectal bleeding
   C. numbness of hands and feet
   D. melena
3. Headaches occur frequently in pregnancy due to
   A. standing for prolonged periods
   B. sitting for prolonged periods
   C. hormonal changes
   D. the enlarging uterus
4. Possible causes of dyspnea in pregnancy include all of the following EXCEPT
   A. pulmonary edema
   B. acidosis
   C. polyhydramnios
   D. polycythemia
5. A decrease in FHR variability can be attributed to all of the following EXCEPT
   A. fetal sleep
   B. $MgSO_4$
   C. congenital anomalies
   D. maternal weight gain
6. Symptoms of pulmonary edema include
   A. shortness of breath, dyspnea, and tachypnea
   B. chest pain radiating down left arm
   C. cramping
   D. hypertension
7. Symptoms of amniotic fluid embolism include all of the following EXCEPT
   A. acute respiratory distress
   B. shock out of proportion with blood loss
   C. chills, shivering, and sweating
   D. hematemesis
8. Supportive care for a patient with ARDS includes
   A. oxygen infused at 10 L/min
   B. intubation and mechanical ventilation
   C. Valium to decrease anxiety
   D. low flow oxygen
9. Complications that predispose to ARDS include
   A. DIC, abruptio placentae, hemorrhagic shock
   B. premature labor
   C. febrile illness
   D. drug abuse
10. A predisposing factor that increases the risk of preeclampsia is
    A. diabetes
    B. twin gestation
    C. multiple spontaneous abortions
    D. increased stress
11. The drug of choice for preventing eclamptic seizures is
    A. hydralazine
    B. $MgSO_4$
    C. phenytoin
    D. aspirin
12. To infuse $MgSO_4$ safely, the nurse should do all of the following EXCEPT

A. infuse $MgSO_4$ on infusion pump
B. infuse as a piggyback or secondary line
C. auscultate lungs and check DTRs prior to bolus
D. check maternal vital signs each shift

13. If a patient complains of chest pain or shortness of breath during an $MgSO_4$ infusion, the nurse should
A. explain to the patient that this is normal
B. stop the infusion immediately
C. change the patient's position
D. have the patient cough

14. The H in the anagram HELLP syndrome stands for
A. high blood pressure
B. hematocrit
C. hemolytic anemia
D. hemolytic abnormalities

15. Abruptio placentae can occur in association with
A. trauma to the abdomen
B. hypertension
C. cocaine use
D. hypotension

16. Postpartum hemorrhage occurs most frequently
A. 12 hours after delivery
B. 1 month after delivery
C. within 1 hour after delivery
D. immediately before delivery

17. After delivery, the nurse notes that the patient's fundus is deviated to the right and that bleeding is moderate. The nurse should
A. call a physician immediately
B. examine the lower genitourinary tract for active bleeding
C. empty the patient's bladder with an in-and-out catheter and then reexamine fundus and bleeding
D. prepare patient for immediate surgery

18. The goal of management of hemorrhagic shock is
A. maintaining the patient's LOC
B. volume replacement
C. maintaining UO
D. maintenance of vital signs

19. In a pregnant patient, clinical signs of shock are present with a loss of approximately
A. 20 percent to 25 percent of blood volume
B. 10 percent of blood volume
C. 50 percent of blood volume
D. 15 percent to 20 percent of blood volume

20. The MOST common effect of severe abdominal trauma in pregnancy is
A. placenta previa
B. premature labor
C. pulmonary edema
D. postpartum hemorrhage

21. The MOST frequent cause of blunt trauma is
A. MVCs
B. burns
C. falls
D. stabbings

22. An AFP is performed at 16 weeks' gestation to
A. rule out IUGR
B. determine metabolic control of the fetus
C. help rule out fetal defects
D. confirm Down syndrome

23. Genetic testing is performed only if there are all EXCEPT
A. an abnormal AFP
B. advanced maternal age
C. a history that includes a high genetic risk
D. multiple elective abortions

24. The laboring diabetic patient requires
A. hourly fingersticks
B. hourly insulin injections
C. intermittent glucose
D. continuous insulin

25. The neonate of a diabetic patient is at risk for all EXCEPT
A. poor glycemia control
B. RDS
C. macrosomia
D. underweight for gestational age

26. A patient who presents with uterine contractions and no cervical change is managed by
A. $MgSO_4$ infusion
B. bedrest and IV hydration
C. weekly NSTs
D. terbutaline

27. The agents used to induce fetal lung maturity include
A. surfactant
B. corticosteroids
C. terbutaline
D. $MgSO_4$

28. The nurse's initial intervention in the presence of a prolapsed cord is to
A. call a physician
B. place the patient in the knee–chest position
C. tell the patient to push
D. place patient on her left side

29. Prior to every delivery, the nurse should do all of the following EXCEPT
A. check the emergency equipment to ensure it is functioning effectively
B. select a mask size suitable for the infant's gestational age
C. have suction equipment available
D. administer oxygen to the mother

30. After delivery of an infant the first step in infant resuscitation is
A. assessing color
B. opening the airway
C. drying the skin
D. providing tactile stimulation

POSTTEST ANSWERS

Question	Answer	Section	Question	Answer	Section
1	A	One	16	C	Six
2	A	One	17	C	Six
3	C	One	18	B	Seven
4	D	One	19	A	Seven
5	D	Two	20	B	Eight
6	A	Three	21	A	Eight
7	D	Three	22	C	Nine
8	B	Three	23	D	Nine
9	A	Three	24	A	Nine
10	A	Four	25	D	Nine
11	B	Four	26	B	Ten
12	D	Four	27	B	Ten
13	B	Four	28	B	Twelve
14	C	Five	29	D	Twelve
15	C	Six	30	C	Fourteen

REFERENCES

American Diabetes Association. (1993). Medical management of pregnancy complicated by diabetes. Alexandria, Virginia: Author.

CDC (Centers for Disease Control and Prevention). (1997). Alcohol consumption among pregnant and childbearing women—United States: 1991 and 1995. MMWR *(Morbidity Mortality Weekly Report)* 46:346.

Cowet, R.M. (1991). *Neonatal glucose metabolism: Principles of perinatal–neonatal metabolism* (pp. 356–389). New York: Springer-Verlag.

Creasy, R., & Resnick, R. (1999). *Maternal–fetal medicine: Principles and practice* (4th ed.). Philadelphia: W.B. Saunders.

Crosby, E.T. (1991). Obstetrical anesthesia for patients with HELLP. *Can J Anaesth 38*:227.

Cunningham, F.G., Gant, N.F., MacDonald, P.C. et. al. (1997). *Williams Obstetrics*, 20th ed. McGraw Hill.

Cunningham, F., MacDonald, P., & Gant, N. (1989). *Williams obstetrics: Dystocia due to abnormalities of the expulsive forces and precipitous labor*. Norwalk, CT: Appleton & Lange.

Deihl, K. (1998). Thyroid dysfunction in pregnancy. *J Perinat Neonat Nurs 1*(4):1–12.

Feller, C. M., & Franko-Filiposie, K.J. (1993). Headaches during pregnancy: Diagnosis and management. *J Perinat Neonat Nurs 7*(1):1–10.

Harvey, C. (1991). Critical care obstetrical nursing. Rockville, MD: Aspen.

Jones, M.W., & Stone, L.C. (1998). Management of the woman with gestational diabetes. *J Perinat Neonat Nurs 11*(4):13–24.

Jovanovic, L., & Peterson, C.M. (1982). Optimal insulin delivery for the pregnant diabetic patient. *Diabetes Care 5*:24–35.

Mahlmeister, L. (1996). Perinatal group B streptococcal infections: The nurses's role in identification and prophylaxsis. *J Perinat Neonat Nurs 10*(2):1–16.

Marcovici, J., & Scoccia, F. (1999). Postpartum hemorrhage and intrauterine balloon tamponade. *J Reproduc Med 44*:122–126.

Pastore, L.M., et al. (1999). Association between bacterial vaginosis and fetal fibronectin at 24–29 weeks' gestation. *Obstet Gynecol 93*(1):117–122.

Ritchie, J., & Green, N. (1985). Local anesthetics. In A.G. Gilman, et al. (eds). *The pharmacological basis of therapeutics* (7th ed.) (pp. 309–310). New York: Macmillan.

Shannon, D. (1987). HELLP syndrome: A severe consequence of pregnancy-induced hypertension. *Obstet Gynecol Neonatal Nurs 16*(6):395–402.

Simpson, K.R. (1998). Fetal oxygen saturation monitoring during labor. *J Perinat Neonatal Nurs 12*(3):26–37.

Stone, M.L. (1971). Narcotic addiction in pregnancy. *Am J Obstet Gynecol 109*:717.

Van Beek, E., & Peeters, L.L.H. (1998). Pathogenesis of preeclampsia: A comprehensive model. *Obstetrical and Gynecological Survey, 53*(4):233–239.

Viamontes, C.M. (1996). Pharmacologic intervention in the management of preterm labor: An update. *J Perinat Neonatal Nurs 9*(4):13–30.

Weinstein, L. (1982). Syndrome of hemolysis, elevated liver enzymes, and low platelet count, a consequence of hypertension in pregnancy. *Am J Obstet Gynecol 142*:159.

Module 38

Nursing Care of the Acutely Ill Elderly Patient

Pamela Stinson Kidd, Deborah Kitchen

This self-study module is written at the core knowledge level for individuals who provide nursing care for elderly patients regardless of the practice setting. It is not a comprehensive review; rather, the module focuses on frequently encountered situations and issues relevant to the elderly patient. There are nine sections in the module. Section One introduces physiologic and anatomic changes associated with aging. Section Two discusses general assessment of the elderly, with an emphasis on analyzing functional decline. Section Three explains the effects of aging on drug metabolism. Common ventilation and perfusion concerns in the acutely ill elderly patient are discussed in Sections Four and Five, respectively. Cognitive impairments in the elderly are explained in Section Six. The manifestation of infection in the elderly is discussed in Section Seven. Traumatic injury and perioperative nursing care of the elderly patient are addressed in Sections Eight and Nine, respectively. Each section includes a set of review questions to help the learner evaluate his or her understanding of the section's content before moving on to the next section. All Section Reviews and the module Pretest and Posttest include answers. It is suggested that the learner review those concepts answered incorrectly in the review questions before proceeding to the next section.

OBJECTIVES

Following completion of this module, the learner will be able to

1. Describe age-associated anatomic and physiologic changes.
2. Discuss focal assessment areas for elderly patients.
3. Describe assessment of functional decline.
4. Discuss implications of mechanical ventilation in the elderly.
5. Explain signs and symptoms of cardiac ischemia in the elderly.
6. Differentiate between dementia, delirium, and depression.
7. Explain sources of and responses to infection in the elderly.
8. Discuss high-risk injuries in the elderly.
9. Identify issues in resuscitating the elderly trauma patient.
10. Discuss factors that increase the elderly patient's surgical risk.

PRETEST

1. Hypoxia may occur in the elderly patient because of which of the following physiologic changes associated with aging?
   A. hyperventilation
   B. decreased alveolar surface area
   C. ineffective airway clearance
   D. decreased anterior–posterior chest diameter
2. The elderly patient is at higher risk for incontinence because of
   A. increased glomelular filtration rate
   B. diuretic use
   C. decreased bladder capacity
   D. dilated urethra
3. Which of the following should the nurse assess in an immunization history?
   A. pneumococcal vaccine
   B. chickenpox exposure
   C. measles vaccine
   D. flu vaccine
4. Instrumental activities of daily living include all of the following EXCEPT
   A. toileting
   B. shopping
   C. telephone use
   D. meal preparation
5. Functional decline is
   A. normal aging
   B. a symptom of multiple organ dysfunction
   C. a symptom of drug toxicity
   D. a gradual process
6. Mary Wagner, age 81, is complaining of dizziness when she stands up. This may indicate
   A. drug toxicity
   B. a visual problem
   C. dementia
   D. functional decline
7. Which of the following is a complication of mechanical ventilation in the elderly?
   A. pneumothorax
   B. hypercapnea
   C. lacerated trachea
   D. congestive heart failure
8. A 67-year-old patient's vital signs have changed during the weaning process from mechanical ventilation. His blood pressure has decreased by 20 mm Hg. His heart rate has increased by 24 beats per minute. These findings indicate
   A. normal reaction to weaning for his age
   B. weaning failure
   C. patient anxiety
   D. adequate respiratory muscle training
9. Cardiac ischemia in an elderly patient usually produces
   A. very high creatine kinase levels
   B. acute confusion
   C. ST-T wave changes
   D. chest pain radiating to the left arm
10. Bill Mott, age 76, complains of an appetite change and acute inability to concentrate. These symptoms suggest
    A. sundowner syndrome
    B. delirium
    C. normal aging
    D. depression
11. The most dependable sign of infection in the elderly is
    A. fever
    B. change in mental status
    C. pain
    D. decreased breath sounds with crackles
12. Priorities in caring for the elderly trauma patient are
    A. circulation, airway, breathing
    B. disability (neurologic), circulation, breathing
    C. airway, breathing, circulation
    D. airway, breathing, disability (neurologic)

Mr. Moore, age 74, was in a motor vehicle crash and had a positive loss of consciousness. He is confused at present. Questions 13 through 15 pertain to Mr. Moore.

13. All of the following may explain his confusion EXCEPT
    A. preexisting sensory deficit
    B. closed head injury
    C. hypovolemia
    D. decreased reflexes
14. Because of his age, Mr. Moore is at risk for a(n)
    A. epidural hematoma
    B. subdural hematoma
    C. subarachnoid bleed
    D. skull fracture
15. Mr. Moore is taken to the operating suite for a craniotomy. He is given a general anesthesia. He is at greater risk for
    A. prolonged absorption and elimination of the anesthetic agent
    B. breakthrough pain
    C. hyperthermia
    D. hypoglycemia

Pretest answers: 1. B, 2. C, 3. A, 4. A, 5. C, 6. A, 7. D, 8. B, 9. B, 10. D, 11. D, 12. C, 13. D, 14. B, 15. A

GLOSSARY

Delirium. A reversible disorder of acute onset characterized by short-term memory impairment, hallucinations, perceptual disturbances, and incoherent speech

Dementia. An irreversible disorder characterized by gradual onset, disorientation, repetitive speech, and an inability to perform self-care

Depression. A reversible disorder of acute onset characterized by self-neglect, decreased appetite, and decreased ability to concentrate

Pressure support. Positive pressure applied to the patient's airway during the patient's spontaneous inspiratory efforts for the purpose of decreasing the work of breathing

Synchronized intermittent mandatory ventilation (SIMV). Intermittent ventilator breaths synchronized with the patient's breaths to reduce competition between the ventilator and the patient (Stillwell, 1992)

ABBREVIATIONS

ADL. Activities of daily living

AMI. Acute myocardial infarction

DPT. Diphtheria, pertussis, and tetanus vaccine

IADL. Instrumental activities of daily living

MMSE. Mini-Mental State Examination

SIMV. Synchronous intermittent mandatory ventilation

SECTION ONE: Anatomic and Physiologic Changes

At the completion of this section, the learner will be able to describe anatomic and physiologic changes associated with aging.

There are changes associated with aging; however, the degree to which these changes occur is dependent on lifestyle. It is important not to assume that total body function has declined in an elderly patient and that all elderly patients have the same degree of decline. Rather, the nurse should focus on the patient's "physiologic" age and not chronologic age.

The physiologic changes of aging affect the total body. Major changes are presented in Table 38–1.

Cardiovascular Changes

Cardiac output decreases while blood pressure increases. Anatomic changes promoting these changes are ventricular hypertrophy, valve incompetence, and arteriosclerosis. Orthostatic hypotension occurs due to decreased vasomotor tone and baroreceptor response.

Respiratory Changes

The diaphragm flattens, the chest wall becomes more rigid, and the anterior–posterior diameter of the chest increases. All these factors contribute to decreased vital capacity and air trapping. Alveolar surface area decreases, lowering the PO_2.

Central Nervous System Changes

Neurotransmitters are not synthesized at the same rate, producing a decline in sympathetic response (catecholamine release) and causing decreased cardiac compensation in hypovolemia. There is a decline in nerve conduction producing slow reflex responses. It is important to note that a change in mentation is not associated with aging and usually indicates malnutrition, a medication-related problem, depression, or dehydration (Saleh, 1993).

Gastrointestinal Changes

Hepatic blood flow declines. Thus, drugs metabolized by the liver will remain present and active for a longer period of time. Peristalsis slows while gastric acidity decreases. Both of these factors impede digestion.

Renal Changes

Bladder capacity decreases, predisposing the patient to incontinence. Glomerular filtration rate decreases, prolonging the clearance of most drugs.

Metabolic Changes

The ability to metabolize glucose decreases with aging. The pancreas secretes less insulin. T_3 and T_4 secretion decreases, producing hypothyroidism in some elderly. The

TABLE 38–1. AGE-RELATED PHYSIOLOGIC CHANGES

Cardiovascular	**Metabolic**
Decreased cardiac output/index	Decreased production of immunoglobulin M
Increased heart wall rigidity	Decreased functioning of the thymus gland (cell-mediated immunity)
Loss of vasomotor tone	Decreased production of norepinephrine
Increased systolic blood pressure	Decreased response to norepinephrine
Increased peripheral vascular resistance	Decreased metabolic rate
Slowed myocardial contraction rate	Insulin resistance
	Decreased insulin secretion
Respiratory	Decreased TSH
Increased work of breathing by 10%	
Ventilation/perfusion mismatch due to 4 mm Hg decrease in PO_2 per decade of life	**Body Composition**
Structural changes	Decreased subcutaneous fat
59% reduction in the response to hypercapnea and hypoxia	Increased fat stores
Decreased alveolar surface area (increased alveolar–arterial gradient)	Decreased total body water
Drop in 2, 3-diphosphoglycerate (oxyhemoglobin curve shift to the left)	Decreased vascularity of skin
	Decreased skin elasticity
Central Nervous System	**Musculoskeletal**
Decreased brain tissue weight	Increased joint stiffness
Decreased conduction velocity	Osteoporosis (increased parathyroid hormone secretion, decreased vitamin D GI absorption, decreased estrogen production
Loss of functioning neurons	Vertebral compression
Shorter attention span, poor short-term memory	
Decreased psychomotor speed	
Renal	
Decreased glomerular filtration	
Decreased ability to concentrate and dilute urine	
Decreased kidney mass	

overall basal metabolic rate decreases, also prolonging the excretion of drugs.

Body Composition

Overall body fat increases, providing a greater reservoir for fat-soluble drugs (most anesthetic agents). The number and efficiency of sweat glands decreases, predisposing the patient to hyperthermia. Skin pigmentation declines, making pallor a less reliable sign of anemia or distress.

Musculoskeletal Changes

Decreased muscle mass, bone demineralization, and increased joint stiffness predispose the elderly to fractures and falls.

In summary, the physiologic and anatomic changes of aging may contribute to decreased cardiac output, hypertension, hypoxia, indigestion, incontinence, hypothyroidism, drug toxicity, fractures, and falls.

SECTION ONE REVIEW

1. A change in the elderly patient's mentation or level of consciousness
   - **A.** is produced by an age-associated decline in nerve conduction
   - **B.** is related to a decrease in neurotransmitters
   - **C.** usually indicates a non–central nervous system (CNS) problem
   - **D.** reflects slow reflex responses
2. Hyperglycemia is a common condition in the elderly patient because
   - **A.** the pancreas secretes a poorer grade of insulin
   - **B.** the elderly tend to eat nonbalanced meals
   - **C.** glucose is metabolized faster causing more rapid release of glucagon from the liver
   - **D.** the pancreas secretes less insulin

Answers: 1. C, 2. D

SECTION TWO: General Assessment and Functional Decline

At the completion of this section, the learner will be able to describe assessment of the elderly patient and what information is useful for analyzing functional impairment.

The initial assessment of the elderly patient should include observation of general grooming, movement, and nourishment. This will provide information regarding the patient's functional status. Their speech may clue you to a cerebrovascular problem or a previous stroke. The content of the speech may indicate if the patient is alert and cognitively intact.

When eliciting a history, pace the questions to allow the patient time to think and to respond. Be very specific with questions and relate questions to specific organ systems. A social history should be obtained to identify caregiver issues (if pertinent) and support systems. Internal and external environmental hazards should be assessed. Internal hazards may include steps, floor rugs, and heating devices. External hazards may include steps, safety of the neighborhood, and integrity of curbs and sidewalks. Personal habits should be assessed including caffeine and alcohol intake as well as tobacco use. Exercise patterns may also be obtained. A nutritional history is elicited to determine use of food groups and to assess money and cooking problems. Immunizations are extremely important to assess and include DPT (or tetanus toxoid), pneumococcal, and influenza vaccines. Medications, both over-the-counter and prescribed, should be asked about (see Section Three for more details on how to elicit a drug history). This helps clue the nurse to drug absorption problems (see Section Three). Questions about medications should include ease of dosing schedule, affordability, ability to swallow, and obtainability (Khanna & Geller, 1992).

Functional decline is the recent difficulty or the inability to perform tasks that are necessary or desirable for independent living (Lachs, 1995). These tasks involve activities of daily living (ADLs) and instrumental activities (such as using the telephone, shopping, etc.). The inability to perform these tasks usually indicates an underlying physiologic change from a new illness or decompensation of a chronic disease. There is a direct relationship between the number of functional impairments and patient outcome from hospitalization: the greater the number of impairments, the poorer the outcome. Since the elderly may present with atypical signs of ischemia and hypoxia, functional decline should alert the nurse to conduct further assessment. For example, cardiac ischemia may cause the patient to complain of immobility and/or fatigue instead of chest pain. The most frequent complaint among the elderly when seeking emergency care is a problem of self care. Since the majority of elderly patients are admitted through the emergency department, nurses in a variety of settings will need to be familiar with the concept of functional decline.

Whenever the patient complains of a functional impairment, the nurse should assess ADLs and instrumental ADLs using standardized scales. The Katz ADL scale is most frequently used to record changes in ADLs (Katz, 1983) (Fig. 38–1). Any change in an ADL is a positive finding. The Instrumental ADL (IADL) Scale provides additional information regarding the functioning of the individual with the environment (Lawton, 1988) (Fig. 38–2). The higher the score on the IADL, the more independently functioning the individual. While information is gained from the patient regarding IADLs, it is appropriate for the nurse to ask whether the patient needs additional community services and family assistance. Table 38–2 is a list of referral resources.

If a functional impairment is present, the nurse must assess the following:

- How long has it been present (acute versus chronic in origin)? In cases in which the patient is transferred from an extended care facility, the nurse should obtain functional decline data, as a functional impairment may be a major reason for placement in this type of facility.
- If multiple ADLs are impaired, in what order did they appear? If IADLs are intact but ADLs are impaired, the etiology is most likely physical rather than cognitive.
- Is the patient capable of performing the activities or is it a motivation problem?
- Is the impairment present because of environmental factors (e.g., location of home)?

Impaired functional status and dependency in ADLs at the time of hospital admission are better than age or mental status for predicting complications of hospitalization and subsequent institutionalization or services needed (Gudmundsson & Carnes, 1996).

Functional decline may occur because the patient is cognitively impaired, in pain, depressed, or experiencing drug toxicity. Thus, a Mini-Mental State Examination (MMSE) should be performed. A confusion assessment method scale should be administered (see Section Six). An environmental and drug history should be obtained.

In summary, functional impairment may be a sign of an acute disorder and reflect hypoxia and ischemia. A formal assessment of ADLs and IADLs gives a baseline from which the effectiveness of interventions can be evaluated. The greater the functional decline, the more at risk the patient is for poor treatment outcomes.

Activities of Daily Living (ADL) Scale
Evaluation Form

Name ______________________ Day of evaluation ______________________

For each area of functioning listed below, check description that applies. (The word "assistance" means supervision, direction, or personal assistance.)

Bathing—either sponge bath, tub bath, or shower

☐	☐	☐
Receives no assistance (gets in and out of tub by self, if tub is usual means of bathing)	Receives assistance in bathing only one part of the body (such as back or a leg)	Receives assistance in bathing more than one part of the body (or not bathed)

Dressing—gets clothes from closets and drawers, including underclothes, outer garments, and using fasteners (including braces, if worn)

☐	☐	☐
Gets clothes and gets completely dressed without assistance	Gets clothes and gets dressed without assistance, except for assistance in tying shoes	Receives assistance in getting clothes or in getting dressed, or stays partly or completely undressed

Toileting—going to the "toilet room" for bowel and urine elimination; cleaning self after elimination and arranging clothes

☐	☐	☐
Goes to "toilet room," cleans self, and arranges clothes without assistance (may use object for support such as cane, walker, or wheelchair and may manage night bedpan or commode, emptying same in morning)	Receives assistance in going to "toilet room" or in cleansing self or in arranging clothes after elimination or in use of night bedpan or commode	Doesn't go to room termed "toilet" for elimination process

Transfer

☐	☐	☐
Moves in and out of bed as well as in and out of chair without assistance (may be using object for support, such as cane or walker)	Moves in and out of bed or chair with assistance	Doesn't get out of bed

Continence

☐	☐	☐
Controls urination and bowel movement completely by self	Has occasional "accidents"	Supervision helps keep urine or bowel control; catheter is used or person is incontinent

Feeding

☐	☐	☐
Feeds self without assistance	Feeds self except for getting assistance in cutting meat or buttering bread	Receives assistance in feeding or is fed partly or completely by using tubes or intravenous fluids

Figure 38–1. *Activities of Daily Living Scale. (From Katz, S., Ford, A., Moskowitz, R., et al. [1963]. Studies in illness in the aged. The index of ADL: Standardized measurement of biologic and psychosocial function. JAMA 185:914–919. Copyright © 1963, American Medical Association.)*

Instrumental Activities of Daily Living (IADL) Scale
Self-Rated Version Extracted from the Multilevel Assessment Instrument (MAI)

1. Can you use the telephone:	
without help,	3
with some help, or	2
are you completely unable to use the telephone?	1
2. Can you get to places out of walking distance:	
without help,	3
with some help or,	2
are you completely unable to travel unless special arrangements are made?	1
3. Can you go shopping for groceries:	
without help,	3
with some help, or	2
are you completely unable to do any shopping?	1
4. Can you prepare your own meals:	
without help,	3
with some help, or	2
are you completely unable to prepare any meals?	1
5. Can you do your own housework:	
without help,	3
with some help, or	2
are you completely unable to do any housework?	1
6. Can you do your own handyman work:	
without help,	3
with some help, or	2
are you completely unable to do any handyman work?	1
7. Can you do your own laundry:	
without help,	3
with some help, or	2
are you completely unable to do any laundry at all?	1
8a. Do you take medicines or use any medications?	
Yes (If yes, answer Question 8b)	1
No (If no, answer Question 8c)	2
8b. Do you take your own medicine:	
without help (in the right doses at the right time),	3
with some help (take medicine if someone prepares it for you and/or reminds you to take it), or	2
(are you/would you be) completely unable to take your own medicine?	1
8c. If you had to take medicine, could you do it:	
without help (in the right doses at the right time),	3
with some help (take medicine if someone prepares it for you and/or reminds you to take it), or	2
(are you/would you be) completely unable to take your own medicine?	1
9. Can you manage your own money:	
without help	3
with some help, or	2
are you completely unable to handle money?	1

Figure 38–2. *Instrumental Activities of Daily Living Scale. (From Lawton, M., & Brody, E. [1969]. Assessment of older people: Self-maintaining and instrumental activities of daily living.* Gerontologist 9:179–185.)

TABLE 38–2. COMMON SOCIAL PROBLEMS OF THE ELDERLY: REFERRAL RESOURCES

PROBLEM	RESOURCE
Isolation	Senior citizen's centers Senior grandparent program Friendly visitor program Telephone reassurance services Medical alert systems
Transportation	Senior citizen paratransit services Volunteer agencies County assistance office Medical transportation services
Medication assistance	Senior citizen's discounts Pharmacy assistance programs Pharmaceutical company sample
Access to medical care	Neighborhood health centers Health maintenance organizations Senior wellness programs Listing of physicians accepting Medicare
Nutrition	Meals on Wheels program Senior citizen lunch programs County assistance—food stamps
Housing	Senior citizen's housing Retirement communities Emergency shelters
Residential care	Nursing home directory Boarding home listings
Financial assistance	Tax rebate program Social Security Energy assistance relief Volunteer agencies
Emotional problems	Psychiatric emergency services In-home counseling programs Support groups Religious counseling services Community mental health services
Caretaking issues	Area Agency on Aging Homemaker/companion services Chore services Shopping services Area home health agencies Visiting nursing services
Caregiver relief	Adult day care centers Respite programs
Terminal illness	Hospice programs Bereavement support services
Alcohol/drug dependence	Geriatric treatment programs Alcoholics Anonymous
Inactivity/boredom	Senior employment programs Foster grandparent program Retired senior volunteer program Voluntary agencies
Abuse, neglect, exploitation	Adult protective services Department of Human Services Victim assistance program Area Agency on Aging

From McDonald, A., & Abrahams, S. (1990). Social emergencies in the elderly. Emerg Med Clin North Am 8:447.

SECTION TWO REVIEW

Mr. Hazard, age 77, is admitted with a diagnosis of functional decline. He is unable to perform bathing and dressing activities. Questions 1 through 3 pertain to Mr. Hazard.

1. When assessing Mr. Hazard's decline, the nurse should consider all of the following EXCEPT
   A. Mr. Hazard is not motivated
   B. Mr. Hazard cannot perform bathing and dressing due to environmental factors
   C. Mr. Hazard is not physically capable of performing these activities
   D. Mr. Hazard is exhibiting regression to childlike behavior
2. Because Mr. Hazard exhibits two functional impairments, the nurse should question
   A. in what order did they appear
   B. were they associated with a particular time of day
   C. has he had an injury
   D. which of the two worry Mr. Hazard the most
3. Mr. Hazard tells you that he is unable to balance his checkbook anymore. This indicates
   A. an impairment of ADLs
   B. a physical origin to his problem
   C. the need to perform a Mini-Mental State Exam
   D. a separate problem unrelated to his bathing and dressing difficulty

Answers: 1. D, 2. A, 3. C

SECTION THREE: Pharmacology and Aging

At the completion of this section, the learner will be able to describe the relationship between aging and drug metabolism.

The elderly are at risk for drug toxicity for a variety of reasons (Fig. 38–3). Drug reactions may be dose related or the result of the drug's interaction at the cellular level. The elderly may have several chronic illnesses that require medication for management. These medications

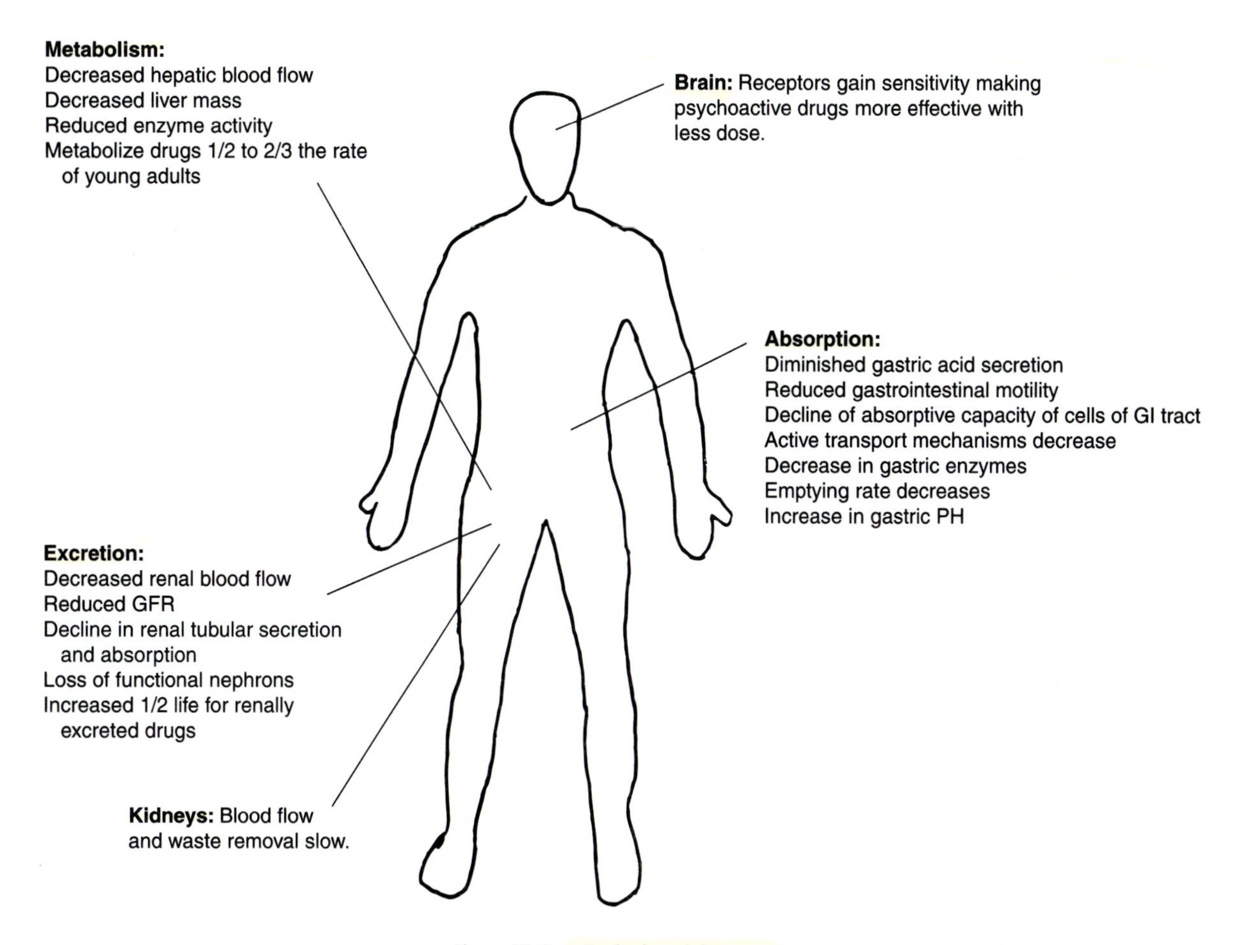

Figure 38–3. Aging body and drug use.

may interact, producing symptoms. Short-term memory impairment may cause a person to take incorrect dosages, multiple doses, or skip doses. Impaired vision may lead to overdosage. Impaired agility in opening containers may encourage a patient to miss a dose. Financial factors as well as limited transportation may keep the patient from filling prescriptions.

In obtaining a medication history, the nurse should ask about prescription and over-the-counter preparations; vitamins and minerals; alcohol, caffeine, and tobacco use; and home remedies. Diuretics, anticholinergics, and sedatives have the greatest number of undesirable side effects in the elderly (Evans et al., 1995). Some of the drugs with very narrow therapeutic windows in the elderly include: digoxin, theophylline, warfarin, lithium, lidocaine, and aminoglycosides. Factors such as those listed in the preceding paragraph, should also be assessed (e.g., vision, memory, transportation, finances).

Several physiologic changes associated with aging affect drug metabolism. These are summarized in Table 38–3 and Figure 38–3. Symptoms of drug toxicity in the elderly frequently include delirium, depression, worsening dementia, orthostatic hypotension, falls, and incontinence, rather than the more commonly seen nausea, vomiting, diarrhea, and rash.

TABLE 38–3. PHYSIOLOGIC CHANGES ASSOCIATED WITH DRUG EFFECT

CHANGE	EFFECT
Heart is dependent upon endogenous catecholamines for effective pumping	Beta-blocking agents may precipitate heart failure
Dopamine-making capacity of neurons decreases	Phenothiazines further block dopamine uptake, precipitating Parkinson-like symptoms
Dependence on prostacyclin-mediated renal vasodilation to maintain glomerular blood flow	Nonsteroidal anti-inflammatory agents that block prostacyclin may decrease renal blood flow and precipitate acute renal failure
Dependence on elevated renin levels to maintain renal perfusion	Angiotensin-converting enzyme inhibitors may decrease renal blood flow and precipitate acute renal failure
Increased body fat	Prolonged effects of fat-soluble drugs (e.g., sedatives/hypnotics) due to increased distribution volume in fat tissue
Less body water	Higher blood levels of water-soluble drugs (e.g., alcohol) due to decreased distribution volume

The mass of functional liver tissue decreases and blood flow to the liver declines. Microsomal enzymes which oxidize and reduce drugs act slower. Drugs and active metabolites may remain in the system for longer periods. Renal function declines with age. After age 40, creatine clearance falls by 10 percent for every decade of life (Lee, 1996).

Hepatic breakdown of drugs involves two types of reactions: synthetic (not influenced by aging) and nonsynthetic. Nonsynthetic reactions are influenced by aging. These reactions may affect drugs within the same drug classification. For example, diazepam (Valium) and lorazepam (Ativan) are both benzodiazepines, but diazepam undergoes nonsynthetic reactions while lorazepam is broken down in synthetic reactions. Thus, diazepam will have more sedative effects in the elderly than lorazepam. In patients with hepatic or renal insufficiency, drugs metabolized by these organs will have a prolonged half-life, increasing their likelihood to produce side effects. Glucocorticoids, because of a prolonged half-life, may produce greater osteoporosis, gastric irritation, and higher blood glucose levels. Cimetidine may produce central nervous system side effects such as delirium, hallucinations, and slurred speech owing to its prolonged half-life in the elderly.

In summary, it is essential to obtain a medication history in elderly patients. Nursing care includes monitoring drug levels, evaluating the effects of medications, and anticipating side effects and interactions. When drug doses are increased or other drugs added, the nurse should increase surveillance in these areas. Typical signs of drug toxicity in the elderly involve CNS changes.

SECTION THREE REVIEW

1. Which of the following drugs have the greatest number of undesirable side effects in the elderly?
   A. anti-inflammatory agents
   B. beta-blocking agents
   C. vitamins and minerals
   D. sedatives
2. Mrs. Todd, age 82, is to receive an IV glucocorticoid for her acute asthma attack. The nurse should observe her for
   A. hyperglycemia
   B. nausea and vomiting
   C. hypotension
   D. stress fractures
3. An elderly patient is more susceptible to the effects of alcohol because
   A. alcohol is fat soluble
   B. the elderly patient has less body water
   C. the elderly patient has an increased distribution volume
   D. alcohol may precipitate acute renal failure

Answers: 1. D, 2. A, 3. B

SECTION FOUR: Ventilation

At the completion of this section, the learner will be able to discuss issues related to weaning the elderly patient from mechanical ventilation.

Owing to the physiologic changes associated with aging discussed in Section One, it is not clear from research which mechanical ventilation mode (see Module 7) is best suited for the elderly patient. Regardless of the ventilation mode used, the elderly patient is at higher risk for nosocomial pneumonia and congestive heart failure from mechanical ventilation (Stiesmeyer, 1992). A decrease in gastric acidity and intestinal motility allows proliferation of bacteria. This proliferation occurs at the same time that immunoglobulin production is decreasing. Thus, the elderly may benefit greatly from the use of sucralfate in preventing gastric bleeding without decreasing gastric acidity. Sucralfate indirectly decreases nosocomial pneumonia by decreasing the amount of bacteria present for possible translocation across the diaphragm. Histamine H_2 blocking agents increase the risk for nosocomial pneumonia because they further decrease gastric acidity, which encourages bacterial proliferation.

The elderly acutely ill patient may be prescribed oxygen more frequently because, as a group, they are at greater risk to develop respiratory problems due to age-related decline in pulmonary function. The elderly also have a higher prevalence of respiratory diseases (Kleinpell & Ferrans, 1998).

Heart failure may be one reason why the elderly patient requires mechanical ventilation. However, the greater the pressure and volume generated by the ventilator to expand the patient's lungs, regardless of the ventilatory mode, the more resistance the heart must fill and pump against to maintain cardiac output. The smallest tidal volume and pressure support needed to achieve cellular oxygenation (as measured by flow-dependent oxygen consumption, base deficit, or mixed venous oxygen saturation) should be used in the elderly patient.

The elderly may need respiratory muscle conditioning in order to be sucessfully weaned from mechanical ventilation. This conditioning is often completed by using **synchronized intermittent mandatory ventilation (SIMV)** mode for a longer period of time to allow for spontaneous patient inspiratory efforts. **Pressure support** ventilation also increases endurance by delivering a preset airway pressure that is proportional to the patient's effort, which encourages "airway toning." For successful weaning, the elderly patient must be hemodynamically stable and have good left ventricular function.

Nursing care includes monitoring for indications of poor left ventricular function, such as increasing pulmonary arterial systolic, diastolic, and wedge pressures with decreasing cardiac output. An increase or decrease in heart rate and blood pressure by 20 from baseline after initiating weaning indicates weaning failure (Stiesmeyer, 1992). Tidal volumes of less than 300 mL and an increase in minute elevation of ≥ 5 L/min also suggests weaning failure. Generally, the patient will exhibit signs of respiratory fatigue (e.g., rapid shallow breathing, accessory muscle use, diaphoresis, and restlessness), while the patient's PO_2 will be less than 60 mm Hg. Oxygen saturation will be less than 90 percent. The aim of nursing is to prevent or anticipate weaning failure in order to stop weaning prior to patient exhaustion, since weaning failure produces anxiety for the patient and requires resting periods before future attempts.

In summary, elderly patients with a history of congestive heart failure (CHF), or those receiving histamine H_2 blocking agents are at greater risk for weaning failure. Prior to weaning elderly patients, the nurse should assess the patient's ability to ventilate in SIMV mode and with pressure support (as per physician's order). Baseline measurements of both hemodynamic function and oxygenation status should be obtained. If the patient appears compromised during the weaning attempt, the attempt should be stopped prior to patient exhaustion.

SECTION FOUR REVIEW

1. The aim of mechanical ventilation in the elderly is to
   - **A.** administer the smallest tidal volume needed to achieve cellular oxygenation
   - **B.** administer high levels of pressure support to decrease the work of breathing
   - **C.** achieve synchronous patient and ventilator breathing
   - **D.** achieve an oxygen saturation level of 90 percent

2. Respiratory muscle toning in the elderly is accomplished by
   - **A.** removing the patient from the ventilator for increasingly longer times
   - **B.** using pressure support or SIMV mode
   - **C.** maintaining excellent pulmonary hygiene
   - **D.** having the patient cough and deep breathe

Answers: 1. A, 2. B

SECTION FIVE: Perfusion

At the completion of this section, the learner will be able to describe manifestations and treatment of cardiac ischemia in the elderly patient.

Acute myocardial infarction (AMI) accounts for 66 percent of all deaths over the age of 65 (Kalbfleisch, 1995). Risk factors for AMI include age, male gender, tobacco use, and history of hypertension, diabetes, or hypercholesterolemia.

Elderly patients with cardiac ischemia and AMI may present atypically (30 percent). The patient may complain of abdominal, shoulder, throat, or back pain. The elderly patient may have associated symptoms of syncope, acute confusion, flulike syndrome, and/or fall. These additional symptoms often confuse and delay their diagnosis and treatment. It is important for the nurse to suspect cardiac ischemia anytime an elderly patient presents with one of the above complaints.

Diagnostic tests can be deceiving in the elderly patient. A normal electrocardiogram does not rule out cardiac ischemia since 50 percent of elderly patients do not have ST-T wave changes in ischemia. Creatine kinase levels are lower in the elderly; therefore, in ischemia, even though they may elevate, the elevation may not be greater than the upper limits of normal, particularly if the patient delays seeking help.

The risk/benefit ratio of thrombolytic therapy in the elderly has not been explored because in many of the clinical trials, patients were excluded if they were over the age of 75. The trend is to assess the patient's physiologic, not chronologic, age (e.g., previous history of stroke) and to administer thrombolytics to the elderly patient if other contraindications are not present. (For more information about contraindications, refer to module 15).

Percutaneous transluminal coronary angioplasty and coronary artery bypass grafts may be used to treat elderly patients who have a good surgical risk (see Section Nine). If the patient experiences sustained or symptomatic ventricular ectopy, requiring IV lidocaine, the bolus, maintenance, and total dosage should be cut in half to avoid acute mental status changes.

In summary, nursing care of the elderly patient with cardiac ischemia involves recognizing that ischemia produces different symptoms in the elderly, traditional diagnostic tests of cardiac ischemia may be less reliable, and the treatments used in a younger patient with AMI are applicable to the older patient although some modifications may be needed.

SECTION FIVE REVIEW

An elderly patient presents with an acute onset of back pain and fatigue. An AMI is diagnosed by the electrocardiogram (ECG). Questions 1 and 2 pertain to this patient.

1. The patient's creatine kinase levels will be
   - **A.** extremely elevated
   - **B.** below normal
   - **C.** at the upper limits of normal
   - **D.** inaccurate
2. The patient undergoes coronary angioplasty and experiences multifocal premature ventricular contractions. A decision is made to give the patient a lidocaine IV bolus followed by a continuous IV infusion. Which of the following statements is true?
   - **A.** lidocaine should not be used
   - **B.** the bolus dosage must be cut in half
   - **C.** the bolus and total dosage must be cut in half
   - **D.** the dosage must be increased to have a therapeutic effect

Answers: 1. C, 2. C

SECTION SIX: Cognition/Perception

At the completion of this section, the learner will be able to differentiate dementia, depression, and delirium.

The elderly are at risk for cognitive impairment in cases of preexisting chronic illness, polypharmacy, malnutrition, and sensory deficits (Guin & Freudenberger, 1992). Up to 80 percent of elderly patients with terminal illness develop delirium near death (Breitbart et al., 1997). Sensory–perceptual alterations may occur from placement in a critical care setting (see Module 1). Patients who experience sensory alterations are five times more likely to die (Foreman, 1992). Statistics indicate the elderly patient experiencing acute confusion is three to five times more likely to die than the nonconfused elderly patient (Ribby & Cox, 1996).

Acute confusion develops abruptly and the symptoms fluctuate throughout the day. Table 38–4 lists etiologies of acute confusion. It is a potentially reversible state. **Delirium** is an acute confusional state. Delirium may be due to altered cerebral perfusion related to decreased cardiac output (e.g., AMI, dehydration, CHF). Hypoxia may also produce acute confusion. Medications and alcohol use may also contribute to confusion (Pierre, 1996).

Dementia is a disorder of memory that is insidious, progressive, and irreversible. **Depression** is a disorder of mood. It develops abruptly, usually in relation to a major life event (Kozak-Campbell & Hughes, 1996). Table 38–5 compares dementia, delirium, and depression. The elderly patient should have cognition and behavior assessed. An MMSE should be performed to assess the elderly patient's appearance, orientation, judgment, memory, behavior, mood, and speech. This type of assessment helps the nurse determine whether a cognitive problem exists, and if it does exist, whether the problem is acute or chronic in nature. The MMSE (Fig. 38–4) includes items related to time, place, registration of three words, attention and calculation, short-term memory, language ability, and reconstruction of a geometric design. The maximum score on the MMSE is 30 points. A score between 18 and 23 points indicates mild impairment. Scores between 0 and 17 indicate severe impairment.

Behavior is assessed using a behavior rating scale such as the Confusion Assessment Method (Fig. 38–5). This allows for evaluation of the patient's ability to function in their environment. Delirium is suggested by items in Box 1 being checked and at least one item in Box 2 being checked.

Nursing care of a patient experiencing dementia or delirium includes positioning and actively using objects within the patient's environment that provide cues about time and place. Diurnal variation is promoted by altering light and noise. Personal objects are placed in the patient's line of vision and reach. Sensory aids should be accessible and in working order. The nurse should speak slowly while facing the patient and repeat key phrases (Banazak, 1996; Foreman, 1992). The patient should be monitored for adverse effects of medications (see Section Three). Assistance may be necessary during meals to encourage nutritional intake. The major difference between these two disorders is that in cases of delirium the nurse should assess possible cause of acute confusion (e.g., oxy-

TABLE 38–4. ETIOLOGIES OF ACUTE CONFUSIONAL STATES IN THE HOSPITALIZED ELDERLY ORGANIZED WITHIN THE FUNCTIONAL CONSEQUENCES THEORY

Age-Related Changes
- Decreased ability of the brain to adapt to metabolic disturbances
- Sensory/perceptual deficits
- Lowered resistance and ability to cope with stress related to changes in hypothalamus
- Reduced ability to regulate body temperature
- Reduction in cerebral blood flow and glucose metabolism

Risk Factors
Physiological Functioning
  Nutritional deficiencies
    A. B vitamins
    B. Vitamin C
    C. Hypoproteinemia
  Cardiovascular abnormalities
    A. Decreased cardiac output states: myocardial infarction, arrhythmias, congestive heart failure, cardiogenic shock
    B. Alterations in peripheral vascular resistance: increased and decreased states.
    C. Vascular occlusion: disseminated intravascular coagulopathy, emboli
  Cerebral disease
    A. Vascular insufficiency: transient ischemic attacks, cerebral vascular accidents, thrombosis
    B. Central nervous system infection: acute and chronic meningitis, neurosyphilis, brain abscess
    C. Trauma: subdural hematoma, concussion, contusion, intracranial hemorrhage
    D. Tumors: primary and metastatic
    E. Normal pressure hydrocephalus
  Endocrine disturbance
    A. Hypo- and hyperthyroidism
    B. Diabetes mellitus
    C. Hypopituitarism
    D. Hypo- and hyperparathyroidism
Alterations in Temperature Regulation: Hypo- and Hyperthermia
  Pulmonary abnormalities
    A. Inadequate gas exchange states: pulmonary disease, alveolar hypoventilation
    B. Infection: pneumonia
  Systemic infective processes: acute and chronic
    A. Viral
    B. Bacterial: endocarditis, pyelonephritis, cystitis
  Metabolic disturbances
    A. Electrolyte abnormalities: hypercalcemia, hypo- and hypernatremia, hypo- and hyperkalemia, hypo- and hyperchloremia, hyperphosphatemia
    B. Acidosis/alkalosis
    C. Hypo- and hyperglycemia
    D. Acute and chronic renal failure
    E. Volume depletion: hemorrhage, inadequate fluid intake, diuretics
    F. Hepatic failure
  Drug intoxications: therapeutic and substance abuse
    A. Misuse of prescribed medications
    B. Side effects of therapeutic medications
    C. Drug–drug interactions
    D. Improper use of over-the-counter medications
    E. Ingestion of heavy metals and industrial poisons
    F. Alcohol intoxication or withdrawal
Immobilization: Therapeutic, Physical, Pharmacologic
  Psychosocial functioning
- Emotional stress: postoperative states, relocation, hospitalization
- Depression
- Anxiety
- Grief
- Dementia
- Social supports
- Unfamiliar environment creating a lack of meaning in the environment
- Nursing care delivery method
- Knowledge and attitudes of caregivers

  Comfort and pleasure
- Pain: acute and chronic
- Fatigue/sleep deprivation
- Hypo/hyperthermia
- Sensory deprivation/environmental monotony creating a lack of meaning in the environment
- Sensory overload
- Lack of meaningful routines

From Kozak-Campbell, C., & Hughes, A. (1996). The use of functional consequence theory in acutely confused hospitalized elderly. J Gerontol Nurs *22(1):32–33.*

gen saturation, hemoglobin levels, albumin levels) and collaborate with the physician in treating predisposing conditions. For depressed elderly patients, a psychiatric referral and suicide appraisal should be made.

In summary, delirium and depression are considered acute disorders with reversible causes. Dementia is chronic, progressive, and irreversible. An experience with life-threatening illness or injury may precipitate acute disorders, as may a critical care unit experience.

TABLE 38–5. DIFFERENTIATING DEMENTIA, DEPRESSION, AND DELIRIUM

	DEMENTIA	DEPRESSION	DELIRIUM
Thought	Disoriented, irrelevant	Seems disoriented	Disoriented
Memory	Impaired (recent)	Decreased ability to concentrate	Possible impairment of short-term
Behavior	Unable to perform self care/ agitation/ apathy	Self neglect; appetite change	Perceptual disturbances, illusions, hallucinations, changes in sleep
Onset	Months to years	Rapid but at least 2 weeks	Hours to days
Mood/ speech	Sparse, repetitive	Understandable, hopeless, worried	Possibly incoherent, sparse or fluent

Mini-Mental State Examination (MMSE)

Add points for each correct response.

Orientation		Score	Points
1. What is the:	Year?	____	1
	Season?	____	1
	Date?	____	1
	Day?	____	1
	Month?	____	1
2. Where are we?	State?	____	1
	County?	____	1
	Town or city?	____	1
	Hospital?	____	1
	Floor?	____	1

Item	Score	Points
Registration		
3. Name three objects, taking one second to say each. Then ask the patient to repeat all three after you have said them. Give one point for each correct answer. Repeat the answers until patient learns all three.	____	3
Attention and calculation		
4. Serial sevens. Give one point for each correct answer. Stop after five answers. Alternate: Spell WORLD backwards.	____	5
Recall		
5. Ask for names of three objects learned in question 3. Give one point for each correct answer.	____	3
Language		
6. Point to a pencil and a watch. Have the patient name them as you point.	____	2
7. Have the patient repeat "No ifs, ands, or buts."	____	1
8. Have the patient follow a three-stage command: "Take a paper in your right hand. Fold the paper in half. Put the paper on the floor."	____	3
9. Have the patient read and obey the following: "CLOSE YOUR EYES." (Write it in large letters.)	____	1
10. Have the patient write a sentence of his or her choice. (The sentence should contain a subject and an object and should make sense. Ignore spelling errors when scoring.)	____	1
11. Have the patient copy the design. (Give one point if all sides and angles are preserved and if the intersecting sides form a quadrangle.)	____	1
	____ = Total	30

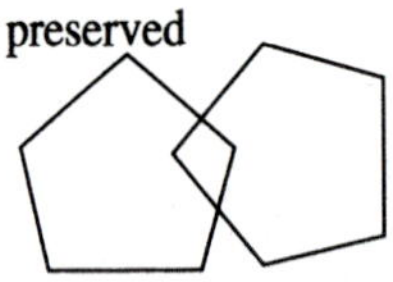

In validation studies using a cut-off score of 23 or below, the MMSE has a sensitivity of 87%, a specificity of 82%, a false positive ratio of 39.4%, and a false negative ratio of 4.7%. These ratios refer to the MMSE's capacity to accurately distinguish patients with clinically diagnosed dementia or delirium from patients without these syndromes.

Figure 38–4. *Mini-Mental State Examination. (From Folstein, M.F., Folstein, S., & McHugh, P.R. (1975). Mini-Mental State: A practical method for grading the cognitive state of patients for the clinician.* J Psych Res 12:*189–198.)*

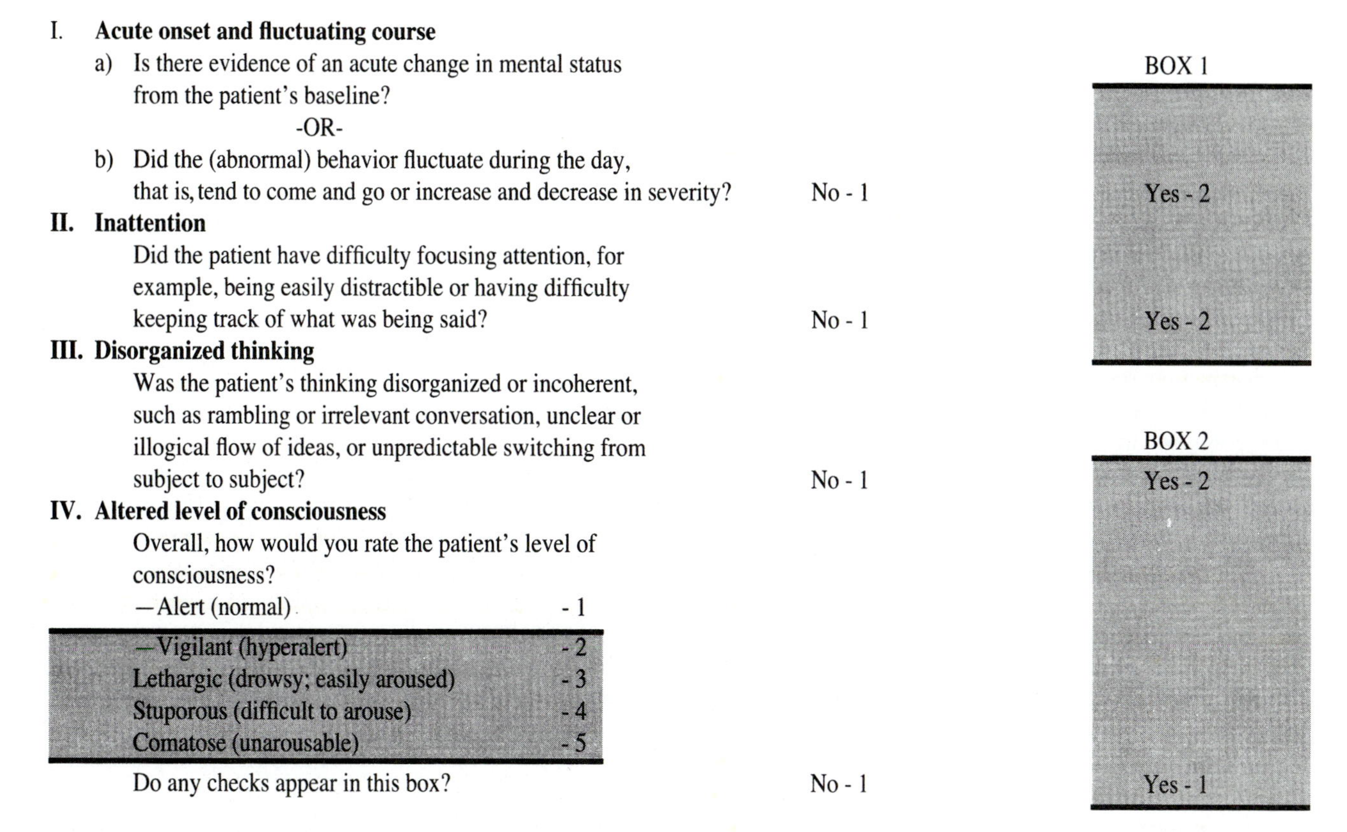

Confusion Assessment Method (CAM) Worksheet

I. **Acute onset and fluctuating course**
   a) Is there evidence of an acute change in mental status from the patient's baseline?
   -OR-
   b) Did the (abnormal) behavior fluctuate during the day, that is, tend to come and go or increase and decrease in severity? — No - 1 — BOX 1: Yes - 2

II. **Inattention**
   Did the patient have difficulty focusing attention, for example, being easily distractible or having difficulty keeping track of what was being said? — No - 1 — BOX 1: Yes - 2

III. **Disorganized thinking**
   Was the patient's thinking disorganized or incoherent, such as rambling or irrelevant conversation, unclear or illogical flow of ideas, or unpredictable switching from subject to subject? — No - 1 — BOX 2: Yes - 2

IV. **Altered level of consciousness**
   Overall, how would you rate the patient's level of consciousness?
   —Alert (normal) - 1
   —Vigilant (hyperalert) - 2
   Lethargic (drowsy; easily aroused) - 3
   Stuporous (difficult to arouse) - 4
   Comatose (unarousable) - 5
   Do any checks appear in this box? — No - 1 — BOX 2: Yes - 1

If all items in Box 1 are checked yes and at least 1 item in Box 2 is checked yes then, the diagnosis of delirium is suggested.

Figure 38–5. *Confusion Assessment Method Worksheet.* (*From Inouye, S., Van Dyck, C., Alessi, C., et al. [1990]. Clarifying confusion: The confusion assessment method.* Ann Intern Med 113:*941–948.*)

Section Six Review

Mary Kidd, age 70, is admitted to your unit for repair of a fractured left hip and femur from being hit by a motor vehicle while crossing the street. She is 2 days postop and is being transferred out of surgical intensive care to the trauma step-down floor. Questions 1 through 3 pertain to Mary.

1. Mary becomes disoriented to place. She complains of seeing the car that hit her. She is exhibiting signs of
   A. posttraumatic stress disorder
   B. depression
   C. delirium
   D. dementia
2. An MMSE is performed and she receives a score of 20. This score indicates
   A. no impairment
   B. mild impairment
   C. severe impairment
   D. inconclusive, perform the test again
3. An appropriate nursing intervention for Mary's disorientation is to
   A. keep her in the ICU until her symptoms improve
   B. create diurnal rhythms by altering light intensity
   C. begin patient teaching
   D. provide pain medication

Answers: 1. C, 2. B, 3. B

SECTION SEVEN: Infection

At the completion of this section, the learner will be able to discuss the sources of infection in the elderly and associated nursing care.

The elderly patient who lives with multiple persons (e.g., in an extended care facility) has a higher risk of contracting pneumonia, hepatitis, tuberculosis, and urinary tract and soft tissue infections (Mick, 1997). Crowded living conditions as well as incontinence of some individuals increase the risk. Community dwelling elderly have a higher risk of contracting upper respiratory infections.

Sepsis is a leading cause of death in the elderly (Stengle & Dries, 1994). Gram-negative pneumonias are more common in elderly debilitated patients (Fraser, 1997). Table 38–6 describes age-related changes that predispose the patient to infection. Some believe this high mortality is influenced by a delay in diagnosis of infection. Signs of infection in the elderly consist of change in mental status, functional decline, history of a fall, hypothermia, unexplained hypo- or hyperglycemia, acidosis, and tachycardia. Fever may not be present but when it is, it usually indicates a bacterial infection.

Elderly patients have a decreased basal temperature and experience heat loss following infection. It is believed that the elderly may have a significant temperature rise initially but the temperature fails to reach fever levels owing to a decreased basal rate. Infection in the elderly often involves multiple organisms and antibiotic resistance due to previous years of use. Treatment of infection is the same in the elderly as it is in younger patients: the goal is to remove the source of infection if possible (as in cases of abscesses), administer intravenous antibiotics and/or fungal agents, and provide inotropic support to maintain perfusion. (For more information, refer to Module 11.) Because infection is difficult to assess and treat in the elderly, prevention of infection through administration of immunizations is important (Miller, 1997) (Table 38–7).

The older adult experiencing intra-abdominal pain most likely has an infection or inflammatory disorder. Acute cholecystitis, diverticulitis, or intestinal obstruction may be present (Abi-Hanna & Gleckman, 1997). Because the elderly may not be febrile or experience pain, the nurse must access infection by carefully examining sputum, urine, and wounds for color and texture changes. Breath sound assessment and monitoring of oxygen saturation is vital to identifying pneumonia early. Signs of consolidation (crackles), wheezing, pleuritic chest pain, and bronchial breath sounds are absent in 30 percent of older patients (Fraser, 1997). A knowledge of preexisting illness is important in assessing infection risk (e.g., diabetes, benign prostatic hypertrophy). Diagnostic tests and treatments may predispose the elderly patient to infection. The placement of pulmonary arterial and urinary catheters are examples of treatments with infection risk. A vaccination history is important to obtain since influenza and pneumoccal vaccines decrease one's risk for pneumonia.

In summary, infection is a major killer of the elderly. Nurses must anticipate patients at high risk for infection and assess them appropriately. This assessment involves examining preexisting illness, diagnostic tests, and treatment for their infection risk as well as observing clinical signs.

TABLE 38–6. AGE-RELATED CHANGES THAT PREDISPOSE TO INFECTION

- Urinary retention
- Prostatic hypertrophy
- Decreased bladder tone
- Delayed gastric emptying
- Decreased cough strength
- Reduced ciliary action
- Flattened diaphragm
- Reduced muscle mass
- Stiffened thoracic cage
- Decreased skin elasticity
- Increased insulin resistance
- Decreased insulin secretion
- Decreased serum albumin (depending on nutritional status)

TABLE 38–7. GUIDELINES FOR IMMUNIZATIONS FOR OLDER ADULTS

IMMUNIZATION	INDICATIONS	FREQUENCY
Influenza	Aged 65 years and older, long-term care residents, anyone with chronic respiratory or cardiovascular disorders, health care workers	Annually, preferably between September and November (but they can be administered as late as January)
Pneumonia	Same groups as influenza, except for health care workers	Once in a lifetime, but people at very high risk may be revaccinated after 6 years
Tetanus toxoid	All adults, particularly debilitated adults with pressure ulcers	Initial series of three, then booster shot every 10 years (or after 5 years if at high risk)
Hepatitis B	Homosexual men, recipients of various blood products, patients receiving hemodialysis, people in health care–related jobs where exposure to hepatitis B is probable	A series of three doses should last for several years

Source: Miller, C.A. (1997). Preventive care should address the immunizations for older adults. Geriatr Nurs 18:*42–43.*

Section Seven Review

1. When assessing an elderly patient's infection risk, it is important to elicit a(n)
   A. medication history
   B. family history
   C. vaccination history
   D. allergy history

2. The best way to assess early an elderly patient for pneumonia is to
   A. monitor the patient's temperature
   B. monitor the patient's white blood cell count and differential
   C. auscultate breath sounds
   D. assess sputum production

Answers: 1. C, 2. C

SECTION EIGHT: Traumatic Injury

At the completion of this section, the learner will be able to describe common etiologies of injury for the elderly and resuscitation issues.

Injury is the fifth leading cause of death in persons 65 years and older (Dandan, 1992). Falls are the most common cause of injury, but motor vehicle crashes (MVCs) account for the most fatalities. Burns have a high mortality rate in the elderly.

Initial Assessment

Priorities in caring for the elderly trauma patient are the same as those for the younger trauma patient; airway, breathing, and circulation (refer to Module 34 for more information on conducting a primary and secondary survey). Because the elderly are less tolerant of the effects of shock, it is essential to monitor oxygenation (via peripheral oxygen saturation, lactic acid level, arterial blood gases, and mixed venous oxygen saturation [when available]) and hemodynamic status (via urine output, level of consciousness [LOC], and cardiac output measurements [when available]).

Once the patient is stabilized, an in-depth history is obtained. Immunization status is important to assess. Antecedent events such as syncope, palpitations, or chest pain may help identify why the traumatic event occurred. The patient's past medical history is important since chronic renal failure, chronic obstructive pulmonary disease, cirrhosis, diabetes, ischemic heart disease, and previous myocardial infarction are associated with poor outcome posttraumatic injury (Morris, MacKenzie, & Edelstein, 1990; Zietlow et al., 1994).

Preexisting cardiovascular disease and treatment for hypertension may precipitate a syncopal episode while the person is operating machinery, either from decreased cardiac output or inadequate cerebral circulation. Anemia and hormonal and electrolyte imbalances, such as hypothyroidism, may produce cardiac dysrhythmias. Diminished senses (e.g., vision, hearing) may place the elderly patient at greater injury risk. Reflexes, agility, and coordination also diminish, increasing the risk for falls.

A complete medication history is essential as certain medications may increase the risk of injury. For example, antihypertensives and oral hypoglycemic agents may induce syncope. Diuretics without potassium replacement may precipitate dysrhythmias and hypotension. Another reason for a thorough medication history is medications may alter the patient's compensatory response to injury. Beta-blocking agents will decrease the patient's sympathetic nervous system response to hypovolemia.

The elderly patient may be agitated or confused not only because of hypovolemia or head injury but also due to preexisting sensory deficits. The patient may not understand questions health care providers are asking or recognize the setting to which they are transported.

High-Risk Injuries

Falls

Falls typically produce fractures of the hip, femur, humerus, and wrist, and head injuries (Bobb, 1993). It is estimated that 50 percent of older adults with significant injury from a fall will die within one year. Preexisting disease, consequences of hospitalization, and lifestyle changes are usually the cause of death (Robins & Courts, 1997). Falls may be due to intrinsic (e.g., diminished visual acuity, decreased coordination) or extrinsic (e.g., poor lighting, loose rugs) factors. Syncope, orthostatic hypotension, and dizziness account for up to 45 percent of falls (McNamara, 1995). A patient who presents with a history of syncope needs additional assessment. Syncope may mean there is a preexisting illness or condition that requires treatment in addition to the injuries sustained during the syncopal episode. Table 38–8 lists focus assessment areas for patients with a history of syncope. Therefore, if a trauma patient presents with the mechanism of injury being a fall, the patient may not respond as posi-

TABLE 38–8. ASSESSMENT OF SYNCOPE

Focus Area: Decreased Perfusion
1. History of palpitations, SOB, diaphoresis, chest pain?
2. History of previous AMI, CVA?
3. Dizziness upon arising or changing position?
4. History of vomiting, diarrhea, gastrointestinal bleeding?
5. Lack of food and/or fluid intake?

Focus Area: Neurologic
1. Any weakness, tingling, or numbness?
2. Prior trouble with walking or balance?
3. Trouble completing ADLs?
4. Any difficulty with speech or communication?

Focus Area: Illness
1. Any history of diabetes; if so, how treated? Last meal, activity, and medication.
2. Any history of cancer; if so, how treated? Last radiation, chemotherapy treatment, CBC, platelet count.
3. Any infection: fever, respiratory symptoms, change in urination and/or urine output?

Focus Area: Medications
1. Use of alcohol or recreational drugs?
2. Use of antihypertensives?
3. Use of antihistamines?
4. Use of sedatives?
5. Use of pain medications?

SOB = shortness of breath; AMI = acute myocardial infarction; CVA = cerebrovascular accident; ADLs = activities of daily living; CBC = complete blood count.

tively to resuscitation efforts due to preexisting cardiac and vascular disease. The nurse must assess for pulmonary, cerebral, and peripheral edema. Because metabolic derangements and hypoxia may precipitate falls, diagnostic tests may include complete blood count (CBC), electrolyte panel, glucose and creatinine levels, toxicology screens, and an ECG.

Head and Spine Injury

Epidural hematomas occur less frequently in the elderly because the dura adheres tightly to the skull. There is a volume loss of the brain that increases the space between the brain and dura. Subdural hematomas occur more frequently and neurologic symptoms may manifest slowly, even weeks after injury. Acute subdural hematomas will usually manifest symptoms within 48 hours of the injury (Robins & Courts, 1997). A computed tomographic (CT) scan of the head is indicated with a history of loss of consciousness, decreased LOC, and/or lateralizing neurologic signs (sensory and motor changes in an extremity). The classic features (such as headache and vomiting) of increased cranial pressure (ICP) may be absent due to age-related cerebral atrophy. Subdural hematomas occur three times more frequently in the elderly who can have large amounts of bleeding into this increased space with minimal clinical symptoms (Robins & Courts, 1997). Increased ICP may appear as subtle changes in LOC or as cranial nerve deficits. Accurately documenting a Glasgow Coma Scale (GCS) score in the elderly may be difficult. Cataracts and glaucoma may alter pupillary response. Muscle fatigue may prevent strength testing of the extremities.

Head injuries in the elderly have a high risk of poor outcome. Outcome is strongly related to the patient age and early GCS scores. In one study, patients over the age of 65 had a 25 percent chance of surviving a major head injury defined as traumatic coma or an intracranial hematoma treated surgically (Ross, Pitts, & Kobayashi, 1992). Of this group, only 13 percent recovered to function independently. Head injury reduces the body's immunologic competence by increasing the permeability of the blood–brain barrier, increases leukocyte infiltration into the brain, and stimulates mediator release.

Older people have a higher incidence of cervical spine fractures due to degenerative spine changes (Robins & Courts, 1997). Immobilization of the cervical spine is necessary until injury is ruled out. However, prolonged backboard use in a malnourished patient increases the incidence of pressure sores. Clinical guidelines for "clearing C-spine films" may need to include shorter time ranges for the elderly.

Chest Injuries

Chest injury has a high association with fractured ribs in the elderly because of osteoporosis. If the patient has preexisting pulmonary disease and less pulmonary reserve, he or she is at higher risk for acute respiratory failure and subsequent intubation and mechanical ventilation. In one study, elderly persons involved in MVCs as a lap–shoulder-belted (3-point restrained) driver had greater injury severity to the chest region (as measured by the Abbreviated Injury Scale) but less injury to other body regions (Martinez, Sharieff, & Hooper, 1994). Chest injuries included myocardial contusions, lacerated aorta, and heart avulsions. Therefore, it is important to note restraint status in the history.

Abdominal Injuries

Abdominal trauma in the elderly has a high mortality rate due to postoperative, pulmonary, and infectious complications. The elderly have diminished sensation and abdominal wall muscle tone, so the typical signs of peritoneal irritation, such as involuntary guarding and muscular rigidity, may be missing. Because of the lack of positive signs on the physical exam, the use of diagnostic peritoneal lavage or CT scanning is recommended in blunt abdominal trauma (Pepe & Lane, 1993). CT scanning is preferred because a higher proportion of elderly have had previous abdominal operative procedures, which increases the rate of adhesions (Mitchell, Gallo, & Turnes, 1992). Fragile ribs and a weakened abdominal wall increase the likelihood of abdominal injury with minor force.

Pelvic Injuries

Pelvic fractures are always associated with great blood loss. However, in the elderly, early control of hemorrhage is essential due to fewer compensatory responses to hypovolemic shock (e.g., decreased heart rate, decreased vascular tone). Embolization of major pelvic arteries may need to be performed as well as early stabilization with external fixation. Early stabilization of any fracture is indicated in the elderly to prevent complications of immobility (e.g., pneumonia, pulmonary emboli).

Burns

The mortality from burn injuries is associated with age, burn size, and the presence of inhalation injury (Staley & Richard, 1993). The elderly tend to have greater depth and size of burn due to their thinner skin, slower reaction times, reduced mobility, and diminished sensation. Loss of elastic fibers and decreased nutrient transfer to dermis cells may delay healing, particularly if the patient is malnourished prior to injury. The elderly are predisposed to flame burns and scalding associated with cooking and bathing, respectively (Lewandowski et al., 1993). The elderly do not scar as much as younger patients; thus, pressure garments are not essential.

Resuscitation Issues

Aggressive resuscitation appears warranted in the elderly. In one study, 50 percent of elderly trauma patients were discharged to the home and were able to function independently (Zietlow et al., 1994). It is difficult to use the same parameters to measure the success of resuscitation in the elderly trauma patient as is used in the younger trauma patient. Resuscitation protocols have been developed based on the assumption of normal function prior to injury. Some authors advocate that all elderly trauma patients should be treated with invasive monitoring and placed in intensive care in order to decrease morbidity and mortality (Pellicane, Byrne, & DeMaria, 1992). A patient over the age of 65 with a trauma score of less than 15 is a candidate for ICU admission.

Because usual hemodynamic values may not be normal in the elderly, the goal of treatment is not to return values to normal but rather to prevent or stop any oxygen deficit (Dandan, 1992). Two-thirds of elderly trauma patients with initial systolic blood pressures over 90 mm Hg died, as compared with less than one-third of younger trauma patients (Finelli, Jonsson, & Champion, 1989). Oxygen deficits are usually produced by low blood flow or a maldistribution of blood flow during shock states.

Elderly patients may be hypokalemic and hypovolemic prior to injury from diuretic use. Their renal function deteriorates with aging. Although lactated Ringer's solution is the solution of choice for initial resuscitation, resuscitation with crystalloids is not as aggressive as in the younger patient. A higher hemoglobin level is needed to deliver oxygen to the tissues as one ages because atherosclerosis decreases venous return. Thus, oxygen delivery is greatly dependent on hemoglobin since the volume of blood ejected to the tissues is more limited. Colloids, such as packed red blood cells, may be administered until a hemoglobin level of 10 g/dL is achieved (Dandan, 1992). Normal saline solution (NS) should be avoided since renal function deteriorates with age and metabolic acidosis may occur with NS infusion. Sodium displaces hydrogen within the cell, causing hydrogen ion to shift into the vascular space. If left untreated, this acidosis could lead to an anaerobic metabolic state with decreased production of adenosine triphosphate (ATP) for metabolic pathways.

The aged heart has less of a chronotropic response; therefore, tachycardia may not occur in hypovolemia. The elderly trauma patient may have a dangerously low cardiac output despite a normal blood pressure and heart rate. In elderly patients with cardiac disease, vasopressors (e.g., dobutamine) may be needed to increase cardiac output. It is speculated that a cardiac index that is 50 percent greater than normal is needed to oxygenate tissues adequately posttraumatic injury (Dandan, 1992).

Hypothermia must be prevented during resuscitation. Elderly patients are unable to increase their metabolic rates in proportion to the metabolic demands of increased heat production. Decreased muscle mass and decreased peripheral vasoconstriction prevent heat conservation in the elderly. They require a warm environment (heating lamps) and warmed intravenous fluids. Core rewarming (e.g., IV fluids, fluids through the nasogastric tube, dialysis) is much more efficient than peripheral warming (e.g., heating blanket).

Hyperglycemia is an immediate response to injury (refer to Modules 11 and 22 for more information). Elevated blood glucose levels are present during the postresuscitation phase despite elevated serum insulin levels. In addition, carbohydrate metabolism in aging results in impaired glucose tolerance and higher fasting blood glucose levels related to decreased insulin secretion. This normal physiologic response of aging coupled with the normal response to injury produces even less insulin secretion posttrauma and higher blood glucose levels. The age-associated decline in renal clearance of glucose also contributes to higher serum glucose levels. Elderly trauma patients should be closely monitored for changes in blood glucose; intravenous insulin may need to be administered. The use of glucose as a principal calorie source posttrauma may be hazardous in the elderly and needs further study (Watters et al., 1994).

Complications of Trauma

Infection and pulmonary, cardiac, and renal complications are the most common sequelae in elderly trauma patients (Smith, Enderson, & Maull, 1990). The presence of shock (systolic blood pressure less than 80 mm Hg for longer than 15 minutes) is a strong predictor of mortality in the elderly (Osler et al., 1988; Zietlow et al., 1994). Severe closed head injury (GCS score of 8 or less), bradycardia at admission, and the need for ventilatory and inotropic support are other predictors of poor outcomes in the elderly trauma patient (Zietlow et al., 1994).

If the elderly patient is malnourished prior to injury, delayed wound healing, organ failure, and immunosuppression may occur. The hypermetabolism posttrauma requires protein catabolism for wound repair. Cell-mediated and humoral responses to antigens are delayed in the elderly (for more information refer to Module 24). Inadequate body mass and protein stores also contribute to decreased immunoglobulin production. Early nutritional assessment (e.g., total lymphocyte count, prealbumin and transferrin levels, and skin-fold measurements) is indicated. Herpes zoster also occurs more frequently after trauma in the elderly (Mitchell, Gallo, & Turnes, 1992).

Nursing Management in the High-Acuity Phase

The challenge for the nurse is to discriminate normal changes in function from those associated with injury or the complications from injury. Section One discusses normal declines in aging. Table 38–9 summarizes facts related to aging relevant to nursing care of the trauma patient.

TABLE 38–9. FACTS IN ELDERLY TRAUMA CARE

1. The severity of injury should not be underestimated. Elderly patients with mild to moderate trauma scores may have poorer outcomes than their younger counterparts.
2. Trauma mortality increases at age 50 (Bobb, 1993). We must think of trauma patients in age-related subgroups and not arbitrarily divide patients on the basis of age 65. Mortality increases at age 50.
3. There are fundamental differences in patients who suffer injury from different causes. For example, patients who fall have lower Injury Severity Scores than those who are involved in MVCs. People who fall may be healthier overall and more active.
4. Overall, elderly trauma patients have good outcomes.
5. The health status of the elderly trauma patient cannot be judged by age.
6. The elderly have well developed coping resources from life experiences. They can help problem solve.
7. The elderly suffer different types of injuries and they respond differently to their injuries (Osler et al., 1988).
8. Trauma patients older than 70 years of age are treated less aggressively than younger trauma patients (Marx, Campbell, & Harder, 1989). Our practice patterns may actually be producing the complications.
9. Of the trauma scoring devices, the Injury Severity Score most accurately reflects probability of survival in the elderly. The Trauma score is not sensitive in the elderly; elderly patients who score 13 out of a possible 16 points have a 10 times higher mortality rate than younger trauma patients with the same score (Finelli, Jonsson, & Champion, 1989).

Adapted from Marx, A., Campbell, R., & Harder, F. (1989). Polytrauma in the elderly. World J Surg *10:330–335.*

Ventilator dependence for more than 5 days is associated with mortality in elderly trauma patients (DeMaria et al., 1987). Aggressive pulmonary toilet is necessary in any elderly patient with a history of chest trauma. Patients should be turned frequently, suctioned regularly, and encouraged to use incentive spirometers once extubated. Vital capacity and rib cage expansion decrease with aging. If the patient is a smoker, mucociliary action is diminished, leading to ineffective airway clearance. All of these factors increase the incidence of pneumonia. The aspiration of tube feedings is a preventable complication that predisposes the patient to pneumonia. Decreased gastric motility is associated with aging; in addition, the administration of opioid narcotics may further impair peristalsis. All tube feedings should be given with the head of the bed elevated after placement of the tube is confirmed. Suction should be available.

Renal function must be closely monitored for several reasons. Glomerular filtration rate and the ability to concentrate and dilute urine diminishes with age. Myoglobin is released with tissue injury, increasing renal workload. Nephrotoxic antibiotics may be given (e.g., aminoglycosides). Aggressive fluid resuscitation combined with decreased serum albumin (if the patient is malnourished prior to injury) may produce pulmonary edema, requiring diuretics for correction. Careful assessment of breath sounds, urine output, and central venous pressure and pulmonary artery wedge pressure are warranted. However, the inability of the kidneys to concentrate urine because of age-related changes, may precipitate an inappropriately high urine output during hypovolemia. As a result urine output may be a poor measure of perfusion (Robins & Courts, 1997).

Survivors of head injury tend to recover from a comatose state within 72 hours of admission (Ross, Pitts, & Kobayashi, 1992). Intracranial pressure monitoring is sensitive in predicting survivors of head injury. ICP values > 20 mm Hg in the first 92 hours postinjury are associated with mortality. ICU nurses should counsel families regarding a realistic appraisal of outcome of their family member.

Burn patients are particularly vulnerable to thrombosis due to immobilization, infection, and inflammation. Ankle pumps, gluteal seats, or ambulation should be attempted every hour for 5 minutes (Staley & Richard, 1993). Continuous passive motion devices may be effective in mobilizing an elderly patient.

The amount of rapid eye movement sleep decreases beginning at age 60. This normal decline compounded by the noise and lighting in the ICU may contribute to sleep deprivation and confusion. Thus, the nurse should adjust noise and light levels to reflect diurnal variations.

The most frequent nursing diagnoses appropriate for the elderly trauma patient are summarized in Table 38–10.

TABLE 38–10. NURSING DIAGNOSES APPROPRIATE FOR THE ELDERLY TRAUMA PATIENT

Relevant for the Emergency Nurse
- Pain
- Impaired verbal communication[a]
- Acute confusion
- Ineffective breathing patterns
- Impaired gas exchange
- Decreased cardiac output
- Impaired tissue integrity
- Altered immune response[a]
- Risk for altered body temperature
- Risk for decreased adaptive capacity: Intracranial
- Risk for fluid volume deficit

Relevant for the Perioperative Nurse
- Ineffective breathing patterns
- Impaired gas exchange
- Decreased cardiac output
- Risk for perioperative positioning injury
- Altered immune response[a]
- Risk for altered body temperature
- Impaired tissue integrity
- Risk for decreased adaptive capacity: Intracranial
- Risk for fluid volume deficit

Relevant for the Critical Care Nurse
- Pain
- Impaired verbal communication[a]
- Acute confusion
- Sleep pattern disturbance
- Altered thought processes: Impaired intellectual functioning, concentration
- Ineffective breathing patterns
- Impaired gas exchange
- Decreased cardiac output
- Altered nutrition: Less than body requirements
- Impaired tissue integrity
- Impaired physical mobility
- Altered immune response[a]
- Risk for fluid volume deficit
- Risk for dysfunctional ventilatory weaning response
- Risk for decreased adaptive capacity: Intracranial

[a] Indicates nursing diagnosis still under development by NANDA.

In summary, the elderly may be at higher risk of injury due to physiologic changes associated with aging, medications, and/or preexisting illness. After initial stabilization, a detailed history should be obtained to help determine whether the patient is experiencing an illness exacerbation in addition to injuries. Resuscitation efforts are aimed at increasing oxygen delivery and involve greater colloid administration than in younger patients. Complications posttrauma occur more frequently in patients with respiratory compromise (due to preexisting respiratory problems as well as severity of injury) and nutritional deficits.

SECTION EIGHT REVIEW

Don White, age 75, presents to the emergency department after falling down a flight of five stairs. Questions 1 through 4 pertain to Mr. White.

1. Based on the physiologic changes of aging, what head injury is Mr. White most likely to sustain?
   - A. epidural hematoma
   - B. subarachnoid bleed
   - C. subdural hematoma
   - D. intracerebral bleed
2. In anticipation of the need for medication and of additional injuries, you insert an intravenous line. Which of the following fluids is most appropriate to use in Mr. White's situation?
   - A. lactated Ringer's
   - B. packed red blood cells
   - C. normal saline
   - D. intermittent intravenous infusion (heparin lock)
3. Mr. White's level of consciousness deteriorates and he becomes combative. The decision is made to chemically paralyze and intubate him. Vecuronium is administered. Because of his age-related changes in body composition, you expect
   - A. Mr. White to not react to the medicine unless a larger than normal dose is given
   - B. the medicine to remain biologically active longer than in the younger patient
   - C. the medicine to cause paradoxical excitement
   - D. the medicine to cause hallucinations upon awakening
4. Mr. White has an ICP monitoring catheter inserted and the opening pressure is 20 mm Hg. Which of the following statements is true?
   - A. this is a normal reading for his age
   - B. this indicates he needs immediate surgery
   - C. he has a high risk for a poor outcome
   - D. ICP readings over the next 96 hours will predict outcome

Answers: 1. C, 2. A, 3. B, 4. D

SECTION NINE: Surgery in the Elderly

At the completion of this section, the learner will be able to describe nursing care appropriate for the elderly surgical patient.

The elderly patient may be at higher surgical risk because of physiologic aging or because of preexisiting disease. Risk factors for surgery in the elderly are described in Table 38–11. The best predictors of perioperative death are cardiac failure, impaired renal function, and angina (Saleh, 1993).

Physiologic Changes Relevant to Perioperative Nursing

Physiologic changes that increase surgical risk are several. The elderly surgical patient is at higher risk for hypothermia due to decreased body fat and the inability to retain heat. Hypothermia is also induced by prolonged surgery, vasodilation due to drugs, and decreased metabolic rate associated with paralysis. Total body water decreases, thus anesthesia induction may precipitate hypotension. In addition, decreased vascular tone and sluggish circulation may prolong drug action. Local and regional anesthesia is preferred to general anesthesia to avoid pulmonary and vascular complications of surgery (Russo & Johnson, 1991). If spinal anesthesia is used, it will take longer for the medication to be absorbed and eliminated due to slowed pia and arachnid circulation. Table 38–12 lists the half-life of common anesthetic agents used in the elderly. Decreased skin elasticity predisposes the elderly patient to injury from electrodes, tape, and movement. Bone demineralization and joint stiffness produce positioning and intubation challenges. Fractures occur easily with little force. Protective airway reflexes diminish, predisposing the patient to aspiration.

Intraoperative Nursing Care

A careful medication history is important preoperatively. If the patient is receiving steroids preoperatively, intravenous steroids must be administered immediately prior to and after surgery. Intravenous steroids may be necessary for a longer period of time if the patient develops postoperative infection (Nolan, 1992).

TABLE 38–11. RISK FACTORS IN ELDERLY SURGICAL PATIENTS

RISK FACTOR	INDICATION
Serum creatinine level greater than 3 mg/dL	Renal failure
Elevated AST or ALT level	Liver failure
Serum albumin level less than 2.7 g/dL	Malnutrition
Total lymphocyte count less than 1,000/μL	Malnutrition
Cardiac dysrhythmia	Cardiac ischemia
More than five PVCs per minute	Cardiac ischemia
Myocardial infarction in the preceding 6 months	Heart failure
S_3 gallop or jugular venous distention	Heart failure

TABLE 38–12. HALF-LIFE IN THE ELDERLY OF COMMON ANESTHETIC/ANALGESIA AGENTS

AGENT	HALF-LIFE
Fentanyl	15.4 hours
Alfentanyl	2.1 hours
Vecuronium	45 minutes
Midazolam	4.3 hours
Diazepam	72 hours

Adapted from Saleh, K. (1993). The elderly patient in the postanesthesia care unit. Nurs Clin North Am *28:510.*

Hypertensive patients may have hypertensive episodes during surgery even if they are well controlled preoperatively. Patients receiving angiotensin-converting enzyme inhibitors (e.g., captopril) and calcium channel blockers (e.g., Cardizem) for control of hypertension should receive these medications preoperatively. Patients with an ejection fraction of less than 30 percent need hemodynamic monitoring intraoperatively (Nolan, 1992). Diabetic patients who receive insulin may benefit from a constant infusion of regular insulin during surgery.

Nursing care intraoperatively includes padding pressure points and performing extremity circulation checks (with use of a Doppler as needed). Body temperature is monitored and a warming blanket or device used as needed. Inhalation gases may be warmed as well.

Immediate Postoperative Nursing Care

Postoperative care priorities are to promote optimal gas exchange by providing high-humidity oxygen, protecting against aspiration, and stimulating the patient to breathe deeply. Pulmonary problems may occur in the first 48 hours postoperatively. Prior to elective surgery, baseline spirometric studies and arterial blood gas values should be obtained. Patients with a baseline P_{CO_2} of > 45 mm Hg or a PO_2 of less than 70 mm Hg have a higher risk for pulmonary complications. A forced vital capacity of < 1 L is associated with ventilator dependency (Nolan, 1992). Patients with a smoking history of > 40 pack-years (calculated by number of packs smoked per day times the number of years smoked) have more pulmonary complications. Hypotension, cardiac dysrhythmias, and hypothermia may occur postoperatively as well.

The patient may have been NPO prior to surgery, had episodes of nausea and vomiting preoperatively, or been on diuretics. All of these factors lead to dehydration postoperatively. The nurse must consider physiologic changes of aging and other preoperative factors when administering IV fluids. Decreased bladder capacity, sphincter tone, and glomerular filtration rate may alter urine output. Breath sounds should be assessed and documented prior to surgery to detect the presence of wet crackles. Anesthetic gases induce bronchial airway hyperactivity, increasing inflammation, and edema. Patient with wet crackles preoperatively have greater perioperative complications regardless of fluid administration. Mobilization of IV fluids administered intraoperatively occurs 36 to 48 hours postoperatively. Monitoring of breath sounds and urine output is important at this time as pulmonary edema and congestive heart failure may occur.

Because of decreased nerve conduction, the elderly patient may require greater stimulation to wake up postoperatively.

In summary, the priority in perioperative nursing care is to promote oxygenation. This may require baseline breath sound assessment immediately prior to surgery; careful documentation of intake and output; monitoring oxygen saturation postoperatively and comparing this reading with a preoperative reading; and stimulation postoperatively to breathe deeply.

SECTION NINE REVIEW

1. Postoperative fluid shifts in the elderly tend to occur
   A. in the postanesthesia recovery area
   B. upon awakening from anesthesia
   C. 36 to 48 hours postoperatively
   D. within the first postoperative day
2. Which of the following is associated with pulmonary complications postoperatively in the elderly?
   A. $\geq$ 40 pack-year history of smoking
   B. patients who receive > 1 L of intraoperative IV fluid
   C. preoperative oxygen saturation of $\leq$ 95 percent
   D. preoperative PCO_2 level of $\geq$ 38 mm Hg

Answers: 1. C, 2. A

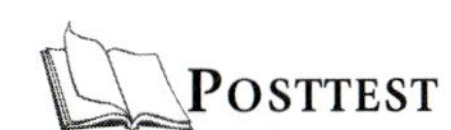

POSTTEST

Mary Williams, age 72, is involved as a restrained driver in a single-vehicle MVC while traveling 40 mph. Questions 1 through 4 pertain to this scenario.

1. Based on the kinetics of injury, her restraint status, and Ms. Williams's age, which injury is she at greater risk for?
   A. head injury
   B. ruptured trachea
   C. lacerated aorta
   D. femur fracture
2. Ms. Williams's systolic blood pressure in the emergency department is 90 mm Hg. You interpret this to mean that she is
   A. normovolemic
   B. compensating for hypovolemia
   C. in shock
   D. receiving too much intravenous fluid
3. Ms. Williams has been in the critical care unit for 6 days and remains intubated on SIMV with pressure support. This is
   A. a normal response for someone her age
   B. an ominous sign
   C. typical preweaning mode
   D. improving her respiratory muscle toning
4. Ms. Williams is transferred to the operating suite for a procedure completed under general anesthesia. Because of her age-associated physiologic changes, you anticipate that she will experience which of the following during the procedure?
   A. hypotension
   B. hyperthermia
   C. hypoglycemia
   D. hyperthyroidism
5. As part of normal aging, the heart rate
   A. decreases
   B. increases
   C. becomes irregular
   D. gallops
6. Difficulty performing an ADL suggests a
   A. financial problem
   B. cognitive problem
   C. emotional problem
   D. physical problem
7. Functional decline in the elderly
   A. indicates an underlying physical problem
   B. eventually occurs in all persons
   C. occurs slowly and insidiously
   D. is defined as organ malfunction

8. Alcohol in the elderly has a pronounced effect due to decreased
   A. vasomotor tone
   B. distribution volume
   C. conduction velocity
   D. glomerular filtration rate
9. A complication of beta-blocking agents in the elderly is
   A. dehydration
   B. hypokalemia
   C. bronchodilation
   D. congestive heart failure
10. Sedatives and hypnotics have prolonged effects in the elderly because
    A. the glomerular filtration rate decreases
    B. of increased body fat
    C. of decreased systemic perfusion
    D. catecholamine production decreases
11. Which of the following indicates a weaning failure in the elderly?
    A. tidal volume of < 300 mL
    B. respiratory rate > 26
    C. oxygen saturation of 92 percent
    D. $PO_2 < 90$ mm Hg
12. Cardiac ischemia in the elderly patient produces
    A. ST segment changes on the ECG
    B. an elevation in creatine kinase levels from baseline
    C. tachycardia
    D. chest pain
13. The factor that separates dementia from depression and delirium is
    A. onset
    B. disorientation
    C. impaired memory/concentration
    D. self-care deficit/self-neglect
14. When assessing an elderly patient who has experienced syncope, the nurse should consider all of the following etiologies EXCEPT
    A. medications
    B. functional decline
    C. current illness
    D. decreased perfusion
15. Which of the following is a risk factor in elderly surgical patients?
    A. elevated white blood cell count
    B. elevated liver enzymes (AST/ALT)
    C. stroke in the preceding 6 months
    D. elevated albumin level

POSTTEST ANSWERS

Question	Answer	Section
1	C	Eight
2	C	Eight
3	B	Eight
4	A	Nine
5	A	One
6	D	Two
7	A	Two
8	B	Three
9	D	Three
10	B	Three
11	A	Four
12	B	Five
13	A	Six
14	B	Eight
15	B	Nine

REFERENCES

Abi-Hanna, P., & Gleckman, R. (1997). Acute abdominal pain: A medical emergency in older patients. *Geriatrics* 52:72.

Banazak, D. (1996). Difficult dementia: Six steps to control problem behavior. *Geriatrics* 51:36–42.

Bobb, J. (1993). Chest trauma in the elderly. *Crit Care Nurs Clin North Am* 5:735–740.

Breitbart, W., et al. (1997). The Memorial Delirium Assessment Scale. *J Pain Symptom Management* 13:128.

Dandan, I. (1992). Trauma in the elderly patient. *Top Emerg Medi* 14(3):39–46.

DeMaria, E., Kenney, P., Merriam, M., et al. (1987). Aggressive trauma care benefits elderly. *J Trauma* 27:1200.

Evans, R., Ireland, G., Morley, J., & Sheahan, S. (1995). Pharmacology and aging. In *Geriatric emergency medicine core curriculum*. Ann Arbor, MI: Society for Academic Emergency Medicine.

Finelli, F., Jonsson, J., & Champion, H. (1989). A case control study for major trauma in geriatric patients. *J Trauma* 29:541.

Foreman, M. (1992). Adverse psychologic responses of the elderly to critical illness. *AACN Clin Issues* 3:64–72.

Fraser, D. (1997). Assessing the elderly for infection. *J Gerontol Nurs* 23:6.

Guin, P., & Freudenberger, K. (1992). The elderly neuroscience patient: Implications for the critical care nurse. *AACN Clin Issues* 3:98–105.

Gudmundsson, A., & Carnes, M. (1996). Geriatric assessment: Making it work in primary care practice. *Geriatrics* 51:62.

Kalbfleisch, N. (1995). Acute myocardial infarction in the elderly. In *Geriatric emergency medicine core curriculum*. Ann Arbor, MI: Society for Academic Emergency Medicine.

Katz, S. (1983). Assessing self maintenance: Activities of daily living, mobility, and instrumental activities of daily living. *JAGS 31*:721–727.

Khanna, P., & Geller, J. (1992). Clinical implications in the elderly. *Top Emerg Med 14*:1–9.

Kleinpell, R.M., & Ferrans, C.E. (1998). Factors influencing intensive care unit survival for critically ill elderly patients. *Heart Lung 27*:337.

Kozak-Campbell, C., & Hughes, A. (1996). The use of functional consequences theory in acutely confused hospitalized elderly. *JAGS 22*:32–33.

Lachs, M. (1995). Recognizing and managing functional decline in the older emergency department patient. In *Geriatric emergency medicine core curriculum*. Ann Arbor, MI: Society for Academic Emergency Medicine.

Lawton, M.P. (1988). Scales to measure competence in everyday activities. *Psychopharmacol Bull 24*:609–614.

Lee, M. (1996). Drug and the elderly: Do you know the risks? *Am J Nurs 96*(7):26–28.

Lewandowski, R., Pegg, S., Fortier, K., & Skimmings, A. (1993). Burn injuries in the elderly. *Burns 19*:513–515.

Martinez, R., Sharieff, G., & Hooper, J. (1994). Three-point restraints as a risk factor for chest injury in the elderly. *J Trauma 37*:980–984.

Marx, A., Campbell, R., & Harder, F. (1989). Polytrauma in the elderly. *World J Surg 10*:330–335.

McNamara, R. (1995). Acute abdominal pain in the older person. In *Geriatric emergency medicine core curriculum*. Ann Arbor, MI: Society for Academic Emergency Medicine.

Mick, D.J. (1997). Pneumonia in elders. *Geriatr Nurs 18*: 99–102.

Miller, C.A. (1997). Preventive care should address the immunizations for older adults. *Geriatr Nurs 18*:42.

Mitchell, C., Gallo, K., & Turnes, C. (1992, July/August). Geriatric trauma: A case study. *Geriatr Nurs 13*:210–213.

Morris, J., MacKenzie, E., & Edelstein, S. (1990). The effect of preexisting conditions on mortality in trauma patients. *JAMA 263*:1942.

Nolan, T. (1992). Surgery in the elderly. *Postgrad Med 91*:199–208.

Osler, T., Hales, K., Baack, B., et al. (1988). Trauma in the elderly. *Am J Surg 156*:537.

Pellicane, J., Byrne, K., & DeMaria, E. (1992). Preventable complications and death from multiple organ failure among geriatric trauma victims. *J Trauma 33*:440–444.

Pepe, J., & Lane, V. (1993). Abdominal trauma in the elderly. *Top Emerg Med 15*(2):48–54.

Pierre, J. (1996). Delirium in hospitalized elderly patients. *Crit Care Nurs Clin North Am 8*:53–59.

Ribby, K., & Cox, K. (1996). Development, implementation, and evaluation of a confusion protocol. *Clin Nurse Specialist 10*:241.

Robins, L.M., & Courts, N.F. (1997). Care of the traumatized older adult. *Geriatr Nurs 18*:210–212.

Ross, A., Pitts, L., & Kobayashi, S. (1992). Prognosticators of outcome after major head injury in the elderly. *J Neurosci Nurs 24*:88–93.

Russo, K., & Johnson, H. (1991). The nursing care of the elderly patient during anesthesia and recovery. *ACORN J 4*(4):21–22, 26, 28, 30–33.

Saleh, K. (1993). The elderly patient in the postanesthesia care unit. *Nurs Clin North Am 28*:507–517.

Smith, D., Enderson, B., & Maull, K. (1990). Trauma in the elderly: Determinants of outcome. *South Med J 83*:171.

Staley, M., & Richard, R. (1993). The elderly patient with burns: Treatment considerations. *J Burn Care Rehab 14*: 559–565.

Stengle, J., & Dries, D. (1994). Sepsis in the elderly. *Crit Care Nurs Clin North Am 6*:421–427.

Stiesmeyer, J. (1992). Care of the elderly mechanically ventilated patient: Preserving the fragile environment. *AACN Clin Issues 3*:129–136.

Stillwell, S. (1992). *Mosby's critical care nursing reference*. St. Louis: C.V. Mosby.

Watters, J., Moulton, S., Clancey, S., Blakslee, J., & Monaghan, R. (1994). Aging exaggerates glucose intolerance following injury. *J Trauma 37*:786–791.

Zietlow, S., Capizzi, P., Bannon, M., & Farnell, M. (1994). Multisystem geriatric trauma. *J Trauma 37*:985–988.

INDEX

B

C

D

F

H

J

K

L

M

P

U